SIXTH EDITION

Clinical Manifestations and Assessment of Respiratory Disease

Terry Des Jardins, MEd, RRT
Former Direct, Professor Emeritus
Department of Respiratory Care
Parkland College
Champagne, Illinois
Faculty/Staff Member
University of Illinois College of Medicine
Urbana-Champagne, Illinois

George G. Burton, MD, FACP, FCCP, FAARC
Associate Dean for Medical Affairs
Kettering College of Medical Arts
Kettering, Ohio
Clinical Professor of Medicine and Anesthesiology
Wright State University School of Medicine
Dayton, Ohio

Medical Illustrations By
Timothy H. Phelps, MS, FAMI, CMI
Associate Professor
Johns Hopkins University School of Medicine
Baltimore, Maryland

MOSBY

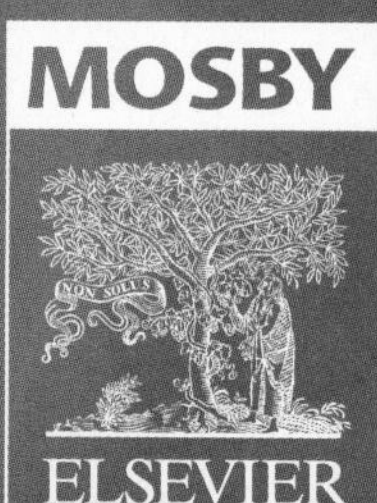

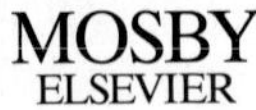

3251 Riverport Lane
Maryland Heights, Missouri 63043

CLINICAL MANIFESTATIONS AND ASSESSMENT OF RESPIRATORY DISEASE
ISBN: 978-0-323-05727-1

Notice

Knowledge and best practice in this field are constantly changing. As new research and experience broaden our knowledge, changes in practice, treatment and drug therapy may become necessary or appropriate. Readers are advised to check the most current information provided (i) on procedures featured or (ii) by the manufacturer of each product to be administered, to verify the recommended dose or formula, the method and duration of administration, and contraindications. It is the responsibility of the practitioner, relying on their own experience and knowledge of the patient, to make diagnoses, to determine dosages and the best treatment for each individual patient, and to take all appropriate safety precautions. To the fullest extent of the law, neither the Publisher nor the Authors assumes any liability for any injury and/or damage to persons or property arising out of or related to any use of the material contained in this book.

The Publisher

Previous editions copyrighted 1984, 1990, 1995, 2002, 2006

Library of Congress Cataloging-in-Publication Data
Des Jardins, Terry R.
Clinical manifestations and assessment of respiratory disease / Terry Des Jardins, George G. Burton; medical illustrations by Timothy H. Phelps.—6th ed.
p. ; cm.
Includes bibliographical references and index.
ISBN 978-0-323-05727-1 (pbk. : alk. paper) 1. Respiratory organs—Diseases. 2. Respiratory organs—Diseases—Diagnosis. I. Burton, George G., 1934- II. Title.
[DNLM: 1. Respiratory Tract Diseases. WF 140 D441c 2011]
RC731.D47 2011
616.2—dc22

2009051883

Managing Editor: Billie Sharp
Developmental Editor: Betsy Stream McCormac
Publishing Services Manager: Julie Eddy
Senior Project Manager: Celeste Clingan

Design Direction: Amy Buxton

Printed in the United States of America

Last digit is the print number: 9 8 7 6 5 4 3 2

Consultant for Newborn and Early Childhood Respiratory Disorders

Nestor A. Ramirez, MD, MPH, FAAP
Specialist in Neonatal-Perinatal Medicine
Diplomate of the American Board of Pediatrics
Advocate Illinois Masonic Medical Center NICU
Chicago, Illinois

Reviewers

Kelly K. Cummins, RRT, RPSGT, BS
Respiratory Care Program
Southeast Community College
Lincoln, Nebraska

Christine A. Hamilton, DHSc, RRT, AE-C
Respiratory Care Program Director
Nebraska Methodist College
The Josie Harper Campus
Omaha, Nebraska

Julie A. Hopwood, MS, RRT, RCP
Respiratory Therapy Program
Central Piedmont Community College
Charlotte, North Carolina

James R. Sills, MEd, CPFT, RRT
Professor Emeritus
Former Director, Respiratory Care Program
Rock Valley College
Rockford, Illinois

Richard B. Wettstein, MMEd, cTTS, RRT
Assistant Professor
University of Texas Health Science Center at San Antonio
San Antonio, Texas

to

Wenda and Jean

"(There is a) manpower shortage of health-care providers who care for the critically ill. This is one of the most pressing issues affecting the future of our aging population and American medicine ... it has been generally acknowledged...that the shortages in nursing, respiratory care practitioners, and pharmacists have already reached crisis levels...a severe shortage of (pulmonary/critical care physicians) can be expected by 2007."[1]

"... respiratory therapists are important for patient outcome *and their roles might even be expanded beyond traditional boundaries.* More research is needed to define the ICU multidisciplinary staffing that matches patient needs and optimizes patient outcomes."[2]

These issues will drive the growth of the respiratory care profession in to the twenty-first century: an aging population with complex health-care issues, ever more complex and expensive respiratory care technologies, and concern to find the most cost-effective way to face these challenges.

---

[1]Irwin RS, Marcus L, Lever A: The Critical Care Professional Societies address the critical care crisis in the United States, *Chest* 125:1512-1513, 2004.

[2]Kelly MA, Angus D, Chalfin DB, et al: The critical care crisis in the United States, *Chest* 125: 1514-1517, 2004.

Preface

The use of therapist-driven protocols (TDPs) is now an integral part of respiratory health services. TDPs provide the much-needed flexibility to respiratory care practitioners and increase the quality of health care. This is because the respiratory therapy can be modified easily and efficiently according to the needs of the patient.

Essential cornerstones to the success of a TDP program are (1) the quality of the respiratory therapist's assessment skills at the bedside and (2) the ability to transfer objective clinical data into a treatment plan that follows agreed-on guidelines. This textbook is designed to provide the student with the fundamental knowledge and understanding necessary to assess and treat patients with respiratory diseases in order to meet these objectives.

Part I of the textbook, entitled *Assessment of Respiratory Disease,* consists of the following three sections:

- Section I, entitled *Clinical Data Obtained at the Patient's Bedside,* consists of two chapters. Chapter 1 describes the knowledge and skills involved in the patient interview. Chapter 2 provides the knowledge and skills needed for the physical examination. This chapter also presents a more in-depth discussion of the pathophysiologic basis for the clinical manifestations associated with respiratory diseases.
- Section II, entitled *Clinical Data Obtained from Laboratory Tests and Special Procedures,* is composed of Chapters 3 to 8. Collectively these chapters provide the reader with the essential knowledge and understanding basis for the assessment of pulmonary function studies, arterial blood gases, oxygenation, the cardiovascular system (including hemodynamic monitoring), the radiologic examination of the chest, and important laboratory tests and procedures.
- Section III, entitled *The Therapist-Driven Protocol Program—The Essentials,* consists of Chapters 9 and 10.

  Chapter 9, entitled *The Therapist-Driven Protocol Program and the Role of the Respiratory Care Practitioner,* provides the reader with the essential knowledge base and the step-by-step process needed to assess and implement respiratory care protocols in the clinical setting. The student is provided with the basic knowledge and helpful tools to (1) gather clinical data systematically, (2) formulate an assessment (i.e., the cause and severity of the patient's condition), (3) select an appropriate and cost-effective treatment plan, and (4) document these essential steps clearly and precisely. At the end of each respiratory disorder chapter, one or more representative case studies demonstrate appropriate TDP assessment and treatment strategies. In addition, students can also visit the Student Resource Evolve website at http://evolve.elsevier.com/DesJardins/respiratory to test their (1) knowledge base and (2) assessment and treatment selection skills in additional case studies. Chapter 9 is a cornerstone chapter to the fundamentals necessary for good assessment and critical thinking skills. The case studies presented at the end of each respiratory disorder chapter often direct the reader back to Chapter 9.

  Chapter 10, entitled *Recording Skills: The Basis for Data Collection, Organization, Assessment Skills, and Treatment Plans,* provides the basic foundation needed to collect and record respiratory assessments and treatment plans.

Parts II to XII (Chapters 11 to 42) provide the reader with essential information regarding common respiratory diseases. Each chapter adheres to the following format: anatomic alterations of the lungs, etiology of the disease process, an overview of the cardiopulmonary clinical manifestations associated with the disorder, management of the respiratory disorder, one or more case studies, and a brief set of self-assessment questions.

Anatomic Alterations of the Lungs

Each respiratory disease chapter begins with a detailed, colored illustration showing the major anatomic alterations of the lungs associated with the disorder. Although a serious effort has been made to illustrate each disorder accurately at the beginning of each chapter, artistic license has been taken to emphasize certain anatomic points and pathologic processes. The material that follows this section in each respiratory disorder chapter discusses the disease in terms of the following:

1. The common pathophysiologic mechanisms activated throughout the respiratory system as a result of the anatomic alterations
2. The clinical manifestations that develop as a result of the pathophysiologic mechanisms
3. The basic respiratory therapy modalities used to improve the anatomic alterations and pathophysiologic mechanisms caused by the disease

When the anatomic alterations and pathophysiologic mechanisms caused by the disorder are improved, the clinical manifestations also should improve.

Etiology

A discussion of the etiology of the disease follows the presentation of anatomic alterations of the lungs. Various causes and predisposing conditions are described.

Overview of the Cardiopulmonary Clinical Manifestations Associated with the Disorder

This section comprises the central theme of the text. The reader is provided with the clinical manifestations commonly associated with the disease under discussion. In essence the student is given a general "overview" of the signs and symptoms commonly demonstrated by the patient. By having a working knowledge—and therefore a predetermined expectation—of the clinical manifestations associated with a specific respiratory disorder, the practitioner is in a better position to do the following:

1. Gather clinical data relevant to the patient's respiratory status
2. Formulate an objective—and measurable—respiratory assessment
3. Select an effective and safe treatment plan that is based on a valid assessment

If the appropriate data are not gathered and assessed correctly, the ability to treat the patient effectively is lost. As mentioned earlier, the case studies presented at the end of each respiratory disorder chapter frequently refer the reader back to Chapter 9 for a broader discussion of the of the signs and symptoms commonly associated with the disease under discussion—the "clinical scenario." When a particular clinical manifestation is unique to the respiratory disorder, however, a discussion of the pathophysiologic mechanisms responsible for the signs and symptoms is presented in the respective chapter.

Because of the dynamic nature of many respiratory disorders, the reader should note the following regarding this section:

- Because the severity of the disease is influenced by a number of factors (e.g., the extent of the disease, age, the general health of the patient), the clinical manifestations may vary remarkably from one patient to another. In fact, they may vary in the same patient from one *time* to another. Therefore the practitioner should understand that the patient may demonstrate *all* the clinical manifestations presented or just a *few*.

  In addition, many of the clinical manifestations associated with a respiratory disorder may never appear in some patients (e.g., digital clubbing, cor pulmonale, increased hemoglobin level). As a general rule, however, the prototypic patient usually demonstrates most of the manifestations presented during the advanced stages of the disease.
- Some of the clinical manifestations presented in each chapter may not actually be measured (or measurable) in the clinical setting for a variety of practical reasons (e.g., age, mental status, severity of the disorder). They are nevertheless conceptually important and therefore are presented here through extrapolation. For example, the newborn with severe infant respiratory distress syndrome who obviously has a restrictive lung disorder as a result of the anatomic alterations associated with the disease cannot actually perform the maneuvers necessary for a pulmonary function study.
- The clinical manifestations presented in each chapter are based only on the one respiratory disorder under discussion. In the clinical setting, the patient often has a combination of respiratory problems (e.g., emphysema compounded by pneumonia) and may have manifestations related to each of the pulmonary disorders.

This section does not attempt to present the "absolute" pathophysiologic basis for the development of a particular clinical manifestation. Because of the dynamic nature of many respiratory diseases, the precise cause of some of the manifestations presented by the patient is not always clear. In most cases, however, the primary pathophysiologic mechanisms responsible for the various signs and symptoms are known and understood and are described herein.

Management or Treatment of the Disease

Each chapter provides a general overview of the more common therapeutic modalities (treatment protocols) used to offset the anatomic alterations and pathophysiologic mechanisms activated by a particular disorder.

Although several respiratory therapy modalities may be safe and effective in treating a respiratory disorder, the respiratory care practitioner must have a clear conception of the following:

1. How the therapies work to offset the anatomic alterations of the lungs caused by the disease
2. How the correction of the anatomic alterations of the lungs works to offset the pathophysiologic mechanisms
3. How the correction of the pathophysiologic mechanisms works to offset the clinical manifestations demonstrated by the patient

Without this understanding, the practitioner merely goes through the motions of performing therapeutic tasks with no anticipated or measurable outcomes.

Case Study

The case study at the end of each respiratory disease chapter provides the reader with a realistic example of (1) the manner in which the patient may arrive in the hospital with the disorder under discussion, (2) the various clinical manifestations commonly associated with the disease, (3) the way the clinical manifestations can be gathered, organized, and documented, (4) the way an assessment of the patient's respiratory status is formulated from the clinical manifestations, and (5) the way a comprehensive treatment plan is developed from the assessment.

In essence, the case study provides the reader with a good example of the way in which the respiratory care practitioner would gather clinical data, make an assessment, and treat a patient with the disorder under discussion. In addition, many of the case studies presented in the text describe a respiratory care practitioner assessing and treating the patient several times—demonstrating the importance of assessment skills and the way therapy is often up-regulated or down-regulated on a moment-to-moment basis in the clinical setting.

References

A list of literature references for each chapter is provided on the Student Resource Evolve website. The student is encouraged to review selected references, especially the "state of the art" references regarding the respiratory disorders discussed throughout the textbook.

Self-Assessment Questions

Each disease chapter concludes with a set of self-assessment questions. At the end of self-assessment section, the student is provided the following message:

> To access additional student assessment questions—and additional case studies—for application of text material to real-life scenarios, visit the Student Resource Evolve website: http://evolve.elsevier.com/DesJardins/respiratory.

Glossary and Appendixes

Finally, a glossary and appendixes are provided at the end of the text. The appendixes include the following:

- A table of symbols and abbreviations commonly used in respiratory physiology
- Medications commonly used in the treatment of cardiopulmonary disorders, including the following:
  - Aerosolized bronchodilators
  - Mucolytic agents
  - Aerosolized antiinflammatory agents
  - Xanthine bronchodilators
  - Expectorants
  - Antibiotic agents
  - Positive inotropic agents
  - Diuretics
- The ideal alveolar gas equation
- Physiologic dead space calculation
- Units of measurement
- Poiseuille's law
- $P_{CO_2}/HCO_3^-/pH$ nomogram
- Calculated hemodynamic measurements
- DuBois body surface area chart
- Cardiopulmonary profile

Approach

Finally, in writing this textbook, we have tried to present a realistic balance between the esoteric language of pathophysiology and the simple, straight-to-the-point approach generally preferred by busy students.

Terry Des Jardins
George G. Burton

Acknowledgments

A number of exceptional people have provided key contributions to the development of the sixth edition of this textbook. First, we extend a very special thank-you to Wenda Speers for the artwork she provided for this book. Especially noteworthy is the art she rendered for the $PCO_2/HCO_3^-/pH$ nomogram, which is also provided as a handy, pocket-sized reference tool in Appendix XII. For his reviews and consultation for newborn and early childhood respiratory disorders, our appreciation goes to Dr. Nestor Ramirez, specialist in Neonatal-Perinatal Medicine, Advocate Illinois Masonic Medical Center. A special thank you goes to Chad Goveia, Director of Respiratory Care, BroMenn Health Care Center, Bloomington, Illinois, for providing radiology material to croup syndrome chapter of this new addition. For her contributions and help in preparing the cystic fibrosis chapter, our thanks goes to Janice Douglas, RRT, Pediatric Respiratory Specialist, Carle Clinic Pediatric Pulmonary and Cystic Fibrosis Clinic, Urbana, Illinois.

We also very much appreciate the outstanding work Robert Wilkins provided in the development of the Instructor's Manual that accompanies this textbook. In addition, for the many hours of work in the development of the additional test questions in the style of the NBRC examinations—both for the instructor and students, a very special thank you goes to James R. Sills, MEd, CPFT, RRT.

For their very extensive and comprehensive reviews and helpful suggestions regarding the depth, breadth, and accuracy of the material presented in this textbook, we thank the following outstanding respiratory care educators: Kelly K. Cummins, RRT, RPSGT, BS; Christine A. Hamilton, DHSc, RRT, AE-C; Julie A. Hopwood, MS, RRT, RCP; and Richard B. Wettstein, MMEd, cTTS, RRT.

Finally, we are very grateful to the team at Elsevier: Managing Editor Billie Sharp, Developmental Editor Betsy Stream McCormac, and Senior Project Manager Celeste Clingan. Their work and helpful coordination during the development of this textbook, and the supplemental student and instructor website packages associated with this book, has been most appreciated.

Terry Des Jardins, Med, RRT
George Burton, MD

Contents

PART XII

Other Important Topics, 477

Introduction

The Assessment Process—An Overview

Assessment is (1) the process of collecting clinical information about the patient's health status, (2) the evaluation of the data and identification of the specific problems, concerns, and needs of the patient, and (3) the development of a treatment plan that can be managed by the health-care provider. The clinical information gathered may consist of subjective and objective data (signs and symptoms) about the patient, the results of diagnostic tests and procedures, the patient's response to therapy, and the patient's general health practices.

The first step in the assessment process is thinking—even before the actual collection of clinical data begins. In other words, the practitioner must first "think" about why the patient has entered the health-care facility and about what clinical data will likely need to be collected. Merely obtaining answers to a specific list of questions does not serve the assessment process well. For example, while en route to evaluate a patient who is said to be having an asthmatic episode, the health-care practitioner might mentally consider the following: What are the likely signs and symptoms that can be observed at the bedside during a moderate or severe asthmatic attack? What are the usual emotional responses? What are the anatomic alterations associated with an asthma episode that would be responsible for the signs and symptoms observed? Table 1 presents a broader overview of what the practitioner might think about before assessing a patient said to be having an asthmatic episode.

To collect data wisely, health-care providers must have well-developed skills in observing and listening. In addition, the practitioner must apply his or her mental skills of translation, reason, intuition, and validation to render the clinical data meaningful. Clinically, the collection of data is more useful when the evaluation process is organized into common problem areas, or categories. As the practitioner gathers information in each problem category, a clustering of related data about the patient will be generated. This framework for collecting clinical information enhances the practitioner's ability to establish priorities of care. Furthermore, any time the health-care provider interacts with the patient, for any reason, an assessment of the patient's problems, needs, and concerns should be made. To efficiently and correctly gather data, the health-care provider must make decisions about what type of assessment is needed, how to obtain the data, the framework and focus of the assessment, and what additional data may be needed before a complete treatment plan can be developed.

Purpose of Assessment

Relative to the purpose, an assessment may involve asking just two or three specific questions or it may involve an in-depth conversation with the patient. An assessment may involve a comprehensive focus (head-to-toe assessment) or a specific or narrow focus. The purpose of the assessment may include any of the following:

- To obtain a baseline databank about the patient's physical and mental status
- To supplement, verify, or refute any previous data
- To identify actual and potential problems
- To obtain data that will help the practitioner establish an assessment and treatment plan
- To focus on specific problems
- To determine immediate needs and to establish priorities
- To determine the cause (etiology) of the problem
- To determine any related or contributing factors
- To identify patient strengths as a basis for changing behavior
- To identify the risk for complications
- To recognize complications

Types of Assessment

There are four major types of assessment: initial, focused, emergency, and ongoing.

The *initial assessment* is conducted at the first encounter with the patient. In the hospitalized patient, the initial assessment is typically performed by the admitting nurse and is more comprehensive than subsequent assessments. It starts with the reasons that prompted the patient to seek care, and it entails a holistic overview of the patient's health-care needs. The general objective of the initial assessment is to rule out as well as to identify (rule in) specific problems. The initial assessment most commonly occurs when the patient has sought medical services for a specific problem or desires a general health status examination. The goals of the initial assessment include prevention, maintenance, restoration, or rehabilitation. In general, the thoroughness of the initial assessment is directly proportional to the length of expected care.

The *focused assessment* consists of a detailed examination of the specific problem areas, or patient complaints. The focused assessment looks at clinical data in detail, considers possible causes, looks at possible contributing factors, and examines the patient's personal characteristics that will help—or hinder—the problem. The focused assessment also is used when the patient describes or manifests a new problem. Common patient complaints include pain, shortness of

TABLE 1 Examples of What Might Be Considered before Evaluation of a Patient Having an Asthmatic Episode

Questions and/or Considerations	Likely Responses
What are the likely initial observations?	Shortness of breath, use of accessory muscles to breathe, intercostal retractions, pursed-lip breathing; cyanosis, barrel chest
What might be the patient's emotional response to his or her asthma?	Anxious, concerned, frightened
What are the anatomic alterations of the lungs associated with asthma?	Bronchospasm; excessive, thick, white, and tenacious bronchial secretions; air trapping; mucous plugging
What are the known causes of asthma?	*Extrinsic factors:* pollen, grass, house dust, animal dander *Intrinsic factors:* infection, cold air, exercise, emotional stress
What are the expected vital signs?	Increased respiratory rate, heart rate, and blood pressure
What are the expected chest assessment findings?	Breath sounds: diminished, wheezing, rhonchi Percussion: hyperresonant
What are the expected pulmonary function study findings?	Decreased: PEFR, FEV_T, FEV_T/FVC Increased: RV, FRC
What are the expected acute arterial blood gas findings?	Increased pH, decreased $Paco_2$, decreased HCO_3^-, decreased Pao_2, decreased Sao_2 and Spo_2
What are the expected chest radiograph findings?	Translucent lung fields; hyperinflated alveoli; depressed diaphragm
What are the usual respiratory treatments?	Bronchodilator therapy, bronchial hygiene therapy; oxygen therapy
What complications can occur?	Poor response to oxygen and bronchodilator therapy Acute ventilatory failure Severe hypoxia Necessity for mechanical ventilation

breath, dizziness, and fatigue. The practitioner must be prepared to evaluate the severity of such problems, assess the possible cause, and determine the appropriate plan of action.

The *emergency assessment* identifies—or rules out—any life-threatening problems or problems that require immediate interventions. When the patient's medical condition is life threatening or when time is of the essence, the emergency assessment will include only key data needed for dealing with the immediate problem. Additional information can be gathered after the patient's condition has stabilized. The emergency assessment always follows the basic "ABCs" of cardiopulmonary resuscitation (i.e., the securing of the patient's *a*irway, *b*reathing, and *c*irculation).

The *ongoing assessment* consists of the data collection that occurs during each contact with the patient throughout the patient's hospital stay. Depending on the patient's condition, ongoing assessments may take place hourly, daily, weekly, or monthly. In fact, for the critically ill patient, assessments often take place continuously via electronic monitoring equipment. Ongoing assessments also take place while a patient is receiving anesthesia, as well as afterward until the effects of the anesthesia have worn off.

Respiratory therapy practitioners routinely make decisions about the frequency, depth, and breadth of the assessment requirements of the patient. To make these decisions effectively, the practitioner must anticipate the potential for a patient's condition to change, the speed at which it could change, and the clinical data that would justify a change. For example, when a patient experiencing an asthmatic episode inhales the aerosol of a selected bronchodilator, assessment decisions are based on the expected onset of drug action, expected therapeutic effects of the medication, and potential adverse effects that may develop.

Types of Data

Clinical information that is provided by the patient, and that cannot be observed directly, is called *subjective data.* When a patient's subjective data describe characteristics of a particular disorder or dysfunction, they are known as *symptoms.* For example, shortness of breath (dyspnea), pain, dizziness, nausea, and ringing in the ears are symptoms because they cannot be observed directly. The patient must communicate to the health-care provider what symptoms he or she is experiencing. The patient is the only source of information about subjective findings.

Characteristics about the patient that can be observed directly by the practitioner are called *objective data.* When a patient's objective data describe characteristics of a particular disorder or dysfunction, they are known as *signs.* For example, swelling of the legs (pedal edema) is a sign of congestive heart failure. Objective data can be obtained through the practitioner's sense of sight, hearing, taste, touch, and smell. Objective information can be measured (or quantified), and it can be replicated from one practitioner to another—a concept called *inter-rater reliability.* For example, the respiratory practitioner can measure the patient's pulse, respiratory rate, blood pressure, inspiratory effort, and arterial blood gases. Because objective data are factual, they have a high degree of certainty.

Sources of Data

Sources of clinical information include the patient, the patient's significant others, other members of the health-care team, the patient's past history, and results of a variety of clinical tests and procedures. The practitioner must confirm that each data source is appropriate, reliable, and valid for the patient's assessment. *Appropriate* means the source is suitable for the specific purpose, patient, or event. *Reliable* means that the practitioner can trust the data to be accurate and honestly reported. *Valid* means that the clinical data can be verified or confirmed.

The Assessment Process—Role of the Respiratory Practitioner

When the lungs are affected by disease or trauma, they are anatomically altered to some degree, depending on the severity of the process. In general, the anatomic alterations caused by an injury or disease process can be classified as resulting in an obstructive lung disorder, a restrictive lung disorder, or a combination of both. Common anatomic alterations associated with obstructive and restrictive lung disorders are illustrated in Figure 1. Common respiratory diseases and their general classifications are listed in Table 2.

When the normal anatomy of the lungs is altered, certain pathophysiologic mechanisms throughout the cardiopulmonary system are activated. These pathophysiologic mechanisms, in turn, produce a variety of clinical manifestations specific to the illness. Such clinical manifestations can be readily—and objectively—identified in the clinical setting (e.g., increased heart rate, depressed diaphragm, increased functional residual capacity). Because differing chains of events happen as a result of anatomic alterations of the lungs, treatment selection is most appropriately directed at the basic causes of the clinical manifestations—that is, the anatomic alterations of the lungs. For example, a clinician prescribes a

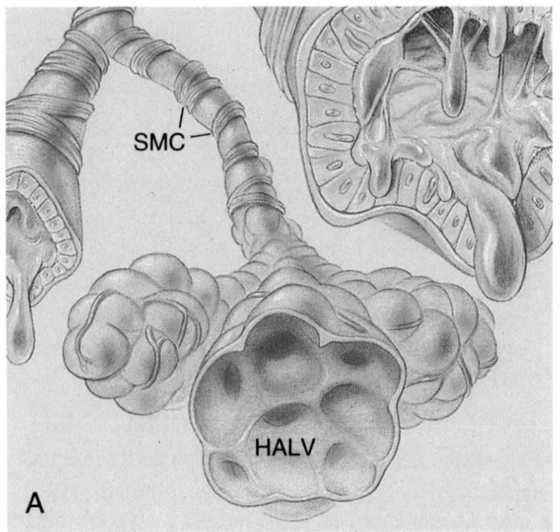

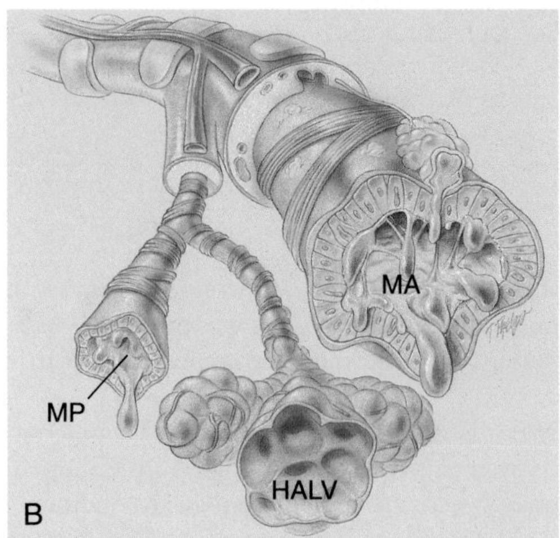

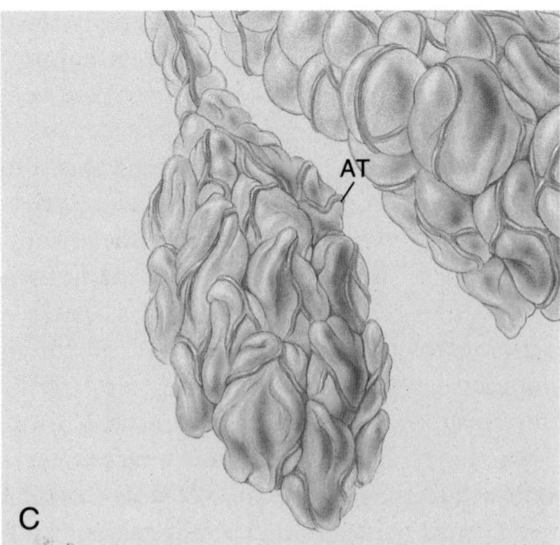

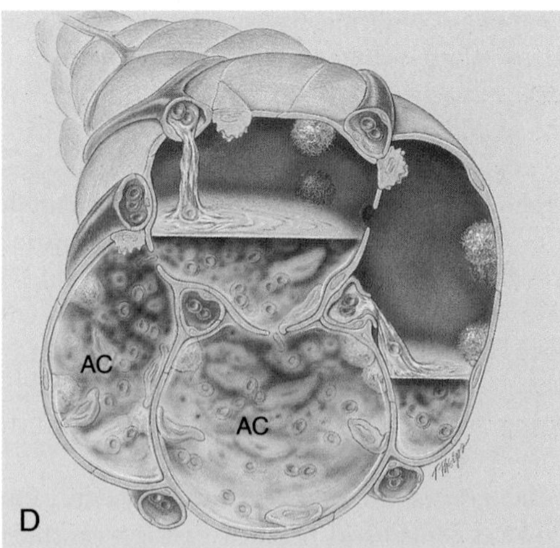

Figure 1 *Common anatomic alterations of the lungs in obstructive lung disorders.* **A**, Bronchial smooth muscle constriction accompanied by air trapping (as seen in asthma). **B**, Tracheobronchial inflammation accompanied by mucous accumulation, partial airway obstruction, and air trapping (as seen in bronchitis). When mucous accumulation causes total airway obstruction, alveolar atelectasis ensues.

Common anatomic alterations of the lungs in restrictive lung disorders. **C**, Alveolar collapse or atelectasis. **D**, Alveolar consolidation (as seen in pneumonia). *AC,* Alveolar consolidation; *AT,* atelectasis; *HALV,* hyperinflated alveoli; *MA,* mucus accumulation; *MP,* mucous plug; *SMC,* smooth muscle constriction.

TABLE 2 General Classification of Respiratory Diseases

	Classification		
Respiratory Disease	**Obstructive**	**Restrictive**	**Combination**
Chronic obstructive pulmonary disease (chronic bronchitis and emphysema)	X		
Asthma	X		
Bronchiectasis			X
Cystic fibrosis			X
Pneumonia		X	
Lung abscess		X	
Tuberculosis		X	
Fungal disease of the lungs		X	
Pulmonary edema		X	
Flail chest		X	
Pneumothorax		X	
Plenural effusion		X	
Kyphoscoliosis		X	
Chronic interstitial lung disease			X
Cancer of the lungs		X	
Acute respiratory distress syndrome		X	
Meconium aspiration syndrome			X
Transient tachypnea of the newborn			X
Idiopathic respiratory distress syndrome		X	
Pulmonary air leak syndrome			X
Respiratory syncytial virus			X
Bronchopulmonary dysplasia			X
Diaphragmatic hernia		X	
Near drowning	X		
Postoperative atelectasis		X	

bronchodilator to offset the bronchospasm associated with an asthmatic episode.

The Knowledge Base

A strong knowledge base of the following four factors is essential to good respiratory care assessment and therapy selection skills:

1. Anatomic alterations of the lungs caused by common respiratory disorders
2. Major pathophysiologic mechanisms activated throughout the respiratory system as a result of the anatomic alterations
3. Common clinical manifestations that develop
4. Treatment modalities used to correct the anatomic alterations and pathophysiologic mechanisms caused by the disorder

Specific Components of the Assessment Process

A respiratory care practitioner with good assessment and treatment selection skills must be competent in performing the actual assessment process, which has the following components:

1. Quick and systematic collection of the important clinical manifestations demonstrated by the patient
2. Formulation of an accurate assessment of the clinical data—that is, identification of the *cause* and *severity* of the data abnormalities
3. Selection of an optimal treatment modality
4. Quick, clear, and precise documentation of this process

Without this basic knowledge and understanding, the respiratory care practitioner merely goes through the motions of performing assigned therapeutic tasks with no short- or long-term anticipated outcomes that can be measured. In such an environment the practitioner works in an unchallenging task-oriented rather than goal-oriented manner.

That goal-oriented (patient-oriented) respiratory care has become the hallmark of practice was suggested in the early 1990s by analyzing the work performance of other health-care disciplines. For example, physical therapists had long been greatly empowered by virtue of the more generic physician's orders under which they work; respiratory therapists, on the other hand, customarily received detailed and specific orders. For example, physical therapists are instructed to "improve back range of motion" or "strengthen quadriceps muscle groups," rather than to "provide warm fomentations to the low back" or "initiate quadriceps setting exercises with 10-pound ankle weights, four times a day, for 10 minutes." In addition, physical therapists are permitted to start, up-regulate, down-regulate, or discontinue the therapy on the basis of the patient's current needs and capabilities—not on the basis of a 2-hour-, 2-day-, or 2-week-old physician assessment. Goal achievement, not task completion, is the way the success of physical therapy is routinely measured.

In the current "sicker in, quicker out" cost-conscious environment, a change has come to respiratory care. Under fixed reimbursement programs, shorter lengths of stay have required hospital administrators and medical staff to examine allocation of health-care resources. Recent data suggest that fully one third of all hospitalized patients receive respiratory care services; therefore such services have come under close scrutiny. Studies using available peer-reviewed clinical practice guidelines have identified tremendous overuse (and, less frequently, underuse) of therapy modalities, and from this misallocation, the now firmly entrenched "therapist-driven protocol" (TDP) approach has emerged as the new gold standard of respiratory care practice. Observing that the patient (and more accurately, the pulmonary pathophysiology!) should set the pace, some centers have called these protocols "patient-driven protocols," but the appellation of TDP has more strongly caught on. Clinical practice guidelines (CPGs) such as those developed by the American Association of Respiratory Care (AARC) are routinely used as the basis for TDPs in respiratory care.

The American College of Chest Physicians defines respiratory care protocols as follows:

> Patient care plans which are initiated and implemented by credentialed respiratory care workers. These plans are designed and developed with input from physicians, and are approved for use by the medical staff and the governing body of the hospitals in which they are used. They share in common extreme reliance on assessment and evaluation skills. Protocols are by their nature dynamic and flexible, allowing up- or down-regulation of intensity of respiratory services. Protocols allow the respiratory care practitioner authority to evaluate the patient, [to] initiate care, to adjust, discontinue, or restart respiratory care procedures on a shift-by-shift or hour-to-hour basis once the protocol is ordered by the physician. They must contain clear strategies for various therapeutic interventions, while avoiding any misconception that they infringe on the practice of medicine.

Numerous studies have now shown beyond a shadow of a doubt that when respiratory care protocol guidelines are followed appropriately, the outcomes of respiratory care services improve. This improvement is noted in both clinical and economic ways (e.g., shorter ventilator weaning time in postoperative coronary artery bypass graft [CABG] patients). Under this paradigm, respiratory care that is inappropriately ordered is either withheld or modified (whichever is appropriate), and patients who *need* respiratory care services (but are not receiving them) should now be able to receive care. (Chapter 9 discusses the implementation of a good TDP program in detail.) The notion that today's respiratory care practitioner "might" practice in the TDP setting has passed. Respiratory practitioners who find that they are working in an archaic setting where TDPs are not in daily use should critically reexamine their employment options and career goals! To practice in today's health-care environment without the cognitive (thinking) skills used in the TDP environment is no longer acceptable.

Experience, however, indicates that at least *some* respiratory care practitioners are not entirely comfortable with the new role and responsibility the TDP paradigm has thrust on them. These workers have difficulty separating the contents of *their* "little black bag" of diagnostic and therapeutic modalities from the one traditionally carried and used by the physician. The choice to be a "protocol safe and ready therapist," however, is no longer elective. The profession of respiratory care has changed and moved on. The Clinical Simulation Examination portion of the National Board for Respiratory Care (NBRC) Advanced Practitioner Examination reflects the actual, no longer just "simulated," bedside practice of respiratory care.

Similar to their physical therapist colleagues, today's respiratory care practitioners are now routinely asked to participate actively in the appropriate allocation of respiratory care services. Modern respiratory care practitioners must possess the basic knowledge, skills, and personal attributes to collect and assess clinical data and treat their patients effectively. Under the TDP paradigm, specific clinical indicators (clinical manifestations) for a particular respiratory care procedure must first be identified. In other words, a specific treatment plan is only started, up-regulated, down-regulated, or discontinued on the basis of the following:

1. The presence and collection of specific clinical indicators, and
2. An assessment made from the clinical data (i.e., the cause of the clinical data) that justifies the therapy order or change

In addition, after a particular treatment has been administered to the patient, all treatment outcomes must be measured and documented. Clearly, the success or failure of protocol work depends on accurate and timely patient assessment.

In view of these considerations, it must be stressed that today's respiratory care practitioner must have competent bedside pulmonary assessment skills. Fundamental to this process is the ability to systematically gather clinical data, make an assessment, and develop an appropriate, safe, and effective action plan. Typically, once a treatment regimen has been implemented, the patient's progress is monitored on an ongoing assessment basis. In other words, clinical data are, again, collected, evaluated, and acted on based on the patient's progress toward a predefined goal.

To be fully competent in the assessment of respiratory disorders, the respiratory care practitioner must first have a strong academic foundation in the areas presented in Part I of this textbook. Part I is divided into three sections:

I. Clinical Data Obtained at the Patient's Bedside
II. Clinical Data Obtained from Laboratory Tests and Special Procedures
III. The Therapist-Driven Protocol Program—The Essentials

These three sections provide the reader with the essential knowledge base to assess and treat the patient with respiratory disease. The respiratory care practitioner must master the material in these sections to work efficiently and safely in a good TDP program.

PART I

Assessment of Respiratory Disease

The Patient Interview 1

Chapter Objectives

After reading this chapter, you will be able to:

- Describe the major items found on a patient history form.
- Explain the primary tasks performed during the patient interview.
- Describe the internal factors the practitioner brings to the interview.
- Discuss the external factors that provide a good physical setting for the interview.
- Differentiate between open-ended questions and closed or direct questions.
- Describe the following nine types of verbal responses:
  - Facilitation
  - Silence
  - Reflection
  - Empathy
  - Clarification
  - Confrontation
  - Interpretation
  - Explanation
  - Summary
- Describe why the following are nonproductive verbal messages:
  - Providing assurance or reassurance
  - Giving advice
  - Using authority
  - Using avoidance language
  - Distancing
  - Professional jargon
  - Asking leading or biased questions
  - Talking too much
  - Interrupting and anticipating
  - Using "why" questions
- List positive and negative nonverbal messages of the interview, including:
  - Physical appearance
  - Posture
  - Gestures
  - Facial expression
  - Eye contact
  - Voice
  - Touch
- Describe how to close the interview.
- Define key terms and complete self-asessment questions at the end of the chapter and on Evolve.

Key Terms

Clarification
Closed or Direct Questions
Confrontation
Empathy
Explanation
External Factors
Facilitation
Internal Factors
Interpretation
Nonproductive Verbal Messages
Nonverbal Skills
Open-Ended Questions
Reflection
Silence
Summary

Chapter Outline

Patient History

A complete patient assessment includes the patient interview. The purpose of the patient history is to gather pertinent subjective and objective data, which in turn can be used to develop a more complete picture of the patient's past and present health. In most clinical settings the patient is asked to fill out a printed history form or checklist. The patient should be allowed ample time to recall important dates, health-related landmarks, and family history. The patient interview is then used to validate what the patient has written and collect additional data on the patient's health status and lifestyle. Although history forms vary, most contain the following:

- Biographic data (age, gender, occupation)
- The patient's chief complaint or reason for seeking care, including the onset, duration, and characteristics of the signs and symptoms
- Present health or history of present illness
- Past health, including childhood illnesses, accidents or injuries, serious or chronic illnesses, hospitalizations, operations, obstetric history, immunizations, last examination date, allergies, current medications, and history of smoking or other habits
- The patient's family history
- Review of each body system, including skin, head, eyes, ears and nose, mouth and throat, respiratory system, cardiovascular system, gastrointestinal system, urinary system, genital system, and endocrine system
- Functional assessment (activities of daily living), including activity and exercise, work performance, sleep and rest, nutrition, interpersonal relationships, and coping and stress management strategies

Patient Interview

The interview is a meeting between the respiratory care practitioner and the patient. It allows the collection of subjective data about the patient's feelings regarding the condition. During a successful interview, the practitioner performs the following tasks:

1. Gathers complete and accurate data about the patient's impressions about his or her health, including a description and chronology of any symptoms
2. Establishes rapport and trust so the patient feels accepted and comfortable in sharing all relevant information
3. Develops and shows an understanding about the patient's health state, which in turn enhances the patient's participation in identifying problems
4. Builds rapport to secure a continuing working relationship, which facilitates future assessments, evaluations, and treatment plans

Interview skills are an art form that takes time—and experience—to develop. The most important components of a successful interview are communication and understanding. Understanding the various signals of communication is the most difficult part. When understanding (conveying of meaning) breaks down between the practitioner and the patient, no communication can occur. Communication cannot be assumed just because two people have the ability to speak and listen. Communication is about behaviors—conscious and unconscious, verbal and nonverbal. All these behaviors convey meaning. The following paragraphs describe important factors that enhance the sending and receiving of information during communication.

Internal Factors

Internal factors encompass what the practitioner brings to the interview—a genuine concern for others, **empathy,** understanding, and the ability to listen. A genuine liking of other people is essential in developing a strong rapport with the patient. It requires a generally optimistic view of people, a positive view of their strengths, and an acceptance of their weaknesses. This affection generates an atmosphere of warmth and caring. The patient must feel accepted unconditionally.

Empathy is the art of viewing the world from the patient's point of view while remaining separate from it. Empathy entails recognition and acceptance of the patient's feelings without criticism. It is sometimes described as feeling with the patient rather than feeling like the patient. To have empathy the practitioner needs to listen. Listening is not a passive process. Listening is active and demanding. It requires the practitioner's complete attention. If the examiner is preoccupied with personal needs or concerns, he or she will invariably miss something important. Active listening is a cornerstone to understanding. Nearly everything the patient says or does is relevant.

During the interview the examiner should observe the patient's body language and note the patient's facial expressions, eye movement (e.g., avoiding eye contact, looking into space, diverting gaze), pain grimaces, restlessness, and sighing. The examiner should listen to the way things are said. For example, is the tone of the patient's voice normal? Does the patient's voice quiver? Are there pitch breaks in the patient's voice? Does the patient say only a few words and then take a breath?

External Factors

External factors such as a good physical setting enhances the interviewing process. Regardless of the interview's setting (the patient's bedside, an office in the hospital or clinic, or the patient's home), efforts should be made to (1) ensure privacy, (2) prevent interruptions, and (3) secure a comfortable physical environment (e.g., comfortable room temperature, sufficient lighting, absence of noise).

Techniques of Communication

During the interview the patient should be addressed by his or her surname, and the examiner should introduce himself or herself and state the purpose for being there. The following introduction serves as an example: "Good morning, Mr. Jones. I'm Mrs. Smith, and I'm from Respiratory Care. I want to ask you some questions about your breathing so that we can plan your respiratory care here in the hospital."

Verbal skills and techniques used by the examiner to facilitate the interview may include **open-ended questions, closed or direct questions,** and responses.

Open-Ended Questions

An open-ended question asks the patient to provide narrative information. The examiner identifies the topic to be discussed but only in general terms. This technique is commonly used (1) to begin the interview, (2) to introduce a new section of questions, or (3) to gather further information whenever the patient introduces a new topic. The following are examples of open-ended questions:

"What brings you to the hospital today?"

"Tell me why you have come to the hospital today."

"How has your breathing been getting along?"

"You said that you have been short of breath. Tell me more about that."

The open-ended question is unbiased; it allows the patient freedom to answer in any way. This type of question encourages the patient to respond at greater length and give a spontaneous account of the condition. As the patient answers, the examiner should stop and listen. Patients often answer in short phrases or sentences and then pause, waiting for some kind of direction from the examiner. What the examiner does next is often the key to the direction of the interview. If the examiner presents new questions on other topics, much of the initial story may be lost. Ideally, the examiner should first respond by saying such things as "Tell me about it" and "Anything else?" The patient will usually add important information to the story.

Closed or Direct Questions

A closed or direct question asks the patient for specific information. This type of question elicits a short one- or two-word answer, a yes or no, or a forced choice. The closed question is commonly used after the patient's narrative to fill in any details the patient may have left out. Closed questions also are used to obtain specific facts, such as "Have you ever had this chest pain before?" Closed or direct questions speed up the interview. The use of only open-ended questions is unwieldy and takes an unrealistic amount of time, causing undue stress in the patient. Box 1-1 compares closed and open-ended questions.

Box 1-1 Comparison of Closed and Open-Ended Questions

Open-Ended	Closed
Used for narrative	Used for specific information
Call for long answers	Call for short one- or two-word answers
Elicit feelings, options, ideas	Elicit "cold facts"
Build and enhance rapport	Limit rapport and leave interaction neutral

Responses—Assisting the Narrative

As the patient answers the open-ended questions, the examiner's role is to encourage free expression but not to let the patient digress. The examiner's responses work to clarify the story. There are nine types of verbal responses. In the first five responses the patient leads; in the last four responses the examiner leads.

The first five responses require the examiner's reactions to the facts or feelings the patient has communicated. The examiner's response focuses on the patient's frame of reference; the examiner's frame of reference is not relevant. For the last four responses the examiner's reaction is not required. The frame of reference shifts from the patient's perspective to the examiner's. These responses include the examiner's thoughts or feelings. The examiner should use these responses only when the situation calls for them. If these responses are used too often, the interview becomes focused more on the examiner than on the patient. The nine responses are described in the following sections.

Facilitation

Facilitation encourages patients to say more, to continue with the story. Examples of facilitating responses include the following: "Mm hmm," "Go on," "Continue," "Uh-huh." This type of response shows patients that the examiner is interested in what they are saying and will listen further. Nonverbal cues, such as maintaining eye contact and shifting forward in the seat, also encourage the patient to continue talking.

Silence

Silent attentiveness is effective after an open-ended question. **Silence** communicates that the patient has time to think and organize what he or she wishes to say without interruption by the examiner.

Reflection

Reflection is used to echo the patient's words. The examiner repeats a part of what the patient has just said to clarify or stimulate further communication. Reflection helps the patient focus on specific areas and continue in his or her own way. The following is a good example:

PATIENT: "I'm here because of my breathing. It's blocked."

EXAMINER: "It's blocked?"

PATIENT: "Yes, every time I try to exhale, something blocks my breath and prevents me from getting all my air out."

Reflection also can be used to express the emotions implicit in the patient's words. The examiner focuses on these emotions and encourages the patient to elaborate:

PATIENT: "I have three little ones at home. I'm so worried they're not getting the care they need."

EXAMINER: "You feel worried and anxious about your children."

The examiner acts as a mirror reflecting the patient's words and feelings. This technique helps the patient elaborate on the problem.

Empathy

Empathy is defined as the identification of oneself with another and the resulting capacity to feel or experience sensations, emotions, or thoughts similar to those being experienced by another person. It is often characterized as the ability to "put oneself into another's shoes." A physical symptom, condition, or disease frequently has accompanying emotions. Patients often have trouble expressing these feelings. An empathic response recognizes these feelings and allows expression of them:

PATIENT: "This is just great! I used to work out every day, and now I don't have enough breath to walk up the stairs!"

EXAMINER: "It must be hard—you used to exercise every day, and now you can't do a fraction of what you used to do."

The examiner's response does not cut off further communication, which would occur by giving false reassurance (e.g., "Oh, you'll be back on your feet in no time"). Also, it does not deny the patient's feelings, nor does it suggest that the patient's feelings are unjustified. An empathic response recognizes the patient's feelings, accepts them, and allows the patient to express them without embarrassment. It strengthens rapport.

Clarification

Clarification is used when the patient's choice of words is ambiguous or confusing:

"Tell me what you mean by bad air."

Clarification also is used to summarize and simplify the patient's words. When simplifying the patient's words, the examiner should ask whether the paraphrase is accurate. The examiner is asking for agreement, and this allows the patient to confirm or deny the examiner's understanding.

Confrontation

In using **confrontation,** the examiner notes a certain action, feeling, or statement made by the patient and focuses the patient's attention on it:

"You said it doesn't hurt when you cough, but when you cough you grimace."

Alternatively, the examiner may focus on the patient's affect:

"You look depressed today."

"You sound angry."

Interpretation

Interpretation links events and data, makes associations, and implies causes. It provides the basis for inference or conclusion:

"It seems that every time you have a serious asthma attack, you have had some kind of stress in your life."

The examiner runs the risk of making an incorrect inference. However, even if the patient corrects the inference, the patient's response often serves to prompt further discussion of the topic.

Explanation

Explanation provides the patient with factual and objective information:

"It is very common for your heart rate to increase a bit after a bronchodilator treatment."

Summary

The **summary** is the final overview of the examiner's understanding of the patient's statements. It condenses the facts and presents an outline of the way the examiner perceives the patient's respiratory status. It is a type of validation in that the patient can agree or disagree with the examiner's summary. Both the examiner and the patient should participate in the summary. The summary signals that the interview is about to end.

Nonproductive Verbal Messages

In addition to the verbal techniques commonly used to enhance the interview, the examiner must refrain from making **nonproductive verbal messages.** These defeating messages restrict the patient's response. They act as barriers to obtaining data and establishing rapport.

Providing Assurance or Reassurance

Providing assurance or reassurance gives the examiner the false sense of having provided comfort. In fact, this type of response probably does more to relieve the examiner's anxiety than that of the patient.

PATIENT: "I'm so worried about the mass the doctor found on my chest x-ray. I hope it doesn't turn out to be cancer! What happens to your lung?"

EXAMINER: "Now, don't worry. I'm sure you will be all right. You have a very good doctor."

The examiner's response trivializes the patient's concern and effectively halts further communication about the topic. Instead, the examiner might have responded in a more empathic way:

"You are really worried about that mass on your x-ray, aren't you? It must be very hard to wait for the lab results."

This response acknowledges the patient's feelings and concerns and, more important, keeps the door open for further communication.

Giving Advice

A key step in professional growth is to know when to give advice and when to refrain from it. Patients will often seek the examiner's professional advice and opinion on a specific topic:

"What types of things should I avoid to keep my asthma under control?"

This is a straightforward request for information that the examiner has and the patient needs. The examiner should respond directly, and the answer should be based on knowledge and experience. The examiner should refrain from dispensing advice that is based on a hunch or feeling. For example, consider the patient who has just seen the doctor:

"Dr. Johnson has just told me I may need an operation to remove the mass they found in my lungs. I just don't know. What would you do?"

If the examiner answers, the accountability for the decision shifts from the patient to the examiner. The examiner is not the patient. The patient must work this problem out. In fact, the patient probably does not really want to know what the examiner would do. In this case, the patient is worried about what he or she might have to do. A better response is reflection:

EXAMINER: "Have an operation?"

PATIENT: "Yes, and I've never been put to sleep before. What do they do if you don't wake up?"

Now the examiner knows the patient's real concern and can work to help the patient deal with it. For the patient to accept advice, it must be meaningful and appropriate. For example, in planning pulmonary rehabilitation for a male patient with severe emphysema, the respiratory therapist advises him to undertake a moderate walking program. The patient may treat the therapist's advice in one of two ways—either follow it or not. Indeed, the patient may choose to ignore it, feeling that it is not appropriate for him (e.g., he feels he gets plenty of exercise at work anyway).

On the other hand, if the patient follows the therapist's advice, three outcomes are possible: The patient's condition stays the same, improves, or worsens. If the walking strengthens the patient, the condition improves. However, if the patient was not part of the decision-making process to initiate a walking program, the psychologic reward is limited, promoting further dependency. If the walking program does not improve his condition or compromises it, the advice did not work. Because the advice was not the patient's, he can avoid any responsibility for the failure:

"See, I did what you advised me to do, and it didn't help. In fact, I feel worse! Why did you tell me to do this anyway?"

Although giving advice might be faster, the examiner should take the time to involve the patient in the problem-solving process. A patient who is an active player in the decision-making process is more likely to learn and modify behavior.

Using Authority

The examiner should avoid responses that promote dependency and inferiority:

"Now, your doctor and therapist know best."

Although the examiner and the patient cannot have equality in terms of professional skills and experience, both are equally worthy human beings and owe each other respect.

Using Avoidance Language

When talking about potentially frightening topics, people often use euphemisms (e.g., "passed on" rather than "died") to avoid reality or hide their true feelings. Although the use of euphemisms may appear to make a topic less frightening, it does not make the topic or the fear go away. In fact, not talking about a frightening subject suppresses the patient's feelings and often makes the patient more fearful. The use of direct and clear language is the best way to deal with potentially uncomfortable topics.

Distancing

Distancing is the use of impersonal conversation that places space between a frightening topic and the speaker. For example, a patient with a lung mass may say, "A friend of mine has a tumor on her lung. She is afraid that she may need an operation" or "There is a tumor in the left lung." By using "the" rather than "my," the patient can deny any association with the tumor. Occasionally, health-care workers also use distancing to soften reality. As a general rule, this technique does not work because it communicates to the patient that the health-care practitioner also is afraid of the topic. The use of frank, specific terms usually helps defuse anxiety rather than causing it.

Professional Jargon

What a health-care worker calls a myocardial infarction, a patient calls a heart attack. The use of professional jargon can sound exclusionary and paternalistic to the patient. Health-care practitioners should always try to adjust their vocabulary to the patient's understanding without sounding condescending. Even if patients use medical terms, the examiner cannot assume that they fully understand the meaning. For example, patients often think the term *hypertension* means that they are very tense and therefore take their medication only when they are feeling stressed, not when they feel relaxed.

Asking Leading or Biased Questions

Asking a patient "You don't smoke anymore, do you?" implies that one answer is better than another. The patient is forced either to answer in a way corresponding to the examiner's values or to feel guilty when admitting the other answer. When responding to this type of question, the patient risks the examiner's disapproval and possible alienation, which are undesirable responses from the patient's point of view.

Talking Too Much

Some examiners feel that helpfulness is directly related to verbal productivity. If they have spent the session talking, they leave feeling that they have met the patient's needs. In fact, the opposite is true. The patient needs time to talk. As a general rule, the examiner should listen more than talk.

Interrupting and Anticipating

While patients are speaking, the examiner should refrain from interrupting them, even when the examiner believes that she or he knows what is about to be said. Interruptions do not facilitate the interview. Rather, they communicate to the patient that the examiner is impatient or bored with the interview. Another trap is thinking about the next question while the patient is answering the last one, or anticipating the answer. Examiners who are overly preoccupied with their role as interviewer are not really listening to the patient. As a general rule the examiner should allow a second or so of silence between the patient's statement and the next question.

Using "Why" Questions

The examiner should be careful in presenting "why" questions. The use of "why" questions often implies blame; it puts the patient on the defensive:

"Why did you wait so long before calling your doctor?"

"Why didn't you take your asthma medication with you?"

The only possible answer to a "why" question is "because...," and this places the patient in an uncomfortable position. To avoid this trap, the examiner might say, "I noticed you didn't call your doctor right away when you were having trouble breathing. I'd like to find out what was happening during this time."

Nonverbal Skills

Nonverbal skills of communication include physical appearance, posture, gestures, facial expression, eye contact, voice, and touch. Nonverbal messages are important in establishing rapport and conveying feelings. Nonverbal messages may either support or contradict verbal messages. Therefore an awareness of the nonverbal messages that may be conveyed by either the patient or the examiner during the interview process is important. Box 1-2 provides an overview of nonverbal messages that may occur during an interview.

Physical Appearance

The examiner's general personal appearance, grooming, and choice of clothing send a message to the patient. Professional dress codes vary among hospitals and clinical settings. Depending on the setting, a professional uniform can project a message that ranges from comfortable or casual to formal or distant. Regardless of one's personal choice in clothing and general appearance, the aim should be to convey a competent and professional image.

Box 1-2 Nonverbal Messages of the Interview

Positive	Negative
Professional appearance	Nonprofessional appearance
Sitting next to patient	Sitting behind a desk
Close proximity to patient	Far away from patient
Turned toward patient	Turned away from patient
Relaxed, open posture	Tense, closed posture
Leaning toward patient	Slouched away from patient
Facilitating gestures	Nonfacilitating gestures
• Nodding of head	• Looking at watch
Positive facial expressions	Negative facial expressions
• Appropriate smiling	• Frowning
• Interest	• Yawning
Good eye contact	Poor eye contact
Moderate tone of voice	Strident, high-pitched voice
Moderate rate of speech	Speech too fast or too slow
Appropriate touch	Overly frequent or inappropriate touch

Posture

An open position is one in which a communicator extends the large muscle groups (i.e., arms and legs are not crossed). An open position shows relaxation, physical comfort, and a willingness to share information. A closed position, with arms and legs crossed, sends a defensive and anxious message. The examiner should be aware of any posture changes. For example, if the patient suddenly shifts from a relaxed to a tense position, it suggests discomfort with the topic. In addition, the examiner should try to sit comfortably next to the patient during the interview. Sitting too far away or standing over the patient often sends a negative nonverbal message.

Gestures

Gestures send nonverbal messages. For example, pointing a finger may show anger or blame. Nodding of the head or an open hand with the palms turned upward can show acceptance, attention, or agreement. Wringing the hands suggests worry and anxiety. The patient often describes a crushing chest pain by holding a fist in front of the sternum. When a patient has a sharp, localized pain, one finger is commonly used to point to the exact spot.

Facial Expression

An individual's face can convey a wide range of emotions and conditions. For example, facial expressions can reflect alertness, relaxation, anxiety, anger, suspicion, and pain. The examiner should work to convey an attentive, sincere, and interested expression. Patient rapport will deteriorate if the examiner exhibits facial expressions that suggest boredom, distraction, disgust, criticism, and disbelief.

Eye Contact

Lack of eye contact suggests that a person may be insecure, intimidated, shy, withdrawn, confused, bored, apathetic, or depressed. The examiner should work to maintain good eye contact but not stare the patient down with a fixed, penetrating look. Generally, an easy gaze toward the patient's eyes with occasional glances away works well. The examiner, however, should be aware that this approach may not work when interviewing a patient from a culture in which direct eye contact is generally avoided. For example, Asian, Native American, Indochinese, Arab, and some Appalachian people may consider direct eye contact impolite or aggressive, and they may avert their own eyes during the interview.

Voice

Nonverbal messages are reflected through the tone of voice, intensity and rate of speech, pitch, and long pauses. These messages often convey more meaning than the spoken word. For example, a patient's voice may show sarcasm, anxiety, sympathy, or hostility. An anxious patient frequently talks in a loud and fast voice. A soft voice may reflect shyness and fear. A patient with hearing impairment generally speaks in a loud voice. Long pauses may have important meanings. For instance, when a patient pauses for a long time before answering an easy and straightforward question, the honesty of the answer may be questionable. Slow speech with long and frequent pauses, combined with a weak and monotonous voice, suggests depression.

Touch

The meaning of touch is often misinterpreted; it can be influenced by an individual's age, gender, cultural background, past experiences, and the present setting. As a general rule, the examiner should not touch patients during interviews unless he or she knows the patient well and is sure that the gesture will be interpreted correctly. When appropriate, touch (such as a touch of the hand or arm) can be effective in conveying empathy.

To summarize, extensive nonverbal messages, communicated by both the examiner and patient, may be conveyed during the interview. Therefore the examiner must be aware of the patient's various nonverbal messages while working to communicate nonverbal messages that are productive and enhancing to the examiner-patient relationship.

Closing the Interview

The interview should end gracefully. If the session has an abrupt or awkward closing, the patient may be left with a negative impression. This final moment may destroy any rapport gained during the interview. To ease into the closing, the examiner might ask the patient one of the following questions:

"Is there anything else that you would like to talk about?"
"Do you have any questions that you would like to ask me?"
"Are there any other problems that we have not discussed?"

These types of questions give the patient an opportunity for self-expression. The examiner may choose to summarize or repeat what was learned during the interview. This serves as a final statement of the examiner's and the patient's assessment of the situation. Finally, the examiner should thank the patient for the time and cooperation provided during the interview.

SELF-ASSESSMENT QUESTIONS

evolve See Evolve Resources for answers. To access additional student assessment questions and case studies for application of text material to real-life scenarios, visit **http://evolve.elsevier.com/DesJardins/respiratory.**

1. During the patient interview, the practitioner states: "You are worried about your child." This is known as:
   a. Reflection
   b. An open-ended question
   c. Confrontation
   d. Facilitation

2. Which of the following is a closed or direct question?
   a. You look depressed today. Are you angry?
   b. Have you had this pain before?
   c. Now, don't you think your doctor knows best?
   d. Why did you wait so long before calling your doctor?

3. Which of the following is or are considered negative nonverbal messages of the interview?
   1. Nodding of head
   2. Sitting behind a desk
   3. Moderate tone of voice
   4. Sitting next to the patient
      a. 2 only
      b. 3 and 4 only
      c. 1, 2, and 3 only
      d. 2, 3, and 4 only

4. Which of the following is or are likely to be found on a patient history form?
   1. The patient's family history
   2. Activities of daily living
   3. The patient's chief complaint
   4. Review of each body system
      a. 2 and 3 only
      b. 1 and 4 only
      c. 2, 3, and 4 only
      d. 1, 2, 3, and 4

5. Which of the following is considered a "facilitation" response?
   a. "You feel anxious about your children."
   b. "It must be hard to not be able to do that now."
   c. "Mm hmmm, go on."
   d. "Tell me what you mean by bad air."

The Physical Examination and Its Basis in Physiology 2

Chapter Objectives

After reading this chapter, you will be able to:

- Describe the major components of a patient's vital signs, including:
  - Body temperature
  - Pulse
  - Respiration
  - Blood pressure
  - Oxygen saturation
- Describe the systematic examination of the chest and lungs, including:
  - Lung and chest topography
  - Inspection
  - Palpation
  - Percussion
  - Auscultation
- Discuss in more depth the common clinical manifestations observed during inspection, including normal ventilatory pattern and the common pathophysiologic mechanisms that affect the ventilatory pattern.
- Describe the function of the following accessory muscles of inspiration:
  - Scalene
  - Sternocleidomastoid
  - Pectoralis major
  - Trapezius
- Describe the function of the following accessory muscles of expiration:
  - Rectus abdominis
  - External oblique
  - Internal oblique
  - Transversus abdominis
- Discuss the effects of pursed-lip breathing.
- Describe the pathophysiologic basis for substernal and intercostal retractions.
- Explain nasal flaring.
- Discuss splinting caused by chest pain or decreased chest expansion including pleuritic chest pain and nonpleuritic chest pain.
- List abnormal chest shape and configuration.
- List abnormal extremity findings, and include:
  - Altered skin color (e.g., cyanotic, pale, with prominent venous distention)
  - Presence or absence of digital clubbing
  - Presence or absence of peripheral edema
  - Presence or absence of distended neck veins
- Describe how the following correlates to normal and abnormal sputum production, including:
  - Normal histology and mucous production of the tracheobronchial tree
  - Abnormal sputum production
  - Cough
- Define key terms and complete self-assessment questions at the end of the chapter and on Evolve.

Key Terms

Abnormal Ventilatory Patterns
Absolute Shunts
Accessory Muscles of Expiration
Accessory Muscles of Inspiration
Adventitious (Abnormal) Breath Sounds
Afebrile
Airway Resistance
Anatomic Shunts
Anterior Axillary Line
Aortic and Carotid Sinus Baroreceptor Reflexes
Apical Pulse
Apnea
Auscultation
Biot's Respiration
Blood Pressure (BP)
Body Temperature (T)
Brachial Pulse
Bradycardia
Bradypnea
Bronchial
Bronchial Breath Sounds
Bronchovesicular
Capillary Shunts
Cardiac Diastole
Cardiac Output (CO)
Cardiac Systole
Carotid Pulse
Central Chemoreceptors
Central Cyanosis
Chest Excursion

Cheyne-Stokes Respiration
Constant Fever
Core Temperature
Crackles and Rhonchi
Crepitus
Deflation Reflex
Diaphragm
Diaphragmatic Excursion
Diastole
Diastolic Blood Pressure
Diminished Breath Sounds
Dull Percussion Note
External Oblique
Febrile
Femoral Pulse
Hemoptysis
Hering-Breuer Reflex
Horizontal Fissure
Hyperpyrexia
Hyperresonant note
Hypertension
Hyperthermia
Hyperventilation
Hypotension
Hypoventilation
Inspection
Inspiratory-to-Expiratory Ratio (I:E Ratio)
Intermittent Fever
Internal Oblique
Irritant Reflex
Juxtapulmonary-Capillary Receptors (J Receptors) Reflex
Kussmaul's Respiration
Lung and Chest Topography
Lung Compliance
Midaxillary Line
Midclavicular Lines
Midscapular Line
Midsternal Line
Mild Hypoxemia
Moderate Hypoxemia
Normal Breath Sounds
Normal Ventilatory Pattern
Oblique Fissure
Palpation
Pectoralis Major
Pedal (Dorsalis Pedis) Pulse
Percussion
Peripheral Chemoreceptors
Pleural Friction Rub
Popliteal Pulse
Posterior Axillary Line
Posterior Tibial Pulse
Pulmonary Reflexes
Pulmonary Shunting
Pulse (P)
Pulse Oximetry (Spo_2)
Pulse Pressure
Pulsus Alternans
Pulsus Paradoxus
Pyrexia
Radial Pulse
Rectus Abdominis
Refractory
Relapsing Fever
Relative Shunt
Remittent Fever
Respiration
Scalene
Severe Hypoxemia
Shuntlike Effect
Sinus Arrhythmia
Sternocleidomastoid
Stridor
Stroke Volume
Subcutaneous Emphysema
Systole
Systolic Blood Pressure
Tachycardia
Tachypnea
Tactile Fremitus
Temporal Pulse
Thebesian Veins
Tidal Volume (V_T)
Transversus Abdominis
Trapezius
True Shunts
Ultrasonic Doppler
Vasoconstriction
Vasodilation
Ventilatory Rate
Vertebral Line
Vesicular Breath Sounds
Vocal Fremitus
Wheezing
Whispering Pectoriloquy

Chapter Outline

Vital Signs

The four major vital signs—**body temperature (T), pulse (P), respiratory rate (R)**, and **blood pressure (BP)**—are excellent bedside clinical indicators of the patient's physiologic and psychologic health. In many patient care settings, the oxygen saturation as measured by **pulse oximetry (Spo_2)** is considered to be the fifth vital sign. Table 2-1 shows the normal values that have been established for various age groups.

During the initial measurement of a patient's vital signs, the values are compared with these normal values. After several vital signs have been documented, these data are then used as a baseline for subsequent measurements. Isolated vital sign measurements are not as valuable as a series of measurements. By evaluating a series of values, the practitioner can identify important vital sign trends for the patient. The identification of vital sign trends that deviate from the patient's normal measurements is often more significant than an isolated measurement.

Although the skills involved in obtaining the vital signs are easy to learn, interpretation and clinical application require knowledge, problem-solving skills, critical thinking, and experience. Even though vital sign measurements are part of routine bedside care, they provide important information and should always be considered as an important part of the assessment process. The frequency with which vital signs should be assessed depends on the individual needs of each patient.

Body Temperature

Body temperature is routinely measured to assess for signs of inflammation or infection. Even though the body's skin temperature varies widely in response to environmental conditions and physical activity, the temperature inside the body, the **core temperature,** remains relatively constant—about 37° C (98.6° F), with a daily variation of ±0.5° C (1° to 2° F). Under normal circumstances the body is able to maintain this constant temperature through various physiologic compensatory mechanisms, such as the autonomic nervous system and special receptors located in the skin, abdomen, and spinal cord.

In response to temperature changes the receptors sense and send information through the nervous system to the hypothalamus. The hypothalamus, in turn, processes the information and activates the appropriate response. For example, an increase in body temperature causes the blood vessels near the skin surface to dilate—a process called **vasodilation.** Vasodilation, in turn, allows more warmed blood to flow near the skin surface, thereby enhancing heat loss. In contrast, a decrease in body temperature causes **vasoconstriction,** which works to keep warmed blood closer to the center of the body—thus working to maintain the core temperature.

At normal body temperature, the metabolic functions of all body cells are optimal. When the body temperature increases or decreases significantly from the normal range, the metabolic rate and therefore the demands on the cardiopulmonary system also change. For example, during a fever

TABLE 2-1 Average Range for Vital Signs According to Age Group

Age Group	Temperature (F°)	Pulse (bpm)	Respirations (breaths/min)	Blood Pressure (mm Hg)	
				Systolic	Diastolic
Newborn	96-99.5	100-180	30-60	60-90	20-60
Infant (1 mo.-1 yr)	99.4-99.7	80-160	30-60	75-100	50-70
Toddler (1-3 yrs)	99.4-99.7	80-130	25-40	80-110	55-80
Preschooler (3-6 yrs)	98.6-99	80-120	20-35	80-110	50-80
Child (6-12 yrs)	98.6	65-100	20-30	100-110	60-70
Adolescent (12-18 yrs)	97-99	60-90	12-20	110-120	60-65
Adult	97-99	60-100	12-20	110-140	60-90
Older adult (>70 yrs)	95-99	60-100	12-20	120-140	70-90

the metabolic rate increases. This action leads to an increase in oxygen consumption and to an increase in carbon dioxide production at the cellular level. According to estimates, for every 1° C increase in body temperature, the patient's oxygen consumption increases about 10%. As the metabolic rate increases, the cardiopulmonary system must work harder to meet the additional cellular demands. Hypothermia reduces the metabolic rate and cardiopulmonary demand.

As shown in Figure 2-1, the normal body temperature is positioned within a relatively narrow range. A patient who has a temperature within the normal range is said to be **afebrile.** A body temperature above the normal range is called **pyrexia** or **hyperthermia.** When the body temperature rises above the normal range, the patient is said to have a *fever* or to be **febrile.** An exceptionally high temperature, such as 41° C (105.8° F), is called **hyperpyrexia.**

The four common types of fevers are **intermittent fever, remittent fever, relapsing fever,** and **constant fever.** An intermittent fever is said to exist when the patient's body temperature alternates at regular intervals between periods of fever and periods of normal or below-normal temperatures. In other words, the patient's temperature undergoes peaks and valleys, with the valleys representing normal or below-normal temperatures. During a remittent fever, the patient has marked peaks and valleys (more than 2° C or 3.6° F) over a 24-hour period, all of which are above normal—that is, the body temperature does not return to normal between the spikes. A relapsing fever is said to exist when short febrile periods of a few days are interspersed with 1 or 2 days of normal temperature. A continuous fever is present when the patient's body temperature remains above normal with minimal or no fluctuation.

Hypothermia is a core temperature below normal range. Hypothermia may occur as a result of (1) excessive heat loss, (2) inadequate heat production to counteract heat loss, and (3) impaired hypothalamic thermoregulation. Box 2-1 lists the clinical signs of hypothermia.

Hypothermia may be caused accidentally or may be induced. Accidental hypothermia is commonly seen in the patient who (1) has had an excessive exposure to a cold environment; (2) has been immersed in a cold liquid environment for a prolonged time; or (3) has inadequate clothing, shelter, or heat. A reduced metabolic rate may compound hypothermia in older patients. In addition, older patients often take sedatives, which further depress the metabolic rate. Box 2-2 lists common therapeutic interventions for patients with hypothermia.

Induced hypothermia refers to the intentional lowering of a patient's body temperature to reduce the oxygen demand of the tissue cells. Induced hypothermia may involve only a portion of the body or the whole body. Induced hypothermia is often indicated before certain surgeries, such as heart or brain surgery.

Factors Affecting Body Temperature

Table 2-2 lists several factors that affect body temperature. Knowing these factors can help the practitioner to better assess the significance of expected or normal variations in a patient's body temperature.

Box 2-1 Clinical Signs of Hypothermia

- Below normal body temperature
- Decreased pulse and respiratory rate
- Severe shivering (initially)
- Patient indicating coldness or presence of chills
- Pale or bluish cool, waxy skin
- Hypotension
- Decreased urinary output
- Lack of muscle coordination
- Disorientation
- Drowsy or unresponsive
- Coma

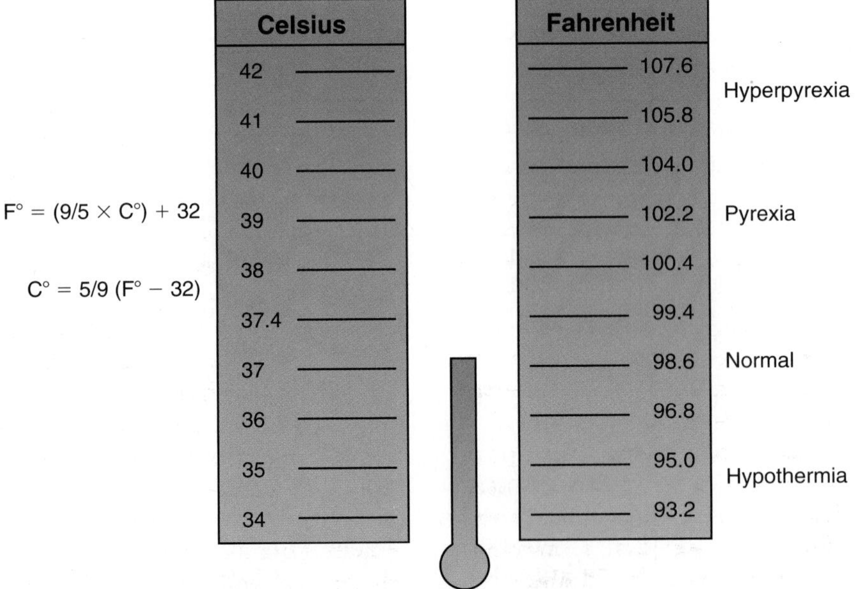

FIGURE 2-1 Range of normal body temperature and alterations in body temperature on the Celsius and Fahrenheit scales. See conversion formulas for Fahrenheit and Celsius scales on left side of figure.

TABLE 2-2 Factors Affecting Body Temperature

Age	Temperature varies with age. For example, the temperature of the newborn infant is unstable because of immature thermoregulatory mechanisms. However, it is not uncommon for the elderly person to have a body temperature below 36.4° C (97.6° F). The normal temperature decreases with age.
Environment	Normally, variations in environmental temperature do not affect the core temperature. However, exposure to extreme hot or cold temperatures can alter body temperature. If an individual's core temperature falls to 25° C (77° F), death may occur.
Time of day	Body temperature normally varies throughout the day. Typically, an individual's temperature is lowest around 3:00 am and highest between 5:00 pm and 7:00 pm. Approximately 95% of patients have their highest temperature around 6:00 pm. Body temperature often fluctuates by as much as 2° C (1.8° F) between early morning and late afternoon.
Exercise	Body temperature increases with exercise because exercise increases heat production as the body breaks down carbohydrates and fats to provide energy. During strenuous exercise, the body temperature can increase to as high as 40° C (104° F).
Stress	Physical or emotional stress may increase body temperature because stress can stimulate the sympathetic nervous system, causing the epinephrine and norepinephrine levels to increase. When this occurs, the metabolic rate increases, causing an increased heat production. Stress and anxiety may cause a patient's temperature to increase without underlying disease.
Hormones	Women normally have greater fluctuations in temperature than do men. The female hormone progesterone, which is secreted during ovulation, causes the temperature to increase 0.3° to 0.6° C (0.5° to 1° F). After menopause, women have the same mean temperature norms as men.

Box 2-2 Common Therapeutic Interventions for Hypothermia

- Remove wet clothing
- Provide dry clothing
- Place patient in a warm environment (eg, slowly increase room temperature)
- Cover patient with warm blankets or electric heating blanket
- Apply warming pads (increase temperature slowly)
- Keep patient's limbs close to body
- Cover patient's head with a cap or towel
- Supply warm oral or intravenous fluids

Body Temperature Measurement

The measurement of body temperature establishes an essential baseline for clinical comparison as a disease progresses or as therapies are administered. To ensure the reliability of a temperature reading, the practitioner must (1) select the correct measuring equipment, (2) choose the most appropriate site, and (3) use the correct technique or procedure. The four most commonly used sites are the mouth, rectum, ear (tympanic), and axilla. Any of these sites is satisfactory when proper technique is used.

Additional measurement sites include the esophagus and pulmonary artery. Temperatures measured at these sites and in the rectum and at the tympanic membrane are considered core temperatures. The skin, typically that of the forehead or abdomen, may also be used for general temperature purposes. However, practitioners must remember that although skin temperature–sensitive strips or disposable paper thermometers may be satisfactory for general temperature measurements, the patient's precise temperature should always be confirmed—when indicated—with a glass or tympanic thermometer.

Because body temperature is usually measured orally, the practitioner must be aware of certain external factors that can lead to false oral temperature measurements. For example, drinking hot or cold liquids can cause small changes in oral temperature measurements. The most significant temperature changes have been reported after a patient drinks ice water. Drinking ice water may lower the patient's actual temperature by 0.2° to 1.6° F. Before taking an oral temperature, the practitioner should wait 15 minutes after a patient has ingested ice water. Oral temperature may increase in the patient receiving heated oxygen aerosol therapy and decrease in the patient receiving a cool mist aerosol. Table 2-3 lists the body temperature sites, their advantages and disadvantages, and the equipment used.

Pulse

A pulse is generated through the vascular system with each ventricular contraction of the heart **(systole).** Thus a pulse is a rhythmic arterial blood pressure throb created by the pumping action of the ventricular muscle. Between contractions, the ventricle rests **(diastole)** and the pulsation disappears. The pulse can be assessed at any location where an artery lies close to the skin surface and can be palpated against a firm underlying structure, such as muscle or bone. Nine common pulse sites are the temporal, carotid, apical, brachial, radial, femoral, popliteal, pedal (dorsalis pedis), and posterior tibial area (Figure 2-2).

In clinical settings the pulse is usually assessed by **palpation.** Initially the practitioner uses the first, second, or third finger and applies light pressure to any one of the pulse sites (e.g., carotid or radial artery) to detect a pulse with a strong pulsation. After locating the pulse, the practitioner may apply a more forceful palpation to count the rate, determine the rhythm, and evaluate the quality of pulsation. The practitioner then counts the number of pulsations for 15, 30, or 60 seconds and then multiplies appropriately to determine the

TABLE 2-3 Body Temperature Measurements: Sites, Normal Values, Advantages and Disadvantages, and Equipment Used

Site and Temperature	Advantages and Disadvantages	Equipment
Oral (most common) Average 37° C or 98.6° F	**Advantages:** Convenient. Easy access and patient comfort. **Disadvantages:** Affected by hot or cold liquids. Contraindicated in patients who cannot follow directions to keep mouth closed, who are mouth breathing, or who might bite down and break thermometer. Smoking, drinking, and eating can slightly alter the oral temperature. About 1° F lower than rectal temperature.	Glass mercury thermometer, electronic thermometers
Rectal Average 0.7° C or 0.4° F higher than oral	**Advantages:** Very reliable. Considered most accurate. **Disadvantages:** Contraindicated in patients with diarrhea, patients who have undergone rectal surgery, or patients who have diseases of the rectum. **General Comment:** Used less often now that tympanic thermometers are available.	Glass mercury thermometer
Ear (tympanic) Reflects core temperature. Also calibrated to oral or rectal scales	**Advantages:** Convenient, readily accessible, fast, safe, and noninvasive. Does not require contact with any mucous membrane. Infection control is less of a concern. With the advent of the tympanic membrane thermometer, the ear is now a site where a temperature can be easily and safely measured. Reflects the core body temperature because it measures the tympanic membrane blood supply—the same vascular system that supplies the hypothalamus. Smoking, drinking, and eating do not affect tympanic temperature measurements. Allows rapid temperature measurements in the very young, confused, or unconscious patient. **Disadvantages:** No remarkable disadvantages, assuming site is available.	Tympanic thermometer
Axillary Average 0.6° C or 1° F lower than oral	**Advantages:** Safe and noninvasive. Recommended for infants and children, this is the route of choice in patients whose temperature cannot be measured at other sites. **Disadvantages:** Considered the least accurate and least reliable site because a number of factors can adversely affect the measurement. For example, if the patient has recently been given a bath, the temperature may reflect the temperature of the bath water. Similarly, friction applied to dry the patient's skin may influence the temperature.	Glass mercury thermometer

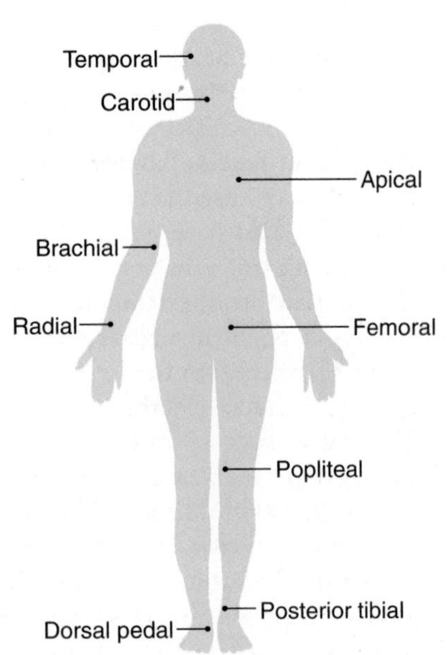

FIGURE 2-2 The nine common pulse sites.

pulse per minute. Shorter time intervals may be used for patients with normal rates or regular cardiac rhythms.

In patients with irregular, abnormally slow, or fast cardiac rhythms, the pulse rates should be counted for 1 minute. To prevent overestimation for any time interval, the practitioner should count the first pulsation as zero and not count pulses at or after the completion of a selected time interval. Counting even one extra pulsation during a 15-second interval leads to an overestimation of the pulse rate by 4. The characteristics of the pulse are described in terms of rate, rhythm, and strength.

Rate

The normal pulse rate (or heart rate) varies with age. For example, in the newborn the normal pulse rate range is 100 to 180 beats per minute (bpm). In the toddler the normal range is 80 to 130 bpm. The normal range for the child is 65 to 100 bpm, and the normal adult range is 60 to 100 bpm (see Table 2-1).

A heart rate lower than 60 bpm is called **bradycardia.** Bradycardia may be seen in patients with hypothermia and in physically fit athletes. The pulse may also be lower than expected when the patient is at rest or asleep or as a result of head injury, vomiting, or advanced age. A pulse rate greater than 100 bpm in adults is called **tachycardia.** Tachycardia may occur as a result of hypoxemia, anemia, fever, anxiety, emotional stress, fear, hemorrhage, hypotension, dehydration, shock, and exercise. Tachycardia also is a common side effect in patients receiving certain medications, such as sympathomimetic agents (e.g., adrenaline or dobutamine).

Rhythm

Normally the ventricular contraction is under the control of the sinus node in the atrium, which generates a normal rate and regular rhythm. Certain conditions and chemical disturbances, such as inadequate blood flow and oxygen supply to the heart or an electrolyte imbalance, can cause the heart to beat irregularly. In children and young adults it is not uncommon for the heart rate to increase during inspiration and decrease during exhalation. This is called **sinus arrhythmia.**

Strength

The quality of the pulse reflects the strength of left ventricular contraction and the volume of blood flowing to the peripheral tissues. A normal left ventricular contraction combined with an adequate blood volume will generate a strong, throbbing pulse. A weak ventricular contraction combined with an inadequate blood volume will result in a weak, thready pulse wave. An increased heart rate combined with a large blood volume will generate a full, bounding pulse.

Several conditions may alter the strength of a patient's pulse. For example, heart failure can cause the strength of the pulse to vary every other beat while the rhythm remains regular. This condition is called **pulsus alternans.** The practitioner may detect a pulse that decreases markedly in strength during inspiration and increases back to normal during exhalation, a condition called **pulsus paradoxus** that is common among patients experiencing a severe asthmatic episode. This phenomenon can also be heard when blood pressure is measured.

Finally, the stimulation of the sympathetic nervous system increases the force of ventricular contraction, increasing the volume of blood ejected from the heart and creating a stronger pulse. Stimulation of the parasympathetic nervous system decreases the force of the ventricular contraction, thus leading to a decreased volume of blood ejected from the heart and a weaker pulse. Clinically the strength of the pulse may be recorded on a scale of 0 to 4+ (Box 2-3).

Box 2-3 Scale to Rate Pulse Quality

0: Absent or no pulse detected
1+: Weak, thready, easily obliterated with pressure; difficult to feel
2+: Pulse difficult to palpate; may be obliterated by strong pressure
3+: Normal pulse
4+: Bounding, easily palpated and difficult to obliterate

For peripheral pulses that are difficult to detect by palpation, an **ultrasonic Doppler** device may also be used. A transmitter attached to the Doppler is placed over the artery to be assessed. The transmitter amplifies and transmits the pulse sounds to an earpiece or to a speaker attached to the Doppler device. The heart rate can also be obtained through **auscultation** by placing a stethoscope over the apex of the heart.

Respiration

The **diaphragm** is the primary muscle of respiration. Inspiration is an active process whereby the diaphragm contracts and causes the intrathoracic pressure to decrease. This action, in turn, causes the pressure in the airways to fall below the atmospheric pressure, and air flows in. At the end of inspiration, the diaphragm relaxes and the natural lung elasticity (recoil) causes the pressure in the lung to increase. This action, in turn, causes air to flow out of the lung. Under normal circumstances, expiration is a passive process.

The normal respiratory rate varies with age. For example, in the newborn the normal respiratory rate varies between 30 and 60 breaths per minute. In the toddler, the normal range is 25 to 40 breaths per minute. The normal range for the preschool child is 20 to 25 breaths per minute, and the normal adult range is 12 to 20 breaths per minute (see Table 2-1).

Ideally the respiratory rate should be counted when the patient is not aware. One good method is to count the respiratory rate immediately after taking the pulse, while leaving the fingers over the patient's artery. As respirations are being counted, the practitioner should observe for variations in the pattern of breathing. For example, an increased breathing rate is called **tachypnea.** Tachypnea is commonly seen in patients with fever, metabolic acidosis, hypoxemia, pain, or anxiety. A respiratory rate below the normal range is called **bradypnea.** Bradypnea may occur with hypothermia, head injuries, and drug overdose. Table 2-4 provides an overview of common normal and **abnormal breathing patterns**.

Blood Pressure

The arterial blood pressure is the force exerted by the circulating volume of blood on the walls of the arteries. The pressure peaks when the ventricles of the heart contract and eject blood into the aorta and pulmonary arteries. The blood pressure measured during ventricular contraction **(cardiac systole)** is the **systolic blood pressure.** During ventricular relaxation **(cardiac diastole),** blood pressure is generated by the elastic recoil of the arteries and arterioles. This pressure is called the normal and **diastolic blood pressure**.

The normal blood pressure in the aorta and large arteries varies with age. For example, in the newborn the normal systolic blood pressure range is 60 to 180 mm Hg. In the toddler the normal range is 80 to 110 mm Hg. The normal range for the child is 100 to 110 mm Hg, and the normal adult range is 110 to 140 mm Hg (see Table 2-1). The numeric difference between the systolic and diastolic blood pressure is the **pulse pressure**. For example, a systolic pressure of 120 mm Hg and a diastolic pressure of 80 mm Hg equal a pulse pressure of 40 mm Hg.

TABLE 2-4 Common Normal and Abnormal Breathing Patterns

Pattern	Graphic Overview	Description
Eupnea	Volume / Time (15 seconds)	Normal rate and rhythm; between 12 and 20 breaths per minute in regular rhythm and of moderate depth for an adult
Bradypnea	Volume / Time (15 seconds)	Regular rhythm of less than 12 breaths per minute
Tachypnea	Volume / Time (15 seconds)	Regular rhythm of more than 20 breaths per minute for an adult
Apnea	Volume / Apnea / Time (15 seconds)	Absence of breathing that leads to respiratory arrest and death
Hypoventilation	Volume / Time (15 seconds)	Decreased rate and depth, decreasing alveolar ventilation and leading to an increased Pa_{CO_2}
Hyperventilation	Volume / Time (15 seconds)	Increased rate and depth, which increases alveolar ventilation and leads to a decreased Pa_{CO_2}

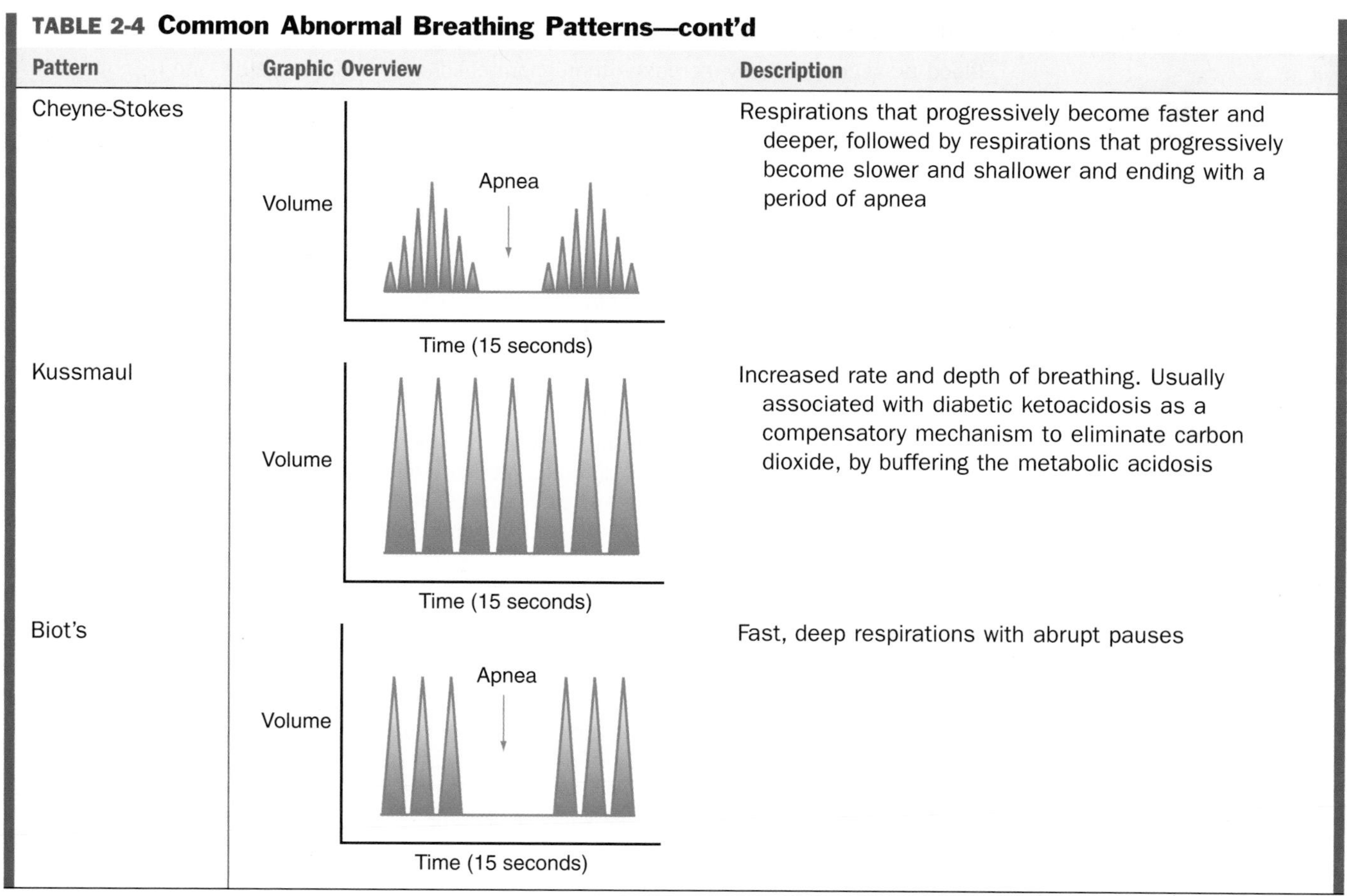

TABLE 2-4 Common Abnormal Breathing Patterns—cont'd

Pattern	Graphic Overview	Description
Cheyne-Stokes	Volume; Apnea; Time (15 seconds)	Respirations that progressively become faster and deeper, followed by respirations that progressively become slower and shallower and ending with a period of apnea
Kussmaul	Volume; Time (15 seconds)	Increased rate and depth of breathing. Usually associated with diabetic ketoacidosis as a compensatory mechanism to eliminate carbon dioxide, by buffering the metabolic acidosis
Biot's	Volume; Apnea; Time (15 seconds)	Fast, deep respirations with abrupt pauses

Blood pressure is a function of (1) the blood flow generated by ventricular contraction and (2) the resistance to blood flow caused by the vascular system. Thus blood pressure (BP) equals flow ($\dot{V}$) multiplied by resistance: $BP = \dot{V} + R$.

Blood Flow

Blood flow is equal to cardiac output. Cardiac output is equal to the product of (1) the volume of blood ejected from the ventricles during each heartbeat **(stroke volume)** multiplied by (2) the heart rate. Thus a stroke volume (SV) of 75 mL and a heart rate (HR) of 70 bpm produce a **cardiac output (CO)** of 5250 mL/minute, or 5.25 L/min ($CO = SV \times HR$). The average cardiac output in the resting adult is about 5 L/min.

A number of conditions can alter stroke volume and therefore blood flow. For instance, a decreased stroke volume may develop as a result of poor cardiac pumping (e.g., ventricular failure) or as a result of a decreased blood volume (e.g., during severe hemorrhage). Bradycardia may also reduce cardiac output and blood flow. Conversely, an increased heart rate or blood volume will likely increase cardiac output and blood flow. In addition, an increased heart rate in response to a decreased blood volume (or stroke volume) may also occur as a compensatory mechanism to maintain normal cardiac output and blood flow.

Resistance

The friction between the components of the blood ejected from the ventricles and the walls of the arteries results in a natural resistance to blood flow. Friction between the blood components and the vessel walls is inversely related to the dimensions of the vessel lumen (size). Thus as the vessel lumen narrows (or constricts), resistance increases. As the vessel lumen widens (or relaxes), the resistance decreases. The autonomic nervous system monitors and regulates the vascular tone.

Table 2-5 presents factors that affect the blood pressure.

Abnormalities

Hypertension. Hypertension is the condition in which an individual's blood pressure is chronically above normal range. Whereas blood pressure normally increases with aging, hypertension is considered a dangerous disease and is associated with an increased risk of morbidity and mortality. According to the Joint National Committee on Detection, Evaluation, and Treatment of High Blood Pressure, the physician may make the diagnosis of hypertension in the adult when an average of two or more diastolic readings on at least two different visits is 90 mm Hg or higher or when the average of two or more systolic readings on at least two visits is consistently higher than 140 mm Hg.

An elevated blood pressure of unknown cause is called *primary hypertension.* An elevated blood pressure of a known cause is called *secondary hypertension.* Factors associated with hypertension include arterial disease, obesity, a high serum sodium level, pregnancy, obstructive sleep apnea, and a family history of high blood pressure. The incidence of hypertension

TABLE 2-5 Factors Affecting Blood Pressure

Age	Blood pressure gradually increases throughout childhood, and correlates with height, weight, and age. In the adult, the blood pressure tends to gradually increase with age.
Exercise	Vigorous exercise increases cardiac output and thus blood pressure.
Autonomic nervous system	Increased sympathetic nervous system activity causes an increased heart rate, an increased cardiac contractility, changes in vascular smooth muscle tone to enhance blood flow to vital organs and skeletal muscles, and an increased blood volume. Collectively, these actions cause an increased blood pressure.
Stress	Stress stimulates the sympathetic nervous system and thus can increase blood pressure.
Circulating blood volume	A decreased circulating blood volume, either from blood or fluid loss, causes blood pressure to decrease. Common causes of fluid loss include abnormal, unreplaced fluid losses such as in diarrhea or diaphoresis, and overenthusiastic use of diuretics. Inadequate oral fluid intake can also result in a fluid volume deficit. Excess fluid, such as in congestive heart failure, can cause the blood pressure to increase.
Medications	Any medication that affects one or more of the previous conditions may cause blood pressure changes. For example, diuretics reduce blood volume; cardiac pharmaceuticals may increase or decrease heart rate and contractility; pain medications may reduce sympathetic nervous system stimulation; and specific antihypertension agents may exert their effects as well.
Normal fluctuations	Under normal circumstances, blood pressure varies from moment to moment in response to a variety of stimuli. For example, an increased environmental temperature causes blood vessels near the skin surface to dilate, causing blood pressure to decrease. In addition, normal respirations alter blood pressure: Blood pressure increases during expiration and decreases during inspiration. Blood pressure fluctuations caused by inspiration and expiration may be significant during a severe asthmatic episode.
Race	Black males over 35 years of age often have elevated blood pressures.
Obesity	Blood pressure is often higher in overweight and obese individuals.
Daily variations	Blood pressure is usually lowest early in the morning, when the metabolic rate is lowest.

is higher in men than in women and is twice as common in blacks as in whites. People with mild or moderate hypertension may be asymptomatic or may experience suboccipital headaches (especially on rising), tinnitus, light-headedness, easy fatigability, and cardiac palpitations. With sustained hypertension, arterial walls become thickened, inelastic, and resistant to blood flow. This process in turn causes the left ventricle to distend and hypertrophy. Hypertension may lead to congestive heart failure.

Hypotension. *Hypotension* is said to be present when the patient's blood pressure falls below 90/60 mm Hg. It is an abnormal condition in which the blood pressure is not adequate for normal perfusion and oxygenation of vital organs. Hypotension is associated with peripheral vasodilation, decreased vascular resistance, hypovolemia, and left ventricular failure. Hypotension can also be caused by analgesics such as meperidine hydrochloride (Demerol) and morphine sulfate, severe burns, prolonged diarrhea, and vomiting. Signs and symptoms include pallor, skin mottling, clamminess, blurred vision, confusion, dizziness, syncope, chest pain, increased heart rate, and decreased urine output. Hypotension is life threatening.

Orthostatic hypotension, also called *postural hypotension,* occurs when blood pressure quickly drops as the individual rises to an upright position or stands. Orthostatic hypotension develops when the peripheral blood vessels—especially in central body organs and legs—are unable to constrict or respond appropriately to changes in body positions. Orthostatic hypotension is associated with decreased blood volume, anemia, dehydration, prolonged bed rest, and antihypertensive medications. The assessment of orthostatic hypotension is made by obtaining pulse and blood pressure readings when the patient is in the supine, sitting, and standing positions.

Pulsus Paradoxus

Pulsus paradoxus is defined as a systolic blood pressure that is more than 10 mm Hg lower on inspiration than on expiration. This exaggerated waxing and waning of arterial blood pressure can be detected with a sphygmomanometer or, in severe cases, by palpating the pulse at the wrist or neck. Commonly associated with severe asthmatic episodes, pulsus paradoxus is believed to be caused by the major intrapleural pressure swings that occur during inspiration and expiration. The reason for this phenomenon is described in the following sections.

Decreased blood pressure during inspiration. During inspiration the asthmatic patient frequently relies on **accessory muscles of inspiration.** The accessory muscles help produce an extremely negative intrapleural pressure, which in turn enhances intrapulmonary gas flow. The increased negative intrapleural pressure, however, also causes blood vessels in the lungs to dilate, creating pooled blood. Consequently the volume of blood returning to the left ventricle decreases, causing a reduction in cardiac output and arterial blood pressure during inspiration.

TABLE 2-6 Spo_2 and Pao_2 Relationship for the Adult and Newborn

	Adult		Newborn	
Oxygen Status	Spo_2	Pao_2	Spo_2	Pao_2
Normal	95-99%	75-100	91-96%	60-80
Mild hypoxemia	90-95%	60-75	88-90%	55-60
Moderate hypoxemia	85-90%	50-60	85-89%	50-58
Severe hypoxemia	<85%	<50	<85%	<50

Note: The Spo_2 will be lower than predicted when the following are present: low pH, high $Paco_2$, and high temperature.

Increased blood pressure during expiration. During expiration, the patient often activates the **accessory muscles of expiration** in an effort to overcome an increased **airway resistance** (R_{aw}). The increased power produced by these muscles generates a greater positive intrapleural pressure. Although increased positive intrapleural pressure helps offset R_{aw}, it also works to narrow or squeeze the blood vessels of the lung. This increased pressure on the pulmonary blood vessels enhances left ventricular filling and results in increased cardiac output and arterial blood pressure during expiration.

Oxygen Saturation

Oxygen saturation, often considered the fifth vital sign, is used to establish an immediate baseline Spo_2 value. It is an excellent monitor by which to assess the patient's response to respiratory care interventions. In the adult, normal Spo_2 values range from 95% to 99%. Spo_2 values of 91% to 94% indicate **mild hypoxemia.** Mild hypoxemia warrants additional evaluation by the respiratory practitioner but does not usually require supplemental oxygen. Spo_2 readings of 86% to 90% indicate **moderate hypoxemia.** These patients often require supplemental oxygen. Spo_2 values of 85% or lower indicate **severe hypoxemia** and warrant immediate medical intervention, including the administration of oxygen, ventilatory support, or both. Table 2-6 presents the relationship of Spo_2 to Pao_2 for the adult and newborn. Table 2-7 provides an overview of the signs and symptoms of inadequate oxygenation.

TABLE 2-7 Signs and Symptoms of Inadequate Oxygenation

Central Nervous System	
Apprehension	Early
Restlessness or irritability	Early
Confusion or lethargy	Early or late
Combativeness	Late
Coma	Late
Respiratory	
Tachypnea	Early
Dyspnea on exertion	Early
Dyspnea at rest	Late
Use of accessory muscles	Late
Intercostal retractions	Late
Takes a breath between each word or sentence	Late
Cardiovascular	
Tachycardia	Early
Mild hypertension	Early
Arrhythmias	Early or late
Hypotension	Late
Cyanosis	Late
Skin is cool or clammy	Late
Other	
Diaphoresis	Early or late
Decreased urinary output	Early or late
General fatigue	Early or late

Systematic Examination of the Chest and Lungs

The physical examination of the chest and lungs should be performed in a systematic and orderly fashion. The most common sequence is as follows:

- **Inspection**
- **Palpation**
- **Percussion**
- **Auscultation**

Before the practitioner can adequately inspect, palpate, percuss, and auscultate the chest and lungs, however, he or she must have a good working knowledge of the topographic landmarks of the lung and chest. Various anatomic landmarks and imaginary vertical lines drawn on the chest are used to identify and document the location of specific abnormalities.

Lung and Chest Topography

Thoracic Cage Landmarks

Anteriorly, the first rib is attached to the manubrium just beneath the clavicle. After the first rib is identified, the rest of the ribs can easily be located and numbered. The sixth rib and its cartilage are attached to the sternum just above the xiphoid process (Figure 2-3).

Posteriorly, the spinous processes of the vertebrae are useful landmarks. For example, when the patient's head is extended forward and down, two prominent spinous processes can usually be seen at the base of the neck. The top one is the spinous process of the seventh cervical vertebra (C-7); the bottom one is the spinous process of the thoracic vertebra (T-1). When only one spinous process can be seen, it is usually C-7 (see Figure 2-3).

Imaginary Lines

Various imaginary vertical lines are used to locate abnormalities on chest examination (Figure 2-4). The **midsternal line,** which is located in the middle of the sternum, equally divides the anterior chest into left and right hemithoraces. The **midclavicular lines,** which start at the middle of either the right or left clavicle, run parallel to the sternum.

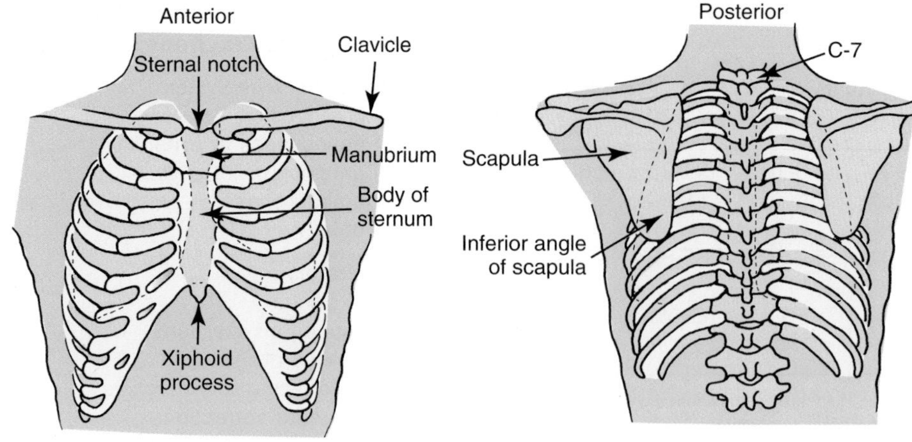

FIGURE 2-3 Anatomic landmarks of the chest.

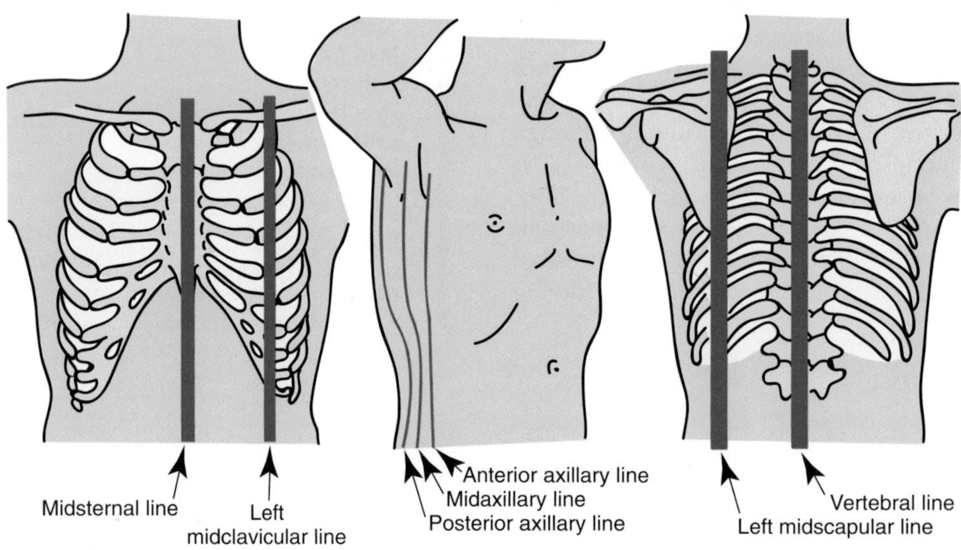

FIGURE 2-4 Imaginary vertical lines in the chest.

On the lateral portion of the chest, three imaginary vertical lines are used. The **anterior axillary line** originates at the anterior axillary fold and runs down along the anterolateral aspect of the chest, the **midaxillary line** divides the lateral chest into two equal halves, and the **posterior axillary line** runs parallel to the midaxillary line along the posterolateral wall of the thorax.

Posteriorly, the **vertebral line** (also called the *midspinal line*) runs along the spinous processes of the vertebrae. The **midscapular line** runs through the middle of either the right or the left scapula parallel to the vertebral line.

Lung Borders and Fissures

Anteriorly, the apex of the lung extends about 2 to 4 cm above the medial third of the clavicle. Under normal conditions the lungs extend down to about the level of the sixth rib. Posteriorly, the superior portion of the lung extends to about the level of T-1 and down to about the level of T-10 (Figure 2-5).

The right lung is separated into the upper, middle, and lower lobes by the **horizontal fissure** and the **oblique fissure.** The horizontal fissure runs anteriorly from the fourth rib at the sternal border to the fifth rib at the midaxillary line. The horizontal fissure separates the right anterior upper lobe from the middle lobe. The oblique fissure runs laterally from the sixth or seventh rib and the midclavicular line to the fifth rib at the midaxillary line. From this point the oblique fissure continues to run around the chest posteriorly and upward to about the level of T-3. Anteriorly, the oblique fissure divides the lower lobe from the lower border of the middle lobe. Posteriorly, the oblique fissure separates the upper lobe from the lower lobe.

The left lung is separated into the upper and lower lobes by the oblique fissure. Anteriorly, the oblique fissure runs laterally from the sixth or seventh rib and the midclavicular line to the fifth rib at the midaxillary line. The fissure continues to run around the chest posteriorly and upward to about the level of T-3.

Inspection

The inspection of the patient is an ongoing observational process that begins with the history and continues throughout the patient interview, taking of vital signs, and physical examination. The inspection consists of a series of observa-

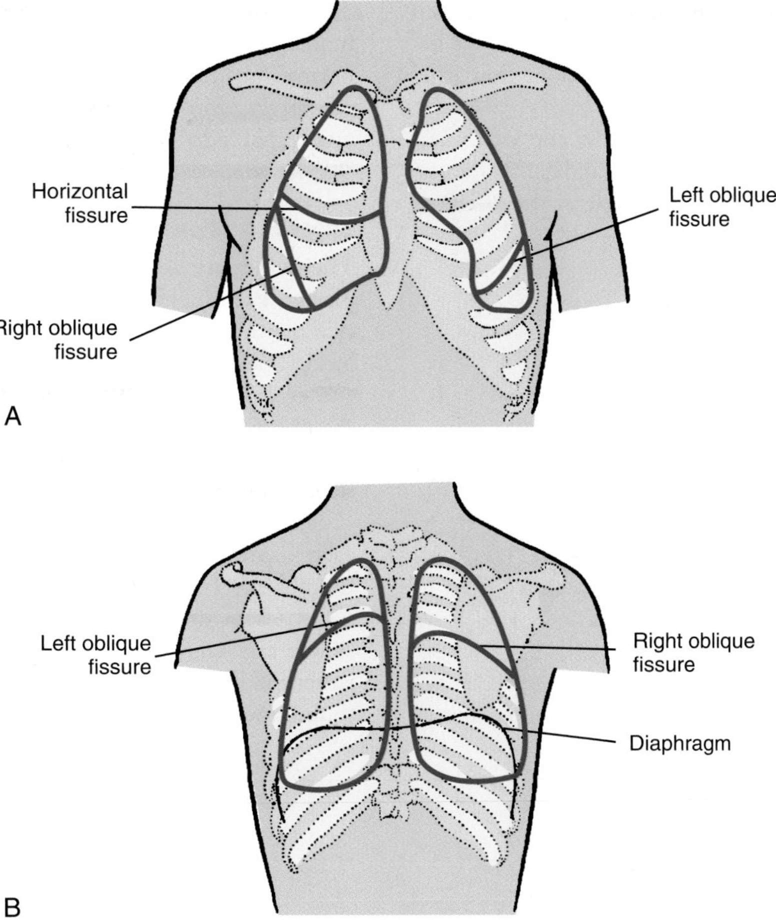

FIGURE 2-5 Topographic location of lung fissures projected on the anterior chest (**A**) and posterior chest (**B**).

tions to gather clinical manifestations—signs and symptoms—that are directly or indirectly related to the patient's respiratory status. Although many visual observations are based on the practitioner's professional judgment (subjective information), the information gathered is nevertheless considered important objective clinical data when gathered by a trained respiratory care practitioner.

Common Clinical Manifestations Observed during Inspection

Box 2-4 lists common clinical manifestations observed during the inspection of the patient with a pathologic respiratory condition. For example, during a systematic visual inspection, the respiratory practitioner might note the patient's ventilatory pattern. Is the patient using accessory muscles of inspiration? Is the patient engaging in pursed-lip breathing? Are substernal or intercostal retractions occurring during inspiration? Does the patient appear to be splinting or to have decreased chest expansion because of chest pain? Are the shape and configuration of the chest normal? Do the patient's skin, lips, fingers, or toenails appear cyanotic? Does the patient have digital clubbing, pedal edema, or distended neck veins? Is the patient coughing? How strong is the patient's cough? What are the characteristics of the patient's sputum? A more **in-depth discussion of common clinical manifestations observed during inspection** can be found later in this chapter (see page 28).

Box 2-4 Common Clinical Manifestations Observed during Inspection

- Abnormal ventilatory pattern findings
- Use of accessory muscles of inspiration
- Use of accessory muscles of expiration
- Pursed-lip breathing
- Substernal or intercostal retractions
- Nasal flaring
- Splinting due to chest pain or decreased chest expansion
- Abnormal chest shape and configuration
- Abnormal extremity findings:
  - Altered skin color
  - Digital clubbing
  - Pedal edema
  - Distended neck veins
- Cough (note characteristics)

Palpation

Palpation is the process of touching the patient's chest to evaluate the symmetry of chest expansion, the position of the trachea, skin temperature, muscle tone, areas of tenderness, lumps, depressions, and **tactile and vocal fremitus.** When palpating the chest, the clinician may use the heel or ulnar side of the hand, the palms, or the fingertips. As shown in Figure 2-6, both the anterior and posterior chest should be palpated from side to side in an orderly fashion, from the apices of the chest down.

To evaluate the position of the trachea, the examiner places an index finger over the sternal notch and gently moves it from side to side. The trachea should be in the midline directly above the sternal notch. A number of abnormal pulmonary conditions can cause the trachea to deviate from its normal position. For example, a tension pneumothorax, pleural effusion, or tumor mass may push the trachea to the unaffected side, whereas atelectasis and pulmonary fibrosis pull the trachea to the affected side.

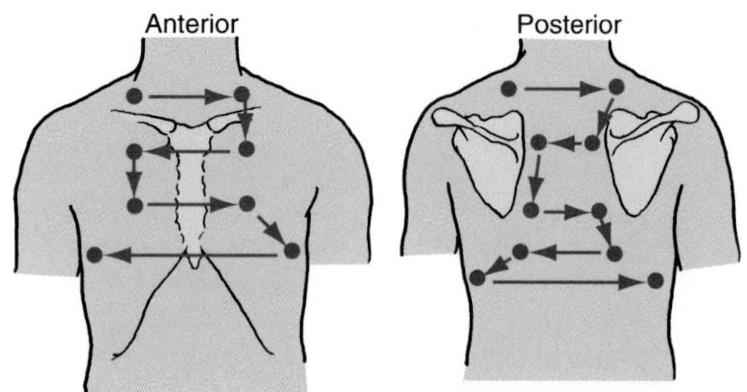

FIGURE 2-6 Path of palpation for vocal or tactile fremitus.

Chest Excursion

The symmetry of chest expansion is evaluated by lightly placing each hand over the patient's posterolateral chest so that the thumbs meet at the midline at about the T-8 to T-10 level. The patient is instructed to exhale slowly and completely and then to inhale deeply. As the patient is inhaling, the examiner evaluates the distance that each thumb moves from the midline. Normally, each thumb tip moves equally about 3 to 5 cm from the midline (Figure 2-7).

The examiner next faces the patient and lightly places each hand on the patient's anterolateral chest so that the thumbs meet at the midline along the costal margins near the xiphoid process. The patient is again instructed to exhale slowly and completely and then to inhale deeply. As the patient is inhaling, the examiner observes the distance each thumb moves from the midline.

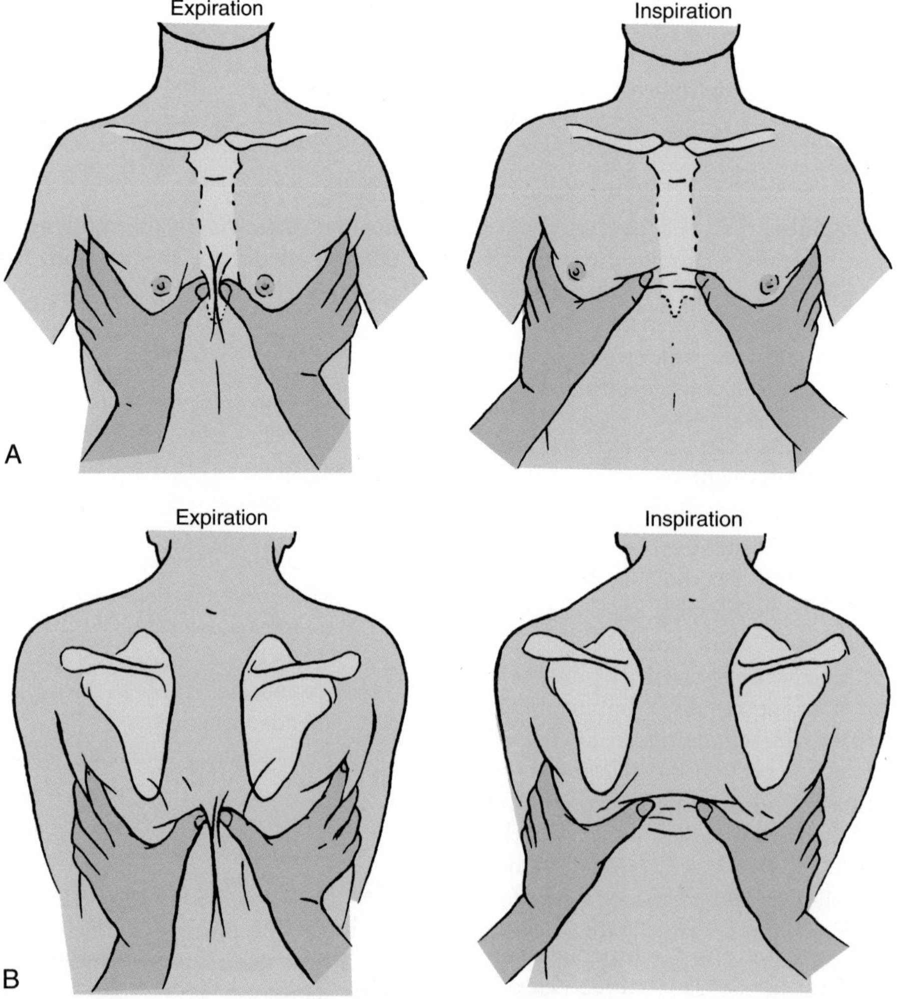

FIGURE 2-7 Assessment of chest excursion. **A**, Anterior. **B**, Posterior. Note that the thumbs move apart on inspiration as the volume of the thorax increases.

A number of pulmonary disorders can alter the patient's **chest excursion.** For example, a bilaterally decreased chest expansion may be caused by both obstructive and restrictive lung disorders. An unequal chest expansion may be caused by alveolar consolidation (e.g., pneumonia), lobar atelectasis, pneumothorax, large pleural effusions, and chest trauma (e.g., fractured ribs).

Tactile and Vocal Fremitus

Vibrations that can be perceived by palpation over the chest are called **tactile fremitus.** This condition is commonly caused by gas flowing through thick secretions that are partially obstructing the large airways. Vibrations that can be perceived by palpation or auscultation over the chest during phonation are called **vocal fremitus.** Sounds produced by the vocal cords are transmitted down the tracheobronchial tree and through the lung parenchyma to the chest wall, where the examiner can feel the vibration. Vocal fremitus can often be elicited by having the patient repeat the phrase "ninety-nine" or "blue moon." These are resonant phrases that produce strong vibrations. Normally, fremitus is most prominent between the scapulae and around the sternum, sites where the large bronchi are closest to the chest wall.

Tactile and vocal fremitus decrease when anything obstructs the transmission of vibration. Such conditions include chronic obstructive pulmonary disease, tumors or thickening of the pleural cavity, pleural effusion, pneumothorax, and a muscular or obese chest wall. Tactile and vocal fremitus increase in patients with alveolar consolidation, atelectasis, pulmonary edema, lung tumors, pulmonary fibrosis, and thin chest walls.

Crepitus (also called **subcutaneous emphysema**) is a coarse, crackling sensation that may be palpable over the skin surface. It occurs when air escapes from the thorax and enters the subcutaneous tissue. It may occur after a tracheostomy and mechanical ventilation, open thoracic injury, or thoracic surgery.

Percussion

Percussion over the chest wall is performed to determine the size, borders, and consistency of air, liquid, or solid material in the underlying lung. When percussing the chest, the examiner firmly places the distal portion of the middle finger of the nondominant hand between the ribs over the surface of the chest area to be examined. No other portion of the hand should touch the patient's chest. With the end of the middle finger of the dominant hand, the examiner quickly strikes the distal joint of the finger positioned on the chest wall and then quickly withdraws the tapping finger (Figure 2-8). The examiner should perform the chest percussion in an orderly fashion from top to bottom, comparing the sounds generated on both sides of the chest, both anteriorly and posteriorly (Figure 2-9).

In the normal lung the sound created by percussion is transmitted throughout the air-filled lung and is typically described as loud, low in pitch, and long in duration. The sounds elicited by the examiner vibrate freely throughout the large surface area of the lungs and create a sound similar to that elicited by knocking on a watermelon (Figure 2-10).

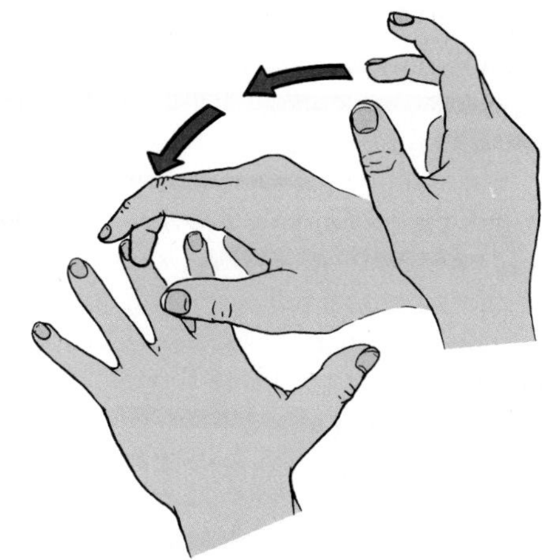

FIGURE 2-8 Chest percussion technique.

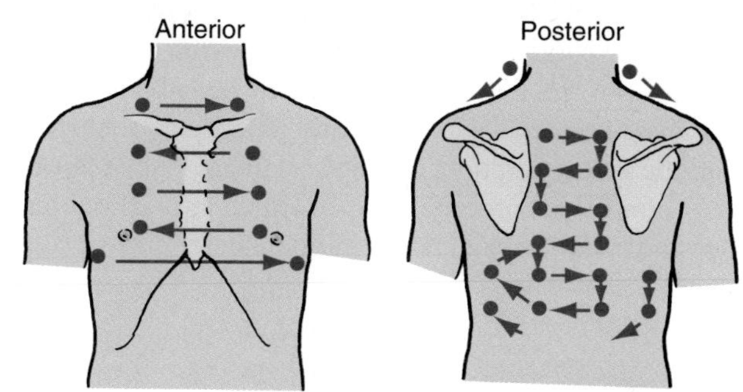

FIGURE 2-9 Path of systematic percussion to include all important areas.

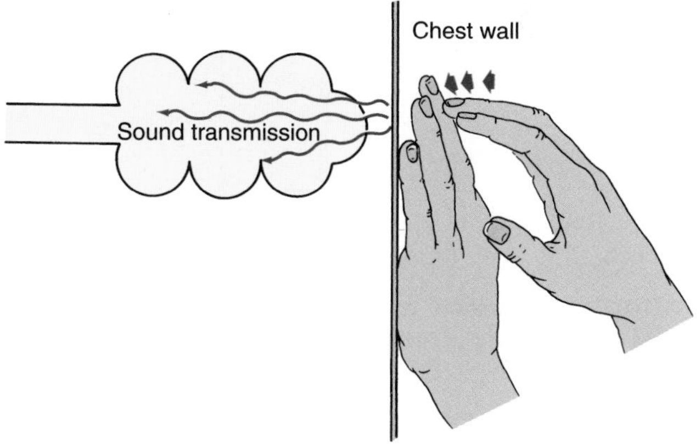

FIGURE 2-10 Chest percussion of a normal lung.

Resonance may be muffled somewhat in the individual with a heavily muscular chest wall and in the obese person. When percussing the anterior chest, the examiner should take care not to confuse the normal borders of cardiac dullness with pulmonary pathology. In addition, the upper border of liver dullness is normally located in the right fifth intercostal space and midclavicular line. Over the left side of the chest, tympany is produced over the gastric space. When percussing the posterior chest, the examiner should avoid the damping effect of the scapulae.

Abnormal Percussion Notes

A **dull percussion note** is heard when the chest is percussed over areas of pleural thickening, pleural effusion, atelectasis, and consolidation. When these conditions exist, the sounds produced by the examiner do not freely vibrate throughout the lungs. A dull percussion note is described as flat or soft, high in pitch, and short in duration, similar to the sound produced by knocking on a full barrel (Figure 2-11).

When the chest is percussed over areas of trapped gas, a **hyperresonant note** is heard. These sounds are described as very loud, low in pitch, and long in duration, similar to the sound produced by knocking on an empty barrel (Figure 2-12). A hyperresonant note is commonly elicited in the patient with chronic obstructive pulmonary disease or pneumothorax.

Diaphragmatic Excursion

The relative position and range of motion of the diaphragms also can be determined by percussion. Clinically, this evaluation is called the *determination of* **diaphragmatic excursion.** To assess the patient's diaphragmatic excursion, the examiner first maps out the lower lung borders by percussing the posterior chest from the apex down and identifying the point at which the percussion note definitely changes from a resonant to flat sound. This procedure is performed at maximal inspiration and again at maximal expiration. Under normal conditions the diaphragmatic excursion should be equal bilaterally and should measure about 4 to 8 cm in the adult.

When severe alveolar hyperinflation is present (e.g., severe emphysema, asthma), the diaphragm is low and flat in position and has minimal excursion. Lobar collapse of one lung may pull the diaphragm up on the affected side and reduce excursion. The diaphragms may be elevated and immobile in neuromuscular diseases that affect them.

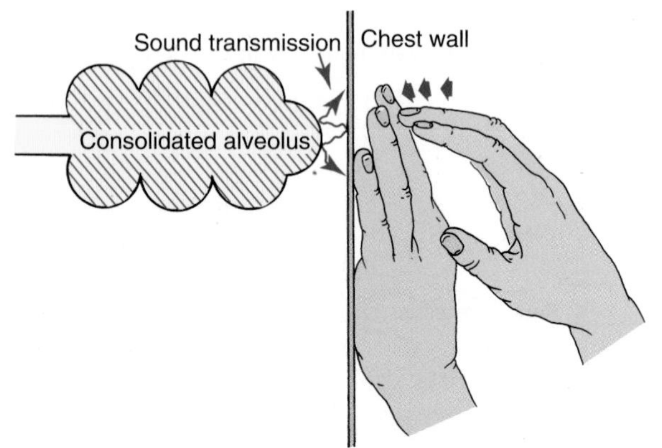

FIGURE 2-11 A short, dull, or flat percussion note is typically produced over areas of alveolar consolidation.

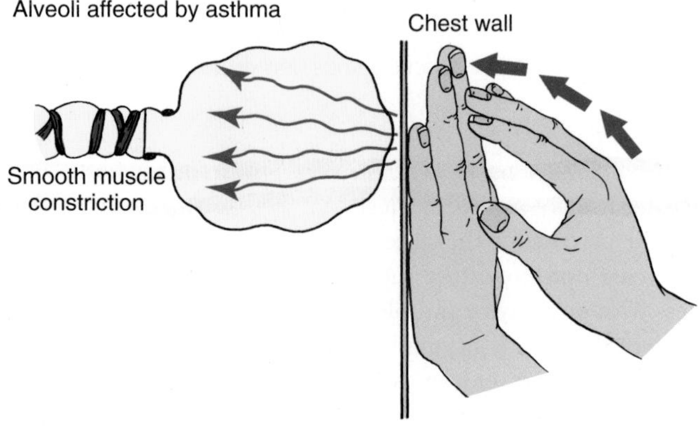

FIGURE 2-12 Percussion becomes more hyperresonant with alveolar hyperinflation.

Auscultation

Auscultation of the chest provides information about the heart, blood vessels, and air flowing in and out of the tracheobronchial tree and alveoli. A stethoscope is used to evaluate the frequency, intensity, duration, and quality of the sounds. During auscultation the patient should ideally be in the upright position and instructed to breathe slowly and deeply through the mouth. The anterior and posterior chest should be auscultated in an orderly fashion from the apex to base while the right side of the chest is compared with the left (Figure 2-13). When examining the posterior chest, the examiner should ask the patient to rotate the shoulders forward so that a greater surface area of the lungs can be auscultated.

Normal Breath Sounds

Three different **normal breath sounds** can be auscultated over the normal chest. They are called **bronchial, bronchovesicular,** and **vesicular breath sounds.**

Bronchial breath sounds. Bronchial breath sounds have a harsh, hollow, or tubular quality. They are loud, high in pitch, and about equal in duration in length of inspiration and expiration. A slight pause occurs between these two components. Bronchial breath sounds are normally auscultated directly over the trachea and are caused by the turbulent flow of gas through the upper airway. Clinically, these sounds are also called *tracheal, tracheobronchial,* and *tubular breath sounds.*

Bronchovesicular breath sounds. Bronchovesicular breath sounds are auscultated directly over the mainstem bronchi. They are softer and lower in pitch than bronchial breath sounds and do not have a pause between the inspiratory and expiratory phase. These sounds are reduced in intensity and

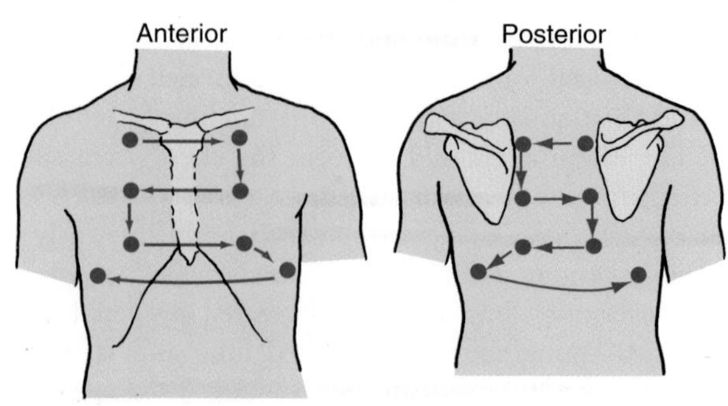

FIGURE 2-13 Path of systematic auscultation to include all important areas. Note the exact similarity of this pathway to Figure 2-6.

pitch as a result of the filtering of sound that occurs as gas moves between the large airways and alveoli.

Anteriorly, bronchovesicular breath sounds can be heard directly over the mainstem bronchi between the first and second ribs. Posteriorly, they are heard between the scapulae near the spinal column between the first and sixth ribs, especially on the right side (Figure 2-14, *A*).

Vesicular breath sounds. Vesicular breath sounds are the normal sounds of gas rustling or swishing through the small bronchioles and possibly the alveoli. Under normal conditions, vesicular breath sounds are auscultated over most of the lung field, both anteriorly and posteriorly (see Figure 2-14, *B*). Vesicular breath sounds are described as soft and low in pitch and are primarily heard during inspiration. As the gas molecules enter the alveoli, they are able to spread out over a large surface area and, as a result of this action, create less gas turbulence. As gas turbulence decreases, the breath sounds become softer and lower in pitch, similar to the sound of the wind in the trees. Vesicular breath sounds also are heard during the initial third of exhalation as gas leaves the alveoli and bronchioles and moves into the large airways (Figure 2-15).

Adventitious (Abnormal) Breath Sounds

Adventitious (abnormal) breath sounds are additional or different sounds that are not *normally* heard over a particular area of the thorax. Bronchial breath sounds heard over an area of the chest that normally demonstrates vesicular breath sounds are one example. Several different types of adventitious breath sounds exist, each indicating a particular pulmonary abnormality.

Bronchial breath sounds. If gas molecules are not permitted to dissipate throughout the parenchymal areas (because of alveolar consolidation or atelectasis, for example) the gas molecules have no opportunity to spread out over a larger surface area and therefore become less turbulent. Consequently, the sounds produced in this area are louder because the gas sounds are coming mainly from the tracheobronchial tree and not the lung parenchyma. These sounds are called *bronchial breath sounds.*

It is commonly believed that breath sounds in patients with alveolar consolidation should be diminished because the consolidation acts as a sound barrier. Although alveolar collapse or consolidation does act as a sound barrier and reduces bronchial breath sounds, the reduction is not as great as it would be if the gas molecules were allowed to dissipate throughout normal lung parenchyma. In addition, liquid and solid materials transmit sounds more readily than air-filled spaces and therefore may further contribute to the bronchial quality of the breath sound. Therefore when disease causes alveolar collapse or consolidation, harsher, bronchial-type sounds rather than the normal vesicular sounds are heard over the affected areas (Figure 2-16).

Diminished breath sounds. Breath sounds are diminished or distant in respiratory disorders that lead to alveolar **hypoventilation,** regardless of the cause. For example, patients with chronic obstructive pulmonary disease often have **diminished breath sounds.** These patients hypoventilate because of air trapping and increased functional residual capacity. In addition, when the functional residual capacity is increased, the gas that enters the enlarged alveoli during each breath spreads out over a greater-than-normal surface area, resulting in less gas turbulence and a softer sound (Figure 2-17). Heart sounds also may be diminished in patients with air trapping.

Diminished breath sounds also are found in respiratory disorders that cause hypoventilation by compressing the lung. Such disorders include flail chest, pleural effusion, and pneumothorax. Diminished breath sounds also are characteristic of neuromuscular diseases that cause hypoventilation. Such

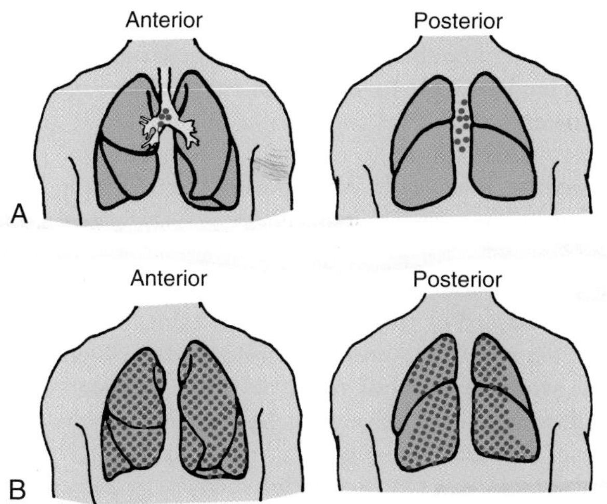

FIGURE 2-14 The location at which bronchovesicular breath sounds **(A)** and vesicular breath sounds **(B)** are normally auscultated.

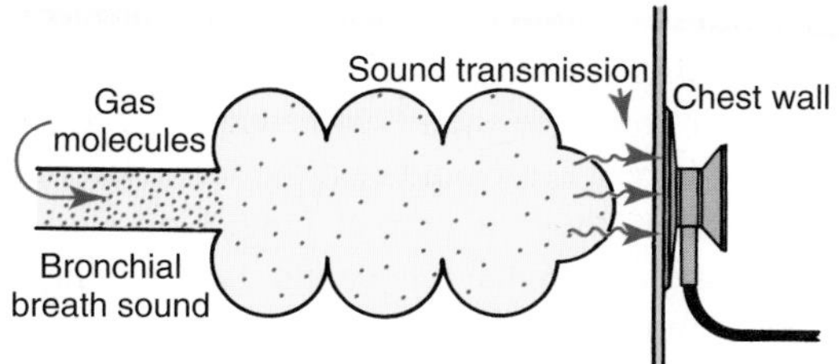

FIGURE 2-15 Auscultation of vesicular breath sounds over a normal lung unit.

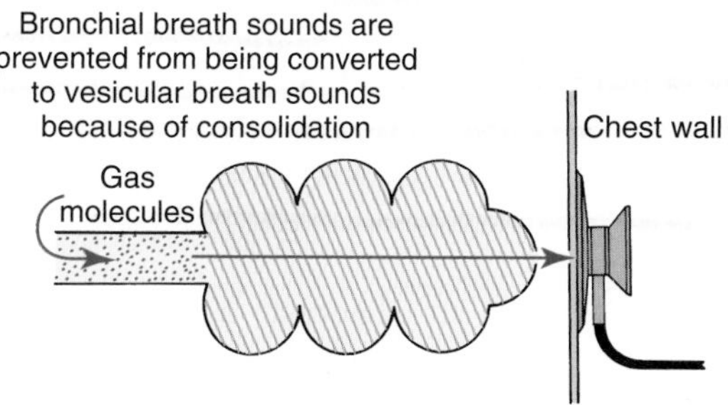

FIGURE 2-16 Auscultation of bronchial breath sounds over a consolidated lung unit.

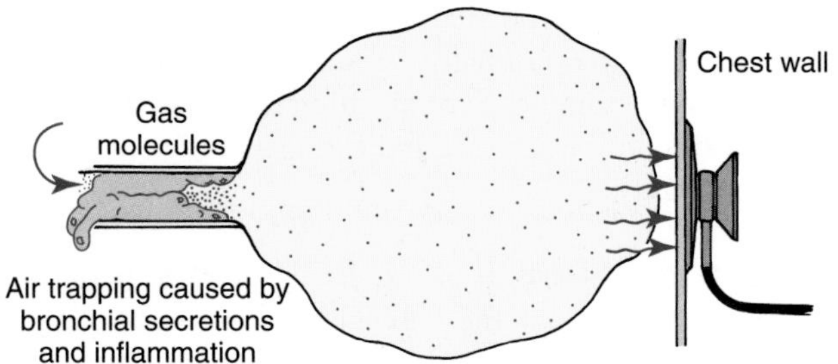

FIGURE 2-17 As air trapping and alveolar hyperinflation develop in obstructive lung diseases, breath sounds progressively diminish.

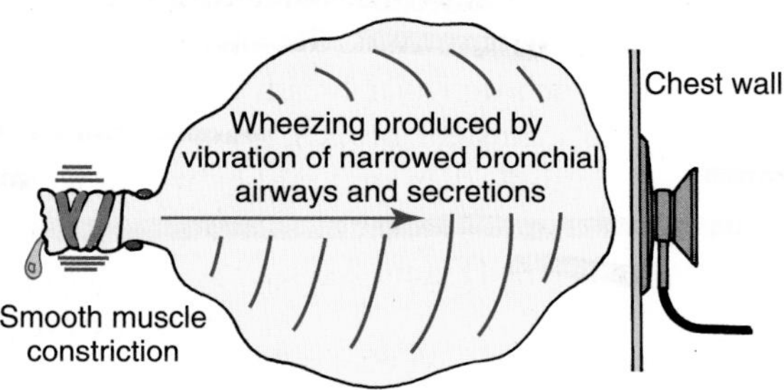

FIGURE 2-18 Wheezing and rhonchi often develop during an asthmatic episode because of smooth muscle constriction, wall edema, and mucous accumulation.

disorders include Guillain-Barré syndrome and myasthenia gravis.

Crackles and rhonchi. Adjectives used in the older literature to describe **crackles and rhonchi** (moist, wet, dry, crackling, sibilant, coarse, fine, crepitant) depend largely on the auditory acuity and experience of the examiner. Descriptions have little value because only the presence or absence of crackles or rhonchi is important. When fluid accumulation is present in a respiratory disorder, some crackles or rhonchi are almost always present (i.e., "bubbly" or "slurpy" sounds accompanying the breath sounds).

Crackles (rales) are usually fine or medium crackling wet sounds that are typically heard during inspiration. They are formed in the small and medium-sized airways and may or may not change in nature after a strong, vigorous cough.

Rhonchi, on the other hand, usually have a coarse, "bubbly" quality and are typically heard during expiration. They are formed in the larger airways and often change in nature or disappear after a strong, vigorous cough.

Wheezing. Wheezing is the characteristic sound produced by airway obstruction. Found in all bronchospastic disorders, it is one of the cardinal findings in bronchial asthma. The sounds are high-pitched and whistling and generally last throughout the expiratory phase. The mechanism of a wheeze is similar to the vibrating reed of a woodwind instrument. The reed, which partially occludes the mouthpiece of the instrument, vibrates and produces a sound when air is forced through it (Figure 2-18). The softest, higher-pitched wheezes occur in the tightest airway obstruction.

Pleural friction rubs. If pleurisy accompanies a respiratory disorder, the inflamed pleural membranes resist movement during breathing and create a peculiar and characteristic sound known as a **pleural friction rub.** The sound is reminiscent of that made by a creaking shoe and is usually heard in the area where the patient complains of pain.

Stridor. Stridor is an abnormal audible high-pitched musical sound caused by an obstruction in the trachea or larynx. It is generally heard during inspiration. Stridor indicates a neoplastic or inflammatory condition, including glottic edema, asthma, diphtheria, laryngospasm, and papilloma (a benign epithelial neoplasm of the larynx). Stridor is usually loud enough to hear without a stethoscope, as in infantile croup.

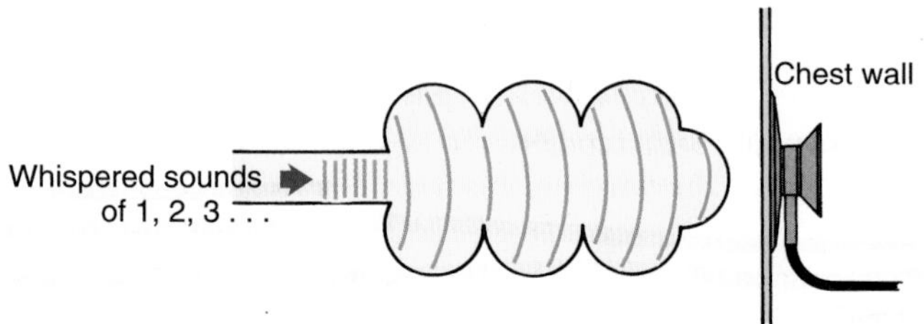

FIGURE 2-19 Whispered voice sounds auscultated over a normal lung are usually faint and unintelligible.

Whispering pectoriloquy. Whispering pectoriloquy is the term used to describe the unusually clear transmission of the whispered voice of a patient as heard through the stethoscope. When the patient whispers "one, two, three," the sounds produced by the vocal cords are transmitted not only toward the mouth and nose but throughout the lungs as well. As the whispered sounds travel down the tracheobronchial tree, they remain relatively unchanged, but as the sound disperses throughout the large surface area of the alveoli, it diminishes sharply. Consequently, when the examiner listens with a stethoscope over a normal lung while a patient whispers "one, two, three," the sounds are diminished, distant, muffled, and unintelligible (Figure 2-19).

When a patient who has atelectasis or consolidated lung areas whispers "one, two, three," the sounds produced are prevented from spreading out over a large alveolar surface area. Even though the consolidated area may act as a sound barrier and diminish the sounds somewhat, the reduction in sound is not as great as it would be if the sounds were allowed to dissipate throughout a normal lung. Consequently the whispered sounds are much louder and more intelligible over the affected lung areas (Figure 2-20).

Table 2-8 provides an overview of the common assessment abnormalities found during inspection, palpation, percussion, and auscultation.

TABLE 2-8 Common Assessment Abnormalities

Finding	Description	Possible Etiology and Significance
Inspection		
Pursed-lip breathing	Exhalation through mouth with lips pursed together to slow exhalation.	COPD, asthma. Suggests ↑ breathlessness. Strategy taught to slow expiration, ↓ dyspnea.
Tripod position; inability to lie flat	Leaning forward with arms and elbows supported on overbed table.	COPD, asthma in exacerbation, pulmonary edema. Indicates moderate to severe respiratory distress.
Accessory muscle use; intercostal retractions	Neck and shoulder muscles used to assist breathing. Muscles between ribs pull in during inspiration.	COPD, asthma in excerbation, secretion retention. Indicates severe respiratory distress, hypoxemia.
Splinting	Voluntary ↓ in tidal volume to ↓ pain on chest expansion.	Thoracic or abdominal incision. Chest trauma, pleurisy.
↑ AP diameter	AP chest diameter equal to lateral. Slope of ribs more horizontal (90 degrees) to spine.	COPD, asthma, cystic fibrosis. Lung hyperinflation. Advanced age.
Tachypnea	Rate >20 breaths/min; >25 breaths/min in elderly.	Fever, anxiety, hypoxemia, restrictive lung disease. Magnitude of ↑ above normal rate reflects increased work of breathing.
Kussmaul's respirations	Regular, rapid, and deep respirations.	Metabolic acidosis; ↑ in rate aids body in ↑ CO_2 excretion.
Cyanosis	Bluish color of skin best seen in earlobes, under the eyelids, or in nail beds.	↓ Oxygen transfer in lungs, ↓ cardiac output. Nonspecific, unreliable indicator.
Clubbing of fingers	↑ Depth, bulk, sponginess of distal digit of finger.	Chronic hypoxemia. Cystic fibrosis, lung cancer, bronchiectasis.
Peripheral edema	Pitting edema.	Congestive heart failure, cor pulmonale.
Distended neck veins	Jugular venous distention.	Cor pulmonale, flail chest, pneumothorax.
Cough	Productive or non-productive.	Bronchial airway and alveolar disease.
Sputum	See Table 2-11	COPD, asthma, cystic fibrosis.
Abdominal paradox	Inward (rather than normal outward) movement of abdomen during inspiration.	Inefficient and ineffective breathing pattern. Nonspecific indicator of severe respiratory distress.
Palpation		
Tracheal deviation	Leftward or rightward movement of trachea from normal midline position.	Nonspecific indicator of change in position of mediastinal structures. Medical emergency if caused by tension pneumothorax.
Altered tactile fremitus	Increase or decrease in vibrations.	↑ In pneumonia, atelectasis; pulmonary edema; ↓ in pleural effusion, lung hyperinflation; absent in pneumothorax.
Altered chest movement	Unequal or equal but diminished movement of two sides of chest with inspiration.	Unequal movement caused by atelectasis, pneumothorax, pleural effusion, splinting; equal but diminished movement caused by barrel chest, restrictive disease, neuromuscular disease.
Percussion		
Hyperresonance	Loud, lower-pitched sound over areas that normally produce a resonant sound.	Lung hyperinflation (COPD), lung collapse (pneumothorax), air trapping (asthma).
Dullness/Flatness	Medium-pitched sound over areas that normally produce a resonant sound.	↑ Density (pneumonia, large atelectasis), ↑ fluid pleural space (pleural effusion).
Auscultation		
Fine crackles	Series of short, explosive, high-pitched sounds heard just before the end of inspiration; result of rapid equalization of gas pressure when collapsed alveoli or terminal bronchioles suddenly snap open; similar sound to that made by rolling hair between fingers just behind ear.	Interstitial fibrosis (asbestosis), interstitial edema (early pulmonary edema), alveolar filling (pneumonia), loss of lung volume (atelectasis), early phase of congestive heart failure.

Continued

TABLE 2-8 Common Assessment Abnormalities—cont'd

Finding	Description	Possible Etiology and Significance
Coarse crackles	Series of short, low-pitched sounds caused by air passing through airway intermittently occluded by mucus, unstable bronchial wall, or fold of mucosa; evident on inspiration and, at times, expiration; similar sound to blowing through straw under water; increase in bubbling quality with more fluid.	Congestive heart failure, pulmonary edema, pneumonia with severe congestion, COPD.
Rhonchi	Continuous rumbling, snoring, or rattling sounds from obstruction of large airways with secretions; most prominent on expiration; change often evident after coughing or suctioning.	COPD, cystic fibrosis, pneumonia, bronchiectasis.
Wheezes	Continuous high-pitched squeaking sound caused by rapid vibration of bronchial walls; first evident on expiration but possibly evident on inspiration as obstruction of airway increases; possibly audible without stethoscope.	Bronchospasm (caused by asthma), airway obstruction (caused by foreign body, tumor), COPD.
Stridor	Continuous musical sound of constant pitch; result of partial obstruction of larynx or trachea.	Croup, epiglottitis, vocal cord edema after extubation, foreign body.
Absent breath sounds	No sound evident over entire lung or area of lung.	Pleural effusion, mainstem bronchi obstruction, large atelectasis, pneumonectomy, lobectomy.
Pleural friction rub	Creaking or grating sound from roughened, inflamed surfaces of the pleura rubbing together; evident during inspiration, expiration, or both and no change with coughing; usually uncomfortable, especially on deep inspiration.	Pleurisy, pneumonia, pulmonary infarct.
Bronchophony, whispered pectoriloquy	Spoken or whispered syllable more distinct than normal on auscultation.	Pneumonia.
Egophony	Spoken "e" similar to "a" on auscultation because of altered transmission of voice sounds.	Pneumonia, pleural effusion.

Modified from Lewis S, Heitkemper MM, Dirksen SR: *Medical-surgical nursing: Assessment and management of clinical problems*, ed 7, vol. 1, St. Louis, 2007, Mosby.

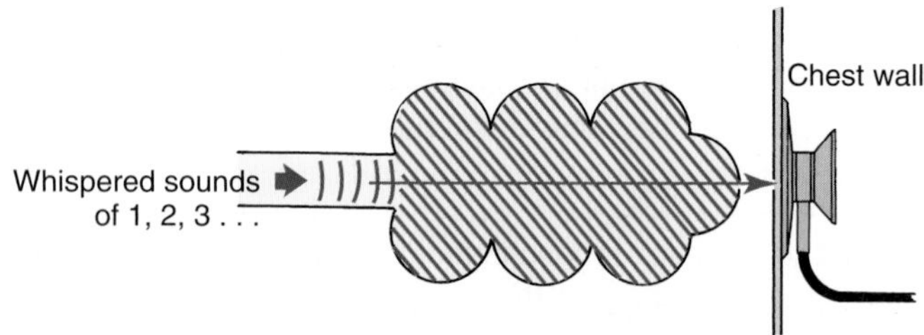

FIGURE 2-20 Whispering pectoriloquy. Whispered voice sounds heard over a consolidated lung are often louder and more intelligible compared with those of a normal lung.

In-Depth Discussion of Common Clinical Manifestations Observed during Inspection

Normal Ventilatory Pattern

An individual's **normal breathing pattern** is composed of a **tidal volume (V_T),** a **ventilatory rate** and **an inspiratory-to-expiratory ratio (I:E ratio).** In normal adults the V_T is about 500 mL (7 to 9 mL/kg), the ventilatory rate is about 15 (with a range of 12 to 18) breaths per minute, and the I:E ratio is about 1 : 2. In patients with respiratory disorders, however, an abnormal ventilatory pattern is often present (see Table 2-4 for common abnormal ventilatory patterns).

Abnormal Ventilatory Patterns

Although the precise cause of an **abnormal ventilatory pattern** may not always be known, it frequently is related to (1) the anatomic alterations of the lungs associated with a specific disorder and (2) the pathophysiologic mechanisms that develop because of the anatomic alterations. Therefore to evaluate and assess the various abnormal ventilatory patterns (rate and volume relationships) seen in the clinical setting, the following pathophysiologic mechanisms that can alter the ventilatory pattern must first be understood:

- **Lung compliance**
- **Airway resistance**

- **Peripheral chemoreceptors**
- **Central chemoreceptors**
- **Pulmonary reflexes:**
  - **Hering-Breuer reflex**
  - **Deflation reflex**
  - **Irritant reflex**
  - **Juxtapulmonary-capillary receptors (J receptors) reflex**
  - **Reflexes from the aortic and carotid sinus baroreceptors**
- **Pain, anxiety, and fever**

Common Pathophysiologic Mechanisms That Affect the Ventilatory Pattern

Lung Compliance and Its Effect on the Ventilatory Pattern

The ease with which the elastic forces of the lungs accept a volume of inspired air is known as *lung compliance (C_L)*. C_L is measured in terms of unit volume change per unit pressure change. Mathematically it is written as liters per centimeter of water pressure. In other words, compliance determines how much air in liters the lungs will accommodate for each centimeter of water pressure change in distending pressure.

For example, when the normal individual generates a negative intrapleural pressure change of –2 cm H_2O during inspiration, the lungs accept a new volume of about 0.2 L gas. Therefore the C_L of the lungs is 0.1 L/cm H_2O:

$$\begin{aligned} C_L &= \frac{\Delta V\,(L)}{\Delta P\,(cm\ H_2O)} \\ &= \frac{0.2\ L\ gas}{2\ cm\ H_2O} \\ &= 0.1\ L/cm\ H_2O \end{aligned}$$

The normal compliance of the lungs is graphically illustrated by the volume-pressure curve (Figure 2-21). When C_L increases, the lungs accept a greater volume of gas per unit pressure change. When C_L decreases, the lungs accept a smaller volume of gas per unit pressure change (Figure 2-22).

Although the precise mechanism is not clear, the fact that certain ventilatory patterns occur when lung compliance is altered is well documented. For example, when C_L decreases, the patient's breathing rate generally increases while the tidal volume simultaneously decreases (Figure 2-23). This type of breathing pattern is commonly seen in restrictive lung disorders such as pneumonia, pulmonary edema, and adult respiratory distress syndrome. This breathing pattern also is commonly seen during the early stages of an acute asthmatic attack when the alveoli are overinflated; C_L progressively decreases as the alveolar volume increases (see Figure 2-21) at high lung volumes.

Airway Resistance and Its Effect on the Ventilatory Pattern

R_{aw} is defined as the pressure difference between the mouth and the alveoli (transairway pressure) divided by the flow rate. Therefore the rate at which a certain volume of gas flows through the airways is a function of the pressure gradient and the resistance created by the airways to the flow of gas. Mathematically, R_{aw} is calculated as follows:

$$R_{aw} = \frac{\Delta P\,(cm\ H_2O)}{\dot{V}\,(L/sec)}$$

For example, if a patient produces a flow rate of 6 L/sec during inspiration by generating a transairway pressure difference of 12 cm H_2O, R_{aw} would be 2 cm H_2O/L/sec:

$$\begin{aligned} R_{aw} &= \frac{\Delta P}{\dot{V}} \\ &= \frac{12\ cm\ H_2O}{6\ L/sec} \\ &= 2\ cm\ H_2O/L/sec \end{aligned}$$

Under normal conditions the R_{aw} in the tracheobronchial tree is about 1.0 to 2.0 cm H_2O/L/sec. However, in large airway obstructive pulmonary diseases (e.g., bronchitis, asthma), the R_{aw} may be extremely high. An increased R_{aw} has a profound effect on the patient's ventilatory pattern.

When airway resistance increases significantly, the patient's ventilatory rate usually decreases while the tidal volume simultaneously increases (see Figure 2-23). This type of breathing pattern is commonly seen in large airway obstructive lung diseases (e.g., chronic bronchitis, bronchiectasis, asthma, cystic fibrosis) during the advanced stages.

The ventilatory pattern adopted by the patient in either a restrictive or an obstructive lung disorder is thought to be based on minimum work requirements rather than gas exchange efficiency. In physics, work is defined as the force multiplied by the distance moved (work = force × distance). In respiratory physiology the change in pulmonary pressure (force) multiplied by the change in lung volume (distance) may be used to quantify the amount of work required to breathe (work = pressure × volume).

The patient's usual adopted ventilatory pattern may not be seen in the clinical setting because of secondary heart or lung problems. For example, a patient with chronic bronchitis who has adopted a decreased ventilatory rate and an increased tidal volume because of the increased airway resistance associated with the disorder demonstrates an increased ventilatory rate and decreased tidal volume in response to a secondary pneumonia (a restrictive lung disorder superimposed on a chronic obstructive lung disorder).

Because the patient may adopt a ventilatory pattern based on the expenditure of energy rather than on the efficiency of ventilation, the examiner cannot assume that the ventilatory pattern acquired by the patient in response to a certain respiratory disorder is the most efficient one in terms of physiologic gas exchange.

Peripheral Chemoreceptors and Their Effect on the Ventilatory Pattern

The peripheral chemoreceptors (also called *carotid* and *aortic bodies*) are oxygen-sensitive cells that react to a reduction of oxygen in the arterial blood (Pa_{O_2}). The peripheral chemoreceptors are located at the bifurcation of the internal and external carotid arteries (Figure 2-24) and on the aortic arch

FIGURE 2-21 Normal volume-pressure curve. The curve shows that lung compliance progressively decreases as the lungs expand in response to more volume. For example, note the greater volume change between 5 and 10 cm H_2O (small and medium alveoli) than between 30 and 35 cm H_2O (large alveoli).

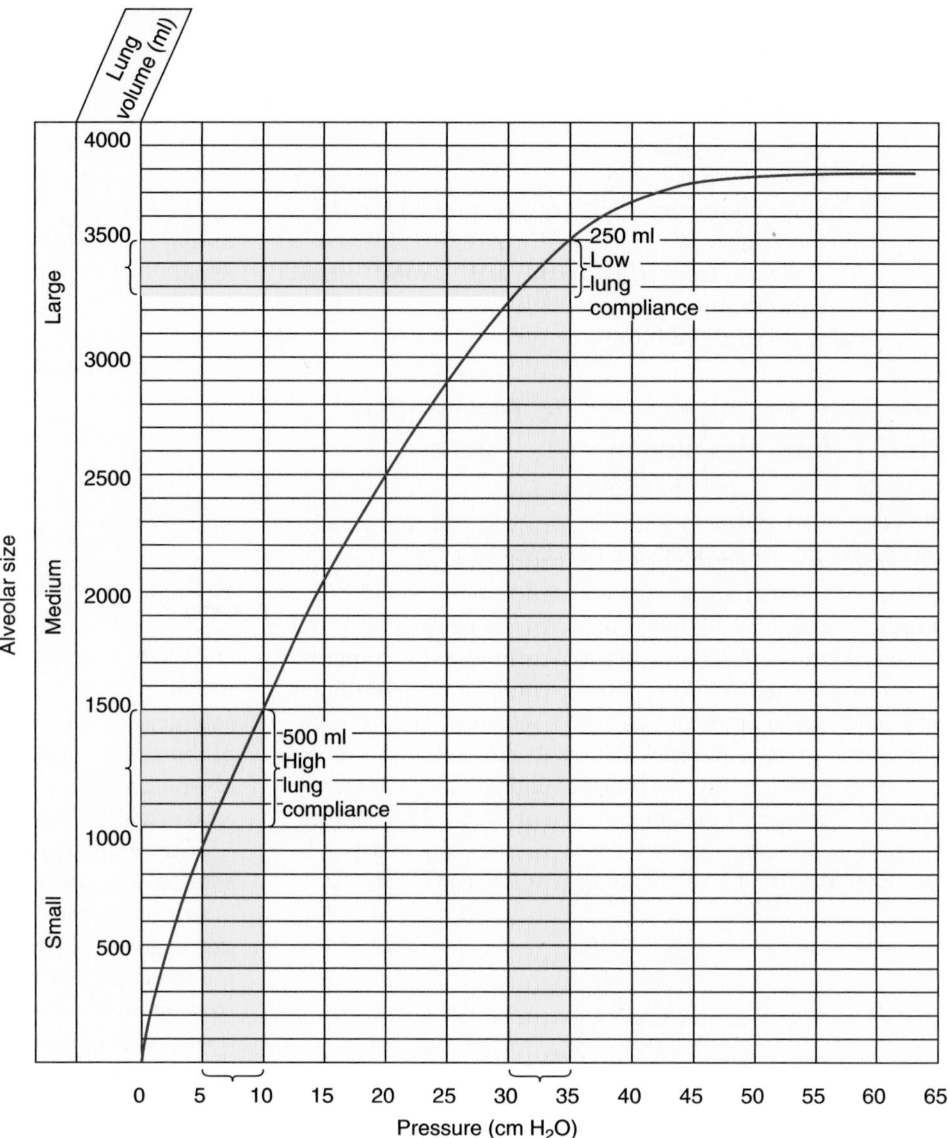

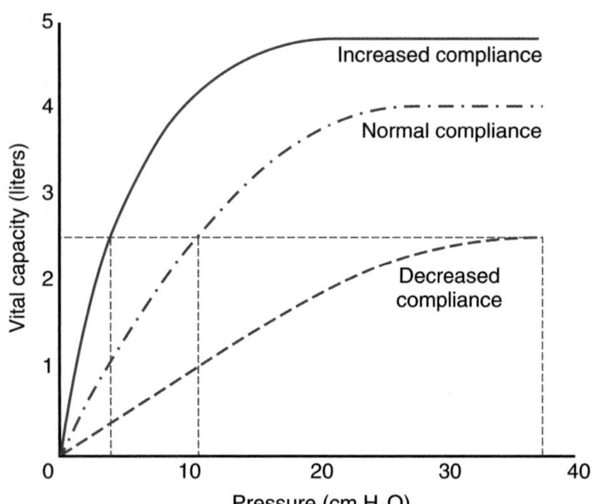

FIGURE 2-22 The effects of increased and decreased compliance on the volume-pressure curve. As the lung compliance decreases, greater pressure change is required to obtain the same volume of 2.5 L *(dotted lines).*

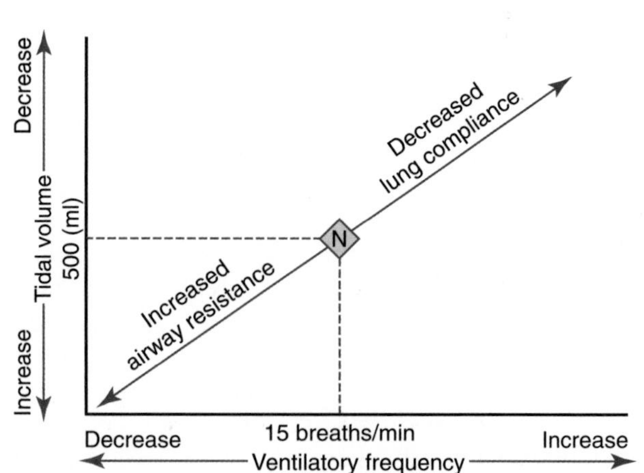

FIGURE 2-23 The effects of increased airway resistance and decreased lung compliance on ventilatory frequency and tidal volume. *N,* Normal resting tidal volume and ventilatory frequency.

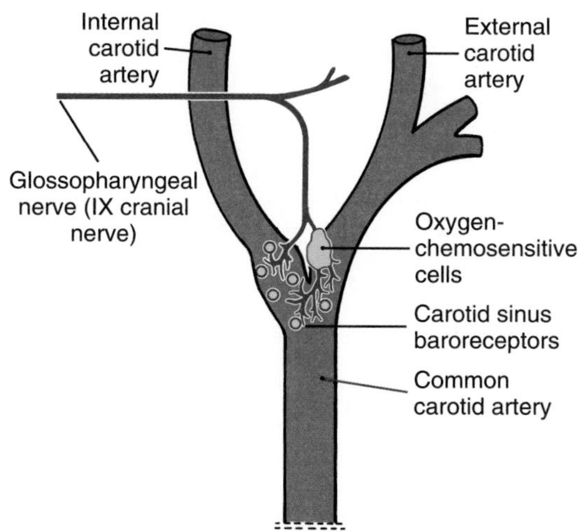

FIGURE 2-24 Oxygen-chemosensitive cells and the carotid sinus baroreceptors are located on the carotid artery.

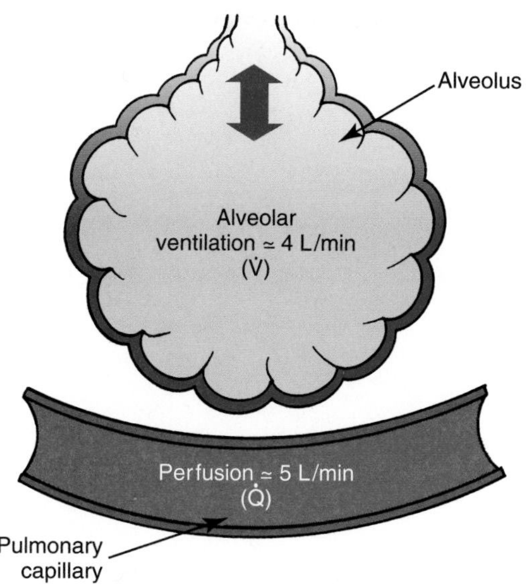

FIGURE 2-26 The normal overall pulmonary ventilation-perfusion ratio ($\dot{V}/\dot{Q}$) is appropriately 0.8.

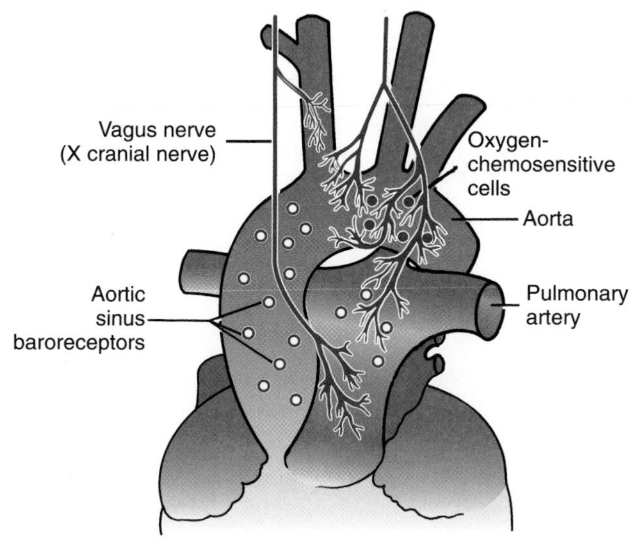

FIGURE 2-25 Oxygen-chemosensitive cells and the aortic sinus baroreceptors are located on the aortic notch and pulmonary artery.

(Figure 2-25). Although the peripheral chemoreceptors are stimulated whenever the Pa_{O_2} is less than normal, they are generally most active when the Pa_{O_2} falls below 60 mm Hg (Sa_{O_2} of about 90%). Suppression of these chemoreceptors, however, is seen when the Pa_{O_2} falls below 30 mm Hg.

When the peripheral chemoreceptors are activated, an afferent (sensory) signal is sent to the respiratory centers of the medulla by way of the glossopharyngeal nerve (cranial nerve IX) from the carotid bodies and by way of the vagus nerve (cranial nerve X) from the aortic bodies. Efferent (motor) signals are then sent to the respiratory muscles, which results in an increased rate of breathing.

In patients who have a chronically low Pa_{O_2} and a high Pa_{CO_2} (e.g., during the advanced stages of emphysema), the peripheral chemoreceptors may be totally responsible for the control of ventilation because a chronically high CO_2 concentration in the cerebrospinal fluid (CSF) inactivates the hydrogen ion (H^+) sensitivity of the **central chemoreceptors.**

Causes of hypoxemia. In respiratory disease, a decreased arterial oxygen level (hypoxemia) is the result of a decreased **ventilation-perfusion ratio, pulmonary shunting,** and **venous admixture** (see Chapter 5 for a broader discussion of hypoxemia).

Decreased ventilation-perfusion ratios. Ideally, each alveolus should receive the same ratio of ventilation and pulmonary capillary blood flow. In reality, however, this is not the case. Alveolar ventilation is normally about 4 L/min, and the pulmonary capillary blood flow is about 5 L/min, which makes the overall ratio of ventilation to blood flow 4 : 5, or 0.8. This relationship is referred to as the *ventilation-perfusion* ($\dot{V}/\dot{Q}$) *ratio* (Figure 2-26).

In some disorders, such as pulmonary embolism, the lungs receive less blood flow in relation to ventilation. When this condition develops, the $\dot{V}/\dot{Q}$ ratio increases. A larger portion of the alveolar ventilation therefore will not be physiologically effective and will be said to demonstrate "wasted" or dead-space ventilation (Figure 2-27).

In most lung disorders (e.g., asthma, emphysema, pulmonary edema, or pneumonia), the lungs receive less ventilation in relation to blood flow. When this condition develops, the $\dot{V}/\dot{Q}$ ratio decreases. A larger portion of the pulmonary blood flow is not physiologically effective in terms of molecular gas exchange and is said to be "shunted" blood (see the following section on pulmonary shunting). Generally, when the $\dot{V}/\dot{Q}$ ratio decreases, the Pa_{O_2} decreases and the Pa_{CO_2} increases.

FIGURE 2-27 Dead-space ventilation (V_D).

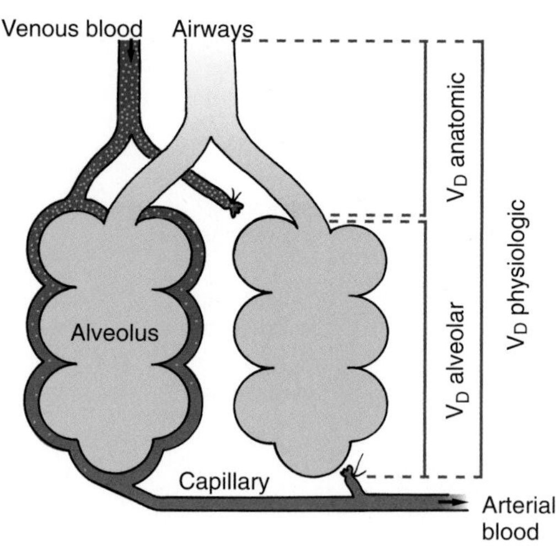

Only the inspired air that reaches the alveoli is physiologically effective. This portion of the inspired gas is referred to as *alveolar ventilation.* The volume of inspired air that does not reach the alveoli is not physiologically effective. This portion of gas is referred to as *dead-space ventilation.* There are three types of dead spaces: anatomic, alveolar, and physiologic.

Anatomic dead space. Anatomic dead space is the volume of gas in the conducting airways: the nose, mouth, pharynx, larynx, and lower portions of the airways down to but not including the respiratory bronchioles. The volume of the anatomic dead space is approximately equal to 1 ml/lb (2.2 ml/kg) of normal body weight.

Alveolar dead space. When an alveolus is ventilated but not perfused with blood, the volume of air in the alveolus is dead space, that is, the air within the alveolus is not physiologically effective in terms of gas exchange. The amount of alveolar dead space is unpredictable.

Physiologic dead space. The physiologic dead space is the sum of the anatomic dead space and the alveolar dead space. Because neither of these two forms of dead space is physiologically effective in terms of gas exchange, the two forms are combined and are referred to as *physiologic dead space.* (See Physiologic Dead Space Calculation, Appendix IX.)

Pulmonary shunting. Pulmonary shunting is defined as that portion of the cardiac output that moves from the right side to the left side of the heart without being exposed to alveolar oxygen (P_{AO_2}). Clinically, pulmonary shunting can be subdivided into absolute shunts and relative shunts.

Absolute shunts. **Absolute shunts** (also called **true shunts**) are divided into the following two major groups: **anatomic shunts** and **capillary shunts.**

ANATOMIC SHUNTS. An anatomic shunt exists when blood flows from the right side of the heart to the left side without coming in contact with an alveolus for gas exchange (Figure 2-28, *B*). In the healthy individual, the normal anatomic shunt is about 3% of the cardiac output. This normal shunting is caused by nonoxygenated blood completely bypassing the alveoli and entering (1) the pulmonary vascular system by means of the bronchial venous drainage, and (2) the left atrium by way of the **thebesian veins.** Common causes of anatomic shunts include the following:

- Congenital heart diseases
- Intrapulmonary fistulas
- Pulmonary vascular tumors

CAPILLARY SHUNTS. A capillary shunt is commonly caused by (1) alveolar collapse or atelectasis, (2) alveolar fluid accumulation, or (3) alveolar consolidation or pneumonia (see Figure 2-28, *C*).

The sum of the anatomic shunt and capillary shunt is called the **absolute,** or **true, shunt**. Patients with absolute shunting respond poorly to oxygen therapy. This is because alveolar oxygen does not come in contact with the shunted blood. As a result, absolute shunting is **refractory** to oxygen therapy. In short, the reduced arterial oxygen level caused by absolute shunting cannot be easily treated by increasing the concentration of oxygen for these two major reasons: (1) because of the alveolar pathology associated with an absolute shunt, the alveoli are unable to accommodate any form of ventilation, and (2) the blood that bypasses the normal, functional alveoli is unable to carry more oxygen once it has become fully saturated—except for a very small amount that dissolves in the plasma ($P_{O_2} \times 0.003$ = dissolved O_2).

Relative shunts. When pulmonary capillary perfusion is in excess of alveolar ventilation, a **relative shunt**, or **shunt-like effect**, is said to be present (see Figure 2-28, *D*). Common causes of a relative shunt include (1) hypoventilation, (2) decreased $\dot{V}/\dot{Q}$ ratios (e.g., emphysema, chronic bronchitis, asthmatic episode, excessive airway secretions), and (3) increased alveolar-capillary membrane thickness disorders (e.g., pulmonary edema, acute respiratory distress syndrome, pneumoconiosis, chronic interstitial lung disease).

Even though the alveolus may be ventilated in the presence of an alveolar-capillary defect, the blood passing by the

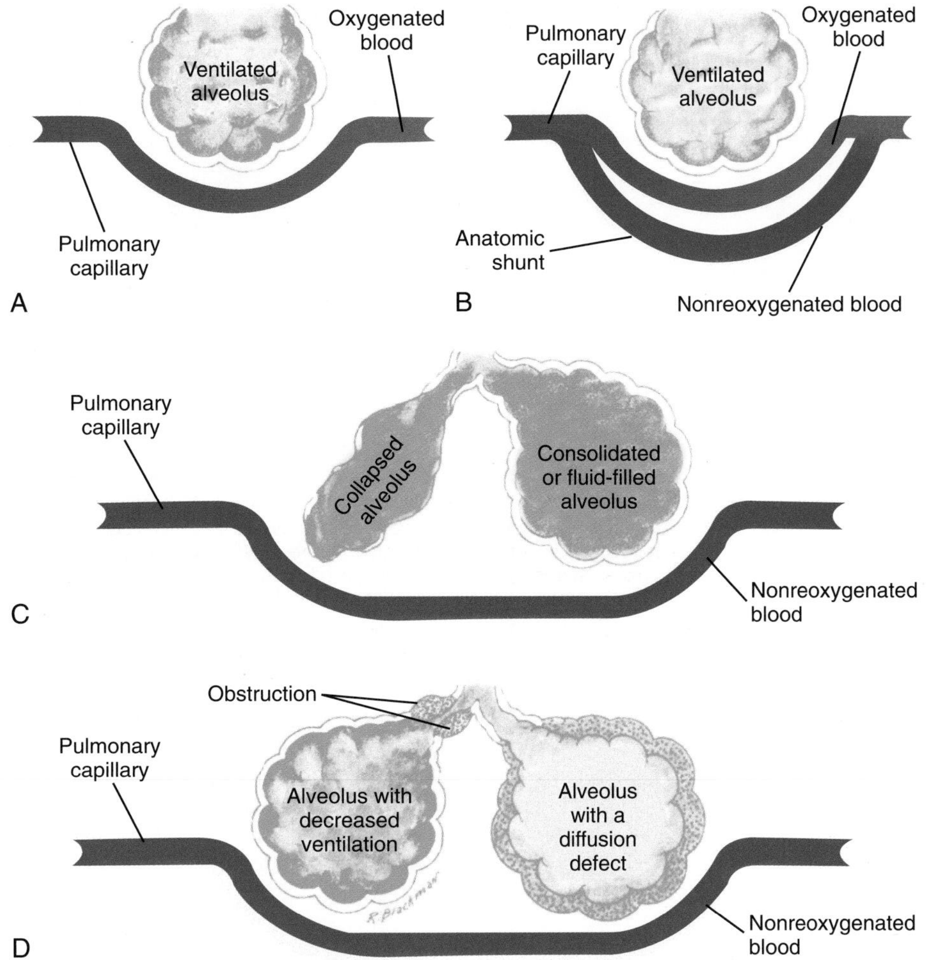

FIGURE 2-28 Pulmonary shunting. **A**, Normal alveolar-capillary unit. **B**, Anatomic shunt. **C**, Types of capillary shunts. **D**, Types of relative or shuntlike effects.

alveolus does not have enough time to equilibrate with the alveolar oxygen tension. If the diffusion defect is severe enough to completely block gas exchange across the alveolar-capillary membrane, the shunt is called an *absolute* or *true shunt* (see earlier discussion). A relative shunt may also develop after the administration of drugs that cause an increase in cardiac output or the dilation of the pulmonary blood vessels. Unlike an absolute shunt, which is refractory to oxygen therapy, conditions that cause a relative shunt (shuntlike effect) are readily corrected by oxygen therapy.

Table 2-9 illustrates the type of pulmonary shunting associated with common diseases.

Venous admixture. The result of pulmonary shunting is venous admixture, which is the mixing of shunted nonreoxygenated blood with reoxygenated blood distal to the alveoli (i.e., downstream in the pulmonary circulatory system; Figure 2-29). When venous admixture occurs, the shunted nonreoxygenated blood gains oxygen molecules while the reoxygenated blood loses oxygen molecules. The result is a blood mixture that has (1) higher Po_2 and Cao_2 values than the nonreoxygenated blood and (2) lower Po_2 and Cao_2 values than the reoxygenated blood—in other words, a blood mixture with Pao_2 and Cao_2 values somewhere between the original values of the reoxygenated and nonreoxygenated blood. Clinically, this mixed blood is sampled downstream (e.g., from the radial artery) to assess the patient's arterial blood gases.

The peripheral chemoreceptors are frequently stimulated in respiratory disease because they respond to hypoxemia caused by decreased $\dot{V}/\dot{Q}$ ratios, pulmonary shunting, and venous admixture. The decreased arterial oxygen tension then stimulates the peripheral chemoreceptors to send a signal to the medulla to increase ventilation (Figure 2-30).

Other factors that stimulate the peripheral chemoreceptors. Although the peripheral chemoreceptors are primarily activated by a decreased arterial oxygen level, they also are stimulated by a decreased pH (increased H^+ concentration). For example, the accumulation of lactic acid (from anaerobic

TABLE 2-9 Type of Pulmonary Shunting Associated with Common Respiratory Diseases

Respiratory Diseases	Capillary Shunt	Relative or Shuntlike Effect
Chronic bronchitis		X
Emphysema		X
Asthma		X
Croup/epiglottitis		X
Bronchiectasis*	X	X
Cystic fibrosis*	X	X
Pneumoconiosis*	X	X
Pneumonia	X	
Lung abscess	X	
Pulmonary edema	X	
Near-drowning	X	
Adult respiratory distress syndrome	X	
Chronic interstitial lung disease	X	
Flail chest	X	
Pneumothorax	X	
Pleural diseases	X	
Kyphoscoliosis	X	
Tuberculosis	X	
Fungal diseases	X	
Idiopathic (infant) respiratory distress syndrome	X	
Smoke inhalation	X	

* Relative or shuntlike effect is most common.

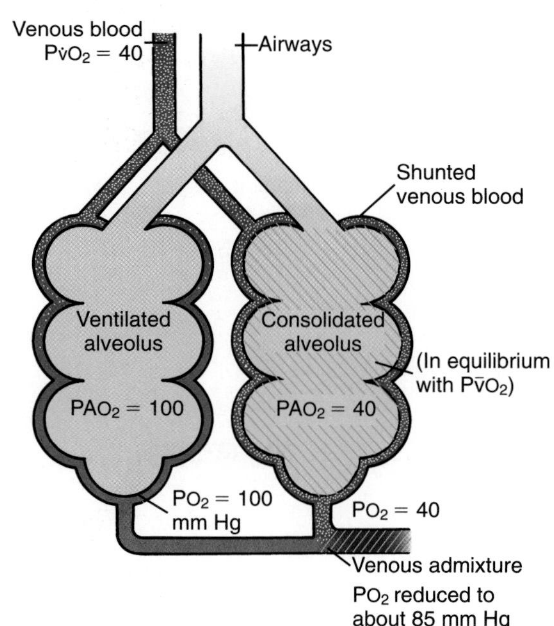

FIGURE 2-29 Venous admixture occurs when reoxygenated blood mixes with nonreoxygenated blood distal to the alveoli. Technically, the Po_2 in the pulmonary capillary system will not equilibrate completely because of the normal $P(A\text{-}a)O_2$. The Po_2 in the pulmonary capillary system is normally a few millimeters of mercury less than the Po_2 in the alveoli.

FIGURE 2-30 Schematic illustration showing the way a low Pao_2 stimulates the respiratory components of the medulla to increase alveolar ventilation. As shown, alveolar hypoventilation (decreased $\dot{V}/\dot{Q}$ ratio) leads to shunting and venous admixture. This process causes the Pao_2 to fall. The low Pao_2 stimulates the carotid and aortic bodies to send signals to the medulla. The medulla then sends out signals to increase ventilation.

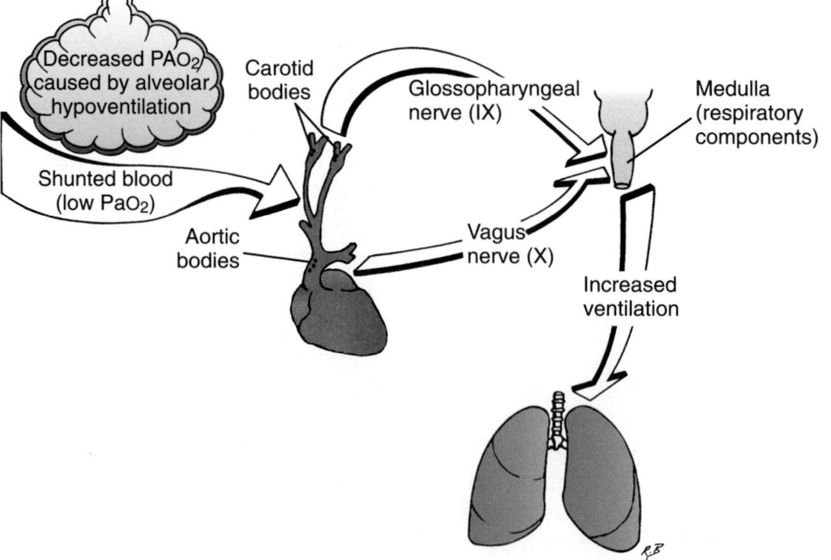

metabolism) or ketoacids (diabetic acidosis) in the blood increases ventilatory rate almost entirely through the peripheral chemoreceptors. The peripheral chemoreceptors also are activated by hypoperfusion, increased temperature, nicotine, and the direct effect of $Paco_2$. The response of the peripheral chemoreceptors to $Paco_2$ stimulation, however, is relatively small compared with the response generated by the central chemoreceptors.

Central Chemoreceptors and Their Effect on the Ventilatory Pattern

Although the mechanism is not fully understood, it is now believed that two special respiratory centers in the medulla, the dorsal respiratory group (DRG) and the ventral respiratory group (VRG), are responsible for coordinating **respiration** (Figure 2-31). Both the DRG and VRG are stimulated by an increased concentration of H^+ in the CSF. The H^+

concentration of the CSF is monitored by the central chemoreceptors, which are located bilaterally and ventrally in the substance of the medulla. A portion of the central chemoreceptor region is actually in direct contact with the CSF. The central chemoreceptors transmit signals to the respiratory neurons by the following mechanism:

1. When the CO_2 level increases in the blood (e.g., during periods of hypoventilation), CO_2 molecules readily diffuse across the blood-brain barrier and enter the CSF. The blood-brain barrier is a semipermeable membrane that separates circulating blood from the CSF. The blood-brain barrier is relatively impermeable to ions such as H^+ and HCO_3^- but is very permeable to CO_2.
2. After CO_2 crosses the blood-brain barrier and enters the CSF, it forms carbonic acid:

$$CO_2 + H_2O \Leftrightarrow H_2CO_3^- \Leftrightarrow H^+ + HCO_3^-$$

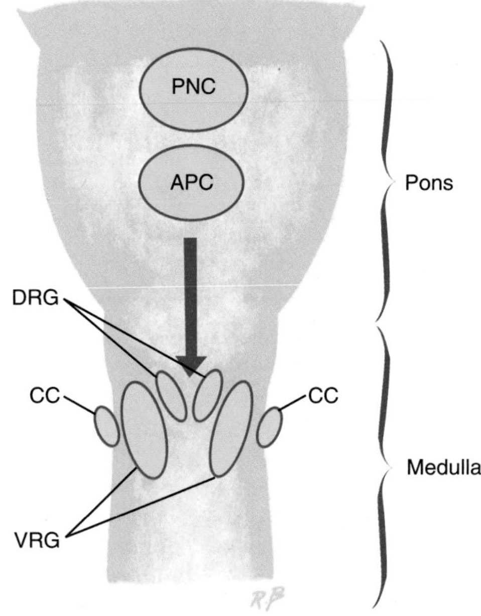

FIGURE 2-31 Schematic illustration of the respiratory components of the lower brain stem (pons and medulla). *APC,* Apneustic center; *CC,* central chemoreceptors; *DRG,* dorsal respiratory group; *PNC,* pneumotaxic center; *VRG,* ventral respiratory group.

3. Because the CSF has an inefficient buffering system, the H^+ produced from the previous reaction rapidly increases and causes the pH of the CSF to decrease.
4. The central chemoreceptors react to the liberated H^+ by sending signals to the respiratory components of the medulla, which in turn increases the ventilatory rate.
5. The increased ventilatory rate causes the Pa_{CO_2} and subsequently the P_{CO_2} in the CSF to decrease. Therefore the CO_2 level in the blood regulates ventilation by its indirect effect on the pH of the CSF (Figure 2-32).

Pulmonary Reflexes and Their Effect on the Ventilatory Pattern

Several reflexes may be activated in certain respiratory diseases and influence the patient's ventilatory rate.

Deflation reflex. When the lungs are compressed or deflated (e.g., atelectasis), an increased rate of breathing is seen. The precise mechanism responsible for this reflex is not known. Some investigators suggest that the increased rate of breathing may simply result from reduced stimulation of the receptors (the Hering-Breuer reflex) rather than the stimulation of specific deflation receptors. Receptors for the Hering-Breuer reflex are located in the walls of the bronchi and bronchioles. When these receptors are stretched (e.g., during a deep inspiration), a reflex response is triggered to decrease the ventilatory rate. Other investigators, however, feel that the deflation reflex does not result from the absence of receptor stimulation of the Hering-Breuer reflex because the deflation reflex is still seen when the bronchi and bronchioles are below a temperature of 8° C. The Hering-Breuer reflex does not occur when the bronchi and bronchioles are below this temperature.

Irritant reflex. When the lungs are compressed, deflated, or exposed to noxious gases, the irritant receptors are stimulated. The irritant receptors are subepithelial mechanoreceptors located in the trachea, bronchi, and bronchioles. When the receptors are activated, a reflex causes the ventilatory rate to increase. Stimulation of the irritant reflex also may produce a cough and bronchoconstriction.

Juxtapulmonary capillary receptors. The juxtapulmonary capillary receptors, or J receptors, are located in the interstitial

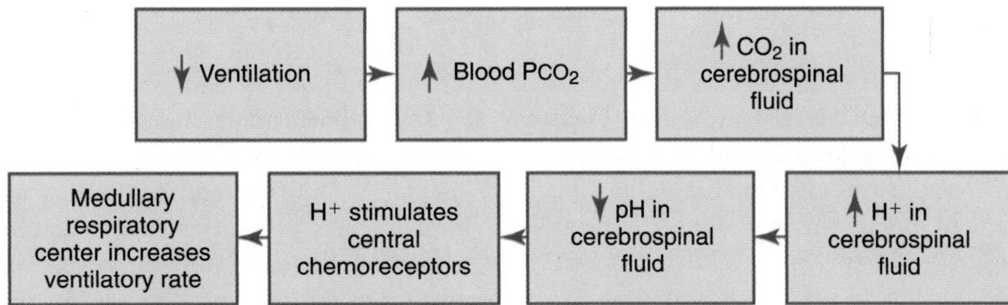

FIGURE 2-32 Sequence of events in alveolar hypoventilation. The central chemoreceptors are stimulated by hydrogen ions (H^+), which increase in concentration as CO_2 moves into the cerebrospinal fluid.

tissues between the pulmonary capillaries and the alveoli. Their precise mechanism of action is not known. When the J receptors are stimulated, a reflex triggers rapid, shallow breathing. The J receptors may be activated by the following:

- Pulmonary capillary congestion
- Capillary hypertension
- Edema of the alveolar walls
- Humoral agents (e.g., serotonin)
- Lung deflation
- Emboli in the microcirculation

Reflexes from the aortic and carotid sinus baroreceptors. The normal function of the **aortic and carotid sinus baroreceptors**, located near the aortic and carotid peripheral chemoreceptors, is to activate reflexes that cause (1) decreased heart rate and ventilatory rate in response to increased systemic blood pressure and (2) increased heart rate and ventilatory rate in response to decreased systemic blood pressure.

Pain, Anxiety, and Fever

An increased respiratory rate may result from the chest pain or fear and anxiety associated with the patient's inability to breathe. Chest pain and fear occur in a number of cardiopulmonary pathologies, such as pleurisy, rib fractures, pulmonary hypertension, and angina. An increased respiratory rate also may be caused by fever. Fever is commonly associated with infectious lung disorders such as pneumonia, lung abscess, tuberculosis, and fungal disease.

Use of the Accessory Muscles of Inspiration

During the advanced stages of chronic obstructive pulmonary disease, the accessory muscles of inspiration are activated when the diaphragm becomes significantly depressed by the increased residual volume and functional residual capacity. The accessory muscles assist or largely replace the diaphragm in creating subatmospheric pressure in the pleural space during inspiration. The major accessory muscles of inspiration are as follows:

- **Scalene**
- **Sternocleidomastoid**
- **Pectoralis major**
- **Trapezius**

Scalenes

The anterior, medial, and posterior scalene muscles are separate muscles that function as a unit. They originate on the transverse processes of the second to sixth cervical vertebrae and insert into the first and second ribs (Figure 2-33). These muscles normally elevate the first and second ribs and flex the neck. When they are used as accessory muscles of inspiration, their primary role is to elevate the first and second ribs.

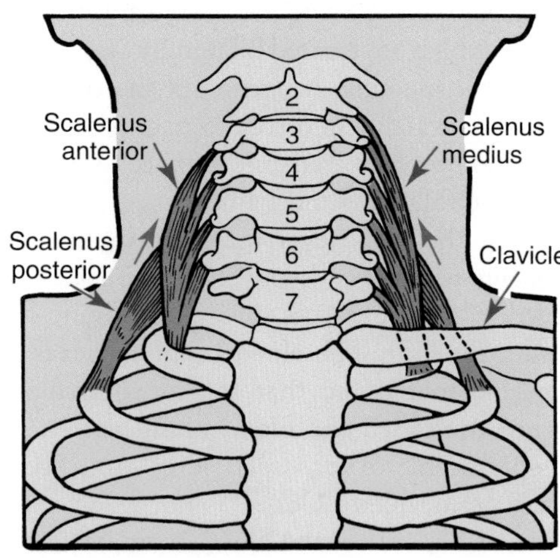

FIGURE 2-33 The scalene muscles. Red arrows indicate upward movement of the ribs.

Sternocleidomastoids

The sternocleidomastoid muscles are located on each side of the neck (Figure 2-34), where they rotate and support the head. They originate from the sternum and clavicle and insert into the mastoid process and occipital bone of the skull.

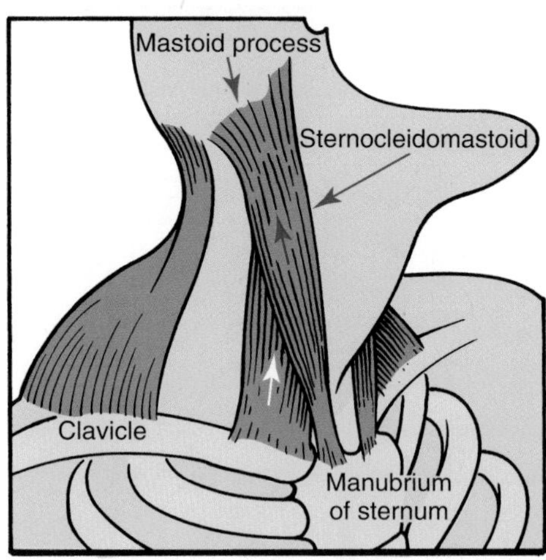

FIGURE 2-34 The sternocleidomastoid muscle. White arrow indicates upward movement of the sternum.

Normally, the sternocleidomastoid pulls from its sternoclavicular origin, rotates the head to the opposite side, and turns it upward. When the sternocleidomastoid muscle functions as an accessory muscle of inspiration, the head and neck are fixed by other muscles, and the sternocleidomastoid pulls from its insertion on the skull and elevates the sternum. This action increases the anteroposterior diameter of the chest.

Pectoralis Major Muscles

The pectoralis major muscles are powerful, fan-shaped muscles that originate from the clavicle and sternum and insert into the upper part of the humerus. The primary function of the pectoralis muscles is to pull the upper part of the arm to the body in a hugging motion (Figure 2-35).

When operating as an accessory muscle of inspiration, the pectoralis pulls from the humeral insertion and elevates the chest, resulting in an increased anteroposterior diameter. Patients with chronic obstructive pulmonary disease usually secure their arms to something stationary and use the pectoralis major muscles to increase the anteroposterior diameter of the chest (Figure 2-36). This braced position is called the *emphysematous habitus.*

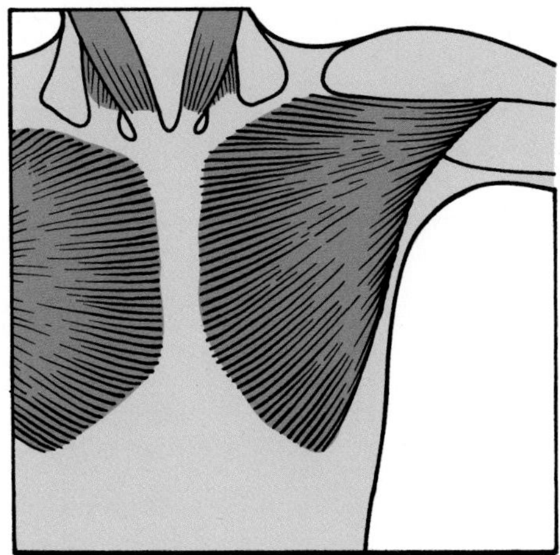

FIGURE 2-35 The pectoralis major muscles.

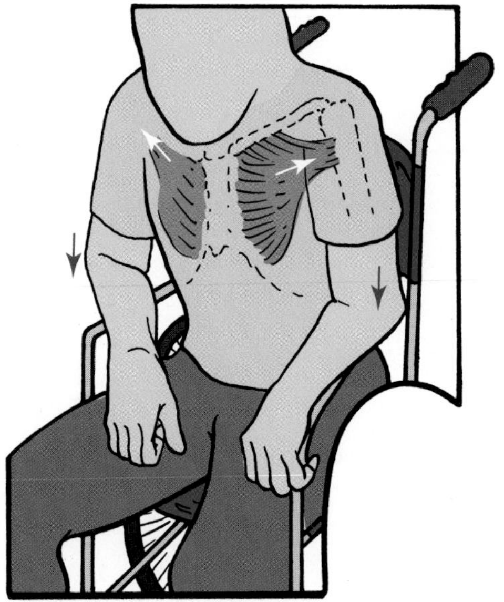

FIGURE 2-36 The way a patient may appear when using the pectoralis major muscles for inspiration. White arrows indicate the elevation of the chest. Downward arrows near the patient's elbows indicate how the patient may fix the arms to a stationary object.

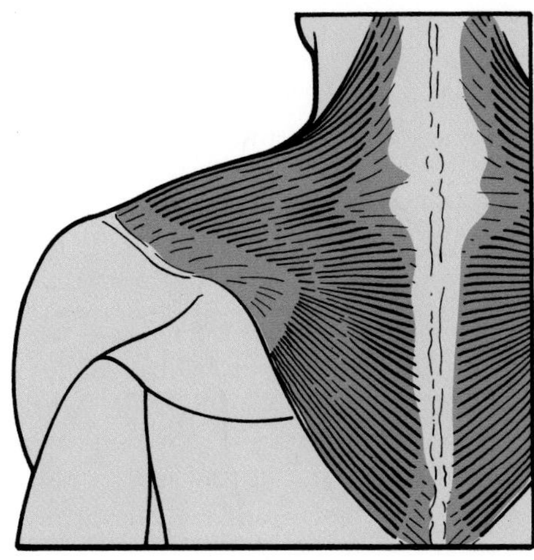

FIGURE 2-37 The trapezius muscles.

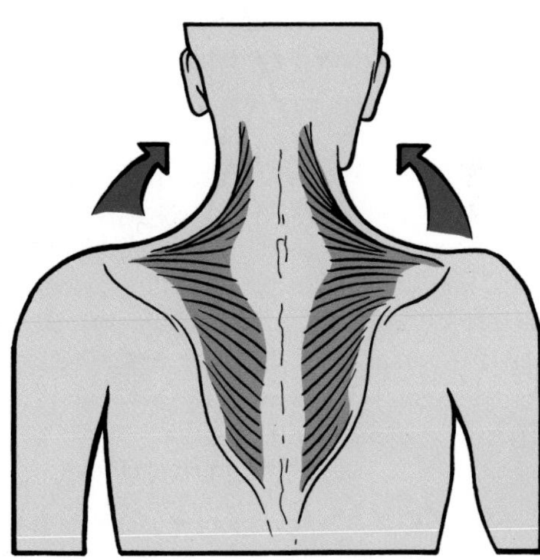

FIGURE 2-38 The action of the trapezius muscle is typified in shrugging the shoulders.

Trapezius

The trapezius is a large, flat, triangular muscle that is situated superficially in the upper part of the back and the back of the neck. The muscle originates from the occipital bone, the ligamentum nuchae, the spinous processes of the seventh cervical vertebra, and all the thoracic vertebrae. It inserts into the spine of the scapula, the acromion process, and the lateral third of the clavicle (Figure 2-37). The trapezius muscle rotates the scapula, raises the shoulders, and abducts and flexes the arm. Its action is typified in shrugging the shoulders (Figure 2-38). When used as an accessory muscle of inspiration, the trapezius helps elevate the thoracic cage.

Use of the Accessory Muscles of Expiration

Because of the airway narrowing and collapse associated with chronic obstructive pulmonary disorders, the accessory muscles of exhalation are often recruited when airway resistance becomes significantly elevated. When these muscles actively contract, intrapleural pressure increases and offsets the increased airway resistance. The major accessory muscles of exhalation are as follows:

- **Rectus abdominis**
- **External oblique**
- **Internal oblique**
- **Transversus abdominis**

Rectus Abdominis

A pair of rectus abdominis muscles extends the entire length of the abdomen. Each muscle forms a vertical mass about 4 inches wide, separated by the linea alba. It arises from the iliac crest and pubic symphysis and inserts into the xiphoid process and the fifth, sixth, and seventh ribs. When activated, the muscle assists in compressing the abdominal contents, which in turn push the diaphragm into the thoracic cage (Figure 2-39).

External Obliques

The broad, thin, external oblique muscle is on the anterolateral side of the abdomen. The muscle is the longest and most superficial of all the anterolateral muscles of the abdomen.

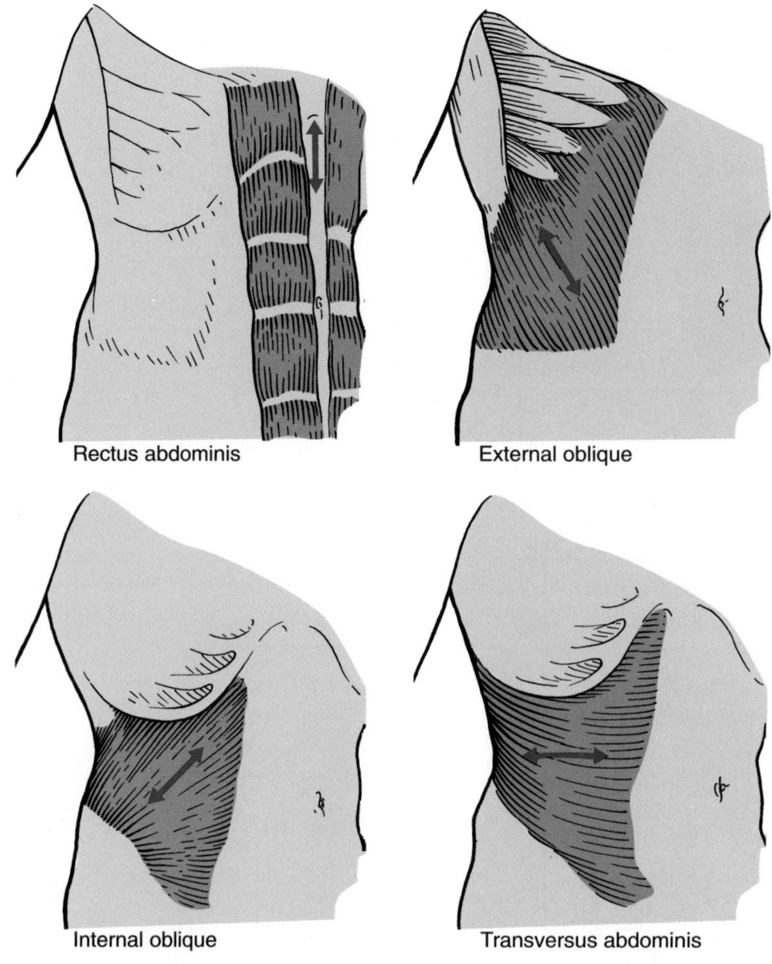

FIGURE 2-39 Accessory muscles of expiration. Arrows indicate the action of these muscles in enlarging the volume of the lungs.

It arises by eight digitations from the lower eight ribs and the abdominal aponeurosis. It inserts in the iliac crest and into the linea alba. The muscle assists in compressing the abdominal contents. This action also pushes the diaphragm into the thoracic cage during exhalation (see Figure 2-39).

Internal Obliques

The internal oblique muscle is in the lateral and ventral part of the abdominal wall directly under the external oblique muscle. It is smaller and thinner than the external oblique. It arises from the inguinal ligament, the iliac crest, and the lower portion of the lumbar aponeurosis. It inserts into the last four ribs and the linea alba. The muscle assists in compressing the abdominal contents and pushing the diaphragm into the thoracic cage (see Figure 2-39).

Transversus Abdominis

The transversus abdominis muscle is found immediately under each internal oblique muscle. It arises from the inguinal ligament, the iliac crest, the thoracolumbar fascia, and the lower six ribs. It inserts into the linea alba. When activated, it constricts the abdominal contents (see Figure 2-39).

When all four pairs of accessory muscles of exhalation contract, the abdominal pressure increases and drives the diaphragm into the thoracic cage. As the diaphragm moves into the thoracic cage during exhalation, the intrapleural pressure increases and enhances expiratory gas flow (Figure 2-40).

Pursed-Lip Breathing

Pursed-lip breathing occurs in patients during the advanced stages of obstructive pulmonary disease. It is a relatively simple technique that many patients learn without formal instruction. During pursed-lip breathing the patient exhales through lips that are held in a position similar to that used for whistling, kissing, or blowing through a flute. The positive pressure created by retarding the airflow through pursed lips provides the airways with some stability and an increased ability to resist surrounding intrapleural pressures. This action offsets early airway collapse and air trapping during exhalation. In addition, pursed-lip breathing has been shown to slow the patient's ventilatory rate and generate a ventilatory pattern that is more effective in gas mixing (Figure 2-41).

Substernal and Intercostal Retractions

Substernal and intercostal retractions may be seen in patients with severe restrictive lung disorders such as pneumonia or

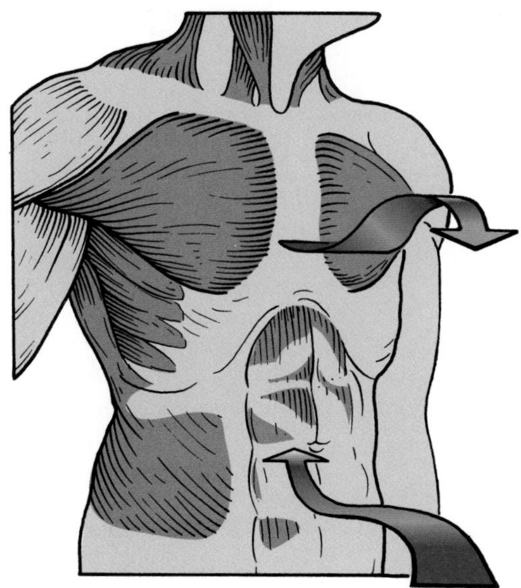

FIGURE 2-40 When the accessory muscles of expiration contract, intrapleural pressure increases, the chest moves outward, and airflow increases.

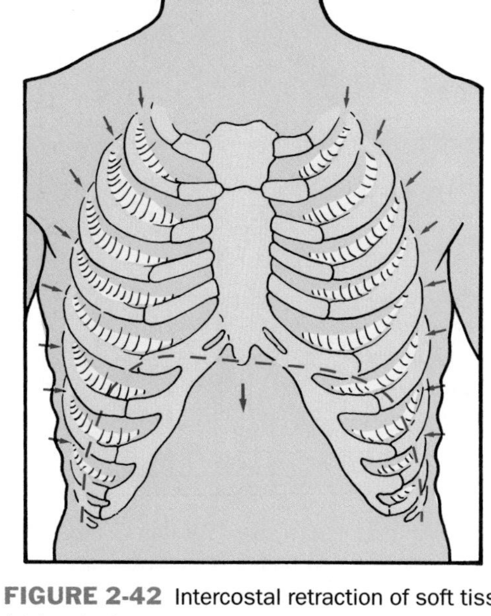

FIGURE 2-42 Intercostal retraction of soft tissues during forceful inspiration.

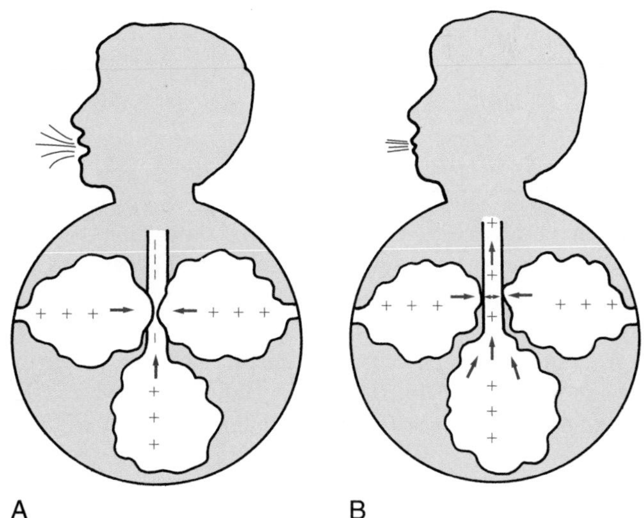

FIGURE 2-41 **A**, Schematic illustration of alveolar compression of weakened bronchiolar airways during normal expiration in patients with chronic obstructive pulmonary disease (e.g., emphysema). **B**, Effects of pursed-lip breathing. The weakened bronchiolar airways are kept open by the effects of positive pressure created by pursed lips during expiration.

adult respiratory distress syndrome. In an effort to overcome the low lung compliance, the patient must generate a greater-than-normal negative intrapleural pressure during inspiration. This greater negative intrapleural pressure causes the tissues between the ribs and the substernal area to retract during inspiration (Figure 2-42). Because the thorax of the newborn is quite flexible (as a result of the large amount of cartilage found in the skeletal structure), substernal and intercostal retractions are seen in infants with idiopathic respiratory distress syndrome (IRDS).

Nasal Flaring

Nasal flaring is often seen during inspiration in infants experiencing respiratory distress. It is likely a facial reflex that enhances the movement of gas into the tracheobronchial tree. The dilator naris, which originates from the maxilla and inserts into the ala of the nose, is the muscle responsible for this clinical manifestation. When activated the dilator naris pulls the alae laterally and widens the nasal aperture, providing a larger orifice for gas to enter the lungs during inspiration (see Chapter 31).

Splinting Caused by Chest Pain or Decreased Chest Expansion

Chest pain is one of the most common complaints among patients with cardiopulmonary problems. It can be divided into two categories: pleuritic and nonpleuritic.

Pleuritic Chest Pain

Pleuritic chest pain is usually described as a sudden, sharp, or stabbing pain. The pain generally intensifies during deep inspiration and coughing and diminishes during breath holding or splinting. The origin of the pain may be the chest wall, muscles, ribs, parietal pleura, diaphragm, mediastinal structures, or intercostal nerves. Because the visceral pleura, which covers the lungs, does not have any sensory nerve supply, pain originating in the parietal region signifies extension of inflammation from the lungs to the contiguous parietal pleura lining the inner surface of the chest wall. This condition is known as *pleurisy* (Figure 2-43). When a patient with pleurisy inhales, the lung expands, irritating the inflamed parietal pleura and causing pain.

Because of the nature of the pleuritic pain, the patient usually prefers to lie on the affected side to allow greater expansion of the uninvolved lung and help splint the chest.

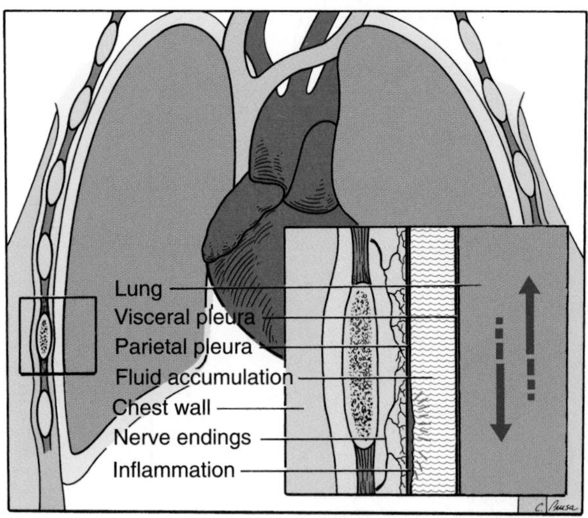

FIGURE 2-43 When the parietal pleura is irritated, the nerve endings in the parietal pleura send pain signals to the brain.

Pleuritic chest pain is a characteristic feature of the following respiratory diseases:

- Pneumonia
- Pleural effusion
- Pneumothorax
- Pulmonary infarction
- Lung cancer
- Pneumoconiosis
- Fungal diseases
- Tuberculosis

Nonpleuritic Chest Pain

Nonpleuritic chest pain is usually described as a constant pain that is located centrally. The pain also may radiate. Nonpleuritic chest pain is associated with the following disorders:

- Myocardial ischemia
- Pericardial inflammation
- Pulmonary hypertension
- Esophagitis
- Local trauma or inflammation of the chest cage, muscles, bones, or cartilage

Abnormal Chest Shape and Configuration

During inspection the respiratory care practitioner systematically observes the patient's chest for both normal and abnormal findings. Is the spine straight? Are any lesions or surgical scars evident? Are the scapulae symmetric? Common chest deformities are listed in Table 2-10.

Abnormal Extremity Findings

The inspection of the patient's extremities should include the following:

- Altered skin color (e.g., cyanotic, pale, with prominent venous distention)
- Presence or absence of digital clubbing
- Presence or absence of peripheral edema
- Presence or absence of distended neck veins

TABLE 2-10 Common Abnormal Chest Shapes and Configurations

Condition	Description
Kyphosis	A "hunchbacked" appearance caused by posterior curvature of the spine
Scoliosis	A lateral curvature of the spine that results in the chest protruding posteriorly and the anterior ribs flattening out
Kyphoscoliosis	The combination of kyphosis and scoliosis (see Figure 25-1)
Pectus carinatum	The forward projection of the xiphoid process and lower sternum (also known as "pigeon breast" deformity)
Pectus excavatum	A funnel-shaped depression over the lower sternum (also called "funnel chest")
Barrel chest	In the normal adult, the anteroposterior diameter of the chest is about half its lateral diameter, or 1 : 2. When the patient has a barrel chest, the ratio is nearer to 1 : 1 (Figure 2-44)

Altered Skin Color

A general observation of the patient's skin color should be routinely performed. For example, does the patient's skin color appear normal—pink, tan, brown, or black? Is the skin cold or clammy? Does the skin appear ashen or pallid? This appearance could be caused by anemia or acute blood loss. Do the patient's eyes, face, trunk, and arms have a yellow, jaundiced appearance (caused by increased bilirubin in the blood and tissue)? Is there redness of the skin, or erythema (often caused by capillary congestion, inflammation, or infection)? Does the patient appear cyanotic?

Cyanosis

Cyanosis is common in severe respiratory disorders. *Cyanosis* is the term used to describe the blue-gray or purplish discoloration of the mucous membranes, fingertips, and toes whenever the blood in these areas contains at least 5 g/dL of reduced hemoglobin. When the normal 14 to 15 g/dL of hemoglobin is fully saturated, the Pa_{O_2} is about 97 to 100 mm Hg, and there is about 20 vol% of oxygen in the blood. In a cyanotic patient with one third (5 g/dL) of the hemoglobin reduced, the Pa_{O_2} is about 30 mm Hg and there is 13 vol% of oxygen in the blood (Figure 2-45).

The detection and interpretation of cyanosis are difficult, and wide individual variations occur among observers. The recognition of cyanosis depends on the acuity of the observer, the light conditions in the examining room, and the pigmentation of the patient. Cyanosis of the nail beds also is influenced by temperature because vasoconstriction induced by cold may slow circulation to the point at which

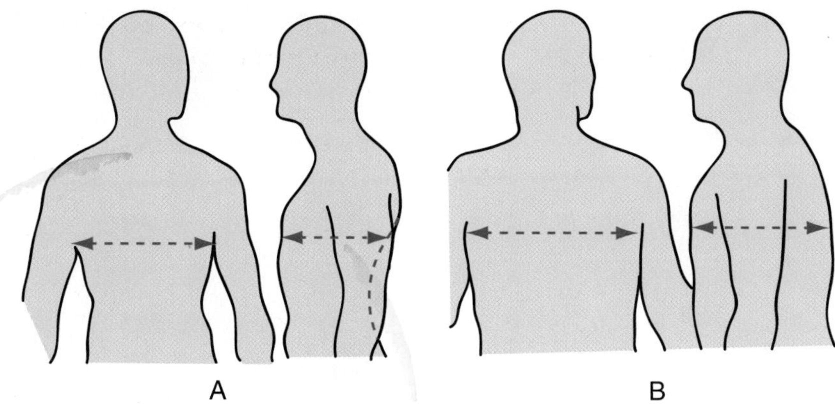

FIGURE 2-44 **A**, Normally, the anteroposterior diameter is about half the lateral diameter (a ratio of 1 : 2). Because of the air trapping and lung hyperinflation in obstructive pulmonary diseases, the natural tendency of the lungs to recoil is decreased and the normal tendency of the chest to move outward prevails. This condition results in an increased anteroposterior diameter and is referred to as the *barrel chest deformity.* The ratio is nearer to 1 : 1. **B**, The anteroposterior diameter commonly increases with aging. Therefore older individuals may have a slight barrel chest appearance in the absence of any pulmonary disease. Normal infants also usually have an anteroposterior diameter near 1 : 1.

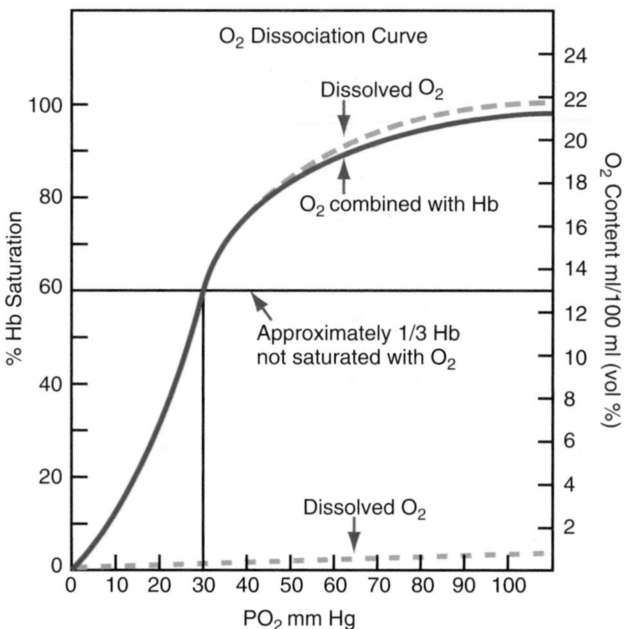

FIGURE 2-45 Cyanosis is likely whenever the blood contains at least 5 g of reduced hemoglobin. In the normal individual who has about 15 g of hemoglobin per 100 mL of blood, a Po_2 of about 30 mm Hg produces 5 g of reduced hemoglobin. The hemoglobin, however, is still approximately 60% saturated with oxygen.

the blood becomes hypoxic (bluish) in the surface capillaries even though the arterial blood in the major vessels is not lacking in oxygen.

Central cyanosis, as observed on the mucous membranes of the lips and mouth, is almost always a sign of hypoxemia and therefore has a definite diagnostic value.

In the patient with polycythemia, cyanosis may be present at a Pao_2 well above 30 mm Hg because the amount of reduced hemoglobin is often greater than 5 g/dL in these patients, even when their total oxygen content is within normal limits. In respiratory disease, cyanosis is the result of (1) a decreased $\dot{V}/\dot{Q}$ ratio, (2) pulmonary shunting, (3) venous admixture, and (4) hypoxemia.

Digital Clubbing

Digital clubbing is sometimes noticed in patients with chronic respiratory disorders. Clubbing is characterized by a bulbous swelling of the terminal phalanges of the fingers and toes. The contour of the nail becomes rounded both longitudinally and transversely, which results in an increase in the angle between the surface of the nail and the terminal phalanx (Figure 2-46).

The specific cause of clubbing is unknown. It is a normal hereditary finding in some families without any known history of cardiopulmonary disease. It is believed that the following factors may be causative: (1) circulating vasodilators, such as bradykinin and the prostaglandins, that are released from normal tissues but are not degraded by the lungs because of intrapulmonary shunting; (2) chronic infection; (3) unspecified toxins; (4) capillary stasis from increased venous backpressure; (5) arterial hypoxemia; and (6) local hypoxia. Successful treatment of the underlying disease may result in resolution of the clubbing and return of the digits to normal.

Peripheral Edema

Bilateral, dependent, pitting edema is commonly seen in patients with congestive heart failure, cor pulmonale, and hepatic cirrhosis. To assess the presence and severity of pitting edema, the health-care practitioner places a finger or fingers over the tibia or medial malleolus (2 to 4 inches above the foot), firmly depresses the skin for 5 seconds, and then releases. Normally, this procedure leaves no indentation, although a pit may be seen if the person has been standing all day or is pregnant. If pitting is present, it is graded on the following subjective scale: 1+ (mild, slight depression) to 4+ (severe, deep depression) (Figure 2-47).

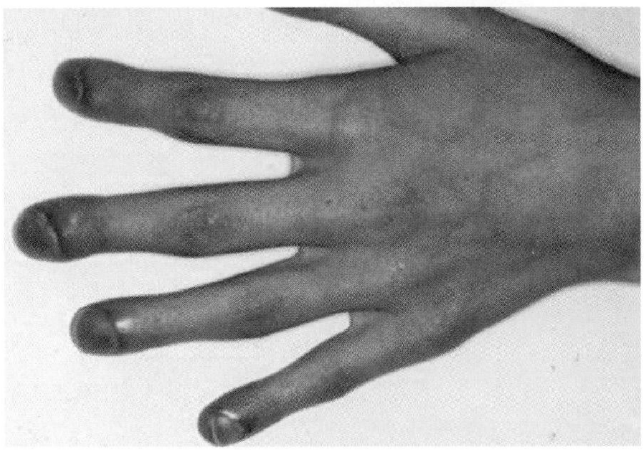

A

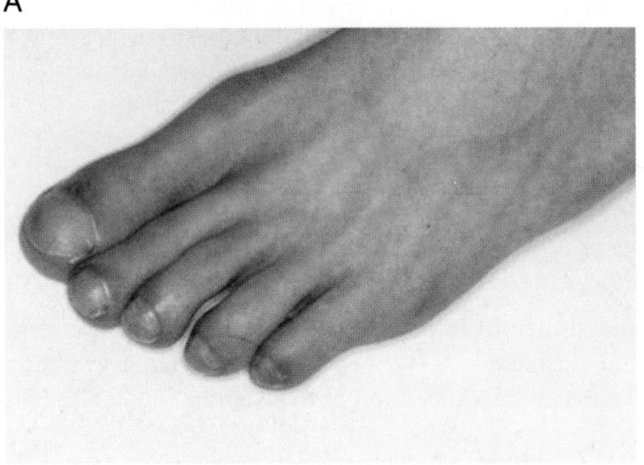

B

FIGURE 2-46 Digital clubbing.

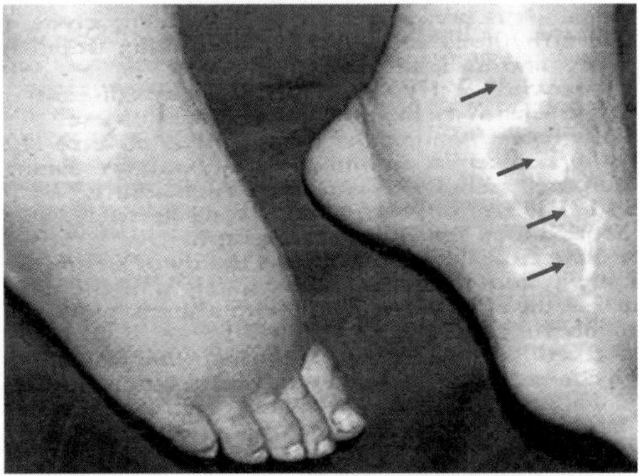

FIGURE 2-47 Pitting edema. (From Bloom A, Ireland J: *Color atlas of diabetes,* ed 2, London, 1992, Mosby-Wolfe.)

Distended Neck Veins

In patients with cor pulmonale, severe flail chest, pneumothorax, or pleural effusion, the major veins of the chest that return blood to the right side of the heart may be compressed. When this happens, venous return decreases and central venous pressure (CVP) increases. This condition is manifested by distended neck veins (also called *jugular venous distention;* Figure 2-48). The reduced venous return also may

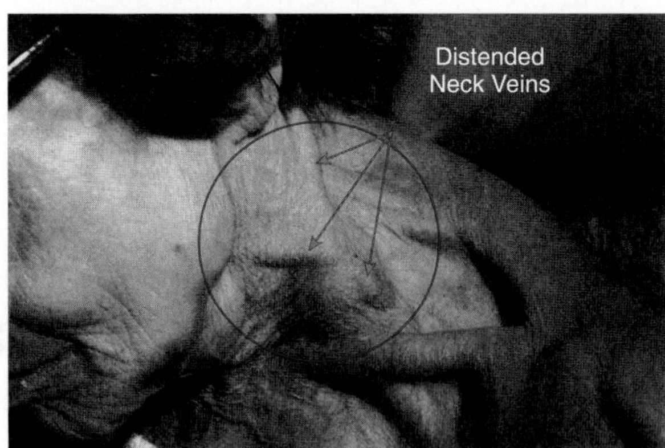

FIGURE 2-48 Distended neck veins *(arrows).*

cause the patient's cardiac output and systemic blood pressure to decrease. In severe cases the veins over the entire upper anterior thorax may be dilated.

Normal and Abnormal Sputum Production

Normal Histology and Mucous Production of the Tracheobronchial Tree

The wall of the tracheobronchial tree is composed of three major layers: an epithelial lining, the lamina propria, and a cartilaginous layer (Figure 2-49).

The epithelial lining, which is separated from the lamina propria by a basement membrane, is predominantly composed of pseudostratified, ciliated, columnar epithelium interspersed with numerous mucus-secreting glands and serous cells. The ciliated cells extend from the beginning of the trachea to—and sometimes including—the respiratory bronchioles. As the tracheobronchial tree becomes progressively smaller, the columnar structure of the ciliated cells gradually decreases in height. In the terminal bronchioles the epithelium appears more cuboidal than columnar. These cells flatten even more in the respiratory bronchioles (see Figure 2-49).

A mucous layer, commonly referred to as the *mucous blanket,* covers the epithelial lining of the tracheobronchial tree (Figure 2-50). The viscosity of the mucous layer progressively increases from the epithelial lining to the inner luminal surface and has two distinct layers: (1) the sol layer, which is adjacent to the epithelial lining, and (2) the gel layer, which is the more viscous layer adjacent to the inner luminal surface. The mucous blanket is 95% water. The remaining 5% consists of glycoproteins, carbohydrates, lipids, DNA, some cellular debris, and foreign particles.

The mucous blanket is produced by the goblet cells and the submucosal, or bronchial, glands. The goblet cells are located intermittently between the pseudostratified, ciliated columnar cells distal to the terminal bronchioles.

Most of the mucous blanket is produced by the submucosal glands, which extend deeply into the lamina propria and are composed of different cell types: serous cells, mucous cells, collecting duct cells, mast cells, myoepithelial cells, and

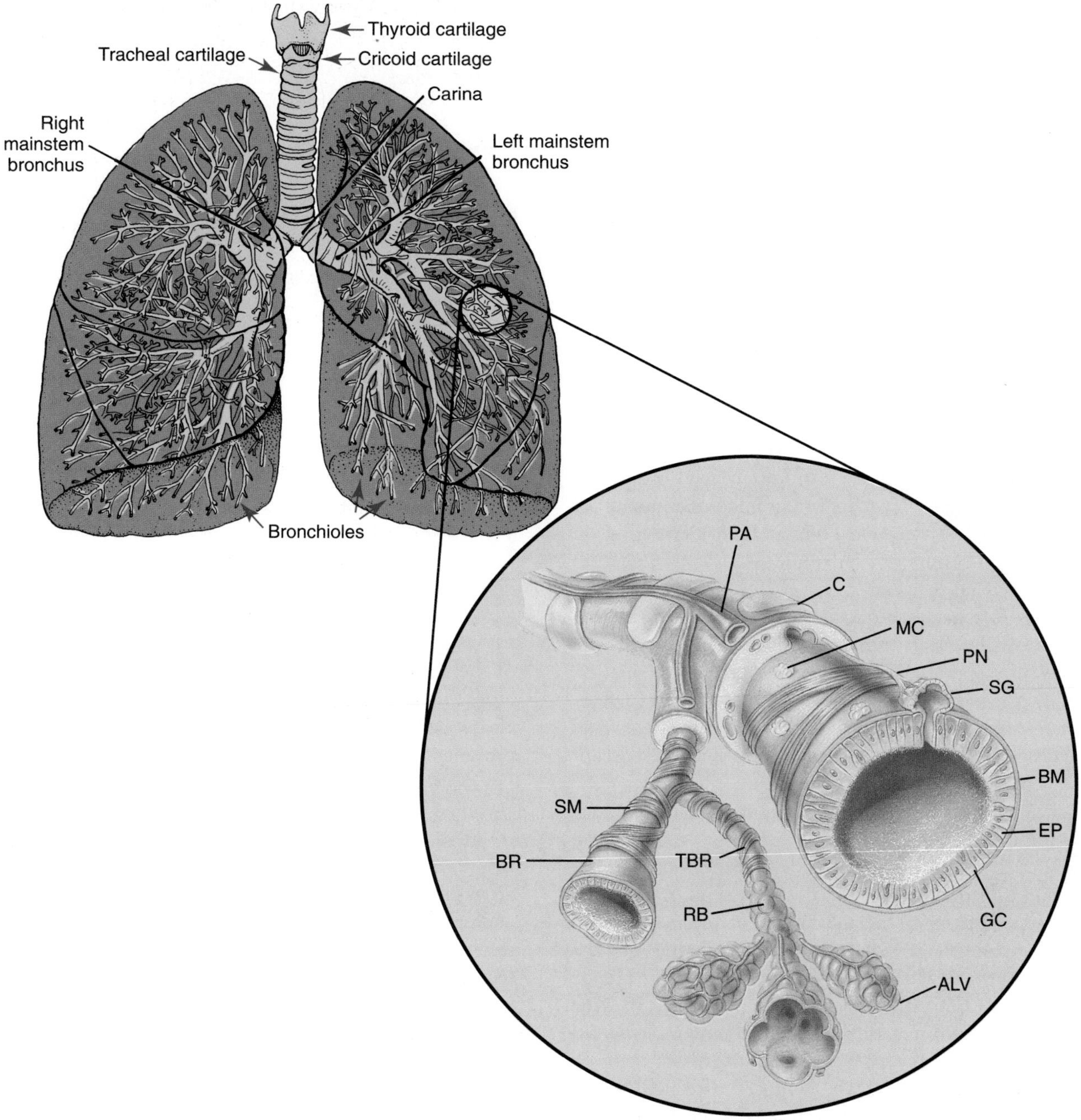

FIGURE 2-49 The normal lung. *ALV,* Alveoli; *BM,* basement membrane; *BR,* bronchioles; *C,* cartilage; *EP,* epithelium; *GC,* goblet cell; *MC,* mast cell; *PA,* pulmonary artery; *PN,* parasympathetic nerve; *RB,* respiratory bronchioles; *SG,* submucosal gland; *SM,* smooth muscle; *TBR,* terminal bronchioles.

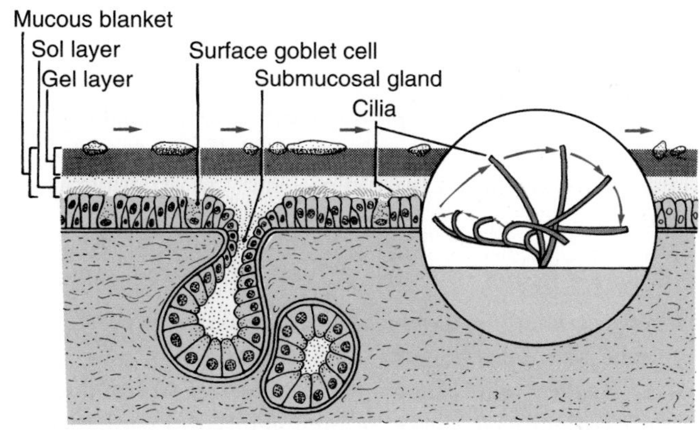

FIGURE 2-50 The epithelial lining of the tracheobronchial tree.

clear cells, which are probably lymphocytes. The submucosal glands are particularly numerous in the medium-sized bronchi and disappear in the bronchioles. These glands are innervated by parasympathetic (cholinergic) nerve fibers and normally produce about 100 mL of clear, thin bronchial secretions per day.

The mucous blanket is an important cleansing mechanism of the tracheobronchial tree. Inhaled particles stick to the mucus. The distal ends of the cilia continually strike the innermost portion of the gel layer and propel the mucous layer, along with any foreign particles, toward the larynx. At this point, the cough mechanism moves secretions beyond the larynx and into the oropharynx. This mucociliary mechanism is commonly referred to as the *mucociliary transport* or the *mucociliary escalator.* The cilia move the mucous blanket at an estimated average rate of 2 cm/min.

The submucosal layer of the tracheobronchial tree is the lamina propria. Within the lamina propria is a loose, fibrous tissue that contains tiny blood vessels, lymphatic vessels, and branches of the vagus nerve. A circular layer of smooth muscle also is found within the lamina propria. It extends from the trachea down to and including the terminal bronchioles.

The cartilaginous structures that surround the tracheobronchial tree progressively diminish in size as the airways extend into the lungs. The cartilaginous layer is completely absent in bronchioles less than 1 mm in diameter (see Figure 2-49).

Abnormal Sputum Production

Excessive sputum production is commonly seen in respiratory diseases that cause an acute or chronic inflammation of the tracheobronchial tree (see Figure 11-1). Depending on the severity and nature of the respiratory disease, sputum production may take several forms. For example, during the early stages of tracheobronchial tree inflammation, the sputum is usually clear, thin, and odorless. As the disease intensifies, the sputum becomes yellow-green and opaque. The yellow-green appearance results from an enzyme (myeloperoxidase) that is released during the cellular breakdown of leukocytes. It may also be caused by retained or stagnant secretions or secretions caused by an acute infection.

Thick and tenacious sputum is commonly seen in patients with chronic bronchitis, bronchiectasis, cystic fibrosis, and asthma. Patients with pulmonary edema expectorate a thin, frothy, pinkish sputum. Technically, this fluid is not true sputum. It results from the movement of plasma and red blood cells across the alveolar-capillary membrane into the alveoli. **Hemoptysis** is the coughing up of blood or blood-tinged sputum from the tracheobronchial tree. In true hemoptysis the sputum is usually bright red and interspersed with air bubbles.

Clinically, hemoptysis may be confused with hematemesis, which is blood that originates from the upper gastrointestinal tract and usually has a dark, coffee-ground appearance. Repeated expectoration of blood-streaked sputum is seen in chronic bronchitis, bronchiectasis, cystic fibrosis, pulmonary embolism, lung cancer, necrotizing infections, tuberculosis, and fungal diseases. A small amount of hemoptysis is common after bronchoscopy, particularly when biopsies are performed. *Massive hemoptysis* is defined as coughing up 400 to 600 mL of blood within a 24-hour period. Death from exsanguination resulting from hemoptysis is rare. Table 2-11 provides a general overview and analysis of the types of sputum commonly seen in the clinical setting.

TABLE 2-11 Analysis of Sputum Color

Color	Indications and Conditions
Brown/dark	Old blood
Bright red (hemoptysis)	Fresh blood (bleeding tumor, tuberculosis)
Clear and translucent	Normal
Copious	Large amount
Frank hemoptysis	Massive amount of blood
Green	Stagnant sputum or gram-negative bacteria
Green and foul smelling	Pseudomonas or anaerobic infection
Mucoid (white/gray)	Asthma, chronic bronchitis
Pink, frothy	Pulmonary edema
Tenacious	Secretions that are sticky or adhesive or otherwise tend to hold together
Viscous	Thick, viscid, sticky, or glutinous
Yellow or opaque	Presence of white blood cells, bacterial infection

Cough

A cough is a sudden, audible expulsion of air from the lungs. It is commonly seen in respiratory disease, especially in disorders that cause inflammation of the tracheobronchial tree. In general, a cough is preceded by (1) a deep inspiration, (2) partial closure of the glottis, and (3) forceful contraction of the accessory muscles of expiration to expel air from the lungs. In essence, a cough is a protective mechanism that clears the lungs, bronchi, or trachea of irritants. A cough also prevents the aspiration of foreign material into the lungs. For example, a cough is a common symptom associated with chronic sinusitis and postnasal drip. The effectiveness of a cough depends largely on (1) the depth of the preceding inspiration and (2) the extent of dynamic compression of the airways.

Although a cough may be voluntary, it is usually a reflex response that arises when an irritant stimulates the irritant receptors (also called *subepithelial mechanoreceptors*). The irritant receptors are located in the pharynx, larynx, trachea, and large bronchi. When stimulated, the irritant receptors send a signal by way of the glossopharyngeal nerve (cranial nerve IX) and vagus nerve (cranial nerve X) to the cough reflex center located in the medulla. The medulla then causes the glottis to close and the accessory muscles of expiration to contract. Box 2-5 lists common factors that stimulate the irritant receptors.

Clinically, a cough is termed *productive* if sputum is produced and *nonproductive* if no sputum is produced.

Nonproductive Cough

Common causes of a nonproductive cough include (1) irritation of the airway, (2) inflammation of the airways, (3) mucous accumulation, (4) tumors, and (5) irritation of the pleura.

Productive Cough

When the cough is productive, the respiratory practitioner should assess the following:

- Is the cough strong or weak? In other words, does the patient have a good or poor ability to mobilize bronchial secretions? A good, strong cough may indicate

Box 2-5 Common Factors that Stimulate the Irritant Receptors

- Inflammation
- Infectious agents
- Excessive secretions
- Noxious gases (e.g., cigarette smoke, chemical inhalation)
- Very hot or very cold air
- A mass of any sort compressing the lungs
- Mechanical stimulation (e.g., endotracheal suctioning, compression of the airways)

only deep breath and cough therapy, whereas an inadequate cough may indicate chest physical therapy or postural drainage.

- A productive cough should be evaluated in terms of its frequency, pitch, and loudness. A brassy cough may indicate a tumor, whereas a barking or hoarse cough indicates croup.
- Finally, the sputum of a productive cough should be monitored and evaluated continuously in terms of amount (teaspoons, tablespoons, cups), consistency (thin, thick, tenacious), odor, and color (see Table 2-11).

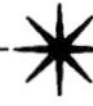

SELF-ASSESSMENT QUESTIONS

evolve Answers to questions can be found on Evolve. To access additional student assessment questions and case studies for application of text material to real-life scenarios, visit **http://evolve.elsevier.com/DesJardins/respiratory**.

1. Which of the following pathologic conditions increases vocal fremitus?
1. Atelectasis
2. Pleural effusion
3. Pneumothorax
4. Pneumonia
   a. 3 only
   b. 4 only
   c. 2 and 3 only
   d. 1 and 4 only

2. A dull or soft percussion note would likely be heard in which of the following pathologic conditions?
1. Chronic obstructive pulmonary disease
2. Pneumothorax
3. Pleural thickening
4. Atelectasis
   a. 1 only
   b. 2 only
   c. 2 and 3 only
   d. 3 and 4 only

3. Bronchial breath sounds are likely to be heard in which of the following pathologic conditions?
1. Alveolar consolidation
2. Chronic obstructive pulmonary disease
3. Atelectasis
4. Fluid accumulation in the tracheobronchial tree
   a. 3 only
   b. 4 only
   c. 1 and 3 only
   d. 2 and 4 only

4. Wheezing is:
1. Produced by bronchospasm
2. Generally auscultated during inspiration
3. A cardinal finding of bronchial asthma
4. Usually heard as high-pitched sounds
   a. 1 only
   b. 1 and 3 only
   c. 2 and 4 only
   d. 1, 3, and 4 only

5. In which of the following pathologic conditions is transmission of the whispered voice of a patient through a stethoscope unusually clear?
1. Chronic obstructive pulmonary disease
2. Alveolar consolidation
3. Atelectasis
4. Pneumothorax
   a. 1 only
   b. 2 and 3 only
   c. 1 and 4 only
   d. 1, 2, and 3 only

6. An individual's ventilatory pattern is composed of which of the following?
1. Inspiratory and expiratory force
2. Ventilatory rate
3. Tidal volume
4. Inspiratory and expiratory ratio
   a. 1 and 3 only
   b. 2 and 3 only
   c. 2, 3, and 4 only
   d. 1, 2, and 3 only

7. Which of the following abnormal breathing patterns is commonly associated with diabetic acidosis?
   a. Orthopnea
   b. Kussmaul's respiration
   c. Biot's respiration
   d. Hypoventilation

8. What is the average compliance of the lungs and chest wall combined?

a. 0.05 L/cm H_2O
b. 0.1 L/cm H_2O
c. 0.2 L/cm H_2O
d. 0.3 L/cm H_2O

9. When lung compliance decreases, which of the following is seen?

1. Ventilatory rate usually decreases.
2. Tidal volume usually decreases.
3. Ventilatory rate usually increases.
4. Tidal volume usually increases.

a. 1 only
b. 2 only
c. 3 and 4 only
d. 2 and 3 only

10. What is the normal airway resistance in the tracheobronchial tree?

a. 0.5 to 1.0 cm H_2O/L/sec
b. 1.0 to 2.0 cm H_2O/L/sec
c. 2.0 to 3.0 cm H_2O/L/sec
d. 3.0 to 4.0 cm H_2O/L/sec

11. What is the normal overall ventilation-perfusion ratio ($\dot{V}/\dot{Q}$ ratio)?

a. 0.2
b. 0.4
c. 0.6
d. 0.8

12. When venous admixture occurs, which of the following occur(s)?

1. The Po_2 of the nonreoxygenated blood increases.
2. The Cao_2 of the reoxygenated blood decreases.
3. The Po_2 of the reoxygenated blood increases.
4. The Cao_2 of the nonreoxygenated blood decreases.

a. 1 only
b. 4 only
c. 2 and 3 only
d. 1 and 2 only

13. The pathophysiology of some respiratory disorders cause relative shunt or a shuntlike effect, whereas some disorders feature a capillary shunt and others a combination of both. Which of the following respiratory diseases causes a shuntlike effect?

1. Pneumonia
2. Asthma
3. Pulmonary edema
4. Adult respiratory distress syndrome

a. 2 only
b. 3 only
c. 1 and 3 only
d. 2, 3, and 4 only

14. What percentage is the normal anatomic shunt?

a. 2 to 5
b. 6 to 8
c. 9 to 10
d. 11 to 15

15. When the systemic blood pressure increases, the aortic and carotid sinus baroreceptors initiate reflexes that cause which of the following?

1. Increased heart rate
2. Decreased ventilatory rate
3. Increased ventilatory rate
4. Decreased heart rate

a. 1 only
b. 2 only
c. 3 only
d. 2 and 4 only

16. What is the anteroposterior-transverse chest diameter ratio in the normal adult?

a. 1 : 0.5
b. 1 : 1
c. 1 : 2
d. 1 : 3
e. 1 : 4

17. Which of the following muscles originate from the clavicle?

1. Scalene muscles
2. Sternocleidomastoid muscles
3. Pectoralis major muscles
4. Trapezius muscles

a. 1 only
b. 2 only
c. 4 only
d. 2 and 3 only

18. Which of the following muscles inserts into the xiphoid process and into the fifth, sixth, and seventh ribs?

a. Rectus abdominis muscle
b. External oblique muscle
c. Internal oblique muscle
d. Transversus abdominis muscle

19. Which of the following is associated with digital clubbing?

1. Chronic infection
2. Local hypoxia
3. Circulating vasodilators
4. Arterial hypoxia

a. 2 only
b. 2 and 4 only
c. 2, 3, and 4 only
d. 1, 2, 3, and 4

20. Which of the following is associated with pleuritic chest pain?

1. Lung cancer
2. Pneumonia
3. Myocardial ischemia
4. Tuberculosis

a. 1 only
b. 2 only
c. 1 and 3 only
d. 1, 2, and 4 only

Pulmonary Function Study Assessments 3

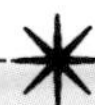

Chapter Objectives

After reading this chapter, you will be able to:

- Describe the following lung volumes and capacities:
  - Tidal volume (V_T)
  - Inspiratory reserve volume (IRV)
  - Expiratory reserve volume (ERV)
  - Residual volume (RV)
  - Vital capacity (VC)
  - Inspiratory capacity (IC)
  - Functional residual capacity (FRC)
  - Total lung capacity (TLC)
  - Residual volume/total lung capacity ratio (RV/TLC)
- List the normal lung volumes and capacities of normal recumbent subjects who are 20 to 30 years of age.
- Identify lung volumes and capacity findings characteristic of restrictive lung disorders.
- Describe the anatomic alterations of the lungs associated with restrictive lung disorders.
- Identify lung volumes and capacity findings characteristic of obstructive lung disorders.
- Describe the anatomic alterations of the lungs associated with obstructive lung disorders.
- List the indirect measurements of the residual volume and lung capacities containing the residual volume.
- Describe expiratory flow rate and volume measurements and their respective normal values:
  - Forced vital capacity (FVC)
  - Forced expiratory volume timed (FEV_T)
  - Forced expiratory volume in 1 second/forced vital capacity ratio (FEV_1/FVC)
  - Forced expiratory flow at 25% to 75% ($FEF_{25\%-75\%}$)
  - Forced expiratory flow at 50% ($FEF_{50\%}$)
  - Forced expiratory flow between 200 and 1200 mL of FVC ($FEF_{200-1200}$)
  - Peak expiratory flow rate (PEFR)
  - Maximum voluntary ventilation (MVV)
  - Flow-volume loop
- Describe how the FVC, FEV_1, and FEV_1/FVC are used to differentiate restrictive and obstructive lung disorders.
- Identify forced expiratory flow rate findings characteristic of restrictive lung disorders.
- Identify forced expiratory flow rate findings characteristic of obstructive lung disorders.
- Describe the pulmonary diffusion capacity (DLCO).
- Identify DLCO findings characteristic of restrictive lung disorders.
- Identify DLCO findings characteristic of obstructive lung disorders.
- Define key terms and complete self-assessment questions at the end of the chapter and on Evolve.

Key Terms

Air Trapping
Body Plethysmography
Closed Circuit Helium Dilution Test
Expiratory Reserve Volume (ERV)
Flow-Volume Loop
Forced Expiratory Flow 200-1200 mL of FVC ($FEF_{200-1200}$)
Forced Expiratory Flow 25%-75% ($FEF_{25\%-75\%}$)
Forced Expiratory Flow at 50% ($FEF_{50\%}$)
Forced Expiratory Volume in 1 second (FEV_1)
Forced Expiratory Volume in 1 second/Forced Vital Capacity Ratio (FEV_1/FVC)
Forced Expiratory Volume in 1 second Percentage ($FEV_{1\%}$)
Forced Expiratory Volume Timed (FEV_T)
Forced Vital Capacity (FVC)
Functional Residual Capacity (FRC)
Inspiratory Capacity (IC)
Inspiratory Reserve Volume (IRV)
Lung Capacities
Lung Volumes
Maximum Voluntary Ventilation (MVV)
Obstructive Lung Disorders
Open Circuit Nitrogen Washout Test
Peak Expiratory Flow Rate (PEFR)
Pulmonary Diffusion Capacity of Carbon Monoxide (DLCO)
Residual Volume (RV)
Residual Volume/Total Lung Capacity Ratio (RV/TLC)
Restrictive Lung Disorders
Tidal Volume (V_T)
Total Expiratory Time (TET)
Total Lung Capacity (TLC)
Vital Capacity (VC)

Chapter Outline

Pulmonary function studies play a major role in the assessment of pulmonary disease. The results of pulmonary function studies are used to (1) evaluate pulmonary causes of dyspnea, (2) differentiate between obstructive and restrictive pulmonary disorders, (3) assess severity of the pathophysiologic impairment, (4) follow the course of a particular disease, (5) evaluate the effectiveness of therapy, and (6) assess the patient's preoperative status. Pulmonary function studies are commonly subdivided into the following three categories: (1) **lung volumes** and **lung capacities, (2) forced expiratory flow rate and volume measurements,** and **(3) pulmonary diffusion capacity measurements**.

Normal Lung Volumes and Capacities

As shown in Table 3-1, gas in the lungs is divided into four lung volumes and four lung capacities. The lung capacities represent different combinations of lung volumes. The amount of air the lungs can accommodate varies with age, weight, height, gender, and, to a much lesser extent, race. Prediction formulas for normal values exist that take these variables into account. Lung volumes and capacities change as a result of pulmonary disorders. These changes are classified as either **restrictive lung disorders** or **obstructive lung disorders.**

Restrictive Lung Disorders: Lung Volume and Capacity Findings

Table 3-2 presents an overview of the lung volume and capacity findings characteristic of restrictive lung disorders. Restrictive lung volumes and capacities are associated with pathologic conditions that alter the anatomic structures of

TABLE 3-2 Restrictive Lung Disorders: Lung Volume and Capacity Findings

V_T	IRV	ERV	RV	
N or ↓	↓	↓	↓	
VC	**IC**	**FRC**	**TLC**	**RV/TLC**
↓	↓	↓	↓	N

N, Normal.

TABLE 3-1 Lung Volumes and Capacities of Normal Recumbent Subjects 20 to 30 Years of Age

	Male (in milliliters)	Female (in milliliters)
Lung Volume Measurements		
Tidal volume (V_T): The volume of gas that normally moves into and out of the lungs in one quiet breath.	500	400-500
Inspiratory reserve volume (IRV): The volume of air that can be forcefully inspired after a normal tidal volume.	3100	1900
Expiratory reserve volume (ERV): The volume of air that can be forcefully exhaled after a normal tidal volume exhalation.	1200	800
Residual Volume (RV): The amount of air remaining in the lungs after a forced exhalation.	1200	1000
Lung Capacity Measurements		
Vital capacity (VC): VC = IRV + V_T + ERV. The volume of air that can be exhaled after a maximal inspiration.	4800	3200
Inspiratory capacity (IC): IC = V_T + IRV. The volume of air that can be inhaled after a normal exhalation.	3600	2400
Functional residual capacity (FRC): FRC = ERV + RV. The lung volume at rest after a normal tidal volume exhalation.	2400	1800
Total lung capacity (TLC): TLC = IC + ERV + RV. The maximal amount of air that the lungs can accommodate.	6000	4200
Residual volume/total lung capacity ratio (RV/TLC × 100): The percentage of TLC occupied by the RV.	$\frac{1200}{6000}$ = 20% (approx)	$\frac{1000}{4200}$ = 25% (approx)

the lungs distal to the terminal bronchioles (i.e., the alveoli or the lung parenchyma). Table 3-3 provides some of the more common restrictive anatomic alterations of the lungs and examples of respiratory disorders that cause them. Restrictive lung disorders result in an increased lung rigidity, which in turn decreases lung compliance. When lung compliance decreases, the ventilatory rate increases and the **tidal volume (V_T)** decreases (see Figure 2-23).

Obstructive Lung Disorders: Lung Volume and Capacity Findings

Table 3-4 provides an overview of the lung volumes and capacity findings characteristic of obstructive lung disorders. These lung volume and capacity findings are associated with pathologic conditions that alter the tracheobronchial tree. Table 3-5 provides some of the more common obstructive anatomic alterations of the lungs and examples of respiratory disorders that cause them.

In obstructive lung disorders, the gas that enters the alveoli during inspiration (when the bronchial airways are naturally wider) is prevented from leaving the alveoli during expiration (when the bronchial airways narrow). As a result, the alveoli become overdistended with gas, a condition known as **air trapping**. Figure 3-1 provides a visual comparison of obstructive and restrictive lung disorders.

TABLE 3-3 Anatomic Alterations of the Lungs Associated with Restrictive Lung Disorders: ***(Pathology of the Alveoli or Lung Parenchyma)***

Pathology (Anatomic Alteration of the Alveoli)	Examples of Respiratory Disorders Associated with Specific Pathology
Atelectasis	Pneumothorax, pleural effusion, flail chest, or mucous plugging
Consolidation	Pneumonia, acute respiratory distress syndrome, lung abscess, tuberculosis
Increased alveolar-capillary membrane thickness	Pulmonary edema, pneumoconiosis, tuberculosis, fungal disease

TABLE 3-4 Obstructive Lung Disorders: ***(Lung Volume and Capacity Findings)***

V_T	IRV	ERV	RV	
N or ↑	N or ↓	N or ↓	↑	
VC	**IC**	**FRC**	**TLC**	**RV/TLC ratio**
↓	N or ↓	↑	N or ↑	N or ↑

N, Normal.

TABLE 3-5 Anatomic Alterations of the Lungs Associated with Obstructive Lung Disorders: ***(Pathology of the Tracheobronchial Tree)***

Pathology (Anatomic Alteration of the Bronchial Airways)	Examples of Respiratory Disorders Associated with Specific Pathology
Excessive mucous production and accumulation	Chronic bronchitis, asthma, respiratory syncytial virus
Bronchospasm	Asthma
Distal airway weakening	Emphysema

Indirect Measurements of the Residual Volume and Lung Capacities Containing the Residual Volume

Because the **residual volume (RV)** cannot be exhaled, the RV and the lung capacities that contain the RV (**functional residual capacity [FRC]** and **total lung capacity [TLC]**) are measured indirectly in the clinical setting by one of the following methods:

- **Closed circuit helium dilution test**
- **Open circuit nitrogen washout test**
- **Body plethysmography**

Forced Expiratory Flow Rate and Volume Measurements

In addition to the volumes and capacities that can be measured by pulmonary function testing, the flow rate and volume at which gas flows out of the lungs also can be measured. Such measurements provide data on the patency of the airways and the severity of the airway impairment.

Forced Vital Capacity

The **forced vital capacity (FVC)** is the total volume of gas that can be exhaled as forcefully and rapidly as possible after a maximal inspiration. In the healthy individual, the **total expiratory time (TET)** necessary to perform a FVC is 4 to 6 seconds. In obstructive lung disease (e.g., chronic bronchitis or emphysema), the TET increases because of the increased airway resistance and air trapping associated with the disorder. TETs of more than 10 seconds have been reported in these patients. In the normal individual the FVC equals the **vital capacity (VC).** Clinically, the lungs are considered normal if the FVC and the VC are within 200 mL of each other. In the patient with obstructive lung disease the FVC is lower than the VC because of increased airway resistance and air trapping with maximal effort (Figure 3-2).

A decreased FVC also is a common clinical manifestation in the patient with a restrictive lung disorder (e.g., pneumonia, acute respiratory distress syndrome, atelectasis). This decrease is mainly a result of the fact that restrictive lung disorders reduce the patient's ability to fully expand the lungs, thus reducing the VC necessary to generate a good FVC exhalation. However, the TET required to perform an FVC exhalation is usually normal or even less than normal because of the high lung elasticity (low lung compliance) associated with restrictive disorders.

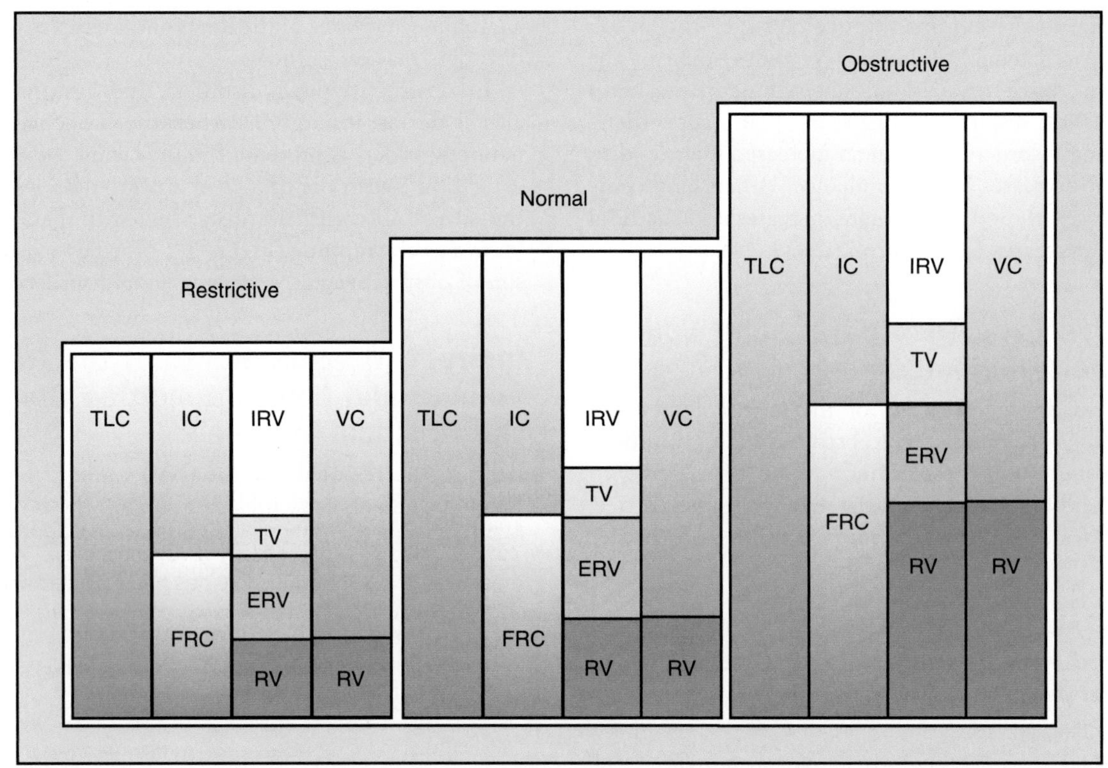

FIGURE 3-1 Visual comparison of lung volumes and capacities in obstructive and restrictive lung disorders. (From Wilkins RL, Stoller JK, Kacmarek RM: *Egan's fundamentals of respiratory care,* ed 9, St Louis, 2009, Elsevier.)

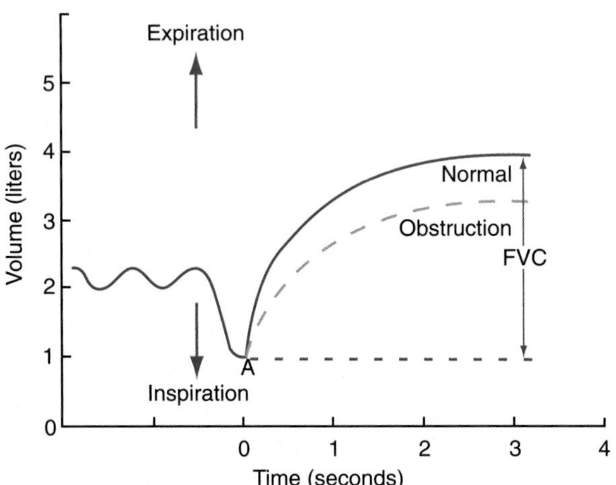

FIGURE 3-2 Forced vital capacity (FVC). A is the point of maximal inspiration and the starting point of an FVC maneuver. Note the reduction in FVC in obstructive pulmonary disease.

A number of pulmonary function tests can be extrapolated from a single FVC maneuver. The most common tests are as follows:

- **Forced expiratory volume timed (FEV_T)**
- **Forced expiratory volume in 1 second/forced vital capacity ratio (FEV_1/FVC)**
- **Forced expiratory flow between 200 and 1200 mL of FVC ($FEF_{200\text{-}1200}$)**
- **Forced expiratory flow at 25% to 75% ($FEF_{25\%\text{-}75\%}$)**
- **Peak expiratory flow rate (PEFR)**

Forced Expiratory Volume Timed

The maximum volume of gas that can be exhaled over a specific period is the **forced expiratory volume timed (FEV_T).** This measurement is obtained from an FVC measurement. Commonly used time periods are 0.5, 1.0, 2.0, 3.0, and 6.0 seconds. The most commonly used time period is 1 second **(forced expiratory volume in 1 second [FEV_1]).** In the normal adult the percentages of the total volume exhaled during these time periods are as follows: $FEV_{0.5}$, 60%; FEV_1, 83%; FEV_2, 94%; and FEV_3, 97%. In obstructive disease the FEV_T is decreased because the time necessary to exhale a certain volume forcefully is increased (Figure 3-3). Although the FEV_T may be normal in restrictive lung disorders (e.g., pneumonia, acute respiratory distress syndrome, atelectasis), it is commonly decreased because of the decreased VC associated with restrictive disorders (similar to the FVC in restrictive disorders). The FEV_T progressively decreases with age.

Forced Expiratory Volume in 1 second/Forced Vital Capacity (FEV_1/FVC) Ratio

The FEV_1/FVC ratio compares the amount of air exhaled in 1 second with the total amount exhaled during an FVC maneuver. Because the FEV_1/FVC ratio is expressed as a percentage, it is commonly referred to as the **forced expiratory volume in 1 second percentage ($FEV_{1\%}$).** Simply stated, the FEV_1/FVC ratio provides the percentage of the patient's total volume of air forcefully exhaled (FVC) in 1 second. As

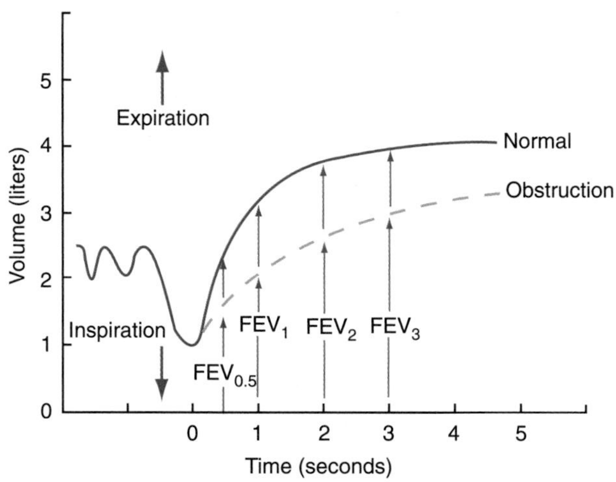

FIGURE 3-3 Forced expiratory volume timed (FEV_T). In obstructive pulmonary disease, more time is needed to exhale a specified volume.

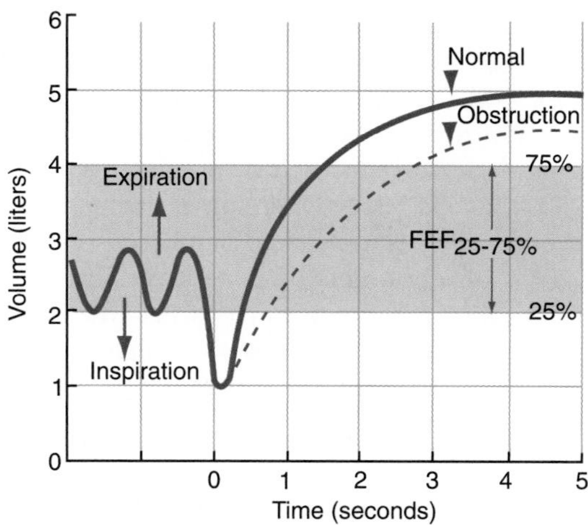

FIGURE 3-4 Forced expiratory flow at 25% to 75% ($FEF_{25\%-75\%}$). This test measures the average rate of flow between 25% and 75% of a forced vital capacity (FVC) maneuver. The flow rate is measured when 25% of the FVC has been exhaled and again when 75% of the FVC has been exhaled. The average rate of flow is derived by dividing the combined flow rates by 2. Note that expiration (in this figure) starts at 1.0 L on the upward axis.

discussed earlier in the FEV_T section, the normal adult exhales 83% or more of the FVC in 1 second (FEV_1). Therefore the FEV_1/FVC ratio should also be 83% or greater under normal circumstances. The $FEV_{1\%}$ progressively decreases with age.

Clinically, the **FVC, FEV_1, and $FEV_{1\%}$** are commonly used to (1) assess the severity of a patient's pulmonary disorder and (2) to determine whether the patient has either an obstructive or a restrictive lung disorder. The primary pulmonary function study differences between an obstructive and a restrictive lung disorder are as follows:

- In an obstructive disorder the FEV_1 and $FEV_{1\%}$ are both decreased.
- In a restrictive disorder the FEV_1 is decreased and the $FEV_{1\%}$ is normal or increased.

Forced Expiratory Flow 25%-75% ($FEF_{25\%-75\%}$)

The **$FEF_{25\%-75\%}$** is the average flow rate generated by the patient during the middle 50% of an FVC measurement (Figure 3-4). This expiratory maneuver is used to evaluate the status of medium-to-small airways in obstructive lung disorders. The normal $FEF_{25\%-75\%}$ in a healthy man 20 to 30 years of age is about 4.5 L/sec (270 L/min). The normal $FEF_{25\%-75\%}$ in a healthy woman 20 to 30 years of age is about 3.5 L/sec (210 L/min). The $FEF_{25\%-75\%}$ is somewhat effort-dependent because it depends on the FVC exhaled.

The $FEF_{25\%-75\%}$ progressively decreases in obstructive diseases and with age. The $FEF_{25\%-75\%}$ may also be decreased in moderate or severe restrictive lung disorders. This decrease is believed to be caused primarily by the reduced cross-sectional area of the small airways associated with restrictive lung problems. Clinically, the $FEF_{25\%-75\%}$ is often used to further confirm—or rule out—the presence of an obstructive pulmonary disease in the patient with a borderline $FEV_{1\%}$ value.

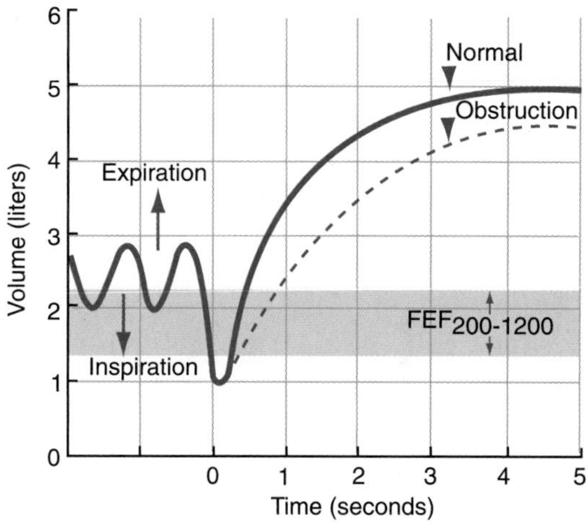

FIGURE 3-5 Forced expiratory flow between 200 and 1200 mL of forced vital capacity (FVC) ($FEF_{200-1200}$). This test measures the average rate of flow between 200 mL and 1200 mL of the FVC. The flow rate is measured when 200 mL have been exhaled and again when 1200 mL have been exhaled. The average rate of flow is derived by dividing the combined flow rates by 2. Note that expiration (in this figure) starts at 1.0 L on the upward axis.

Forced Expiratory Flow 200-1200 ($FEF_{200-1200}$)

The **$FEF_{200-1200}$** measures the average flow rate between 200 and 1200 mL of an FVC (Figure 3-5). The first 200 mL of the FVC is usually exhaled more slowly than at the average flow rate because of (1) the normal inertia involved in the respiratory maneuver and (2) the initial slow response time of the pulmonary function equipment. Because the $FEF_{200-1200}$ measures expiratory flows at high lung volumes (i.e., the initial part of the FVC), it provides a good assessment of the large upper airways. The $FEF_{200-1200}$ is relatively effort-dependent.

The normal $FEF_{200\text{-}1200}$ for the average healthy man 20 to 30 years of age is approximately 8 L/sec (480 L/min). The normal $FEF_{200\text{-}1200}$ in the average healthy woman 20 to 30 years of age is approximately 5.5 L/sec (330 L/min). The $FEF_{200\text{-}1200}$ decreases in obstructive lung disorders. The $FEF_{200\text{-}1200}$ is a good test to determine the patient's response to bronchodilator therapy. In restrictive lung disorders the $FEF_{200\text{-}1200}$ is usually normal because it measures the early expiratory flow rates during the first part of an FVC maneuver (i.e., when the patient's VC is at its highest level). The $FEF_{200\text{-}1200}$ progressively decreases with age.

Peak Expiratory Flow Rate (PEFR)

The **PEFR** (also known as the *peak flow rate*) is the maximum flow rate generated during an FVC maneuver (Figure 3-6). The PEFR provides a good assessment of the large upper airways. It is quite effort-dependent. The normal PEFR in the average healthy man 20 to 30 years of age is approximately 10 L/sec (600 L/min). The normal PEFR in the average healthy woman 20 to 30 years of age is approximately 7.5 L/sec (450 L/min). The PEFR decreases in obstructive lung diseases. In restrictive lung disorders, the PEFR is usually normal because it measures the early expiratory flow rates during the first part of an FVC maneuver (i.e., when the patient's VC is at its highest level). The PEFR progressively decreases with age.

The PEFR also can easily be measured at the patient's bedside with a hand-held peak flowmeter (e.g., Wright peak flowmeter). The hand-held peak flowmeter is used to monitor the degree of airway obstruction on a moment-to-moment basis and is relatively small, inexpensive, accurate, reproducible, and easy for the patient to use. In addition, the mouthpieces are disposable, thus allowing the safe use of the same peak flowmeter from one patient to another. PEFR measurements should routinely be performed at the patient's bedside to assess the degree of bronchospasm, effect of bronchodilators, and day-to-day progress. The PEFR results generated by the patient before and after bronchodilator therapy can serve as excellent objective data by which to assess the effectiveness of therapy.

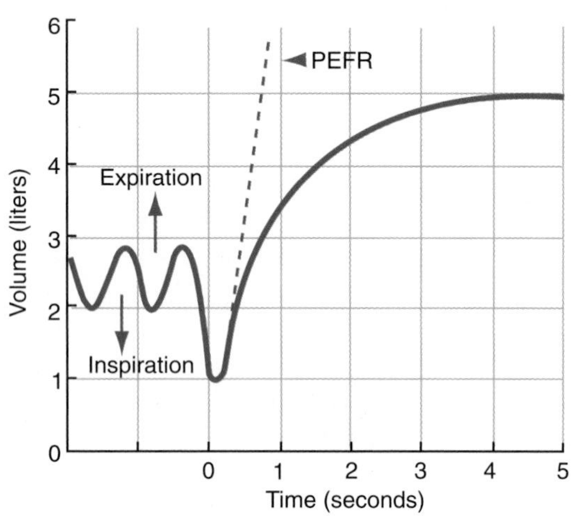

FIGURE 3-6 Peak expiratory flow rate (PEFR). The steepest slope of the $\Delta\dot{V}/\Delta T$ line is the PEFR ($\dot{V}$).

Maximum Voluntary Ventilation (MVV)

The **MVV** is the largest volume of gas that can be breathed voluntarily in and out of the lungs in 1 minute (Figure 3-7). The normal MVV in the average healthy man 20 to 30 years of age is approximately 170 L/min. The normal MVV in the average healthy woman 20 to 30 years of age is approximately 110 L/min. The MVV progressively decreases in obstructive pulmonary disorders. In restrictive pulmonary disorders, the MVV may be normal or decreased.

Flow-Volume Loop

The flow-volume loop is a graphic illustration of both a forced vital capacity (FVC) maneuver and a forced inspiratory volume (FIV) maneuver. The FVC and FIV are plotted

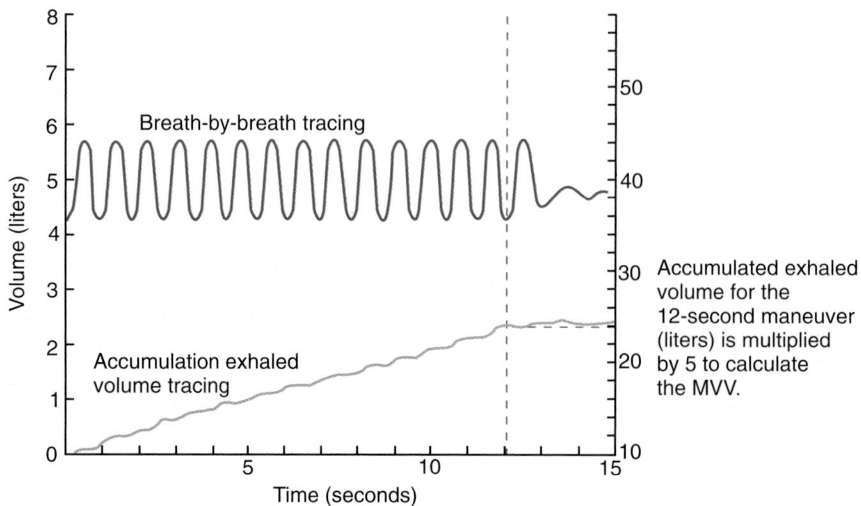

FIGURE 3-7 Volume-time tracing for a maximum voluntary ventilation (MVV) maneuver. Note: the patient actually performs the MVV maneuver for only 12 sec, not 60 sec.

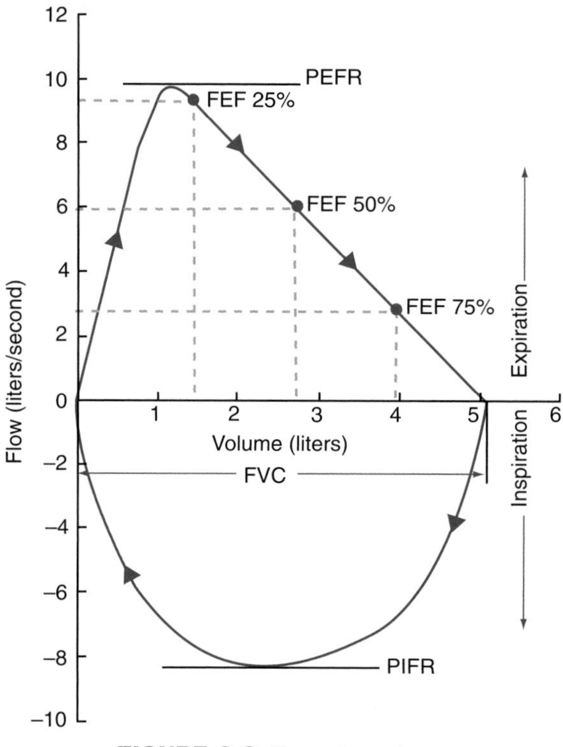

FIGURE 3-8 Flow-volume loop.

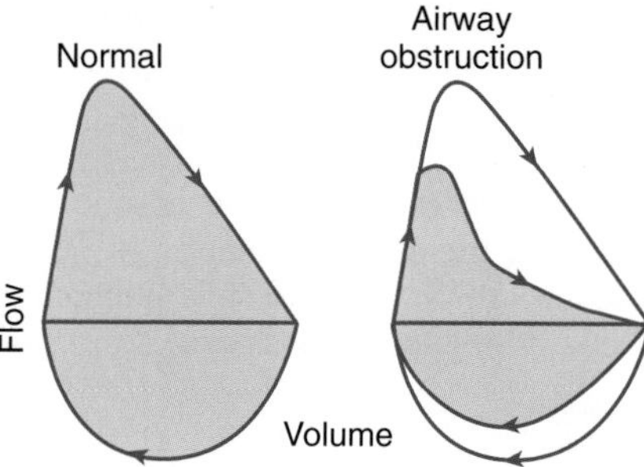

FIGURE 3-9 Flow-volume loop demonstrating the shape change that results from an obstructive lung disorder. The curve on the right represents intrathoracic airway obstruction.

together as two curves that form what is called a **flow-volume loop.** As shown in Figure 3-8, the upper half of the flow-volume loop (above the zero flow axis) represents the maximum expiratory flow generated at various lung volumes during an FVC maneuver plotted against volume. This portion of the curve shows the flow generated between the TLC and RV.

The lower half of the flow-volume loop (below the zero flow axis) illustrates the maximum inspiratory flow generated at various lung volumes during a forced inspiration (called a *forced inspiratory volume [FIV]*) plotted against the volume inhaled. This portion of the curve shows the flow generated between the RV and TLC. Depending on the sophistication of the equipment, several important pulmonary function study measurements can be obtained, including the following:

- FVC
- FEV_T
- $FEF_{25\%-75\%}$
- $FEF_{200-1200}$
- PEFR
- Peak inspiratory flow rate (PIFR)
- **Forced expiratory flow at 50% ($FEF_{50\%}$)**
- Instantaneous flow at any given lung volume during forced inhalation and exhalation

In the normal subject the expiratory flow rate decreases linearly during an FVC maneuver, immediately after the PEFR has been achieved. In the patient with an obstructive lung disease, however, the flow rate decreases in a nonlinear fashion after the PEFR has been reached. This nonlinear flow rate causes a cuplike or scooped-out appearance in the expiratory flow curve when 50% of the FVC has been exhaled. This portion of the flow curve is the $FEF_{50\%}$, or $\dot{V}_{max50}$ (Figure 3-9). Table 3-6 summarizes (1) the forced expiratory flow rate and volume measurements and (2) the normal values found in healthy men and women ages 20 to 30 years.

Table 3-7 provides an overview of the expiratory flow rate measurements characteristic of restrictive lung disorders. In restrictive lung disorders, flow and volume are, in general, reduced equally. Clinically, this phenomenon is referred to as *symmetric reduction* in flows and volumes. The flow-volume loop therefore is a small version of normal in restrictive pulmonary disease (Figure 3-10).

Table 3-8 provides an overview of the expiratory flow rate measurements characteristic of obstructive lung disorders. Obstructive lung disorders cause increased airway resistance (R_{aw}) and airway closure during expiration. When R_{aw} becomes high, the patient's ventilatory rate decreases and the V_T increases. This ventilatory pattern is thought to be an adaptation to reduce the work of breathing (see Figure 2-23).

Pulmonary Diffusion Capacity

The **pulmonary diffusion capacity of carbon monoxide (DLCO)** measures the amount of carbon monoxide (CO) that moves across the alveolar-capillary membrane. When the patient has a normal hemoglobin concentration, pulmonary capillary blood volume, and ventilatory status, the only limiting factor to the diffusion of CO is the alveolar-capillary membrane. Under normal conditions the average DLCO value for the resting man is 25 mL/min/mm Hg (STPD). This value is slightly lower in women, presumably because of their smaller normal lung volumes. Table 3-9 provides a general guide to conditions that alter the patient's DLCO.

TABLE 3-6 Normal Forced Expiratory Flow Rate Measurements in Healthy Men and Women 20 to 30 Years of Age

Forced Expiratory Flow Rate Measurement	Men	Women
Forced vital capacity (FVC). *A* is the point of maximal inspiration and the starting point of an FVC maneuver. Note the reduction in FVC in obstructive pulmonary disease, caused by dynamic compression of the airways. 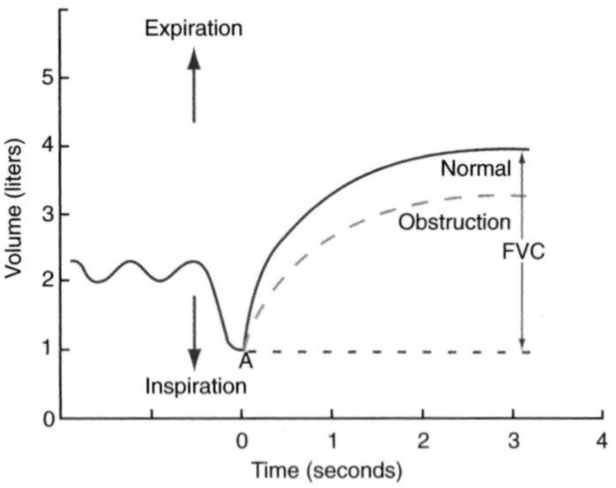	Usually equals vital capacity (VC) (FVC and VC should be within 200 mL of each other)	Usually equals VC (FVC and VC should be within 200 mL of each other)
Forced expiratory volume timed (FEV_T): $FEV_{0.5}$, $FEV_{1.0}$, $FEV_{2.0}$, $FEV_{3.0}$. In obstructive disorders, more time is needed to exhale a specified volume. 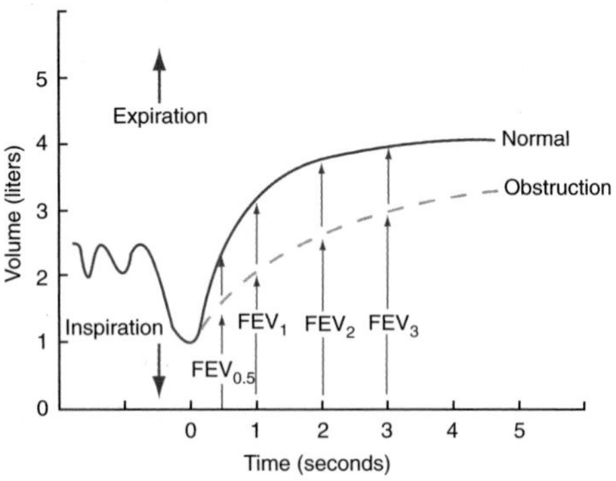	$FEV_{0.5}$: 60% $FEV_{1.0}$: 83% $FEV_{2.0}$: 94% $FEV_{3.0}$: 97%	$FEV_{0.5}$: 60% $FEV_{1.0}$: 83% $FEV_{2.0}$: 94% $FEV_{3.0}$: 97%
Forced expiratory volume in 1 second/forced vital capacity ratio (FEV_1/FVC); commonly called *forced expiratory volume in 1 second percentage* ($FEV_{1\%}$).	Derived by dividing the predicted FEV_1 by the predicted FVC Should be $>$ 70%	Derived by dividing the predicted FEV_1 by the predicted FVC Should be $>$ 70%
Forced expiratory flow 25%-75% ($FEF_{25\%-75\%}$). This test measures the average rate of flow between 25% and 75% of an FVC maneuver. The flow rate is measured when 25% of the FVC has been exhaled and again when 75% of the FVC has been exhaled. The average rate of flow is derived by dividing the combined flow rates by 2. 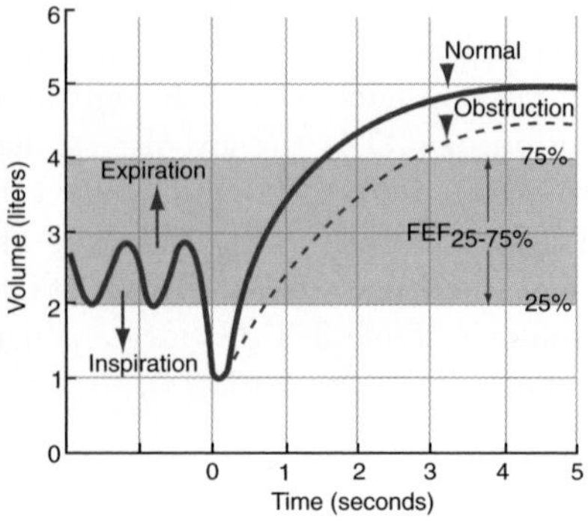	4.5 L/sec (270 L/min)	3.5 L/sec (210 L/min)

TABLE 3-6 Normal Forced Expiratory Flow Rate Measurements in Healthy Men and Women 20 to 30 Years of Age—cont'd

Forced Expiratory Flow Rate Measurement	Men	Women
Forced expiratory flow 200-1200 ($FEF_{200\text{-}1200}$). This test measures the average rate of flow between 200 mL and 1200 mL of an FVC maneuver. The flow rate is measured when 200 mL have been exhaled and again when 1200 mL have been exhaled. The average rate of flow is derived by dividing the combined flow rates by 2. 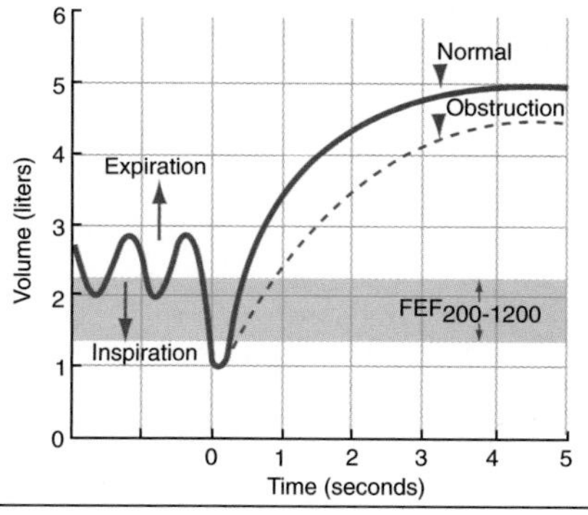	8 L/sec (480 L/min)	5.5 L/sec (330 L/min)
Peak expiratory flow rate (PEFR). The maximum flow rate (steepest slope of the volume-time trace) generated during an FVC maneuver. 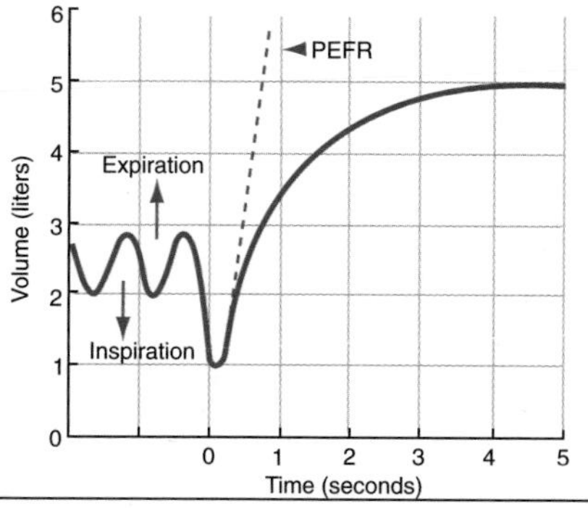	8-10 L/sec (500-600 L/min)	7.5 L/sec (450 L/min)
Maximum voluntary ventilation (MVV). The largest volume of gas that can be breathed voluntarily in and out of the lungs in 1 minute. 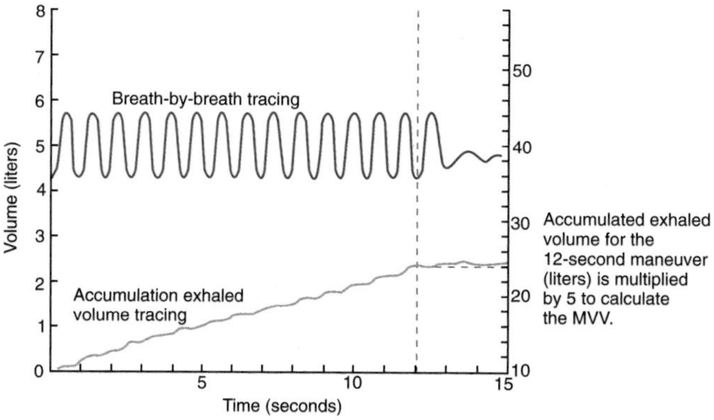	170 L/min	110 L/min

TABLE 3-7 Restrictive Lung Disease: Forced Expiratory Flow Rate and Volume Findings

FVC	FEV_T	FEV_1/FVC	$FEF_{25\%-75\%}$
↓	N or ↓	N or ↑	N or ↓
$FEF_{50\%}$	$FEF_{200-1200}$	PEFR	MVV
N or ↓	N or ↓	N or ↓	N or ↓

TABLE 3-8 Obstructive Lung Diseases: Forced Expiratory Flow Rate and Volume Findings

FVC	FEV_T	FEV_1/FVC	$FEF_{25\%-75\%}$
↓	↓	↓	↓
$FEF_{50\%}$	$FEF_{200-1200}$	PEFR	MVV
↓	↓	↓	↓

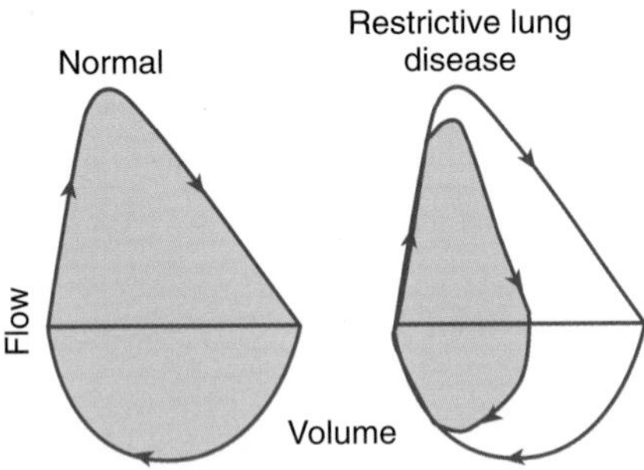

FIGURE 3-10 Flow-volume loop demonstrating the shape change that results from a restrictive lung disorder. Note the symmetric loss of flow and volume.

TABLE 3-9 Pulmonary Diffusion Capacity of Carbon Monoxide (DLCO)

Obstructive Lung Disorders*	Restrictive Lung Disorders†
N or ↓	N or ↓

N, Normal.
*A decreased DLCO is a hallmark clinical manifestation in emphysema (because of the destruction of the alveolar pulmonary capillaries and decreased surface area for gas diffusion associated with the disease). The DLCO is usually normal in all other obstructive lung disorders.
†This is usually decreased when moderate to severe alveolar atelectasis, alveolar consolidation, or increased alveolar-capillary membrane thickness is present in the restrictive lung disorder.

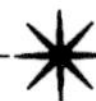

SELF-ASSESSMENT QUESTIONS

evolve Answers to questions can be found on Evolve. To access additional student assessment questions and case studies for application of text material to real-life scenarios, visit **http://evolve.elsevier.com/DesJardins/respiratory.**

1. What is the PEFR in the normal healthy woman 20 to 30 years of age?
   a. 250 L/min
   b. 350 L/min
   c. 450 L/min
   d. 550 L/min

2. A restrictive lung disorder is confirmed when the:
   1. FEV_1 is decreased
   2. FVC is increased
   3. FEV_1/FVC ratio is normal or increased
   4. FEV_1 is increased
      a. 1 only
      b. 4 only
      c. 1 and 3 only
      d. 2 and 4 only

3. Which of the following expiratory maneuver findings are characteristic of restrictive lung disease?
   1. Normal FVC
   2. Decreased $FEF_{25\%-75\%}$
   3. Increased PEFR
   4. Decreased FEV_T
      a. 1 and 3 only
      b. 2 and 4 only
      c. 3 and 4 only
      d. 2 and 3 only

4. In an obstructive lung disorder, which of the following occurs?
   1. FRC is decreased
   2. RV is increased
   3. VC is decreased
   4. IRV is increased
      a. 1 and 3 only
      b. 2 and 3 only
      c. 2 and 4 only
      d. 2, 3, and 4 only

5. Under normal conditions, the average DLCO value for the resting man is which of the following?
   a. 10 mL/min/mm Hg
   b. 15 mL/min/mm Hg
   c. 20 mL/min/mm Hg
   d. 25 mL/min/mm Hg

6. What is the vital capacity of the normal recumbent man 20 to 30 years of age?
   a. 2700 mL
   b. 3200 mL
   c. 4000 mL
   d. 4800 mL

7. What is the normal percentage of the total volume exhaled during an FEV_1?

a. 60%
b. 83%
c. 94%
d. 97%

8. Which of the following can be obtained from a flow-volume loop study?

1. FVC
2. PEFR
3. FEV_T
4. $FEF_{25\%-75\%}$

a. 4 only
b. 1 and 2 only
c. 1, 3, and 4 only
d. 1, 2, 3, and 4

9. An obstructive lung disorder is confirmed when the:

1. FEV_1 is decreased
2. FVC is increased
3. FEV_1 is increased
4. FEV_1/FVC ratio is decreased

a. 3 only
b. 4 only
c. 1 and 3 only
d. 1 and 4 only

10. Which of the following anatomic alterations of the lungs is or are associated with a restrictive lung disorder?

1. Bronchospasm
2. Atelectasis
3. Distal airway weakening
4. Consolidation

a. 1 only
b. 3 only
c. 2 and 4 only
d. 1 and 3 only

Arterial Blood Gas Assessments

4

Chapter Objectives

After reading this chapter, you will be able to:

- Identify the following respiratory acid-base disturbances:
  - Acute alveolar hyperventilation (acute respiratory alkalosis)
  - Acute alveolar hyperventilation with partial renal compensation (partially compensated respiratory alkalosis)
  - Chronic alveolar hyperventilation with complete renal compensation (compensated respiratory alkalosis)
  - Acute ventilatory failure (acute respiratory acidosis)
  - Acute ventilatory failure with partial renal compensation (partially compensated respiratory acidosis)
  - Chronic ventilatory failure with complete renal compensation (compensated respiratory acidosis)
  - Acute alveolar hyperventilation superimposed on chronic ventilatory failure
  - Acute ventilatory failure superimposed on chronic ventilatory failure
- Identify the following metabolic acid-base disturbances:
  - Metabolic acidosis
  - Metabolic acidosis with partial respiratory compensation
  - Metabolic acidosis with complete respiratory compensation
  - Metabolic alkalosis
  - Metabolic alkalosis with partial respiratory compensation
  - Metabolic alkalosis with complete respiratory compensation
- Identify the following combined acid-base disturbances:
  - Combined metabolic and respiratory acidosis
  - Combined metabolic and respiratory alkalosis
- Describe the pH, $Paco_2$, and HCO_3^- relationship, and include the following:
  - How acute Pco_2 increases affect the pH and HCO_3^- values
  - How acute Pco_2 decreases affect the pH and HCO_3^- values
  - The quick clinical calculation commonly used for acute Pco_2 changes on pH and HCO_3^- values
  - The general rule of thumb for the $Paco_2/HCO_3^-/pH$ relationship
- Describe the following six most common acid-base abnormalities seen in the clinical setting:
  - Acute alveolar hyperventilation (acute respiratory alkalosis)
  - Acute ventilatory failure (acute respiratory acidosis)
  - Chronic ventilatory failure (compensated respiratory acidosis)
  - Acute alveolar hyperventilation superimposed on chronic ventilatory failure
  - Acute ventilatory failure superimposed on chronic ventilatory failure
  - Lactic acidosis (metabolic acidosis)
- Describe the metabolic acid-base abnormalities including metabolic acidosis, anion gap, and metabolic alkalosis.
- List the causes of metabolic acidosis and metabolic alkalosis.
- Describe the potential hazards of oxygen therapy in patients with chronic ventilatory failure with hypoxemia.
- Define key terms and complete self-assessment questions at the end of the chapter and on Evolve.

Key Terms

Acute Alveolar Hyperventilation
Acute Alveolar Hyperventilation with Partial Renal Compensation
Acute Alveolar Hyperventilation Superimposed on Chronic Ventilatory Failure
Acute Respiratory Acidosis
Acute Respiratory Alkalosis
Acute Ventilatory Failure
Acute Ventilatory Failure with Partial Renal Compensation
Acute Ventilatory Failure Superimposed on Chronic Ventilatory Failure
Anaerobic Metabolism
Anion Gap
Chronic Alveolar Hyperventilation with Complete Renal Compensation
Chronic Ventilatory Failure
Chronic Ventilatory Failure with Complete Renal Compensation
Combined Metabolic and Respiratory Acidosis
Combined Metabolic and Respiratory Alkalosis
Compensated Respiratory Acidosis
Compensated Respiratory Alkalosis
Hyperchloremic Metabolic Acidosis
Hypoxemia
Lactic Acidosis
Law of Electroneutrality
Metabolic Acidosis
Metabolic Acidosis with Complete Respiratory Compensation
Metabolic Acidosis with Partial Respiratory Compensation
Metabolic Alkalosis
Metabolic Alkalosis with Complete Respiratory Compensation

Metabolic Alkalosis with Partial Respiratory Compensation
Partially Compensated Respiratory Acidosis
Partially Compensated Respiratory Alkalosis
$Pco_2/HCO_3^-/pH$ nomogram
$Pco_2/HCO_3^-/pH$ relationship

Chapter Outline

Acid-Base Abnormalities

As the pathologic processes of a respiratory disorder intensify, the patient's arterial blood gas (ABG) values are usually altered to some degree. Table 4-1 lists the normal ABG values. Box 4-1 provides an overview of the respiratory and metabolic acid-base disturbances. In the profession of respiratory care, a basic knowledge and understanding of the acid-base disturbances is an absolute—and unconditional—prerequisite to the assessment and treatment of the patient with a respiratory disorder. Because of the fundamental importance of this subject, this chapter provides the following review:

- **The $Pco_2/HCO_3^-/pH$ relationship—an essential cornerstone of ABG interpretations**
- **The six most common acid-base abnormalities seen in the clinical setting**
- **The metabolic acid-base abnormalities**
- **The hazards of oxygen therapy in patients with chronic ventilatory failure with hypoxemia**

The $Pco_2/HCO_3^-/pH$ Relationship

To fully understand the clinical significance of the acid-base disturbances listed in Box 4-1, a fundamental knowledge base of the $Pco_2/HCO_3^-/pH$ relationship is essential. The $Pco_2/HCO_3^-/pH$ relationship is graphically illustrated in the **$Pco_2/HCO_3^-/pH$ nomogram** shown in Figure 4-1.*

*The $PCO_2/HCO_3^-/pH$ nomogram is an excellent clinical tool to identify acid-base disturbances. See Appendix xiv for a pocket-size $Pco_2/HCO_3^-/pH$ nomogram card that can be cut out, laminated, and used as a handy arterial blood gas reference tool in the clinical setting.

TABLE 4-1 Normal Blood Gas Values

Blood Gas Value*	Arterial	Venous
pH	7.35 to 7.45	7.30 to 7.40
Pco_2	35 to 45 mm Hg	42 to 48 mm Hg
HCO_3^-	22 to 28 mEq/L	24 to 30 mEq/L
Po_2	80 to 100 mm Hg	35 to 45 mm Hg

*Technically, only the oxygen (Po_2) and carbon dioxide (Pco_2) pressure readings are true blood gas values. The pH indicates the balance between the bases and acids in the blood. The bicarbonate (HCO_3^-) reading is an indirect measurement that is calculated from the pH and Pco_2 levels.

How to Read the $Pco_2/HCO_3^-/pH$ Nomogram

The thick red bar moving from left to right across the **$Pco_2/HCO_3^-/pH$ nomogram** represents the normal Pco_2 blood buffer line. This red bar is used to identify the pH and HCO_3^- changes that occur immediately in response to an **acute increase or decrease in Pco_2**. The purple bar is used to identify the pH and HCO_3^- changes that occur in response to acute **metabolic acidosis** and **metabolic alkalosis** conditions. The colored areas that surround the red and purple

Box 4-1 Acid-Base Disturbance Classifications

Respiratory Acid-Base Disturbances
- Acute alveolar hyperventilation (acute respiratory alkalosis)
- Acute alveolar hyperventilation with partial renal compensation (partially compensated respiratory alkalosis)
- Chronic alveolar hyperventilation with complete renal compensation (compensated respiratory alkalosis)
- Acute ventilatory failure (acute respiratory acidosis)
- Acute ventilatory failure with partial renal compensation (partially compensated respiratory acidosis)
- Chronic ventilatory failure with complete renal compensation (compensated respiratory acidosis)
  - Acute alveolar hyperventilation superimposed on chronic ventilatory failure
  - Acute ventilatory failure superimposed on chronic ventilatory failure

Metabolic Acid-Base Disturbances
- Metabolic acidosis
- Metabolic acidosis with partial respiratory compensation
- Metabolic acidosis with complete respiratory compensation
- Metabolic alkalosis
- Metabolic alkalosis with partial respiratory compensation
- Metabolic alkalosis with complete respiratory compensation

Combined Acid-Base Disturbances
- Combined metabolic and respiratory acidosis
- Combined metabolic and respiratory alkalosis

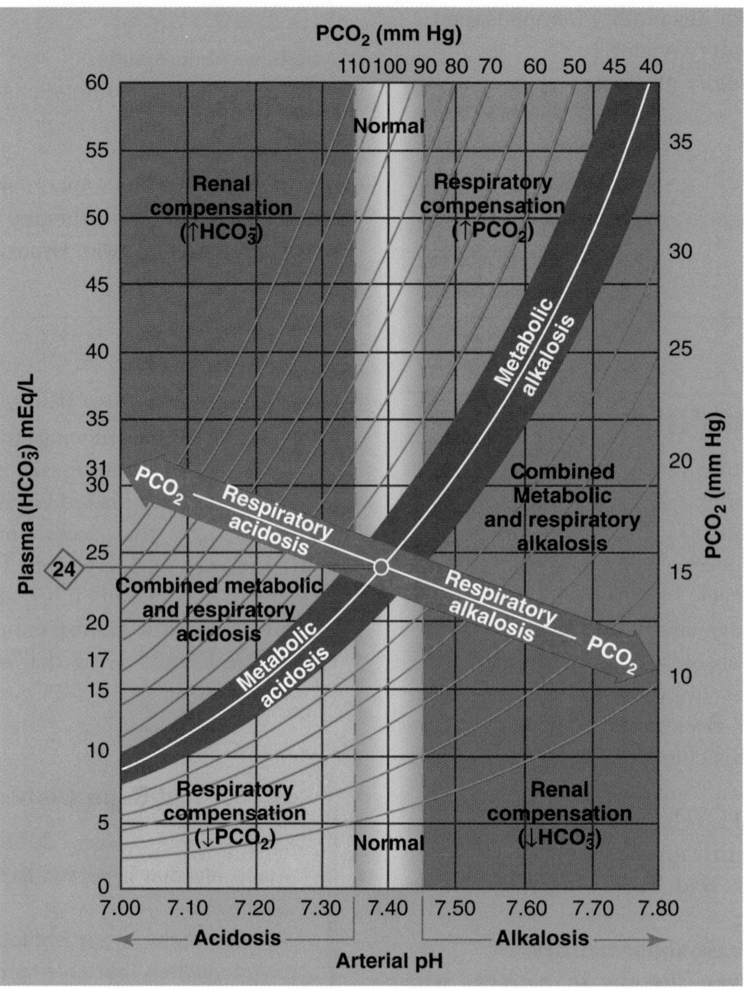

FIGURE 4-1 Nomogram of $Pco_2/HCO_3^-/pH$ relationship. For explanation see text. (Used with permission from author, Terry DesJardins.)

bars are used to identify (1) partial and complete renal compensation, (2) partial and complete respiratory compensation, and (3) combined metabolic and respiratory acid-base disturbances (see Figure 4-1).

For example, when the pH, Pco_2, and HCO_3^- values all intersect in the light purple area—shown in the upper left hand corner of the $Pco_2/HCO_3^-/pH$ nomogram—partial renal compensation has occurred in response to a chronically high Pco_2 level. When the HCO_3^- increases enough to move the pH into the light-blue normal bar, complete renal compensation is confirmed. When the pH, Pco_2, and HCO_3^- values all intersect in the in the green area—shown in the lower right hand corner of the $Pco_2/HCO_3^-/pH$ nomogram—partial renal compensation has occurred in response to a chronically low Pco_2 level. When the HCO_3^- decreases enough to move the pH into the light-blue normal bar, complete renal compensation is confirmed.

When the pH, Pco_2, and HCO_3^- values all intersect in the in the orange area—shown immediately below the red bar on the left side of the $Pco_2/HCO_3^-/pH$ nomogram—a combined respiratory and metabolic acidosis is confirmed. When the pH, Pco_2, and HCO_3^- values all intersect in the in the blue area—shown immediately above the red bar on the right side of the $Pco_2/HCO_3^-/pH$ nomogram—a combined respiratory and **metabolic alkalosis** is confirmed.

Finally, when the pH, Pco_2, and HCO_3^- values all intersect in the yellow area—shown in the lower left corner of the $Pco_2/HCO_3^-/pH$ nomogram—respiratory compensation has occurred in response to metabolic acidosis. When the pH, Pco_2, and HCO_3^- values all intersect in the pink area—shown in the upper right corner of the $Pco_2/HCO_3^-/pH$ nomogram—respiratory compensation has occurred in response to metabolic alkalosis.

Although it is beyond the scope of this textbook to fully explain how each of the acid-base disturbances listed in Box 4-1 can be identified on the $Pco_2/HCO_3^-/pH$ nomogram, a basic understanding of the following two most commonly encountered $Pco_2/HCO_3^-/pH$ relationships is important: (1) an acute Pco_2 increase and its effects on the pH and HCO_3^- values, and (2) an acute Pco_2 decrease and its effects on the pH and HCO_3^- values.*

How Acute Pco_2 Increases Affect the pH and HCO_3^- Values

As mentioned previously, the red normal Pco_2 blood buffer bar shown on the $Pco_2/HCO_3^-/pH$ nomogram is used to

*For a complete review of the role of the $PCO_2/HCO_3^-/pH$ relationship in acid-base balance, see Des Jardins T: *Cardiopulmonary anatomy and physiology: essentials of respiratory care,* ed 5, 2008, Delmar/Cengage Learning.

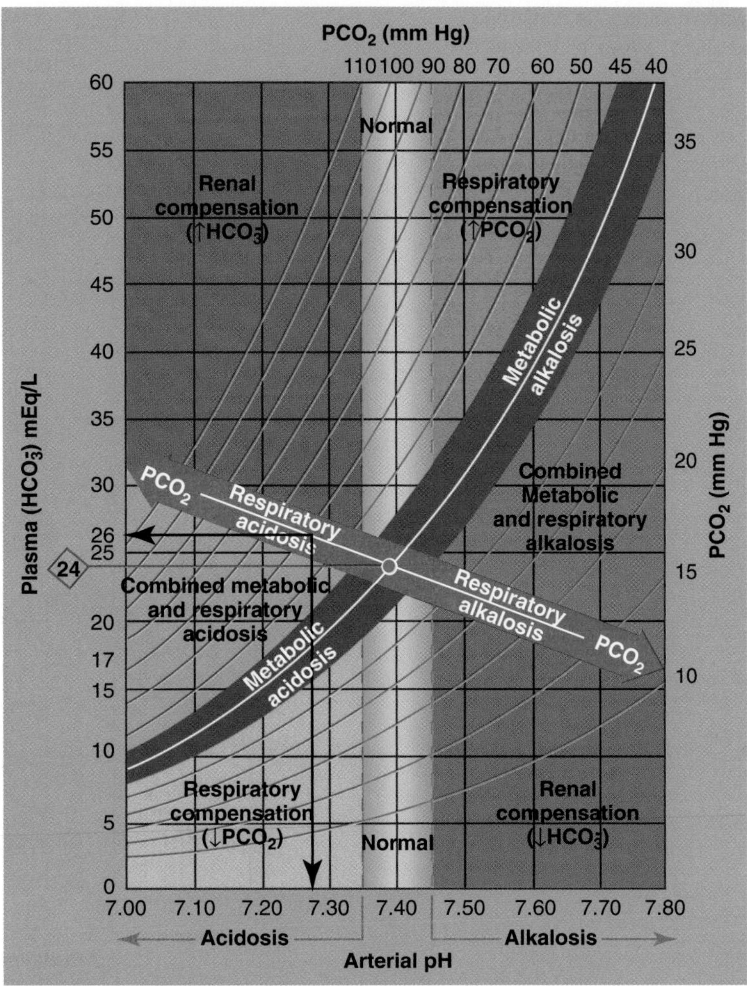

FIGURE 4-2 Acute ventilatory failure is confirmed when the reported Pco_2, pH, and HCO_3^- values all intersect within the red-colored respiratory acidosis bar to the left of the light blue, vertical bar labeled "normal". For example, when the Pco_2 is 60 mm Hg at a time when the pH is 7.28 and the HCO_3^- is 26 mEq/L, acute ventilatory failure is confirmed. (Used with permission from author, Terry DesJardins.)

identify the pH and HCO_3^- values that will result immediately in response to a sudden increase in Pco_2. For example, if the patient's $Paco_2$ were to suddenly increase to, say, 60 mm Hg, the pH would immediately fall to about 7.28 and the HCO_3^- level would increase to about 26 mEq/L. Furthermore, the $Pco_2/HCO_3^-/pH$ nomogram shows that these ABG values represent **acute ventilatory failure (acute respiratory acidosis).** This is because (1) all of the ABG values (i.e., Pco_2, HCO_3^-, and pH) intersect within the red normal Pco_2 blood buffer bar, and (2) the pH and HCO_3^- readings are precisely what is expected for an acute increase in the Pco_2 of 60 mm Hg (Figure 4-2).

How Acute Pco_2 Decreases Affect the pH and HCO_3^- Values

On the other hand, the red normal Pco_2 blood buffer bar shown on the $Pco_2/HCO_3^-/pH$ nomogram is also used to identify the pH and HCO_3^- values that will result immediately in response to a sudden decrease in Pco_2. For example, if the patient's $Paco_2$ were suddenly to decrease to, say, 25 mm Hg, the pH would immediately increase to about 7.55 and the HCO_3^- level would decrease to about 21 mEq/L. In addition, the $Pco_2/HCO_3^-/pH$ nomogram shows that these ABG values represent **acute alveolar hyperventilation (acute respiratory alkalosis).** This is because (1) all of the ABG values (i.e., Pco_2, HCO_3^-, and pH) intersect within the red normal Pco_2 blood buffer bar, and (2) the pH and HCO_3^- readings are precisely what is expected for an acute increase in the Pco_2 of 25 mm Hg (Figure 4-3).

A Quick Clinical Calculation for the Effect of Acute $Paco_2$ Changes on pH and HCO_3^-

In addition to using the graphic $Pco_2/HCO_3^-/pH$ nomogram (see Figure 4-1), the following simple calculations can also be used to estimate the expected pH and HCO_3^- value changes that will immediately occur in response to a sudden increase or decrease in $Paco_2$.

Acute increases in $Paco_2$ (e.g., acute hypoventilation). Using the normal ABG values as a baseline (i.e., pH 7.40, $Paco_2$ 40 mm Hg, and HCO_3^- 24 mEq/L), for every 10 mm Hg the $Paco_2$ increases, the pH will decrease about 0.06 units (from 7.4) and the HCO_3^- will increase about 1 mEq/L (from 24). Or, by way of another example, for every 20 mm Hg the $Paco_2$ increases, the pH will decrease about 0.12 units (from 7.4), and the HCO_3^- will increase about

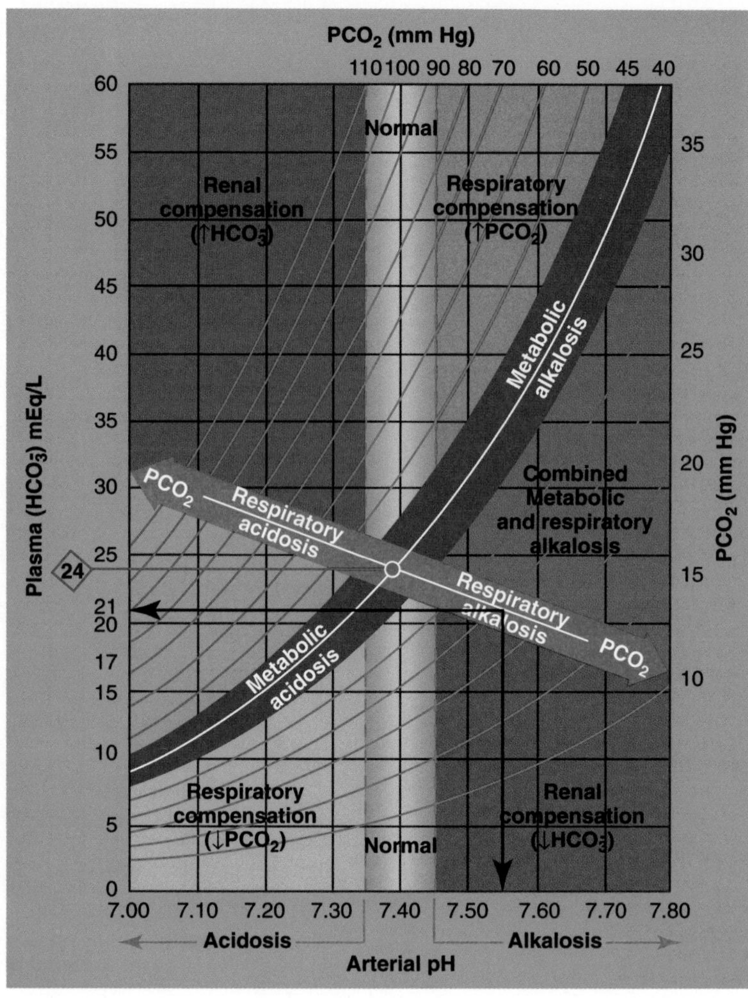

FIGURE 4-3 Acute alveolar hyperventilation is confirmed when the reported P_{CO_2}, pH, and HCO_3^- values all intersect within the red-colored "Respiratory alkalosis" bar. For example, when the reported P_{CO_2} is 25 mm Hg at a time when the pH is 7.55 and the HCO_3^- is 21 mEq/L, acute alveolar hyperventilation is confirmed. (Used with permission from author, Terry DesJardins.)

2 mEq/L (from 24). Thus, if the patient's Pa_{CO_2} suddenly increases to, say, 60 mm Hg, the expected pH change would be about 7.28 and the HCO_3^- would be about 26 mEq/L.

It should be noted, however, that if the patient's Pa_{O_2} is severely low, lactic acid may also be present; resulting in **a combined metabolic and respiratory acidosis.** In such cases, the patient's pH and HCO_3^- values would both be lower than expected for a particular Pa_{CO_2} level.

Acute decreases in Pa_{CO_2} (e.g., acute hyperventilation). Using the normal ABG values as a baseline (i.e., pH 7.40, Pa_{CO_2} 40 mm Hg, and HCO_3^- 24 mEq/L), for every 5 mm Hg the Pa_{CO_2} decreases, the pH will increase about 0.06 unit (from 7.4), and the HCO_3^- will decrease about 1 mEq/L. Or, by way of another example, for every 10 mm Hg the Pa_{CO_2} decreases, the pH will increase about 0.12 units (from 7.4), and the HCO_3^- will decrease about 2 mEq/L. Thus, if a patient's Pa_{CO_2} suddenly decreases to, say, 30 mm Hg, the expected pH change would be around 7.52 and the HCO_3^- would be about 22 mEq/L.

Again, it should be noted that if the patient's Pa_{O_2} is also very low, lactic acid may also be present. In such cases, the patient's pH and HCO_3^- values would both be lower than expected for a particular Pa_{CO_2} level.

Using these calculations, Table 4-2 provides a general rule of thumb for the expected pH and HCO_3^- changes that occur in response to an acute increase or decrease in the P_{CO_2} level.

TABLE 4-2 General Rule of Thumb for the Pa_{CO_2}/HCO_3^-/pH Relationship

pH (Approximate)	Pa_{CO_2} (Approximate)	HCO_3^- mEq/L (Approximate)
7.55	25	21
7.50	30	22
7.45	35	23
7.40	**40**	**24**
7.35	50	25
7.30	60	26
7.25	70	27

The Six Most Common Acid-Base Abnormalities Seen in the Clinical Setting

The most common acid-base abnormalities associated with the respiratory disorders presented in this textbook are (1) **acute alveolar hyperventilation** (acute respiratory alkalosis),

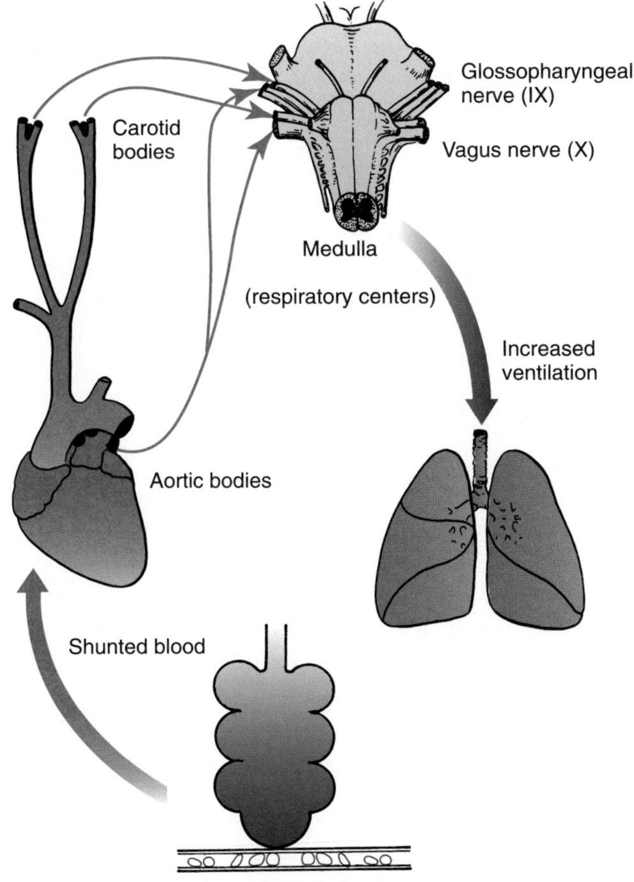

FIGURE 4-4 Relationship of venous admixture to the stimulation of peripheral chemoreceptors in response to alveolar consolidation.

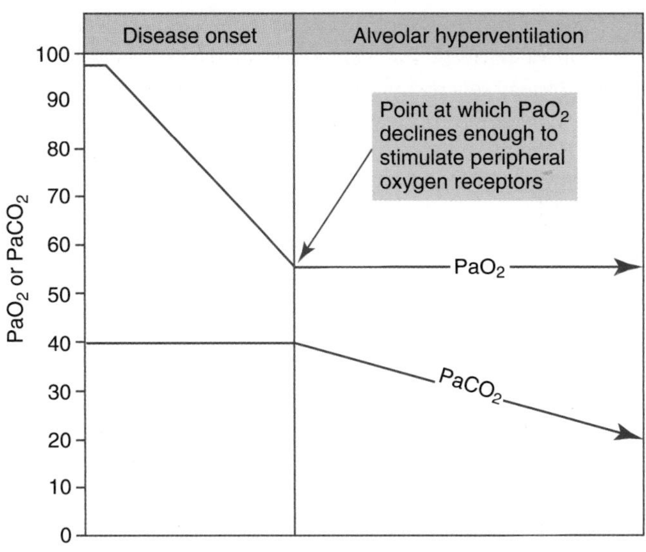

FIGURE 4-5 Pao_2 and $Paco_2$ trends during acute alveolar hyperventilation.

(2) **acute ventilatory failure** (acute respiratory acidosis), (3) **chronic ventilatory failure** (compensated respiratory acidosis), (4) **acute alveolar hyperventilation superimposed on chronic ventilatory failure,** (5) **acute ventilatory failure superimposed on chronic ventilatory failure,** and (6) **lactic acidosis** (metabolic acidosis).

Acute Alveolar Hyperventilation (Acute Respiratory Alkalosis)

ABG Changes	Example
pH: increased	7.55
$Paco_2$: decreased	29 mm Hg
HCO_3^-: decreased	22 mEq/L
Pao_2: decreased	61 mm Hg (when pulmonary pathology is present)

The most common cause of **acute alveolar hyperventilation** is hypoxemia. The decreased Pao_2 seen during acute alveolar hyperventilation usually develops from the decreased ventilation-perfusion ratio ($\dot{V}/\dot{Q}$ ratio), capillary shunting (or a relative shunt or shuntlike effect), and venous admixture associated with the pulmonary disorder. The Pao_2 continues to drop as the pathologic effects of the disease intensify.

Box 4-2 Pathophysiologic Mechanisms That Lead to a Reduction in the $Paco_2$

- Decreased lung compliance
- Stimulation of the central chemoreceptors
- Activation of the deflation reflex
- Activation of the irritant reflex
- Stimulation of the J receptors
- Pain and anxiety

Eventually the Pao_2 may decline to a point sufficiently low (a Pao_2 of about 60 mm Hg) to stimulate the peripheral chemoreceptors, which in turn causes the ventilatory rate to increase (Figure 4-4). The increased ventilatory response in turn causes the $Paco_2$ to decrease and the pH to increase (Figure 4-5). Box 4-2 lists additional pathophysiologic mechanisms in respiratory disorders that can contribute to an increased ventilatory rate and a reduction in the $Paco_2$.

Acute Ventilatory Failure (Acute Respiratory Acidosis)

ABG Changes	Example
pH: decreased	7.21
$Paco_2$: increased	79 mm Hg
HCO_3^-: increased (slightly)	28 mEq/L
Pao_2: decreased	57 mm Hg

Acute ventilatory failure is a condition in which the lungs are unable to meet the metabolic demands of the body in terms of CO_2 homeostasis. In other words, the patient is unable to provide the muscular, mechanical work necessary to move gas into and out of the lungs to meet the normal CO_2 production of the body. This condition leads to an increased P_{ACO_2} and decreased P_{AO_2} and, subsequently, to an increased $Paco_2$ and decreased Pao_2 in the arterial blood.

Acute ventilatory failure is not associated with a typical ventilatory pattern. For example, the patient may demonstrate apnea, severe hyperpnea, or tachypnea. The bottom line is that acute ventilatory failure can develop in response to any ventilatory pattern that does not provide adequate *alveolar* ventilation. When an increased Pa_{CO_2} is accompanied by acidemia (decreased pH), then acute ventilatory failure, or respiratory acidosis, is said to exist. Clinically, this is a medical emergency that requires mechanical ventilation.

Chronic Ventilatory Failure (Compensated Respiratory Acidosis)

ABG Changes	Example
pH: normal	7.38
Pa_{CO_2}: increased	66 mm Hg
HCO_3^-: increased (significantly)	35 mEq/L
Pa_{O_2}: decreased	63 mm Hg

Chronic ventilatory failure is defined as a greater-than-normal Pa_{CO_2} level with a normal pH status. Although chronic ventilatory failure is most commonly seen in patients with severe chronic obstructive pulmonary disease, it is also seen in several chronic restrictive lung disorders (e.g., severe tuberculosis, kyphoscoliosis). Box 4-3 lists common respiratory diseases associated with chronic ventilatory failure during the advanced stages of the disorder.

The basic pathophysiologic mechanisms that produce ABGs associated with chronic ventilatory failure are these: As a respiratory disorder gradually worsens, the work of breathing progressively increases to a point at which more oxygen is consumed than is gained. Although the exact mechanism is unclear, the patient slowly develops a breathing pattern that uses the least amount of oxygen for the energy expended. In essence, the patient selects a breathing pattern based on *work efficiency* rather than *ventilatory efficiency*.* As a result, the patient's alveolar ventilation slowly decreases, which in turn causes the Pa_{O_2} to decrease and the Pa_{CO_2} to increase further (Figure 4-6). As the Pa_{CO_2} increases, the pH falls.

When an individual hypoventilates for a long period of time, the kidneys work to correct the decreased pH by retaining HCO_3^- in the blood. Renal compensation in the presence of chronic hypoventilation can be shown when the calculated HCO_3^- and pH readings are higher than expected for a particular P_{CO_2} level. For example, in terms of the absolute $P_{CO_2}/HCO_3^-/pH$ relationship, when the P_{CO_2} level is about 70 mm Hg, the HCO_3^- level should be about 27 mEq/L and the pH should be about 7.22, according to the normal blood buffer line (see Figure 4-2).

*See the discussion of airway resistance and its effect on the ventilatory pattern in Chapter 2.

Box 4-3 Respiratory Diseases Associated with Chronic Ventilatory Failure during the Advanced Stages

Chronic Obstructive Pulmonary Disorders (Most Common)

- Chronic bronchitis
- Emphysema
- Bronchiectasis
- Cystic fibrosis

Restrictive Respiratory Disorders

- Tuberculosis
- Fungal diseases
- Kyphoscoliosis
- Chronic interstitial lung diseases
- Bronchopulmonary dysplasia

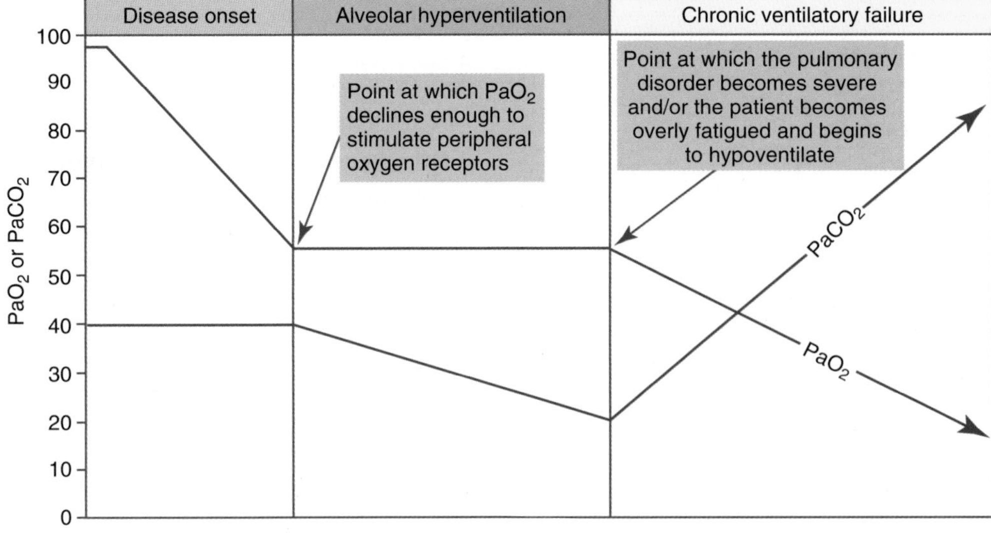

FIGURE 4-6 Pa_{O_2} and Pa_{CO_2} trends during acute or chronic ventilatory failure.

If the HCO_3^- and pH levels are greater than these values (i.e., the pH and HCO_3^- readings cross a PCO_2 isobar[†] above the normal blood buffer line in the upper left-hand corner of the nomogram), renal retention of HCO_3^- (partial renal compensation) has occurred. When the HCO_3^- level increases enough to return the acidic pH to normal, complete renal compensation is said to have occurred (chronic ventilatory failure).

Thus, the following should be understood: The lungs play an important role in maintaining the Pa_{CO_2}, HCO_3^-, and pH levels on a moment-to-moment basis. The kidneys play an important role in maintaining the HCO_3^- and pH levels during long periods of hyperventilation or hypoventilation.

Acute Ventilatory Changes Superimposed on Chronic Ventilatory Failure

Because acute ventilatory changes (i.e., hyperventilation or hypoventilation) are frequently seen in patients who have chronic ventilatory failure (compensated respiratory acidosis), the respiratory care practitioner must be familiar with and be on the alert for (1) **acute alveolar hyperventilation superimposed on chronic ventilatory failure**, and (2) **acute ventilatory failure superimposed on chronic ventilatory failure**.

Acute Alveolar Hyperventilation Superimposed on Chronic Ventilatory Failure (Acute Hyperventilation on Compensated Respiratory Acidosis)

ABG Changes	Example
pH: increased	7.53
Pa_{CO_2}: increased	51 mm Hg
HCO_3^-: increased	37 mEq/L
Pa_{O_2}: decreased	46 mm Hg

Like any other person (healthy or unhealthy), the patient with chronic ventilatory failure can also acquire an acute shunt-producing disease (e.g., pneumonia). Some of these patients have the mechanical reserve to increase their alveolar ventilation significantly in an attempt to maintain their baseline Pa_{O_2}. However, in regard to the patient's baseline Pa_{CO_2} level, the increased alveolar ventilation is often excessive.

When excessive alveolar ventilation occurs, the patient's P_{ACO_2} rapidly decreases. This action causes the patient's Pa_{CO_2} to decrease from its normally high baseline level. As the Pa_{CO_2} decreases, the arterial pH increases. As this condition intensifies, the patient's baseline ABG values can quickly change from chronic ventilatory failure to **acute alveolar hyperventilation superimposed on chronic ventilatory failure** (Table 4-3).

If the clinician does not know the past history of the patient with acute alveolar hyperventilation superimposed on chronic ventilatory failure, he or she might initially interpret the ABG values as signifying partially compensated metabolic alkalosis with severe hypoxemia (see Box 4-1). However, the clinical situation that offsets this interpretation is the presence of marked hypoxemia. A low oxygen level is not normally seen in patients with pure metabolic alkalosis. Thus, whenever the ABG values appear to reflect partially compensated metabolic alkalosis but the condition is accompanied by significant hypoxemia, the respiratory care practitioner should be alert to the possibility of acute alveolar hyperventilation superimposed on chronic ventilatory failure.

Acute Ventilatory Failure Superimposed on Chronic Ventilatory Failure (Acute Hypoventilation on Compensated Respiratory Acidosis)

ABG Changes	Example
pH: decreased	7.21
Pa_{CO_2}: increased	110 mm Hg
HCO_3^-: increased	43 mEq/L
Pa_{O_2}: decreased	34 mm Hg

Often patients with chronic ventilatory failure do not have the mechanical reserve to meet the hypoxemic challenge of a respiratory disorder. When these patients attempt to maintain their baseline Pa_{O_2}, by increasing alveolar ventilation, they consume more oxygen than is gained. When this happens, the patient begins to breathe less. This action causes the Pa_{CO_2} to increase and eventually to rise above the patient's normally high Pa_{CO_2} baseline level. This action causes the patient's arterial pH level to fall, or become acidic. In short, the patient's baseline ABG values shift from chronic ventilatory failure to **acute ventilatory failure superimposed on chronic ventilatory failure** (see Table 4-3).

TABLE 4-3 Examples of Acute Changes in Chronic Ventilatory Failure

Acute Ventilatory Failure on Chronic Ventilatory Failure		Chronic Ventilatory Failure (Baseline Values)		Acute Alveolar Hyperventilation on Chronic Ventilatory Failure
7.21	←--------	pH 7.39	--------→	7.53
110	←--------	Pa_{CO_2} 76	--------→	51
43	←--------	HCO_3^- 41	--------→	37
34	←--------	Pa_{O_2} 61	--------→	46

[†]The isobars on the PCO_2/HCO_3^-/pH nomogram illustrate the pH changes that develop in the blood as a result of (1) metabolic changes (i.e., HCO_3^- changes) or (2) a combination of metabolic and respiratory (CO_2) changes.

Lactic Acidosis (Metabolic Acidosis)	
ABG Changes	**Example**
pH: decreased	7.21
Pa_{CO_2}: Normal or decreased	35 mm Hg
HCO_3^-: decreased	19 mEq/L
Pa_{O_2}: decreased	34 mm Hg

Because acute hypoxemia is commonly associated with all of the respiratory disorders presented in this textbook, **acute metabolic acidosis** (caused by **lactic acid**) often further compromises the patient's ABG status. This is because oxygenation is inadequate to meet tissue metabolism, so alternate biochemical reactions that do not use oxygen are activated. This is called **anaerobic metabolism** (non–oxygen-using). Lactic acid is the end-product of this process. When acidic ions move into the blood, the pH decreases. Thus, whenever acute hypoxemia is present, the possible presence of lactic acid should be suspected. For example, when acute alveolar hyperventilation is caused by a sudden drop in Pa_{O_2}, the patient's pH may be lower than expected for a particular decrease in Pa_{CO_2} level.

As shown in Box 4-1, metabolic acid-base disturbances are subdivided into the following two categories: metabolic acidosis and metabolic alkalosis. An overview of the metabolic acid-base disturbances are presented in the following section.

Metabolic Acid-Base Abnormalities

Metabolic Acidosis	
ABG Changes	**Example**
pH: decreased	7.26
Pa_{CO_2}: normal	37 mm Hg
HCO_3^-: decreased	18 mEq/L
Pa_{O_2}: normal (or decreased if lactic acidosis is present)	94 mm Hg (or 52 mm Hg if lactic acidosis is present)

Metabolic Acidosis

The presence of other acids not related to an increased Pa_{CO_2} level or renal compensation can be identified by using the isobars of the $P_{CO_2}/HCO_3^-/pH$ nomogram shown in Figure 4-1. The presence of other acids is verified when the calculated HCO_3^- reading and pH level are both lower than expected for a particular Pa_{CO_2} level in terms of the absolute $P_{CO_2}/HCO_3^-/pH$ relationship. For example, according to the normal blood buffer line, an HCO_3^- reading of 15 mEq/L and a pH of 7.20 would both be less than expected in a patient who has a P_{CO_2} of 40 mm Hg. This condition is referred to as **metabolic acidosis.**

Anion Gap

The **anion gap** is used to assess if a patient's metabolic acidosis is caused by either (1) the accumulation of fixed acids (lactic acids, keto acids, or salicylate intoxication) or (2) an excessive loss of HCO_3^-.

The **law of electroneutrality** states that the total number of plasma positively charged ions (cations) must equal the total number of plasma negatively charged ions (anions) in the body fluids. To calculate the anion gap, the most commonly measured cations are sodium (Na^+) ions. The most commonly measured anions are the chloride (Cl^-) ions and bicarbonate (HCO_3^-) ions. The normal plasma concentrations of these cations and anions are the following:

Na^+: 140 mEq/L
Cl^-: 105 mEq/L
HCO_3^-: 24 mEq/L

The anion gap is the calculated difference between the Na^+ ions and the sum of the HCO_3^- and Cl^- ions:

$$\begin{aligned}\text{Anion gap} &= Na^+ - (Cl^- + HCO_3^-)\\ &= 140 - (105 + 24)\\ &= 140 - 129\\ &= 11\,\text{mEq/L}\end{aligned}$$

The normal range for the anion gap is 9 to 14 mEq/L. When the anion gap is greater than 14 mEq/L, metabolic acidosis is present. An elevated anion gap is frequently caused by the accumulation of fixed acids (e.g., lactic acids, keto acids, or salicylate intoxication) in the blood. Fixed acids produce H^+ ions that chemically react with—and are buffered by—the plasma HCO_3^-. This action causes (1) the HCO_3^- level to fall, and (2) the anion gap to rise.

Clinically, when the patient demonstrates both metabolic acidosis and an increased anion gap, the source of the fixed acids must be identified for the patient to be appropriately treated. For example, metabolic acidosis caused by lactic acids requires oxygen therapy to reverse the accumulation of the lactic acids. Metabolic acidosis caused by ketone acids requires insulin therapy to reverse the accumulation of the ketone acids.

It is interesting to note that metabolic acidosis caused by an excessive loss of HCO_3^- (e.g., from renal disease or severe diarrhea) does not cause an increase in the anion gap. This is because as the HCO_3^- level decreases, the Cl^- level usually increases to maintain electroneutrality. In short, for every HCO_3^- ion that is lost, a Cl^- anion takes its place (i.e., the law of electroneutrality). This action maintains a normal anion gap. Metabolic acidosis caused by decreased HCO_3^- is commonly called **hyperchloremic metabolic acidosis.**

Thus, when metabolic acidosis is accompanied by an increased anion gap, the most likely cause of the acidosis is fixed acids (e.g., lactic acids, keto acids, or salicylate intoxication). When metabolic acidosis is seen with a normal anion gap, the most likely cause of the acidosis is an excessive loss of HCO_3^- (e.g., caused by renal failure or severe diarrhea).

Metabolic Alkalosis	
ABG Changes	**Example**
pH: increased	7.56
Pa_{CO_2}: normal	44 mm Hg
HCO_3^-: increased	27 mEq/L
Pa_{O_2}: normal	94 mm Hg

Box 4-4 Common Causes of Metabolic Acid-Base Abnormalities

Metabolic Acidosis
- Lactic acidosis (most common)
- Ketoacidosis (most commonly associated with diabetes mellitus)
- Salicylate intoxication (aspirin overdose)
- Renal failure
- Chronic diarrhea

Metabolic Alkalosis
- Hypokalemia
- Hypochloremia
- Gastric suctioning
- Vomiting
- Excessive administration of corticosteroids
- Excessive administration of sodium bicarbonate
- Diuretic therapy
- Hypovolemia

Metabolic Alkalosis

The presence of other bases not related to either a decreased Pa_{CO_2} level or renal compensation also can be identified by using the $P_{CO_2}/HCO_3^-/pH$ nomogram illustrated in Figure 4-1. The presence of metabolic alkalosis is verified when the calculated HCO_3^- and pH readings are both higher than expected for a particular Pa_{CO_2} level in terms of the absolute $P_{CO_2}/HCO_3^-/pH$ relationship. For example, according to the normal blood buffer line, an HCO_3^- reading of 35 mEq/L and a pH level of 7.54 would both be higher than expected in a patient who has a Pa_{CO_2} level of 40 mm Hg (see Figure 4-1). This condition is known as **metabolic alkalosis**.

Clinically, metabolic alkalosis is seen more often than metabolic acidosis. Box 4-4 provides common causes of the metabolic abnormalities.

The Hazards of Oxygen Therapy in Patients with Chronic Ventilatory Failure with Hypoxemia

In some patients with chronic ventilatory failure and hypoxemia, the administration of moderate to high concentrations of oxygen may suppress ventilation, causing the patient's arterial carbon dioxide (Pa_{CO_2}) to increase and the pH to decrease. This means that when a patient with chronic hypercapnia is given too much oxygen, the patient may develop acute ventilatory failure, superimposed on the already chronic condition. In other words, patients with chronically high CO_2 levels may experience acute oxygen-induced hypercapnia—on top of their already high CO_2 levels—when breathing high concentrations of oxygen. In severe cases the sudden increase in carbon dioxide and acidemia may depress the patient's central nervous system, cause lethargy, and ultimately lead to coma. Clinically, oxygen-induced hypoventilation is most commonly seen in the relaxed, unstimulated patient with chronic hypercapnia. *Patients who are experiencing oxygen-induced hypoventilation are often described as sleepy, lethargic, and hard to arouse, with slow and shallow breathing.*

Although the precise mechanism for this phenomenon is not known, one prominent theory suggests that the administration of high concentrations of oxygen may suppress the patient's so-called "hypoxic drive to breathe." According to this theory, the sensitivity of the central chemoreceptors (CO_2 sensors), which are located in the medulla, is blunted—or rendered insensitive—when the carbon dioxide level is chronically high. As a result, the patient's primary stimulus to breathe on a moment-to-moment basis falls to the peripheral chemoreceptors (oxygen sensors), which are located near the bifurcation of the common carotid arteries and ascending aorta. Presumably, the excessive administration of oxygen depresses the oxygen peripheral chemoreceptors, which in turn depresses the patient's ventilatory drive. When this occurs, the Pa_{CO_2} increases and the pH decreases.

Other investigators have suggested that the excessive oxygen administration somehow causes the patient's $\dot{V}/\dot{Q}$ relationships to deteriorate, leading to an acute rise in P_{CO_2} and a decrease in pH. Most researchers agree, however, that the oxygen-induced hypercapnia phenomenon most likely results from a combination of both mechanisms—the oxygen-induced peripheral chemoreceptor depression and the oxygen-induced redistribution of the $\dot{V}/\dot{Q}$ ratio. Regardless of the precise cause of oxygen-induced hypercapnia, the respiratory care practitioner must always exercise caution when providing oxygen therapy to patients with chronic hypercapnia. Clinically, patients with chronic hypercapnia (e.g., obstructive pulmonary disease) are typically oxygenated with low and precisely controlled concentrations of oxygen. In such patients, oxygen devices that provide a fixed F_{IO_2} regardless of the patient's ventilatory pattern should be used.

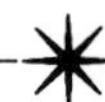

SELF-ASSESSMENT QUESTIONS

evolve Answers to questions can be found on Evolve. To access additional student assessment questions and case studies for application of text material to real-life scenarios, visit **http://evolve.elsevier.com/DesJardins/respiratory.**

1. During acute alveolar hyperventilation, which of the following occurs?
1. HCO_3^- decreases.
2. $Paco_2$ increases.
3. HCO_3^- increases.
4. P_{ACO_2} decreases.
   a. 2 only
   b. 3 only
   c. 1 and 4 only
   d. 2, 3, and 4 only

2. When lactic acidosis is present, which of the following will occur?
1. pH will likely be lower than expected for a particular $Paco_2$.
2. HCO_3^- will likely be higher than expected for a particular P_{ACO_2}.
3. pH will likely be higher than expected for a particular $Paco_2$.
4. HCO_3^- will likely be lower than expected or a particular $Paco_2$.
   a. 2 only
   b. 3 only
   c. 2 and 3 only
   d. 1 and 4 only

3. What is the clinical interpretation of the following ABG values (in addition to hypoxemia)?
pH: 7.17
$Paco_2$: 77 mm Hg
HCO_3^-: 28 mEq/L
Pao_2: 54 mm Hg
   a. Acute alveolar hyperventilation superimposed on chronic ventilatory failure
   b. Acute ventilatory failure
   c. Acute alveolar hyperventilation
   d. Acute ventilatory failure superimposed on chronic ventilatory failure

4. A 74-year-old man with a long history of emphysema and chronic bronchitis enters the emergency room in respiratory distress. His respiratory rate is 34 breaths per minute and labored. His heart rate is 115 beats per minute, and his blood pressure is 170/120. What is the clinical interpretation of the following ABG values (in addition to hypoxemia)?
pH: 7.51
$Paco_2$: 68 mm Hg
HCO_3^-: 52 mEq/L
Pao_2: 49 mm Hg
   a. Acute alveolar hyperventilation superimposed on chronic ventilatory failure
   b. Acute ventilatory failure
   c. Acute alveolar hyperventilation
   d. Acute ventilatory failure superimposed on chronic ventilatory failure

5. Which of the following is classified as metabolic acidosis?
   a. pH 7.23; $Paco_2$ 63; HCO_3^- 26; Pao_2 52
   b. pH 7.16; $Paco_2$ 38; HCO_3^- 14; Pao2 86
   c. pH 7.56; $Paco_2$ 27; HCO_3^- 23; Pao_2 101
   d. pH 7.64; $Paco_2$ 49; HCO_3^- 47; Pao_2 91

6. Which of the following cause metabolic acidosis?
1. Hypokalemia
2. Renal failure
3. Excessive administration of sodium bicarbonate
4. Hypochloremia
   a. 1 only
   b. 2 only
   c. 1 and 4 only
   d. 2 and 3 only

7. Using the general rule of thumb for the $Paco_2/HCO_3^-/pH$ relationship, if the $Paco_2$ suddenly increased to 90 mm Hg in a patient who normally has a pH of 7.40, a $Paco_2$ of 40 mm Hg, and an HCO_3^- of 24 mEq/L, the pH will decrease to approximately what level?
   a. 7.15
   b. 7.10
   c. 7.05
   d. 7.00

8. Which of the following is classified as metabolic alkalosis?
   a. pH 7.23; $Paco_2$ 63; HCO_3^- 26; Pao_2 52
   b. pH 7.16; $Paco_2$ 38; HCO_3^- 14; Pao_2 86
   c. pH 7.56; $Paco_2$ 27; HCO_3^- 23; Pao_2 101
   d. pH 7.64; $Paco_2$ 44; HCO_3^- 47; Pao_2 91

9. Lactic acidosis develops from which of the following?
1. Inadequate tissue oxygenation
2. Renal failure
3. An inadequate insulin level
4. Anaerobic metabolism
5. An inadequate glucose level
   a. 1 only
   b. 2 only
   c. 1 and 4 only
   d. 3 and 5 only

10. Metabolic alkalosis can develop from which of the following?
1. Hyperchloremia
2. Hypokalemia

3. Hypochloremia
4. Hyperkalemia
   a. 4 only
   b. 1 and 3 only
   c. 1 and 4 only
   d. 2 and 3 only

11. During acute alveolar hypoventilation, the blood:
1. HCO_3^- increases
2. pH decreases
3. Pco_2 increases
4. HCO_3^- decreases
   a. 2 only
   b. 4 only
   c. 2 and 3 only
   d. 1, 2, and 3 only

12. During acute alveolar hyperventilation, the blood
1. Pco_2 increases
2. HCO_3^- increases
3. HCO_3^- decreases
4. pH increases
   a. 2 only
   b. 4 only
   c. 1 and 3 only
   d. 3 and 4 only

13. In chronic hypoventilation, kidney compensation has likely occurred when the
1. HCO_3^- is higher than expected for a particular $Paco_2$
2. pH is lower than expected for a particular $Paco_2$
3. HCO_3^- is lower than expected for a particular $Paco_2$
4. pH is higher than expected for a particular $Paco_2$
   a. 1 only
   b. 2 only
   c. 1 and 4 only
   d. 3 and 4 only

14. Which of the following represents acute alveolar hyperventilation?
   a. pH 7.56; $Paco_2$ 51; HCO_3^- 43
   b. pH 7.45; $Paco_2$ 37; HCO_3^- 37
   c. pH 7.53; $Paco_2$ 46; HCO_3^- 29
   d. pH 7.54; $Paco_2$ 21; HCO_3^- 22

15. Which of the following represents compensated metabolic alkalosis?
   a. pH 7.55; $Paco_2$ 21; HCO_3^- 17
   b. pH 7.52; $Paco_2$ 45; HCO_3^- 29
   c. pH 7.45; $Paco_2$ 26; HCO_3^- 19
   d. pH 7.45; $Paco_2$ 61; HCO_3^- 41

Oxygenation Assessments

5

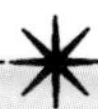

Chapter Objectives

After reading this chapter, you will be able to:

- Write the equation for the following common oxygen transport calculations:
  - Oxygen dissolved in the blood plasma
  - Oxygen bound to hemoglobin
  - Total oxygen content
  - Oxygen content of arterial blood (Ca_{O_2})
  - Oxygen content of venous blood ($C\bar{v}_{O_2}$)
  - Oxygen content of pulmonary capillary blood (Cc_{O_2})
- Calculate the following oxygen tension–based indices:
  - Alveolar-arterial oxygen tension difference ($P[A\text{-}a]_{O_2}$)
  - Ideal alveolar gas equation (P_{AO_2})
- Calculate the following oxygen saturation– and content–based indices:
  - Total oxygen delivery (D_{O_2})
  - Arterial-venous oxygen content difference ($C[a\text{-}\bar{v}]_{O_2}$)
  - Oxygen consumption ($\dot{V}_{O_2}$)
  - Oxygen extraction ratio (O_2ER)
  - Mixed venous oxygenation saturation ($S\bar{v}_{O_2}$)
  - Pulmonary shunt fraction ($\dot{Q}_S/\dot{Q}_T$)
- Describe the clinical significance of pulmonary shunting.
- List factors that increase and decrease the previously listed oxygen transport calculations.
- Discuss how specific respiratory diseases alter the oxygen transport studies.
- Differentiate between hypoxemia and hypoxia.
- Distinguish the classification differences between mild, moderate, and severe hypoxemia.
- Describe the following types of hypoxia:
  - Hypoxic hypoxia
  - Anemic hypoxia
  - Circulatory hypoxia
  - Histotoxic hypoxia
- List common causes for each of the listed types of hypoxia.
- Describe the following pathophysiologic conditions associated with chronic hypoxia:
  - Cor pulmonale
  - Polycythemia
  - Hypoxic vasoconstriction of the lungs
- Define key terms and complete self-assessment questions at the end of the chapter and on Evolve.

Key Terms

Alveolar-Arterial Oxygen Tension Difference ($P[A\text{-}a]_{O_2}$)
Anemic Hypoxia
Arterial-Venous Oxygen Content Difference ($C[a\text{-}\bar{v}]_{O_2}$)
Circulatory Hypoxia
Cor Pulmonale
Histotoxic Hypoxia
Hypoxemia
Hypoxia
Hypoxic Hypoxia
Hypoxic Vasoconstriction of the Lungs
Ideal Alveolar Gas Equation (P_{AO_2})
Lactic Acid
Mild Hypoxemia
Mixed Venous Oxygenation Saturation ($S\bar{v}_{O_2}$)
Moderate Hypoxemia
Oxygen Consumption ($\dot{V}_{O_2}$)
Oxygen Content of Arterial Blood (Ca_{O_2})
Oxygen Content of Pulmonary Capillary Blood (Cc_{O_2})
Oxygen Content of Venous Blood ($C\bar{v}_{O_2}$)
Oxygen Extraction Ratio (O_2ER)
Polycythemia
Pulmonary Shunt Fraction ($\dot{Q}_S/\dot{Q}_T$)
Severe Hypoxemia
Total Oxygen Delivery (D_{O_2})

Chapter Outline

Oxygen Transport Review

Oxygen transport between the lungs and the tissue cells is a function of the blood and the heart. Oxygen is carried in the blood in two ways: (1) as dissolved oxygen in the blood plasma, and (2) bound to the hemoglobin (Hb). Most oxygen is carried to the tissue cells bound to the hemoglobin.

Oxygen Dissolved in the Blood Plasma

A small amount of oxygen that diffuses from the alveoli to the pulmonary capillary blood remains in the dissolved form. The term *dissolved* means that the gas molecule (in this case oxygen) maintains its exact molecular structure and freely moves throughout the plasma of the blood in its normal gaseous state. Clinically, it is the dissolved oxygen that is measured to assess the patient's partial pressure of oxygen (Po_2).

At normal body temperature, approximately 0.003 mL of oxygen will dissolve in each 100 mL of blood for every 1 mm Hg of Po_2. Therefore in the normal individual with an arterial oxygen partial pressure (Pao_2) of 100 mm Hg, about 0.3 mL of oxygen exists in the dissolved form in every 100 mL of plasma (0.003 × 100 mm Hg = 0.3 mL). Clinically, this is written as 0.3 volumes percent (vol%), or as 0.3 vol% oxygen. Relative to the total oxygen transport, only a small amount of oxygen is carried to the tissue cells in the form of dissolved oxygen.

Oxygen Bound to Hemoglobin

In the healthy individual, over 98% of the oxygen that diffuses into the pulmonary capillary blood chemically combines with hemoglobin (Hb). The normal hemoglobin value for men is 14 to 16 g/100 mL of blood. Clinically, the weight measurement of hemoglobin, in reference to 100 mL of blood, is known as the *grams percent of hemoglobin* (g% Hb). The normal hemoglobin value for women is 12 to 15 g%. The normal hemoglobin value for infants is 14 to 20 g%.

Each gram of Hb (1 g% Hb) is capable of carrying about 1.34 mL of oxygen. Therefore if the hemoglobin level is 12 g% and the hemoglobin is fully saturated with oxygen (i.e., carrying all the oxygen that is physically possible), about 15.72 vol% will be bound to the hemoglobin:

$$\begin{aligned} O_2 \text{ bound to Hb} &= 1.34 \text{ mL } O_2 \times 12 \text{ g\% Hb} \\ &= 15.72 \text{ vol\% } O_2 \text{ (15.72 mL of oxygen/} \\ &\quad \text{100 mL of blood)} \end{aligned}$$

Because of normal physiologic shunts (e.g., thebesian venous drainage and bronchial venous drainage), however, the actual normal hemoglobin saturation is only about 97%. Therefore the amount of arterial oxygen shown in the calculation must be adjusted to 97% as follows:

$$15.72 \text{ (vol\% } O_2) \times 0.97 = 15.24 \text{ vol\% } O_2$$

Total Oxygen Content

To calculate the total amount of oxygen in each 100 mL of blood, the dissolved oxygen and the oxygen bound to the hemoglobin must be added together. The following case example summarizes the mathematics required to determine an individual's total oxygen content.

Case Example

A 44-year-old woman with a long history of asthma arrives in the emergency room in severe respiratory distress. Her vital signs are as follows: respiratory rate 36 breaths/min, heart rate 130 beats/minute, and blood pressure 160/95 mm Hg. Her hemoglobin concentration is 10 g%, and her Pao_2 is 55 mm Hg (Sao_2 85%). On the basis of these data, the patient's total oxygen content is determined as follows:

1. Dissolved O_2

$$\begin{array}{r} 55 \text{ } Pao_2 \\ \times 0.003 \text{ (dissolved } O_2 \text{ factor)} \\ \hline 0.165 \text{ (vol\% } O_2) \end{array}$$

2. Oxygen bound to hemoglobin

$$\begin{array}{r} 10 \text{ g\% Hb} \\ \times 1.34 \text{ (} O_2 \text{ bound to Hb factor)} \\ \hline 13.4 \text{ vol\% } O_2 \text{ (at } Sao_2 \text{ of 100\%)} \end{array}$$

$$\begin{array}{r} 13.4 \text{ vol\% } O_2 \\ \times 0.85 \text{ } Sao_2 \\ \hline 11.39 \text{ vol\% } O_2 \text{ (at } Sao_2 \text{ of 85\%)} \end{array}$$

3. Total oxygen content

$$\begin{array}{r} 11.39 \text{ vol\% } O_2 \text{ (bound to hemoglobin)} \\ + 0.165 \text{ vol\% } O_2 \text{ (dissolved } O_2) \\ \hline 11.555 \text{ vol\% } O_2 \text{ (total amount of } O_2\text{/100 mL of blood)} \end{array}$$

The total oxygen content can be calculated in the patient's arterial blood (Cao_2), venous blood ($C\bar{v}o_2$), and pulmonary capillary blood, also known as the *oxygen content of capillary blood* (Cco_2). The mathematics for these calculations are as follows:

Cao_2: Oxygen content of arterial blood
$(Hb \times 1.34 \times Sao_2) + (Pao_2 \times 0.003)$

$C\bar{v}o_2$: Oxygen content of mixed venous blood
$(Hb \times 1.34 \times S\bar{v}o_2) + (P\bar{v}o_2 \times 0.003)$

Cco_2: Oxygen content of pulmonary capillary blood
$(Hb \times 1.34^{*}) + (Pao_2^{\dagger} \times 0.003)$

As it will be shown later in this chapter, various mathematical manipulations of the Cao_2, $C\bar{v}o_2$, and Cco_2 values are used in several different oxygen transport studies that provide excellent clinical information regarding the patient's ventilatory and cardiac status.

*It is assumed that the hemoglobin saturation with oxygen in the pulmonary capillary blood is 100%.

†See Ideal Alveolar Gas Equation, Appendix VIII.

Oxygenation Indices

A number of oxygen transport measurements are available to assess the oxygenation status of the critically ill patient. Results from these studies can provide important information to adjust therapeutic interventions. The oxygen transport studies can be divided into (1) the oxygen tension–based indices, and (2) the oxygen saturation– and content–based indices.[‡]

Oxygen Tension–Based Indices

Arterial Oxygen Tension (Pa_{O_2})

The Pa_{O_2} has withstood the test of time as a good indicator of the patient's oxygenation status. In general, an appropriate Pa_{O_2} on an inspired low oxygen concentration almost always indicates good tissue oxygenation. The Pa_{O_2}, however, can be misleading in a number of clinical situations. For example, the Pa_{O_2} may give a "falsely normal" oxygenation reading when the patient (1) has a low hemoglobin concentration, (2) has a decreased cardiac output, (3) has peripheral shunting, or (4) has been exposed to carbon monoxide or cyanide.

Alveolar-Arterial Oxygen Tension Difference ($P[A\text{-}a]_{O_2}$)

The **alveolar-arterial oxygen tension difference ($P[A\text{-}a]_{O_2}$)** is the oxygen tension difference between the alveoli and arterial blood. The $P(A\text{-}a)_{O_2}$ also is known as the *alveolar-arterial oxygen tension gradient.* Clinically, the information required for the $P(A\text{-}a)_{O_2}$ is obtained from (1) the patient's calculated alveolar oxygen tension (PA_{O_2}), which is derived from the **ideal alveolar gas equation (PA_{O_2})**, and (2) the patient's Pa_{O_2} and Pa_{CO_2}, which are obtained from an arterial blood gas analysis.

The ideal alveolar gas equation is written as follows:

$$PA_{O_2} = FI_{O_2}(P_B - P_{H_2O}) - Pa_{CO_2}(1.25)$$

where P_B is the barometric pressure, PA_{O_2} is the partial pressure of oxygen within the alveoli, P_{H_2O} is the partial pressure of water vapor in the alveoli (which is 47 mm Hg), FI_{O_2} is the fractional concentration of inspired oxygen, Pa_{CO_2} is the partial pressure of arterial carbon dioxide, and the number 1.25 is a factor that adjusts for alterations in oxygen tension resulting from variations in the respiratory exchange ratio, or respiratory quotient (RQ). The RQ is the ratio of carbon dioxide production ($\dot{V}_{CO_2}$) divided by **oxygen consumption ($\dot{V}_{O_2}$)**. Under normal circumstances, approximately 250 mL of oxygen per minute are consumed by the tissue cells and approximately 200 mL of carbon dioxide are excreted into the lung. Thus, the RQ is normally about 0.8.

Accordingly, if a patient is receiving an FI_{O_2} of 0.30 on a day when the barometric pressure is 750 mm Hg, and if the patient's Pa_{CO_2} is 70 mm Hg and Pa_{O_2} is 60 mm Hg, the $P(A\text{-}a)_{O_2}$ can be calculated as follows:

$$\begin{aligned} PA_{O_2} &= FI_{O_2}(P_B - P_{H_2O}) - Pa_{CO_2}(1.25) \\ &= 0.30(750-47) - 70(1.25) \\ &= (703)\,0.30 - 87.5 \\ &= (210.9) - 87.5 \\ &= 123.4 \text{ mm Hg} \end{aligned}$$

Using the Pa_{O_2} obtained from the arterial blood gas, the $P(A\text{-}a)_{O_2}$ can now easily be calculated as follows:

$$\begin{array}{r} 123.4 \text{ mm Hg } (PA_{O_2}) \\ -\ 60.0 \text{ mm Hg } (Pa_{O_2}) \\ \hline = 63.4 \text{ mm Hg } [P(A\text{-}a)_{O_2}] \end{array}$$

The normal $P(A\text{-}a)_{O_2}$ on room air at sea level ranges from 7 to 15 mm Hg, and it should not exceed 30 mm Hg. The $P(A\text{-}a)_{O_2}$ increases in response to (1) oxygen diffusion disorders (e.g., chronic interstitial lung diseases), (2) decreased ventilation-perfusion ratio disorders (e.g., chronic obstructive pulmonary diseases, atelectasis, consolidation), (3) right-to-left intracardiac shunting (e.g., a patent ventricular septum), and (4) age.

Although the $P(A\text{-}a)_{O_2}$ may be useful in patients breathing a low FI_{O_2}, it loses some of its sensitivity in patients breathing a high FI_{O_2}. The $P(A\text{-}a)_{O_2}$ increases at high oxygen concentrations. Because of this, the $P(A\text{-}a)_{O_2}$ has less value in the critically ill patient who is breathing a high oxygen concentration.

Oxygen Saturation– and Content–Based Indices

The oxygen saturation– and content–based indices can serve as excellent indicators of an individual's cardiac and ventilatory status. These oxygenation studies are derived from the patient's total **oxygen content in the arterial blood (Ca_{O_2}) mixed venous blood ($C\bar{v}_{O_2}$)**, and **pulmonary capillary blood (Cc_{O_2})**. As explained earlier in this chapter, the Ca_{O_2}, $C\bar{v}_{O_2}$, and Cc_{O_2} are calculated using the following formulas*:

$$Ca_{O_2} = (Hb \times 1.34 \times Sa_{O_2}) + (Pa_{O_2} \times 0.003)$$

$$C\bar{v}_{O_2} = (Hb \times 1.34 \times S\bar{v}_{O_2}) + (P\bar{v}_{O_2} \times 0.003)$$

$$Cc_{O_2} = (Hb \times 1.34) + (PA_{O_2} \times 0.003)$$

Clinically, the most common oxygen saturation– and content–based indices are (1) **total oxygen delivery (D_{O_2})**, (2) **arterial-venous oxygen content difference**, (3) **oxygen consumption**, (4) **oxygen extraction ratio (O_2ER)**, (5) **mixed venous oxygen saturation**, and (6) **pulmonary shunt fraction ($\dot{Q}_S/\dot{Q}_T$)**.

Total Oxygen Delivery

Total oxygen delivery (D_{O_2}) is the amount of oxygen delivered to the peripheral tissue cells. The D_{O_2} is calculated as follows:

$$D_{O_2} = \dot{Q}_T \times (Ca_{O_2} \times 10)$$

[‡]See Appendix X for a representative example of a cardiopulmonary profile sheet used to monitor the oxygen transport status of the critically ill patient.

where $\dot{Q}_T$ is total cardiac output (L/min), Ca_{O_2} is oxygen content of arterial blood (milliliters of oxygen per 100 mL of blood), and the factor 10 is used to convert the Ca_{O_2} to milliliters of oxygen per liter of blood.

Therefore if a patient has a cardiac output of 4 L/min and a Ca_{O_2} of 15 vol%, the D_{O_2} is 600 mL of oxygen per minute:

$$\begin{aligned} D_{O_2} &= \dot{Q}_T \times (Ca_{O_2} \times 10) \\ &= 4\ \text{L/min} \times (15\ \text{vol\%} \times 10) \\ &= 600\ \text{mL}\ O_2/\text{min} \end{aligned}$$

Normally, the D_{O_2} is approximately 1000 mL of oxygen per minute. Clinically, a patient's D_{O_2} decreases when blood oxygen saturation, hemoglobin concentration, or cardiac output declines. The D_{O_2} increases in response to an increase in blood oxygen saturation, hemoglobin concentration, or cardiac output.

Arterial-Venous Oxygen Content Difference

The **arterial-venous oxygen content difference ($C[a\text{-}\bar{v}]O_2$)** is the difference between the Ca_{O_2} and the $C\bar{v}_{O_2}$ ($Ca_{O_2} - C\bar{v}_{O_2}$). Therefore if a patient's Ca_{O_2} is 15 vol% and the $C\bar{v}_{O_2}$ is 8 vol%, the $C(a\text{-}\bar{v})O_2$ is 7 vol%:

$$\begin{aligned} C(a\text{-}\bar{v})O_2 &= Ca_{O_2} - C\bar{v}_{O_2} \\ &= 15\ \text{vol\%} - 8\ \text{vol\%} \\ &= 7\ \text{vol\%} \end{aligned}$$

Normally the $C(a\text{-}\bar{v})O_2$ is about 5 vol%. The $C(a\text{-}\bar{v})O_2$ is useful in assessing the patient's cardiopulmonary status because oxygen changes in the mixed venous blood ($C\bar{v}_{O_2}$) often occur earlier than oxygen changes in arterial blood gas. Clinically, the patient's $C(a\text{-}\bar{v})O_2$ increases in response to such factors as decreased cardiac output, exercise, seizures, and hyperthermia. The $C(a\text{-}\bar{v})O_2$ decreases in response to increased cardiac output, skeletal relaxation (e.g., induced by drugs), peripheral shunting (e.g., sepsis), certain poisons (e.g., cyanide), and hypothermia.

Oxygen Consumption

Oxygen consumption ($\dot{V}_{O_2}$), also known as *oxygen uptake,* is the amount of oxygen consumed by the peripheral tissue cells during a 1-minute period. The $\dot{V}_{O_2}$ is calculated as follows:

$$\dot{V}_{O_2} = \dot{Q}_T [C(a\text{-}\bar{v})O_2 \times 10]$$

where $Q_{\dot{T}}$ is the total cardiac output (L/min), $C(a\text{-}\bar{v})O_2$ is the arterial-venous oxygen content difference, and the factor 10 is used to convert the $C(a\text{-}\bar{v})O_2$ to mL O_2/L.

Therefore if a patient has a cardiac output of 4 L/min and a $C(a\text{-}\bar{v})O_2$ of 6 vol%, the total amount of oxygen consumed by the tissue cells in 1 minute would be 240 mL:

$$\begin{aligned} \dot{V}_{O_2} &= \dot{Q}_T [C(a\text{-}\bar{v})O_2 \times 10] \\ &= 4\ \text{L/min} \times 6\ \text{vol\%} \times 10 \\ &= 240\ \text{mL}\ O_2/\text{min} \end{aligned}$$

Normally, the $\dot{V}_{O_2}$ is about 250 mL of oxygen per minute. Clinically, the $\dot{V}_{O_2}$ increases in response to seizures, exercise, hyperthermia, and body size. The $\dot{V}_{O_2}$ decreases in response to skeletal muscle relaxation (e.g., induced by drugs), peripheral shunting (e.g., sepsis), certain poisons (e.g., cyanide), and hypothermia. It is often as a function of body weight (i.e., mL/kg or mL/lb).

Oxygen Extraction Ratio

The **oxygen extraction ratio (O_2ER)**, also known as the *oxygen coefficient ratio* or *oxygen utilization ratio,* is the amount of oxygen consumed by the tissue cells divided by the total amount of oxygen delivered. The O_2ER is calculated by dividing the $C(a\text{-}\bar{v})O_2$ by the Ca_{O_2}. Therefore if a patient has a Ca_{O_2} of 15 vol% and a $C\bar{v}_{O_2}$ of 10 vol%, the O_2ER would be 33%:

$$\begin{aligned} O_2ER &= \frac{Ca_{O_2} - C\bar{v}_{O_2}}{Ca_{O_2}} \\ &= \frac{15\ \text{vol\%} - 10\ \text{vol\%}}{15\ \text{vol\%}} \\ &= \frac{5\ \text{vol\%}}{15\ \text{vol\%}} \\ &= 0.33 \end{aligned}$$

Normally, the O_2ER is about 25%. Clinically, the patient's O_2ER increases in response to (1) a decreased cardiac output, (2) periods of increased oxygen consumption (e.g., exercise, seizures, hyperthermia), (3) anemia, and (4) decreased arterial oxygenation. The O_2ER decreases in response to (1) increased cardiac output, (2) skeletal muscle relaxation (e.g., induced by drugs), (3) peripheral shunting (e.g., sepsis), (4) certain poisons (e.g., cyanide), (5) hypothermia, (6) increased hemoglobin, and (7) increased arterial oxygenation.

Mixed Venous Oxygen Saturation

When a patient has a normal arterial oxygen saturation (Sa_{O_2}) and hemoglobin concentration, the **mixed venous oxygen saturation ($S\bar{v}_{O_2}$)** is often used as an early indicator of changes in the patient's $C(a\text{-}\bar{v})O_2$, $\dot{V}_{O_2}$, and O_2ER. The $S\bar{v}_{O_2}$ can signal changes in the patient's $C(a\text{-}\bar{v})O_2$, $\dot{V}_{O_2}$, and O_2ER earlier than arterial blood gases because the Pa_{O_2} and Sa_{O_2} levels are often normal during early $C(a\text{-}\bar{v})O_2$, $\dot{V}_{O_2}$, and O_2ER changes.

Normally the $S\bar{v}_{O_2}$ is approximately 75%. Clinically, the $S\bar{v}_{O_2}$ decreases in response to (1) a decreased cardiac output, (2) exercise, (3) seizures, and (4) hyperthermia. The $S\bar{v}_{O_2}$ increases in response to (1) an increased cardiac output, (2) skeletal muscle relaxation (e.g., induced by drugs), (3) peripheral shunting (e.g., sepsis), (4) certain poisons (e.g., cyanide), and (5) hypothermia.

Over the past several years, there has been a move away from the oxygen tension–based indices to the oxygen saturation– and content–based indices when the oxygenation status of the critically ill patient is monitored. Table 5-1 summarizes the way various clinical factors alter the patient's D_{O_2}, $\dot{V}_{O_2}$, $C(a\text{-}\bar{v})O_2$, O_2ER, and $S\bar{v}_{O_2}$.

TABLE 5-1 Clinical Factors That Affect Oxygen Transport Calculations

Oxygen Transport Study	Equation	Factors That Increase Value	Factors That Decrease Value
Total oxygen delivery (DO_2)	$DO_2 = \dot{Q}_T \times (CaO_2 \times 10)$	Increased blood oxygenation Increased hemoglobin Increased cardiac output	Increased blood oxygenation Increased hemoglobin Increased cardiac output
Arterial-venous oxygen content difference ($C(a\text{-}\bar{v})O_2$)	$C(a\text{-}\bar{v})O_2$	Decreased cardiac output Increased O_2 consumption Exercise Seizures Shivering Hyperthermia	Increased cardiac output Skeletal muscle relaxation Induced by drugs Peripheral shunting Sepsis Trauma Certain poisons Cyanide Hypothermia
Oxygen consumption ($\dot{V}O_2$)	$\dot{V}O_2 = \dot{Q}_T[C(a\text{-}\bar{v})O_2 \times 10$	Exercise Seizures Shivering Hyperthermia	Skeletal muscle relaxation induced by drugs Peripheral shunting Sepsis Trauma Certain poisons Cyanide Hypothermia
Oxygen extraction ratio (O_2ER)	$O_2ER = \frac{CaO_2 - C\bar{v}O_2}{CaO_2}$	Decreased cardiac output Increased O_2 consumption Exercise Seizures Shivering Hyperthermia Anemia Decreased arterial oxygenation	Increased cardiac output Skeletal muscle relaxation induced by drugs Peripheral shunting Sepsis Trauma Certain poisons Cyanide Hypothermia Increased hemoglobin Increased arterial oxygenation
Mixed venous oxygen saturation ($S\bar{v}O_2$)	N/A	Decreased cardiac output Increased O_2 consumption Exercise Seizures Shivering Hyperthermia	Increased cardiac output Skeletal muscle relaxation induced by drugs Peripheral shunting Sepsis Trauma Certain poisons Cyanide Hypothermia
Pulmonary shunt fraction ($\dot{Q}_S/\dot{Q}_T$)	$\frac{\dot{Q}_S}{\dot{Q}_T} = \frac{CcO_2 - CaO_2}{CcO_2 - C\bar{v}O_2}$	See Table 5-3	N/A

Pulmonary Shunt Fraction

Because pulmonary shunting and venous admixture are frequent complications in respiratory disorders, knowledge of the degree of shunting is desirable in developing patient care plans. The amount of intrapulmonary shunting can be calculated by using the classic shunt equation:

$$\frac{\dot{Q}_S}{\dot{Q}_T} = \frac{CcO_2 - CaO_2}{CcO_2 - C\bar{v}O_2}$$

where $\dot{Q}_S$ is the cardiac output that is shunted, $\dot{Q}_T$ is the total cardiac output, CcO_2 is the oxygen content of pulmonary capillary blood, CaO_2 is the oxygen content of arterial blood, and $C\bar{v}O_2$ is the oxygen content of mixed venous blood.

To obtain the data necessary to calculate the patient's intrapulmonary shunt, the following information must be gathered:

- Barometric pressure
- PaO_2
- $PaCO_2$
- $P\bar{v}O_2$
- Hb concentration
- P_AO_2 (partial pressure of alveolar oxygen)*
- F_IO_2 (fractional concentration of inspired oxygen)

A clinical example of the shunt calculation follows.

*See Ideal Alveolar Gas Equation, Appendix VIII.

Shunt Study Calculation in an Automobile Accident Victim

A 22-year-old man is on a volume-cycled mechanical ventilator on a day when the barometric pressure is 755 mm Hg. The patient is receiving an F_{IO_2} of 0.60. The following clinical data are obtained:

- Hb: 15 g/dL
- Pa_{O_2}: 65 mm Hg ($Sa_{O_2} \times 90\%$)
- Pa_{CO_2}: 56 mm Hg
- $P\bar{v}_{O_2}$: 35 mm Hg ($S\bar{v}_{O_2} \times 65\%$)

With this information the patient's PA_{O_2}, Cc_{O_2}, Ca_{O_2}, and $C\bar{v}_{O_2}$ can now be calculated. (The clinician should remember that P_{H_2O} represents alveolar water vapor pressure and is always 47 mm Hg.)

1. $$\begin{aligned} PA_{O_2} &= (PB - P_{H_2O})F_{IO_2} - Pa_{CO_2}(1.25) \\ &= (755 - 47)\,0.60 - 56\,(1.25) \\ &= (708)\,0.60 - 70 \\ &= 424.8 - 70 \\ &= 354.8 \end{aligned}$$
2. $$\begin{aligned} Cc_{O_2} &= (Hb \times 1.34)(PA_{O_2} \times 0.003) \\ &= (15 \times 1.34)(354.8 \times 0.003) \\ &= 20.1 + 1.064 \\ &= 21.164\ (\text{vol\% } O_2) \end{aligned}$$
3. $$\begin{aligned} Ca_{O_2} &= (Hb \times 1.34 \times Sa_{O_2})(Pa_{O_2} \times 0.003) \\ &= (15 \times 1.34 \times 0.90)(65 \times 0.003) \\ &= 18.09 + 0.195 \\ &= 18.285\ (\text{vol\% } O_2) \end{aligned}$$
4. $$\begin{aligned} C\bar{v}_{O_2} &= (Hb \times 1.34 \times S\bar{v}_{O_2})(P\bar{v}_{O_2} \times 0.003) \\ &= (15 \times 1.34 \times 0.65)(35 \times 0.003) \\ &= 13.065 + 0.105 \\ &= 13.17\ (\text{vol\% } O_2) \end{aligned}$$

With this information the patient's intrapulmonary shunt fraction can now be calculated:

$$\begin{aligned} \frac{\dot{Q}_S}{\dot{Q}_T} &= \frac{Cc_{O_2} - Ca_{O_2}}{Cc_{O_2} - C\bar{v}_{O_2}} \\ &= \frac{21.164 - 18.285}{21.164 - 13.17} \\ &= \frac{2.879}{7.994} \\ &= 0.36 \end{aligned}$$

Therefore 36% of the patient's pulmonary blood flow is perfusing lung alveoli that are not being ventilated.

With the proliferation of inexpensive personal computers, much of the shunt equation is now being written in simple programs. What was once a rather esoteric, error-prone procedure is now readily and accurately available to respiratory therapy practitioners.

Table 5-2 shows the clinical significance of pulmonary shunting. Table 5-3 summarizes how specific respiratory diseases alter the oxygen saturation– and content–based indices.*

*Note in Table 5-3 that virtually every respiratory disorder presented in this textbook causes the $\dot{Q}_S/\dot{Q}_T$ to increase and the DO_2 to decrease.

TABLE 5-2 Clinical Significance of Pulmonary Shunting

Degree of Pulmonary Shunting (%)	Clinical Significance
Below 10%	Normal lung status
10% to 20%	Indicates a pulmonary abnormality but is not significant in terms of cardiopulmonary support
20% to 30%	May be life threatening, possibly requiring cardiopulmonary support
Greater than 30%	Serious life-threatening condition, almost always requiring cardiopulmonary support

Hypoxemia versus Hypoxia

Hypoxemia refers to an abnormally low arterial oxygen tension (Pa_{O_2}) and is frequently associated with **hypoxia,** which is an inadequate level of tissue oxygenation (see following discussion). Although the presence of hypoxemia strongly suggests tissue hypoxia, it does not necessarily mean the absolute existence of tissue hypoxia. For example, the reduced level of oxygen in the arterial blood may be offset by an increased cardiac output. Hypoxemia is commonly classified as **mild hypoxemia, moderate hypoxemia,** or **severe hypoxemia** (Table 5-4). Clinically, the presence of mild hypoxemia generally stimulates the oxygen peripheral chemoreceptors to increase the patient's breathing rate and heart rate (see Figure 2-25).

Hypoxia refers to low or inadequate oxygen for aerobic cellular metabolism. Hypoxia is characterized by tachycardia, hypertension, peripheral vasoconstriction, dizziness, and metal confusion. Table 5-5 provides an overview of the four main types of hypoxia. When hypoxia exists, alternate anaerobic mechanisms are activated in the tissues that produce dangerous metabolites—such as **lactic acid**—as waste products. Lactic acid is a nonvolatile acid and causes the pH to decrease.

Pathophysiologic Conditions Associated with Chronic Hypoxia

Cor Pulmonale

Cor pulmonale is the term used to denote pulmonary arterial hypertension, right ventricular hypertrophy, increased right ventricular work, and ultimately right ventricular failure. The three major mechanisms involved in producing cor pulmonale in chronic pulmonary disease are (1) the increased viscosity of the blood associated with **polycythemia,** (2) the increased pulmonary vascular resistance caused by hypoxic vasoconstriction, and (3) the obliteration of the pulmonary capillary bed, particularly in emphysema. Items 1 and 2 are discussed in greater depth in the following paragraphs.

Polycythemia

When pulmonary disorders produce chronic hypoxia, the hormone erythropoietin responds by stimulating the bone marrow to increase red blood cell (RBC) production. RBC

TABLE 5-3 Oxygenation Index Changes Commonly Seen in Respiratory Diseases

Pulmonary Disorder	Oxygenation Indices					
	$S\bar{v}O_2$	DO_2*	$\dot{V}O_2$	$C(a-\bar{v})O_2$	O_2ER	$\dot{Q}_S/\dot{Q}_T$
Obstructive airway diseases	↑	↓	~†	~	↑	↓
Chronic bronchitis						
Emphysema						
Bronchiectasis						
Asthma						
Cystic fibrosis						
Croup syndrome						
Infectious pulmonary diseases	↑	↓	~	~	↑	↓
Pneumonia						
Lung abscess						
Fungal disorders						
Tuberculosis			~			
Pulmonary edema	↑	↓	~	↑‡	↑	↓
Pulmonary embolism	↑	↓	~	↑‡	↑	↓
Lung collapse	↑	↓		↑‡	↑	↓
Flail chest						
Pneumothorax						
Pleural disease (e.g., hemothorax)						
Kyphoscoliosis	↑	↓	~	~	↑	↓
Pneumoconiosis	↑	↓	~	~	↑	↓
Cancer of the lung	↑	↓	~	~	↑	↓
Adult respiratory distress syndrome	↑	↓	~	~	↑	↓
Idiopathic (infant) respiratory distress syndrome	↑	↓	~	~	↑	↓
Chronic interstitial lung disease	↑	↓	~	~	↑	↓
Sleep apnea	↑	↓	~	↑‡	↑	↓
Smoke inhalation						
Without surface burns	↑	↓	~	~	↑	↓
With surface burns	↑	↓	↑	↑	↑	↓
Near drowning (wet)	↑	↓	↑	↑	↑	↓

*The DO_2 may be normal in patients with an increased cardiac output, an increased hemoglobin level (polycythemia), or a combination of both. For example, a normal DO_2 is often seen in patients with chronic obstructive pulmonary disease and polycythemia. When the DO_2 is normal, the patient's O_2ER is usually normal.

†~, Unchanged.

‡The increased $C(a-\bar{v})O_2$ is associated with a decreased cardiac output.

TABLE 5-4 Hypoxemia Classifications*

Classification	PaO_2 (mm Hg) (Rule of Thumb)
Normal	80-100
Mild hypoxemia	60-80
Moderate hypoxemia	40-60
Severe hypoxemia	<40

*The hypoxemia classifications provided in this table are generally accepted clinical values. Minor variations of these classifications are found in the literature. In addition, a number of clinical factors may mandate some degree of changes in the listed values (e.g., a PaO_2 of 55 mm Hg may be called "severe" in the patient with a very low hemoglobin level or carbon monoxide poisoning). As a general rule of thumb, however, the hypoxemia classifications and PaO_2 range(s) presented in this table are useful guidelines.

production is known as *erythropoiesis.* An increased level of RBCs is called *polycythemia.* The polycythemia that results from hypoxia is an adaptive mechanism that increases the oxygen-carrying capacity of the blood.

Unfortunately, the advantage of the increased oxygen-carrying capacity in polycythemia is at least partially offset by the increased viscosity of the blood when the hematocrit reaches 50% to 60%. Because of the increased viscosity of the blood, a greater driving pressure is needed to maintain a given flow. The work of the right ventricle must increase to generate the pressure needed to overcome the increased viscosity. This can lead to right ventricular hypertrophy, or cor pulmonale.

Hypoxic Vasoconstriction of the Lungs

Hypoxic vasoconstriction of the pulmonary vascular system **(hypoxic vasoconstriction of the lungs)** commonly develops in response to the decreased P_AO_2 that occurs in chronic respiratory disorders. The decreased P_AO_2 causes the smooth muscles of the pulmonary arterioles to constrict. The exact mechanism of this phenomenon is unclear. However, the P_AO_2 (and not the PaO_2) is known to chiefly control this response.

TABLE 5-5 Types of Hypoxia

Hypoxia	Descriptions	Common Causes
Hypoxic hypoxia (also called *hypoxemic hypoxia*)	Inadequate oxygen at the tissue cells caused by low arterial oxygen tension (Pa_{O_2})	Low P_{AO_2} caused by: • Hypoventilation • High altitude Diffusion impairment • Interstitial fibrosis • Interstitial lung disease • Pulmonary edema • Pneumonconiosis Ventilation-perfusion mismatch Pulmonary shunting
Anemic hypoxia	Pa_{O_2} is normal, but the oxygen-carrying capacity of the hemoglobin is inadequate	Decreased hemoglobin concentration • Anemia • Hemorrhage Abnormal hemoglobin • Carboxyhemoglobin • Methemoglobin
Circulatory hypoxia (also called *stagnant* or *hypoperfusion hypoxia*)	Blood flow to the tissue cells is inadequate; therefore oxygen is not adequate to meet tissue needs	Slow or stagnant (pooling) peripheral blood flow Arterial-venous shunts
Histotoxic hypoxia	Impaired ability of the tissue cells to metabolize oxygen	Cyanide poisoning

The early effect of hypoxic vasoconstriction is to direct blood away from the hypoxic regions of the lungs and thereby offset the shunt effect. However, when the number of hypoxic regions becomes significant—as during the advanced stages of emphysema or chronic bronchitis—a generalized pulmonary vasoconstriction develops, causing the pulmonary vascular resistance to increase substantially. Increased pulmonary vascular resistance leads to pulmonary hypertension, increased work of the right side of the heart, right ventricular hypertrophy, and cor pulmonale.

The cor pulmonale associated with chronic respiratory disorders may develop from the combined effects of polycythemia and pulmonary arterial vasoconstriction. Both of these conditions occur as a result of chronic hypoxia. Clinically, cor pulmonale leads to the accumulation of venous blood in the large veins. This condition causes (1) the neck veins to become distended (see Figure 2-46), (2) the extremities to show signs of peripheral edema and pitting edema (see Figure 2-45), and (3) the liver to become enlarged and tender.

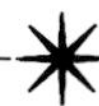

SELF-ASSESSMENT QUESTIONS

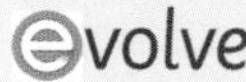

Answers to questions can be found on Evolve. To access additional student assessment questions and case studies for application of text material to real-life scenarios, visit **http://evolve.elsevier.com/DesJardins/respiratory.**

1. A 46-year-old woman with severe asthma arrives in the emergency room with the following clinical data:

Hb: 11 g%
Pa_{O_2}: 46 mm Hg
Sa_{O_2}: 70%

Based on these clinical data, what is the patient's Ca_{O_2}?

a. 6.75 vol% O_2
b. 10.50 vol% O_2
c. 12.30 vol% O_2
d. 15.25 vol% O_2

2. If a patient has a cardiac output of 6 L/min and a Ca_{O_2} of 12 vol%, what is the D_{O_2}?

a. 210 mL O_2/min
b. 345 mL O_2/min
c. 540 mL O_2/min
d. 720 mL O_2/min

3. If a patient's Ca_{O_2} is 11 vol% and the $C\bar{v}_{O_2}$ is 7 vol%, what is the $C(a-\bar{v})_{O_2}$?

a. 4 vol%
b. 7 vol%
c. 11 vol%
d. 15 vol%

4. Clinically, the patient's $C(a-\bar{v})O_2$ increases in response to which of the following?

1. Hypothermia
2. Decreased cardiac output
3. Seizures
4. Cyanide poisoning
   a. 2 only
   b. 4 only
   c. 2 and 3 only
   d. 1 and 4 only

5. If a patient has a cardiac output of 6 L/min and a $C(a-\bar{v})O_2$ of 4 vol%, what is the $\dot{V}O_2$?

a. 160 mL O_2/min
b. 180 mL O_2/min
c. 200 mL O_2/min
d. 240 mL O_2/min

6. Clinically, the $\dot{V}O_2$ decreases in response to which of the following?

1. Exercise
2. Hyperthermia
3. Body size
4. Peripheral shunting
   a. 2 only
   b. 4 only
   c. 1 and 3 only
   d. 2, 3, and 4 only

7. If a patient's CaO_2 is 12 vol% and the $C\bar{v}O_2$ is 7 vol%, what is the O_2ER?

a. 0.27
b. 0.33
c. 0.42
d. 0.53

8. Clinically, the $S\bar{v}O_2$ decreases in response to which of the following?

1. Increased cardiac output
2. Peripheral shunting
3. Hypothermia
4. Seizures
   a. 1 only
   b. 4 only
   c. 2 and 3 only
   d. 1, 2, and 3 only

9. In the patient with severe emphysema, which of the following oxygenation indices are commonly seen?

1. Decreased $S\bar{v}O_2$
2. Increased $\dot{V}O_2$
3. Decreased $C(a-\bar{v})O_2$
4. Increased O_2ER
   a. 1 only
   b. 3 only
   c. 1 and 4 only
   d. 2 and 3 only

10. In the patient with pulmonary edema, which of the following oxygenation indices are commonly seen?

1. Increased O_2ER
2. Decreased $S\bar{v}O_2$
3. Increased $\dot{V}O_2$
4. Decreased $\dot{V}O_2$
   a. 2 only
   b. 4 only
   c. 1 and 2 only
   d. 1, 2, and 3 only

Case Study: Gunshot Victim (Questions 11-15)

A 37-year-old woman is on a volume-cycled mechanical ventilator on a day when the barometric pressure is 745 mm Hg. The patient is receiving an FIO_2 of 0.50. The following clinical data are obtained:

Hb: 11 g%
PaO_2: 60 mm Hg (SaO_2 90%)
$P\bar{v}O_2$: 35 mm Hg ($S\bar{v}O_2$ 65%)
$PaCO_2$: 38 mm Hg
Cardiac output: 6 L/minute

11. Based on this information, calculate the patient's total oxygen delivery.

a. 510 mL O_2/min
b. 740 mL O_2/min
c. 806 mL O_2/min
d. 930 mL O_2/min

12. Based on this information, calculate the patient's arterial-venous oxygen content difference.

a. 2.45 vol% O_2
b. 3.76 vol% O_2
c. 4.20 vol% O_2
d. 5.40 vol% O_2

13. Based on this information, calculate the patient's intrapulmonary shunt fraction.

a. 22%
b. 26%
c. 33 %
d. 37%

14. Based on this information, calculate the patient's oxygen consumption.

a. 170 mL O_2/min
b. 200 mL O_2/min
c. 230 mL O_2/min
d. 280 mL O_2/min

15. Based on this information, calculate the patient's oxygen extraction ratio:

a. 16%
b. 24%
c. 26%
d. 28%

Cardiovascular System Assessments 6

Chapter Objectives

After reading this chapter, you will be able to:

- Describe the ECG pattern of a normal cardiac cycle, and include the following:
  - P wave
  - QRS complex
  - T wave
  - Normal heart rate
- Describe the characteristics of the following arrhythmias:
  - Sinus bradycardia
  - Sinus tachycardia
  - Sinus arrhythmia
  - Atrial flutter
  - Atrial fibrillation
  - Premature ventricular contractions
  - Ventricular tachycardia
  - Ventricular flutter
  - Ventricular fibrillation
  - Asystole (cardiac standstill)
- Describe the noninvasive hemodynamic monitoring assessments, and include the following:
  - The definition of hemodynamics
  - The evaluation of the patient's heart rate, cardiac output, blood pressure, and perfusion state
- Describe the basic pathophysiologic mechanisms for the following hemodynamic changes that frequently develop during the acute stages of respiratory disease:
  - Increased heart rate (pulse), cardiac output, and blood pressure
  - Decreased perfusion state
- Describe the invasive hemodynamic monitoring assessments, and include the following:
  - Pulmonary artery catheter measurements
  - Arterial catheter measurements
  - Central venous pressure catheter measurements
- Describe how the hypoxemia, acidemia, or pulmonary vascular obstruction associated with respiratory disease alters the hemodynamic status.
- Define key terms and complete self-assessment questions at the end of the chapter and on Evolve.

Key Terms

Arterial Catheter
Asystole (Cardiac Standstill)
Atrial Fibrillation
Atrial Flutter
Central Venous Pressure (CVP) Catheter
ECG Patterns
Invasive Hemodynamic Monitoring Assessments
Noninvasive Hemodynamic Monitoring Assessments
Normal Heart Rate
P Wave
Premature Ventricular Contraction (PVC)
Pulmonary Artery Catheter
QRS Complex
Sinus Arrhythmia
Sinus Bradycardia
Sinus Tachycardia
T wave
Ventricular Fibrillation
Ventricular Flutter
Ventricular Tachycardia

Chapter Outline

Because the transport of oxygen to the tissue cells and the delivery of carbon dioxide to the lungs are functions of the cardiovascular system, a basic knowledge and understanding of (1) **normal electrocardiogram (ECG) patterns,** (2) **common heart arrhythmias,** (3) **noninvasive hemodynamic monitoring assessments,** (4) **invasive hemodynamic monitoring assessments,** and (5) **determinants of cardiac output** are essential components of patient assessment.*

The Electrocardiogram

Because the respiratory care practitioner frequently works with critically ill patients who are on cardiac monitors, a basic understanding of normal and common abnormal **ECG patterns** is important. An ECG monitors, both visually and on recording paper, the electrical activity of the heart. Figure 6-1 illustrates the ECG pattern of a **normal cardiac cycle.** The **P wave** reflects depolarization of the atria. The **QRS complex** represents the depolarization of the ventricles, and the **T wave** represents ventricular repolarization.

In normal adults the **heart rate** is between 60 and 100 beats per minute (bpm). In normal infants the heart rate is 130 to 150 bpm. A number of methods can be used to calculate the heart rate. For example, when the rhythm is regular, the heart rate can be determined at a glance by counting the number of large boxes (on the ECG strip) between two QRS complexes and then dividing this number into 300. Therefore if an ECG strip consistently shows four large boxes between each pair of QRS complexes, the heart rate is 75 bpm (300 ÷ 4 = 75). When the rhythm is irregular, the heart rate can be determined by counting the QRS complexes on a 6-second strip and multiplying by 10. The following heart arrhythmias are commonly seen and should be recognized by the respiratory care practitioner.

*See Appendix XV for an example of a cardiopulmonary profile sheet used to monitor the hemodynamic status of the critically ill patient.

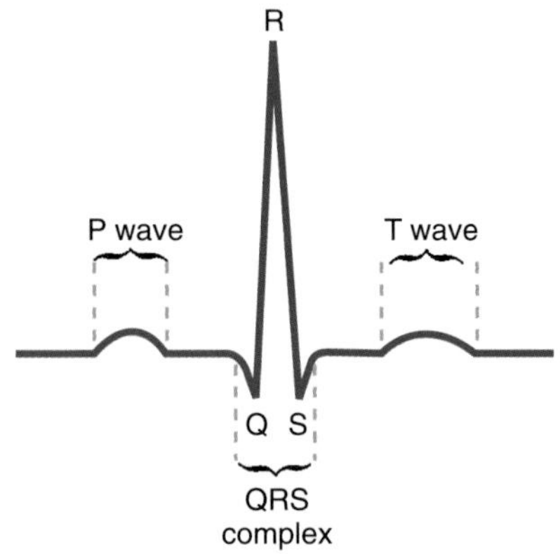

FIGURE 6-1 Electrocardiographic pattern of a normal cardiac cycle.

Common Heart Arrhythmias[†]

Sinus Bradycardia

In **sinus bradycardia** the heart rate is less than 60 bpm. *Bradycardia* means "slow heart." Sinus bradycardia has a normal P-QRS-T pattern, and the rhythm is regular (Figure 6-2). Athletes often normally demonstrate this finding because of increased cardiac stroke volume and other poorly understood mechanisms. Common pathologic causes of sinus bradycardia include a weakened or damaged sinoatrial (SA) node, severe or chronic hypoxemia, increased intracranial pressure, obstructive sleep apnea, and certain drugs (most notably the beta-blockers). Sinus bradycardia may lead to decreased cardiac output and blood pressure. In severe cases, sinus bradycardia may lead to a decreased vascular perfusion state and tissue hypoxia. The patient may demonstrate a weak or absent pulse, poor capillary refill, cold and clammy skin, and a depressed sensorium.

Sinus Tachycardia

In **sinus tachycardia** the heart rate is greater than 100 bpm. Tachycardia means "fast heart." Sinus tachycardia has a normal P-QRS-T pattern, and the rhythm is regular (Figure 6-3). Sinus tachycardia is the normal physiologic response to stress and exercise. Common causes of sinus tachycardia include hypoxemia, severe anemia, hyperthermia, massive hemorrhage, pain, fear, anxiety, hyperthyroidism, and sympathomimetic or parasympatholytic drug administration.

Sinus Arrhythmia

In **sinus arrhythmia** the heart rate varies by more than 10% from beat to beat. The P-QRS-T pattern is normal (Figure 6-4), but the interval between groups of complexes (i.e., the R-R interval) varies. Sinus arrhythmia is a normal rhythm in children and young adults. The patient's pulse will often increase during inspiration and decrease during expiration. No treatment is required unless significant alteration occurs in the patient's arterial blood pressure.

[†]For a complete review of common heart arrhythmias see Des Jardins T: *Cardiopulmonary anatomy and physiology: essentials of respiratory care,* ed 5, 2008, Cengage/Delmar Learning.

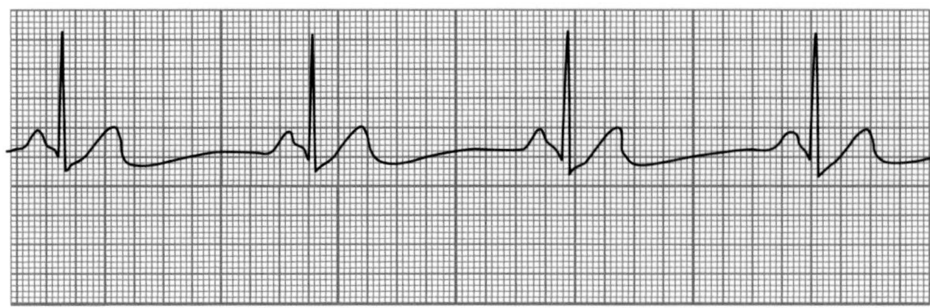

FIGURE 6-2 Sinus bradycardia. Rate is about 37 beats per minute.

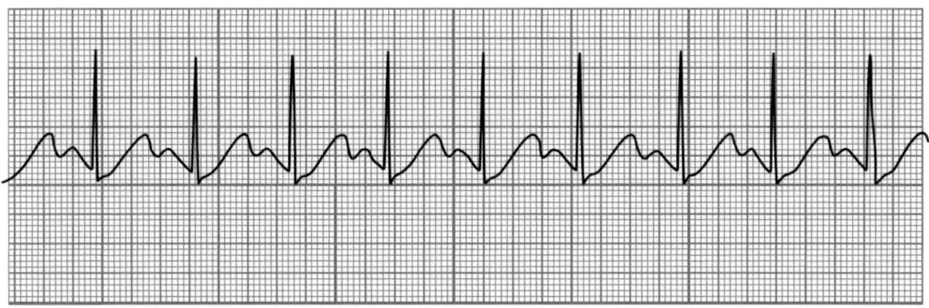

FIGURE 6-3 Sinus tachycardia. Rate is about 100 beats per minute.

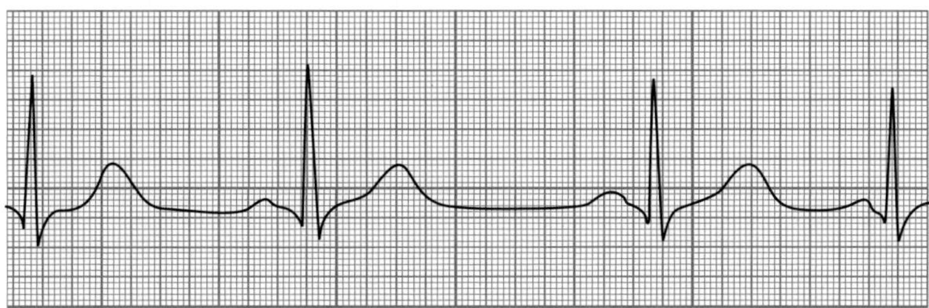

FIGURE 6-4 Sinus arrhythmia. Note the varying R-R interval.

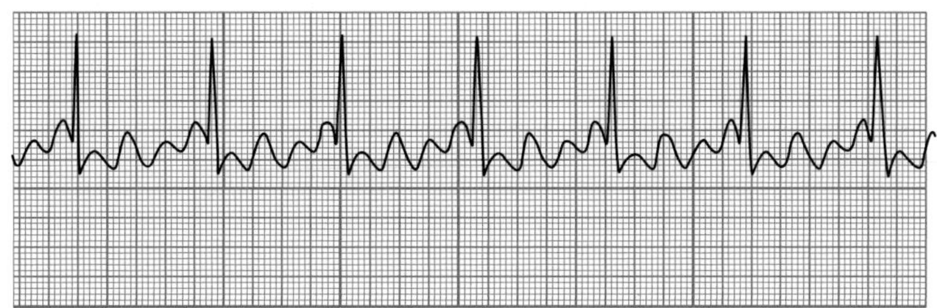

FIGURE 6-5 Atrial flutter. Atrial rate is greater than 300 beats per minute; ventricular rate is about 60 beats per minute and regular.

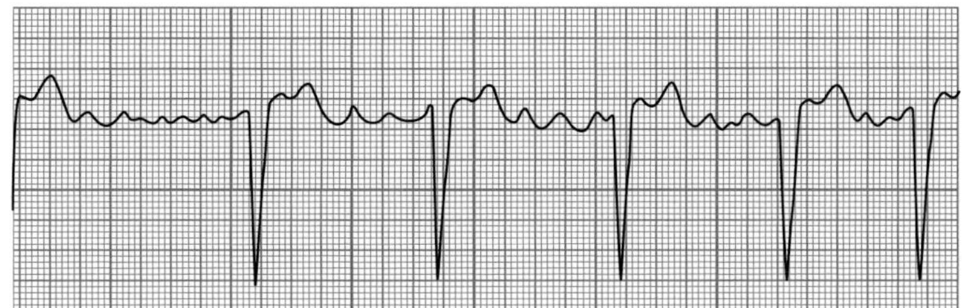

FIGURE 6-6 Atrial fibrillation. Note: the ventricular rate is irregular.

Atrial Flutter

In **atrial flutter** the normal P wave is absent and replaced by two or more regular sawtooth waves. The QRS complex is normal and the ventricular rate may be regular or irregular, depending on the relationship of the atrial to the ventricular beats. Figure 6-5 shows an atrial flutter with a regular rhythm with a 4 : 1 conduction ratio (i.e., four atrial beats for every ventricular beat). The atrial rate is usually constant, between 250 and 350 bpm, whereas the ventricular rate is in the normal range. Causes of atrial flutter include hypoxemia, a damaged SA node, and congestive heart failure.

Atrial Fibrillation

In **atrial fibrillation** the atrial contractions are disorganized and ineffective, and the normal P wave is absent (Figure 6-6). The atrial rate ranges from 350 to 700 bpm. The QRS complex is normal, and the ventricular rate ranges from 100 to 200 bpm. Causes of atrial fibrillation include hypoxemia and a damaged SA node. Atrial fibrillation may reduce the cardiac output by 20% because of a loss of atrial filling (the so-called "atrial kick").

Premature Ventricular Contractions

The **premature ventricular contraction (PVC)** is not preceded by a P wave. The QRS complex is wide, bizarre, and unlike the normal QRS complex (Figure 6-7). The regular heart rate is altered by the PVC. The heart rhythm may be quite irregular when there are many PVCs. PVCs can occur at any rate. They often occur in pairs, after every normal

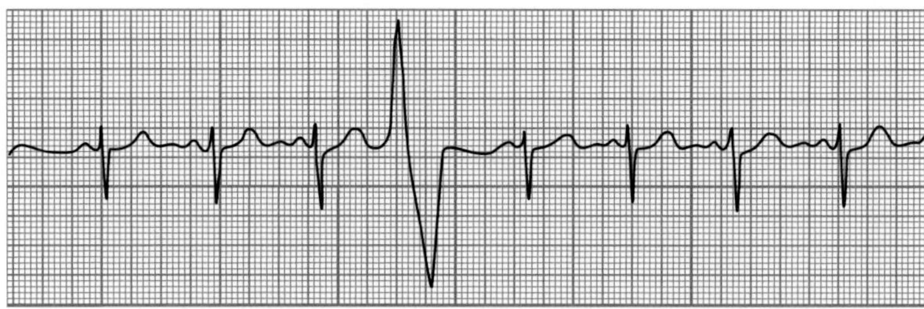

FIGURE 6-7 Premature ventricular contraction.

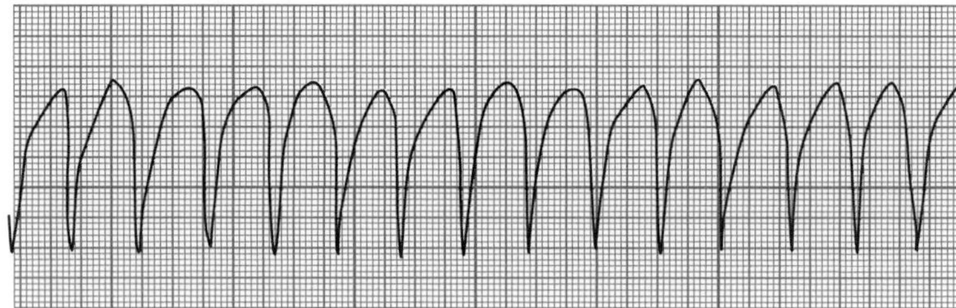

FIGURE 6-8 Ventricular tachycardia.

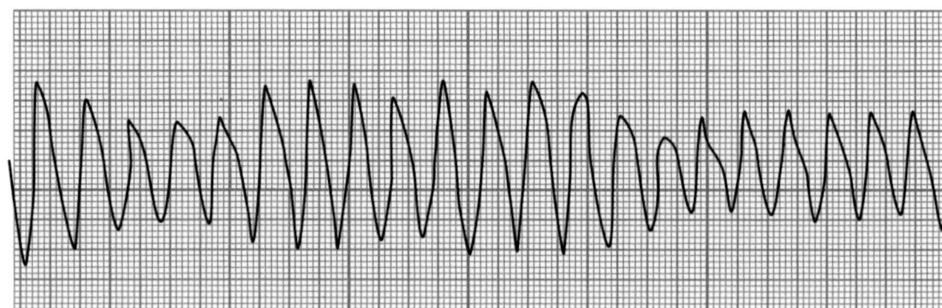

FIGURE 6-9 Ventricular flutter.

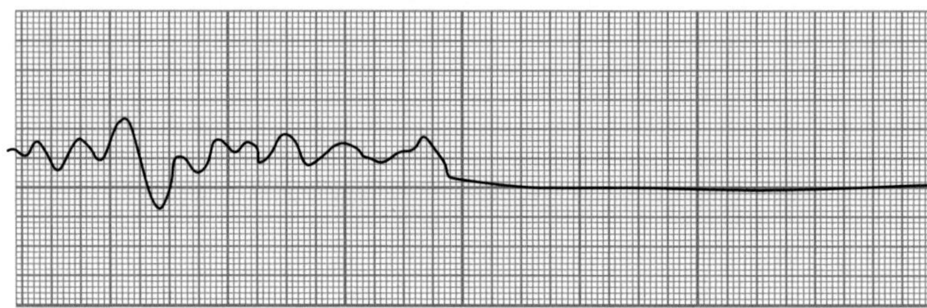

FIGURE 6-10 Ventricular fibrillation and asystole.

heartbeat (bigeminal PVCs), and after every two normal heartbeats (trigeminal PVCs). Common causes of PVCs include intrinsic myocardial disease, hypoxemia, acidemia, hypokalemia, and congestive heart failure. PVCs also may be a sign of theophylline or alpha- or beta-agonist toxicity.

Ventricular Tachycardia

In **ventricular tachycardia** the P wave is generally indiscernible, and the QRS complex is wide and bizarre in appearance (Figure 6-8). The T wave may not be separated from the QRS complex. The ventricular rate ranges from 150 to 250 bpm, and the rate is regular or slightly irregular. The patient's blood pressure is often decreased during ventricular tachycardia.

Ventricular Flutter

In **ventricular flutter** the QRS complex has the appearance of a wide sine wave (regular, smooth, rounded ventricular wave; Figure 6-9). The rhythm is regular or slightly irregular. The rate is 250 to 350 bpm. There is usually no discernible peripheral pulse associated with ventricular flutter.

Ventricular Fibrillation

Ventricular fibrillation is characterized by chaotic electrical activity and cardiac activity. The ventricles literally quiver out of control with no perfusion beat-producing rhythm (Figure 6-10). During ventricular fibrillation, there is no cardiac output or blood pressure, and the patient will die in minutes without treatment.

Asystole (Cardiac Standstill)

Asystole (cardiac standstill) is the complete absence of electrical and mechanical activity. As a result the cardiac output stops and the blood pressure falls to zero. The ECG tracing appears as a flat line and indicates severe damage to the heart's electrical conduction system (see Figure 6-10). Occasionally, periods of disorganized electrical and mechanical activity may be generated during long periods of asystole; this is referred to as an *agonal rhythm* or a *dying heart.*

Noninvasive Hemodynamic Monitoring Assessments

Hemodynamics is the study of forces that influence the circulation of blood. The general hemodynamic status of the patient can be monitored noninvasively at the bedside by assessing the heart rate (via an ECG monitor, auscultation, or pulse), blood pressure, and perfusion state. During the acute stages of respiratory disease, the patient frequently demonstrates the hemodynamic changes described in the following paragraphs.

Increased Heart Rate (Pulse), Cardiac Output, and Blood Pressure

Increased heart rate, pulse, and blood pressure develop frequently during the acute stages of pulmonary disease. This can result from the indirect response of the heart to hypoxic stimulation of the peripheral chemoreceptors, primarily the carotid bodies. When the carotid bodies are stimulated, reflex signals are sent to the respiratory muscles, which in turn activate the so-called *pulmonary reflex,* which triggers tachycardia and an increased cardiac output and blood pressure. The increased cardiac output is a compensatory mechanism that at least partially counteracts the hypoxemia produced by the pulmonary shunting in respiratory disorders.

This process is perhaps best understood by assuming that the body's oxygen use remains relatively constant over time. When the cardiac output increases during a period of steady metabolic requirements, oxygen transport increases, and the amount of oxygen extracted from each 100 mL of blood decreases. This results in an increase in the oxygen saturation of the returning venous blood, which in turn reduces the hypoxemia produced by the shunted blood. In other words, venous blood that perfuses underventilated alveoli will have less of a shunt effect if the oxygen content of the systemic venous blood is 13 vol% compared with, say, 10 vol%.

Other causes of increased heart rate, pulse, and blood pressure include severe anemia, high fever, anxiety, massive hemorrhage, certain cardiac arrhythmias, and hyperthyroidism. When the heart rate increases beyond 150 to 175 bpm, cardiac output and blood pressure begin to decline (the Starling relationship).

Decreased Perfusion State

The perfusion state can be evaluated by examining the patient's color, capillary refill, skin, and sensorium. Under normal conditions the patient's nail beds and oral mucosa are pink. If these areas appear cyanotic or mottled, poor perfusion and tissue hypoxia are likely present. When the nail beds are compressed to expel blood, they should normally refill quickly and turn pink when the pressure is released. If the nail beds remain white, perfusion is inadequate. Under normal conditions a patient's skin should be dry and warm. When the skin is diaphoretic (wet), cool, or clammy, local perfusion is inadequate. Finally, when the patient is disoriented as to person, place, and time, a decreased perfusion state and cerebral hypoxia may be present.

Invasive Hemodynamic Monitoring Assessments

Invasive hemodynamic monitoring is used in the assessment and treatment of critically ill patients. Invasive hemodynamic monitoring includes the measurement of (1) intracardiac pressures and flows via a **pulmonary artery catheter,** (2) arterial pressure via an **arterial catheter,** and (3) central venous pressure via a **central venous catheter**. Monitoring of these values provides rapid and precise measurements (assessment data) of the patient's cardiovascular function—which in turn are used to down-regulate or up-regulate the patient's treatment plan in a timely manner.

Pulmonary Artery Catheter

The pulmonary artery catheter (Swan-Ganz catheter) is a balloon-tipped, flow-directed catheter that is inserted at the patient's bedside; the respiratory care professional monitors the pressure waveform as the catheter, with the balloon inflated, is guided by blood flow through the right atrium and right ventricle into the pulmonary artery (Figure 6-11). The pulmonary artery catheter is used directly to measure the right atrial pressure (via the proximal port), pulmonary artery pressure (via the distal port), left atrial pressure (indirectly via the pulmonary capillary wedge pressure), and cardiac output (via the thermodilution technique).

Arterial Catheter

The arterial catheter (line) is the most commonly used mode of invasive hemodynamic monitoring. It is generally inserted in the radial artery for patient comfort and convenient access reasons. The indwelling arterial catheter allows (1) continuous and precise measurements of systolic, diastolic, and mean blood pressure; (2) accurate information regarding fluctuations in blood pressure; and (3) guidance in the decision to up-regulate or down-regulate therapy for hypotension or hypertension. The arterial catheter also is useful in patients who require frequent or repeated arterial blood gas samples (e.g., the patient being mechanically ventilated). The blood samples are readily available, and the patient is not subjected to the pain of repeated arterial punctures.

Central Venous Pressure Catheter

The **central venous pressure (CVP) catheter** readily measures the CVP and the right ventricular filling pressure. It serves as an excellent monitor of right ventricular function.

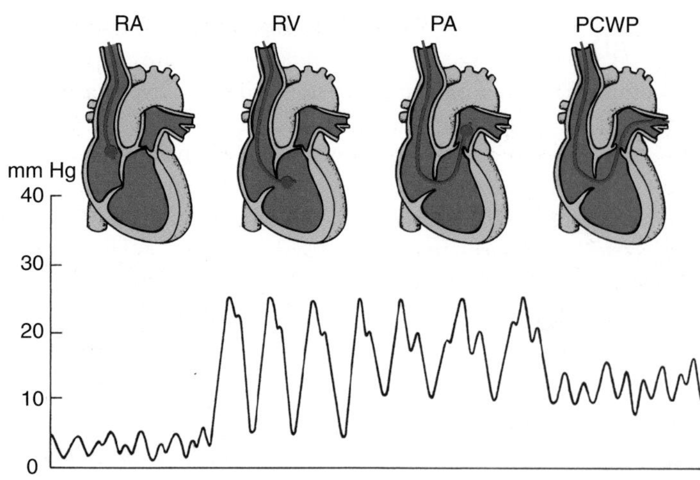

FIGURE 6-11 Insertion of the pulmonary catheter. The insertion site of the pulmonary catheter may be the basilic, brachial, femoral, subclavian, or internal insertion sites. As the catheter advances, pressure readings and waveforms are monitored to determine the catheter's position as it moves through the right atrium (RA), right ventricle (RV), pulmonary artery (PA), and finally into a pulmonary capillary wedge pressure (PCWP) position. Immediately after a PCWP reading, the balloon is deflated to allow blood to flow past the tip of the catheter. When the balloon is deflated, the catheter continuously monitors the pulmonary artery pressure.

An increased CVP reading is commonly seen in patients who (1) have left ventricular heart failure (e.g., pulmonary edema), (2) are receiving excessively high positive pressure mechanical breaths, (3) have cor pulmonale, or (4) have a severe flail chest, pneumothorax, or pleural effusion.

Table 6-1 summarizes the hemodynamic parameters that can be measured directly. Table 6-2 lists the hemodynamic parameters that can be calculated from results obtained from the direct measurements.

Hemodynamic Monitoring in Respiratory Diseases

Because respiratory disorders can have a profound effect on the structure and function of the pulmonary vascular bed, right side of the heart, left side of the heart, or a combination of all three, the data generated by the previously described invasive hemodynamic monitors are commonly used in the assessment and treatment of these patients. For example, respiratory diseases associated with severe or chronic hypoxemia, acidemia, or pulmonary vascular obstruction can increase the pulmonary vascular resistance (PVR) significantly. An increased PVR, in turn, can lead to a variety of secondary hemodynamic changes such as increased CVP, RAP, $\overline{PA}$, RVSWI, and decreased CO, SV, SVI, CI, and LVSWI (see Tables 6-1 and 6-2 for abbreviation definitions). Table 6-3 lists common hemodynamic changes seen in pulmonary diseases known to alter the patient's hemodynamic status.

TABLE 6-1 Hemodynamic Values Measured Directly

Hemodynamic Value	Abbreviation	Normal Range
Central venous pressure	CVP	0-8 mm Hg
Right atrial pressure	RAP	0-8 mm Hg
Mean pulmonary artery pressure	$\overline{PA}$	10-20 mm Hg
Pulmonary capillary wedge pressure (also called *pulmonary artery wedge; pulmonary artery occlusion*)	PCWP PAW PAO	4-12 mm Hg
Cardiac output	CO	4-6 L/min

TABLE 6-2 Hemodynamic Values Calculated from Direct Hemodynamic Measurements

Hemodynamic Value	Abbreviation	Normal Range
Stroke volume	SV	40-80 ml
Stroke volume index	SVI	40 ± ml/beat/m^2
Cardiac index	CI	3.0 ± 0.5 L/min/m^2
Right ventricular stroke work index	RVSWI	7-12 g/m^2
Left ventricular stroke work index	LVSWI	40-60 g/m^2
Pulmonary vascular resistance	PVR	50-150 dynes × sec × cm^{-5}
Systemic vascular resistance	SVR	800-1500 dynes × sec × cm^{-5}

TABLE 6-3 Hemodynamic Changes Commonly Seen in Respiratory Diseases

Disorder	Hemodynamic Indices											
	CVP	RAP	$\overline{PA}$	PCWP	CO	SV	SVI	CI	RVSWI	LVSWI	PVR	SVR
COPD Chronic bronchitis Emphysema Cystic fibrosis Bronchiectasis	↑	↑	↑↑	~*	~	~	~	~	↑	~	↑	~
Pulmonary edema (cardiogenic)	~	↑	↑	↑↑	↓	↓	↓	↓	↑	↓	↑	↓
Pulmonary embolism	↑	↑	↑↑	↓	↓	↓	↓	↓	↑	↓	↑	~
Adult respiratory distress syndrome (ARDS)—severe	~↑	~↑	~↑	~	~	~	~	~	~↑	~	~↑	~
Lung collapse Flail chest Pneumothorax Pleural disease (e.g., hemothorax)	↑	↑	↑	↓	↓	↓	↓	↓	↑	↓	↑	↓
Kyphoscoliosis	↑	↑	↑	~	~	~	~	~	↑	~	↑	~
Pneumoconiosis	↑	↑	↑↑	~	~	~	~	~	↑	~	↑	~
Chronic interstitial lung diseases	↑	↑	↑↑	~	~	~	~	~	↑	~	↑	~
Cancer of the lung (tumor mass)	↑	↑	↑	↓	↓	↓	↓	↓	↑	~	↑	~
Hypovolemia	↓↓	↓	↓	↓	↓	↓	↓	↓	↓	↓	~	↑
Hypervolemia (burns)	↑↑	↑	↑	↑	↑	↑	↑	↑	↑	↑	~	~
Right heart failure (cor pulmonale)	↑↑	↑↑	↓	↓	~	~	~	~	~	~	~	~

* ~, Unchanged.

SELF-ASSESSMENT QUESTIONS

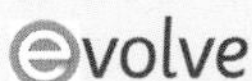

Answers to questions can be found on Evolve. To access additional student assessment questions and case studies for application of text material to real-life scenarios, visit **http://evolve.elsevier.com/DesJardins/respiratory.**

1. In which of the following arrhythmias is there no cardiac output or blood pressure?
  a. Ventricular flutter
  b. Arial fibrillation
  c. Premature ventricular contractions
  d. Ventricular fibrillation

2. The general hemodynamic status of the patient can be monitored noninvasively at the patient's bedside by assessing which of the following?
  1. Perfusion state
  2. Heart rate
  3. Pulse
  4. Blood pressure
    a. 4 only
    b. 2 and 3 only
    c. 2, 3, and 4 only
    d. 1, 2, 3, and 4

3. Cardiac output and blood pressure begin to decline when the heart rate increases beyond which of the following?
  a. 125 to 150 bpm
  b. 150 to 175 bpm
  c. 175 to 200 bpm
  d. 200 to 250 bpm

4. An increased CVP reading is commonly seen in the patient who:
  1. Has a severe pneumothorax
  2. Is receiving high positive pressure breaths
  3. Has cor pulmonale
  4. Is in left-sided heart failure
    a. 3 only
    b. 4 only
    c. 2, 3, and 4 only
    d. 1, 2, 3, and 4

5. What is the normal range of the mean pulmonary artery pressure?
  a. 0 to 5 mm Hg
  b. 5 to 10 mm Hg
  c. 10 to 20 mm Hg
  d. 20 to 30 mm Hg

6. What is the normal range for the PCWP?
a. 0 to 4 mm Hg
b. 4 to 12 mm Hg
c. 12 to 20 mm Hg
d. 20 to 25 mm Hg

7. The hemodynamic indices in patients with COPD commonly show which of the following?
1. Increased CVP
2. Decreased RAP
3. Increased $\overline{PA}$
4. Decreased PCWP
5. Increased CO
   a. 3 only
   b. 1 and 3 only
   c. 2 and 4 only
   d. 3, 4, and 5 only

8. The hemodynamic indices in patients with pulmonary edema commonly show which of the following?
1. Decreased CVP
2. Increased RAP
3. Decreased $\overline{PA}$
4. Increased PCWP
5. Decreased CO
   a. 1 and 3 only
   b. 2, 3, and 5 only
   c. 2, 4, and 5 only
   d. 1, 2, 4, and 5

9. Atrial flutter is defined as a constant atrial rate of:
a. 100 to 150 bpm
b. 150 to 250 bpm
c. 350 and 350 bpm
d. 350 and 350 bpm

10. In sinus arrhythmia, the heart rate varies by more than:
a. 5%
b. 10%
c. 15%
d. 20%

Radiologic Examination of the Chest 7

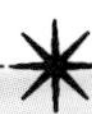

Chapter Objectives

After reading this chapter, you will be able to:

- Describe the fundamentals of radiography.
- Differentiate among the following standard positions and techniques of chest radiography:
  - Posteroanterior radiograph
  - Anteroposterior radiograph
  - Lateral radiograph
  - Lateral decubitus radiograph
- Define the following radiologic terms commonly used during inspection of the chest radiograph:
  - Air cyst
  - Bleb
  - Bronchogram
  - Bulla
  - Cavity
  - Consolidation
  - Homogeneous density
  - Honeycombing
  - Infiltrate
  - Interstitial density
  - Lesion
  - Opacity
  - Pleural density
  - Pulmonary mass
  - Pulmonary nodule
  - Radiodensity
  - Radiolucency
  - Translucent
- Describe the three steps to evaluate technical quality of the radiograph.
- Describe the sequence of examination, and include the following:
  - Mediastinum
  - Trachea
  - Heart
  - Hilar region
  - Lung parenchyma (tissue)
  - Pleura
  - Diaphragm
  - Gastric air bubble
  - Bony thorax
  - Extrathoracic soft tissues
- Describe the diagnostic values of the following radiologic procedures:
  - Computed tomography (CT)
  - Positron emission tomography (PET)
  - Positron emission tomography and computed tomography scan (PET/CT scan)
  - Magnetic resonance imaging (MRI)
  - Pulmonary angiography
  - Ventilation-perfusion scan
  - Fluoroscopy
  - Bronchography
- Define key terms and complete self-assessment questions at the end of the chapter and on Evolve.

Key Terms

Air Cyst
Anteroposterior (AP) Radiograph
Bleb
Bronchogram
Bronchography
Bulla
Cardiothoracic Ratio
Cavity
Computed Tomography (CT)
Consolidation
Fluoroscopy
High Resolution CT (HRCT) Scans
Homogeneous Density
Honeycombing
Infiltrates
Interstitial Density
Lateral Decubitus Radiograph
Lateral Radiograph
Lesion
Lung Window CT Scan
Magnetic Resonance Imaging (MRI)
Mediastinal Window CT Scan
Opacity
Pleural Density
Pleural Mass
Pleural Nodule
Positron Emission Tomography (PET)
Positron Emission Tomography and Computed Tomography Scan (PET/CT Scan)
Posteroanterior (PA) Projection
Pulmonary Angiography
Pulmonary Mass
Pulmonary Nodule
Radiodensity

Radiolucency
Translucent
Ventilation-Perfusion Scan

Chapter Outline

Radiography is the making of a photographic image of the internal structures of the body by passing x-rays through the body to an x-ray film, or radiograph. In patients with respiratory disease, radiography plays an important role in the diagnosis of lung disorders, the assessment of the extent and location of the disease, and the evaluation of the subsequent progress of the disease.

Fundamentals of Radiography

X-rays are created when fast-moving electrons with sufficient energy collide with matter in any form. Clinically, x-rays are produced by an electronic device called an *x-ray tube.*

The x-ray tube is a vacuum-sealed glass tube that contains a cathode and a rotating anode. A tungsten plate approximately ½-inch square is fixed to the end of the rotating anode at the center of the tube. This tungsten block is called the *target.* Tungsten is an effective target metal because of its high melting point, which can withstand the extreme heat to which it is subjected, and because of its high atomic number, which makes it more effective in the production of x-rays.

When the cathode is heated, electrons "boil off." When a high voltage (70 to 150 kV) is applied to the x-ray tube, the electrons are driven to the rotating anode where they strike the tungsten target with tremendous energy. The sudden deceleration of the electrons at the tungsten plate converts energy to x-rays. Although most of the electron energy is converted to heat, a small amount (less than 1%) is transformed to x-rays and allowed to escape from the tube through a set of lead shutters called a *collimator.* From the collimator the x-rays travel through the patient to the x-ray film.

The ability of the x-rays to penetrate matter depends on the density of the matter. For chest radiographs the x-rays may pass through bone, air, soft tissue, and fat. Dense objects such as bone absorb more x-rays (preventing penetration) than objects that are not as dense, such as the air-filled lungs.

After passing through the patient, the x-rays strike the x-ray film. X-rays that pass through low-density objects strike the film at full force and produce a black image on the film. X-rays that are absorbed by high-density objects (such as bone) either do not reach the film at all or strike the film with less force. Relative to the density of the object, these objects appear as light gray to white on the film.

Standard Positions and Techniques of Chest Radiography

Clinically, the standard radiograph of the chest includes two views: a **posteroanterior (PA) projection** and a lateral projection (either a left or right **lateral radiograph**) with the patient in the standing position. When the patient is seriously ill or immobilized, an upright radiograph may not be possible. In such cases a supine **anteroposterior (AP) radiograph** is obtained at the patient's bedside. A lateral radiograph is rarely obtainable under such circumstances.

Posteroanterior Radiograph

The standard PA chest radiograph is obtained by having the patient stand (or sit) in the upright position. The anterior aspect of the patient's chest is pressed against a film cassette holder, with the shoulders rotated forward to move the scapulae away from the lung fields. The distance between the x-ray tube and the film is 6 feet. The x-ray beam travels from the x-ray tube, through the patient, and to the x-ray film.

The x-ray examination is usually performed with the patient's lungs in full inspiration to show the lung fields and related structures to their greatest possible extent. At full inspiration the diaphragm is lowered to approximately the level of the ninth to eleventh ribs posteriorly (Figure 7-1). For certain clinical conditions, radiographs are sometimes taken at the end of both inspiration and expiration. For example, in patients with obstructive lung disease an expiratory radiograph may be made to evaluate diaphragmatic excursion and the symmetry or asymmetry of such excursion (Figure 7-2).

Anteroposterior Radiograph

The supine AP radiograph may be taken in patients who are debilitated, immobilized, or too young to tolerate the PA procedure. The AP radiograph is usually taken with a portable x-ray machine at the patient's bedside. The film is placed behind the patient's back, with the x-ray machine positioned in front of the patient approximately 48 inches from the film.

Compared with the PA radiograph, the AP radiograph has a number of disadvantages. For example, the heart and superior portion of the mediastinum are significantly magnified in the AP radiograph. This is because the heart is

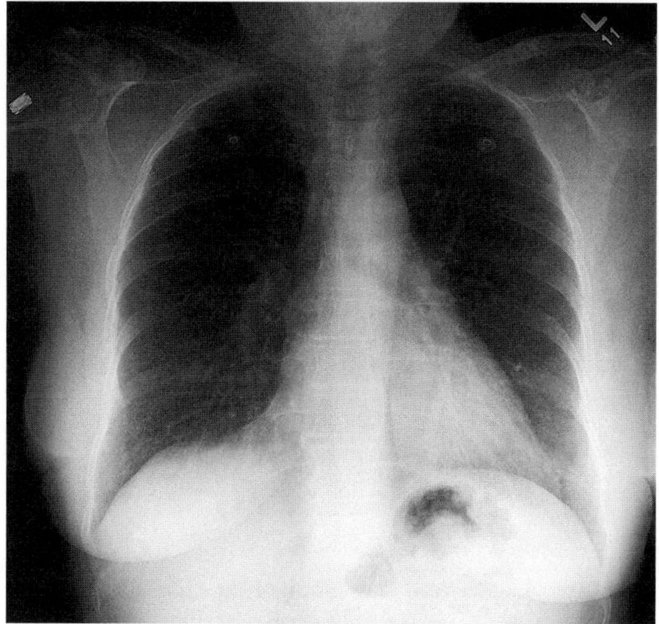

FIGURE 7-1 Standard posteroanterior chest radiograph with the patient's lungs in full inspiration.

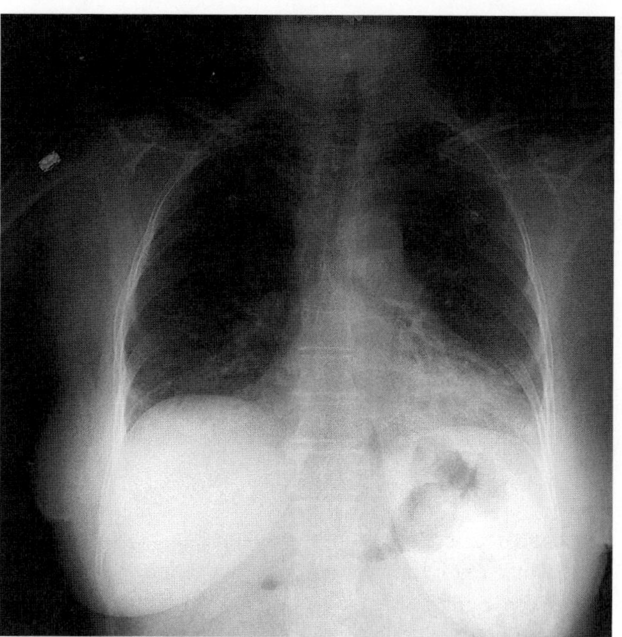

FIGURE 7-2 A posteroanterior chest radiograph of the same patient shown in Figure 7-1 during expiration.

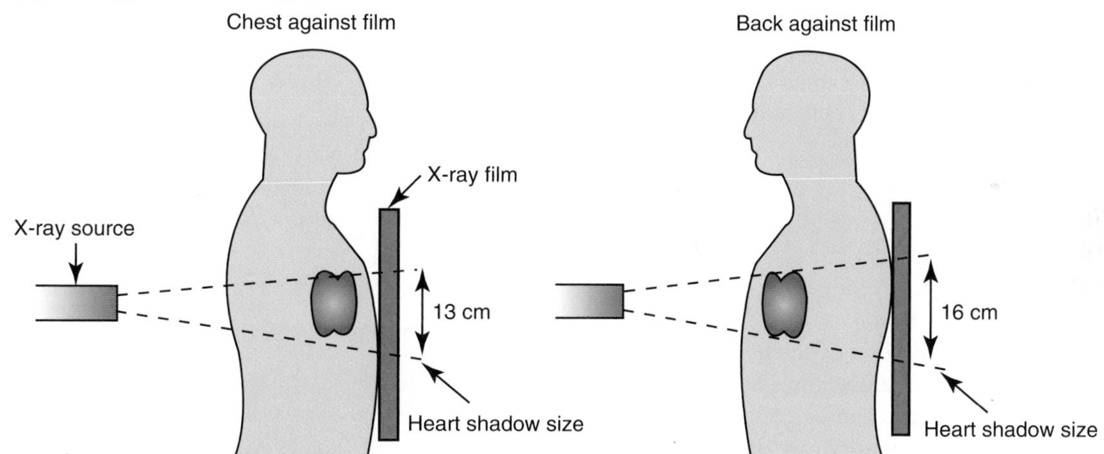

FIGURE 7-3 Compared with the posteroanterior (PA) chest radiograph, the heart is significantly magnified in the anteroposterior (AP) chest radiograph. In the PA radiograph the ratio of the width of the heart to the thorax is normally less than 1 : 2. The reason the heart appears larger in the AP radiograph is that it is positioned in front of the thorax as the x-ray beams pass through the chest in the anterior-to-posterior direction. This allows more space for the heart shadow to "fan out" before it reaches the x-ray film.

positioned in front of the thorax as the x-ray beams pass through the chest in the anterior-to-posterior direction, causing the image of the heart to be enlarged (Figure 7-3).

The AP radiograph also often has less resolution and more distortion. Because the patient is often unable to sustain a maximal inspiration, the lower lung lobes frequently appear hazy, erroneously suggesting pulmonary congestion or pleural effusion. Finally, because the AP radiograph is often taken in the intensive care unit, extraneous shadows, such as those produced by ventilator tubing and indwelling lines, are often present (Figure 7-4).

Lateral Radiograph

The lateral radiograph is obtained to complement the PA radiograph. It is taken with the side of the patient's chest compressed against the cassette. The patient's arms are raised, with the forearms resting on the head.

To view the right lung and heart, the patient's right side is placed against the cassette. To view the left lung and heart, the patient's left side is placed against the cassette. Therefore a right lateral radiograph would be selected to view a density or **lesion** that is known to be in the right lung. If neither lung is of particular interest, a left lateral radiograph is usually

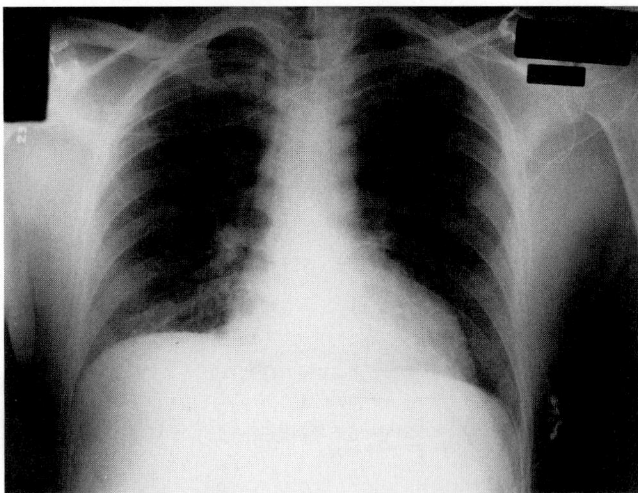

FIGURE 7-4 Anteroposterior (AP) chest radiograph. The diaphragms are elevated, the lower lung lobes appear hazy, the ratio of the width of the heart to the thorax is greater than 2 : 1, and extraneous lines are apparent on the patient's left side. X-ray examinations using portable machines are frequently performed on patients too ill to be transported to the radiology department. These films, in the best of circumstances, are of poorer quality than erect films taken with standard x-ray apparatus. The films are usually AP projections taken with the x-ray unit in front of and the film plate behind the patient. Overexposure, underexposure, malpositioning, marginal cutoffs, and motion artifacts are often present. In this setting, major events such as partial pneumothoraces, pleural effusions, and infiltrates in dependent parts of the lung may go unrecognized. Therefore careful clinical correlation with the patient's pathophysiology and symptomatology is imperative.

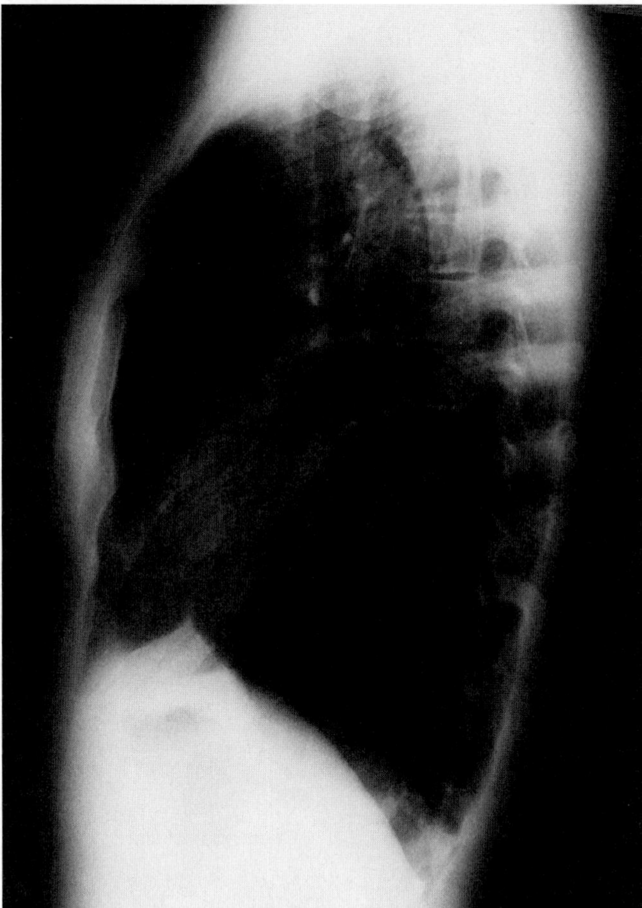

FIGURE 7-5 Lateral radiograph. The patient has an overexpanded lung and chest wall (barrel chest deformity) consistent with his known emphysema.

selected to reduce the magnification of the heart. The lateral radiograph provides a view of the structures behind the heart and diaphragmatic dome. It also can be combined with the PA radiograph to give the respiratory care provider a three-dimensional view of the structures or of any abnormal densities (Figure 7-5).

Lateral Decubitus Radiograph

The **lateral decubitus radiograph** is obtained by having the patient lie on the left or right side rather than standing or sitting in the upright position. The naming of the decubitus radiograph is determined by the side on which the patient lies; thus a right lateral decubitus radiograph means that the patient's right side is down.

The lateral decubitus radiograph is useful in the diagnosis of a suspected or known fluid accumulation in the pleural space (pleural effusion) that is not easily seen in the PA radiograph. A pleural effusion, which is usually more thinly spread out over the diaphragm in the upright position, collects in the gravity-dependent areas while the patient is in the lateral decubitus position, allowing the fluid to be more readily seen (Figure 7-6).

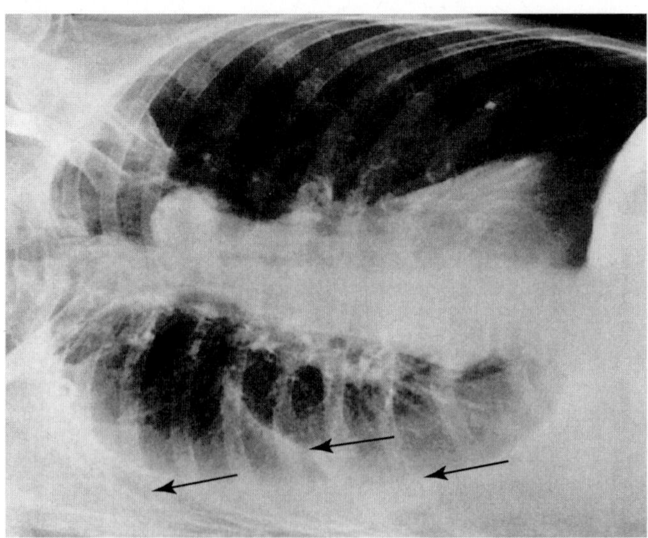

FIGURE 7-6 Subpulmonic pleural effusion. Right lateral decubitus view. Subdiaphragmatic fluid has run up the lateral chest wall, producing a band of soft tissue density. The medial curvilinear shadow *(arrows)* indicates fluid in the lips of the major fissure.

Inspecting the Chest Radiograph

Before the respiratory care practitioner can effectively identify abnormalities on a chest radiograph, he or she must be able to recognize the normal anatomic structures. Figure 7-7 represents a normal PA chest radiograph with identification of important anatomic landmarks. Figure 7-8 labels the anatomic structures seen on a lateral chest radiograph.

Table 7-1 lists some of the more important radiologic terms used to describe abnormal lung findings.

Technical Quality of the Radiograph

The first step in examining a chest radiograph is to evaluate its technical quality. Was the patient in the correct position when the radiograph was taken? To verify the proper position, check the relationship of the medial ends of the clavicles to the vertebral column. For the PA radiograph the vertebral column should be precisely in the center between the medial ends of the clavicles, and the distance between the right and left costophrenic angles and the spine should be equal. Even a small degree of patient rotation relative to the film can create a false image, erroneously suggesting tracheal deviation, cardiac displacement, or cardiac enlargement.

Second, the exposure quality of the radiograph should be evaluated. Normal exposure is verified by determining whether the spinal processes of the vertebrae are visible to the fifth or sixth thoracic level (T-5 to T-6). X-ray equipment is now available that allows the vertebrae to be seen down to the level of the cardiac shadow. The degree of exposure can be evaluated further by comparing the relative densities of the heart and lungs. For example, because the heart has a greater density than the air-filled lungs, the heart appears whiter than the lung fields. The heart and lungs become more radiolucent (darker) with greater exposure of the radiograph. A radiograph that has been overexposed is said to be "heavily penetrated" or "burned out." Conversely, the heart and lungs on an underexposed radiograph may appear denser and whiter. The lungs may erroneously appear to have **infiltrates,** and there may be little or no visibility of the thoracic vertebrae.

Third, the level of inspiration at the moment the radiograph was taken should be evaluated. At full inspiration the diaphragmatic domes should be at the level of the ninth to eleventh ribs posteriorly. On radiographs taken during expiration, the lungs appear denser, the diaphragm is elevated, and the heart appears wider and enlarged (see Figure 7-2).

Sequence of Examination

Although the precise sequence in examining a chest radiograph is not important, the inspection should be done in a

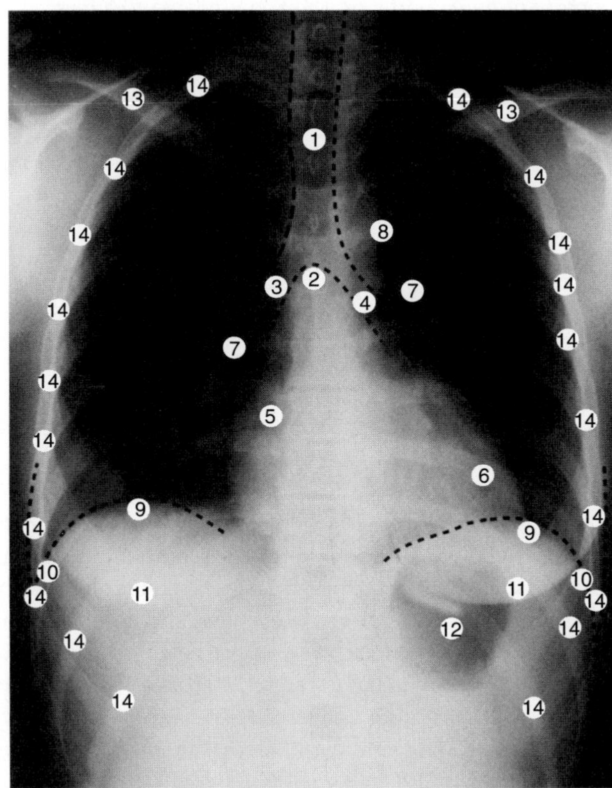

FIGURE 7-7 Normal posteroanterior (PA) chest radiograph. *1,* Trachea (note vertebral column in middle of trachea); *2,* carina; *3,* right main stem bronchus; *4,* left main stem bronchus; *5,* right atrium; *6,* left ventricle; *7,* hilar vasculature; *8,* aortic knob; *9,* diaphragm; *10,* costophrenic angles; *11,* breast shadows; *12,* gastric air bubble; *13,* clavicle; *14,* rib.

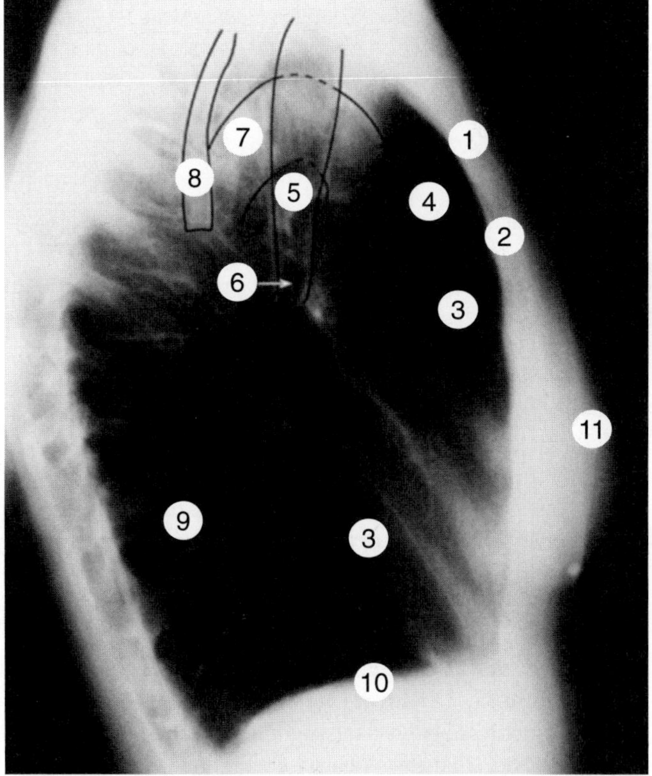

FIGURE 7-8 Normal lateral chest radiograph. *1,* Manubrium; *2,* sternum; *3,* cardiac shadow; *4,* retrosternal air space in the lung; *5,* trachea; *6,* bronchus, on end; *7,* aortic arch (ascending and descending); *8,* scapulae; *9,* vertebral column; *10,* diaphragm; *11,* breast shadow.

TABLE 7-1 Common Radiologic Terms

Term	Definition
Air cyst	A thin-walled radiolucent area surrounded by normal lung tissue
Bleb	A superficial air cyst protruding into the pleura; also called *bulla*
Bronchogram	An outline of air-containing bronchi beyond the normal point of visibility. An air bronchogram develops as a result of an infiltration or consolidation that surrounds the bronchi, producing a contrasting air column on the radiograph—that is, the bronchi appear as dark tubes surrounded by a white area produced by the infiltration or consolidation
Bulla	A large, thin-walled radiolucent area surrounded by normal lung tissue
Cavity	A radiolucent (dark) area surrounded by dense tissue (white). A cavity is the hallmark of a lung abscess. A fluid level may be seen inside a cavity
Consolidation	The act of becoming solid; commonly used to describe the solidification of the lung caused by a pathologic engorgement of the alveoli, as occurs in acute pneumonia
Homogeneous density	Refers to a uniformly dense lesion (white area); commonly used to describe solid tumors, fluid-containing cavities, or fluid in the pleural space
Honeycombing	A coarse reticular (netlike) density commonly seen in pneumoconiosis
Infiltrate	Any poorly defined radiodensity (white area); commonly used to describe an inflammatory lesion
Interstitial density	A density caused by interstitial thickening
Lesion	Any pathologic or traumatic alteration of tissue or loss of function of a part
Opacity	State of being opaque (white); an opaque area or spot; impervious to light rays, or by extension, X-rays; opposite of translucent or radiolucent
Pleural density	A radiodensity caused by fluid, tumor, inflammation, or scarring
Pulmonary mass	A lesion in the lung that is 6 cm or more in diameter; commonly used to describe a pulmonary tumor
Pulmonary nodule	A lesion in the lung that is less than 6 cm in diameter and composed of dense tissue; also called a *solitary pulmonary nodule* or *"coin" lesion* because of its rounded, coinlike appearance
Radiodensity	Dense areas that appear white on the radiograph; the opposite of radiolucency
Radiolucency	The state of being radiolucent; the property of being partly or wholly permeable to X-rays; commonly used to describe darker areas on a radiograph such as an emphysematous lung or a pneumothorax
Translucent	Permitting the passage of light; commonly used to describe darker areas of the radiograph

systematic fashion. Some practitioners prefer an "inside-out" approach to inspecting the chest radiograph, which entails beginning with the mediastinum and proceeding outward to the extrathoracic soft tissue. Some practitioners prefer the reverse. The following is an "inside-out" method.

Mediastinum

The mediastinum should be inspected for width, contour, and shifts from the midline. The respiratory care practitioner should inspect the anatomy of the mediastinum, including the trachea, carina, cardiac borders, aortic arch, and superior vena cava (see Figure 7-7).

Trachea

On the PA projection the trachea should appear as a **translucent column** overlying the vertebral column. The diameter of the bronchi progressively tapers a short distance beyond the carina and then disappears (see Figure 7-7). A number of clinical conditions can cause the trachea to shift from its normal position. For example, fluid or gas accumulation in the pleural space causes the trachea to shift away from the affected area. Lung collapse or fibrosis usually causes the trachea to shift toward the affected area. The trachea also may be displaced by tumors of the upper lung regions.

Anatomic structures in the chest (e.g., the trachea) move out of their normal position because they are either pushed or pulled in a given direction. In other words, they may be moved up or down or from side to side by lesions pulling or pushing in that direction. Table 7-2 lists examples of factors that push or pull the trachea out of its normal position in the chest radiograph.

Heart

On the PA projection the ratio of the width of the heart to the thorax (the **cardiothoracic ratio**) is normally less than 1 : 2. A small portion of the heart should be visible on the right side of the vertebral column. Two bulges should be seen on the right border of the heart. The upper bulge is the superior vena cava; the lower bulge is the right atrium. Three bulges are normally seen on the left side of the heart. The superior bulge is the aorta, the middle bulge is the main pulmonary artery, and the inferior bulge is the left ventricle (see Figure 7-7). See Table 7-2 for examples of factors that push or pull the heart out of its normal position in the chest radiograph.

Hilar Region

The right and left hilar regions should be evaluated for change in size or position. Normally the left hilum is about

TABLE 7-2 Examples of Factors That Pull or Push Anatomic Structures out of Their Normal Position in the Chest Radiograph

Structure	Examples of Abnormal Position	Lesion
Mediastinum and hilar region Trachea Carina Heart Major vessels	Leftward shift	Pulled left by upper lobe tuberculosis, atelectasis, or fibrosis Pushed left by right upper lobe emphysematous bulla, fluid, gas, or tumor
Left diaphragm	Upward shift	Pulled up by left lower lobe atelectasis or fibrosis Pushed up by distended gastric air bubble
Horizontal fissure	Downward shift	Pulled down by right middle lobe or right lower lobe atelectasis Pushed down by right upper lobe neoplasm
Left lung	Rightward shift	Pulled right by right lung collapse, atelectasis, or fibrosis Pushed right by left-sided tension pneumothorax or hemothorax

2 cm higher than the right (see Figure 7-7). An increased density of the hilar region may indicate engorgement of hilar vessels caused by increased pulmonary vascular resistance. Vertical displacement of the hilum suggests volume loss from one or more upper lobes of the lung on the affected side. In infectious lung disorders such as histoplasmosis or tuberculosis the lymph nodes around the hilar region are often enlarged, calcified, or both. Malignant pulmonary lesions, including hilar malignant lymphadenopathy, also may be seen. See Table 7-2 for additional factors that push or pull the hilar region out of its normal position in the chest radiograph.

Lung Parenchyma (Tissue)

The lungs parenchyma should be examined systematically from top to bottom, one lung compared with the other. Normally, tissue markings can be seen throughout the lungs (see Figure 7-7). The absence of tissue markings may suggest a pneumothorax, recent pneumonectomy, or chronic obstructive lung disease (e.g., emphysema) or may be the result of an overexposed radiograph. An excessive amount of tissue markings may indicate fibrosis, interstitial or alveolar edema, lung compression, or an underexposed radiograph. The periphery of the lung fields should be inspected for abnormalities that obscure the lung's interface with the pleural space, mediastinum, or diaphragm. See Table 7-2 for additional examples of factors that push or pull the lung tissue out of its normal position in the chest radiograph.

Pleura

The peripheral borders of the lungs should be examined for pleural thickening, presence of fluid (pleural effusion) or air (pneumothorax) in the pleural space, or mass lesions (see Figure 7-7). The costophrenic angles should be inspected. Blunting of the costophrenic angle suggests the presence of fluid. A lateral decubitus radiograph may be required to confirm the presence of fluid (see Figure 7-6).

Diaphragms

Both the right and left hemidiaphragms should have an upwardly convex, dome-shaped contour. The right and left costophrenic angles should be clear. Normally, the right diaphragm is about 2 cm higher than the left because of the liver below it (see Figure 7-7). Chronic obstructive pulmonary diseases (e.g., emphysema) and diseases that cause gas or fluid to accumulate in the pleural space flatten and depress the normal curvature of the diaphragm. Abnormal elevation of one diaphragm may result from excessive gas in the stomach, collapse of the middle or lower lobe on the affected side, pulmonary infection at the lung bases, phrenic nerve damage, or spinal curvature. See Table 7-2 for additional examples of factors that push or pull the diaphragm out of its normal position in the chest radiograph.

Gastric Air Bubble

The area below the diaphragm should be inspected. A stomach air bubble is commonly seen under the left hemidiaphragm (see Figure 7-7). Free air may appear under either diaphragm after abdominal surgery or in patients with peritoneal abscess.

Bony Thorax

The ribs, vertebrae, clavicles, sternum, and scapulae should be inspected. The intercostal spaces should be symmetric and equal over each lung field (see Figure 7-7). Intercostal spaces that are too close together suggest a loss of muscle tone, commonly seen in patients with paralysis involving one side of the chest. In chronic obstructive pulmonary disease the intercostal spaces are generally far apart because of alveolar hyperinflation. Finally, the ribs should be inspected for deformities or fractures. If a rib fracture is suspected but not seen on the standard chest radiograph, a special rib series (radiographs that focus on the ribs) may be necessary.

Extrathoracic Soft Tissues

The soft tissue external to the bony thorax should be closely inspected. If the patient is a female, the outer boundaries of the breast shadows should be identified (see Figure 7-7). If the patient has undergone a mastectomy, there will be a relative hyperlucency on the side of the mastectomy. Large breasts can create a significant amount of haziness over the lower lung fields, giving the false appearance of pneumonia or pulmonary congestion. Although nipple shadows are easily identified when they are bilaterally symmetric, one may become less visible when the patient is slightly rotated. The other nipple then appears abnormally opaque and may be mistaken for a **pulmonary nodule.** After a tracheostomy or pneumothorax, subcutaneous air bubbles (called *subcutaneous emphysema*) often form in the soft tissue, especially if the patient is on a positive-pressure ventilator.

Computed Tomography

The same basic principles used in film radiography apply to **computed tomography (CT)** scanning—namely the absorption of x-rays by tissues that contain anatomic structures and organs of different atomic number. A CT scan provides a series of cross-sectional (transverse) pictures (called *tomograms*) of the structures within the body at numerous levels. The procedure is painless and noninvasive and requires no special preparation. The patient simply lies on the examination table, and this moves the patient through the opening of the CT scanner. The major components of a CT scanner are (1) an x-ray tube, which rotates in a continuous 360-degree motion around the patient to image the body in cross-sectional slices; (2) an array of x-ray detectors opposite the x-ray tube, which record the x-rays that pass through the body; and (3) a computer, which converts the different x-ray absorption levels to cross-sectional images based on the density of the structures being scanned. This cross-sectional slice is called an *axial view,* or *computerized axial tomogram* (Figure 7-9).

Up to 250 images, approximately 1 mm apart, can be generated on a chest CT scan. These "cuts" are often called **high resolution CT (HRCT) scans** (also called *spiral, volume,* or *helical scans*). In essence, each CT scan provides an image of what a "slice" through the body looks like at specific points—similar to cutting a piece of fruit in half and viewing the cross-section of the structures inside the fruit. Dense structures, such as bone, appear white on the tomogram, whereas structures with a relatively low density, such as the lungs, appear dark or black. Therefore a dense tumor in the lungs would appear as a white object surrounded by dark lungs.

The resolution of a CT scan can be adjusted to primarily view (1) lung tissue—commonly called a **lung window CT scan**—or (2) bone and mediastinal structures—commonly called a **mediastinal window CT scan.** In a mediastinal window CT scan, the lung tissue is overexposed and appears mostly black; the bones and mediastinal organs appear mostly white. Figure 7-10 provides an overview of a normal lung window CT scan. Figure 7-11 shows a close-up of one "slice" of a normal lung window CT scan. Figure 7-12 provides a close-up view of one slice of a normal mediastinal window CT scan.

Finally, for poorly defined lesions evident on the standard radiograph, the CT scan is a useful supplement in determining the precise location, size, and shape of the lesion. The CT scan is especially helpful in confirming the presence of a mediastinal mass, small pulmonary nodules, small lesions of the bronchi, pulmonary cavities, a small pneumothorax, pleural effusion, and small tumors (as small as 0.3 to 0.5 cm). The CT scan can be done with contrast material in the vessels to delineate vascular structures.

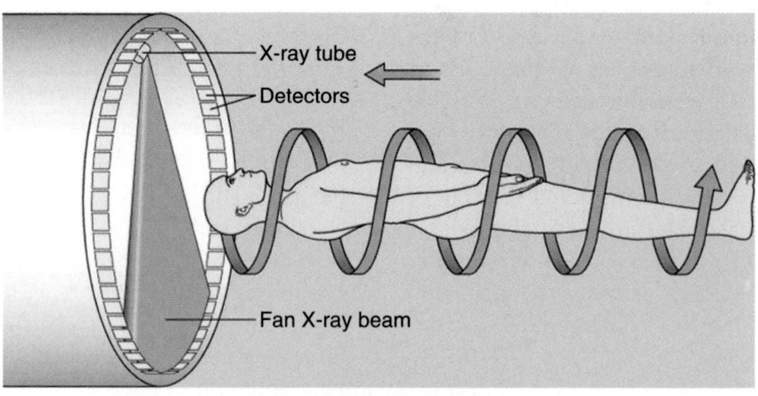

FIGURE 7-9 The principle of spiral computed tomography. The patient moves into the scanner with the x-ray tube continuously rotating and the detectors acquiring information. The rapidity of data acquisition allows a complete examination of the thorax to be performed in a single breath hold. (From Albert RK, Spiro SG, Jett JR: *Clinical respiratory medicine,* ed 3, St Louis, 2008, Mosby.)

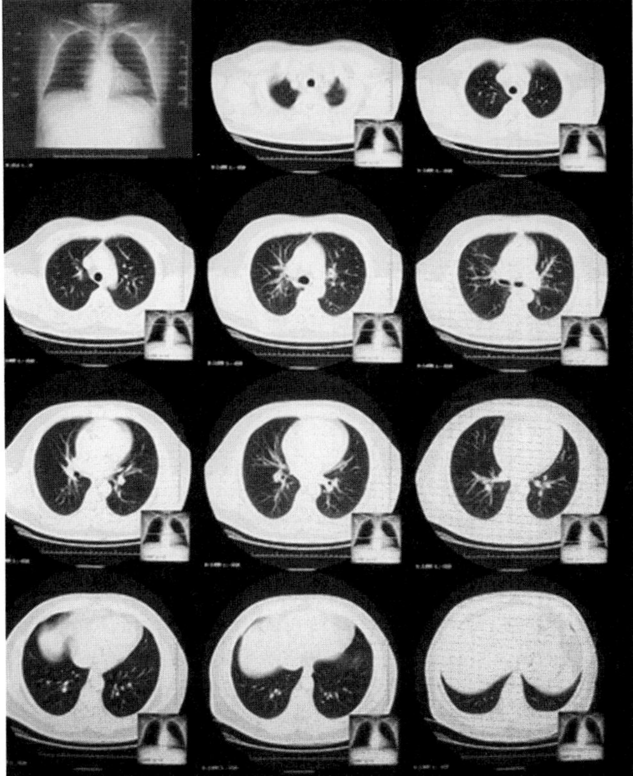

FIGURE 7-10 Overview of normal lung window computed tomography (CT) scan. The apex appears in the two views in the upper right hand corner of this figure; the diaphragm at the base of the lungs appears in the lower right hand view.

Positron Emission Tomography

The **positron emission tomography (PET)** scan shows both the anatomic structures and the metabolic activity of the tissues and organs scanned. Used in conjunction with a chest x-ray and CT scan for comparison, the PET scan is an excellent diagnostic tool for early detection of cancerous lesions. The unique aspect of the PET scan is its ability to evaluate the metabolic rate of certain tissue cells that may be cancerous. In other words, the PET scan is able to detect cancerous cells in the tissues of the body before changes develop in the anatomic shape of the organ.

Before undergoing the scan, the patient is injected intravenously (IV) with a solution of glucose that has been tagged with a radioactive chemical isotope (generally fluorine-18 fluorodeoxyglucose, or F18-FDG compound). Cancer cells metabolize glucose at extremely high rates. The PET scan measures the way cells burn glucose. When present, the cancer cells rapidly consume the tagged glucose. As the glucose molecules break down, end products that emit positrons are produced. The positrons collide with electrons that give off gamma rays. The gamma rays are converted to dark spots on the PET scan image. These dark spots are commonly referred to as "hot spots." The presence of a hot spot on a PET scan likely confirms a rapidly growing tumor.

Clinically, a PET scan is an excellent tool to rule out suspicious findings (i.e., a possible cancerous area) that are identified on either the chest radiograph or CT scan. For

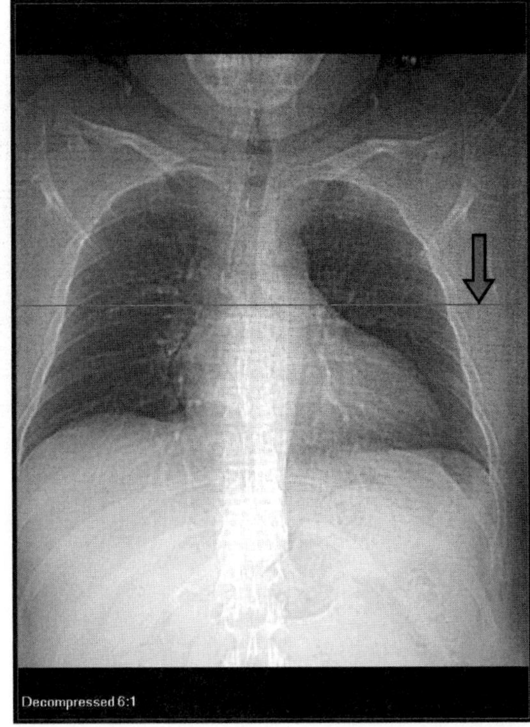

A

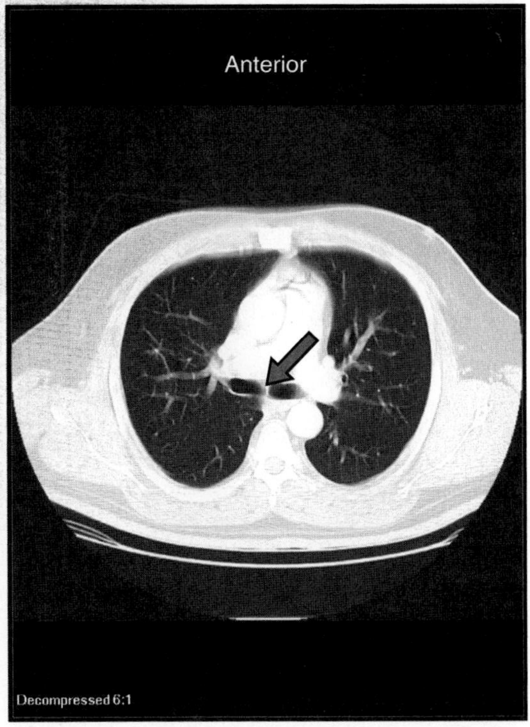

B

FIGURE 7-11 Close-up of a normal lung window computed tomography (CT) scan. **A,** The portion of the chest undergoing CT scanning. **B,** The actual cross-sectional slice, or axial view of the chest. Note the carina and both mainstem bronchi (arrow).

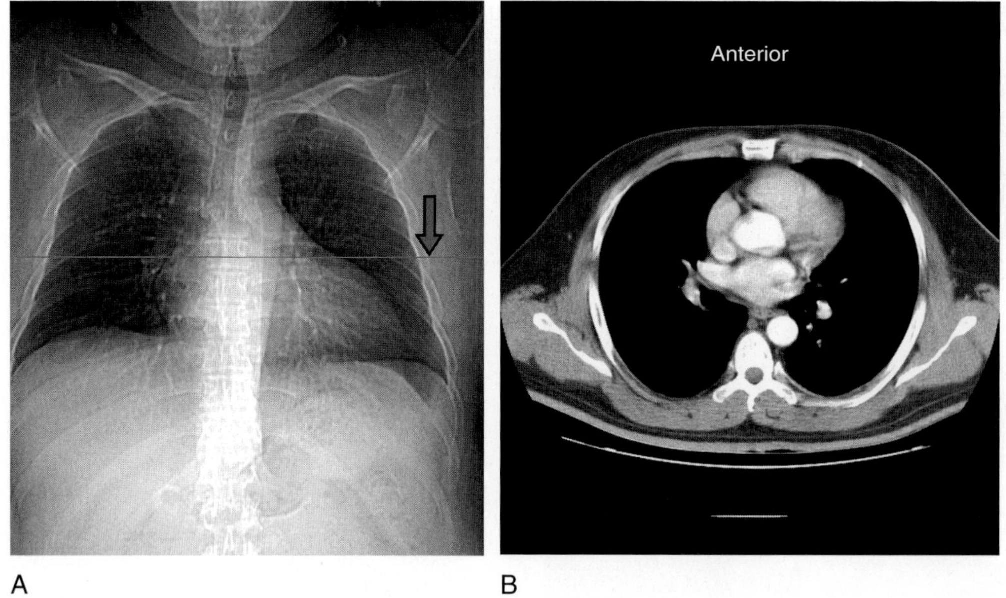

FIGURE 7-12 Close up of normal computed tomography (CT) mediastinal window. **A**, The portion of the chest the CT scan is taken. **B**, The actual cross-sectional slice, or axial view of the chest. Note that the lungs are overexposed and appear mostly black. The bone and mediastinal organs appear mostly white.

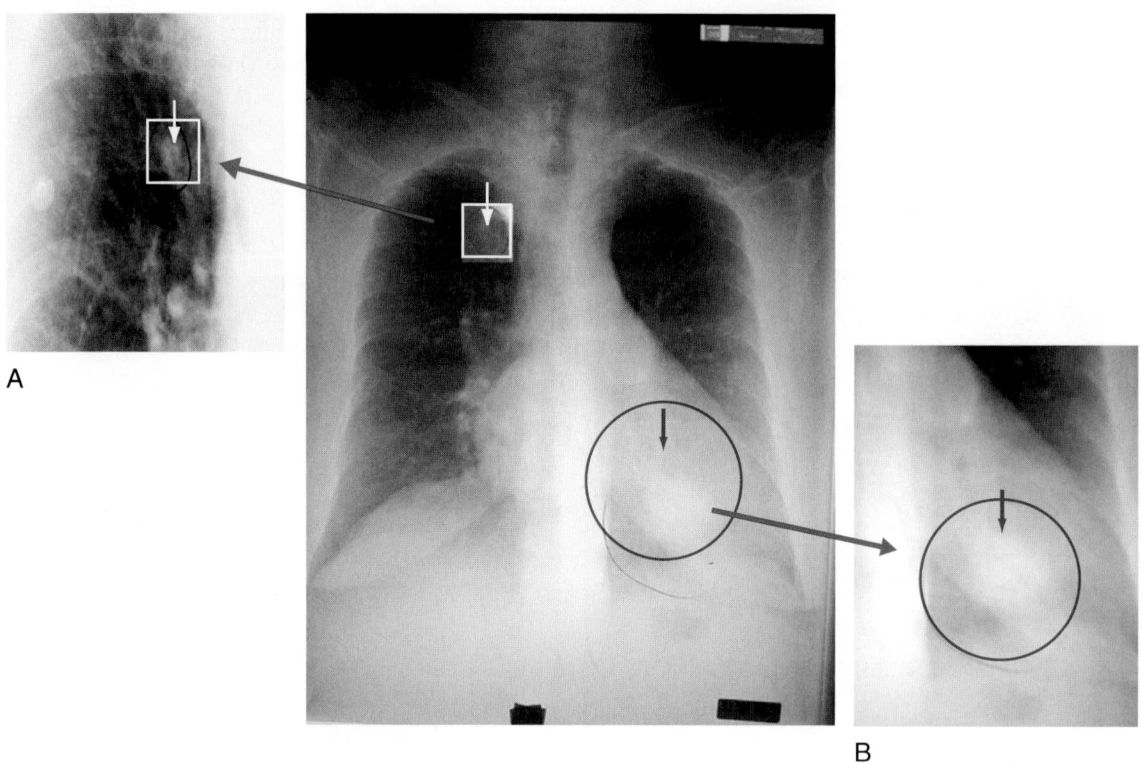

FIGURE 7-13 Chest radiograph identifying two suspicious findings: in the right upper lobe (**A**) and in the left lower lobe (**B**), just behind the heart *(white arrows)*.

example, Figure 7-13 shows a chest radiograph that identifies two suspicious findings—one small nodule in the right upper lung lobe and a larger density in the left lower lung lobe, just behind the heart. Figure 7-14 shows two CT scans that also identify the two suspicious findings and their precise location. Figures 7-15, 7-16 and 7-17 show PET scans that all confirm a hot spot (likely cancer) in the lower left lobe. However, the PET scan shown in Figure 7-18 confirms that the nodule in the right upper lobe is benign (i.e., no hot spot noted).

Although the PET scan is relatively painless (i.e., tantamount to intravenous insertion), it is lengthy. It may take up to 90 minutes to complete the scan. After the injection, the patient quietly rests in a reclining chair for 30 to 60 minutes

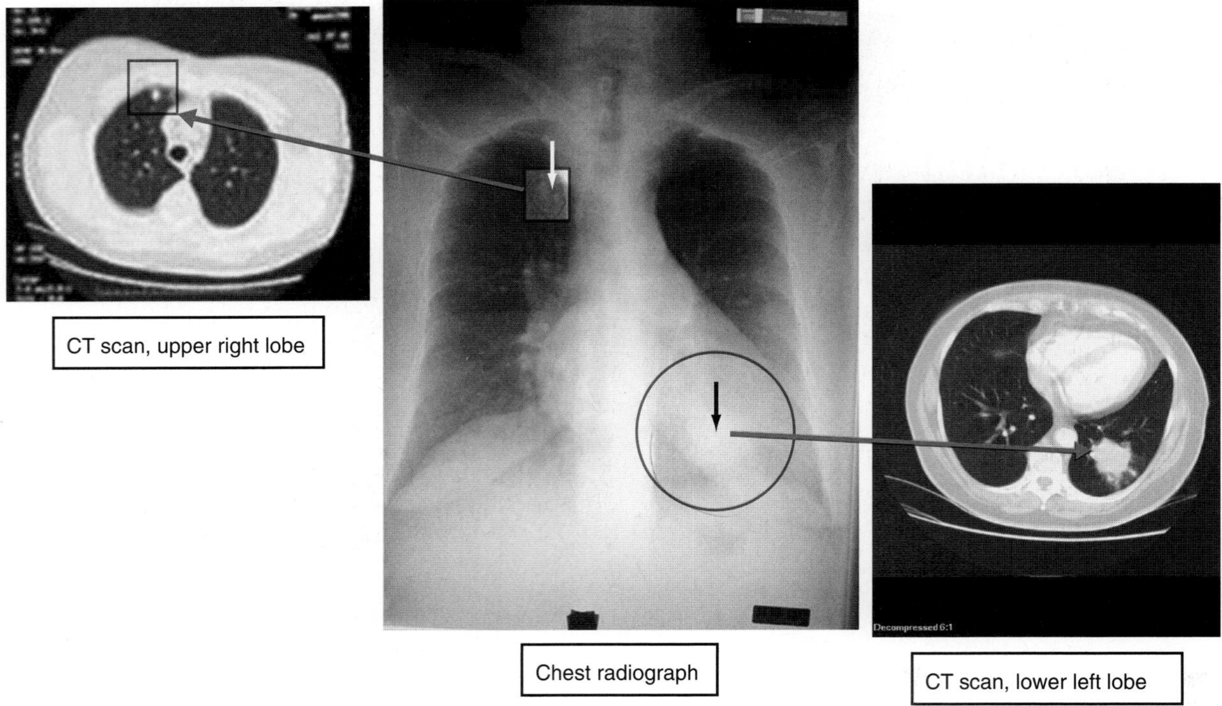

FIGURE 7-14 Same chest radiograph as shown in Figure 7-12. Note that the CT scan also identifies the suspicious nodules and their precise location.

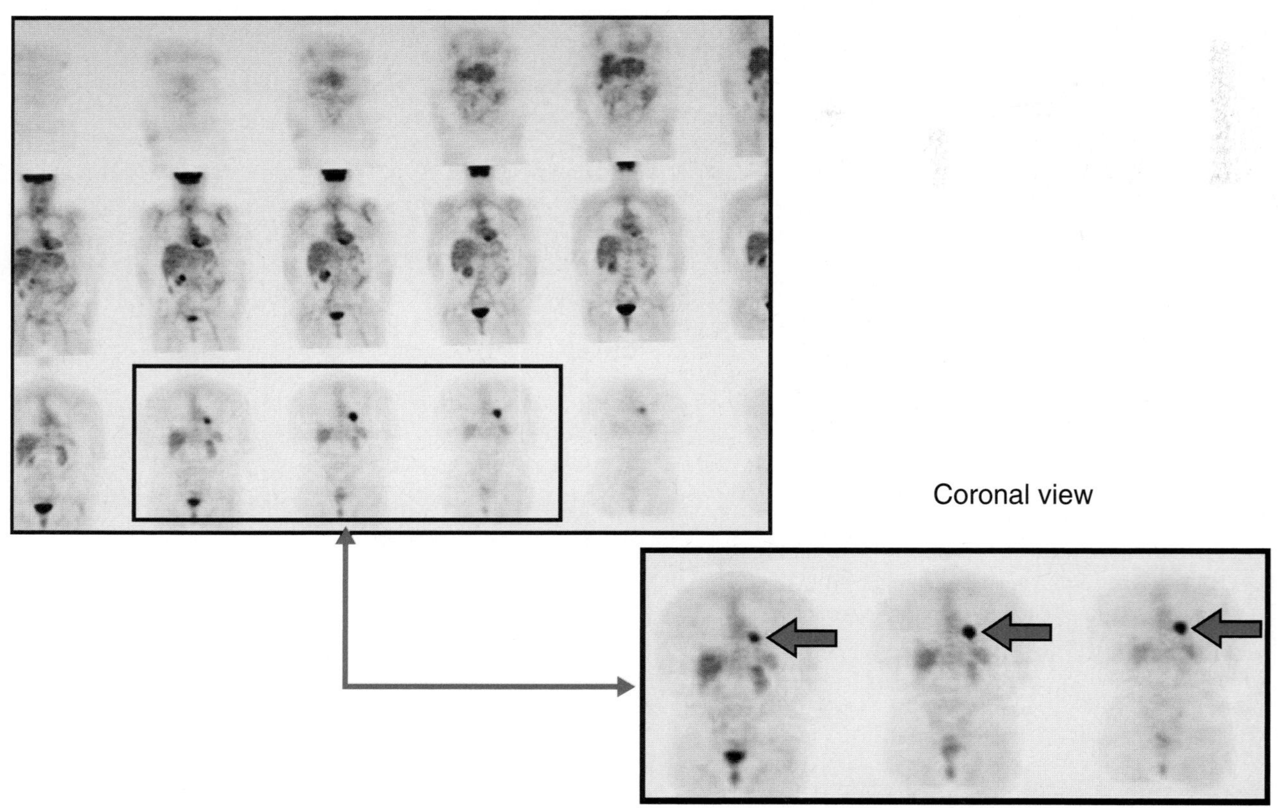

FIGURE 7-15 Positron emission tomography (PET) scan: coronal views. The last three views show a hot spot in left lower lobe.

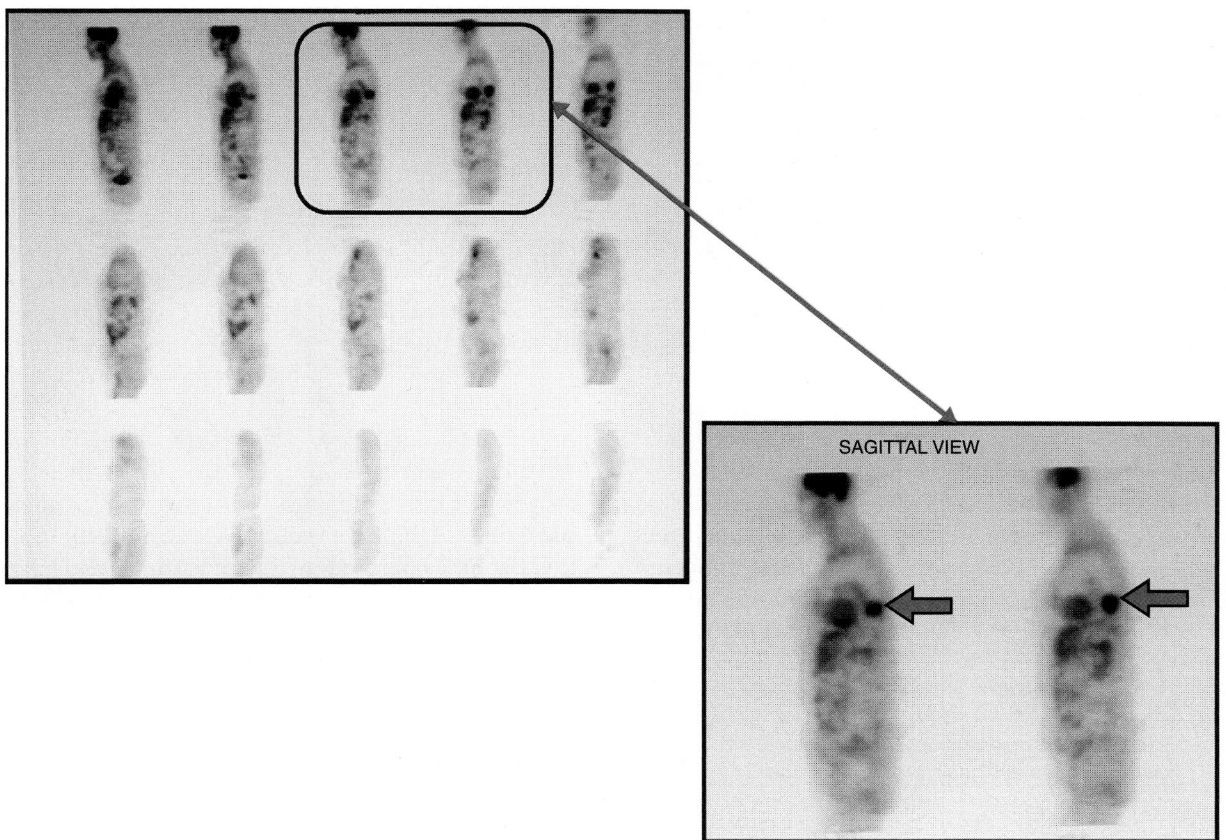

FIGURE 7-16 Positron emission tomography (PET) scan: sagittal views. The encircled images show a hot spot in the lower left lobe.

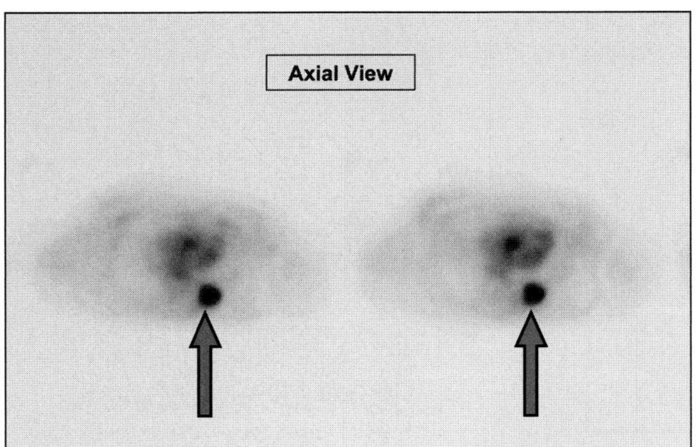

FIGURE 7-17 Positron emission tomography (PET) scan: axial view. A hot spot is further confirmed in left lower lobe.

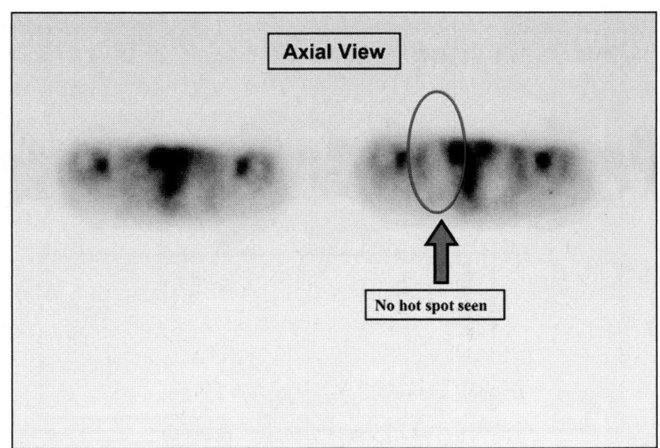

FIGURE 7-18 Positron emission tomography (PET) scan: axial view. This image confirms that the small nodule identified in the upper right lobe in the chest radiograph and computed tomography scan is benign (i.e., no hot spot is evident).

before the scan is performed. This allows time for the body to absorb the compound. This step may be difficult or impossible for patients who are unable to remain motionless for long periods of time. PET scans are very expensive to perform, compared with CT or **magnetic resonance imaging (MRI)** studies.

Positron Emission Tomography and Computed Tomography Scan

As described in the preceding sections, PET and CT are both standard imaging tools used by the radiologist to pinpoint the location of cancer or infection within the body before developing a treatment strategy. Individually, however,

each scan has its own benefits and limitations. For example, the PET scan detects the metabolic activity of growing cancer cells in the body, and the CT scan provides a detailed picture of the internal anatomy that shows the precise location, size, and shape of a tumor or mass. On the other hand, because the PET scan and CT scan are done at different times and locations, variations in the patient's body position often make the interpretation of the two images difficult.

Technology has now been developed that allows both the PET scan and the CT scan to be merged together and performed at the same time. The image produced is called a **positron emission tomography and computed tomography scan (PET/CT scan)** scan (also known as a *PET/CT fusion*). The PET/CT scan provides an image far superior to that afforded by either technology independently. When combined, the CT scan provides the anatomic detail regarding the precise size, shape, and location of the tumor, and the PET scan provides the metabolic activity of the tumor or mass. The PET/CT image provides excellent image quality and high sensitivity and specificity in detecting malignant lesions in the chest. Figure 7-19 shows a PET/CT scan alongside a CT scan and a PET scan; all the images show the same malignant nodule in the right upper lung lobe.

The benefits of a combined PET/CT scan include earlier diagnosis, accurate staging and localization, and precise treatment and monitoring. With the high quality and accuracy of the PET/CT image, the patient has a better chance for a favorable outcome, without the need for unnecessary procedures. In addition, the PET/CT scan provides early detection of the recurrence or metastasis of cancer, revealing tumors that might otherwise be obscured by scars from surgery and radiation therapy. This is because the combined PET/CT scan provides the radiologist with a more complete overview of what is occurring in the patient's body, both anatomically and metabolically at the same time.

Magnetic Resonance Imaging

MRI uses magnetic resonance as its source of energy to take cross-sectional (transverse, sagittal, or coronal) images of the body. It uses no ionizing radiation. The patient is placed in the cylindric imager, and the body part in question is exposed to a magnetic field and radiowave transmission. The MRI produces a high-contrast image that can detect subtle lesions (Figure 7-20).

MRI is superior to CT scanning in identifying complex congenital heart disorders, bone marrow diseases, adenopathy, and lesions of the chest wall. MRI is an excellent supplement to CT scanning for study of the mediastinum and hilar region. For most abnormalities of the chest, however, CT scanning is generally better than MRI for motion (patient motion causes loss of resolution), spatial resolution, and cost reasons.

Because the magnetic resonance imager generates an intense magnetic field, objects made of ferromagnetic material are strongly attracted to it. Therefore patients with ferromagnetic cerebral aneurysm clips or ferromagnetic prosthetic cardiac valves should not undergo MRI because the magnetic force of the imager can cause these devices to heat, shift and harm the patient. The magnetic force of the imager also can interfere with the normal function of cardiac pacemakers and most ventilators.

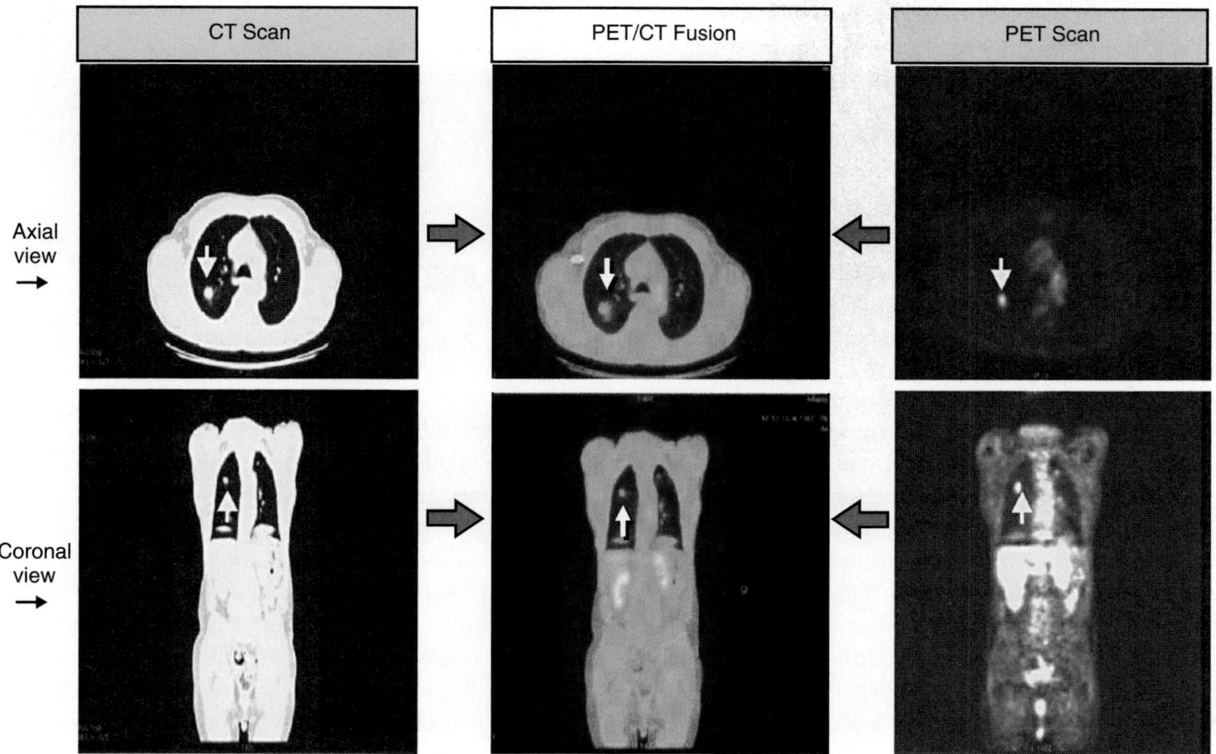

FIGURE 7-19 Positron emission tomography and computed tomography scan (PET/CT scan) *(center)*. The CT scan, PET/CT fusion, and PET scan are all showing the same malignant nodule in right upper lobe *(white arrow)*. Note: The PET/CT fusion is normally presented in color (e.g., red, blue, yellow).

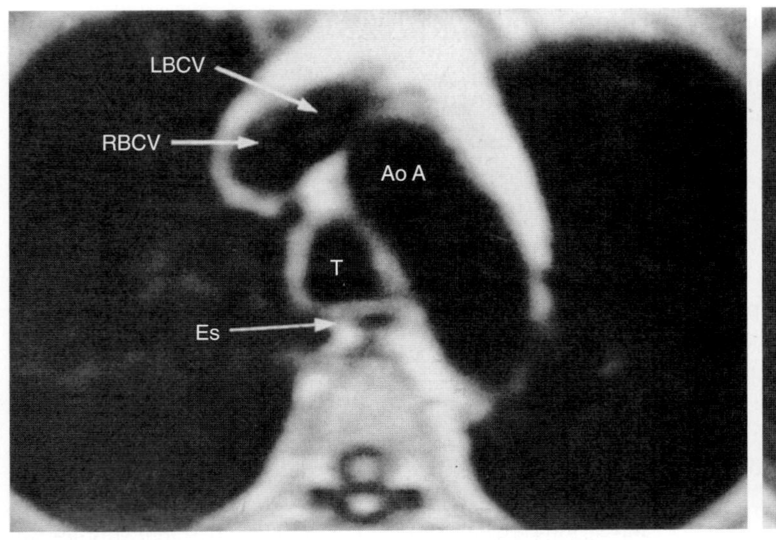

A

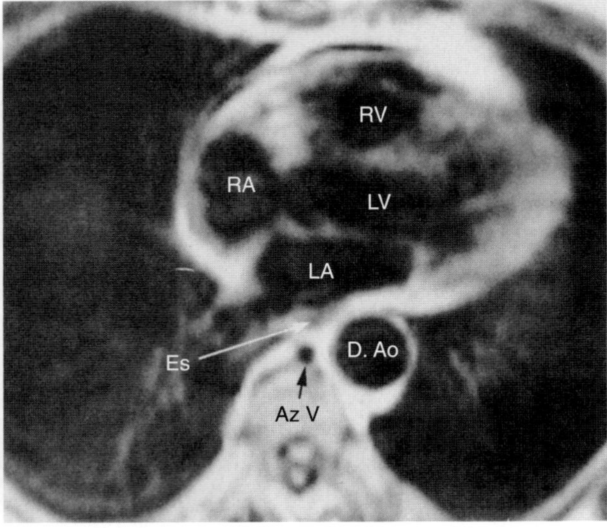

B

FIGURE 7-20 Anatomy of mediastinum on magnetic resonance imaging (MRI) scan. **A,** *Ao A,* Aortic arch; *Es,* esophagus; *LBCV,* left brachiocephalic vein; *RBCV,* right brachiocephalic vein; *T,* trachea. **B,** *Az V,* Azygos vein; *D Ao,* descending aorta; *Es,* esophagus; *LA,* left atrium; *LV,* left ventricle; *RA,* right atrium; *RV,* right ventricle. (From Armstrong P, Wilson AG, Dee P: *Imaging of diseases of the chest,* St Louis, 1990, Mosby.)

Pulmonary Angiography

Pulmonary angiography is useful in identifying pulmonary emboli or arteriovenous malformations. It involves the injection of a radiopaque contrast medium through a catheter that has been passed through the right side of the heart and into the pulmonary artery. The injection of the contrast material into the pulmonary circulation is followed by rapid serial pulmonary angiograms. The pulmonary vessels are filled with radiopaque contrast material and therefore appear white. Figure 7-21 shows an abnormal angiogram in which the major blood vessels appear absent distal to pulmonary emboli in the left lung.

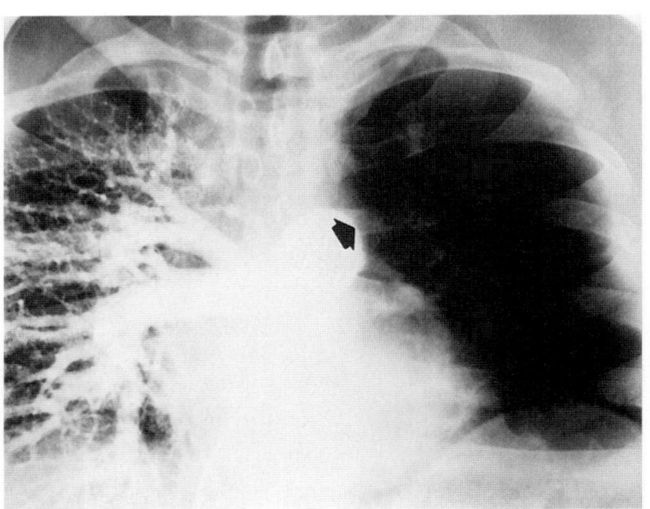

FIGURE 7-21 Abnormal pulmonary angiogram. Radiopaque material injected into the blood is prevented from flowing into the left lung past the pulmonary embolism *(arrow).* No vascular structures are seen distal to obstruction.

Ventilation-Perfusion Scan

A **ventilation-perfusion scan** is useful in determining the presence of a pulmonary embolism. The perfusion scan is obtained by injecting small particles of albumin, called *macroaggregates,* tagged with a radioactive material such as iodine-131 or technetium-99m. After injection the radioactive particles are carried in the blood to the right side of the heart, from which they are distributed throughout the lungs by the blood flow in the pulmonary arteries. The radioactive particles that travel through unobstructed arteries become trapped in the pulmonary capillaries because they are 20 to 50 μm in diameter and the diameter of the average pulmonary capillary is approximately 8 to 10 μm.

The lungs are then scanned with a gamma camera that produces a picture of the radioactive distribution throughout the pulmonary circulation. The dark areas show good blood flow, and the white or light areas represent decreased or complete absence of blood flow. The macroaggregates eventually break down, pass through the pulmonary circulation, and are excreted by the liver. The injection of these radioactive particles has no significant effect on the patient's hemodynamics because the patent pulmonary capillaries far outnumber those "embolized" by the radioactive particles. In addition to pulmonary emboli, a perfusion scan defect (white or light areas) may be caused by a lung abscess, lung compression, loss of the pulmonary vascular system (e.g., emphysema), atelectasis, or alveolar **consolidation.**

The perfusion scan is supplemented with a ventilation scan. During the ventilation scan the patient breathes a radioactive gas such as xenon-133 from a closed-circuit spirometer. A gamma camera is used to create a picture of the gas distribution throughout the lungs. A normal ventilation scan shows a uniform distribution of the gas, with the dark areas reflecting the presence of the radioactive gas and therefore good ventilation. White or light areas represent decreased or complete absence of ventilation. See Figure 7-22 for an

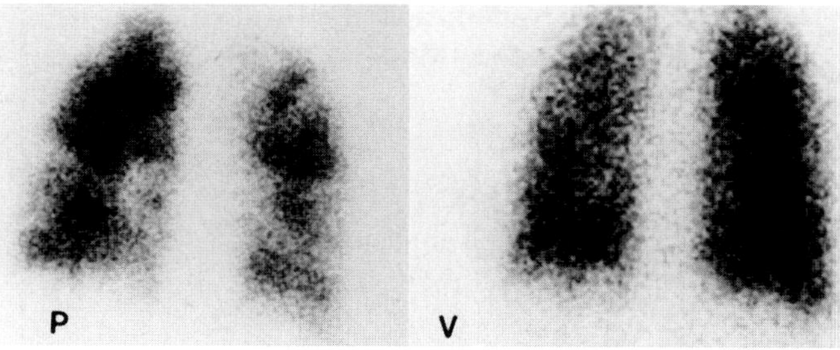

FIGURE 7-22 Fat embolism in a patient with dyspnea and hypoxemia after a recent orthopedic procedure. Perfusion (P) and ventilation (V) radionuclide scans show multiple peripheral subsegmental perfusion defects suggestive of fat embolism. (From Hansell DM, Armstrong P, Lynch DA, McAdams HP: *Imaging of diseases of the chest,* ed 4, Philadelphia, 2005, Elsevier.)

abnormal perfusion scan and a normal ventilation scan of a patient with a severe pulmonary embolism. An abnormal ventilation scan also may be caused by airway obstruction (e.g., mucous plug or bronchospasm), loss of alveolar elasticity (e.g., emphysema), alveolar consolidation, or pulmonary edema.

Fluoroscopy

Fluoroscopy is a technique by which x-ray motion pictures of the chest are taken. Fluoroscopy subjects the patient to a larger dose of x-rays than does standard radiography. Therefore it is used only in selected cases, as in the assessment of abnormal diaphragmatic movement (e.g., unilateral paralysis) or for localization of lesions to be biopsied during fiberoptic bronchoscopy.

Bronchography

Bronchography entails the instillation of a radiopaque material into the lumen of the tracheobronchial tree. A chest radiograph is then taken, providing a film called a **bronchogram.** The contrast material provides a clear outline of the trachea, carina, right and left main stem bronchi, and segmental bronchi. Bronchography is occasionally used to diagnose bronchogenic carcinoma and determine the presence or extent of bronchiectasis (Figure 7-23). CT of the chest has largely replaced this technique.

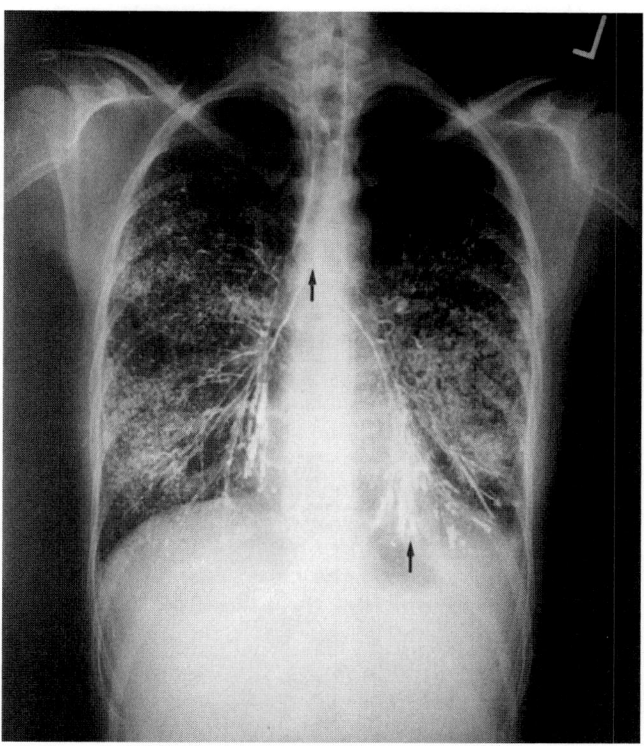

FIGURE 7-23 Bronchogram obtained using contrast medium in a patient with a history of bronchiectasis. Arrows indicate the carina and the dilated bronchi leading to the posterior basilar segment of the left lower lobe. (From Rau JL Jr, Pearce DJ: *Understanding chest radiographs,* Denver, 1984, Multi-Media Publishing.)

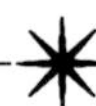

SELF ASSESSMENT QUESTIONS

evolve Answers to questions can be found on Evolve. To access additional student assessment questions and case studies for application of text material to real-life scenarios, visit **http://evolve.elsevier.com/DesJardins/respiratory.**

1. Clinically, the standard radiograph of the chest includes which of the following?
1. AP radiograph
2. Lateral decubitus radiograph
3. Lateral radiograph
4. PA radiograph
   a. 1 only
   b. 4 only
   c. 3 and 4 only
   d. 1 and 2 only

2. Compared with the PA radiograph, the AP radiograph:
1. Magnifies the heart
2. Is usually more distorted
3. Frequently appears more hazy
4. Often has extraneous shadows
   a. 2 only
   b. 3 and 4 only
   c. 1, 3, and 4 only
   d. 1, 2, 3, and 4

3. To view the right lung and the heart in the lateral radiograph, the:

a. Left side of the patient's chest is placed against the cassette
b. Anterior portion of the patient's chest is placed against the cassette
c. Right side of the patient's chest is placed against the cassette
d. Posterior portion of the patent's chest is placed against the cassette

4. A right lateral decubitus radiograph means that the:

a. Right side of the chest is down
b. Posterior side of the chest is up
c. Left side of the chest is down
d. Anterior side of the chest is up

5. A leftward shift of the mediastinum is commonly seen on the chest radiograph in response to which of the following?

1. Left upper lobe atelectasis
2. Right upper lobe gas
3. Left upper lobe fibrosis
4. Right upper lobe tumor

a. 1 and 3 only
b. 3 and 4 only
c. 2, 3, and 4 only
d. 1, 2, 3, and 4

6. The normal exposure of the radiograph is verified by determining whether the spinal processes of the vertebrae are visible to which level?

a. C-1 to C-3
b. C-3 to C-5
c. T-2 to T-4
d. T-5 to T-6

7. The lungs in a radiograph that is described as being "heavily penetrated" is which of the following?

1. Darker in appearance
2. More translucent
3. Whiter in appearance
4. More opaque in appearance

a. 3 only
b. 4 only
c. 3 and 4 only
d. 1 and 2 only

8. When the radiograph is taken at full inspiration, the diaphragmatic domes should be at the level of the:

a. First to fourth ribs posteriorly
b. Fourth to sixth ribs posteriorly
c. Sixth to ninth ribs posteriorly
d. Ninth to eleventh ribs posteriorly

9. Which of the following involves x-ray motion pictures of the chest?

a. Bronchography
b. Fluoroscopy
c. MRI
d. CT

10. MRI is superior to CT scanning for identifying which of the following?

1. Lesions of the chest
2. Bone marrow diseases
3. Congenital heart disorders
4. Adenopathy

a. 3 and 4 only
b. 2 and 3 only
c. 2, 3, and 4 only
d. 1, 2, 3, and 4

Other Important Tests and Procedures 8

Chapter Objectives

After reading this chapter, you will be able to:

- Describe the diagnostic values of the sputum examination, and include common organisms associated with respiratory disorders:
  - Gram-negative organisms *(Klebsiella, Pseudomonas aeruginosa, Haemophilus influenzae, Legionella pneumophila)*
  - Gram-positive organisms *(Streptococcus, Staphylococcus)*
  - Viral organisms (*Mycoplasma pneumoniae,* respiratory syncytial virus)
- Discuss the diagnostic values of the following tests and procedures:
  - Skin tests
  - Endoscopic examinations (bronchoscopy and mediastinoscopy)
  - Lung biopsy
  - Video-assisted thoracoscopy (VATS)
  - Thoracentesis
  - Pleurodesis
- Describe the following components of hematology testing:
  - Complete blood count (CBC)
  - Red blood cell (RBC) count (red blood cell indices and types of anemias)
  - White blood cell (WBC) count, including granular leukocytes and nongranular leukocytes
- Describe the role of platelets, including the following:
  - Causes of platelet deficiency
  - Clinical significance of platelet deficiency
- Identify the following blood chemistry tests commonly monitored in respiratory care:
  - Glucose
  - Lactic dehydrogenase (LDH)
  - Serum glutamic oxaloacetic transaminase (SGOT)
  - Aspartate aminotransferase (AST)
  - Alanine aminotransferase (ALT)
  - Bilirubin
  - Blood urea nitrogen (BUN)
  - Serum creatinine
- Identify the following electrolytes commonly monitored in respiratory care:
  - Sodium (Na^+)
  - Potassium (K^+)
  - Chloride (Cl^-)
  - Calcium (Ca^{++})
- Define key terms and complete self-assessment questions at the end of the chapter and on Evolve.

Key Terms

Acid-Fast Smear and Culture
Alanine Aminotransferase (ALT)
Anergy
Aspartate Aminotransferase (AST)
Basophils
Bilirubin
Blood Chemistry
Blood Urea Nitrogen (BUN)
Bronchoscopy
Calcium (Ca^{++})
Chloride (Cl^-)
Complete Blood Count (CBC)
Cytology
Culture and Sensitivity Study
Electrolytes
Endoscopic Examination
Eosinophils
Exudates
Glucose
Gram-Negative Organisms
Gram-Positive Organisms
Gram Staining
Granular Leukocytes
Haemophilus influenzae
Hematocrit (Hct)
Hematology
Hemoglobin (Hb)
Hypochromic Microcytic Anemia
Klebsiella
Lactic Dehydrogenase (LDH)
Legionella pneumophila
Leukocytosis
Lung Biopsy
Lymphocytes
Macrocytic Anemia
Macrophages
Mean Cell Hemoglobin (MCH)
Mean Cell Volume (MCV)
Mean Corpuscular Hemoglobin Concentration (MCHC)
Mediastinoscopy
Monocytes
Mycoplasma pneumoniae
Neutrophils
Nongranular Leukocytes
Normochromic and Normocytic Anemia

Open Lung Biopsy
Platelets
Pleurodesis
Potassium (K^+)
Pseudomonas aeruginosa
Red Blood Cell (RBC) Count
Red Blood Cell Indices
Respiratory Syncytial Virus
Serum Creatinine
Serum Glutamic Oxaloacetic Transaminase (SGOT)
Skin Tests
Sodium (Na^+)
Sputum Examination
Staphylococcus
Streptococcus
Therapeutic Bronchoscopy
Therapeutic Thoracentesis
Thoracentesis
Thrombocytopenia
Transbronchial Lung Biopsy
Transudates
Video-Assisted Thoracoscopy (VATS)
Viral Organisms
White Blood Cell (WBC) Count (Leukopenia)

Chapter Outline

As already discussed throughout the first seven chapters of this textbook, the correct assessment associated with patients with pulmonary disease depends on a variety of important diagnostic studies and bedside skills. In addition to the clinical data obtained at the patient bedside (i.e., the patient interview and the physical examinations) and from standard laboratory tests and special procedures (i.e., pulmonary function studies, arterial blood gases, hemodynamic monitoring, and the radiologic examination of the chest), a number of other important tests are often required to treat the patient appropriately. Additional important diagnostic studies include the **sputum examination, skin tests, endoscopic examination, lung biopsy, thoracentesis,** and **hematology, blood chemistry, and electrolyte tests.**

Sputum Examination

A sputum sample can be obtained by expectoration, tracheal suction, or **bronchoscopy** (discussed later). In addition to the analysis of the amount, quality, and color of the sputum (previously discussed in Chapter 2, page 44), the sputum sample may be examined for (1) culture and sensitivity, (2) Gram stain, (3) acid-fast smear and culture, and (4) cytology.

For a **culture and sensitivity study,** a single sputum sample is collected in a sterile container. This test is performed to diagnose bacterial infection, select an antibiotic, and evaluate the effectiveness of antibiotic therapy. The turnaround time for this test is 48 to 72 hours. The **Gram staining** of sputum is performed to classify bacteria into **gram-negative organisms** and **gram-positive organisms.** The results of the Gram stain tests guide therapy until the culture and sensitivity results are obtained. Box 8-1 presents common organisms associated with respiratory disorders. All but the viral organisms can be seen on a Gram stain.

The **acid-fast smear and culture** is performed to determine the presence of acid-fast bacilli (e.g., *Mycobacterium tuberculosis*). A series of three early morning sputum samples is tested. **Cytology** examination entails the collection of a single sputum sample in a special container with fixative solution. The sample is evaluated under a microscope for the presence of abnormal cells that may indicate a malignant condition.

The amount, color, and constituents of the sputum are often important in the assessment and diagnosis of many respiratory disorders, including tuberculosis, pneumonia, cancer of the lungs, and pneumoconiosis. For example, yellow sputum indicates an acute infection. Green sputum is

Box 8-1 Common Organisms Associated With Respiratory Disorders

Gram-Negative Organisms
Klebsiella
Pseudomonas aeruginosa
Haemophilus influenzae
Legionella pneumophila

Gram-Positive Organisms
Streptococcus (80% of all bacterial pneumonias)
Staphylococcus

Viral Organisms
Mycoplasma pneumoniae
Respiratory syncytial virus

associated with old, retained secretions. Green and foul-smelling secretions are frequently found in patients with anaerobic or *Pseudomonas* infection. Thick, stringy, and white or mucoid sputum suggests bronchial asthma. Brown sputum suggests the presence of old blood. Red sputum indicates fresh blood.

Skin Tests

Skin tests are commonly performed to evaluate allergic reactions or exposure to tuberculous bacilli or fungi. Skin tests entail the intradermal injection of an antigen. A positive test result indicates that the patient has been exposed to the antigen. However, it does not mean that the disease is actually present. A negative test result indicates that the patient has had no exposure to the antigen. A negative test result also may be seen in patients with a depression of cell-mediated immunity (**anergy**), such as that which develops in human immunodeficiency virus (HIV) infections.

Endoscopic Examinations

Bronchoscopy

A **bronchoscopy** is a well-established diagnostic and therapeutic tool used by a number of medical specialists, including those in intensive care units, special procedure rooms, and outpatient settings. With minimal risk to the patient—and without interrupting the patient's ventilation—the flexible fiberoptic bronchoscope allows direct visualization of the upper airways (nose, oral cavity, and pharynx), larynx, vocal cords, subglottic area, trachea, bronchi, lobar bronchi, and segmental bronchi down to the third or fourth generation. Under fluoroscopic control, more peripheral areas can be examined or treated (Figure 8-1). Bronchoscopy may be diagnostic or therapeutic.

A diagnostic bronchoscopy is usually performed when an infectious disease is suspected and not otherwise diagnosed or to obtain a lung biopsy sample when the abnormal lung tissue is located on or near the bronchi. A diagnostic bronchoscopy is indicated for a number of clinical conditions, including further inspection and assessment of (1) abnormal radiographic findings (e.g., question of bronchogenic carcinoma or the extent of a bronchial tumor or mass lesion), (2) persistent atelectasis, (3) excessive bronchial secretions, (4) acute smoke inhalation injuries, (5) intubation damage, (6) bronchiectasis, (7) foreign bodies, (8) hemoptysis, (9) lung abscess, (10) major thoracic trauma, (11) stridor or localized wheezing, and (12) unexplained cough.

A videotape or colored picture of the procedure may also be obtained to record any abnormalities. When abnormalities are found, additional diagnostic procedures include brushings, biopsies, needle aspirations, and washings. For example, a common diagnostic bronchoscopic technique, termed *bronchoalveolar lavage* (BAL), involves injecting a small amount (30 mL) of sterile saline through the bronchoscope and then withdrawing the fluid for examination of cells. BAL is commonly used to diagnose *Pneumocystis carinii* pneumonia.

Therapeutic bronchoscopy includes (1) suctioning of excessive secretions or mucous plugs, especially when lung atelectasis is forming, (2) the removal of foreign bodies or cancer obstructing the airway, (3) selective lavage (with normal saline or mucolytic agents), and (4) management of life-threatening hemoptysis. Although the virtues of therapeutic bronchoscopy are well established, routine respiratory therapy modalities at the patient's bedside (e.g., chest physical therapy, intermittent percussive ventilation [IPV], postural drainage, deep breathing and coughing techniques, and positive expiratory pressure [PEP] therapy) are considered the first line of defense in the treatment of atelectasis from pooled secretions. Clinically, therapeutic bronchoscopy is commonly used in the management of bronchiectasis, lung abscess, smoke inhalation and thermal injuries, and lung cancer (see Bronchopulmonary Hygiene Therapy Protocol 9-2, page 120).

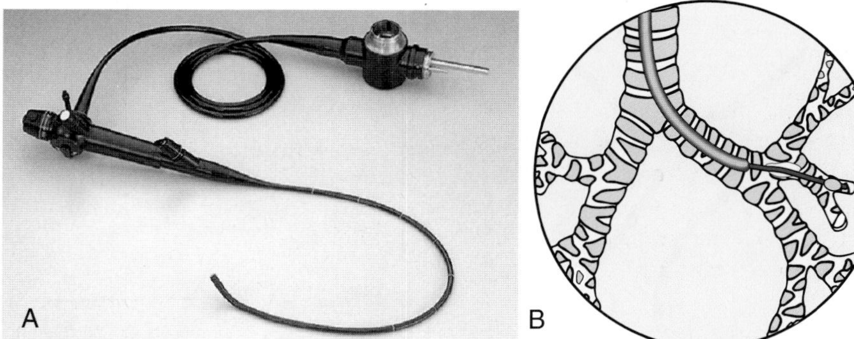

FIGURE 8-1 Fiberoptic bronchoscope. **A**, The transbronchoscopic balloon-tipped catheter and the flexible fiberoptic bronchoscope. Transbronchoscopic tissue biopsies may be obtained with this device. **B**, The catheter is introduced into a small airway and the balloon inflated with 1.5 to 2 mL of air to occlude the airway. Bronchoalveolar lavage is performed by injecting and withdrawing 30-mL aliquots of sterile saline solution, gently aspirating after each instillation. Specimens are sent to the laboratory for analysis. (A from Lewis SM, Heitkemper MM, Dirksen SR: *Medical-surgical nursing: assessment and management of clinical problems,* ed 6, St Louis, 2004, Mosby. B from Meduri GU, Beals DH, Maijub AG, Baselski V: Protected bronchoalveolar lavage. A new bronchoscopic technique to retrieve uncontaminated distal airway secretions, *Am Rev Respir Dis* 143:855, 1991.)

Mediastinoscopy

Mediastinoscopy is the insertion of a scope through a small incision in the suprasternal notch; the scope is then advanced into the mediastinum. The test is used to inspect and biopsy lymph nodes in the mediastinal area. This procedure is performed to diagnose carcinoma, granulomatous infections, and sarcoidosis. Mediastinoscopy is done in the operating room while the patient is under general anesthesia.

Lung Biopsy

A lung biopsy sample can be obtained by means of a transbronchial needle biopsy or an open-lung biopsy. A **transbronchial lung biopsy** entails passing a forceps or needle through a bronchoscope to obtain a specimen (Figure 8-2). An open lung biopsy involves surgery to remove a sample of lung tissue. An incision is made over the area of the lung from which the tissue sample is to be collected. In some cases a large incision may be necessary to reach the suspected problem area. After the procedure a chest tube is inserted for drainage and suction for 7 to 14 days. An **open-lung biopsy** is usually performed when either a bronchoscopic biopsy or a needle biopsy has been unsuccessful or cannot be performed or when a larger piece of tissue is necessary to establish a diagnosis.

An open biopsy requires general anesthesia and is more invasive and thus more likely to cause complications. Overall, the risks include pneumothorax, bleeding, bronchospasm, heart arrhythmias, and infection. A needle lung biopsy is contraindicated in patients with lung bullae, cysts, blood coagulation disorders of any type, severe hypoxia, pulmonary hypertension, or cor pulmonale.

A lung biopsy is usually performed to diagnose abnormalities identified on a chest radiograph or computed tomography (CT) scan that are not readily accessible by other diagnostic procedures, such as bronchoscopy. A lung biopsy is especially useful in investigating peripheral lung abnormalities, such as recurrent infiltrates and pleural or subpleural lesions. Additional conditions under which a lung biopsy may be performed include metastatic cancer to the lung and pneumonia with lung abscess.

The tissues from a lung biopsy are sent to a pathology laboratory for examination of malignant cells. Other samples may be sent to a microbiology laboratory to determine the presence of infection. Lung biopsy results are usually available in 2 to 4 days. In some cases, however, it may take several weeks to confirm (by culture) certain infections, such as tuberculosis.

Video-Assisted Thoracoscopy

In video-assisted thoracoscopy (VATS), a newly developed technique, a small incision is made in the chest wall, and a device called a *thoracoscope* is inserted. This device is equipped with a fiberscope that can examine the pleural cavity. The results are displayed on a video monitor (as in bronchoscopy). When pleural lesions are identified, they can be biopsied under video guidance. This procedure is helpful in the diagnosis of tuberculosis, mesothelioma, and metastatic cancer.

Thoracentesis

Thoracentesis (also called *thoracocentesis*) is a procedure in which excess fluid accumulation (pleural effusion) between the chest cavity and lungs (pleural space) is aspirated through

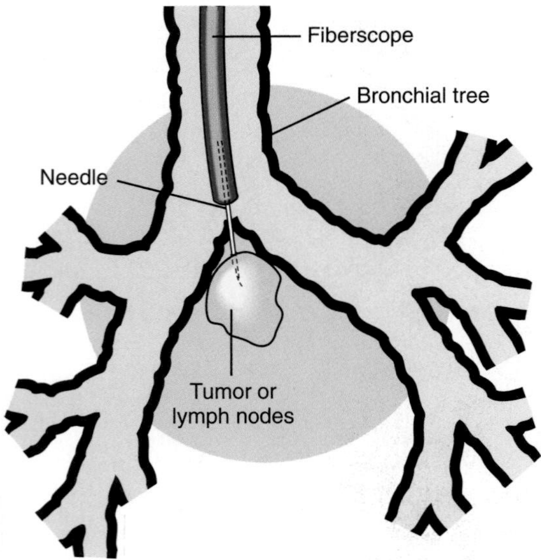

FIGURE 8-2 Transbronchial needle biopsy. The diagram shows a transbronchial biopsy needle penetrating the bronchial wall and entering a mass of subcarinal lymph nodes or tumor. (Redrawn from DuBois RM, Clarke SW: *Fiberoptic bronchoscopy in diagnosis and management,* Orlando, 1987, Grune and Stratton.)

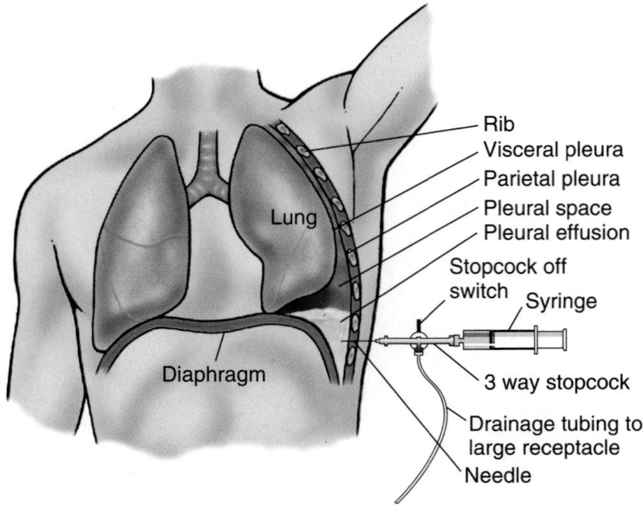

FIGURE 8-3 Thoracentesis. A catheter is positioned in the pleural space to remove accumulated fluid. Pleural fluid is seend as the dark shadow at the base of the left lung. (From Monahan FD, Neighbors M, Sands JK, Marek JF, and Green CJ: Phipps' Medical-surgical nursing health and illness perspectives, ed. 8, St. Louis, 2007, Mosby-Elsevier).

a needle inserted through the chest wall (Figure 8-3). A chest radiograph, CT scan, or ultrasound scan may be used to confirm the precise location of the fluid. Once the fluid has been located, thoracentesis may be performed for diagnostic or therapeutic purposes.

Diagnostic thoracentesis may be performed to identify the cause of a pleural effusion. The analysis of the pleural fluid may be useful in the diagnosis and staging of a suspected or known malignancy. A pleural biopsy may also be performed during a thoracentesis to collect a tissue sample from the inner lining of the chest wall. **Therapeutic thoracentesis** may be performed to relieve shortness of breath or pain caused by a large pleural effusion, to remove air trapped between the lung and chest wall, or to administer medication directly into the lung cavity to treat the cause of the fluid accumulation or to treat cancer. The fluid in the lung cavity is classified as either a transudate or an exudate.

Transudates develop when fluid from the pulmonary capillaries moves into the pleural space. The fluid produced is thin and watery and usually has a low **white blood cell (WBC) count,** a low lactate dehydrogenase (LDH) enzyme level, and a low protein level. The pleural surfaces are not involved in producing the transudate. A transudate may be caused by left ventricular heart failure, cirrhosis, nephrotic syndrome, and peritoneal dialysis.

Exudates may be caused by a variety of conditions, including pulmonary infections (e.g., pneumonia, tuberculosis, and fungal diseases), cancer, chest trauma, pancreatitis, autoimmune disease, or a pulmonary embolism. When an infection is present, the fluid usually has a high WBC count, a high LDH enzyme level, a high protein level, a large amount of cellular debris, and the presence of bacteria or other infectious organisms. When cancer is present, the fluid usually has a high WBC count (often **lymphocytes**), a high LDH enzyme level, and a high protein level. Abnormal cells also may be found. When a pulmonary embolism is present, a large number of red blood cells (RBCs) are usually present and the WBC and protein levels are both low.

The thoracentesis procedure is generally performed while the patient is in an upright position, leaning forward slightly, typically over a bedside table. Using a local anesthetic, the physician inserts a large-bore thoracentesis needle (16 to 19 gauge), or needle-catheter, between the ribs over the fluid accumulation. The needle or catheter is connected to a small tube with a three-way stopcock, which in turn is attached to either a large syringe or a vacuum and collection bottle. Depending on the purpose of the thoracentesis, up to 1500 mL may be withdrawn. Once the fluid has been collected, the needle or catheter is removed and a bandage is placed over the puncture site. The patient is usually instructed to lie on the puncture site side for about an hour to allow the puncture site to seal.

A thoracentesis is usually a safe procedure. However, a chest radiograph is generally obtained shortly after the procedure to ensure that no complications have developed. Complications may include pneumothorax, pulmonary edema (which sometimes occurs when large amounts of fluid are aspirated), infection, bleeding, and organ damage.

Pleurodesis

Pleurodesis is performed to prevent the recurrence of a pneumothorax or pleural effusion. Pleurodesis is achieved by injecting any number of agents (called *sclerosing agents* or *sclerosants*) into the pleural space through a chest tube. There is no one sclerosant that is more effective or safer than the others. Common sclerosant chemicals include a slurry of talc, bleomycin, nitrogen mustard, doxycycline, povidone iodine, or quinacrine. The instilled sclerosing agents cause irritation and inflammation (pleuritis) between the parietal and the visceral layers of the pleura. This action causes the pleurae to stick together and thereby prevents subsequent gas or fluid accumulation.

A chemical pleurodesis is considered to be the standard of care for patients with malignant pleural effusion. Because chemical pleurodesis is a painful procedure, the patient is premedicated with a sedative and analgesics. A local anesthetic may also be instilled into the pleural space or added to the sclerosant. Although complications of pleurodesis are uncommon, risks include the following:

- Infection
- Bleeding
- Acute respiratory distress syndrome
- Collapsed lung (pneumothorax) and respiratory failure

Complications may be specific for each sclerosant.

- Talc and doxycycline can cause fever and pain.
- Quinacrine can cause low blood pressure, fever, and hallucination.
- Bleomycin can cause fever, pain, and nausea.

Pleurodesis may fail because of the following complications:

- Trapped lung, in which the lung is enclosed in scar or tumor tissue
- Formation of isolated pockets (loculation) within the pleural space
- Loss of lung flexibility (elasticity)
- Production of large amounts of pleural fluid
- Extensive spread (metastasis) of pleural cancer
- Improper positioning, blockage, or kinking of the tube

Hematology, Blood Chemistry, and Electrolyte Findings

Abnormal hematology, blood chemistry, or electrolyte values assist the respiratory care practitioner and physician in the assessment of cardiopulmonary disorders. Knowledge of these laboratory tests provides a greater understanding of the clinical manifestations of a particular cardiopulmonary disorder.

Hematology

The most frequent laboratory hematology test is the **complete blood count (CBC).** The CBC provides important information about the patient's diagnosis, prognosis, response to treatment, and recovery. The CBC includes the **red blood**

cell (RBC) count, hemoglobin (Hb), hematocrit (Hct), the total WBC count, and at least an estimate of the platelet count.

Red Blood Cell Count

The RBCs (erythrocytes) constitute the major portion of the blood cells. The healthy man has about 5 million RBCs in each cubic millimeter (mm^3) of blood. The healthy woman has about 4 million RBCs in each cubic millimeter of blood. Clinically, the total number of RBCs and the RBC indices are useful in assessing the patient's overall oxygen-carrying capacity. The RBC indices are helpful in the identification of specific RBC deficiencies. Table 8-1 provides an overview of the **red blood cell indices** and types of anemias.

TABLE 8-1 Red Blood Cell Indices

Index	Description
Hematocrit (Hct)	The Hct is the volume of red blood cells (RBCs) in 100 mL of blood and is expressed as a percentage of the total volume. In the healthy man the Hct is about 45%; in the healthy woman the Hct is about 42%. In the healthy newborn the Hct ranges from 45% to 60%. The Hct also is called the *packed cell volume* (PCV).
Hemoglobin (Hb)	Most of the oxygen that diffuses into the pulmonary capillary blood rapidly moves into the RBCs and chemically attaches to the Hb. Each RBC contains approximately 280 million Hb molecules. The Hb value is reported in grams per 100 mL of blood (also referred to as grams percent of hemoglobin [g% Hb]). The normal Hb value for men is 14 to 16 g%. The normal Hb value for women is 12 to 15 g%. Hb constitutes about 33% of the RBC weight.
Mean cell volume (MCV)	The MCV is the actual size of the RBCs and is used to classify anemias. It is an index that expresses the volume of a single red cell and is measured in cubic microns. The normal MCV is 87 to 103 cubic microns for both men and women.
Mean corpuscular hemoglobin concentration (MCHC)	The MCHC is a measure of the concentration or proportion of Hb in an average (mean) RBC. The MCHC is derived by dividing the g% Hb by the Hct. For example, if a patient has 15 g% Hb and an Hct of 45%, the MCHC is 33%. The normal MCHC for men and women ranges from 32% to 36%. The MCHC is most useful in assessing the degree of anemia because the two most accurate hematologic measurements (Hb and Hct—not RBC) are used for the test.
Mean cell hemoglobin (MCH)	The MCH is a measure of weight of Hb in a single RBC. This value is derived by dividing the total Hb (g% Hb) by the RBC count. The MCH is useful in diagnosing severely anemic patients but not as good as the MCHC because the RBC is not always accurate. The normal range for the MCH is 27 to 32 picograms per RBC.
Types of Anemias	
Normochromic (normal Hb) and normocytic (normal cell size) anemia	Normochromic anemia is most commonly caused by excessive blood loss. The amount of Hb and the number of RBCs are decreased, but the individual size and content remain normal. Clinically, the laboratory report reveals the following: Hct: below normal Hb: below normal MCV: normal MCHC: normal MCH: normal
Hypochromic (decreased Hb) microcytic (small cell size) anemia	In hypochromic anemia the size of the RBCs and the Hb content are decreased. This form of anemia is commonly seen in patients with chronic blood loss, iron deficiency, chronic infections, and malignancies. Clinically, the laboratory report reveals the following: Hct: below normal Hb: below normal MCV: below normal MCHC: below normal MCH: below normal
Macrocytic (large cell size) anemia	Macrocytic anemia is commonly caused by folic acid and vitamin B_{12} deficiencies. Patients with macrocytic anemia produce fewer RBCs, but the RBCs that are present are larger than normal. Clinically, the laboratory report reveals the following: Hct: below normal Hb: below normal MCV: above normal (because of the larger RBC size) MCHC: above normal (because of the larger RBC size)

White Blood Cell Count

The major functions of the **white blood cell count** (WBCs) (leukocytes) are to (1) fight against infection, (2) defend the body by phagocytosis against foreign substances, and (3) produce (or at least transport and distribute) antibodies in the immune response. The WBCs are far less numerous than the RBCs, averaging 5000 to 10,000 cells per cubic millimeter of blood. There are two types of WBCs: **granular leukocytes** and **nongranular leukocytes.** Because the general function of the leukocytes is to combat inflammation and infection, the clinical diagnosis of an injury or infection often entails a differential count, which is the determination of the number of each type of cell in 100 WBCs. Box 8-2 shows a normal differential count. Table 8-2 provides an overview of cell types and common causes for their increase (**leukocytosis**).

Granular Leukocytes. The granular leukocytes (also called *granulocytes*) are so classified because of the granules present in their cytoplasm. The granulocytes are further divided into the following three types according to the staining properties of the granules: **neutrophils, eosinophils,** and **basophils.** Because these cells have distinctive multilobar nuclei, they are often referred to as *polymorphonuclear leukocytes.*

Neutrophils. The neutrophils comprise about 60% to 70% of the total number of WBCs. They have granules that are neutral and therefore do not stain with an acid or a basic dye. The neutrophils are the first WBCs to arrive at the site of inflammation, usually appearing within 90 minutes of the injury. They represent the primary defense against bacterial organisms through the process of phagocytosis. The neutrophils are one of several types of cells called *phagocytes* that ingest and destroy bacterial organisms and particulate matter. The neutrophils also release an enzyme called *lysozyme,* which destroys certain bacteria. An increased neutrophil count is associated with (1) bacterial infection, (2) physical and emotional stress, (3) tumors, (4) inflammatory or traumatic disorders, (5) some leukemias, (6) myocardial infarction, and (7) burns.

Early forms of neutrophils are nonsegmented and are called "band" forms. They almost always signify infection if elevated above 10% of the differential. More mature forms of neutrophils have segmented nuclei. They may increase even in the absence of infection (e.g., with stress [exercise] or the use of corticosteroid medication).

Eosinophils. The cytoplasmic granules of the eosinophils stain red with the acid dye eosin. These leukocytes comprise 2% to 4% of the total number of WBCs. Although the precise function of the eosinophils is unknown, they are thought to play a role in the breakdown of protein material. It is known, however, that the eosinophils are activated by allergies (such as an allergic asthmatic episode) and parasitic infections. Eosinophils are thought to detoxify the agents or chemical mediators associated with allergic reactions. An increased eosinophil count also may be associated with lung cancer, chronic skin infections (e.g., psoriasis, scabies), polycythemia, and tumors.

Basophils. The basophils comprise only about 0.5% to 1% of the total white blood count. The granules of the basophils stain blue with a basic dye. The precise function of the basophils is not clearly understood. Increased basophils are primarily associated with certain myeloproliferative disorders. It is thought that the basophils are involved in allergic and stress responses. They also are considered to be phagocytic and to contain heparin, histamines, and serotonin.

Box 8-2 Normal Differential White Blood Cell Count

Granular Leukocytes
Neutrophils 60% to 70%
Eosinophils 2% to 4%
Basophils 0.5% to 1%

Nongranular Leukocytes
Lymphocytes 20% to 25%
Monocytes 3% to 8%

TABLE 8-2 Common Causes of WBC Increase

Cell Type	Causes of Increase
Neutrophil	Bacterial infection, inflammation
Eosinophil	Allergic reaction, parasitic infection
Basophil	Myeloproliferative disorders
Monocyte	Chronic infections, malignancies
Lymphocyte	Viral infections

Nongranular Leukocytes. There are two groups of nongranular leukocytes, the **monocytes** and lymphocytes. The term *mononuclear leukocytes* also is used to describe these cells because they do not contain granules but have spheric nuclei.

Monocytes. The monocytes are the second order of cells to arrive at the inflammation site, usually appearing approximately 5 hours or more after the injury. After 48 hours, however, the monocytes are usually the predominant cell type in the inflamed area. The monocytes are the largest of the WBCs and comprise about 3% to 8% of the total leukocyte count. The monocytes are short-lived, phagocytic WBCs, with a half-life of approximately 1 day. They circulate in the bloodstream, from which they move into tissues—at which point they may mature into long-living macrophages (also called *histiocytes*). The **macrophages** are large wandering cells that engulf larger and greater quantities of foreign material than the neutrophils. When the foreign material cannot be digested by the macrophages, the macrophages may proliferate to form a capsule that surrounds and encloses the foreign material (e.g., fungal spores). Although the monocytes and macrophages do not respond as quickly to an inflammatory process as the neutrophils, they are considered one of the first lines of inflammatory defense. Therefore an elevated number of monocytes suggests infection and inflammation. The monocytes play an important role in chronic inflammation and also are involved in the immune response and malignancies.

Lymphocytes. Increased lymphocytes are typically seen in viral infections (e.g., infectious mononucleosis). The lymphocytes also are involved in the production of antibodies, which are special proteins that inactivate antigens. For a better understanding of the importance of the lymphocytes and the clinical significance of their destruction or depletion (e.g., in acquired immunodeficiency syndrome [AIDS]), a brief review of the role and function of the lymphocytes in the immune system is in order.

The lymphocytes can be divided into two categories: B cells and T cells. These cells can be identified with an electron microscope according to certain distinguishing surface marks, called *rosettes:* T cells have a smooth surface; B cells have projections. B cells comprise 10% to 30% of the total lymphocytes; T cells comprise 70% to 90% of the total lymphocytes.

The B cells, which are formed in the bone marrow, further divide into either plasma cells or memory cells. The plasma cells secrete antibodies in response to foreign antigens. The memory cells retain the ability to recognize specific antigens long after the initial exposure and therefore contribute to long-term immunity against future exposures to invading pathogens.

The T cells, which are formed in the thymus, are further divided into four functional categories: (1) cytotoxic T cells (also called *killer lymphocytes* or *natural killer cells*), which attack and kill foreign or infected cells; (2) helper T cells, which recognize foreign antigens and help activate cytotoxic T cells and plasma cells (B cells); (3) inducer T cells, which stimulate the production of the different T-cell subsets; and (4) suppressor T cells, which work to suppress the responses of the other cells and help provide feedback information to the system.

The T cells also may be classified according to their surface antigens (i.e., the T cells may display either T4 antigen or T8 antigen). The T4 surface antigen subset, which comprises 60% to 70% of the circulating T cells, consists mainly of the helper and inducer cells. The T8 surface antigen subset consists mainly of the cytotoxic and suppressor cells.

Sequence of Lymphocyte Responses to Infection. Initially, the macrophages attack and engulf the foreign antigens. This activity in turn stimulates the production of T cells and, ultimately, the antibody-producing B cells (plasma cells). The T4 cells play a pivotal role in the overall modulation of this immune response by (1) secreting a substance called *lymphokine,* which is a potent stimulus to T-cell growth and differentiation; (2) recognizing foreign antigens; (3) causing clonal proliferation of T cells; (4) mediating cytotoxic and suppressor functions; and (5) enabling B cells to secrete specific antibodies.

Because T cells (especially the T4 lymphocytes) have such a central role in this complex immune response, it should not be difficult to imagine the devastating effect that would ultimately follow from the systematic depletion of T lymphocytes. For example, virtually all the infectious complications of AIDS may be explained with reference to the effect that HIV has on the T cells. A decreased number of T cells increases the patient's susceptibility to a wide range of opportunistic infections and neoplasms. In the healthy subject, the T4/T8 ratio is about 2.0. In the HIV-infected patient with AIDS, the T4/T8 ratio is usually 0.5 or less.

Platelet Count. Platelets (also called *thrombocytes*) are the smallest of the formed elements in the blood. They are round or oval, flattened, and disk-shaped in appearance. Platelets are produced in the bone marrow and possibly in the lungs. Platelet activity is essential for blood clotting. The normal platelet count is 150,000 to 350,000/mm^3.

A deficiency of platelets leads to prolonged bleeding time and impaired clot retention. A low platelet count (**thrombocytopenia**) is associated with (1) massive blood transfusion, (2) pneumonia, (3) cancer chemotherapy, (4) infection, (5) allergic conditions, and (6) toxic effects of certain drugs (e.g., heparin, isoniazid, penicillins, prednisone, streptomycin). A high platelet count (thrombocythemia) is associated with (1) cancer, (2) trauma, (3) asphyxiation, (4) rheumatoid arthritis, (5) iron deficiency, (6) acute infections, (7) heart disease, and (8) tuberculosis.

A platelet count of less than 20,000/mm^3 is associated with spontaneous bleeding, prolonged bleeding time, and poor clot retraction. The precise platelet count necessary for hemostasis is not firmly established. Generally, platelet counts greater than 50,000/mm^3 are not associated with spontaneous bleeding. Therefore various diagnostic or therapeutic procedures, such as bronchoscopy or the insertion of an arterial catheter, are usually safe when the platelet count is greater than 50,000/mm^3.

Blood Chemistry

A basic knowledge of blood chemistry, normal values, and common health problems that alter these values is an important cornerstone of patient assessment. Table 8-3 lists the blood chemistry tests usually monitored in respiratory care.

Electrolytes

For the cells of the body to function properly, a normal concentration of **electrolytes** must be maintained. Therefore the monitoring of the electrolytes is extremely important in the patient whose body fluids are being endogenously or exogenously manipulated (e.g., intravenous therapy, renal disease, diarrhea). Table 8-4 lists electrolytes monitored in respiratory care.

TABLE 8-3 Blood Chemistry Tests Commonly Monitored in Respiratory Care

Chemical	Normal Value	Common Abnormal Findings
Glucose	70 to 110 mg/dl	Hyperglycemia (excess glucose level) Diabetes mellitus Acute infection Myocardial infarction Thiazide and loop diuretics Hypoglycemia (low glucose level) Pancreatic tumors or liver disease Pituitary or adrenocortical hyperfunction
Lactic dehydrogenase (LDH)	80 to 120 Wacker units	Increases are associated with the following: Myocardial infarction Chronic hepatitis Pneumonia Pulmonary infarction
Serum glutamic oxaloacetic transaminase (SGOT)	8 to 33 U/ml	Increases are associated with the following: Myocardial infarction Congestive heart failure Pulmonary infarction
Aspartate aminotransferase (AST)	7 to 40 U/L (0.12-067 μKat/L)	Increases are associated with the following: Acute aminotransferase hepatitis Liver disease Myocardial infarction Pulmonary infection
Alanine aminotransferase (ALT) (previously called serum glutamic pyruvic transaminase [SGPT])	5 to 36 U/L (0.08-0.6 μKat/L)	Increases are associated with the following: Liver damage Inflammation Shock
Bilirubin	Adult: 0.1 to 1.2 mg/dl Newborn: 1 to 12 mg/dl	Increases are associated with the following; Massive hemolysis Hepatitis
Blood urea nitrogen (BUN)	8 to 18 mg/dl	Increases are associated with acute or chronic renal failure
Serum creatinine	0.6 to 1.2 mg/dl	Increases are associated with renal failure

TABLE 8-4 Electrolytes Commonly Monitored in Respiratory Care

Electrolyte	Normal Value	Common Abnormal Findings	Clinical Manifestations
Sodium (Na^+)	136 to 142 mEq/L	Hypernatremia (excess Na^+) Dehydration	Desiccated mucous membranes Flushed skin Great thirst Dry tongue
		Hyponatremia (low Na^+) Sweating Burns Loss of gastrointestinal secretions Use of some diuretics Excessive water intake	Abdominal cramps Muscle twitching Poor perfusion Vasomotor collapse Confusion Seizures
Potassium (K^+)	3.8 to 5.0 mEq/L	Hyperkalemia (excess K^+) Renal failure Muscle tissue damage	Irritability Nausea Diarrhea Weakness Ventricular fibrillation

Continued

TABLE 8-4 Electrolytes Commonly Monitored in Respiratory Care—cont'd

Electrolyte	Normal Value	Common Abnormal Findings	Clinical Manifestations
		Hypokalemia (low K^+) Diuretic therapy Endocrine disorder Diarrhea Reduced intake or loss of K^+ Chronic stress	Metabolic alkalosis Muscular weakness Malaise Cardiac arrhythmias Hypotension
Chloride (Cl^-)	95 to 103 mEq/L	Hyperchloremia (excess Cl^-) Renal tubular acidosis Hypochloremia (low Cl^-) Alkalosis	Deep, rapid breathing Weakness Disorientation Metabolic alkalosis Muscle hypertonicity Tetany Depressed ventilation (respiratory compensation)
Calcium (Ca^{++})	4.5 to 5.4 mEq/L	Hypercalcemia (excess Ca^{++}) Malignant tumors Bone fractures Diuretic therapy Excessive use of antacids or milk consumption Vitamin-D intoxication Hyperparathyroidism	Lethargy, weakness Hyporeflexia Constipation, anorexia, renal stones Mental deterioration
		Hypocalcemia (low Ca^{++}) Respiratory alkalosis Pregnancy Vitamin D deficiency Diuretic therapy Hypoparathyroidism	Paresthesia, cramping of muscles, stridor, convulsions, mental disturbance, Chvostek's sign, Trousseau's sign

SELF-ASSESSMENT QUESTIONS

evolve Answers to questions can be found on Evolve. To access additional student assessment questions and case studies for application of text material to real-life scenarios, visit **http://evolve.elsevier.com/DesJardins/respiratory.**

1. In the healthy woman, what is the Hct?
a. 31%
b. 38%
c. 42%
d. 45%

2. Which of the following represent the primary defense against bacterial organisms through phagocytosis?
a. Eosinophils
b. Neutrophils
c. Monocytes
d. Basophils

3. What is the normal Hb value for men?
a. 10 to 12 g%
b. 12 to 14 g%
c. 14 to 16 g%
d. 16 to 18 g%

4. What is the normal differential neutrophil count?
a. 20% to 25%
b. 40% to 50%
c. 60% to 70%
d. 75% to 85%

5. In the healthy man, what is the RBC count?
a. 5,000,000/mm^3
b. 6,000,000/mm^3
c. 7,000,000/mm^3
d. 8,000,000/mm^3

6. What is the normal WBC count?
a. 1000 to 5000/mm^3
b. 5000 to 10,000/mm^3
c. 10,000 to 15,000/mm^3
d. 15,000 to 20,000/mm^3

7. Which of the following are activated by allergies (such as an allergic asthmatic episode)?

a. Eosinophils
b. Neutrophils
c. Monocytes
d. Basophils

8. Various clinical procedures such as bronchoscopy or the insertion of an arterial catheter are generally safe when the platelet count is no lower than which of the following?

a. 100,000/mm^3
b. 75,000/mm^3
c. 50,000/mm^3
d. 20,000/mm^3

9. Which of the following are associated with hyperglycemia?

1. Diabetes mellitus
2. Myocardial infarction
3. Thiazide and loop diuretics
4. Acute infection

a. 2 and 4 only
b. 2, 3, and 4 only
c. 1, 2, and 3 only
d. 1, 2, 3, and 4

10. Which of the following are clinical manifestations associated with hyponatremia?

1. Seizures
2. Confusion
3. Muscle twitching
4. Abdominal cramps

a. 2 and 4 only
b. 2, 3, and 4 only
c. 1, 2, and 3 only
d. 1, 2, 3, and 4

The Therapist-Driven Protocol Program and the Role of the Respiratory Care Practitioner

9

Chapter Objectives

After reading this chapter, you will be able to:

- Describe the Therapist-Driven Protocol (TDP) program and the role of the respiratory care practitioner.
- Discuss the knowledge base required for a successful TDP program.
- Explain the assessment process skills required for a successful TDP program, and include the following:
  - The clinical manifestations, assessments, and treatment selections made by the respiratory care practitioner
  - The frequency at which a respiratory therapy modality can be determined in response to a severity assessment
- Describe the following essential cornerstone respiratory protocols for a successful TDP program:
  - Oxygen therapy protocol
  - Bronchopulmonary hygiene therapy protocol
  - Lung expansion therapy protocol
  - Aerosolized medication therapy protocol
  - Mechanical ventilation protocol
  - Mechanical ventilation weaning protocol
- Describe ventilatory management in catastrophes.
- List the following common anatomic alterations of the lungs:
  - Atelectasis
  - Consolidation
  - Increased alveolar-capillary membrane thickness
  - Bronchospasm
  - Excessive bronchial secretions
  - Distal airway and alveolar weakening
- Analyze the clinical scenarios—chain of events—activated by the common anatomic alterations of the lungs, and include the following:
  - Anatomic alterations of the lungs
  - Pathophysiologic mechanisms activated
  - Clinical manifestations
  - Treatment protocols used to correct the problem
- Identify the most common anatomic alterations associated with the respiratory disorders presented in this textbook.
- Define key terms and complete self-assessment questions at the end of the chapter and on Evolve.

Key Terms

Aerosolized Medication Therapy Protocol
Anatomic Alterations of the Lung
Atelectasis
Bronchopulmonary Hygiene Therapy Protocol
Bronchospasm
Clinical Practice Guidelines (CPGs)
Clinical Scenarios
Consolidation
Distal Airway and Alveolar Weakening
Excessive Bronchial Secretions
Increased Alveolar-Capillary Membrane Thickness
Lung Expansion Therapy Protocol
Mechanical Ventilation Protocol
Mechanical Ventilation Weaning Protocol
Oxygen Therapy Protocol
Pathophysiologic Mechanisms
Therapist-Driven Protocols (TDPs)

Chapter Outline

The "Knowledge Base" Required for a Successful Therapist-Driven Protocol Program
The "Assessment Process Skills" Required for a Successful Therapist-Driven Protocol Program
Severity Assessment
Overview Summary of a Good Therapist-Driven Protocol Program
Common Anatomic Alterations of the Lungs
Clinical Scenarios Activated by Common Anatomic Alterations of the Lungs

Introduction

Therapist-driven protocols (TDPs) are an integral part of respiratory care health services. According to the American Association for Respiratory Care (AARC), the purposes of respiratory TDPs are to:

- Deliver individualized diagnostic and therapeutic respiratory care to patients
- Assist the physician with evaluating patients' respiratory care needs and optimize the allocation of respiratory care services
- Determine the indications for respiratory therapy and the appropriate modalities for providing high-quality, cost-effective care that improves patient outcomes and decreases length of stay
- Empower respiratory care practitioners to allocate care using sign- and symptom-based algorithms for respiratory treatment

To further support the AARC's purpose statement on TDPs, the American College of Chest Physicians (ACCP) defines respiratory therapy protocols as follows:

> *...Patient care plans which are initiated and implemented by credentialed respiratory care workers. These plans are designed and developed with input from physicians, and are approved for use by the medical staff and the governing body of the hospitals in which they are used. They share in common extreme reliance on assessment and evaluation skills. Protocols are by their nature dynamic and flexible, allowing up- or down-regulation of intensity of respiratory services. Protocols allow the respiratory care practitioner authority to evaluate the patient, initiate care, to adjust, discontinue, or restart respiratory care procedures on a shift-by-shift or hour-to-hour basis once the protocol is ordered by the physician. They must contain clear strategies for various therapeutic interventions, while avoiding any misconception that they infringe on the practice of medicine.*

Respiratory TDPs provide the respiratory care practitioner with a wide-ranging flexibility to both assess and treat the patient—but only within preapproved and clearly defined boundaries outlined by the physician and/or the medical staff. In addition, respiratory TDPs give the practitioner specific authority to (1) gather clinical information related to the patient's respiratory status, (2) make an assessment of the clinical data collected, and (3) start, increase, decrease, or discontinue certain respiratory therapies on a moment-to-moment, hour-to-hour, shift-by-shift, or day-to-day basis. The innate beauty of respiratory TDPs is that (1) the physician is always in the "information loop" regarding patient care and (2) therapy can be quickly modified in response to the specific and immediate needs of the patient. Numerous clinical research studies have verified these facts: Respiratory TDPs (1) significantly improve respiratory therapy outcomes and (2) appreciably lower therapy costs.

Unfortunately, the implementation of TDPs throughout the United States has been slow. In 2008 the AARC Protocol Implementation Committee conducted a survey to evaluate the barriers to protocol implementation. Over 450 respiratory managers responded to the survey. Despite the overwhelming evidence that protocols clearly improve outcomes and reduce cost, the survey showed that less than 50% of respiratory care was provided by protocols. About 75% of the respondents had at least one protocol in operation. The majority of the hospitals did not have a comprehensive program in place. According to the managers, the medical directors, managers of the department, nurses, and administrators were not perceived as barriers. The biggest barrier to the implementation of protocols was perceived to be the medical staff. The primary reason for the medical staff's resistance was perceived to be that "staff therapists did not have the skills (e.g., assessment skills) to function under protocols." The AARC Protocol Implementation Committee states that "[this] perception *must* change... ."*

The essential components of a good TDP program do not come easy. This is because a strong TDP program promises that the respiratory care practitioner, who is identified as "TDP safe and ready," be qualified to (1) systematically collect the appropriate clinical data, (2) formulate a uniform and accurate assessment, and (3) select a uniform and optimal treatment within the limits set by the protocol (Figure 9-1). The converse, however, is also true: When the respiratory care practitioner is *not* "TDP safe and ready," the collection of clinical data is not done at all or is incomplete. As a result, nonuniform or inaccurate assessments are made, resulting in nonuniform or inaccurate treatment selections (Figure 9-2). This inappropriate and ineffective type of respiratory therapy leads to the misallocation of care, the administration of unneeded care, and—most important—the nonprovision of needed patient care. The bottom line is poor-quality patient

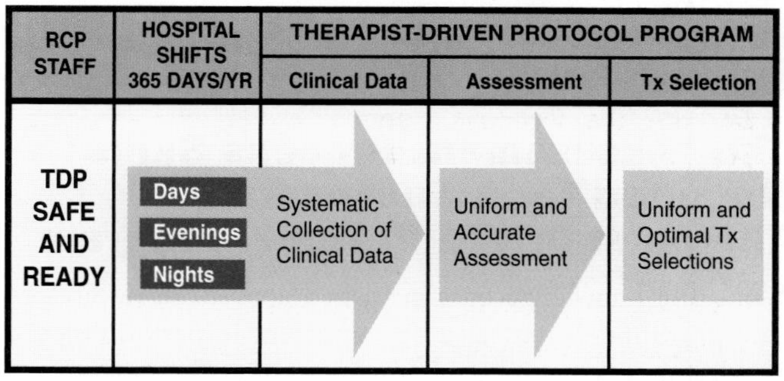

RCP STAFF	HOSPITAL SHIFTS 365 DAYS/YR	THERAPIST-DRIVEN PROTOCOL PROGRAM		
		Clinical Data	Assessment	Tx Selection
TDP SAFE AND READY	Days Evenings Nights	Systematic Collection of Clinical Data	Uniform and Accurate Assessment	Uniform and Optimal Tx Selections

FIGURE 9-1 The promise of a good therapist-driven protocol program.

RCP STAFF	HOSPITAL SHIFTS 365 DAYS/YR	NO THERAPIST-DRIVEN PROTOCOL PROGRAM		
		Clinical Data	Assessment	Tx Selection
			Nonuniform and Inaccurate	Nonuniform and Nonoptimal
NOT TDP SAFE AND READY	Days Evenings Nights	Incomplete or NO Collection of Clinical Data	Assessment Assessment Assessment	Tx Selection Tx Selection Tx Selection

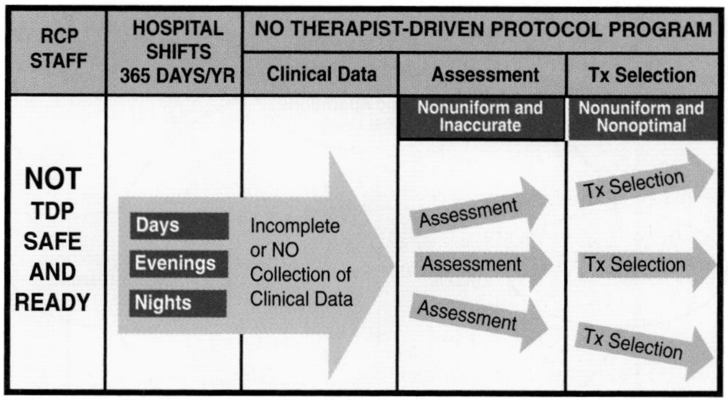

FIGURE 9-2 No assessment program in place.

*The AARC Protocol Implementation Committee has developed a slide presentation of the complete survey, which is intended to assist in understanding the barriers and developing successful strategies to implement protocols (www.aarc.org; search for *AARC Protocol Implementation Committee*).

care and unnecessary costs. To be sure, the development and implementation of a strong TDP program require some fundamental knowledge, training, and practice, but the benefits are worth the price. The essential components of a good TDP program are discussed in the following paragraphs.

The "Knowledge Base" Required for a Successful Therapist-Driven Protocol Program

As shown in Figure 9-3, the essential knowledge base for a successful TDP program includes (1) the anatomic alterations of the lungs caused by common respiratory disorders, (2) the major pathophysiologic mechanisms activated throughout the respiratory and cardiac systems as a result of the anatomic alterations, (3) the common clinical manifestations that develop as a result of the activated pathophysiologic mechanisms, and (4) the treatment modalities used to correct them. *In other words, the clinical manifestations demonstrated by the patient do not arbitrarily appear but are the result of anatomic lung alterations and pathophysiologic events.*

Hence, it is essential that the respiratory practitioner know and understand that certain anatomic alterations of the lung will lead to specific—and often predictable—clinical manifestations. Each respiratory disease chapter presented in this textbook describes these four essential knowledge components necessary for TDP work. In the clinical setting this knowledge base enhances the assessment process essential to a good TDP program.

The "Assessment Process Skills" Required for a Successful Therapist-Driven Protocol Program

Using the knowledge base described above, the respiratory care practitioner must also be competent in performing the actual assessment process. This means that the practitioner can (1) quickly and systematically gather the clinical information demonstrated by the patient, (2) formulate an accurate assessment of the clinical data (i.e., identify the cause and severity of the problem), (3) select an optimal treatment modality, and (4) document this process quickly, clearly, and precisely. In the clinical setting, the practice—and mastery—of the assessment process is absolutely central and essential to the success of a good TDP program (Figure 9-4). In other words, immediately after the respiratory care practitioner identifies the appropriate clinical manifestations (clinical indicators), an assessment of the data must be performed, and a treatment plan must be formulated. For the most part the assessment is primarily directed at the anatomic alterations of the lungs that are causing the clinical indicators (e.g., **bronchospasm**) and the severity of the clinical indicators.

For example, an appropriate assessment for the clinical indicator of wheezing might be bronchospasm—the anatomic alteration of the lungs. If the practitioner assesses the cause of the wheezing correctly as bronchospasm, then the correct treatment selection would be a bronchodilator treatment from the **Aerosolized Medication Therapy Protocol** (see Protocol 9-4, page 122). If, however, the cause of the wheezing is correctly assessed to be excessive airway secretions, then the appropriate treatment plan would entail a specific treatment modality under the **Bronchopulmonary Hygiene Therapy Protocol,** such as cough and deep breathing or chest physical therapy (see Protocol 9-2, page 120).

Table 9-1 illustrates common clinical manifestations (i.e., clinical indicators), assessments, and treatment selections routinely made by the respiratory care practitioner.

Severity Assessment

The frequency at which a respiratory therapy modality is to be administered is just as important as the correct selection of a respiratory therapy treatment. Often the frequency of treatment must be up-regulated or down-regulated on a shift-by-shift, hour-to-hour, minute-to-minute, or even (in life-threatening situations) second-to-second basis. Such frequency changes must be made in response to a severity assessment. In a good TDP program, the well-seasoned

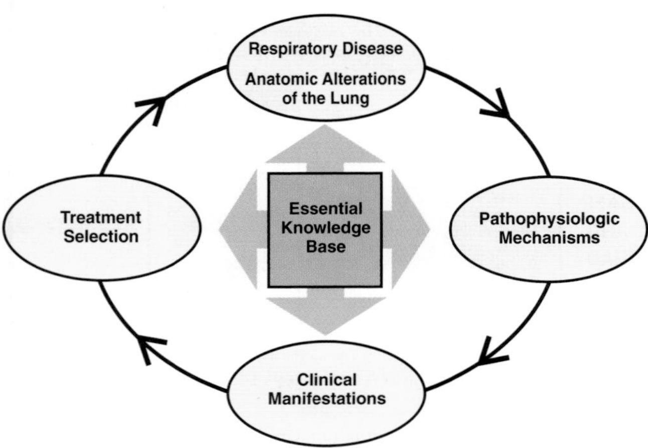

FIGURE 9-3 Foundations for a strong therapist-driven protocol program. Overview of the essential knowledge base for assessment of respiratory disease.

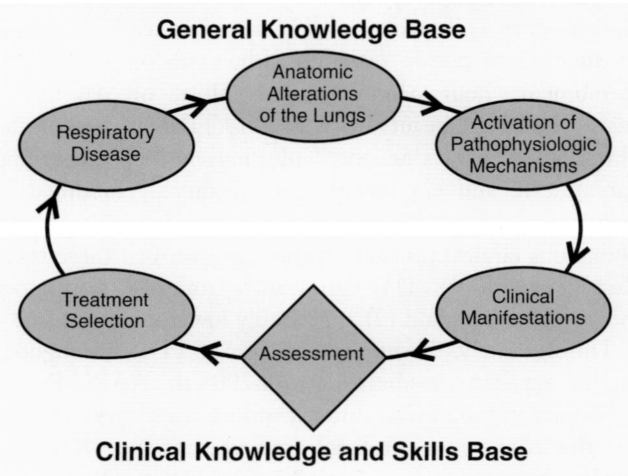

FIGURE 9-4 The way knowledge, assessment, and a therapist-driven protocol program interface.

TABLE 9-1 Clinical Manifestations, Assessments, and Treatment Selections Commonly Made by the Respiratory Care Practitioner

Clinical Data (indicators)	Assessments	Treatment Selections
Vital Signs		
↑Breathing rate, ↑blood pressure, ↑pulse	Respiratory distress	Treat underlying cause
Abnormal Airway Indicators		
Wheezing	Bronchospasm	Bronchodilator treatment
Inspiratory stridor	Laryngeal edema	Cool mist
Rhonchi	Secretions in large airways	Bronchial hygiene treatment
Crackles	Secretions in distal airways	Treat underlying cause—e.g., congestive heart failure (CHF) Hyperinflation treatment
Cough Effectiveness Indicators		
Strong cough	Good ability to mobilize secretions	None
Weak cough	Poor ability to mobilize secretions	Bronchial hygiene treatment
Abnormal Secretion Indicators		
Amount: >30 ml/24 hrs	Excessive bronchial secretions	Bronchial hygiene treatment
White and translucent sputum	Normal sputum	None
Yellow or opaque sputum	Acute airway infection	Treat underlying cause
Green sputum	Old, retained secretions and infections	Bronchial hygiene treatment
Brown sputum		Bronchial hygiene treatment
Red sputum	Old blood	Notify physician
Frothy secretions	Fresh blood Pulmonary edema	Treat underlying cause—e.g., congestive heart failure (CHF) Hyperinflation treatment
Abnormal Lung Parenchyma Indicators		
Bronchial breath sounds	Atelectasis	Hyperinflation treatment, oxygen treatment
Dull percussion note	Infiltrates or effusion	Treat underlying cause
Opacity on chest X-ray	Fibrosis	No specific treatment
Restrictive pulmonary function test values	Consolidation	No specific, effective respiratory care treatment
Depressed diaphragm on X-ray	Air trapping and hyperinflation	Treat underlying cause
Abnormal Pleural Space Indicators		
Hyperresonant percussion note	Pneumothorax	Evacuate air* and hyperinflation treatment
Dull percussion note	Pleural effusion	Evacuate fluid* and hyperinflation treatment
Abnormalities of the Chest Shape and Motion		
Paradoxical movement of the chest wall	Flail chest	Mechanical ventilation*
Barrel chest	Air trapping (hyperinflation)	Treat underlying cause—e.g., asthma
Posterior and lateral curvature of spine	Kyphoscoliosis	Bronchial hygiene treatment
Arterial Blood Gases—Ventilatory		
pH↑, $Paco_2$↓, HCO_3^-↓	Acute alveolar hyperventilation	Treat underlying cause
pH N, $Paco_2$↓, HCO_3^-↓↓	Chronic alveolar hyperventilation	Generally none
pH↓, $Paco_2$↑, HCO_3^-↑	Acute ventilatory failure	Mechanical ventilation*
pH N, $Paco_2$↑, HCO_3^-↑↑	Chronic ventilatory failure	Low-flow oxygen, bronchial hygiene
Sudden Ventilatory Changes on Chronic Ventilatory Failure (CVF)		
pH↑, $Paco_2$↑, HCO_3^-↑↑, Pao_2↓	Acute alveolar hyperventilation on CVF	Treat underlying cause
pH↓, $Paco_2$↑↑, HCO_3^-↑ Pao_2↓	Acute ventilatory failure on CVF	Mechanical ventilation*
Metabolic		
pH↑, $Paco_2$ N, or ↑, HCO_3^-↑, Pao_2 N	Metabolic alkalosis	Give potassium*—Hypokalemia Give chloride*—Hypochloremia

Continued

TABLE 9-1 Clinical Manifestations, Assessments, and Treatment Selections Commonly Made by the Respiratory Care Practitioner—cont'd

Clinical Data (indicators)	Assessments	Treatment Selections
pH↓, $Paco_2$ N or ↓, HCO_3^-↓, Pao_2↓	Metabolic acidosis	Give oxygen—Lactic acidosis
pH↓, $Paco_2$ N or ↓, HCO_3^-↓, Pao_2 N	Metabolic acidosis	Give insulin*—Ketoacidosis
pH↓, $Paco_2$ N or ↓, HCO_3^-↓, Pao_2 N	Metabolic acidosis	Renal therapy*
Indication for Mechanical Ventilation		
pH↑, $Paco_2$↓, HCO_3^-↓, Pao_2↓	Impending ventilatory failure	Mechanical ventilation
pH↓, $Paco_2$↑, HCO_3^-↑, Pao_2↓	Ventilatory failure	
pH↓, $Paco_2$↑, HCO_3^-↑, Pao_2↓	Apnea	
Oxygenation Status		
$Pao_2 < 80$ mm Hg	Mild hypoxemia	Oxygen treatment and treat underlying cause
$Pao_2 < 60$ mm Hg	Moderate hypoxemia	
$Pao_2 < 40$ mm Hg	Severe hypoxemia	
Oxygen Transport Status		
↓Pao_2, anemia, ↓cardiac output	Inadequate oxygen transport	Oxygen treatment and treat underlying cause

* These procedures should be performed only as ordered by the physician.

respiratory care practitioner routinely and systematically documents many severity assessments throughout each working day. For the new practitioner, however, a predesigned Severity Assessment Rating Form may be used to enhance this important part of the assessment process. One excellent, semiquantitative method of accomplishing this is illustrated in Table 9-2. The clinical application of this severity assessment is provided in the following case example.

Severity Assessment Case Example

A 67-year-old man arrived in the emergency room in respiratory distress. The patient was well known to the therapist-driven protocol (TDP) team; he had been diagnosed with chronic bronchitis several years before this admission (3 points). The patient had no recent surgery history, and he was ambulatory, alert, and cooperative (0 points). He complained of dyspnea and was using his accessory muscles of inspiration (3 points). Auscultation revealed bilateral rhonchi over both lung fields (3 points). His cough was weak and productive of thick gray secretions (3 points). A chest x-ray film revealed pneumonia (consolidation) in the left lower lung lobe (3 points). On room air his arterial blood gas values were pH 7.52, $Paco_2$ 54, HCO_3^- 41, and Pao_2 52—acute alveolar hyperventilation on chronic ventilatory failure (3 points).

Using the Severity Assessment Form shown in Table 9-2, the following treatment selection and administration frequency would be appropriate:

Total score: 17

Treatment selection: Chest physical therapy

Frequency of administration: Four times a day; and as needed

*

The Essential Cornerstone Respiratory Protocols for a Successful Therapist-Driven Protocol Program

Although there are many "assess and treat" respiratory care protocols used throughout the health-care industry today, the following respiratory protocol examples provide the "essential foundation" of a successful TDP program:

- **Oxygen Therapy Protocol (Protocol 9-1)**
- **Bronchopulmonary Hygiene Therapy Protocol (Protocol 9-2)**
- **Aerosolized Medication Therapy Protocol (Protocol 9-4)**
- **Lung Expansion Therapy Protocol (Protocol 9-3)**
- **Mechanical Ventilation Protocol (Protocol 9-5 and Protocol 9-6)**
- **Mechanical Ventilation Weaning Protocol (Protocol 9-7)**

The vast majority of the daily work performed by the respiratory practitioner involves assessments and treatments associated with these protocols. Most patients with respiratory problems require care found in one or more of these protocols. These respiratory protocols are the essential cornerstones of a good TDP program. For example, a patient experiencing a severe asthmatic episode would likely demonstrate a variety of objective clinical indicators to justify the assessments that call for the administration of oxygen therapy (e.g., to treat hypoxemia), an aerosolized bronchodilator (e.g., to treat bronchospasm), bronchial hygiene therapy (e.g., to mobilize the thick white secretions associated with asthma), and mechanical ventilation (e.g., to treat acute ventilatory failure).

As shown in the algorithms in Protocols 9-1 through 9-7, a step-by step, branching logic process directs the

Text continued on p. 123

TABLE 9-2 Respiratory Care Protocol Severity Assessment

Item	0 Points	1 Point	2 Points	3 Points	4 Points
Respiratory history	Negative for smoking or history not available	Smoking history <1 pack a day	Smoking history >1 pack a day	Pulmonary disease	Severe or exacerbation
Surgery history	No surgery	General surgery	Lower abdominal	Thoracic or upper abdominal	Thoracic with lung disease
Level of consciousness	Alert, oriented, cooperative	Disoriented, follows commands	Obtunded, uncooperative	Obtunded	Comatose
Level of activity	Ambulatory	Ambulatory with assistance	Nonambulatory	Paraplegic	Quadriplegic
Respiratory pattern	Normal rate 8-20/min	Respiratory rate 20-25/min	Patient complains of dyspnea	Dyspnea, use of accessory muscles, prolonged expiration	Severe dyspnea, use of accessory muscles, respiratory rate >25, and/or swallow
Breath sounds	Clear	Bilateral crackles	Bilateral crackles and rhonchi	Bilateral wheezing, crackles, and rhonchi	Absent and/or diminished bilaterally and/or severe wheezing, crackles, or rhonchi
Cough	Strong, spontaneous, nonproductive	Excessive bronchial secretions and strong cough	Excessive bronchial secretions but weak cough	Thick bronchial secretions and weak cough	Thick bronchial secretions but no cough
Chest X-ray	Clear	One lobe: infiltrates, atelectasis, consolidation, or pleural effusion	Same lung, two lobes: infiltrates, atelectasis, consolidation, or pleural effusion	One lobe in both lungs: infiltrates, atelectasis, consolidation, or pleural effusion	Both lungs, more than one lobe: infiltrates, atelectasis, consolidation, or pleural effusion
Arterial blood gases and/or oxygen saturation measured by pulse oximeter (Spo_2)	Normal	Normal pH and $Paco_2$ but Pao_2 60-80 and/or Spo_2 91-96%	Normal pH and $Paco_2$ but Pao_2 40-60 and/or Spo_2 85-90%	Acute respiratory alkalosis, $Pao_2 < 40$ and/or Spo_2 80-84%	Acute respiratory failure, $Pao_2 < 80$ and/or $Spo_2 < 80\%$

Severity Index

Total Score	Severity Assessment	Treatment Frequency
1-5	Unremarkable	As needed
6-15	Mild	Two or three times a day
16-25	Moderate	Four times a day or as needed
Greater than 26	Severe	Two to four times a day and as needed; Alert attending physician

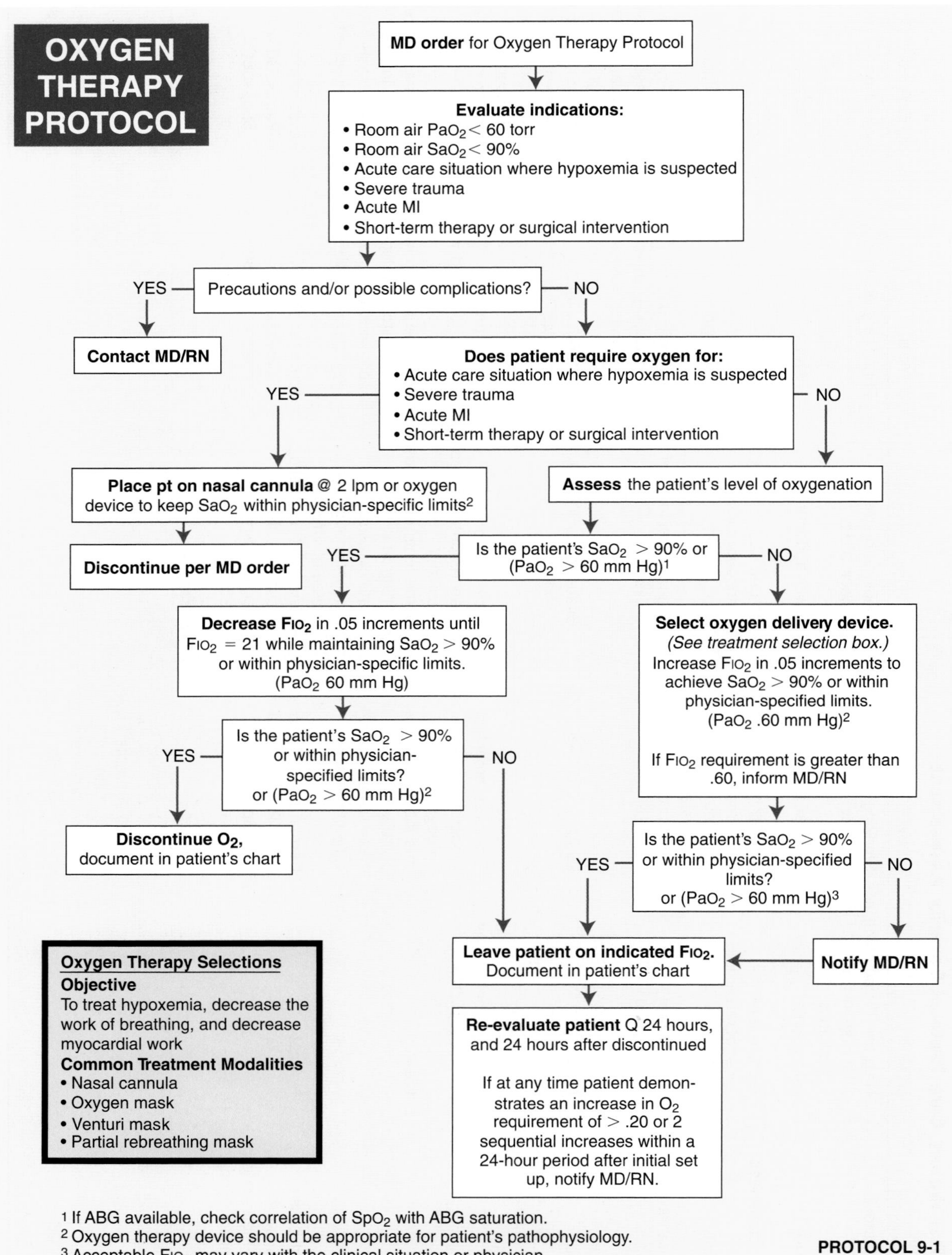
OXYGEN THERAPY PROTOCOL
MD order for Oxygen Therapy Protocol
Evaluate indications:
• Room air $PaO_2 < 60$ torr
• Room air $SaO_2 < 90\%$
• Acute care situation where hypoxemia is suspected
• Severe trauma
• Acute MI
• Short-term therapy or surgical intervention
Precautions and/or possible complications?
YES
Contact MD/RN
NO
Does patient require oxygen for:
• Acute care situation where hypoxemia is suspected
• Severe trauma
• Acute MI
• Short-term therapy or surgical intervention
YES
Place pt on nasal cannula @ 2 lpm or oxygen device to keep SaO_2 within physician-specific limits[2]
Discontinue per MD order
NO
Assess the patient's level of oxygenation
Is the patient's $SaO_2 > 90\%$ or ($PaO_2 > 60$ mm Hg)[1]
YES
Decrease FIO_2 in .05 increments until $FIO_2 = 21$ while maintaining $SaO_2 > 90\%$ or within physician-specific limits. (PaO_2 60 mm Hg)
Is the patient's $SaO_2 > 90\%$ or within physician-specified limits? or ($PaO_2 > 60$ mm Hg)[2]
YES
Discontinue O_2, document in patient's chart
NO
NO
Select oxygen delivery device. (See treatment selection box.) Increase FIO_2 in .05 increments to achieve $SaO_2 > 90\%$ or within physician-specified limits. (PaO_2 .60 mm Hg)[2]
If FIO_2 requirement is greater than .60, inform MD/RN
Is the patient's $SaO_2 > 90\%$ or within physician-specified limits? or ($PaO_2 > 60$ mm Hg)[3]
YES
NO
Leave patient on indicated FIO_2. Document in patient's chart
Notify MD/RN
Re-evaluate patient Q 24 hours, and 24 hours after discontinued
If at any time patient demonstrates an increase in O_2 requirement of > .20 or 2 sequential increases within a 24-hour period after initial set up, notify MD/RN.
Oxygen Therapy Selections
Objective
To treat hypoxemia, decrease the work of breathing, and decrease myocardial work
Common Treatment Modalities
• Nasal cannula
• Oxygen mask
• Venturi mask
• Partial rebreathing mask
1 If ABG available, check correlation of SpO_2 with ABG saturation.
2 Oxygen therapy device should be appropriate for patient's pathophysiology.
3 Acceptable FIO_2 may vary with the clinical situation or physician.
PROTOCOL 9-1

BRONCHOPULMONARY HYGIENE THERAPY PROTOCOL

MD order for Bronchopulmonary Hygiene Therapy Protocol

↓

Evaluate indications:
- Difficulty with secretion clearance with sputum production > 25 ml/day
- Evidence of retained secretions
- Mucous plug-induced atelectasis
- Foreign body in airway
- Diagnosis of cystic fibrosis, bronchiectasis, or cavitating lung disease

↓

Does contraindication or potential hazard exist?

YES → **Address any immediate need and contact MD/RN**

NO →

Select method based on:
- Patient preference/comfort/pain avoidance
- Observation of effectiveness with trial
- History with documented effectiveness

Method may include:
(See treatment selection box)
- Manual chest percussion and positioning
- External chest wall vibration
- Intrapulmonary percussion

↓

Administer therapy no less than QID and PRM, supplemented by suctioning for all patients with artificial airways

↓

Re-evaluate pt every 24 hours, and 24 hours after discontinued

↓

Assess Outcomes — Goals Achieved?
- Optimal hydration with sputum production > 25 ml/day
- Breath sounds from diminished to adventitious with rhonchi cleared by cough.
- Patient subjective impression of less retention and improved clearance
- Resolution/improvement in chest X-ray
- Improvement in vital signs and measures of gas exchange
- If on ventilator, reduced resistance and improved compliance

↓

Care Plan Considerations:
- Discontinue therapy if improvement is observed and sustained over a 24-hour period.
- Patients with chronic pulmonary disease who maintain secretion clearance in their home environment should remain on treatment no less than their home frequency.
- Lung Expansion Therapy Protocol (9-3) should be considered for patients who are at high risk for pulmonary complications as listed in the indications for Lung Expansion Therapy Protocol.

Bronchopulmonary Hygiene Therapy Selections

Objective
To enhance mobilization of bronchial secretions

Common Treatment Modalities
- Increased broncial hydration
  - Increased fluid intake
    (6-10 glasses of water a day)
  - Bland aerosol therapy
  - Ultrasonic nebulization (USN)
- Cough and deep breathing (C & DB)
  Techniques used the enhance C & DB
  - Incentive spirometry (IS)
  - Intermittent positive-pressure breathing (IPPB)
  - Intermittent percussion ventilation (IPV)
  - Positive expiratory pressure (PEP) therapy
  - Flutter valve
- Chest physical therapy (CPT)
- Postural drainage (PD)
- Percussion and vibration with postural drainage
- Suctioning
- Mucolytic therapy (see Protocol 9-4)
  - Acetylcysteine (Mucomyst)—often in combination with a bronchodilator
  - Recombinant human deoxyribonuclease (DNase, Pulmozyme)
  - Sodium bicarbonate (2% solution)
- Assist physician in bronchoscopy

PROTOCOL 9-2

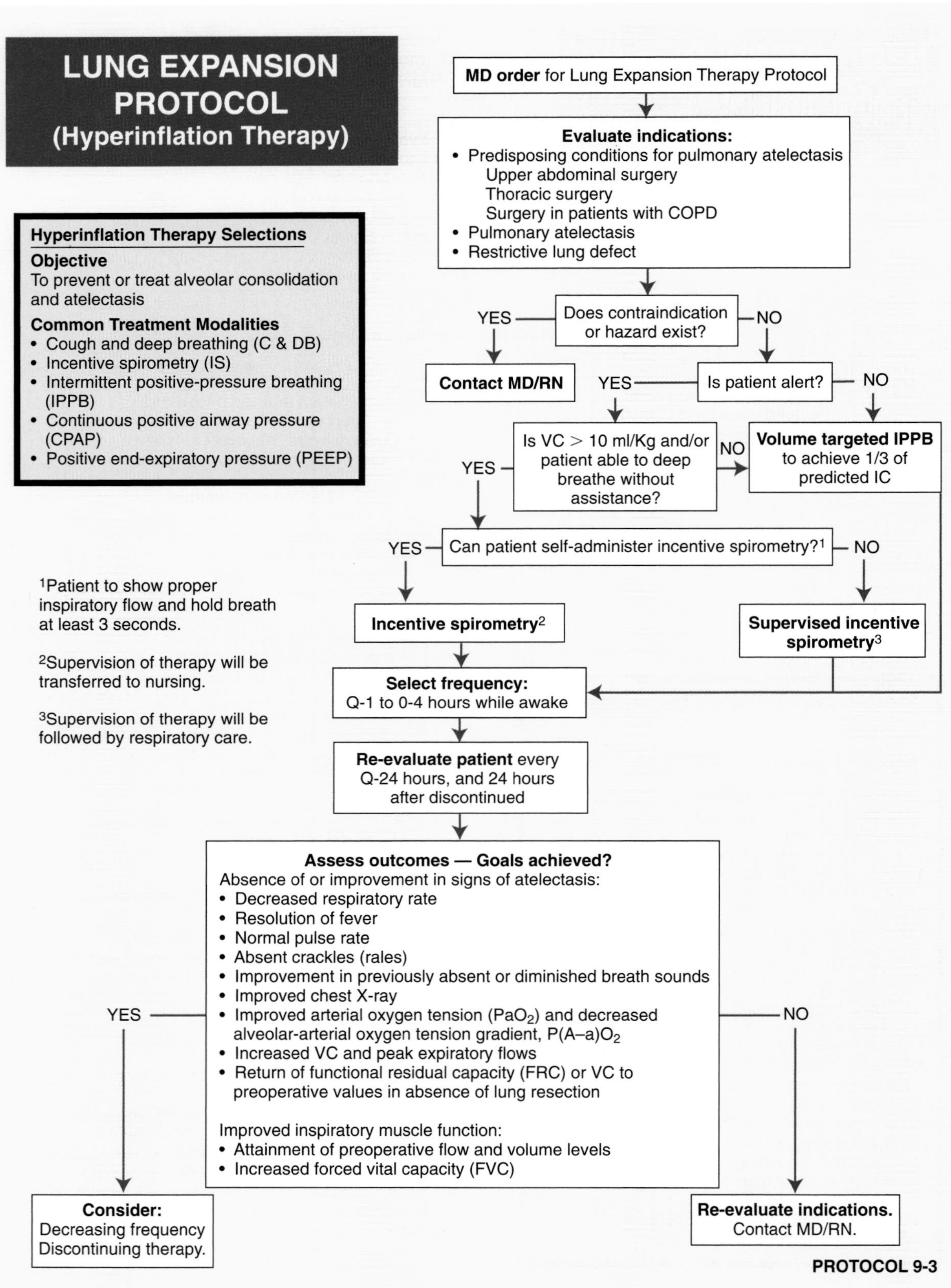

LUNG EXPANSION PROTOCOL
(Hyperinflation Therapy)
Hyperinflation Therapy Selections
Objective
To prevent or treat alveolar consolidation and atelectasis
Common Treatment Modalities
• Cough and deep breathing (C & DB)
• Incentive spirometry (IS)
• Intermittent positive-pressure breathing (IPPB)
• Continuous positive airway pressure (CPAP)
• Positive end-expiratory pressure (PEEP)
MD order for Lung Expansion Therapy Protocol
Evaluate indications:
• Predisposing conditions for pulmonary atelectasis
Upper abdominal surgery
Thoracic surgery
Surgery in patients with COPD
• Pulmonary atelectasis
• Restrictive lung defect
Does contraindication or hazard exist?
YES
NO
Contact MD/RN
Is patient alert?
YES
NO
Is VC > 10 ml/Kg and/or patient able to deep breathe without assistance?
YES
NO
Volume targeted IPPB to achieve 1/3 of predicted IC
Can patient self-administer incentive spirometry?[1]
YES
NO
Incentive spirometry[2]
Supervised incentive spirometry[3]
Select frequency:
Q-1 to 0-4 hours while awake
Re-evaluate patient every Q-24 hours, and 24 hours after discontinued
Assess outcomes — Goals achieved?
Absence of or improvement in signs of atelectasis:
• Decreased respiratory rate
• Resolution of fever
• Normal pulse rate
• Absent crackles (rales)
• Improvement in previously absent or diminished breath sounds
• Improved chest X-ray
• Improved arterial oxygen tension (PaO_2) and decreased alveolar-arterial oxygen tension gradient, $P(A–a)O_2$
• Increased VC and peak expiratory flows
• Return of functional residual capacity (FRC) or VC to preoperative values in absence of lung resection
Improved inspiratory muscle function:
• Attainment of preoperative flow and volume levels
• Increased forced vital capacity (FVC)
YES
NO
Consider:
Decreasing frequency
Discontinuing therapy.
Re-evaluate indications.
Contact MD/RN.
[1]Patient to show proper inspiratory flow and hold breath at least 3 seconds.
[2]Supervision of therapy will be transferred to nursing.
[3]Supervision of therapy will be followed by respiratory care.

PROTOCOL 9-3

AEROSOLIZED MEDICATION THERAPY PROTOCOL

Aerosolized Medication Therapy Selections

AEROSOLIZED BRONCHODILATORS

Objective

Sympathomimetics and parasympatholytics are used to offset bronchial smooth muscle constriction. Common treatment modalities are:

Sympathomimetics

Short-to-Intermediate-Acting

- Metaproterenol (Alupent, Metaprel)
- Terbutaline (Brethine, Brethaire)
- Pirbuterol (Maxair)
- Albuterol (Ventolin, Proventil)
- Levalbuterol (Xopenex)*Long-Acting*
- Salmeterol (Serevent)
- Formoterol (Foradil)

Parasympatholytics (anticholinergics)

- Atropine sulfate (Dey-Dose Atropine Sulfate)
- Ipratropium bromide (Atrovent)
- Tiotroprium (Spiriva)
- Ipratropium bromide and Albuterol (Combivent)

MUCOLYTIC AGENTS

Objective

Mucolytic agents are used to enhance the mobilization and thinning of bronchial secretions. Common treatment modalities are:

- Acetylcysteine (Mucomyst)
- Dornase alfa (Pulmozyme, rhDNase, DNase)
- Sodium bicarbonate (2% solution)

ANTIINFLAMMATORY AGENTS

Objective

Aerosolized corticosteroids are used to suppress bronchial inflammation and edema. They also are used for their ability to enhance the responsiveness of B_2 receptor sites to sympathomimetic agents. Common examples are:

- Beclomethasone dipropionate (Beclovent, Vanceril)
- Triamcinolone acetonide (Azmacort)
- Flunisolide (AeroBid, AeroBid-M)
- Fluticasone propionate (Flovent)
- Budesonide (Pulmicort Turbuhaler, Pulmicort Respules)
- Fluticasone propionate and Salmeterol (Advair Diskus)

MD order for Aerosol Medication Therapy Protocol

↓

Evaluate indications:
The primary general indication for aerosolized bronchodilator therapy is reversible reactive airway disease. This condition is detected through the following symptoms:

- C/O dyspnea
- Wheezing
- Hyperinflation
- Reduction in airflow (peak flow, FEV_1, FVC, prolonged expiration)

↓

Does contraindication or potential hazard exist?

YES → Respond to immediate need and contact MD/RN.

NO → **Select aerosols for bronchospasm:**

- Sympathomimetic agent
- Combine with anti-inflammatory if history of COPD (if used on a daily basis)
- Anticholinergics

Select device: Metered Dose Inhaler (MDI) with accessory device is the preferred delivery method, unless the medication is not available in MDI, or the patient is unable to use the device with proper coaching and instruction. In which case a small volume nebulizer with equivalent dose may be used.

↓

Administer therapy no less than Q4 and PRN.
*Note that MDI dose may be titrated upward to a total of 16 puffs (with 1 minute between activations) if the patient continues to be symptomatic without dose-limiting side effects.

↓

Re-evaluate patient every 24 hours, and 24 hours after discontinued

↓

Assess outcomes — Goals achieved?

- Diminished wheezing and the volume of air moved is increased
- Improvement in airflow (peak expiratory flow rate, PEFR)
- Improved vital signs and measures of gas exchange
- Improved patient appearance with decreased use of accessory muscles

↓

Care Plan Considerations: Discontinue therapy if improvement is observed and sustained over a 24-hour period.

**Note that this protocol is for simple bronchodilator administration for non-ventilated patients. There are a variety of other options such as continuous bronchodilator administration, acute maximum titration of dose, and multiple delivery devices that can be incorporated within this protocol or as a separate protocol depending on site-specific preference.*

PROTOCOL 9-4

practitioner to (1) gather clinical data (clinical indicators), (2) make assessment decisions based on the clinical data, and (3) either start, up-regulate, down-regulate, or discontinue a treatment modality. In fact, the primary reason a good TDP program works is because a specific treatment modality cannot be started, stopped, or modified unless there are specific—and measurable—clinical indicators identified to justify the assessment and treatment decision.

The treatment selections outlined in each of the listed protocols are based on current AARC's **Clinical Practice Guidelines (CPGs),** which provide the most recent scientific evidence that justifies the administration of a specific treatment modality. Using the evidence-based method mandated by the scientific community, CPGs provide the indications, contraindications, hazards and complications, assessment of need, assessment of outcome, and appropriate monitoring techniques used for specific therapy modalities. In other words, the CPGs are the gold standards used by the respiratory care practitioner to start, adjust, or discontinue a specific treatment modality. In Box 9-1, excerpts from the AARC's CPG on oxygen therapy for adults in the acute care facility provide a representative example of a CPG—and, more important, the scientific basis for the Oxygen Therapy Protocol (Protocol 9-1).*

Several different treatment selections are listed under each of the protocols. In essence, the various treatment selections

*See www.aarc.org/ Search Clinical Practice Guidelines for the most recent and complete list of Clinical Practice Guidelines.

Box 9-1 Oxygen Therapy for Adults in the Acute Care Facility

AARC Clinical Practice Guideline (Excerpts)*

Indications

- Documented hypoxemia. Defined as a decreased Pa_{O_2} in the blood below normal range.
  - $Pa_{O_2} < 60$ mm Hg or $Sa_{O_2} < 90\%$ in subjects breathing room air
- Acute care situations in which hypoxemia is suspected
- Severe trauma
- Acute myocardial infarction
- Short-term therapy or surgical intervention (e.g., postanesthesia recovery, hip surgery)

Contraindications

- No specific contraindications to oxygen therapy exist when indications are present.

Precautions and/or Possible Complications

- $Pa_{O_2} > 60$ mm Hg may depress ventilation in some patients with elevated Pa_{CO_2}.
- $F_{IO_2} > 0.5$, may cause absorption atelectasis, oxygen toxicity, and/or ciliary or leukocyte depression.
- Supplemental oxygen should be administered with caution to patients with paraquat poisoning or to those receiving bleomycin.
- During laser bronchoscopy, minimal F_{IO_2} should be used to avoid intratracheal ignition.
- Fire hazard is increased in the presence of increased oxygen concentration.
- Bacterial contamination associated with nebulizers or humidifiers is a possible hazard.

Assessment of Need

- Need is determined by measurement of inadequate oxygen tension and/or saturation, by invasive or noninvasive methods, and/or the presence of clinical indicators.

Assessment of Outcome

- Outcome is determined by clinical and physiologic assessment to establish adequacy of patient response to therapy.

Monitoring

- Patient
  - Clinical assessment including cardiac, pulmonary, and neurologic status
  - Assessment of physiologic parameters (Pa_{O_2}, Sa_{O_2}, Sp_{O_2}) in conjunction with the initiation of therapy or:
    Within 12 hours of initiation with $F_{IO_2} < 40$
    Within 8 hours with $F_{IO_2} \geq 0.40$ (including postanesthesia recovery)
    Within 72 hours in acute myocardial infarction
    Within 2 hours for any patient with principal diagnosis of COPD
- Equipment
  - All oxygen delivery systems should be checked at least once per day.
- More frequent checks are needed in systems:
  Susceptible to variation in oxygen concentration (e.g., hood, high-flow blending systems)
  Applied to patients with artificial airways
  Delivering a heated gas mixture
  Applied to patients who are clinically unstable or who require $F_{IO_2} > 0.50$
- Care should be taken to avoid interruption of oxygen therapy in situations including ambulation or transport for procedure.

*See http://www.aarc.org/ (Clinical Practice Guidelines) for the most recent and complete list of clinical practice guidelines.
From Respir Care 47(6):717-720, 2002. See this article for the complete guidelines.

serve as a "therapy selection menu." When the patient demonstrates the clinical indicators associated with any of these protocols, the respiratory therapist is expected to select and administer the most efficient and most cost-effective treatment to the patient. As already discussed, the treatment selection decision and the frequency with which the therapy is to be administered are based on (1) the identification of the appropriate clinical indicators, (2) the severity suggested by the clinical information, (3) the patient's ability to perform or tolerate the therapy, and (4) the patient's response to the therapy.

For example, the implementation of the **Lung Expansion Therapy Protocol** (Protocol 9-3) would likely be indicated after thoracic surgery to prevent, or correct, **atelectasis.** If the patient were unconscious or unable to follow directions, a continuous positive airway pressure (CPAP) mask would be a more appropriate treatment selection (under the Lung Expansion Therapy Protocol) than, say, incentive spirometry—even though both are designed to treat or prevent atelectasis. In this example, the CPAP mask therapy would be more expensive but more appropriate than the less expensive incentive spirometry.

Remember, the treatment portion of a protocol is based on the therapy that will *best* work to correct or offset the anatomic alterations and pathophysiologic mechanisms caused by the respiratory disorder in a timely and cost-efficient manner. Finally, even when the patient is transferred to the intensive care unit, intubated, and placed on a mechanical ventilator, the respiratory care practitioner must usually still administer one or more of the first four respiratory therapy treatment protocols listed in this section. For example, the patient would likely need CPAP or positive end-expiratory pressure (PEEP) to offset any alveolar atelectasis caused by bronchial airway mucous plugs via the Lung Expansion Therapy Protocol. Or, the patient would likely require a bronchodilator agent to offset bronchospasm via the Aerosolized Medication Therapy Protocol.

The following sections provide an overview of the respiratory care practitioner's most sophisticated and refined protocols—the Mechanical Ventilation Protocol and the Mechanical Ventilation Weaning Protocol.

Mechanical Ventilation Protocol

It is interesting to note that many medical centers have started their TDP programs with a Mechanical Ventilation Protocol rather than with one of the simpler protocols described in this chapter (e.g., Oxygen Therapy Protocol, Bronchial Hygiene Protocol, Lung Expansion Protocol, or Aerosolized Medication Protocol). The decision to proceed in this manner often appears to be based on humanistic, pathophysiologic, and economic grounds. Indeed, who could defend practices that are unnecessary (if not actually harmful), uncomfortable, and costly to patients requiring ventilator support?

Although there are a number of good ventilatory management strategies used to treat specific respiratory disorders, the need for a standardized approach to ventilator management has required the development of Mechanical Ventilation Protocols. Protocol 9-5 provides an example of a Mechanical Ventilation Protocol. Protocol 9-6 further illustrates a more comprehensive—and operational—protocol for Mechanical Ventilator Management, and Protocol 9-7 illustrates an example of a comprehensive operational Mechanical Ventilation Weaning Protocol.*

The primary objectives of mechanical ventilation are (1) to reverse acute ventilatory failure, (2) to maintain normal respiratory balance, or homeostasis—especially the acid-base balance of the blood and the amounts of CO_2 and O_2 exchange, (3) to improve oxygenation and increase lung volume, (4) to reduce the work of breathing, (5) to permit sedation or paralysis (or both), and decrease systemic and/or myocardial oxygen consumption.

Achievement of these objectives reverses acute ventilatory failure (also called *acute respiratory acidosis*) and corrects the patient's acid-base balance and oxygenation status, reverses or prevents atelectasis and stabilizes the chest wall, reverses muscle fatigue, allows sedation and/or neuromuscular blockade, and decreases systemic or myocardial oxygen consumption—a daunting list, indeed! Furthermore, the attainment of these goals and objectives results from an intelligent assessment of the patient's needs, an understanding of the pertinent pathophysiology, and knowledge of ventilator management techniques most likely to meet the needs of the moment. This is the cornerstone of the "assess and treat" paradigm of the Mechanical Ventilation Protocol.

Unquestionably, the high-technology, high-risk, high-visibility portion of respiratory care work is embedded in ventilator management. Much of the success of the TDP movement has occurred because of the dramatic ways in which standardized, data-driven algorithms have improved patient outcomes. Most dramatic are shortened ventilator weaning times, reduction of nosocomial infections, and reduced complication rates of mechanical ventilation (e.g., barotrauma).

Mechanical ventilation may be delivered by endotracheal tube (most common), by tracheostomy, by a face mask, or by a cuirass-type device. Ventilator modes include assist-control (A/C) and synchronized intermittent mandatory ventilation (SIMV) with or without pressure support (PS). Much less commonly used modes include SIMV alone, inverse-ratio ventilation (IRV), and airway pressure release ventilation (APRV). In general, the goal of mechanical ventilation is to totally or partially replace the gas exchange function of the lungs, with as few complications as possible.

Although most Mechanical Ventilation Protocols require the respiratory care practitioner to select a ventilator mode on the basis of specific patient needs, it is not the intent of this textbook to fully review or discuss the various ventilator modes and weaning strategies. Table 9-3, however, does provide an excellent overview of common ventilatory management strategies and good starting points used to treat specific pulmonary disorders.

Text continued on p. 137

*We would like to thank the Respiratory Care Department at the Kettering Medical Center, in Dayton, Ohio, for providing their Ventilator Management Protocol and Ventilator Weaning Protocol.

MECHANICAL VENTILATION PROTOCOL

Patient meets criteria
for Mechanical Ventilation Protocol

↓

Clinical indications for Mechanical Ventilation Protocol:
- Acute ventilatory failure
- Apnea
- Impending ventilatory failure
- Conditions that may require mechanical ventilation
  - Acute exacerbation of COPD
  - Neuromuscular disorders
  - Cardiac or respiratory arrest
  - Postoperative patients requiring ongoing sedation

↓

Reversal of underlying conditions

↓

Adjustment of ventilatory support to meet patient's physical condition:
- Airway establishment (intubation) and management
- Cuff management
- Ventilatory management
  - Respiratory rate (frequency), tidal volume
  - Oxygen concentration (FIO_2) (see Protocol 9-1)

Ventilator System Pressure
- Peak pressure
- Mean airway pressure (MAP)
- Continuous positive airway pressure (CPAP)

Ventilator Mode
- Assist control (A/C)
- Intermittent mandatory ventilation (IMV)
- Synchronized intermittent mechanical ventilation (SIMC)
- Pressure support (PS)
- Pressure regulated control (PRVC)

↓

Ventilatory weaning protocol

↓

Daily assessment of readiness to undergo Spontaneous Breathing Trial (SBT):
- Improvement or resolution of underlying condition
- FIO_2: $< 50\%$ with $SpO_2 > 90\%$
- PEEP: < 8 cm H_2O
- Hemodynamic status: normal or near normal without vasopressors
- Hb: > 8 g%
- Core temperature: $< 38.5°C$
- Nutrition status: normal or near normal serum albumin levels

↓

One minute SBT to determine readiness for prolonged SBT

← Rapid shallow breathing index < 100 → SBT of 30 to 120 minutes as tolerated until patient can tolerate full 120 minutes SBT → **Extubation**

→ Rapid shallow breathing index > 100 → Slow, progressive withdrawal of pressure support until able to tolerate 120 minutes SBT → **Extubation**

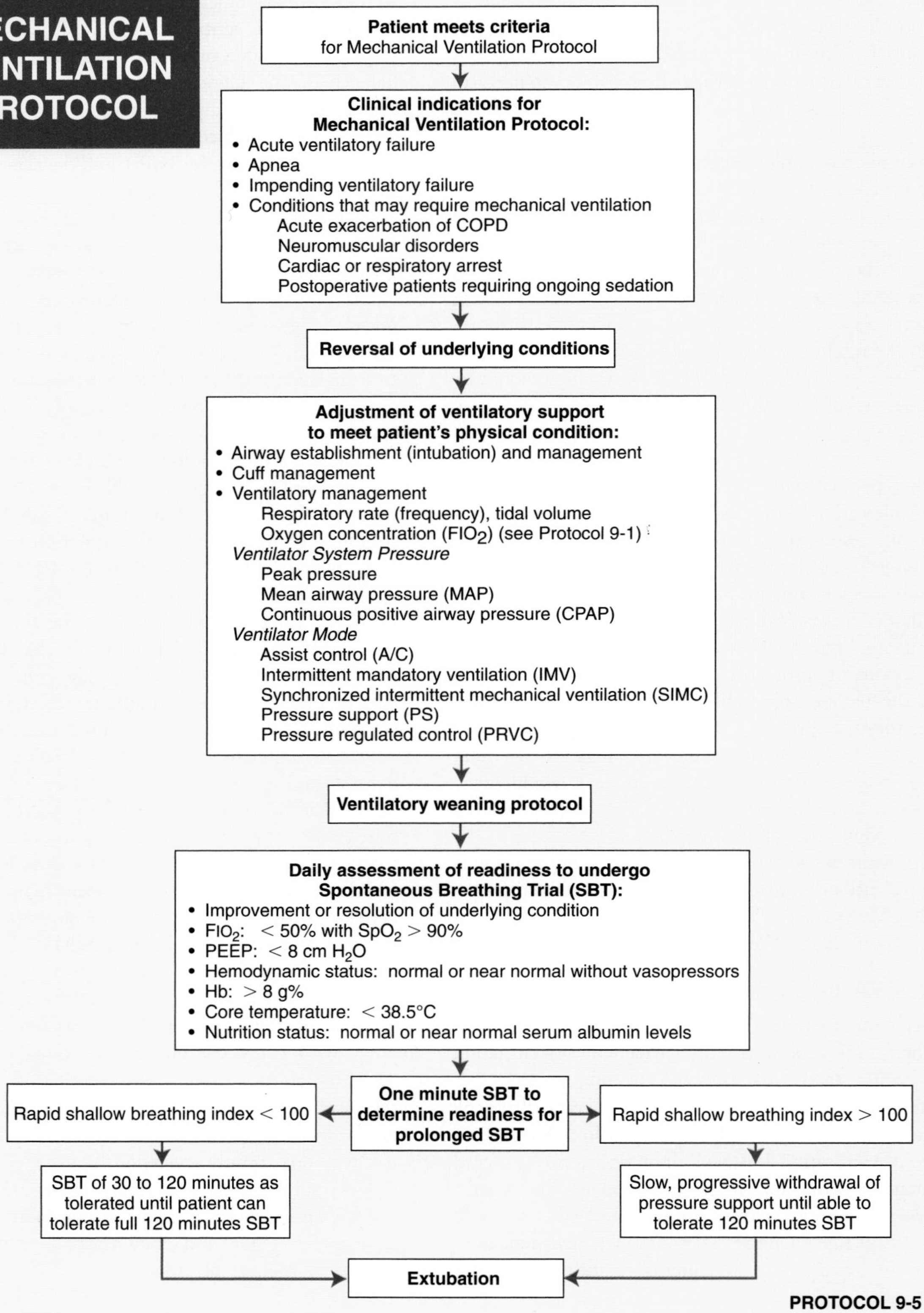

PROTOCOL 9-5

VENTILATOR MANAGEMENT PROTOCOL

PURPOSE:
The Respiratory Care Practitioner will utilize the following protocol to determine the most appropriate settings to maintain and manage oxygenation and ventilation for mechanically ventilated patients.

PATIENT TYPE:
All adult patients requiring mechanical ventilation

EQUIPMENT NEEDED:

- Pulse oximeter
- Ventilator
- Stethoscope
- Oxygen analyzer
- Wright's spirometer
- NIP manometer
- EKG monitor
- Heated aerosol with appropriate attachments
- $ETCO_2$ (if available)

LABORATORY DATA NEEDED:
Recent arterial blood gas results, chest x-ray

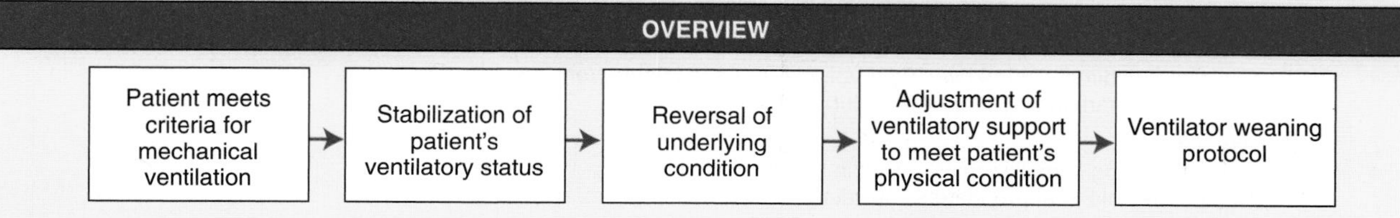

I. Indications for mechanical ventilation include:

A. Basic Indications

1. Acute respiratory failure (ARF)
   a. Acute hypoxic respiratory failure with tachypnea, respiratory distress, and persistent hypoxemia despite administration of high FIO_2 via high flow system or in the presence of any of the following:
      1) acute cardiovascular instability
      2) altered mental status
      3) inability to protect lower airway
   b. Acute hypercarbic ventilatory failure with tachypnea, respiratory distress, and persistent hypoxemia despite administration of high FIO_2 via high flow system or in the presence of any of the following:
      1) pH <7.3
      2) acute cardiovascular instability
      3) altered mental status
      4) inability to protect lower airway
2. Apnea
3. Impending Acute Respiratory Failure: Studies have failed to define impending failure. This remains the judgment call of the attending physician.

B. Clinical Conditions That May Require Mechanical Ventilation

1. Acute exacerbation of COPD if patient has dyspnea, tachycardia, and acute respiratory acidosis plus at least one of the following:
   a. Acute cardiovascular instability
   b. Altered mental status
   c. Inability to protect lower airway
   d. Copious/viscous secretions
   e. Progressive respiratory acidosis despite non-invasive positive pressure ventilation (mask CPAP)

PROTOCOL 9-6P1

B. **Clinical Conditions That May Require Mechanical Ventilation**

2. Neuromuscular disease with any of the following:
   a. Acute respiratory acidosis
   b. Progressive decrease in VC to $<$10-15 ml/kg
   c. Progressive decrease in NIP < -20 to 30 cm H_2O
3. Cardiac or respiratory arrest
4. Postoperative patients requiring ongoing sedation
5. Other complex medical conditions leading to impending acute respiratory failure as determined by the attending physician
6. In the following conditions, Non-Invasive Positive Pressure Ventilation (NIPPV) should be attempted before intubation:
   a. Dyspnea / respiratory distress
   b. Acute exacerbation of COPD without other indicators listed above
   c. Acute hypoxemia in immunocompromised patients
   d. Cardiogenic pulmonary edema

II. The following guidelines will be used in selecting the most appropriate ventilator mode:

A. **Volume Control Ventilation** (although no ventilatory mode has been proven better than another, volume control is generally accepted as a traditional method of ventilation – a good place to start).

1. Benefits
   a. Clinician has direct control over Tidal Volume (V_T) and Minute Ventilation ($\dot{V}_E$)
   b. Appropriate starting place for newly intubated patients
2. Limitations
   a. Decreased lung compliance will result in high airway pressures
   b. May not be able to appropriately ventilate patients with very poor compliance
3. Modes
   a. **Assist Control (A/C)**
      1) Most effective mode for unloading of respiratory muscles
      2) Can be used with patients with no spontaneous respiratory effort
      3) Should be used as long as hyperventilation is necessary to normalize pH (e.g. renal failure with decreased HCO_3^- or metabolic ketoacidosis)
      4) Things to consider with A/C
         a) Alkalosis – if patient assists at high respiratory rate
         b) Auto PEEP if patient assists at high respiratory rate
         c) Increased PIP if lung compliance decreases or if patient assists at high respiratory rate. Both static and dynamic lung compliance should be calculated and documented at least Q8 hours, regardless of the mode of ventilation (formulas to follow in Section B.4.)
   b. **Synchronized Intermittent Mechanical Ventilation (SIMV)**
      1) Normal rate SIMV provides unloading of respiratory muscles with less risk of respiratory alkalosis than A/C.
      2) Prevents respiratory muscle atrophy
      3) Things to consider with SIMV
         a) Fatigue / tachypnea if rate set low
         b) Hypercapnia if rate set too low
         c) High demand valve WOB in older ventilators
      4) Pressure Support (PS) should be used in conjunction with SIMV if the patient has spontaneous respiratory effort above the set ventilator rate. This helps to overcome the resistance to air flow caused by ventilator tubing and ETT, and avoids increased WOB.
      5) The use of SIMV / PS in the clinical setting has not proven as an efficient weaning mode as compared to T-piece trails and pressure support ventilation. Compared to T-piece trials and PSV, it is associated with the longest weaning time and the lowest success rates.

PROTOCOL 9-6P2

B. **Pressure Controlled Ventilation (PCV)**

1. Benefits
   a. In spontaneously breathing patients, the variable flow characteristics of PCV is more comfortable and may actually decrease WOB – especially in patients with variable respiratory demand.
   b. Patients who are air hungry when being ventilated with low tidal volumes in volume ventilation modes may experience less dyspnea in PCV because of the variable flow and patient dependent nature of the mode.
   c. Peak airway pressures are able to be controlled and still ventilate the patient.
2. Limitations
   a. V_T is not pre-set and therefore is not guaranteed.
   b. V_T is dependent on lung compliance and is subject to change quickly.
   c. Alarms are essential in PCV to ensure adequate ventilation.
      1) V_T is set 50-100 ml above and below target V_T
      2) Low exhaled minute ventilation within 1 liter
3. Consider place patient on PCV if:
   a. V_T and V_E are compromised because inspiration terminates when pressure limit is reached in volume control mode.
   b. Patient is spontaneously breathing and appears to be air hungry. PCV may be able to meet patient demand because of its variable flow characteristics.
   c. Patient's oxygenation status requires inverse ratio ventilation (IRV). A physician's order must be received for I:E ratio less than 1:2 (e.g., 1:1.5, 1:1, 2:1, etc.)
4. Compliance
   a. Abnormally low or high lung compliance impairs the lung's ability to effectively exchange gases. Low compliance makes expansion difficult and high compliance induces incomplete exhalation and compromises CO_2 elimination. Changes in lung compliance may greatly impact volumes achieved in pressure control mode.
   b. Dynamic lung compliance should be calculated and documented at least every 6 hours, using the following formula:
      $C_{dyne} = V_T \text{ (in ml)} \div (PIP - PEEP)$
   c. Static lung compliance should be calculated and documented at least every 6 hours using the following formula:
      $C_{st} = V_T \div (P_{plat} - PEEP)$

C. **Bi-Level Ventilation**

1. Benefits
   a. The same as those for PCV
   b. Has been found to result in better gas exchange than CMV (either volume controlled or pressure controlled) in ARDS patients.
   c. Patients requiring Inverse Ratio Ventilation (IRV):
      1) Bi-level may reduce need for sedation and/or paralytics and allow patients to breathe spontaneously.
      2) IRV must be ordered by an attending physician.
2. Limitations
   a. V_T and V_E are not pre-set. They are not guaranteed.
   b. Alarms must be set 50-100 ml above and below target V_T in order to assure adequate ventilation.
   c. Bi-level ventilation is not available on all ventilators.
3. Patients who require PCV may be placed on bi-level as long as an appropriate ventilator is available and the patient's I:E level is 1:2 or greater. It patient requires less than 1:2 I:E (e.g. 1:1.5; 1:1; 2:1, etc.), an order from the attending physician must be obtained.

D. **APRV**

1. Benefits
   a. Airway Pressure Release Ventilation (APRV) has been found to result in better gas exchange than CMV (either volume controlled or pressure controlled) in ARDS patients.
   b. APRV may reduce need for sedation and/or paralytics and allow patients to breathe spontaneously.
2. Limitations
   a. V_T and V_E are not pre-set. They are not guaranteed.
   b. Alarms must be set 50-100 ml above and below target V_T in order to assure adequate ventilation.
   c. APRV is not available on all ventilators.
   d. APRV can only be initiated with the order of the attending physician.

PROTOCOL 9-6P3

E. **Pressure Support Ventilation** (CPAP/PS)

1. Benefits
   a. Peak flow and V_T are entirely patient dependent.
   b. Prevents respiratory muscle atrophy.
2. Limitations
   a. V_T and V_E are not guaranteed, therefore alarms must be set and monitored closely.
   b. Respiratory muscles may become fatigued.
3. Use on patients who
   a. Have stable lung compliance
   b. Are spontaneously breathing
   c. Are hemodynamically stable
4. Things to observe
   a. Sedation levels
   b. Sudden changes in $\dot{V}_E$
   c. Fatigue
   d. Tachypnea
   e. Hypercapnea
   f. Increased WOB

III. The following guidelines will be used in selecting the most appropriate ventilatory settings.

A. **Tidal Volume** (V_T): 6-8 ml/kg ideal body weight.

1. Reasons for using small volumes:
   a. Minimizes ventilator induced lung injury (volutrauma and/or barotrauma)
   b. Improved clinical outcomes for ARDS patient
2. V_T may be increased if:
   a. Patient's demand is not met AND
   b. Plateau pressures are <30 cm H_2O
3. IBW is calculated using the following formulas:
   a. Females – 100 pounds for the first 5 feet in height + 5 pounds for each additional inch of height, divided by 2.2 to convert pounds to kilograms (kg)

      e.g. a 5′5″ female, weighing 250 pounds has an ideal body weight of [100 + (5×5)] / 2.2 100+25 = 125 pounds divided 2.2 = 57 kg and should be placed on V_T of about 340 cc based on 6 ml/kg IBW.

   b. Males – 106 pounds for the first 5 feet of height + 6 pounds for each additional inch in height, divided by 2.2 to convert pounds to kilograms (kg).

      e.g. a 6′1″ male, weighing 310 pounds has an ideal weight of [106 + (6×13)] / 2.2 106+78 = 184 pounds divided 2.2 = 85 kg and should be placed on V_T of about 500 cc based on 6 ml/kg IBW.

B. **Pressure Control Level** (if patient being ventilated in pressure as opposed to volume mode)

1. Inspiratory pressure should be set and adjusted to keep V_T within 50 to 100 ml of the selected target of 6 ml/kg IBW.
2. Setting I:E ratio in pressure control ventilation
   a. I:E ratio should be set between 1:2 and 1:4 for most patients.
   b. When setting I:E, observe patient and waveforms to determine if patient has time for full exhalation.
   c. When traditional I:E ratio has failed to improve patient's ventilation and oxygenation status, inverse ratio ventilation (IRV) may be used, pending physician's approval.[6]
   d. The use of sedation and paralytics may be necessary when a patient is being ventilated with IRV in PC.
   e. If a patient's oxygen status requires ventilation at less than 1:2 I:E ratio (e.g. 1:1.5; 1:1; 2:1, etc), ventilator settings must be ordered by the attending physician.

C. **Respiratory Rate** (RR)

1. Once V_T or PC level is chosen, frequency is set to provide a $\dot{V}_E$ that achieves adequate pH.
2. As a starting point, RR 12-20/min is considered physiological.
   a. When using small V_T per protocol (6 ml/kg IBW), higher RRs will be needed to achieve adequate $\dot{V}_E$.
   b. ABG should be obtained 30 minutes after initiation of mechanical ventilation. The following formula is used to determine the appropriate RR:

PROTOCOL 9-6P4

New Rate $= \dfrac{\text{current vent rate} \times \text{current } P_aCO_2}{\text{*Desired } P_aCO_2}$ *Desired is not necessarily normal P_aCO_2*

For example: 5′8″ male has IBW ~ 75 kg and V_T is set at 450 cc and rate 14.
ABG shows pH = 7.29, PCO_2 = 56. RCP wishes to reduce P_aCO_2 to 45.

New Rate $= \dfrac{14 \times 56}{45} = 17$

c. If RCP determines that both V_T and RR should change as a result of the ABG, use the following formulas, instead:

New $\dot{V}_E = \dfrac{\text{current } \dot{V}_E \times \text{current } P_aCO_2}{\text{Desired } P_aCO_2}$

New RR $= \dfrac{\text{desired } \dot{V}_E}{\text{New } V_T}$

For example: 5′2″ female has IBW ~ 55 kg and is placed on V_T of 330 and RR of 16. ABG shows pH = 7.25, P_aCO_2 = 62. Plateau pressures = 14 cm H_2O; therefore, the RCP decides to increase both V_T and RR. The patient's plateau pressure is 20 at a V_T of 400 cc. The RCP selects V_T of 400 ml. The demand P_aCO_2 in 45 mm Hg.

New $\dot{V}_E = \dfrac{5.28 \times 62}{45} = 7.27$

New RR $= \dfrac{7.27}{.400} = 18$

D. **Positive End Expiratory Pressure (PEEP)**

1. Application of PEEP in patient with ARDS receiving mechanical ventilation may improve oxygenation and increase lung volume.
2. PEEP is especially important in maintaining lung volumes and recruiting alveoli when ventilating at low tidal volumes.
3. Setting Optimal PEEP: Normally, the alveolar and end-expiratory pressure equilibrates with atmospheric pressure (i.e. zero pressure) and the average pleural pressure is approximately −5 cm H_2O. Under these conditions, the alveolar distending pressure is 5 cm H_2O (alveolar-pleural). This distending pressure is sufficient to maintain a normal end-expiratory alveolar volume to overcome the elastic recoil of the alveolar wall.
   a. Patients without expiratory flow limitations (no COPD or asthma).
      1) If ICP and cardiovascular status are **stable**, set PEEP at 5 cm H_2O and make changes based on ABG results, FIO_2 requirements, tolerance of PEEP, and cardiovascular response.
      2) If ICP and/or cardiovascular status is **unstable**, set PEEP at 3 cm H_2O and increase only if attending physician agrees that risk of hypoxemia is greater than risk of increased ICP or cardiovascular collapse.
   b. Patients with expiratory flow limitations (COPD/asthma) are subject to intrinsic PEEP.
      1) Prior to changing PEEP to overcome expiratory flow limitations, adjust RR and peak flow to maximize expiratory time.
      2) If patient is not breathing spontaneously (e.g. sedated), calculate intrinsic PEEP and set PEEP at 85% of that value.
      3) If patient is breathing spontaneously and has PRN sedation ordered, work with RN to coordinate intrinsic PEEP measurement with administration of sedation.
      4) If patient is breathing spontaneously so that intrinsic PEEP measurement is impossible, an optimal PEEP study may be performed.
4. Utilizing PEEP to meet oxygenation goals.
   a. Arterial oxygenation is the driving force behind setting optimal PEEP and FIO_2 levels; however, maximizing oxygenation is not the goal for patients with refractory hyoxemia.
      1) PaO2 of 55-80 with saturation of 88-95% are acceptable therapeutic goals.
      2) The following guide should be used in determining appropriate combined PEEP and FIO_2 levels:

PEEP AND FIO_2 GUIDELINES

PEEP (cm H_2O) Combined with FIO_2	5 → 0.3	5 → 0.4	8 → 0.4	8 → 0.5	10 → 0.5	10 → 0.6	10 → 0.7	12 → 0.7	14 → 0.8	14 → 0.9	14 → 0.9	16 → 1.0	18 → 1.0	18 → 1.0	20 → 1.0	22 → 1.0	24 → 1.0

IF MEASURED VALUE IS BELOW GOAL (PaO_2 55-80 AND/OR SATURATION 88-95%) MOVE UP ONE STEP.

IF PEEP > 10 AND > 0.60, CALL ATTENDING PHYSICIAN BEFORE PROCEEDING THROUGH TABLE.

PROTOCOL 9-6P5

Example using table on previous page:

Patient was intubated yesterday for acute ventilatory failure with hypoxemia. Patient placed on the following settings: V_T 500, A/C rate 12, PEEP +5, FIO_2 0.04. ABG has been within normal limits on those settings. This morning, however, oxygen saturation is dropping and CXR indicates patient is in ARDS. By using the chart on the previous page, the ventilatory changes would be as follows:

Increase PEEP to 8 with FIO_2 at 0.40. If saturation improves, leave on those settings. If saturation continues to drop or does not improve, proceed to next step on the chart.

Increase FIO_2 to 0.50 with PEEP at 8. If saturation improves, leave on those settings. If saturation continues to drop or does not improve, proceed to next step on the chart.

Increase PEEP to 10 with FIO_2 0.50. If saturation improves, leave on those settings. If saturation continues to drop or does not improve, proceed to next step on the chart.

Increase FIO_2 to 0.60 with PEEP at 10. At this point, **call physician.**

E. **Pressure Support (PS)**

1. Pressure support may be used in conjunction with SIMV. In this case, PS increases the patient's spontaneous tidal volume, decreases spontaneous respiratory rate, and decreases work of breathing.
   a. PS can be set to maintain spontaneous V_T to meet the patient's ventilatory requirements while keeping RR <25.
   b. PS can be set to overcome resistance of airflow cause by ETT, thereby decreasing WOB. In this case, PS should be calculated using the following formula:
      1) $\frac{(\text{PIP} - \text{PEEP}) - (\text{Plateau Pressure} - \text{PEEP})}{\text{Peak Flow} \div 60}$

         e.g., PIP 45 cm H_2O P_{plat} 24 cm H_2O, peak flow 70 L/min

         $$\frac{(45-6) - (24-6)}{70 \div 60} = \frac{39 - 18}{1.17} = 17.95 \text{ cm } H_2O$$

         Therefore, PS should be set at 18 for those conditions.
      2) If Tubing Compensation (TC) is available, it may be used instead of PS to compensate for resistance to airflow caused by tubing. TC makes adjustments breath to breath to ensure proper support levels.
   c. If patient's RR >25 or WOB is visibly increased, patient should be returned to A/C until underlying condition resolved.
   d. The use of SIMV/PS in the clinical setting has not proven as an efficient weaning mode as compared to T-piece trials and pressure support ventilation. Compared to T-piece trials and PSV, it is associated with the longest weaning and the lowest success rates.
2. Pressure support may be used as a spontaneous ventilatory mode in conjunction with CPAP in patients who do not require a ventilator rate to ensure adequate ventilation.
   a. The difference between the PS level and the CPAP level is the driving pressure and should be set at a level that meets patient's ventilatory demand with RR <25.
   b. PS may be decreased as the patient's condition and lung compliance improves (see above formula).
   c. Low V_T and/or $\dot{V}_E$ alarms are essential to ensure adequate ventilation in PSV mode.

F. **Peak Inspiratory Flow**

1. Peak inspiratory flow (PF) should be set at the lowest possible flow to maintain I:E ratio and patient comfort.
   a. Normal I:E is 1:2 to 1:4 for mechanically ventilated patients.
   b. Larger I:E ratio should be used on patients needing additional time for exhalation due to air trapping and intrinsic PEEP.
2. Flow rate may be used to change I:E. This should be monitored with each ventilator check.
3. Decelerating flow pattern should be utilized whenever it is available to assure optimal gas distribution, lower inspiratory pressures, improved patient comfort, and reduced WOB.

PROTOCOL 9-6P6

G. **Bi-Level**

1. A form of augmented pressure ventilation that allows for unrestricted spontaneous breathing at any moment of the ventilator cycle, thereby promoting patient/ventilator synchrony.
   a. The initial settings of upper PEEP ($PEEP_H$) and lower PEEP ($PEEP_L$) should be based on the set PEEP and the plateau pressure during volume ventilation.
   b. $PEEP_L$ is adjusted to obtain adequate oxygenation (refer to setting PEEP C-4).
   c. $PEEP_H$ is usually set at 12-16 above $PEEP_{L2}$ depending on patient lung compliance. It should be set to ensure V_T of 6 ml/kg IBW.
   d. PS can be added to assist spontaneous breathing in bi-level.
      1) Since PS is delivered above the $PEEP_L$ level, the RCP must calculate the PS level needed.
         e.g., Patient is set on bi-level of 24/5 ($PEEP_L$ 5) for a driving pressure of 19 cm H_2O (the difference between $PEEP_H$ and $PEEP_L$). You have calculated that you need a PS of 8 to overcome resistance to airflow caused by tubing (see formula on previous page). In order for patient's spontaneous breaths taken at $PEEP_H$ to be supported, PS must be set so that peak pressure on PS breaths is 8 cm H_2O higher than $PEEP_H$.

      $PEEP_H - PEEP_L$ + PS needed to overcome resistance = needed PS

      $24 \text{ cm } H_2O - 5 \text{ cm } H_2O + 8 \text{ cm } H_2O = 27 \text{ cm } H_2O$

   e. If a patient's oxygen status requires ventilation at less than 1:2 I:E ratio (e.g., 1:1.5; 1:1; 2:1, etc), ventilator settings must come from the attending physician.

IV. Ventilator Management

A. **New Ventilator Protocol Orders**

When a new ventilator protocol order is written on a patient who has been on mechanical ventilation for 24 hours or longer and ordered on $V_T > 8$ ml/kg IBW, proceed as follows:

1. Calculate IBW
2. Calculate desired V_T
3. Titrate V_T by 1 ml/kg Q2 hours until 8 ml/kg IBW has been achieved.
4. Increase respiratory rate to ensure that $\dot{V}_E$ remains the same.
5. After achieving 8 ml/kg IBW, obtain an ABG after 30 minutes of last change.

B. Monitoring patient response to therapy

1. RCP will obtain an ABG 30 minutes after the patient has been placed on initial ventilator protocol settings.
2. RCP will obtain an ABG 30 minutes after any significant change in ventilator settings (increase or decrease in $V_T > 100$ ml or increase/decrease respiratory rate ≥ 4 bpm.
3. SpO_2 monitor will be used to titrate PEEP and FIO_2.

C. Maintenance

1. Heat Moisture Exchangers (HMEs) may be used for up to 5 days after initiation of mechanical ventilation as long as patient's core temperature > 32° C, $\dot{V}_E$ <10 L/min, and patient's secretions are not bloody or thick and tenacious. After 5 days, the circuit should be changed to humidified system.
2. In-line suction catheters are to be changed every 7 days. The sticker indicating the day to be changed should be displayed on the suction catheter, and the change date should be documented on the front of each vent sheet.
3. Circuits should be changed every 28 days. Since the circuit is not changed when the humidified system is added, counting should begin when ventilator use was initiated (not when humidified system was added) and continued every 28 days, thereafter.
4. Compliance (both static and dynamic) should be calculated and documented at least every 6 hours. Dramatic changes in compliance should be reported to the attending physician.
5. Cuff pressure should be checked and documented at least every 12 hours. If cuff manometer in not available, minimal leak technique is acceptable, but should be documented.
6. Auto PEEP should be measured and documented every 6 hours if patient is not breathing spontaneously. Newer ventilators calculate this automatically.
7. When pressure support is titrated down to overcome resistance caused by the ETT, documentation of PS calculation should be made.

PROTOCOL 9-6P7

MECHANICAL VENTILATION WEANING PROTOCOL

PURPOSE:
The respiratory care practitioner (RCP) will utilize the following protocol to facilitate timely liberation from mechanical ventilation.

PATIENT TYPE:
All adolescent, adult, and geriatric patients requiring mechanical ventilation

EQUIPMENT NEEDED:
- Pulse oximeter
- Ventilator
- Stethoscope
- Oxygen analyzer
- Wright's spirometer
- NIP manometer
- EKG monitor
- Heated aerosol with appropriate attachments
- $ETCO_2$ (if available)

LABORATORY DATA NEEDED:
Recent arterial blood gas results (if possible) and chest x-ray (if possible).

OVERVIEW

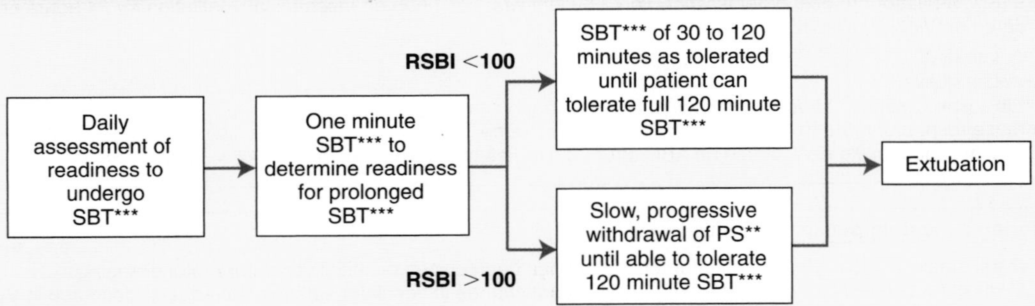

PROTOCOL:
Once clinical improvement has occurred in patients receiving mechanical ventilation for treatment of acute respiratory/ventilatory failure, emphasis must be placed on quickly liberating the patient from the ventilator.
The following guidelines will be followed to liberate patients from mechanical ventilation in a timely manner:

I. Complete patient assessment will be performed on each ventilated patient each morning between 0500 and 1100. The following parameters will be assessed and documented.

A. Improvement or resolution of underlying condition that led to ventilatory failure.
B. FIO_2: Must be $\leq$ 50% with SpO_2 >90% to consider ventilator weaning.
C. PEEP: Must be $\leq$ 8 cm H_2O.
D. Hemodynamic status: Patient should be normotensive without vasopressors or with very low dose dopamine or dobutamine (5 μg/kg/min).
E. Mentation: Patient should be easily arousable with minimal need for sedation.
F. Hgb >8 mg/dL
G. Core temp ≤38.5°C
H. Nutrition Status: Patient should have normal or near normal serum albumin levels.

*RSBI: Rapid Shallow Breathing Index
**PS: Pressure support
***SBT: Spontaneous Breathing Trial

PROTOCOL 9-7P1

II. Readiness testing: Patients who meet the above criteria will be given a readiness test which consists of a one minute spontaneous breathing trial (SBT) using a Wright spirometer.

A. $\dot{V}_E$ should be measured and RR counted during the one minute SBT. Record results on ventilator assessment form.
B. V_T should be calculated using $V_T = \dot{V}_E \div RR$
   - Average spontaeous V_T should be at least 4-6 ml/kg IBW
   - Average spontaneous V_T should be documented on ventilator assessment form
C. Rapid Shallow Breathing Index (RSBI) should be calculated and documented using RSBI $=$ RR $\div$ V_T (in liters).
   - RSBI is the predictor of weaning success that has been most thoroughly researched. It is independent of patient effort, and has been shown to be a better indicator of weaning than V_E or NIP.
   - RSBI must be calculated with patient off the ventilator. Measurements during ventilatory support (even low level CPAP) are less accurate then RSBI calculated during SBT off the ventilator.
   - RSBI $<$100 is considered suitable for continuing in the weaning protocol.
D. When one minute SBT is complete, measure NIP while patient if off the vent. NIP is measured by occluding the airway for $\leq$ 20 seconds. A NIP $\leq$ -20 is considered adequate when combined with other objective weaning data.
E. Subjective Assessment:
   - Assess patient for and document signs of elevated work of breathing such as thoracoabdominal paradox or excessive use of accessory respiratory muscles.
   - Assess patient for and document signs of distress such as diaphoresis, agitation, increased HR, or arrhythmias.
F. If the patient's RSBI is $<$100 breaths/min/L, NIP is $\geq$20 cm H_2O vital signs remain stable (HR, BP, and SpO_2), and patient's subjective assessments is acceptable, proceed to **Prolonged SBT** (section III). If patient DOES NOT tolerate the readiness test, place patient back on the ventilator and proceed to **Prolonged Weaning** (Section IV).

III. Prolonged SBT

A. Patients should be placed on a Spontaneous Breathing Trial (SBT) of 120 minutes to determine readiness to extubate.
B. Methods of providing SBT
   1. Heated, humidified O_2 via T-piece
      a. Recent research indicates that post-extubation WOB is the same as or greater than that imposed by the endortracheal tube.
      b. May be the best option when patients have been intubated for an extended period of time and airway inflammation and/or edema is likely. Breathing unassisted through the ETT may approximate post extubation WOB.
   2. CPAP of $\leq$ 5
   3. CPAP/PS mode
      a. If the CPAP/PS mode is used, the PS level must be calculated and documented to ensure that the patient does not receive more support than is necessary to overcome the work imposed by the ventilator/ventilator tubing/ETT.
      b. Low level PS may be a good option when patient has narrow ETT (high resistance to airflow) or secretions lining the lumen of the tube increasing airway resistance.
         - It is important to note that studies have failed to identify one of these SBT strategies as being statistically better at predicting extubation success than another. What research has proven, however, is the necessity of conducting an SBT. Thirty-seven percent (37%) of patients extubated after satisfying classically applied screening criteria required reintubation. This is up to 3 times greater than that seen among patients extubated after passing SBT.
C. The length of the SBT should be as follows:
   1. Surgical patients or patients with no underlying lung disease a 30 minute SBT. Results must be documented. Weaning parameters, including RSBI should be measured at the end of the trial before placing back on ventilator. Examples of complex medical patients include, but are not limited to, the following.
      a. COPD
      b. ARDS
      c. Multi-System Organ Failure (MSOF)
      d. Patients over 70 years of age (these patients have the highest incidents of reintubation and should complete a full 120 minutes SBT prior to extubation).
D. Use the following to determine response to the SBT.
   1. Criteria to extubate:
      a. RR$<$30
      b. $SpO_2 \geq$ 92% on $\leq$ 50% FIO_2. If patient is a COPD patient, will accept SpO_2 of 88%. An SpO_2 less than 92% (88% in COPD patients) for 5 minutes results in termination of SBT.

PROTOCOL 9-7P2

c. No signs of respiratory distress as evidenced by any two of the following:
    1) Pulse >120% of the rate before initiation of SBT
        a) e.g. if pulse **before** SBT is 70, pulse should not exceed 84 during SBT.
        b) e.g. if **before** SBT is 112, pulse should not exceed 134 during SBT.
    2) Significant change in cardiac rhythm (PVCs, atrial fib, etc.)
    3) Marked use of accessory muscles of respiration
    4) Thoraco-abdominal paradox
    5) Diaphoresis
    6) Marked dyspnea

d. For complex medical patients receiving 120 minutes SBT, RCP should obtain an ABG at the end of the SBT, analyze, and document.
    1) If ABG results are within normal limits and above criteria are met, patient may be extubated.
    2) If ABG results are outside of normal limits, but are normal for the patient, based on documented baseline ABGs and above criteria are met, patient may be extubated.

2. Criteria to call physician before determining if extubation is appropriate.
    a. RR 30-35
    b. ABG results are outside of normal limits but no baseline is available and patient met above criteria.
3. If the patient does not meet the criteria outlined above, place back on ventilator and allow patient to rest for 24 hours. Begin the assessment / SBT process again the following day.

IV. Prolonged Weaning

A. Patients who fail the first SBT should be placed back on the ventilator on full support and reassessed in 24 hours.
B. Patients who fail the second SBT should be weaned using the following guidelines:
    1. Place on CPAP/PS at a PS level that provides the patient with V_T at 6-8 ml/kg and RR <30 bpm.
    2. Rest for 24 hours on those settings and repeat SBT in the a.m.
    3. If SBT failed again, place back on CPAP/PS, but titrate PS level downward by 2 cm H_2O Q12 hours as long as respiratory rate remains <30 bpm.
    4. Repeat SBT daily once every 24 hours.
C. SBTs should be documented daily and reported to the attending physician.

V. Extubation

A. Criteria to extubate. Attending physician must have pre-approved extubation if criteria met (**ALL** 3 criteria must be met to extubate):
    1. Patient tolerates SBT for 120 minutes.
    2. Post SBT parameters are within normal limits.
        a. RSBI <100
        b. RR <30
        c. NIP ≤ -20
        d. VC (is patient able to follow commands) of 10-15 ml/kg IBW
    3. ABG drawn at end of SBT is within normal limits (or normal for the patient based on baseline).
B. Criteria to call physician prior to making the decision to extubate.
    1. Patient tolerated SBT or toleration is marginal (RR 30-35) but one of the following occurs:
        a. Post SBT parameters do not meet above criteria **OR**
        b. Post SBT ABG results are outside of normal limits.
C. Criteria to place back on ventilator and wait 24 hours before attempting another SBT:
    1. Patient does not tolerate SBT
        a. RR >35
        b. SpO_2 <92% (88-90% for COPD patient with chronic hypoxemia)
        c. Exhibits marked dyspnea
        d. Arrhythmia which started after initiation of the SBT.
D. The RCP may obtain a post extubation ABG if (s)he feels it is needed to determine the patient's post extubation status.

PROTOCOL 9-7P3

VI. Following Extubation

A. Place patient on low flow oxygen to approximate the FIO_2 delivered during the SBT. Titrate oxygen for SpO_2 >92% (88-92% for COPD patients with hypoxic drive to breathe).
B. Assess patient's immediate response to extubation by documenting the following:
   1. Vital signs (HR and rhythm, RR and respiratory pattern, SpO_2 BP)
   2. Breath sounds including presence/absence of stridor.
C. If stridor is present, patient should be given stat Vaponephrine med neb and placed on cool mist aerosol.
D. If stridor persists after one Vaponephrine treatment, notify attending physician immediately. A second Vaponephrine treatment should **NOT** be given (may be given Q2 hours).
E. Document extubation and post-extubation assessment on the ventilatory assessment form.

VII. Post operative heart patients (CABG and valve surgeries) in Cardio-Thoracic Care Unit: These patients will be weaned from the ventilator using an expedited form of the SBT process previously outlined.

A. Patient will be received and placed on initial settings as follows:
   1. V_T 6-8
   2. RR 10-20 as needed to keep $ETCO_2$ 35-45
   3. PEEP 3-5 cm H_2O
   4. FIO_2 for SpO_2>92%
   5. May be in AC, PC or SIMV ventilator mode. If patient in SIMV, set PS to match resistance imposed by ventilator tubing and ETT.
B. No ventilator changes should be made until initial ABG has been drawn and analyzed.
C. As soon as patient begins to wake up and has spontaneous respiratory effort, an SBT may be initiated. Any of the following methods may be used:
   1. Heated aerosol
   2. CPAP
   3. CPAP/PS (PS level must be calculated to determine that which overcomes resistance of the ETT and ventilator tubing)
   4. CPAP/TC if patient is ventilated by PB 840.
D. Weaning parameters will be measured and documented when patient has tolerated SBT for 30 minutes.
E. Patient may be extubated when 30 minutes SBT is completed and weaning parameters are within normal limits. The RCP may order an ABG before extubation if (s)he deems it necessary to determine response to SBT.
F. Post extubation ABG will be drawn 30-60 minutes after extubation.

PROTOCOL 9-7P4

Ventilatory Management in Catastrophes

The risk of major catastrophes continues to increase as a result of many factors, including the threat of bioterrorism, the growing mobility of the world's population, and numerous viruses. For example, the events that occurred immediately after September 11, 2001 and the recent reports of the person-to-person transmission of avian influenza identified in Thailand and H1N1 ("swine flu") in the United States are powerful reminders that the population at large is vulnerable to both known and unknown dangers. In addition, it should be understood that because epidemics and bioterrorist attacks can result in conditions that cause acute ventilatory failure, large numbers of mechanical ventilators (which are limited in supply) will certainly be needed should such an unfortunate event occur.

Figure 9-5, a photograph taken during the great poliomyelitis epidemic in the early 1950s (over 50,000 people were stricken), reminds the reader of a need for such intervention. Note the nurse-to-patient ratio of 1 : 2. At the time, each nurse was ready to step in and manually operate the "iron lungs" of two patients in the event of a power outage. Today, it is very unlikely that our health-care system could adequately provide this type of ventilator care and coverage.

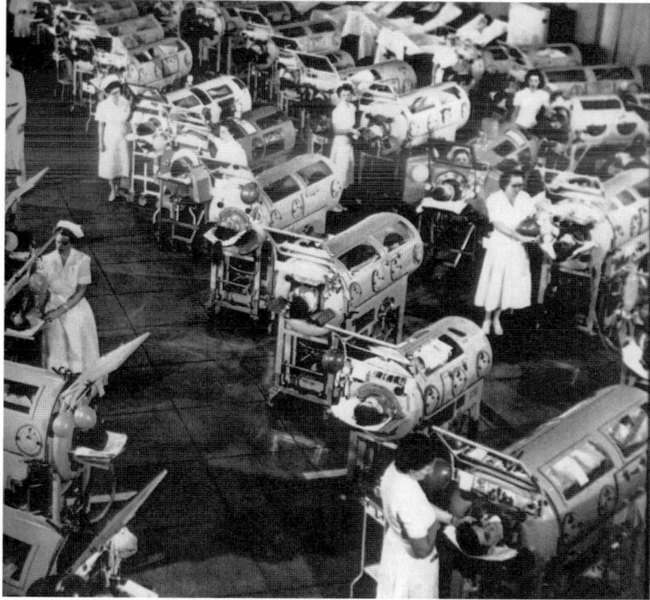

FIGURE 9-5 Iron lungs in gym. Iron lungs were in high demand during the polio epidemic of 1951 to 1953. (Courtesy Rancho Los Amigos National Rehabilitation Center. From http://en.wikipedia.org/wiki/File:Iron_Lung_ward-Rancho_Los_Amigos_Hospital.gif.)

Box 9-2 Three Tiers of Criteria

Tier 1: Do not offer *and* withdraw ventilatory support for patients with any one of the following:

1. Respiratory failure requiring intubation with persistent hypotension (systolic blood pressure <90 mm Hg for adults) unresponsive to adequate fluid resuscitation after 6 to 12 hours of therapy and signs of additional end-organ dysfunction (e.g., oliguria, mental status changes, cardiac ischemia)
2. Failure to respond to mechanical ventilation (no improvement in oxygenation or lung compliance) and antibiotics after 72 hours of treatment for a bacterial pathogen (timeline may be modified based on organism-specific data)
3. Laboratory or clinical evidence of more than four organ systems failing
   a. Pulmonary (acute respiratory distress syndrome, ventilatory failure, refractory hypoxemia)
   b. Cardiovascular (left ventricular dysfunction, hypotension, new ischemia)
   c. Renal (hyperkalemia, diminished urine output despite adequate fluid resuscitation, increasing creatinine level)
   d. Hepatic (transaminase greater than two times normal upper limit, increasing bilirubin or ammonia levels)
   e. Neurologic (altered mental status not related to volume status, metabolic, or hypoxic source, stroke)
   f. Hematologic (clinical or laboratory evidence of disseminated intravascular coagulation)

Tier 2: Do not offer *and* withdraw ventilatory support from patients with respiratory failure requiring intubation with following conditions (in addition to those in Tier 1):

Patients with pre-existing system compromise or failure including the following:

1. Known congestive heart failure with ejection fraction <25% (or persistent ischemia unresponsive to therapy and pulmonary edema)
2. Acute renal failure requiring hemodialysis (related to illness)
3. Severe chronic lung disease including pulmonary fibrosis, obstructive or restrictive diseases requiring continuous home oxygen use before onset of acute illness.
4. Acquired immunodeficiency syndrome (AIDS), other immunodeficiency syndromes at stage of disease susceptible to opportunistic pathogens (e.g., CD4 <200 for AIDS) with respiratory failure requiring intubation
5. Active malignancy with poor potential for survival (e.g., metastatic malignancy, pancreatic cancer)
6. Cirrhosis with ascites, history of variceal bleeding, fixed coagulopathy, or encephalopathy
7. Acute hepatic failure with hyperammonemia
8. Irreversible neurologic impairment that makes patient dependent on personal care (e.g., severe stroke, congenital syndrome, persistent vegetative state)

Tier 3: Specific protocols to be agreed on by guideline development committee. Possibilities include the following:

1. Restriction of treatment based on disease-specific epidemiology and survival data for patient subgroups (may include age-based criteria)
2. Expansion of preexisting disease classes that will not be offered ventilatory support
3. Applying Sequential Organ Failure Assessment scoring to the triage process, and establishing a cutoff score above which mechanical ventilation will not be offered

With the realization that many factors may result in a large demand for ventilator management, some thought is now being offered in the literature that suggests how this might be done. The choices and alternatives are grim ones and are illustrated in a representative three-tier criteria system provided in Box 9-2. As shown, Tier 1 is directed only to acute ventilatory failure with shock and multiple organ dysfunction. Tier 2 presents criteria for high potential for death, prolonged ventilation, and high levels of resource use. Tier 3 criteria may entail additional restrictions or a scoring system and are implemented to maintain consistent standards of care.*

Overview Summary of a Good Therapist-Driven Protocol Program

Figure 9-6 provides an overview of the essential components of a good TDP program. As illustrated, the implementation of every respiratory care plan must be directly linked to (1) a physician's order, (2) the identification and documentation of specific clinical indicators (obtained from both the patient's chart and physical examination), (3) a bedside respiratory assessment and severity assessment, (4) a treatment selection that is both therapeutic and cost-efficient, and (5) the reevaluation of the patient's response to the treatment.

This step-by-step process mandates that the respiratory care practitioner (1) have a strong knowledge base of the major respiratory disorders, and (2) be competent in the actual assessment process (see Figure 9-4). Figure 9-7 provides an assessment form with common examples for each category (i.e., clinical indicators, respiratory assessments, and treatment plans). The examples shown in Figure 9-6 can easily be transferred to the subjective-objective-assessment-plan (SOAP) format. The SOAP format used in the assessment of respiratory diseases is discussed in more detail in Chapter 10.

*See Hicks JL, O'Laughlin DT: Concept of operations for triage of mechanical ventilation in an epidemic, *Acad Emerg Med* 13: 223, 2006.

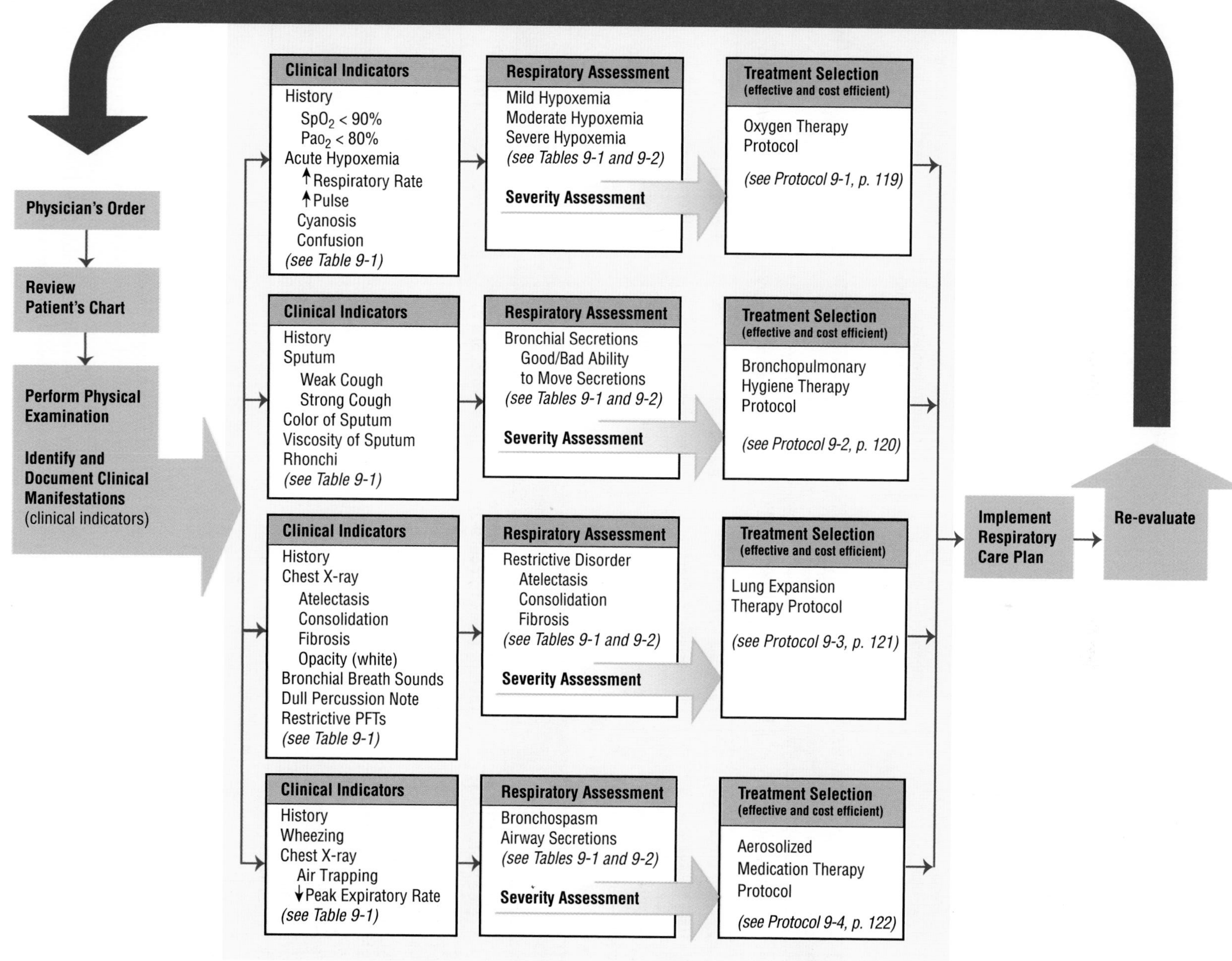

FIGURE 9-6 Overview of the essential components of a good therapist-driven protocol program.

Patient Identification Box	Date:__________ Time:__________	Admitting Diagnosis:__________ Attending Physician:__________	
Clinical Indicators (see Table 9-1)			
Oxygen Therapy	**Bronchopulmonary Hygiene Therapy**	**Lung Expansion Therapy**	**Aerosolized Medication**

Examples:
☐ History
☐ Spo_2 <80%
☐ Pao_2 <80 mm Hg
☐ Acute hypoxemia
  ☐ ≠ Respiratory rate
  ☐ ≠ Pulse
  ☐ Cyanosis
  ☐ Confusion
  ☐ Other
	Examples:
	☐ History
	☐ Sputum
	  ☐ Weak cough
	  ☐ Color of sputum
	  ☐ Viscosity of sputum
	  ☐ Rhonchi
		Examples:
		☐ History
		☐ Chest X-ray
		  ☐ Atelectasis
		  ☐ Consolidation
		  ☐ Fibrosis
		  ☐ Opacity (white)
		☐ Bronchial breath sounds
		☐ Restrictive PFT values
			Examples:
			☐ History
			☐ Wheezing
			☐ Chest X-ray
			  ☐ Air trapping
			☐ Obstructive PFT values

Respiratory Assessments (see Tables 9-1 and 9-2)			
Oxygen Therapy	**Bronchopulmonary Hygiene Therapy**	**Lung Expansion Therapy**	**Aerosolized Medication**
Examples: ☐ Mild hypoxemia ☐ Moderate hypoxemia ☐ Severe hypoxemia Severity Score:_______	Examples: ☐ Excessive sputum production ☐ Thick secretions ☐ Weak cough Severity Score:_______	Examples: ☐ Atelectasis ☐ Consolidation ☐ Weak diaphragm Severity Score:_______	Examples: ☐ Bronchospasm ☐ Thick secretions ☐ Bronchial edema Severity Score:_______
Treatment Plans			
Oxygen Therapy (see Protocol 9-1)	**Bronchopulmonary Hygiene Therapy (see Protocol 9-2)**	**Lung Expansion Therapy (see Protocol 9-3)**	**Aerosolized Medication (see Protocol 9-4)**
Examples: ☐ Nasal cannula ☐ Oxygen mask ☐ 28% Venturi mask Frequency:_______	Examples: ☐ Deep breath and cough ☐ Chest physical therapy ☐ Postural drainage Frequency:_______	Examples: ☐ Incentive spirometry ☐ CPAP ☐ PEEP Frequency:_______	Examples: ☐ Metaproterenol ☐ Albuterol ☐ Acetylcysteine Frequency:_______
Reevaluation Date:__________		Therapist Signature:__________	

FIGURE 9-7 Respiratory care protocol program assessment form.

Common Anatomic Alterations of the Lungs

Although the respiratory care practitioner may at some time treat one or two cases of every respiratory disorder presented in this book, most of the respiratory care practitioner's professional career will be spent caring for patients with only a few of them. For example, the diagnosis-related group (DRG) and International Statistical Classification of Diseases and Related Health Problems (ICD-9) identification systems show that more than 80% of the respiratory care practitioner's work is concerned with intelligent assessment and treatment selection for a relatively short list of respiratory illnesses (Table 9-4).

Therefore the most common anatomic alterations of the lungs treated by the respiratory care practitioner can be derived by recognizing the most common DRG respiratory disorders identified in Table 9-4. The major anatomic alterations include (1) **atelectasis** (e.g., which can occur from mucous plugging, upper abdominal surgery, or pneumothorax), (2) **alveolar consolidation** (e.g., pneumonia), (3) **increased alveolar-capillary membrane thickness** (e.g., acute respiratory distress syndrome [ARDS], pneumoconiosis, or pulmonary edema), (4) **bronchospasm** (e.g., asthma), (5) **excessive bronchial secretions** (e.g., chronic bronchitis, asthma, pulmonary edema), and (6) **distal airway and alveolar weakening** (e.g., emphysema). Each of these anatomic alterations of the lung in turn leads to a chain of events that can be summarized in the following clinical scenarios.

TABLE 9-3 Common Ventilatory Management Strategies Used to Treat Specific Disorders (Good Starting Points)

Disorder	Disease Characteristics	Ventilator Mode	Tidal Volume and Respiratory Rate	Flow Rate	I : E Ratio	FIO_2	General Goals and/or Concerns
Normal Lung Mechanics	Normal compliance & airway resistance	Volume ventilation in the AC or SIMV mode.	10-12 ml/kg of ideal body weight	60-80 L/min	1 : 2	Low to moderate	Care to ensure plateau pressure of 30 cm H_2O or less.
But patient has apnea			10-12 bpm or slower rates (6-10 bpm) when SIMV mode is used				Small tidal volumes (<7 ml/kg) should be avoided, since atelectasis can develop
(e.g., drug overdose or abdominal surgery)		Or pressure ventilation—either PRVC or PC					
Chronic Obstructive Pulmonary Disease	High lung compliance and high airway resistance	Volume ventilation in the AC or SIMV mode	Good starting point: 10 ml/kg and a rate of 10 to 12 bpm	60 L/min	1 : 2 or 1 : 3	Low to moderate	Air trapping and auto-PEEP can occur when expiratory time is too short. The preferred method of managing auto-PEEP is to increase expiratory time.
(e.g., chronic bronchitis or emphysema)		Or pressure ventilation—either PRVC or PC	A smaller tidal volume (8-10 ml/kg) and slightly slower rate (8-10 bpm) with increased flow rates to allow adequate expiratory time	60-100 L/min			In severe cases, the development of auto-PEEP may be inevitable. With controlled ventilation, a small amount of PEEP to offset auto-PEEP may be cautiously applied.
		Noninvasive positive pressure ventilation (NPPV) by nasal or full face mask is a good alternative during acute exacerbation					Inspiratory flow up to 100 L/min may be helpful in decreasing inspiratory time and increasing expiratory time
							Tidal volume or rate may be decreased to reduce inspiratory and increasing expiratory time

Continued

TABLE 9-3 Common Ventilatory Management Strategies Used to Treat Specific Disorders (Good Starting Points)—cont'd

Disorder	Disease Characteristics	Ventilator Mode	Tidal Volume and Respiratory Rate	Flow Rate	I : E Ratio	FIO_2	General Goals and/or Concerns
Chronic Obstructive Pulmonary Disease							Care to avoid overventilating COPD patients with chronically high $PaCO_2$ levels
Acute Asthmatic Episode	High airway resistance (bronchospasm and excessive thick airway secretions)	The SIMV mode is recommended to avoid patient triggering at an increased rate—leading to a decrease in expiratory time and further air trapping	Good starting point: 8 to 10 ml/kg and rate of 10-12 bpm When air trapping is extensive, a lower tidal volume (5-6 ml/kg) and slower rate may be required	60 L/min	1 : 2 or 1 : 3	Start at 100% and titrate downward as pulse oximetric findings and arterial blood gas values permit	In severe cases, the development of auto-PEEP may be inevitable. With controlled ventilation, a small amount of PEEP to offset auto- PEEP may be cautiously applied.
Acute Respiratory Distress Syndrome	Diffuse, uneven alveolar injury	Volume ventilation in the AC or SIMV mode Or pressure ventilation—either PRVC or PC	Typically started at low tidal volumes and higher respiratory rate Initial tidal volume set at 8 ml/kg and adjusted downward to 6 ml/kg May be as low as 4 ml/kg Respiratory rates as high as 35 bpm may be	60-80 L/min	1 : 1 or 1 : 2 Do what is necessary to meet a rapid respiratory rate	FIO_2 less than 0.6 if possible	The goal is to limit transpulmonary pressure and the resultant barotraumas caused by overdistending portions of the lungs Maintaining a plateau pressure of 30 cm H_2O or less is preferred PEEP is usually required with a low tidal volume to prevent atelectasis

							The $Paco_2$ may be allowed to increase (permissive hypercapnia). The hypercapnia is not a therapeutic goal, it is a tradeoff and may be accepted as a lung protective strategy when lower airway pressures are necessary.
Postoperative Ventilatory Support (e.g., coronary artery bypass surgery, heart valve and replacement)	Often normal compliance and airway resisitance	SIMV with pressure support or AC volume ventilation are acceptable modes Or pressure ventilation—either PRVC or PC	Good starting point: 10 to 12 ml/kg and a rate of 10 to 12 bpm However, a larger tidal volume (12-15 ml/kg) and slower rate (6-10 bpm) may be used to maintain lung volume	60 L/min	1 : 2	Low to moderate	PEEP or CPAP of 3 to 5 cm H_2O may be applied to offset the development of atelectasis
Neuromuscular Disorder (e.g., myasthenia gravis or Guillain-Barre syndrome)	Normal compliance and airway resistance	Volume ventilation in the AC or SIMV mode Or pressure ventilation—either PRVC or PC	Good starting point: 12 to 15 ml/kg and a rate of 10 to 12 bpm	60 L/min	1 : 2	Low to moderate	PEEP of 3 to 5 cm H_2O may be applied to offset the development of atelectasis

AC, Assist-control; *SIMV*, synchronous intermittent mandatory ventilation; *PRVC*, pressure regulated volume control; *PC*, pressure control; *CPAP*, continous positive airway pressure; *bpm*, breaths per minute.

TABLE 9-4 Common Respiratory Disorders

Respiratory Disorder	DRG Number*	ICD-10 Code†
Chronic bronchitis	088	491.1, 491.9
Emphysema	088	492.8
Asthma	096	493.0
Acute pneumonia	079, 089, 090	(see below)
Aspiration pneumonia	079	507.0
Atelectasis	101/102	518.89
Adult respiratory distress syndrome	099/102	518.82
Interstitial fibrosis	089	515.0
Pulmonary edema/congestive heart failure	127	402.91
Acute respiratory failure	087	518.81
Respiratory failure with ventilatory support	475	96.7
Respiratory failure/tracheostomy/ventilatory support	483	96.72/31.1

*Respiratory disorders can be identified by their respective diagnosis-related group (DRG). DRG is an identification system used to categorize and document diseases, primarily for use in health care reimbursement (such as Medicaid and Medicare). Patients are routinely assigned a DRG based on their admitting diagnosis, and each DRG communicates information about patients. Because the use of DRGs is prevalent, respiratory care practitioners should recognize and understand the DRGs that they will commonly encounter.

†The ICD-10 code numbers are used for reimbursement with other third party payers. The ICD-10 system is more specific than the DRG system. For example, pneumococcal pneumonia is listed as ICD # 418.0, *Haemophilus influenzae* is ICD # 482.2, etc.

Box 9-3 Pathophysiologic Mechanisms Commonly Activated in Respiratory Disorders

- Decreased ventilation/perfusion ($\dot{V}/\dot{Q}$) ratio
- Alveolar diffusion block
- Decreased lung compliance
- Stimulation of oxygen receptors
- Deflation reflex
- Irritant reflex
- Pulmonary reflex
- Increased airway resistance
- Air trapping and alveolar hyperinflation

Clinical Scenarios Activated by Common Anatomic Alterations of the Lungs

For the purposes of this text, we have chosen to refer to the interrelationship among the major **anatomic alterations of the lung,** the **pathophysiologic mechanisms,** and the **clinical manifestations** that result as "clinical scenarios." Specific anatomic alterations of the lung (such as the ones listed previously) lead to the activation of specific and predictable pathophysiologic mechanisms and to their effects. The more common pathophysiologic mechanisms are listed in Box 9-3. The pathophysiologic mechanisms in turn activate specific and predictable clinical manifestations (see Figure 9-3). To enhance the reader's knowledge and understanding of commonly encountered respiratory disorders, clinical scenarios for the anatomic alterations presented in the following paragraphs are provided.*

*The Case Study Discussion Section at the end of each respiratory disease chapter often refers the reader back to these clinical scenarios, correlating various clinical manifestations to specific pathophysiologic mechanisms and alterations of the lungs.

Key to Abbreviations in Figures 9-8 through 9-13

ABG	=	Arterial blood gas
ARDS	=	Acute respiratory distress syndrome
CPAP	=	Continuous positive airway pressure
CPT	=	Chest physical therapy
Do_2	=	Total oxygen delivery
ERV	=	Expiratory reserve volume
FEF	=	Forced expiratory flow, midexpiratory phase
FEV_1	=	Forced expiratory volume in 1 second
FEV_T	=	Forced expiratory volume timed
FRC	=	Functional residual capacity
FVC	=	Forced vital capacity
IC	=	Inspiratory capacity
MVV	=	Maximum voluntary ventilation
O_2ER	=	Oxygen extraction ratio
PD	=	Postural drainage
PEEP	=	Positive end-expiratory pressure
PEFR	=	Peak expiratory flow rate
PFT	=	Pulmonary function test
$\dot{Q}s/\dot{Q}t$	=	Shunt fraction
RV	=	Residual volume
$S\bar{v}o_2$	=	Mixed venous oxygen saturation
TLC	=	Total lung capacity
VC	=	Vital capacity
$\dot{V}/\dot{Q}$	=	Ventilation-perfusion ratio

Atelectasis

Figure 9-8 shows the pathophysiologic mechanisms caused by atelectasis (e.g., from a pneumothorax), the clinical manifestations that result, and the treatment protocols used to offset them. The hypoxemia that results from atelectasis is caused by capillary shunting. This type of hypoxemia is often refractory to oxygen therapy. Therefore the implementation of the Lung Expansion Therapy Protocol may be more beneficial in the treatment of hypoxemia than the Oxygen Therapy Protocol in such a patient.

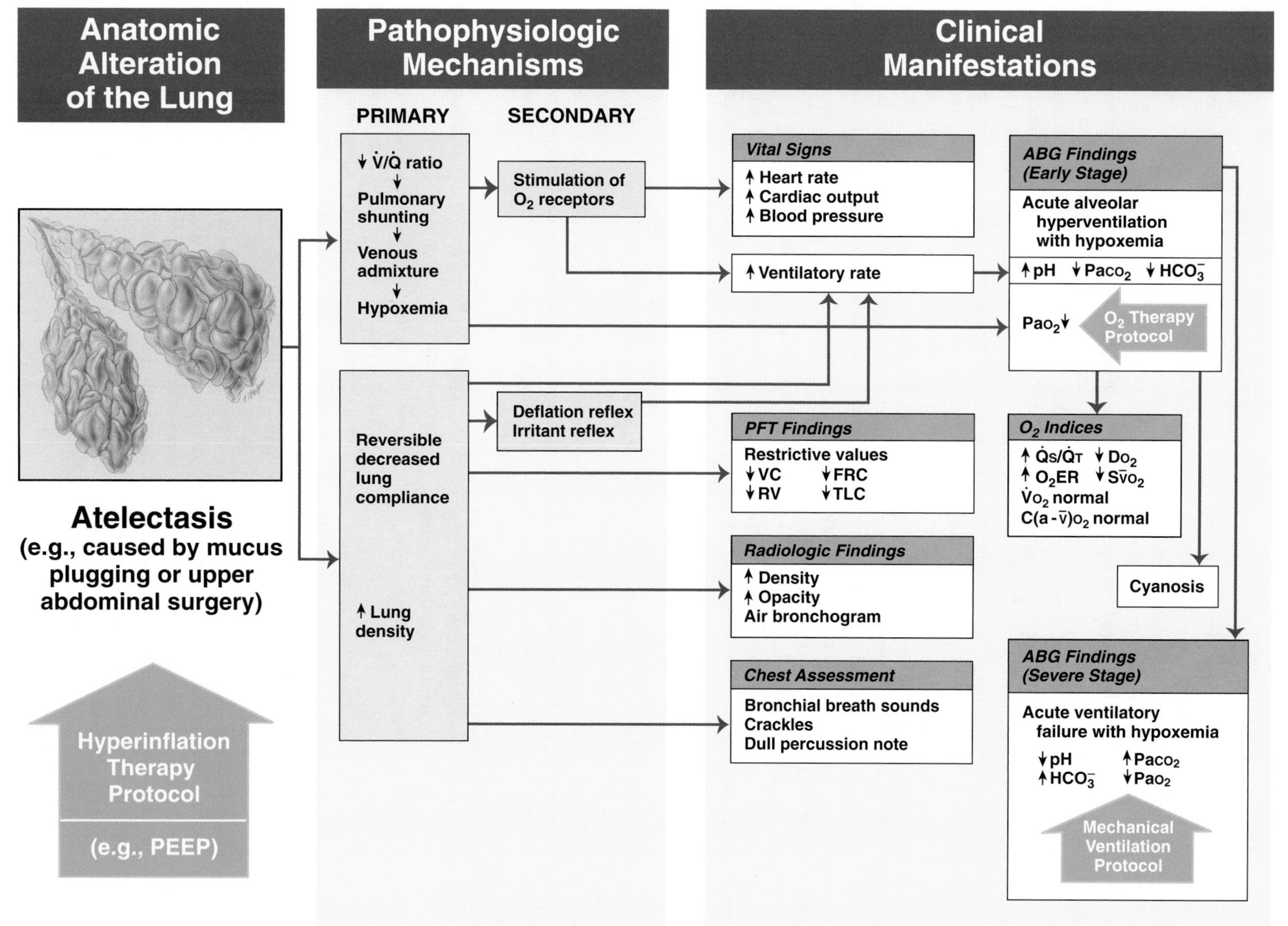

FIGURE 9-8 Atelectasis clinical scenario.

Alveolar Consolidation

Figure 9-9 shows the pathophysiologic mechanisms caused by alveolar consolidation (e.g., pneumonia), the clinical manifestations that result, and the treatment protocols used to offset them. The hypoxemia that develops as a result of consolidation is caused by capillary shunting. This type of hypoxemia is often refractory to oxygen therapy.

Depending on the severity of the alveolar consolidation, the Lung Expansion Therapy Protocol or the Oxygen Therapy Protocol may be beneficial. In general, however, there is no effective, specific respiratory care treatment modality for alveolar consolidation. With pneumonia, the great temptation for the respiratory care practitioner is to do too much, such as instituting lung expansion therapy, bronchodilator therapy, and bronchial hygiene therapy. Such treatment protocols generally are not indicated, especially during the early stages of the disease process. Appropriate antibiotics (prescribed by the physician), bed rest, fluids, and supplementary oxygen are all that is usually needed. When pneumonia is in its resolution stage, however, the patient may experience excessive secretions and atelectasis, accompanied by bronchoconstriction. At this time, other treatment modalities may be indicated.

Increased Alveolar-Capillary Membrane Thickness

Figure 9-10 illustrates the major pathophysiologic mechanisms caused by increased alveolar-capillary membrane thickness (e.g., postoperative ARDS, pulmonary edema, asbestosis, chronic interstitial lung disease), the clinical manifestations that develop, and the treatment protocols used to offset them. The hypoxemia that develops as a result of an increased alveolar-capillary membrane thickness is caused by an alveolar diffusion block. This type of hypoxemia often responds favorably to oxygen therapy.

Bronchospasm

Figure 9-11 shows the major pathophysiologic mechanisms activated by bronchospasm (e.g., asthma), the clinical manifestations that result, and the appropriate treatment protocols used to offset them. The Aerosolized Medication Therapy Protocol (Bronchodilator Therapy) is the primary treatment modality used to offset the anatomic alterations of bronchospasm (the original cause of the pathophysiologic chain of events). The Oxygen Therapy Protocol and Mechanical Ventilation Protocol are secondary treatment modalities used to offset the mild, moderate, or severe clinical manifestations associated with bronchospasm. In other words, when the patient responds favorably to the Aerosolized Medication Therapy Protocol, the need for the Oxygen Therapy Protocol may be minimal and the Mechanical Ventilation Protocol may not be necessary at all.

Excessive Bronchial Secretions

Figure 9-12 illustrates the major pathophysiologic mechanisms caused by excessive bronchial secretions (e.g., chronic bronchitis, asthma), the clinical manifestations that result, and the appropriate treatment protocols used to correct them. The Bronchopulmonary Hygiene Therapy Protocol is the primary treatment modality used to offset the anatomic alterations associated with excessive bronchial secretions. When the patient demonstrates chronic ventilatory failure during the advanced stages of respiratory disorders associated with chronic excessive airway secretions (e.g., chronic bronchitis), caution must be taken not to overoxygenate the patient.

Distal Airway and Alveolar Weakening

Figure 9-13 illustrates the major pathophysiologic mechanisms caused by distal airway and alveolar weakening (e.g., emphysema), the clinical manifestations that result, and the appropriate treatment protocols used to offset them. Pulmonary rehabilitation and oxygen therapy may be all the practitioner can provide to treat the symptoms associated with distal airway and alveolar weakening. When the patient demonstrates chronic ventilatory failure during the advanced stages of the disorder, caution must be taken with the Oxygen Therapy Protocol not to over-oxygenate the patient.

Overview of Common Anatomic Alterations Associated with Respiratory Disorders

When the respiratory therapy practitioner knows and understands the chain of events (clinical scenarios) that develop in response to common anatomic alterations of the lungs, an assessment and an appropriate treatment protocol can be easily determined. Table 9-5 provides an overview of the most common anatomic alterations associated with the respiratory disorders presented in this textbook.

Figure 9-14 provides a three-component overview model of a prototype airway to further enhance the reader's visualization of anatomic alterations of the lungs commonly associated with the obstructive respiratory disorders (e.g., asthma, bronchitis, or emphysema) and the treatment plans commonly used to offset them.

Text continued on p. 153

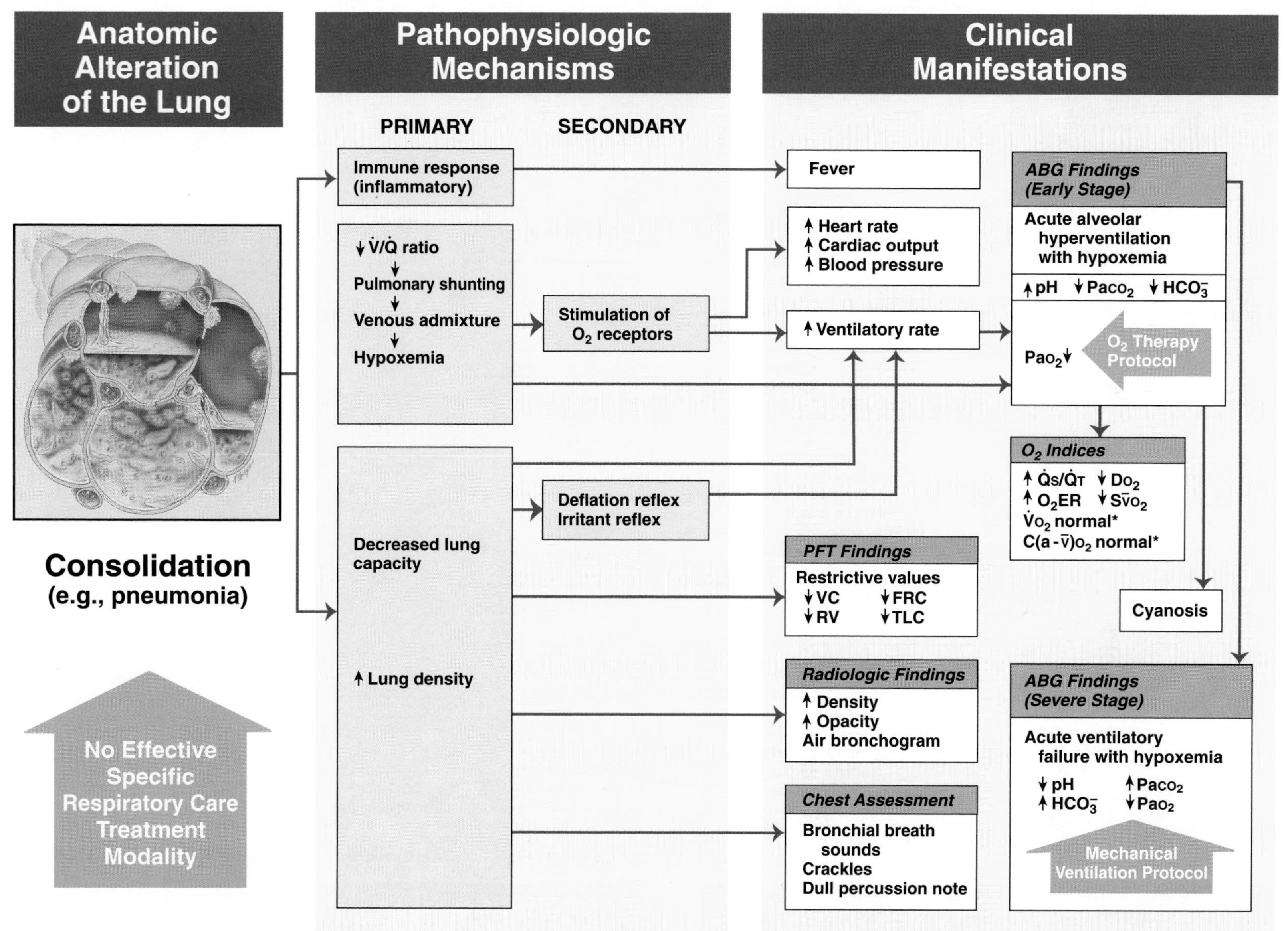

FIGURE 9-9 Alveolar consolidation clinical scenario. *Or increased when a fever is present.

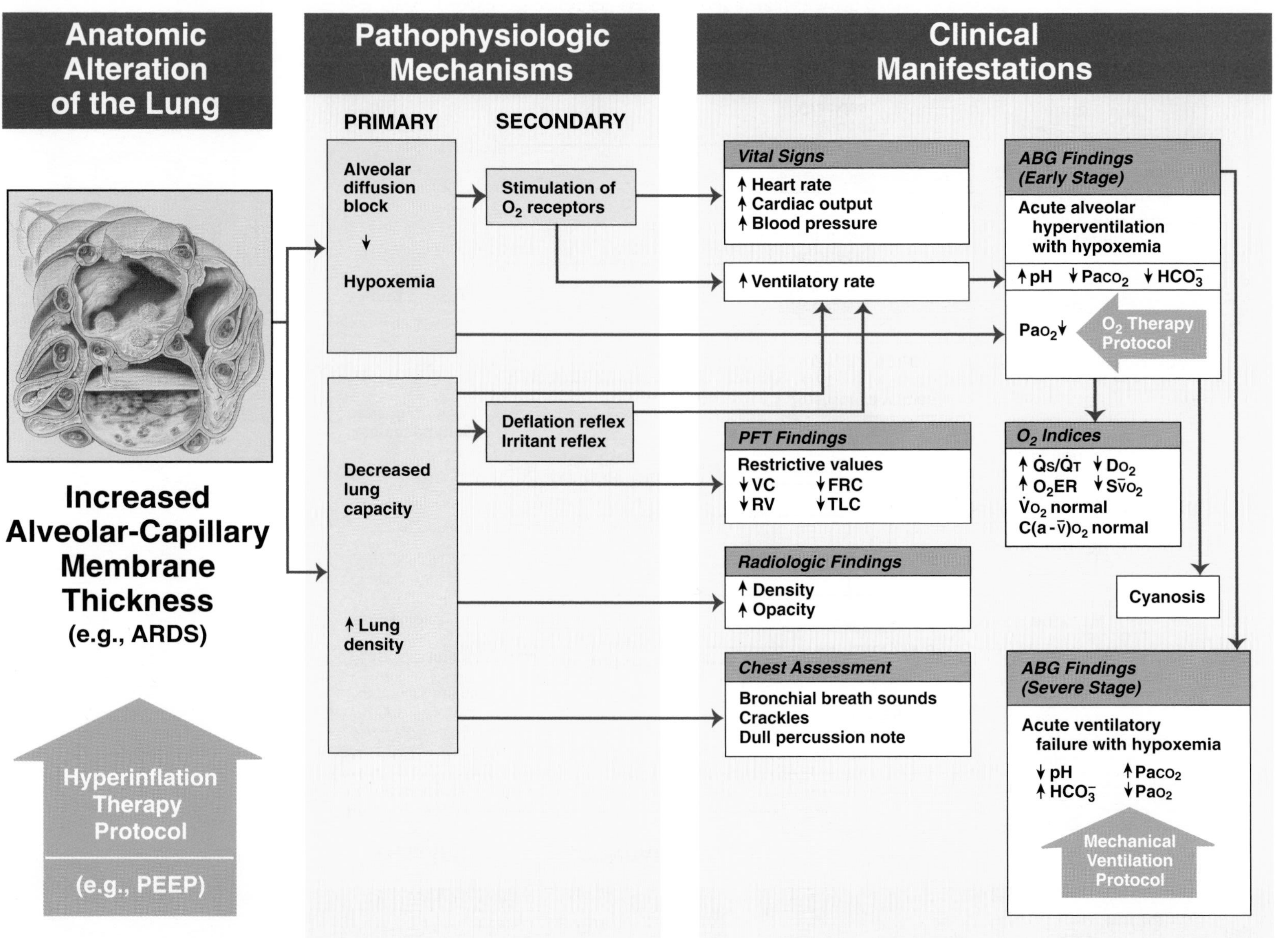

FIGURE 9-10 Increased alveolar-capillary membrane thickness clinical scenario.

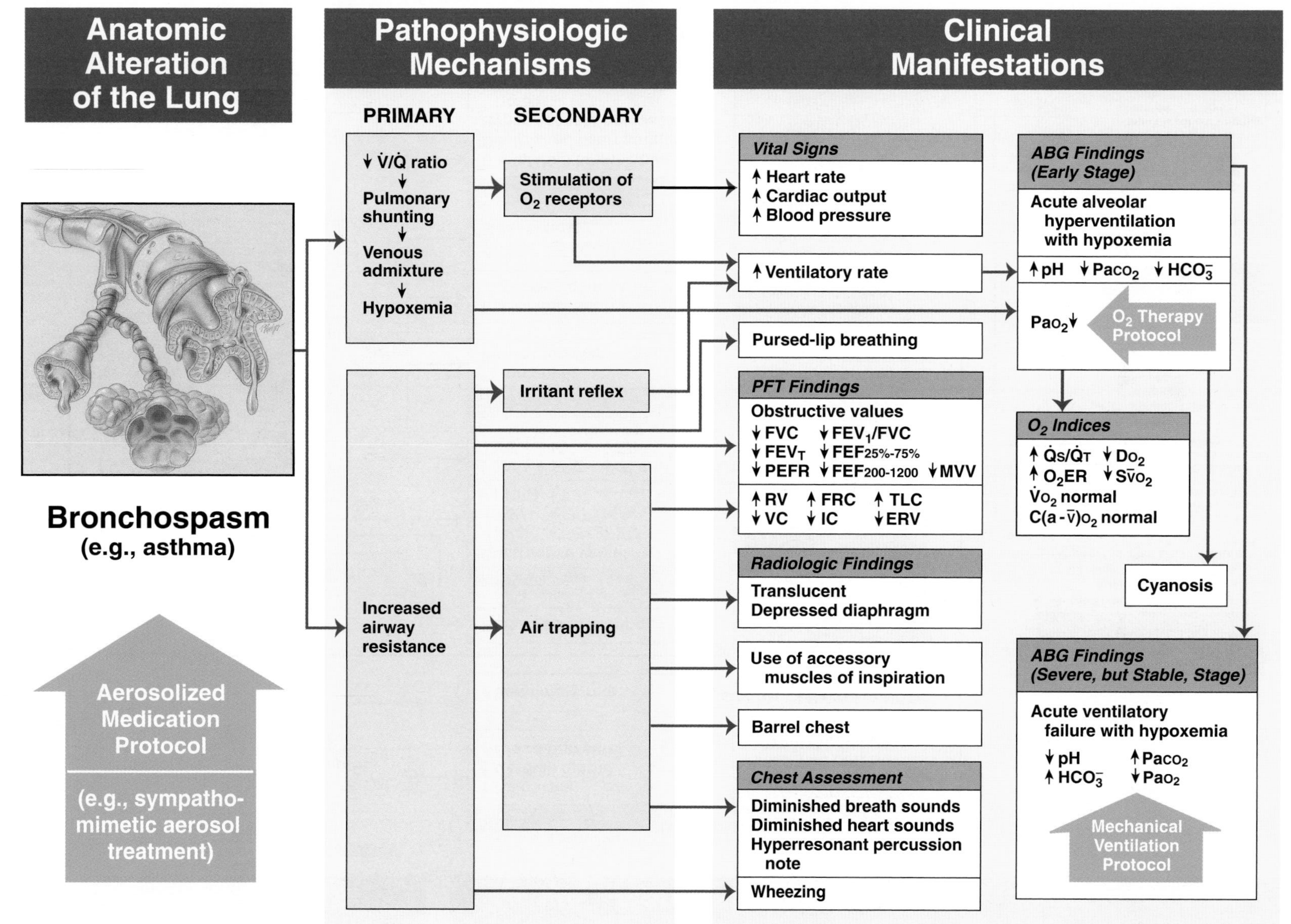

FIGURE 9-11 Bronchospasm clinical scenario.

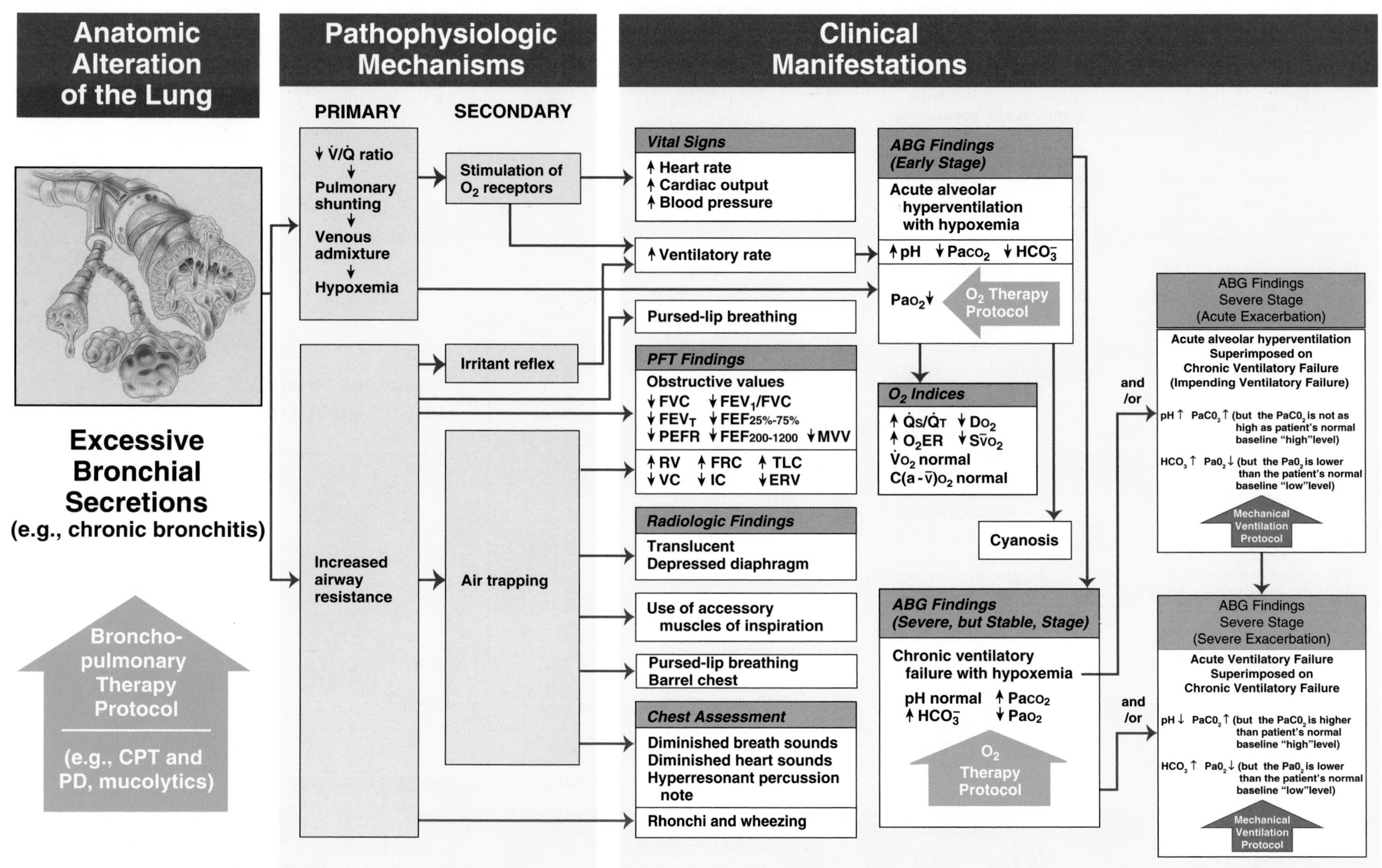

FIGURE 9-12 Excessive bronchial secretions clinical scenario.

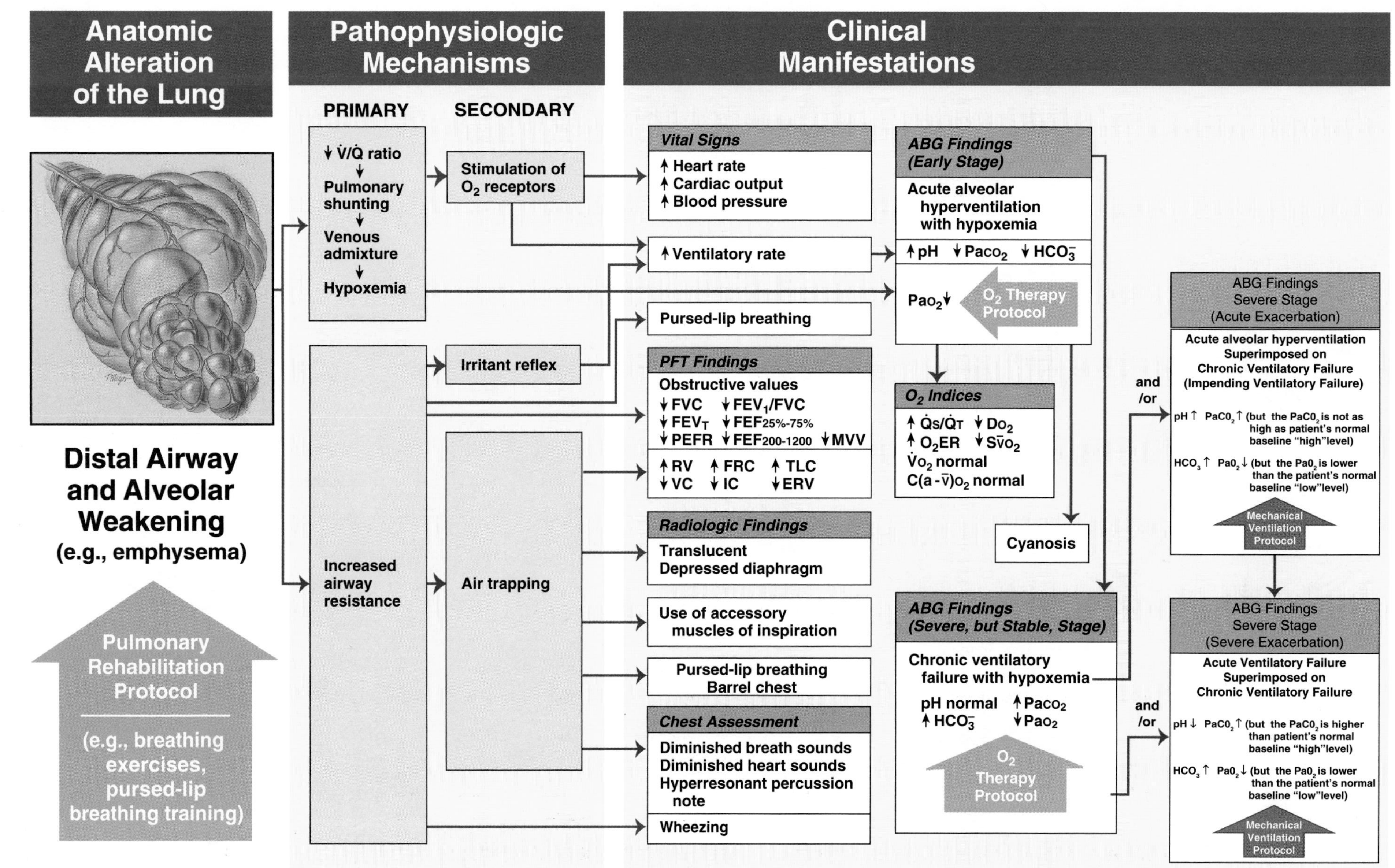

FIGURE 9-13 Distal airway and alveolar weakening clinical scenario. The Pulmonary Rehabilitation Protocol is not covered in the text.

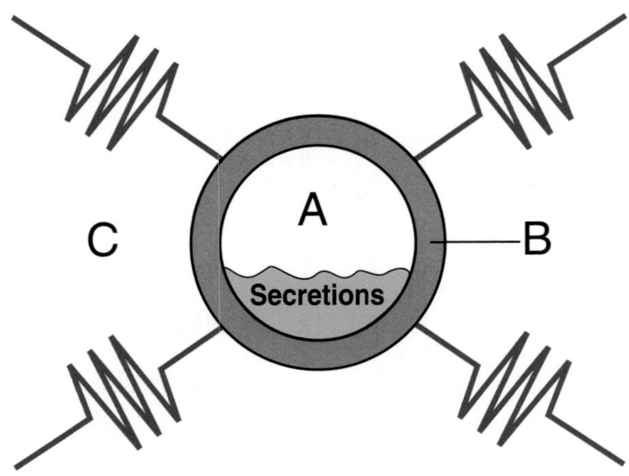

FIGURE 9-14 A three-component model of a prototype airway. Therapy may be directed at any or all components. *A*, Airway lumen; *B*, airway wall; *C*, supporting structures. Therapy for *A* includes deep breathing and coughing, smoking cessation, suctioning, mucolytics, bland aerosols, systemic and parenteral hydration, and therapeutic bronchoscopy. Therapy for *B* includes bronchodilators, aerosolized antiinflammatory agents, aerosolized antibiotics, and aerosolized decongestants. Therapy for *C* includes pursed-lip breathing exercises (e.g., when the elastic recoil of the lungs is absent in emphysema) and removal of external factors compressing the airway (e.g., bullae, pleural effusion, pneumothorax, tumor masses).

TABLE 9-5 Common Anatomic Alterations of the Lungs Associated With Respiratory Disorders

Respiratory Disorder	Atelectasis	Alveolar Consolidation	Increased Alveolar-Capillary Membrane Thickness	Bronchospasm	Excessive Bronchial Secretions	Distal Airway Weakening
Chronic bronchitis				X*	X	
Emphysema				X	X*	X
Bronchiectasis	X	X		X	X	
Asthma				X	X	
Pneumonia		X	X		X*	
Lung abscess		X			X	
Tuberculosis		X	X			
Fungal diseases		X	X			
Pulmonary edema	X		X		X	
Pulmonary embolism	X			X		
Flail chest	X	X				
Pneumothorax	X					
Pleural diseases	X					
Kyphoscoliosis	X				X*	
Pneumoconiosis			X	X		
Cancer of the lung	X	X			X	
Adult respiratory distress syndrome	X*	X	X			
Chronic interstitial lung diseases			X	X*		
Guillain-Barré syndrome	X*	X*			X*	
Myasthenia gravis	X*	X*			X*	
Meconium aspiration syndrome	X	X			X	
Transient tachypnea of newborn			X		X	
Infant respiratory distress syndrome	X	X			X	
Pulmonary air leak syndromes	X					
Respiratory syncytial virus	X	X			X	
Bronchopulmonary dysplasia	X		X		X	
Diaphragmatic hernia	X					
Cystic fibrosis	X*			X*	X	
Near drowning	X	X	X	X		
Smoke inhalation and thermal injuries	X	X	X	X		
Postoperative atelectasis	X					

*Common secondary anatomic alterations of the lungs associated with this disorder.

SELF-ASSESSMENT QUESTIONS

evolve Answers to questions can be found on Evolve. To access additional student assessment questions and case studies for application of text material to real-life scenarios, visit **http://evolve.elsevier.com/DesJardins/respiratory.**

1. Which of the following pathophysiologic mechanism is or are associated with the atelectasis clinical scenario?

1. Air trapping
2. Decreased $\dot{V}/\dot{Q}$ ratio
3. Deflation reflex
4. Increased airway resistance
5. Irritant reflex

A. 1 and 4 only
B. 2 and 3 only
C. 4 and 5 only
D. 2, 3, and 5 only

2. Which of the following clinical manifestations is or are associated with the excessive bronchial secretions clinical scenario?

1. Translucent radiographs
2. Increased FVC
3. Pursed-lip breathing
4. Air bronchograms

A. 1 and 4 only
B. 1 and 3 only
C. 2, 3, and 4 only
D. 1, 2, 3, and 4

3. Which of the following clinical manifestations is or are associated with the atelectasis clinical scenario?

1. Increased opacity in chest x-ray
2. Decreased FRC
3. Bronchial breath sounds
4. Hyperresonant percussion note
5. Diminished heart sounds

A. 1 and 4 only
B. 3 and 5 only
C. 1, 2, and 3 only
D. 2, 3, 4, and 5 only

4. Which of the following pathophysiologic mechanism is or are associated with the bronchospasm clinical scenario?

1. Air trapping
2. Decreased $\dot{V}/\dot{Q}$ ratio
3. Increased PEFR
4. Increased airway resistance
5. Irritant reflex

A. 1 and 4 only
B. 2 and 3 only
C. 4 and 5 only
D. 1, 2, 4, and 5 only

5. Which of the following clinical manifestations is or are associated with the distal airway and alveolar weakening clinical scenario?

1. Diminished breath sounds
2. Decreased RV
3. Pursed-lip breathing
4. Dull percussion note

A. 1 and 4 only
B. 1 and 3 only
C. 2, 3, and 4 only
D. 1, 2, 3, and 4

Recording Skills: The Basis for Data Collection, Organization, Assessment Skills, and Treatment Plans

10

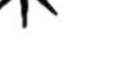

Chapter Objectives

After reading this chapter, you will be able to:

- Describe the clinical importance of good charting skills.
- Differentiate among the following types of patient records:
  - Traditional charting
  - Problem-oriented medical records (POMR), and include SOAPIER progress notes
  - Computer documentation
- Discuss the importance of the Heath Insurance Portability and Accountability Act.
- Define key terms and complete self-assessment questions at the end of the chapter and on Evolve.

Key Terms

Block Chart
Computer-Based Personal Records
Electronic Health Records
Electronic Medical Records
Electronic Patient Medical Charts
Problem-Oriented Medical Record (POMR)
SOAP
SOAPIER
Source-Oriented Record
Traditional Record

Chapter Outline

Types of Patient Records
Traditional Chart
Problem-Oriented Medical Record
Computer Documentation
Health Insurance Portability and Accountability Act

Because all health-care workers share information through written or electronic communication, the respiratory care practitioner must understand the way to document and use the patient's medical records effectively and efficiently. The process of adding documentary information to the patient's chart is called *charting, recording,* or *documenting.* Good charting should provide the basic clinical information necessary for critical thinking, or assessment skills—that is, good charting should be an effective way to summarize pertinent clinical data, analyze and assess it (i.e., determine the cause of the clinical data), record the formulation of an appropriate treatment plan, and document the adjustments of the treatment plan (in response to its effectiveness) after it has been implemented.

Good charting enhances communication and continuity of care among all members of the health-care team. There is a definite and direct relationship between effective charting (communication) and the quality of patient care. Good charting also provides a permanent record of past and current assessment data, treatment plans, therapy given, and the patient's response to various therapeutic modalities. This information may be used by various governmental agencies and accreditation teams to evaluate the hospital's patient care and prove that care was given appropriately. Accurate and legible records are the only means by which hospitals can prove that they are providing appropriate care and meeting established standards.

In addition, many health-care reimbursement plans (e.g., Medicare and Medicaid) are based on diagnosis related groups (DRGs). Under these plans, remuneration is based on disease diagnoses. Many private insurance companies use similar illness categories when setting hospital payment rates.

Before providing reimbursement, insurance companies carefully review the patient's medical record when assessing whether appropriate and efficient care was given.

Finally, the patient's chart is a legal document that can be called into court. Even though the physician or hospital owns the original record, the patient, lawyers, and courts can gain access to it. As an instrument of continuous patient care and as a legal document, the patient's chart therefore should contain all pertinent respiratory care assessments, planning, interventions, and evaluations.

Types of Patient Records

Three basic methods are used to record assessment data: the traditional chart, the **problem-oriented medical record (POMR),** and computer documentation.

Traditional Chart

The **traditional record** (also called **block chart** or **source-oriented record**) is divided into distinct areas or blocks, with emphasis placed on specific information. The traditional record is commonly seen in the patient's chart as full-colored sheets of block information. Typical blocks of information include the admission sheet, physician's order sheet, progress notes, history and physical examination data, medication sheet, nurses' admission information, nursing care plans, nursing notes, graphs and flowsheets, laboratory and x-ray reports, and discharge summary. The order, content, and number of blocks vary among institutions. The traditional chart makes recording easier, but it also makes it more difficult to review a particular event readily and efficiently or to follow the overall progress of the patient.

Problem-Oriented Medical Record (POMR)

The organization of the POMR is based on an objective, scientific, problem-solving method. The POMR is one of the most important medical records used by the health-care practitioner to (1) systematically gather clinical data, (2) formulate an assessment (i.e., the cause of the clinical data), and (3) develop an appropriate treatment plan. A number of good POMR methods are available for recording assessment data. Regardless of the method selected, it is essential that one method be adopted and used consistently.

A good POMR method should take a systematic approach in documenting the following:

- The subjective and objective information collected
- An assessment based on the subjective and objective data
- The treatment plan (with measurable outcomes)
- An evaluation of the patient's response to the treatment plan
- A section to record any adjustments made to the original treatment plan

One of the most common POMR methods is the **SOAPIER** progress note—often abbreviated in the clinical setting to a **SOAP** progress note. *SOAPIER* is an acronym for seven specific aspects of charting that systematically review one health problem.

S *Subjective* information refers to information about the patient's feelings, concerns, or sensations presented by the patient:
"I coughed hard all night long."
"My chest feels very tight."
"I feel very short of breath."
Only the patient can provide subjective information. Some cases may not involve subjective information. For instance, a comatose, intubated patient on a mechanical ventilator is unable to provide subjective data.

O *Objective* information is the data the respiratory care practitioner can measure, factually describe, or obtain from other professional reports or test results. Objective data include the following:

- Heart rate
- Respiratory rate
- Blood pressure
- Temperature
- Breath sounds
- Cough effort
- Sputum production (volume, consistency, color, and odor)
- Arterial blood gas and pulse oximetry data
- Pulmonary function study results
- X-ray reports
- Hemodynamic data
- Chemistry results

A *Assessment* refers to the practitioner's professional conclusion about the cause of the subjective and objective data presented by the patient. In the patient with a respiratory disorder, the cause is usually related to a specific anatomic alteration of the lung. The assessment, moreover, provides the specific reason as to why the respiratory care practitioner is working with the patient. For example, the presence of wheezes are objective data (the clinical indicator) to verify the assessment (the cause) of bronchial smooth muscle constriction; an arterial blood gas with a pH of 7.18, a $PaCO_2$ of 80 mm Hg, an HCO_3^- of 29 mm/L, and a PaO_2 of 54 mm Hg are the objective data to verify the assessment of acute ventilatory failure with moderate hypoxemia. The presence of rhonchi is a clinical indicator to verify the assessment of secretions in the large airways.

P *Plan* is/are the therapeutic procedure(s) selected to remedy the cause identified in the assessment. For example, an assessment of bronchial smooth muscle constriction justifies the administration of a bronchodilator; the assessment of acute ventilatory failure justifies mechanical ventilation.

I *Implementation* is the actual administration of the specific therapy plan. It documents exactly what was done, when, and by whom.

E *Evaluation* is the collection of measurable data regarding the effectiveness of the therapy plan and the patient's response to it. For example, an arterial blood gas assessment may reveal that the patient's PaO_2 did not increase to a safe level in response to oxygen therapy.

R *Revision* refers to any changes that may be made to the original therapy plan in response to the evaluation. For example, if the Pa_{O_2} does not increase appropriately after the implementation of oxygen therapy, the respiratory care practitioner might continue to increase the patient's F_{IO_2} until the desired Pa_{O_2} is reached.

For the new practitioner, a predesigned SOAP form is especially useful in (1) the rapid collection and systematic organization of important clinical data, (2) the formulation of an assessment (i.e., the cause of the clinical data), and (3) the development of a treatment plan. For example, consider the case example and SOAP progress note at the bottom of this page (Figure 10-1).

Although the SOAP form may initially appear long and time-consuming, the experienced respiratory care practitioner and assessor can typically condense and abbreviate SOAP information in a few minutes (primarily at the patient's bedside), in just a few short statements. Typically, a written SOAP form uses only 1 to 3 inches of space in the patient's chart. For example, the information presented in Figure 10-1 may actually be documented in the patient's chart in the following abbreviated form:

SOAP Case Example*

A **26-year-old man** arrived in the emergency room having a **severe asthmatic episode.** On observation, his arms were fixed to the bed rails, he was using his **accessory muscles of inspiration**, and he was using **pursed-lip breathing.** The patient stated that **"it feels like someone is standing on my chest. I just can't seem to take a deep breath."** His **heart rate** was **111 beats per minute**, and his **blood pressure** was **170/110.** His **respiratory rate** was **28 and shallow. Hyperresonant notes** were produced on percussion. **Auscultation** revealed **expiratory wheezing** and **rhonchi bilaterally.** His **chest x-ray film** revealed a **severely depressed diaphragm** and **alveolar hyperinflation.** His **peak expiratory flow** was **165 L/min.** Even though his **cough effort** was **weak,** he produced a **large amount** of **thick white secretions.** His **arterial blood gases** showed a **pH of 7.27**, a **Pa_{CO_2} of 62**, an **HCO_3^-** of 25, and a **Pa_{O_2} of 49** (on room air) (see Figure 10-1).

*Subjective and objective data presented in bold.

Respiratory Assessment Flow Chart

Subjective →	Objective →	Assessment →	Plan →
"It feels like someone is standing on my chest."	Vital signs: RR 28 HR 111 BP 170/110 Temp. — On antipyretic agent? ☐ Yes ☐ No		Present Plan
"I just can't seem to take a deep breath."	Chest assessment: Insp. Use of accessory muscles of inspiration and pursed-lip breathing		None
Anterior (R, L)	Palp. — Perc. Hyperresonant Ausc. Expiratory wheezing and rhonchi bilaterally	Bronchospasm Large airway secretions	Plan Modifications
	Radiography Severely depressed diaphragm	Air trapping	Bronchodilator Tx per protocol
Posterior (L, R)	Bedside spir.: PEFR ā 165 p̄ — Tx SVC FVC NIF		
	Cough: ☐ Strong ☒ Weak Sputum production: ☒ Yes ☐ No Sputum char. Large amt. thick/white secretions	Poor ability to mobilize thick secretions	CPT & PD per protocol Mucolytics per protocol
Pt. name — Age 26 · Male X · Female Date — · Time —	ABG: pH 7.27 PaCO2 62 HCO3- 25 PaO2 49 SaO2 — SpO2 — Neg. O2 transport factors —	Acute ventilatory failure with severe hypoxemia	Mechanical ventilation per protocol
Admitting diagnosis Asthma Therapist — Hospital —	Other: —		ABG in 30 minutes & reassess

FIGURE 10-1 Completed predesigned SOAP form.

S—"It feels like someone is standing on my chest. I can't take a deep breath."

O—Use of acc. mus. of insp.; HR 111, BP 170/110, RR 28 & shallow, pursed-lip; hyperresonance; exp. whz; diaph. & alv. hyperinfl.; PEFR 165; wk. cough; lg. amt. thick/white sec., pH 7.27; Pa_{CO_2} 62; HCO_3^- 25; Pa_{O_2} 49.

A—Bronchospasm; hyperinflation; poor ability to mob. tk. sec.; acute vent. fail. with severe hypox.

P—Bronchodilator Tx/pro., CPT & PD/pro., mucolytic/pro., mech. vent/pro., ABG 30 min.

After the treatment has been administered, another abbreviated SOAP note should be made to determine whether the treatment plan needs to be up-regulated or down-regulated. For example, if the arterial blood gas data obtained after the implementation of the plan (outlined in the SOAP form) showed that the patient's Pa_{O_2} was still too low, it would be appropriate to revise the original treatment plan by increasing the F_{IO_2} on the mechanical ventilator. Figure 10-2 illustrates objective data, assessments, and treatment plans commonly associated with respiratory disorders.

Computer Documentation

Computer-based records (also called **electronic medical records, electronic health records, computer-based personal records,** and **electronic patient medical charts**) are now commonly used throughout the health-care industry. Common uses of computer documentation include ordering supplies and services for the patient; storing admission data; writing and storing patient care plans (e.g., SOAPs and physician progress notes); listing medications, treatments, and procedures; and storing and retrieving diagnostic test results (e.g., x-ray films, pulmonary function studies, and arterial blood gas values). Many health-care facilities have incorporated software for their specific patient care needs. Such computer programs include options for starting individualized patient care plans, using automated Kardex systems, documenting acuity levels, and providing a mechanism to electronically record ongoing assessment data. There are literally hundreds of electronic medical chart solutions available today, targeted at every size and type of medical setting.

With all the patient information in a central location, computer documentation provides easy access to patient data. It greatly reduces the chance for errors, and updated patient information can easily be entered in real time. Computer-based records do away with the need to make phone calls to other departments to gather patient information or to order patient supplies or services. In addition, electronic documentation eliminates the need to read through the entire chart to evaluate the patient's progress or to review specific data such as medication listings, treatments, diagnostic test results, and procedures. The patient's clinical information is permanently recorded, and other health-care departments can review it and communicate with one another.

Basic computer knowledge and skills are usually taught through the hospital's in-service education department. Each nursing station usually has a computer screen to display information, a keyboard to enter and retrieve data, and possibly a printer to produce printed copy. The entire patient record or just a part of it may be retrieved and printed. Today, many health-care practitioners use hand-held bedside computer documentation systems. Bedside computer devices, referred to as *point-of-care (POC) systems,* commonly include specific clinical prompts for data entry, which result in records that are more accurate and complete.

Good charting skills are essential to critical thinking and patient assessment—they provide the basic means to collect clinical data, analyze it, assess it, and formulate a treatment plan. Furthermore, good charting skills document the effectiveness of patient care and adjustments of the treatment plan in response to its effectiveness. Without good charting systems and skills, the practitioner merely administers health care without a predetermined (and recorded) goal.

Historically, respiratory care practitioners have focused on treating patients with specific disease entities and implementing physicians' orders. Little planning was done by respiratory care practitioners to individualize their treatments for a specific patient. Today, a systematic problem-solving approach to respiratory care, based on broad theoretic knowledge, combined with technical expertise and communication skills, is essential.

Health Insurance Portability and Accountability Act

In 2003 the Department of Health and Human Services (HHS) proposed national rules that outlined the ways in which a patient's medical files should be used or shared with others. These rules were adopted as federal standards after the passage of the Health Insurance Portability and Accountability Act (HIPAA). Today HIPAA requires that all health-care practitioners who have access to patient medical records prove that they have a plan to protect the privacy of the records. In essence, the HIPAA regulations protect the patient's privacy with specific rules outlining when, how, and what type of health-care information can be shared. HIPAA gives the patient the right to know about—and to control—how his or her personal medical records will be used. The following provides a general overview of the HIPAA regulations:

- Both the health-care provider and a representative of the insurance company must explain to the patient how they plan to disclose any medical records.
- Patients may request copies of all their medical information and make appropriate changes to it. Patients may also ask for a history of any unusual disclosures.
- The patient must give formal consent should anyone want to share any health information.
- The patient's health information is to be used only for health purposes. Without the patient's consent, medical records cannot be used by either (1) a bank to determine whether to give the patient a loan or (2) a potential employer to determine whether to hire the patient.

A

RESPIRATORY CARE POCKET PROTOCOL CARD

OBJECTIVE DATA Clinical manifestations (clinical indicators) that commonly develop in response to respiratory disease						ASSESSMENT	PLAN
Chest Assessment				Chest Radiograph	Bedside Spirometry	COMMON CAUSES/ SEVERITY OF CLINICAL INDICATORS	TREATMENT SELECTION (PHYSICIAN ORDERED*)
Inspection	Palpation	Percussion	Auscultation				
• Barrel chest • Use of accessory muscles • Pursed-lip breathing • Cyanosis	May show ↓ chest excursion	May be hyper-resonant	• Wheezes • Prolonged exhalation	May be normal or show over expansion	↓ PEFR ↓ FEV_1 ↑ FEV_1/FVC	BRONCHOSPASM e.g., Asthma EXCESSIVE BROCHIAL SECRETIONS e.g., Bronchitis or Cystic Fibrosis BRONCHIAL TUMOR	Bronchodilator therapy Bronchial hygiene therapy General management/ comfort
• Dyspneic • Cyanosis	Usually normal	Usually normal	Inspiratory stridor	Laryngeal narrowing	Not indicated	LARYNGEAL EDEMA e.g., Croup or Post-extubation Edema	Cool, bland aerosol therapy Racemic epinephrine
Sputum production	May be normal	May be normal	Rhonchi	May be normal	↓ PEFR ↓ FEV_1	LARGE AIRWAY SECRETIONS e.g., Bronchitis or Cystic Fibrosis	Bronchial hygiene therapy
• Use of accessory muscles of inspiration • Pursed-lip breathing • Barrel chest • Cyanosis	↓ Tactile and vocal fremitus	Hyper-resonant	• ↓ Breath sounds • ↓ Heart sounds • Prolonged exhalation	• ↓ Diaphragm • Translucency • Over expanded	↓ PEFR ↓ FVC ↓ FEV_1/FVC	AIRTRAPPING (Hyperinflation) e.g., COPD • Asthma • Bronchitis • Emphysema	Treat underlying cause, if possible, e.g., • Bronchospasm • Airway secretions
• May appear dyspneic • Cyanosis	↑ Tactile and vocal fremitus	Dull	• Bronchial breath sounds • Crackles • Whispered pectoriloquy	• Opacity	↓ VC	CONSOLIDATION e.g., Pneumonia ATELECTASIS e.g., Post-op or mucus plugs INFILTRATION e.g., Pneumoconiosis	• Antibiotic agents* • Lung hyperinflation Tx • Bronchial hygiene therapy -when atelectasis is caused by mucus accumulation/ mucus plugs
• Rapid shallow breath • Cyanosis • Frothy pink secretions	Usually normal	Dull	• Crackles • May be: wheezes/ rhonchi	• Enlarged heart • Infiltrates "Butterfly"	↓ VC	PULMONARY EDEMA • Left heart failure	• Lung hyperinflation Tx • Positive inotropic agents* • Diuretics*
• Cyanosis • Rapid shallow breath • Unilateral expansion	• Usually normal • Tracheal shift	Hyper-resonant	Absent or ↓ breath sounds	• Pneumothorax • Translucency • Mediastinum shift • ↓ Diaphragm	Not indicated	AIR PRESSURE IN INTRAPLEURAL SPACE GREATER THAN ATMOSPHERE • Tension pneumothorax	Chest tube to evacuate air* Lung hyperinflation Tx
• Cyanosis • Rapid shallow breath • Unilateral expansion	• Usually normal • May be tracheal shift	Dull	↓ Breath sounds	• Opacity • Obscured diaphragm	↓ VC	FLUID IN INTRAPLEURAL SPACE • Pleural effusion • Empyema	• Treat underlying cause • Thoracentesis* • Lung hyperinflation Tx
Paradoxical chest movement	Tender	Not indicated	Varies	• Rib fractures • Opacity (e.g., ARDS and/or atelectasis	Not possible	DOUBLE FRACTURES OF THREE OR MORE ADJACENT RIBS • Flail chest	• Stabilization of chest-mechanical ventilation* • Lung Hyperinflation Tx

SIMON & KOLZ PUBLISHING

FIGURE 10-2 Respiratory care protocol guide. (Used with permission of Terry DesJardins.)

B

RESPIRATORY CARE POCKET PROTOCOL CARD

Objective Data	ASSESSMENT	Plan
(Clinical manifestations or clinical indicators)	COMMON CAUSES/SEVERITY OF CLINICAL INDICATORS	TREATMENT SELECTION (PHYSICIAN ORDERED*)
Cough effort: ○ Strong ○ Weak Sputum production: ○ No ○ Yes	Patient's abiltily to mobilize secretions: ○ Good ○ Poor	Bronchial hygiene therapy
Sputum characteristics:		
• Amount > 30ml/24 hrs.	• Excessive bronchial secretions	• Bronchial hygiene therapy
• White and translucent sputum	• Normal sputum	• None
• Yellow/opaque sputum	• Acute airway infection	• Treat underlying cause
• Green sputum	• Old, retained secretions and infections	• Bronchial hygiene therapy
• Brown sputum	• Old blood	• Bronchial hygiene therapy
• Red sputum	• Fresh blood	• Notify physician
• Frothy secrection	• Pulmonary edema	• Treat underlying cause, e.g., CHF
Arterial blood gas status - Ventilatory		
• $pH\uparrow$, $PaCO_2\downarrow$, $HCO_3\downarrow$	• Acute alveolar hyperventilation	• Treat underlying cause, if possible. Ex: pneumonia, pain.
• pH normal, $PaCO_2\downarrow$, $HCO_3\downarrow\downarrow$	• Chronic alveolar hyperventilation	• Generally none (occurs normally at high altitude)
• $pH\downarrow$, $PaCO_2\uparrow$, $HCO_3\uparrow$	• Acute ventilatory failure	• Mechanical ventilation*
• pH normal, $PaCO_2\uparrow$, $HCO_3\uparrow\uparrow$	• Chronic ventilatory failure	• Low flow oxygen, bronchial hygiene, nocturnal ventilation
Sudden ventilatory changes or chronic ventilatory failure:		
• $pH\uparrow$, $PaCO_2\uparrow$, $HCO_3\uparrow\uparrow$, $PaO_2\downarrow$	• Acute alveolar hyperventilation on chronic ventilatory failure	• Treat the underlying cause, if possible. Ex: pneumonia
• $pH\uparrow$, $PaCO_2\uparrow\uparrow$, $HCO_3\uparrow$, $PaO_2\downarrow$	• Acute ventilatory failure on chronic ventilatory failure	• Mechanical ventilation*
Indicators for mechanical ventilation:		
• $pH\uparrow$, $PaCO_2\downarrow$, $HCO_3\downarrow$, $PaO_2\downarrow$ but pt is fatigued	• Impending ventilatory failure	• Mechanical ventilation*
• $pH\downarrow$, $PaCO_2\uparrow$, $HCO_3\uparrow$, $PaO_2\downarrow$ hypoventilation	• Ventilatory failure	
• $pH\downarrow$, $PaCO_2\uparrow$, $HCO_3\uparrow$, $PaO_2\downarrow$ apnea	• Apnea	
Metabolic	• Metabolic alkalosis:	
• $pH\uparrow$, $PaCO_2$ normal or $\uparrow$, $HCO_3\uparrow$, PaO_2 normal	• Hypokalemia	• Potassium administration*
	• Hypochloremia	• Chlorine administration*
	•Metabolic acidosis:	
• $pH\downarrow$, $PaCO_2$ normal or $\downarrow$, $HCO_3\downarrow$, $PaO_2\downarrow$	• Lactic acidosis	• Oxygen administration, cardiovascular support*
• $pH\downarrow$, $PaCO_2$ normal or $\downarrow$, $HCO_3\downarrow$, PaO_2 normal	• Ketoacidosis	• Insulin administration*
• $pH\downarrow$, $PaCO_2$ normal or $\downarrow$, $HCO_3\downarrow$, PaO_2 normal	• Renal failure	• Renal failure management*
Ventilatory and metabolic:		
• $pH\downarrow$, $PaCO_2\uparrow$, $HCO_3\downarrow$	• Combined metabolic and respiratory acidosis	• Mechanical ventilation* • Treat the underlying cause of metabolic acidosis (see above)
• $pH\uparrow$, $PaCO_2\downarrow$, $HCO_3\uparrow$	• Combined metabolic and respiratory alkalosis	• Treat the underlying cause for acute alveolar hyperventilation • Treat the underlying cause for metabolic alkalosis (see above)
Oxygenation status:		
• $PaO_2 < 80$mm Hg	• Mild hypoxemia	• Oxygen therapy
• $PaO_2 < 60$mm Hg	• Moderate hypoxemia	• Treat the underlying cause of hypoxemia
• $PaO_2 < 40$mm Hg	• Severe hypoxemia	
Negative oxygen transport indicators: ○ $\downarrow PaO_2$ ○ Anemia ○ Blood loss ○ $\downarrow$Cardiac output ○ CO poisoning ○ Abnormal Hb	Oxygen transport status: ○ Adequate ○ Inadequate	• Treat the underlying cause, if possible, e.g., ○ Oxygen therapy ○ Blood replacement* ○ Positive inotropic agents*

FIGURE 10-2, cont'd

- When the patient's health information is disclosed, only the minimum necessary amount of information should be released.
- Records dealing with a patient's mental health get an extra level of protection.
- The patient has the right to complain to HHS about violations of HIPAA rules.

One disadvantage of the HIPAA regulations, according to many health-care practitioners, is that the health-care provider must allocate large sums of money to comply with the HIPAA rules—dollars that might be better spent elsewhere. Critics also argue that this cost will likely be passed on to the consumer. In addition, many health-care providers believe that the quality of patient care will be compromised as a result of HIPAA, making it more difficult for various health-care practitioners to obtain vital information regarding patient care. For example, consider the potential HIPAA-related problems for a health-care team in a Miami, Florida, hospital that is trying to obtain the pharmaceutical history—in a timely fashion—of an elderly, unconscious car accident victim whose medical records are in a Detroit, Michigan, hospital. Proponents of the HIPAA regulations argue that this is the tradeoff made to ensure the privacy of an individual's health-care information. Regardless of the pros or cons of the HIPAA regulations, the respiratory therapy practitioner—like all other health-care providers—must comply with the current HIPAA regulations.

SELF-ASSESSMENT QUESTIONS

evolve Answers to questions can be found on Evolve. To access additional student assessment questions and case studies for application of text material to real-life scenarios, visit **http://evolve.elsevier.com/DesJardins/respiratory.**

1. What is the process of adding written information to the patient's chart called?

1. Recording
2. Critical thinking
3. Documenting
4. Charting

a. 2 only
b. 3 and 4 only
c. 1 and 3 only
d. 1, 3, and 4 only

2. The admission sheet, physician's order sheet, and history sheet are all what type of patient records?

1. Source-oriented record
2. Problem-oriented medical record
3. Block chart
4. Traditional chart

a. 2 only
b. 4 only
c. 3 and 4 only
d. 1, 3, and 4 only

3. Which of the following is based on a sequential, objective, scientific, problem-solving method?

1. Source-oriented record
2. Problem-oriented medical record
3. Block chart
4. Traditional chart

a. 1 only
b. 2 only
c. 4 only
d. 3 and 4 only

4. According to the respiratory care protocol guide (per Figure 10-2), bronchial breath sounds and dull percussion notes are associated with which of the following clinical assessments?

1. Air trapping
2. Bronchospasm
3. Atelectasis
4. Consolidation

a. 2 only
b. 3 only
c. 1 and 2 only
d. 3 and 4 only

5. Good charting should be an effective way to do the following:

A. ______________________________
____
____

B. ______________________________
____
____

C. ______________________________
____
____

D. ______________________________
____
____

6. A good problem-oriented medical record (POMR) should include a systematic approach that documents the following:

A. ______

B. ______

C. ______

D. ______

E. ______

7. One of the most common POMR methods is the SOAPIER progress note, often abbreviated in the clinical setting to a SOAP progress note. Define the following components of a SOAP progress note, and give one or more examples.

S ______

Example(s): ______

O ______

Example(s): ______

A ______

Example(s): ______

P ______

Example(s): ______

8. According to the respiratory care protocol guide (per Figure 10-2), what are the three major indicators (assessments) for mechanical ventilation?

A. ______

B. ______

C. ______

9. A patient is placed on a mechanical ventilator with arterial blood gas values that reveal a pH of 7.56, a Pa_{CO_2} of 24, an HCO_3^- of 20, and a Pa_{O_2} of 52. Write the indicators for mechanical ventilation that might justify placing the patient on a mechanical ventilator with these arterial blood gas values.

Answer: ______

10. Case: A 36-year-old woman is in the emergency room in respiratory distress. Her heart rate is 136 beats per minute, and her blood pressure is 165/120. Her respiratory rate is 32, and her breathing is labored. The patient states that "It feels like a rope is around my neck." Expiratory wheezing and rhonchi are auscultated bilaterally. Her arterial blood gas values reveal a pH of 7.56, a Pa_{CO_2} of 28, HCO_3^- of 21, and a Pa_{O_2} of 47 mm Hg (on room air). Her cough effort is strong, and she is producing a moderate amount of thin white secretions. Her peak expiratory flow rate is 185 L/min, and her chest x-ray film demonstrates a moderately depressed diaphragm and alveolar hyperinflation.

With this clinical information, provide SOAP documentation for the patient (use Figure 10-2 for assistance).

S ______

O ______

A ______

P ______

PART II

Obstructive Lung Diseases

Obstructive lung diseases are characterized by a variety of pathologic conditions—such as bronchial inflammation, excessive airway secretions, mucous plugging, bronchospasm, and distal airway weakening—that cause a reduction of airflow into and out of the lungs. Gas flow reduction is especially decreased during exhalation.

The most common obstructive lung disorders are **chronic bronchitis, emphysema**, and **asthma**. Although chronic bronchitis, emphysema, and asthma may appear alone, they often appear in combination. When chronic bronchitis and emphysema appear together as one disease complex, the patient is said to have **chronic obstructive pulmonary disease (COPD)**. Although asthma can be chronic, it is usually a more acute and intermittent respiratory disorder. Other obstructive lung disorders include **cystic fibrosis** (presented in newborn and early childhood respiratory disorders) and **bronchiectasis** (less common).

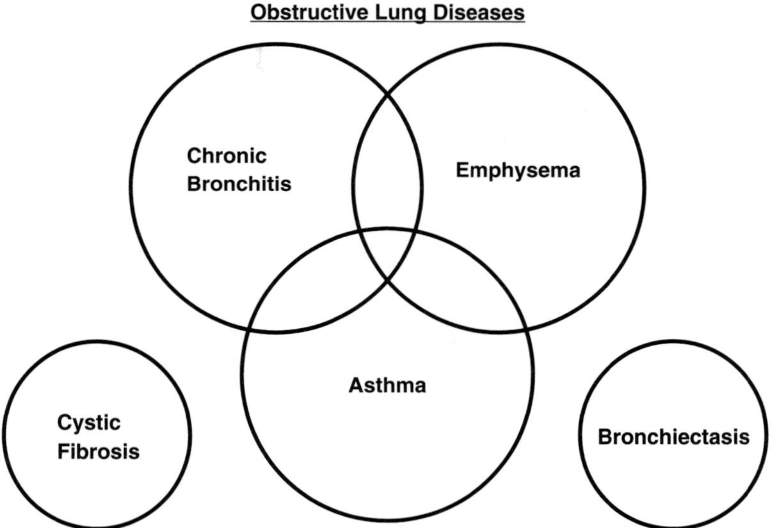

The most common obstructive lung diseases are chronic bronchitis, emphysema, and asthma. They may occur alone or in combination. When chronic bronchitis and emphysema appear together, the patient is said to have chronic obstructive pulmonary diseases (COPD). Other obstructive lung disorders include cystic fibrosis and bronchiectasis.

Chronic Obstructive Pulmonary Disease, Chronic Bronchitis, and Emphysema

11

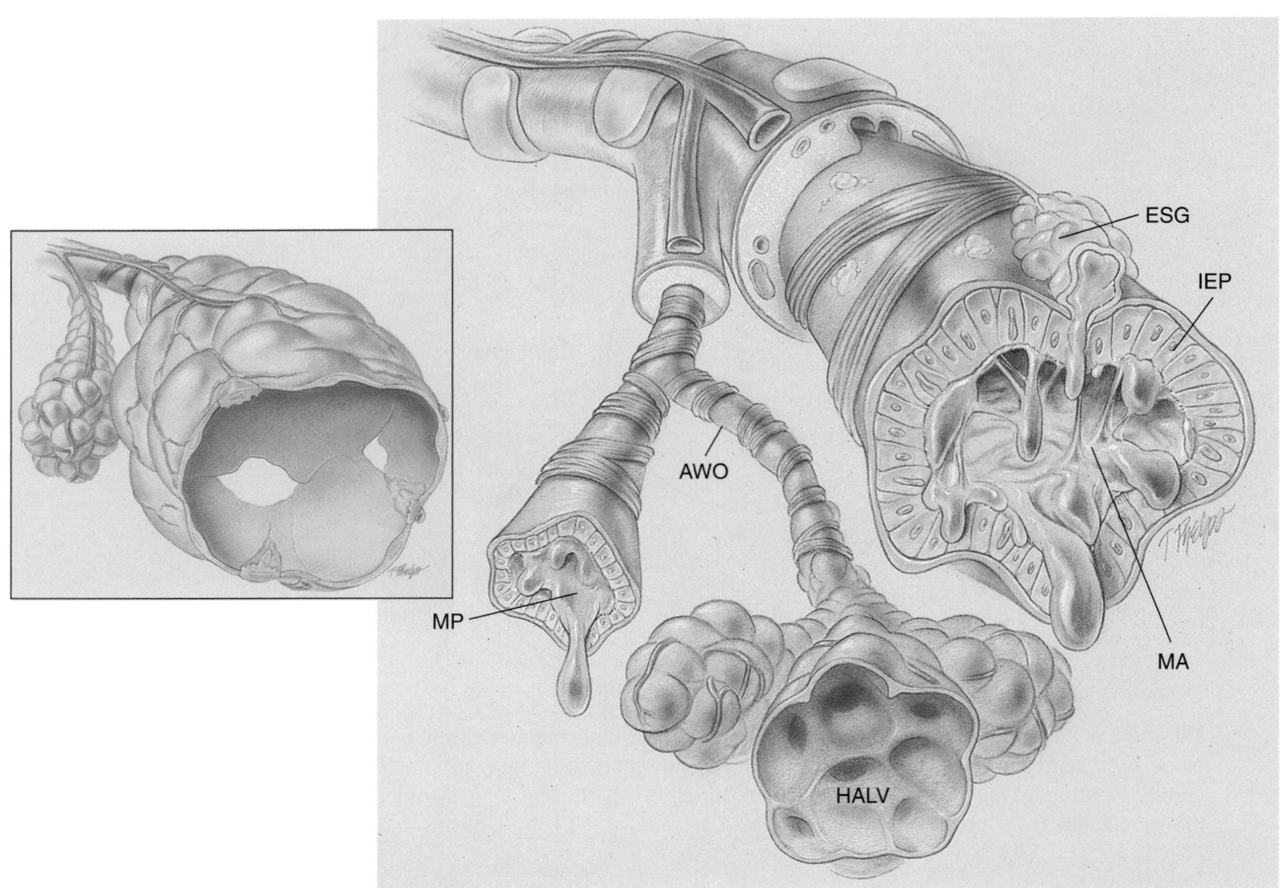

FIGURE 11-1 Chronic bronchitis, one of the most common airway diseases. *AWO,* Airway obstruction; *ESG,* enlarged submucosal gland; *HALV,* hyperinflation of alveoli (distal to airway obstruction); *IEP,* inflammation of epithelium; *MA,* mucous accumulation; *MP,* mucous plug.

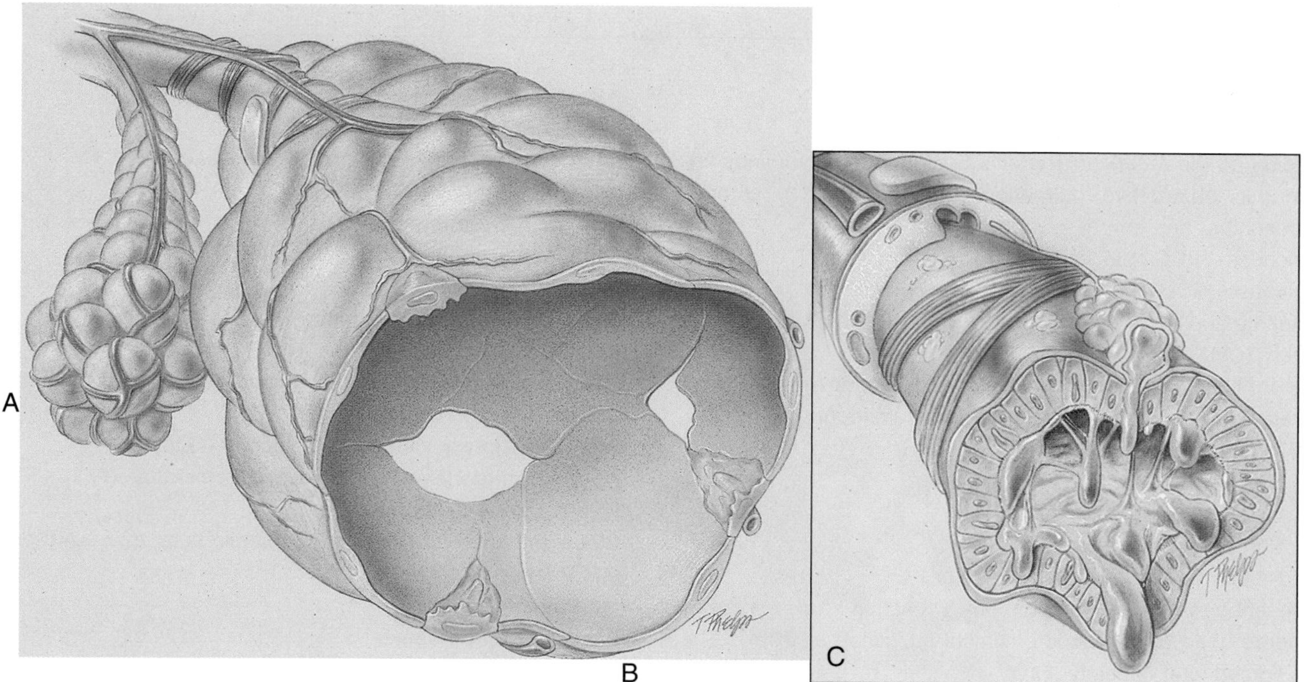

FIGURE 11-2 Panlobular emphysema. **A**, Normal alveoli for comparison purposes. **B**, Panlobular emphysema: abnormal weakening and enlargement of all air spaces distal to the terminal bronchioles. **C**, Excessive bronchial secretions from bronchitis, a common alteration of the lungs.

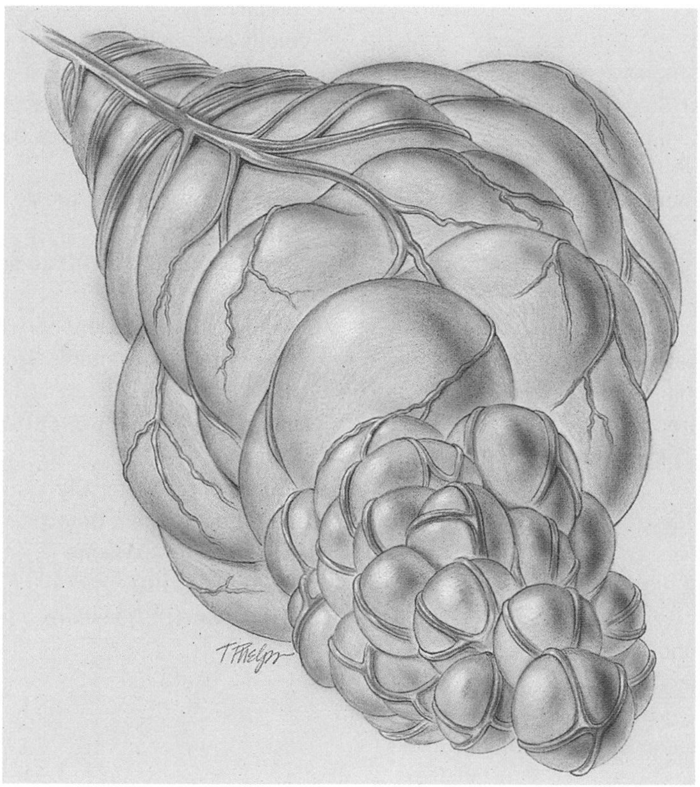

FIGURE 11-3 Centrilobular emphysema. Abnormal weakening and enlargement of the respiratory bronchioles and alveoli in the proximal portion of the acinus.

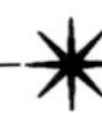

Chapter Objectives

After reading this chapter, you will be able to:

- Describe the American Thoracic Society (ATS) guidelines for chronic obstructive pulmonary disease (COPD), chronic bronchitis, and emphysema.
- Discuss the Global Initiative for Chronic Obstructive Lung Disease (GOLD) definition of COPD.
- List the etiology and epidemiology and risk factors associated with COPD.
- Describe the GOLD global strategy for diagnosing COPD.
- Describe the key indicators for considering a COPD diagnosis.
  - Dyspnea
  - Chronic cough
  - Chronic sputum production
  - History of exposure to risk factors
- Describe the three main pulmonary function study measurements used to confirm the clinical suspicion of COPD:
  - Forced vital capacity (FVC)
  - Forced expiratory volume in 1 second (FEV_1)
  - Forced expiratory volume in 1 second/forced vital capacity ratio (FEV_1/FVC ratio)
- Differentiate the following four stages of COPD as outlined by GOLD:
  - Stage I: Mild COPD
  - Stage II: Moderate COPD
  - Stage III: Severe COPD
  - Stage IV: Very severe COPD
- Identify additional diagnostic studies for patients identified as having Stage II, Stage III, or Stage IV COPD:
  - Bronchodilator reversibility testing
  - Chest x-ray examination
  - Arterial blood gas measurement
  - $Alpha_1$-antitrypsin deficiency screening
- List the anatomic alterations of the lungs caused by both chronic bronchitis and emphysema.
- List the cardiopulmonary clinical manifestations caused by the anatomic alterations and pathophysiologic mechanisms associated with chronic bronchitis and emphysema.
- Identify the key distinctive differences between chronic bronchitis and emphysema—the "pink puffer" and the "blue bloater."
- Describe the GOLD global strategy for the management and prevention of COPD.
- Describe additional treatment considerations for emphysema, including the following:
  - $Alpha_1$-antitrypsin replacement therapy
  - Lung volume reduction surgery
  - Lung transplantation
- Describe the clinical strategies and rationales of the SOAPs presented in the case studies.
- Define key terms and complete self-assessment questions at the end of the chapter and on Evolve.

Key Terms

$Alpha_1$-Antitrypsin Deficiency
American Thoracic Society (ATS) Guidelines
"Blue Bloater"
Centriacinar Emphysema
Centrilobular Emphysema
Chronic Bronchitis
Chronic Obstructive Pulmonary Disease (COPD)
Emphysema
Force Expiratory Volume in 1 Second/Forced Vital Capacity Ratio (FEV_1/FVC Ratio)
Forced Expiratory Volume in 1 Second (FEV_1)
Forced Expiratory Volume 1 Second Percentage ($FEV_{1\%}$)
Forced Vital Capacity (FVC)
Global Initiative for Chronic Obstructive Lung Disease (GOLD)
MM Phenotype
MZ Phenotype
Panacinar Emphysema
Panlobular Emphysema
"Pink Puffer"
ZZ Phenotype

Chapter Outline

Introduction

The **American Thoracic Society (ATS)** guidelines for **chronic obstructive pulmonary disease (COPD), chronic bronchitis,** and **emphysema** provide the following definitions:

> *Chronic obstructive pulmonary disease is a preventable and treatable disease state characterized by airflow limitation that is not fully reversible. The airflow limitation is usually progressive and is associated with an abnormal inflammatory response of the lungs to noxious particles or gases, primarily caused by cigarette smoking. Although COPD affects the lungs, it also produces significant systemic consequences.*
>
> Chronic bronchitis *is defined clinically as chronic productive cough for 3 months in each of 2 successive years in a patient in whom other causes of productive chronic cough have been excluded.*
>
> Emphysema *is defined pathologically as the presence of permanent enlargement of the airspaces distal to the terminal bronchioles, accompanied by destruction of their walls and without obvious fibrosis.*
>
> *In patients with COPD either or both of those conditions may be present. However, the relative contribution of each to the disease process is often difficult to discern.*

Note that the ATS's definition for *chronic bronchitis* is based on the major clinical manifestations associated with the disease. Also note that the ATS's definition for *emphysema* is based on the pathology, or the anatomic alterations of the lung, associated with the disorder.

The **Global Initiative for Chronic Obstructive Lung Disease** (GOLD) now provides the following working definition*:

> *Chronic obstructive pulmonary disease (COPD) is a preventable and treatable disease with some significant extrapulmonary effects that may contribute to the severity in individual patients. Its pulmonary component is characterized by airflow limitation that is not fully reversible. The airflow limitation is usually progressive and associated with an abnormal inflammatory response of the lung to noxious particles or gases.*

Note that the GOLD definition does not use the terms *chronic bronchitis* and *emphysema.* This is because, as GOLD explains, *chronic bronchitis,* which is defined as the presence of cough and sputum production for at least 3 months in each of 2 consecutive years (i.e., clinical manifestations), is not necessarily associated with airflow limitation. GOLD further points out that *emphysema,* which is defined as destruction of the alveoli, is a pathologic term (i.e., anatomic alterations of the lung) that is sometimes—and incorrectly—used to describe only *one* of several structural abnormalities present in patients with COPD.

The bottom line is this: Even though chronic bronchitis and emphysema can each develop alone, they often occur together as one disease complex. When this happens, the disease entity is called *chronic obstructive pulmonary disease.* In other words, *COPD* is a term referring to two lung diseases—chronic bronchitis and emphysema—occurring simultaneously. Patients with COPD demonstrate a variety of clinical manifestations associated with both disorders—although the relative contribution of each respiratory disorder is often difficult to ascertain. This is why, in large part, the treatment of chronic bronchitis, emphysema, or a combination of both disorders (COPD) is essentially the same in the clinical setting.

*GOLD (www.goldcopd.org) is recognized as a worldwide leading authority for the diagnosis, management, and prevention of COPD.

Anatomic Alterations of the Lungs Associated with Chronic Bronchitis

The conducting airways (particularly the bronchi) are the primary structures that undergo change in chronic bronchitis. As a result of chronic inflammation the bronchial walls are narrowed by vasodilation, congestion, and mucosal edema. This condition is often accompanied by bronchial smooth muscle constriction. In addition, continued bronchial irritation causes the submucosal bronchial glands to enlarge and the number of goblet cells to increase, resulting in excessive mucous production. The number and function of cilia lining the tracheobronchial tree are diminished, and the peripheral bronchi are often partially or totally occluded by inflammation and mucous plugs, which in turn leads to hyperinflated alveoli (see Figure 11-1).

The following major pathologic or structural changes are associated with chronic bronchitis:

- Chronic inflammation and swelling of the wall of the peripheral airways
- Excessive mucous production and accumulation
- Partial or total mucous plugging of the airways
- Smooth muscle constriction of bronchial airways (bronchospasm)
- Air trapping and hyperinflation of alveoli—occasionally in late stages

Anatomic Alterations of the Lungs Associated with Emphysema

Emphysema is characterized by a weakening and permanent enlargement of the air spaces distal to the terminal bronchioles and by destruction of the alveolar walls. As these structures enlarge and the alveoli coalesce, many of the adjacent pulmonary capillaries also are affected, and this results in a decreased surface area for gas exchange. Furthermore, the distal airways, weakened in the process, collapse during expiration in response to increased intrapleural pressure. This traps gas in the alveoli. There are two major types of emphysema: panacinar (panlobular) emphysema and centriacinar (centrilobular) emphysema.

In **panacinar emphysema,** or panlobular emphysema, there is an abnormal weakening and enlargement of all alveoli distal to the terminal bronchioles, including the respiratory bronchioles, alveolar ducts, alveolar sacs, and alveoli—the entire acinus is affected by dilatation and destruction. The alveolar-capillary surface area is significantly decreased (see Figure 11-2). Panlobular emphysema commonly is found in the lower parts of the lungs and often is associated with a deficiency of alpha$_1$-antitrypsin. Panlobular emphysema is the most severe type of emphysema and therefore the most likely to produce significant clinical manifestations.

In **centriacinar emphysema,** or **centrilobular emphysema,** the pathology involves the respiratory bronchioles in the proximal portion of the acinus. The respiratory bronchiolar walls enlarge, become confluent, and are then destroyed. A rim of parenchyma remains relatively unaffected (see Figure 11-3). Centriacinar emphysema is the most common form of emphysema and is strongly associated with cigarette smoking and with chronic bronchitis.

The following are the major pathologic or structural changes associated with emphysema:

- Permanent enlargement and destruction of the air spaces distal to the terminal bronchioles
- Destruction of pulmonary capillaries
- Weakening of the distal airways, primarily the respiratory bronchioles
- Air trapping and hyperinflation

Etiology and Epidemiology

Although the precise incidence of COPD is not known, it is estimated that 10 to 15 million people in the United States have chronic bronchitis, emphysema, or a combination of both. Most authorities agree that COPD is underdiagnosed. It is felt that if you take into account the people who have not been "officially" diagnosed with COPD, the incidence would be over 20 million people in the United States. It is generally accepted that more people have chronic bronchitis than emphysema. For example, the National Center for Health Statistics estimates that in the United States about 9.5 million people have chronic bronchitis and 4.1 million people have emphysema. In 2004 the annual cost related to COPD in the United States was about $37.2 billion—including $20.9 billion in direct costs, $7.4 billion in morbidity costs, and $8.9 billion in indirect costs.

COPD is the fourth leading cause of death, claiming more that 100,000 Americans each year. It is estimated that COPD will become the third leading cause of death by 2020. Historically, more men than women have died from COPD each year. Since the year 2000, however, more women than men have died from COPD each year. In 2004, almost 61,000 women died of COPD compared with 57,000 men.

Risk Factors

According to GOLD, COPD risk factors are related to the total burden of inhaled particles a person encounters over his or her lifetime. GOLD recognizes the following as risk factors for COPD:

- Tobacco smoke—including smoke from cigarette, pipe, cigar, and other types of tobacco smoking popular in many countries, as well as environmental tobacco smoke. According to GOLD, cigarette smoking is the most commonly encountered risk factor for COPD worldwide.
- Occupational dusts and chemicals—vapors, irritants, and fumes, when the exposures are sufficiently intense or prolonged.
- Indoor air pollution—from biomass fuel used for cooking and heating in poorly vented dwellings, a risk factor that particularly affects women in developing countries.
- Outdoor air pollution—also contributes to the lungs' total burden of inhaled particles and gases (e.g., silicates, sulfur dioxide, the nitrogen oxides, and ozone), although it appears to have a relatively small effect in *causing* COPD.
- Conditions that affect normal lung growth—any condition that affects lung growth during gestation and childhood (e.g., low birth weight, respiratory infections) has the potential for increasing an individual's risk for developing COPD.
- Genetic predisposition **(alpha$_1$-antitrypsin deficiency)**—in about 1 out of every 50 cases of emphysema, there is a specific hereditary basis for **panlobular emphysema** called *alpha$_1$* (or α_1)-*antitrypsin deficiency.* Alpha$_1$-antitrypsin is a major protein in the blood. It is produced by the liver. Alpha$_1$-antitrypsin protects the lungs by blocking the effects of a powerful enzyme called *elastase.* Elastase is carried by the body's white cells to help kill invading bacteria and to neutralize small particles inhaled into the lung. When old white cells are destroyed in the lungs, elastase is released. Under normal circumstances, alpha$_1$-antitrypsin works to inactivate the released elastase. However, when the alpha$_1$-antitrypsin level is low, the elastase is free to attack and destroy the elastic tissue of the lungs.

  The normal level of alpha$_1$-antitrypsin is 200 to 400 mg/dL. Patients with normal levels of alpha$_1$-antitrypsin are referred to genetically as having an **MM phenotype** or simply an M phenotype (homozygote). The phenotype associated with severely low serum concentrations is the **ZZ phenotype,** or simply Z. The heterozygous offspring of parents with the M and Z phenotypes have an **MZ phenotype.** The MZ phenotype results in an intermediate deficiency of alpha$_1$-antitrypsin. The precise effect of the intermediate level of alpha$_1$-antitrypsin is unclear. It is strongly recommended, however, that individuals with this phenotype not smoke or work in areas having significant environmental air pollution.

New on the list of risk factors is the notion that the remodeling of airways that occurs in asthma may be a harbinger of COPD. It will be interesting to see if this concern plays out.

Diagnosis of Chronic Obstructive Pulmonary Disease

According to GOLD, the diagnosis of COPD should be considered for any patient who is over 40 years of age and has dyspnea, chronic cough or sputum production, and/or a history of exposure to risk factors for the disease, especially cigarette smoking. The key indicators for considering a COPD diagnosis are as follows:

- Dyspnea
- Chronic cough
- Chronic sputum production
- History of exposure to risk factors such as tobacco smoke

Although these indicators are not diagnostic by themselves, the presence of multiple indicators significantly increases the probability of a diagnosis of COPD. When multiple key indicators are present, the diagnosis of COPD should be confirmed by a pulmonary function study.

Pulmonary Function Study in the Diagnosis of Chronic Obstructive Pulmonary Disease

The three main spirometry tests used to identify COPD are the **forced vital capacity (FVC), forced expiratory volume in 1 second (FEV_1),** and **forced expiratory volume in 1 second/forced vital capacity ratio (FEV_1/FVC ratio).** Clinically, the FEV_1/FVC ratio is also commonly called the **forced expiratory volume 1 second percentage ($FEV_{1\%}$).** Figure 11-4 illustrates a normal spirogram and a spirogram typical of patients with mild to moderate COPD.

The presence of COPD is confirmed when the both FEV_1 and FEV_1/FVC ratio are decreased. A postbronchodilator FEV_1 is recommended for both the diagnosis and assessment of the severity of COPD. Although the degree of spirometric abnormality usually determines the severity of COPD, the extent of the symptoms should also be considered when an individualized management program is developed for each patient.

Stages of chronic obstructive pulmonary disease. GOLD now recognizes the following four stages of COPD:

Stage I, mild COPD, consists of mild airflow limitation (FEV_1/FVC < 70%; FEV_1 ≥ 80% predicted). At this stage the symptoms may be so mild that an individual may not recognize abnormal lung function.

Stage II, or moderate COPD consists of worsening airflow limitation (FEV_1/FVC < 70%; FEV_1 50% to <80% of predicted). The patient often complains of shortness of breath upon exertion. The patients usually will seek medical attention at this stage because of their symptoms.)

Stage III, severe COPD, includes further worsening of the airflow limitation (FEV_1/FVC < 70%; FEV_1 30% to <50% of predicted). At this stage the symptoms have an impact on the patient's quality of life.

Stage IV, very severe COPD, includes severe airflow limitation (FEV_1/FVC < 70%; FEV_1 < 30% predicted, or FEV_1 < 50% predicted, plus chronic ventilatory failure). Quality of life is very impaired and exacerbations may be life threatening.

Additional Diagnostic Studies for Chronic Obstructive Pulmonary Disease

In patients who are diagnosed with Stage II: Moderate COPD, Stage III: Severe COPD, and Stage IV: Very Severe COPD, GOLD also recommends the following additional tests for further assessments:

- Bronchodilator reversibility testing: To rule out a diagnosis of asthma, particularly in patients with an atypical history (e.g., asthma in childhood and regular nocturnal night waking with cough and wheeze).
- Chest x-ray examination: Seldom diagnostic in COPD but valuable to exclude alternative and/or additional diagnoses, such as pulmonary tuberculosis, and pneumonia, and to identify comorbidities such as cardiac failure.
- Arterial blood gas measurement: Perform in patients with FEV_1 <50% predicted or with clinical signs suggestive of ventilatory failure or right-sided heart failure. The major clinical sign of ventilatory failure is cyanosis. Clinical signs of right-sided heart failure include ankle edema and an increase in the jugular venous pressure. Ventilatory failure is indicated by a Pa_{O_2} <60 mm Hg, with or without a Pa_{CO_2} >50 mm Hg while breathing room air.
- $Alpha_1$-antitrypsin deficiency screening: Perform when COPD develops in patients of Caucasian descent under 45 years of age or with a strong family history of COPD.

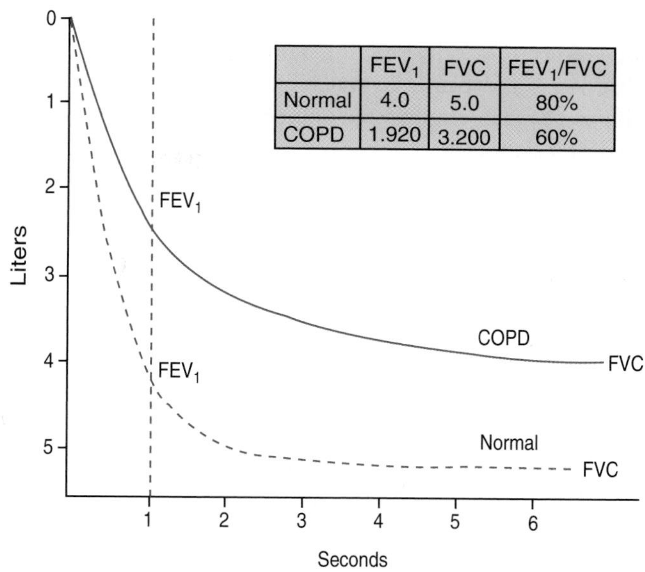

FIGURE 11-4 Normal spirogram and spirogram typical of patients with mild to moderate chronic obstructive pulmonary disease.

Key Distinguishing Features between Emphysema and Chronic Bronchitis

Even though chronic bronchitis and emphysema often occur as one disease complex (COPD), they can develop alone. A complete presentation of all the specific signs and symptoms associated with emphysema and chronic bronchitis are provided in the Overview section on pages 172 and 176. An abbreviated and handy overview of the key distinguishing features between emphysema and chronic bronchitis is provided as follows:

Clinically, the patient with emphysema is sometimes classified as a **"pink puffer,"** or a patient with type A COPD; and the patient with chronic bronchitis is sometimes classified as a **"blue bloater,"** or a patient with type B COPD. These general terms are primarily based on the clinical manifestations commonly associated with each respiratory disorder.

Pink Puffer (Type A Chronic Obstructive Pulmonary Disease)

The term *pink puffer* is derived from the reddish complexion and the "puffing" (pursed-lip breathing) commonly seen in the patient with emphysema. The major pathophysiologic mechanisms responsible for the red complexion and puffing are the following:

- Emphysema is caused by the progressive destruction of the distal airways and pulmonary capillaries.
- The progressive elimination of the pulmonary capillaries leads to a reduced pulmonary blood flow throughout the lungs—that is, an overall increased ventilation-perfusion ratio.
- To compensate for the increased ventilation-perfusion ratio in the patient who has emphysema hyperventilates.
- The increased respiratory rate, in turn, works to maintain a relatively normal arterial oxygenation level and causes a ruddy or flushed skin complexion. During the end stage of emphysema, however, the patient's oxygenation status decreases and the carbon dioxide level increases.
- Thus, the patient with emphysema, who has both a red complexion and a rapid respiratory rate, is called a *pink puffer.*

In addition to the marked dyspnea and ruddy complexion, the pink puffer tends to be thin (because of the muscle wasting and weight loss associated with the increased work of breathing), has a barrel chest (because of overinflated lungs), uses accessory muscles of inspiration, and exhales through pursed lips.

Blue Bloater (Type B Chronic Obstructive Pulmonary Disease)

The term *blue bloater* is derived from the cyanosis—the bluish color of the lips and skin—commonly seen in the patient with chronic bronchitis. The bluish complexion is caused by the following:

- Unlike emphysema, the pulmonary capillaries in the patient with chronic bronchitis are not damaged. The patient with chronic bronchitis responds to the increased airway obstruction by decreasing ventilation and increasing cardiac output—that is, a decreased ventilation-perfusion ratio.
- The chronic hypoventilation and increased cardiac output (decreased ventilation-perfusion ratio) leads to a decreased arterial oxygen level, an increased arterial carbon dioxide level, and a compensated (normal) pH—or chronic ventilatory failure arterial blood gases (also called *compensated respiratory acidosis*). The respiratory drive is depressed in patients with chronic ventilatory failure.
- The persistent low ventilation-perfusion ratio and depressed respiratory drive both contribute to a chronically reduced arterial oxygenation level and polycythemia—which, in turn, causes cyanosis.

In addition, the blue bloater tends to be stocky and overweight, has a chronic productive cough, and frequently has swollen ankles and legs and distended neck veins as a result of right-sided heart failure (cor pulmonale).

Table 11-1 provide an overview of the more common distinguishing features between emphysema and chronic bronchitis.

The clinical features of emphysema and chronic bronchitis are not always clear-cut because many patients have a combined disease process (COPD—this is especially the case during the late stages of emphysema and chronic bronchitis).

Text continued on p. 176

TABLE 11-1 Key Features Distinguishing Emphysema from Chronic Bronchitis*

Clinical Manifestation	Emphysema (Type A COPD: Pink Puffer)	Chronic Bronchitis (Type B COPD: Blue Bloater)
Inspection		
Body build	Thin	Stocky, overweight
Barrel chest	Common—classic sign	Normal
Respiratory pattern	Hyperventilation and marked dyspnea; often occurs at rest Late stage: diminished respiratory drive and hypoventilation	Diminished respiratory drive Hypoventilation common, with resultant hypoxia and hypercapnia
Pursed-lip breathing	Common	Uncommon
Cough	Uncommon	Common—classic sign
Sputum	Uncommon	Common—classic sign Copious amounts, purulent
Cyanosis	Uncommon (reddish skin)	Common
Peripheral edema	Uncommon	Common Right-sided heart failure
Neck vein distention	Uncommon	Common Right-sided heart failure
Use of accessory muscles	Common	Uncommon
Auscultation	Decreased breath sounds, decreased heart sounds, prolonged expiration	Wheezes, crackles, rhonchi, depending on severity of disease
Percussion	Hyperresonance	Normal
Laboratory Tests		
Chest radiograph	Hyperinflation, narrow mediastinum, normal or small vertical heart, low flat diaphragm, presence of blebs or bullae	Congested lung fields, densities, increased bronchial vascular markings, enlarged horizontal heart
Polycythemia	Uncommon	Common
Infections	Occasionally	Common
Pulmonary Function Study		
DLCO and DLCO/VA	Decreased	Often normal
Other		
Pulmonary hypertension	Uncommon	Common
Cor pulmonale	Uncommon	Common Right-sided heart failure

*The clinical features of emphysema and chronic bronchitis are not always clear-cut because many patients have a combined disease process (COPD—this is especially the case during the late stages of emphysema and chronic bronchitis).

OVERVIEW of the Cardiopulmonary Clinical Manifestations Associated with Chronic Bronchitis and Emphysema (COPD)[a]

The following clinical manifestations result from the pathophysiologic mechanisms caused (or activated) by **Excessive Bronchial Secretions** (see Figure 9-12) and **Bronchospasm** (see Figure 9-11)—the major anatomic alterations of the lungs associated with chronic bronchitis (see Figure 11-1); and the clinical manifestations activated by distal airway and alveolar weakening (see Figure 9-13)—the major anatomic alterations of the lungs associated with emphysema (see Figures 11-2 and 11-3).

[a]Chronic bronchitis and emphysema frequently occur together as a disease complex referred to as *chronic obstructive pulmonary disease* (COPD). Patients with COPD typically demonstrate clinical manifestations of both chronic bronchitis and emphysema.

CLINICAL DATA OBTAINED AT THE PATIENT'S BEDSIDE

Vital Signs	Chronic bronchitis and Emphysema
Heart rate and respiratory rate	Stable patients: normal vital signs Exacerbations: usually acute increase in heart rate and respiratory rate (tachypnea) • Classic sign of hypoxemia

Chest Assessment Findings	Emphysema	Chronic Bronchitis
Inspection		
General body build	Thin, underweight	Stocky, overweight
Altered sensorium—anxiety, irritability	Common during severe stage Classic sign of hypoxemia	Common during moderate and severe stage Classic sign of hypoxemia
Barrel chest	Classic sign	Occasionally
Digital clubbing	Late stage	Common
Cyanosis	Uncommon—often reddish skin	Common
Peripheral edema and venous distention	End-stage emphysema	Common Because polycythemia and cor pulmonale are common in chronic bronchitis, the following are often seen: • Distended neck veins • Pitting edema • Enlarged and tender liver
Use of accessory muscles	Common, especially during exacerbations	Uncommon End stage in some chronic bronchitis
Hoover's sign The inward movement of the lower lateral chest wall during each inspiration—indicates severe hyperinflation	Common—severe stage	Uncommon
Pursed-lip breathing	Common	Uncommon
Cough	Uncommon during mild and moderate stage Some coughing during severe stage with infection	Classic sign More severe in the mornings
Sputum	Uncommon Little, mucoid	Common Classic sign; copious amounts, purulent (see sputum examination)
Palpation of the Chest	Decreased tactile fremitus Decreased chest expansion Point of maximal impulse (PMI) often shifts to the epigastric area	Normal
Percussion of the Chest	Hyperresonance Decreased diaphragmatic excursion	Normal
Auscultation of the Chest	Diminished breath sounds Prolonged expirations Diminished heart sounds	Rhonchi Crackles Wheezes

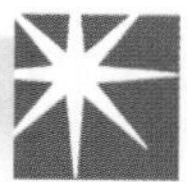

OVERVIEW of the Cardiopulmonary Clinical Manifestations Associated with Chronic Bronchitis and Emphysema (COPD)—cont'd

CLINICAL DATE OBTAINED FROM LABORATORY AND SPECIAL PROCEDURES

Pulmonary Function Test Findings: Moderate to Severe Chronic Bronchitis and Emphysema (Obstructive Lung Pathophysiology)

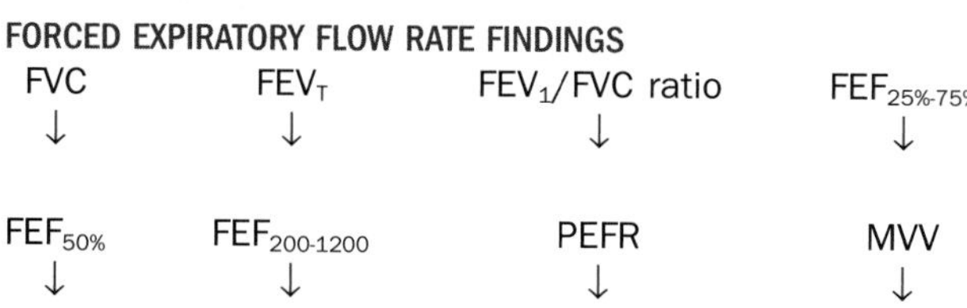

FORCED EXPIRATORY FLOW RATE FINDINGS

FVC	FEV_T	FEV_1/FVC ratio	$FEF_{25\%-75\%}$
↓	↓	↓	↓

$FEF_{50\%}$	$FEF_{200-1200}$	PEFR	MVV
↓	↓	↓	↓

LUNG VOLUME AND CAPACITY FINDINGS

VT	IRV	ERV	RV[b]
N or ↑	N or ↓	N or ↓	↑

VC	IC	FRC[b]	TLC	RV/TLC ratio
↓	N or ↓	↑	N or ↑	N or ↑

[b]Air trapping, and a subsequent increase in the RV and FRC, is uncommon in patients with only chronic bronchitis.

DIFFUSION CAPACITY (DLCO)[c]

Emphysema	Chronic Bronchitis
Decreased	Normal

A decreased DLCO is a classic diagnostic sign of emphysema

[c]The most accurate way to express DLCO as the DLCO corrected for alveolar volume (D_L/V_A). This measure is always reduced in severe emphysema and reflects the loss of alveolar-capillary membrane.

Arterial Blood Gases: Chronic Bronchitis and Emphysema

MILD TO MODERATE STAGES

Acute Alveolar Hyperventilation with Hypoxemia (Acute Respiratory Alkalosis)

pH	$Paco_2$	HCO_3^-	Pao_2
↑	↓	↓ (slightly)	↓

SEVERE STAGE

Chronic Ventilatory Failure with Hypoxemia[d] (Compensated Respiratory Acidosis)

pH	$Paco_2$	HCO_3^-	Pao_2
N	↑	↑ (significantly)	↓

[d]Chronic ventilatory failure is more commonly seen in the patient with chronic bronchitis during the moderate and severe stages. Chronic ventilatory failure usually does not develop in emphysema until the severe stage.

Acute Ventilatory Changes Superimposed on Chronic Ventilatory Failure

Because acute ventilatory changes are frequently seen in patients with chronic ventilatory failure, the respiratory care practitioner must be familiar with and alert for the following:

- Acute alveolar hyperventilation superimposed on chronic ventilatory failure, and/or
- Acute ventilatory failure (acute hypoventilation) superimposed on chronic ventilatory failure

Oxygenation Indices[e] for Chronic Bronchitis and Emphysema, Moderate to Severe Stages

$\dot{Q}_S/\dot{Q}_T$	Do_2[f]	$\dot{V}o_2$	$C(a-\bar{v})O_2$	O_2ER	$S\bar{v}O_2$
↑	↓	N	N	↑	↓

[f]The DO_2 may be normal in patients who have compensated to the decreased oxygenation status with (1) an increased cardiac output, (2) an increased hemoglobin level, or (3) a combination of both. When the DO_2 is normal, the O_2ER is usually normal.

Hemodynamic Indices[g] for Chronic Bronchitis and Emphysema, Moderate to Severe Stages

CVP	RAP	$\overline{PA}$	PCWP	CO	SV
↑	↑	↑	N	N	N

SVI	CI	RVSWI	LVSWI	PVR	SVR
N	N	↑	N	↑	N

LABORATORY TESTS AND PROCEDURES

Test	Emphysema	Chronic Bronchitis
Hematocrit and hemoglobin	Normal—mild to moderate stage Elevated—late stage	Polycythemia common during early and late stage
Electrolytes (abnormal)	Late stage: • Hypochloremia (Cl^-) when chronic ventilatory failure is present • Hypernatremia (Na^+)	Early and late stages: • Hypochloremia (Cl^-) (when chronic ventilatory failure is present) • Hypernatremia (Na^+)
Sputum examination (culture)	Normal	*Streptococcus pneumoniae* *Haemophilus influenzae* *Moraxella catarrhalis*

[e]*Do_2*, Total oxygen delivery; *$C(a-\bar{v})o_2$*, arterial-venous oxygen difference; *O_2ER*, oxygen extraction ratio; *$\dot{Q}_S/\dot{Q}_T$*, pulmonary shunt fraction; *$S\bar{v}o_2$*, mixed venous oxygen saturation; *$\dot{V}o_2$*, oxygen consumption.

[g]*CO*, Cardiac output; *CVP*, central venous pressure; *LVSWI*, left ventricular stroke work index; *$\overline{PA}$*, mean pulmonary artery pressure; *PCWP*, pulmonary capillary wedge pressure; *PVR*, pulmonary vascular resistance; *RAP*, right atrial pressure; *RVSWI*, right ventricular stroke work index; *SV*, stroke volume; *SVI*, stroke volume index; *SVR*, systemic vascular resistance.

OVERVIEW of the Cardiopulmonary Clinical Manifestations Associated with Chronic Bronchitis and Emphysema (COPD)—cont'd

RADIOLOGY FINDINGS

Test	Chronic Bronchitis
Chest Radiograph	Lungs may be clear if only large bronchi are affected Occasionally • Translucent (dark) lung fields • Depressed or flattened diaphragms Common • Cor pulmonale No radiographic abnormalities may be present in chronic bronchitis if only the large bronchi are affected. This often explains why the diagnosis is delayed. Although the situation is uncommon, if the more peripheral bronchi are involved, air trapping may occur. This is revealed on x-ray film as areas of translucency or areas that are darker in appearance. In addition, because of the increased functional residual capacity, the diaphragms may be depressed or flattened and are seen as such on the radiograph (Figure 11-5). Because bronchial wall thickening is common in chronic bronchitis, increased, diffuse, fibrotic-appearing lung markings are often seen. This is commonly referred to as a "dirty chest x-ray." Finally, because right and left ventricular enlargement and failure are commonly associated with chronic bronchitis, in the late stage an enlarged heart may be seen on the chest radiograph.
Bronchogram	Small spikelike protrusions ("train tracks" appearance of airways) from the larger bronchi are often seen on bronchograms of patients with chronic bronchitis. It is believed that the spikes result from pooling of the radiopaque medium in the enlarged ducts of the mucous glands (Figure 11-6). Since the advent of the computed tomography (CT) examination, bronchograms are rarely done today on patients with chronic bronchitis. A "thin-section" CT exam is even more helpful.
	Emphysema
Chest Radiograph	Common • Translucent (dark) lung fields • Depressed or flattened diaphragms • Long and narrow heart (pulled downward by diaphragms) • Increased retrosternal air space (lateral radiograph) Occasionally • Cor pulmonale Because of the decreased lung recoil and air trapping in emphysema, the functional residual capacity increases and the radiographic density of the lungs decreases. Consequently, the resistance to x-ray penetration is not as great, causing areas of translucency or areas that are darker in appearance. Because of the increased functional residual capacity, the diaphragm is depressed or flattened and the heart is often long and narrow (Figure 11-7). The lateral chest radiograph characteristically shows an increased retrosternal air space (more than 3.0 cm from the anterior surface of the aorta to the back of the sternum measured 3.0 cm below the manubriosternal junction) and flattened diaphragms (Figure 11-8). Because right ventricular enlargement and failure sometimes develop as secondary problems during the advanced stages of emphysema, an enlarged heart may be seen on the chest radiograph (Figure 11-9).

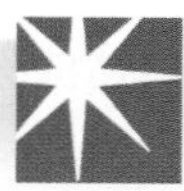

OVERVIEW of the Cardiopulmonary Clinical Manifestations Associated with Chronic Bronchitis and Emphysema (COPD)—cont'd

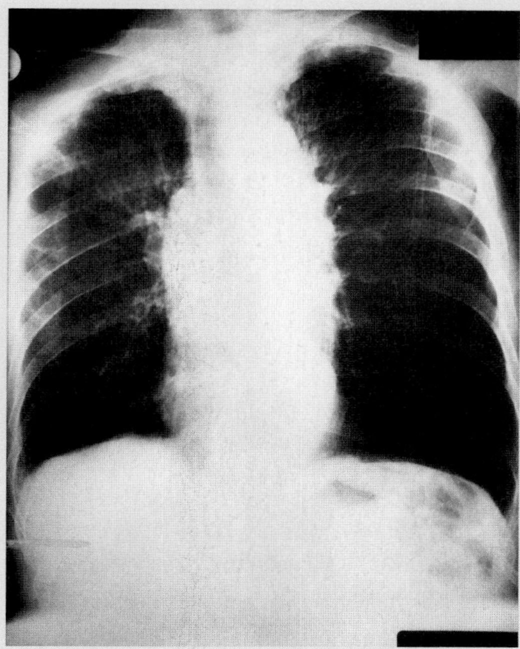

FIGURE 11-5 Chest x-ray film from a patient with chronic bronchitis. Note the translucent (dark) lung fields at the bases, depressed diaphragms, and long and narrow heart.

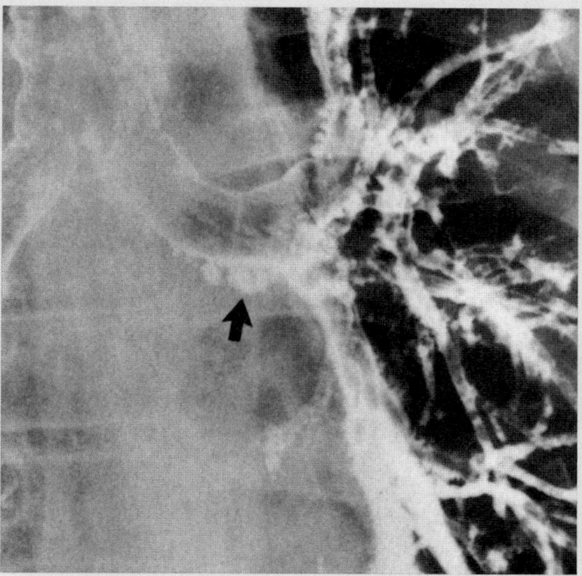

FIGURE 11-6 Chronic bronchitis. Bronchogram with localized view of left hilum. Rounded collections of contrast lie adjacent to bronchial walls and are particularly well demonstrated below the left main stem bronchus *(arrow)* in this film. They are caused by contrast in dilated mucous gland ducts. (From Hansel DM, Armstrong P, Lynch DA, McAdams HP, eds: *Imaging of the diseases of the chest,* ed 4, St Louis, 2005, Mosby.)

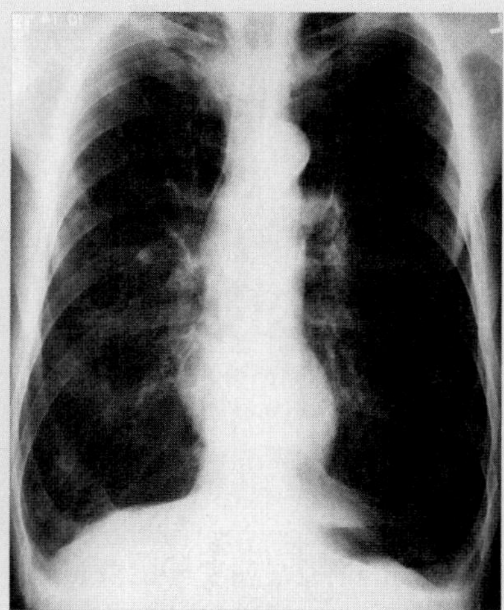

FIGURE 11-7 Chest x-ray film of a patient with emphysema. The heart often appears long and narrow as a result of being drawn downward by the descending diaphragm.

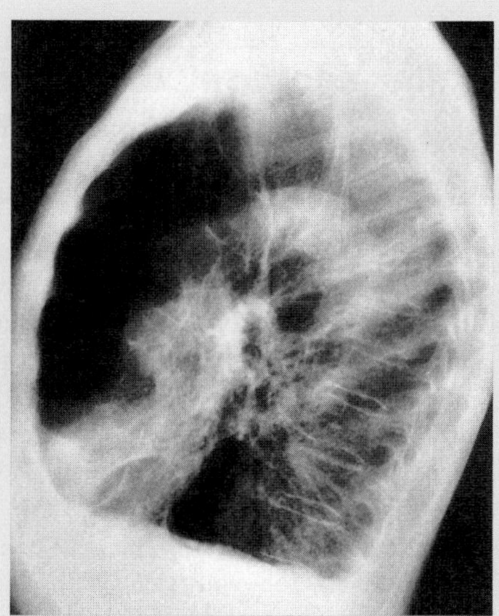

FIGURE 11-8 Emphysema. Lateral chest radiograph demonstrates a characteristically large retrosternal radiolucency with increased separation of the aorta and sternum measuring 4.6 cm, 3 cm below the angle of Louis and extending down to within 3 cm of the diaphragm anteriorly. Both costophrenic angles are obtuse, and both hemidiaphragms are flat. (From Hansel DM, Armstrong P, Lynch DA, McAdams HP, eds: *Imaging of the diseases of the chest,* ed 4, St Louis, 2005, Mosby.)

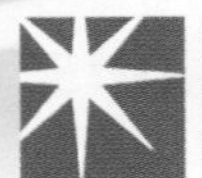

OVERVIEW of the Cardiopulmonary Clinical Manifestations Associated with Chronic Bronchitis and Emphysema (COPD)—cont'd

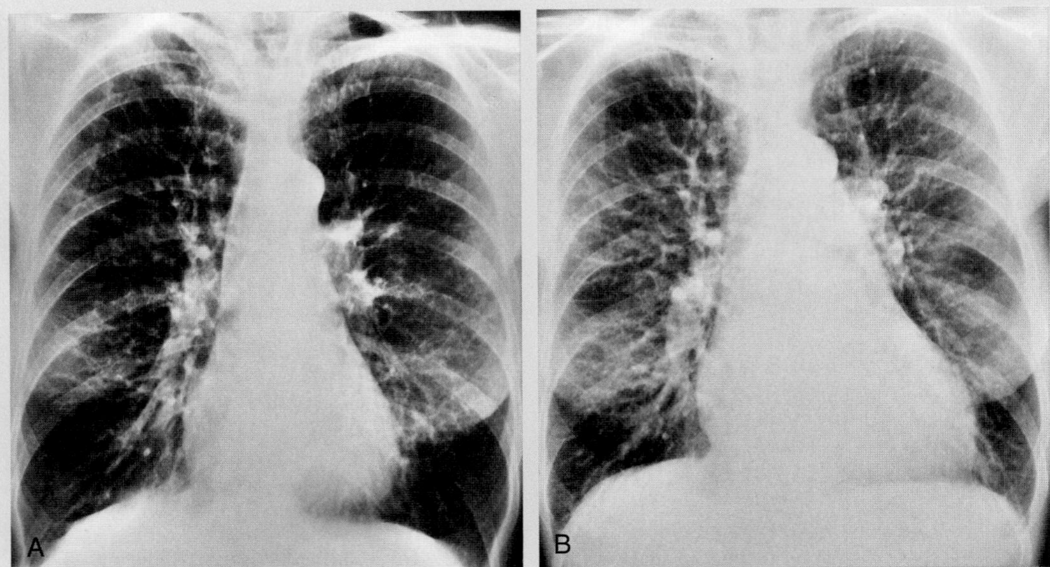

FIGURE 11-9 Cor pulmonale. **A**, A 50-year-old man with chronic airflow obstruction. Lungs are large in volume, the diaphragm is flat, and vascular attenuation is evident at the right apex. These features suggest emphysema, and this diagnosis was supported by a low carbon monoxide diffusion capacity. Lung "markings" are increased peripherally, particularly in the left midzone. **B**, The patient became chronically hypoxic and, with respiratory infections, hypercapnic. One of these episodes was associated with cor pulmonale when the patient became edematous, and the heart and hilar and pulmonary parenchymal vessels became enlarged. The emphysematous right upper zone shows fewer vascular markings and is relatively transradient. The diaphragm is less depressed and more curved than before. (From Hansell DM, Armstrong P, Lynch DA, McAdams HP, eds: *Imaging of the diseases of the chest,* ed 4, St Louis, 2005, Mosby.)

General Management of Chronic Obstructive Pulmonary Disease

Global Initiative for Chronic Obstructive Lung Disease

In 1998, GOLD was created to increase the awareness of COPD among health professionals, public health authorities, and the general public and to improve prevention and management through worldwide efforts. GOLD prepares scientific reports on COPD, encourages dissemination and adoption of the reports, and promotes international collaboration on COPD research.

GOLD provides an outstanding COPD management program that includes the following goals: relieve symptoms, prevent disease progression, improve exercise tolerance, improve health status, prevent and treat complications and exacerbations, reduce mortality and to prevent or minimize side effects from treatment. A COPD management program should help to achieve these goals. The GOLD program consists of (1) **assessing and monitoring the disease**, (2) **reducing risk factors**, (3) **managing stable COPD**, and (4) **managing exacerbations**.

The first component of the COPD management program involves assessing and monitoring the disease. The following should be included in an assessment of a patient known or thought to have COPD:

- exposure to risk factors
- past medical history (including asthma and allergies)
- family history of COPD
- pattern of symptom development
- history of exacerbations
- presence of comorbidities
- appropriateness of current medical treatments
- impact of the disease on patient's life
- social and family support available to the patient
- possibilities of reducing risk factors

The second component, reducing risk factors, is an important step in a COPD management program. Smoking cessation is the single most effective way to reduce the risk of developing COPD as well as slowing its progression. Preventing risks of occupational exposures is also important. Also, patients should avoid indoor and outdoor air pollution.

The third component is to manage the stable COPD patient. In order to achieve this you must determine the disease severity on an individual basis, implement a treatment plan that reflects the severity, and choose treatments according to national and cultural preferences, the patient's abilities and preferences and the availability of medications. Patient education is important to improve skills and the patient's ability to deal with the disease. Pharmacologic treatments used to control and prevent symptoms, reduce exacerbation, and improve exercise tolerance and quality of life can be found in Table 11-2. Bronchodilators are medications that are frequently used in symptom management of COPD. The inhaled method is preferred and these medications are given as needed to relieve and prevent worsening of symptoms. Regular treatment with long-acting bronchodilators is more effective and convenient than treatment with short-acting bronchodilators.

The fourth component is management of exacerbations. An exacerbation is an event in the natural course of the disease that involves a change in the patient's baseline dyspnea, cough or sputum and is beyond the normal day-to-day variations. An exacerbation is acute in onset and may be reason for change in a patient's regular medication. The cause of about one third of severe exacerbations cannot be identified; however, the most common cause is an infection of the tracheobronchial tree and air pollution. In order to assess the severity of an exacerbation a patient must have his or her arterial blood gases measured, chest x-rays examined, and an electrocardiogram must be performed. Home management of an exacerbation consists of use of bronchodilators and glucocorticosteroids. If a patient has any of the following characteristics he or she should be hospitalized:

- marked increase in intensity of signs or symptoms, such as resting dyspnea
- severe history of COPD
- onset of new physical signs (cyanosis, peripheral edema)
- failure of exacerbations to respond to initial medical management
- significant comorbidities
- frequent exacerbations
- newly occurring cardiac arrhythmias
- diagnostic uncertainty
- older age
- insufficient home support

Figure 11-10 provides an overview of a chronic obstructive pulmonary disease (COPD) management algorithm recommended by GOLD.

GOLD provides an excellent framework for the management of COPD that can be adapted to local health care systems and resources. Educational tools, such as laminated cards or computer-based learning programs, can be prepared that are tailored to these systems and resources. As of this writing, the GOLD program includes the following publications:

- *Global Strategy for the Diagnosis, Management, and Prevention of COPD.* Scientific information and recommendations for COPD programs. (November 2008).
- *Pocket Guide to COPD Diagnosis, Management, and Prevention. A Guide for Health Care Professionals.* (2008).

These publications are freely available on the Internet at www.goldcopd.org.

Respiratory Care Treatment Protocols

Oxygen Therapy Protocol

Oxygen therapy is used to treat hypoxemia, decrease the work of breathing, and decrease myocardial work. The hypoxemia that develops in cystic fibrosis is caused by the pulmonary shunting associated with the disorder. When the patient demonstrates chronic ventilatory failure during the advanced stages of COPD, caution must be taken not to overoxygenate the patient (see Oxygen Therapy Protocol, Protocol 9-1).

Bronchopulmonary Hygiene Therapy Protocol

A number of bronchial hygiene treatment modalities may be used to enhance the mobilization of bronchial secretions (see Bronchopulmonary Hygiene Therapy Protocol, Protocol 9-2).

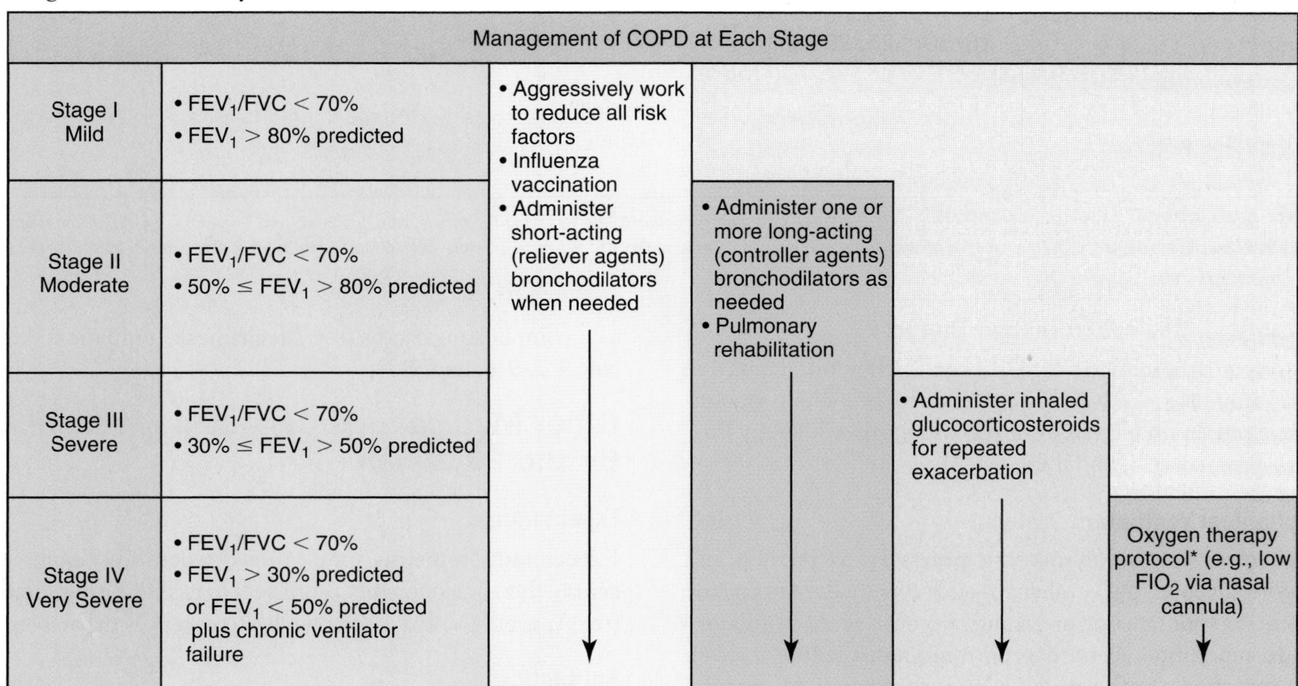

FIGURE 11-10 Chronic obstructive lung disease (COPD) management.

TABLE 11-2 Medications Commonly Used in the Treatment of Chronic Obstructive Pulmonary Disease

Drug	Inhaler (μg)	Solution for Nebulizer (mg/mL)	Oral	Vials for Injection (mg)	Duration of Action (hours)
Beta$_2$-Agonists					
Short-Acting Beta$_2$-Agonists					
Fenoterol	100-200 (MDI)	1	0.05% (syrup)		4-6
Levalbuterol				0.63, 1.25	4-6
Salbutamol (albuterol)	100, 200 (MDI and DPI)	5	5 mg (pill) syrup 0.024%	0.1, 0.5	4-6
Terbutaline	400, 500 (DPI)		2.5, 5 (pill)	0.2, 0.25	4-6
Long-Acting Beta$_2$-Agonists					
Formoterol	4.5-12 (MDI and DPI)				12$^+$
Salmeterol	25-50 (MDI and DPI)				12$^+$
Anticholinergics					
Short-Acting Anticholinergics					
Ipratropium bromide	20, 40 (MDI)	0.25-0.5			6-8
Oxitropium bromide	100 (MDI)	1.5			7-9
Long-Acting Anticholinergics					
Tiotropium	18 (DPI)				24$^+$
Combination Short-Acting Beta$_2$-Agonists Plus Anticholinergic in One Inhaler					
Fenoterol and ipratropium	200/80 (MDI)	1.25/0.5			6-8
Oxitropium bromide	75/15 (MDI)	0.75/4.5			6-8
Methylxanthines					
Aminophylline			200-600 mg (pill)	240 mg	Variable, up to 24
Theophylline (SR)			200-600 mg (pill)		Variable, up to 24
Inhaled Glucocorticosteroids					
Beclomethasone	50-400 (MDI and DPI)	0.2-0.4			
Budesonide	100, 200, 400 (DPI)	0.20, 0.25, 0.5			
Fluticasone	50-500 (MDI and DPI)				
Triamcinolone	100 (MDI)	40		40	
Combination Long-Acting Beta$_2$-Agonists Plus Glucocorticosteroids in One Inhaler					
Formoterol and budesonide	4.5/160, 9/320 (DPI)				
Salmeterol and fluticasone	50/100, 250, 500 (DPI) 25/50, 125, 250 (MDI)				
Systemic Glucocorticosteroids					
Prednisone		5-60 mg (pill)			
Methyl-prednisolone		4, 8, 16 mg (pill)			

Data from *Global Initiative for Chronic Obstructive Lung Disease (GOLD): Pocket Guide to COPD Diagnosis, Management, and Prevention. A Guide for Health Care Professionals*, 2007, GOLD, available at: www.goldcopd.org; and Gardenshire DS: *Rau's respiratory care pharmacology*, ed 7, St. Louis, 2008, Elsevier.

Aerosolized Medication Therapy Protocol

Both sympathomimetic and parasympatholytic agents are commonly used in COPD to induce bronchial smooth muscle relaxation (see Aerosolized Medication Therapy Protocol, Protocol 9-4, and Table 11-2).

Mechanical Ventilation Protocol

Mechanical ventilation may be necessary to provide and support alveolar gas exchange and eventually return the patient to spontaneous breathing. Because acute ventilatory failure superimposed on chronic ventilatory failure is often seen in patients with severe COPD, continuous mechanical ventilation is justified when the acute ventilatory failure is thought to be reversible; e.g., when acute pneumonia exists as a complicating factor (see Mechanical Ventilation Protocols 9-5, 9-6, and 9-7).

Other Medications Commonly Prescribed By the Physician

Expectorants

Expectorants sometimes are ordered when oral liquids and aerosol therapy alone are not sufficient to facilitate expectoration (see Appendix V, Expectorants). Effectiveness is debatable.

Antibiotics

Antibiotics commonly are administered to treat associated respiratory tract infections (see Appendix III, Antibiotics).

CASE STUDY

Chronic Bronchitis

Admitting History and Physical Examination

This 66-year-old man has worked in a cotton mill in South Carolina for the past 37 years. He has a 120 pack/year (3 packs/day for 40 years) history of cigarette smoking, and he also chews tobacco regularly. He sought medical assistance in the chest clinic because of a chronic cough. He described it as a "smoker's cough" and stated that it was present about 4 to 5 months of the year. For the past 3 years, his cough produced grayish-yellow sputum during the winter months. The sputum was thick and yellow. He stated that he was more short of breath during moderate exercise. He attributed this to "getting older." The patient stated he had not been taking any pulmonary medications.

On physical examination the patient was in mild respiratory distress. He was obese (270 lb). He occasionally generated a strong productive cough during the visit. His sputum appeared grayish-yellow. Auscultation of the chest revealed moist rhonchi and scattered wheezes and crackles. An arterial blood gas assessment showed pH 7.36, $Pa{CO_2}$ 87, HCO_3^- 48, and $Pa{O_2}$ 64. The chest radiograph revealed increased markings in the lower lung fields bilaterally. No pulmonary hyperinflation was noticed. Spirometry showed a decrease in the FEV_1/FVC ratio (55% of predicted) and a decreased FEV_1 (35% of predicted). The respiratory care practitioner's assessment at this time was documented in the patient's chart as follows.

Respiratory Assessment and Plan

S "Smoker's cough," sputum production, dyspnea

O Strong productive cough. Sputum: Yellow-gray. Breath sounds: Rhonchi and crackles at lung bases. ABG: pH—7.36, $Pa{CO_2}$—87, HCO_3^-—48, $Pa{O_2}$—64. X-ray: increased markings at bases. PFTs: decreased FEV_1/FVC ratio (55% of predicted), decreased FEV_1 (35% of predicted).

A Severe, Stage III, chronic bronchitis (history, physical exam, and PFT results)
Moderate airway secretions (rhonchi and crackles)
Good ability to mobilize secretions (strong cough and sputum production)
Chronic ventilatory failure with mild hypoxemia (ABG)

P **Bronchopulmonary Hygiene Therapy Protocol** (cough and deep breathing, prn). Patient education on smoking. Refer to Smoking Cessation Clinic. **Aerosolized Medication Protocol** (med. neb. treatment with Levalbuterol q6h).

The patient was advised to stop smoking and seek medical assistance if his sputum became progressively more thick and yellow or his dyspnea became worse. The physician also prescribed a pneumococcal polysaccharide vaccine. Also prescribed was an inhaled glucocorticosteroid (beclomethasone) tid prn, and a formoterol inhaler twice a day. The Smoking Cessation Clinic prescribed slow-release nicotine patches, and the patient attended a week-long smoking cessation program. The patient did well, and at the 6-month follow-up visit he was no longer smoking. At this time, the patient stated that he had not had his "smoker's cough" or produced any sputum in weeks.

A year later, however, the patient came to the emergency room and was clearly not doing well. He was back to his three-packs-per-day cigarette smoking habit, and he had been physically inactive and gained 30 pounds (to a weight of 300 lb) over the past year. He stated that he frequently coughed and it was more troublesome in the early morning. The patient also reported that his cough was now productive—about 3 to 4 tablespoons of thick yellow and green sputum daily. He complained of dyspnea during light exercise (e.g., stair climbing produced shortness of breath). On some days his increased work of breathing was more noticeable than on others. He denied hemoptysis, chest pain, orthopnea, fever, chills, or leg edema to the respiratory care team.

On observation, his ankles were swollen with pitting edema of 3+ and his neck veins were distended. He was cyanotic. Vital signs were as follows: blood pressure 165/90, heart rate 116 beats per minute, and a respiratory rate of 26 breaths per minute. His oral temperature was 98.4° F. Auscultation of the chest revealed bilateral posterior basilar rhonchi and crackles, which partially cleared with coughing. Expectorated sputum was copious, purulent, and yellow and green. A bedside spirometry showed an FEV_1/FVC ratio of 55% and a FEV_1 of 35%. On room air, his arterial blood gas values were pH 7.51, $Pa{CO_2}$ 51, HCO_3^- 39, $Pa{O_2}$ 41. His resting $Sp{O_2}$ on room air was 83% and improved to 89% on 2 L of O_2 per minute. His chest x-ray film showed diffuse, fibrotic-appearing lung markings and a moderately enlarged right side of the heart. His hemoglobin was 17.8 g%. At this time, the respiratory care practitioner reported the following SOAP note in the patient's chart.

Respiratory Assessment and Plan

S Complains of productive cough and exertional dyspnea (history)

O Bibasilar crackles, wheezing, rhonchi, cyanosis, obesity. Vital signs: HR 116, BP 165/90, RR 26/min. Cough: productive with copious yellow green sputum. PFT: FEV_1/FVC 55% and FEV_1 of 35%. CXR: diffuse fibrotic lung markings and cor pulmonale. ABG: pH 7.51, $Pa{CO_2}$ 51, HCO_3^- 39, $Pa{O_2}$ 41. $Sp{O_2}$ 89% on 2 L/min O_2. Hemoglobin 17.8 g%.

A Acute exacerbation of chronic bronchitis (history, physical examination)
Exacerbation of chronic bronchitis (history, PFT)
Excessive mucous accumulation (sputum, rhonchi, and crackles)
Infection (yellow and green sputum)

Acute alveolar hyperventilation superimposed on chronic ventilatory failure with moderate to severe hypoxemia (ABG, Sp_{O_2})

Impending ventilatory failure

Tobacco addiction (history)

P **Aerosolized Medication Therapy Protocol** (MDI with combined albuterol and ipratropium, 2 puffs qid). Inhaled glucocorticosteroid (beclomethasone) qid. **Bronchopulmonary Hygiene Therapy Protocol** (cough and deep breathing under supervision qid, cautious trial of CPT with postural drainage to lower lobes, 3 times a day). Call physician about impending ventilatory failure and chest x-ray report of cor pulmonale. Also check to see whether the doctor wants to schedule complete pulmonary function test. Recheck Sp_{O_2} on room air. Again, advise and facilitate smoking cessation program.

Discussion

In the first portion of this case study, some of the clinical manifestations of chronic **Excessive Airway Secretions** (see Figure 9-11) were present. These findings were clearly documented in the first SOAP note when the therapist charted the presence of productive cough, rhonchi, and crackles sounds and pulmonary function findings that indicated airway obstruction.

The first part of this case also illustrates a definite role for the modern respiratory care practitioner. Such a professional may well be working in outpatient settings that necessitate the evaluation and treatment of patients such as this one. The history of productive cough and the findings of rhonchi and crackles in a smoker who is not seriously ill suggest a diagnosis of Stage III chronic bronchitis or COPD. The patient's history, cough, sputum production, pulmonary function data, and chest x-ray examination confirm this suspicion. The physician's prescription of pneumococcal polysaccharide vaccine and slow-release nicotine patches reflects the key elements of preventive therapy in chronic bronchitis—namely, avoidance of irritant fumes and particles; influenza and pneumococcal vaccines for prevention of those two common complicating diseases; and the need for continued follow-up.

In the second part of this case study, there were more of the classic clinical manifestations associated with chronic bronchitis. For example, the patient's **Excessive Bronchial Secretions** (see Figure 9-11) not only resulted in hypoxia and cyanosis secondary to a decreased $\dot{V}/\dot{Q}$ ratio and pulmonary shunting but also produced increased airway resistance that resulted in rhonchi and crackles and a decreased FEV_1/FVC ratio and FEV_1. In addition, the second part of this case study started with the patient's failure to stop smoking and with increased symptoms and worsening of his obstructive pulmonary disease (dyspnea and productive cough). The findings on the chest x-ray film also suggested cor pulmonale, which often occurs in bronchitis. His pulmonary function was worsening, and he had acute alveolar hyperventilation superimposed on chronic ventilatory failure with moderate to severe hypoxemia. Impending ventilatory failure was a serious concern.

In addition to treating the acute symptoms with a simple MDI bronchodilator regimen (see Protocol 9-4) and **Bronchopulmonary Hygiene Therapy Protocol** (see Protocol 9-2) in the form of cough and deep breathing, a cautious trial of chest physiotherapy, and postural drainage, the respiratory therapist does not give up on the longer-term but extremely important goal of modifying behavior (smoking cessation) in the patient. A complete pulmonary function test in the near future would further define the patient's disease process, both in its nature and severity. Such data are often helpful to the patient's understanding of just how ill he is and may constitute a "teachable moment" for the physician and therapist. Although the patient was discharged from the hospital 5 days later, he unfortunately died from another acute exacerbation of chronic bronchitis, ventilatory failure, and cardiac arrest 7 months later.

CASE STUDY

Emphysema

Admitting History and Physical Examination

This 27-year-old man was admitted to the hospital with the chief complaint of dyspnea on exertion. He had a 3-year history of recurrent respiratory problems that had necessitated several hospitalizations of several days' duration in the past. Recently, his respiratory status had deteriorated to the point where he had to stop working. He had been employed for several years as a cook in a fast-food restaurant, where he was continuously exposed to a smoky environment. He had never smoked. On questioning, the patient related that he had been very short of breath for the past 6 weeks. He further stated that he was unable to walk up one flight of stairs without stopping, and his walking tolerance had decreased to about 100 yards.

On physical examination the patient appeared anxious. He was profusely sweating and was in moderate respiratory distress. He demonstrated a regular heart rate of 120 beats per minute, blood pressure of 140/70, respiratory rate of 32 breaths per minute, and an oral temperature of 100° F. Inspection of the chest revealed suprasternal notch retraction, with some use of the accessory muscles of inspiration. The lungs were hyperresonant to percussion, and breath sounds were diminished. His I : E ratio was 1 : 4. He had a barrel chest and his nail beds were moderately cyanotic. The patient was slightly confused—he was unable to concentrate well. The chest x-ray film showed moderate to severe hyperinflation of the lungs. Some infiltrates were present in the lower lung regions, and possible infiltrates were also noted in the right upper lobe. The radiology report suggested the presence of a pneumonic process superimposed on chronic lung disease.

Bedside spirometry revealed an FEV_1/FVC ratio of 57% and an FEV_1 of 40% of predicted. His arterial blood gases while on a 3 L/min O_2 nasal cannula were pH 7.26, Pa_{CO_2} 82, HCO_3^- 36, and Pa_{O_2} of 48. The Sa_{O_2} was 75%. Laboratory studies revealed a hemoglobin of 16.5 g/dL and a white blood count of 15,000/mm^3. Sputum cultures were positive for a variety of pathogenic and nonpathogenic organisms. The serum alpha$_1$-antitrypsin level was 30 mg/dL (normal = 200 to 400 mg/dL). The remainder of the physical examination findings were not remarkable. The respiratory assessment read as follows.

Respiratory Assessment and Plan

S "I'm short of breath with any exercise at all." Cough for past 6 weeks.

O HR 120, BP 140/70, RR 32, and temp 100° F. Use of accessory muscles of inspiration, increased AP diameter, cyanosis. Hyperresonant percussion note and diminished breath sounds. I:E ratio 1 : 4. Lower lung infiltrates, hyperinflation of lungs on CXR. PFT: FEV_1/FVC ratio of 57% and FEV_1 of 40%. ABGs: pH 7.26, Pa_{CO_2} 82, HCO_3^- 36, and Pa_{O_2} of 48. Sa_{O_2}: 75%. Elevated WBC and gram-positive organisms in the sputum, alpha$_1$-antitrypsin = 30 mg/dL.

A Panacinar emphysema (history, alpha$_1$-antitrypsin deficiency)
Pulmonary hyperinflation (x-ray, diminished breath sounds, barrel chest)
Probable pneumonitis (x-ray)
Acute ventilatory failure on chronic ventilatory failure with moderate/severe hypoxemia (ABGs)

P Notify doctor about acute ventilatory failure. **Oxygen Therapy Protocol** (HAFOE mask at F_{IO_2} = 0.35). Place intubation equipment and ventilator on standby. Monitor and evaluate per ICU standing orders (Sp_{O_2}, vital signs). Check ABG in 30 min.

The hospital course was relatively smooth. The HAFOE oxygen therapy was enough to increase the patient's Pa_{O_2} to an acceptable level and correct the acute-on-chronic ventilatory failure. Within an hour the patient's arterial blood gases were pH 7.36, Pa_{CO_2} 61, HCO_3^- 34, and Pa_{O_2} 76. The patient's heart rate, respiratory rate, and blood pressure returned to normal. Blood serologies suggested *Mycoplasma pneumoniae* infection. Intravenous antibiotics were prescribed. The patient was managed conservatively and improved steadily. When he appeared to have had the maximum benefit from the hospitalization, he was discharged with an oxygen concentrator, a portable "stroller," and an oxygen-conserving device. He was to use O_2 at 1 L/min at rest and 2.5 L/min with exercise for 18 to 24 hours a day. Arrangements were made to have him enroll in an alpha$_1$-antitrypsin therapy trial and attend pulmonary rehabilitation classes. He was urged to secure employment elsewhere.

Discussion

This fascinating (but fortunately rare) form of emphysema is one in which "pure" emphysema is the dominant pathology. In patients with alpha$_1$-antitrypsin deficiency, chronic bronchitis may be present, but it is much less common than is the usual, cigarette smoking–induced COPD. In this condition the patient's deficiency of the protease inhibitor alpha$_1$-antitrypsin resulted in WBC-mediated protease destruction of his pulmonary parenchyma. Note the slow, insidious onset of his symptoms.

The patient's emphysema or **Distal Airway and Alveolar Weakening** (see Figure 9-12) was complicated by additional anatomic alterations of the lungs (i.e., **Alveolar Consolidation** [see Figure 9-8]). The alveolar consolidation was reflected in the patient's immune-inflammatory response (fever and increased WBC), alveolar infiltrates (x-ray), low Pa_{O_2} (caused by a decreased $\dot{V}/\dot{Q}$ ratio and intrapulmonary shunting), and abnormal vital signs (see Figure 9-8).

The effects of distal airway and alveolar weakening were reflected in the patient's increased AP diameter, use of accessory muscles of inspiration, hyperresonant percussion note, diminished breath sounds, PFT results, and the chest x-ray film, which showed *alveolar hyperinflation* (see Figure 9-12).

The selection of a good program of oxygen supplementation was certainly indicated. Note the selection of a HAFOE mask because of the patient's initial significant CO_2 retention. Pneumococcal and influenza prophylaxis were certainly indicated in this case. Frequent intravenous administration of alpha$_1$-antitrypsin replacement represents modern therapy in the treatment of this unusual disease, as does counseling the patient that he should not knowingly expose himself to irritants such as those present in the smoky environment of his workplace.

Replacement alpha$_1$-antitrypsin therapy does not repair the alveolar damage that has already occurred but is thought to stabilize the condition.

CASE STUDY

Chronic Obstructive Pulmonary Disease (COPD)

Admitting History and Physical Examination

This 73-year-old man was brought to this Chicago, Illinois emergency room by his adult son. The son stated that his father had a long history of cardiopulmonary problems with chronic productive cough and had been diagnosed as having COPD about 15 years ago. Over the past 10 years, the patient had been admitted to this hospital three different times for COPD exacerbations. The hospital's electronic records showed that the patient had a long history of Stage III COPD. The patient required mechanical ventilation for 10 days during his last hospital stay. At the time of his last hospital discharge, his baseline FEV_1/FVC ratio was 55% and his FEV_1 was 35% of predicted. His D_{LCO} was 60% of predicted. His baseline arterial blood gas values at his last hospital discharge were as follows: pH 7.37, Pa_{CO_2} 93, HCO_3^- 53, and Pa_{O_2} 63, Sp_{O_2} 90%.

The patient had a long history of cigarette smoking, as well as working many long hours in smoke-filled rhythm-and-blues clubs throughout the Chicago area for over 40 years. The patient had been a rhythm and blues booking agent in the Chicago area since the late 1950s. He had worked with many of the greats—including, Muddy Waters, Buddy Guy, KoKo Taylor, Lonnie Brooks, and Candy Foster and the Shades of Blue. The patient stated that although he no longer worked in smoke-filled bars, he still smoked two to three packs of cigarettes per day. The patient's son stated that when he checked in on his father earlier that day, he realized that his father was very confused and disoriented. The son immediately transported his father to the emergency room.

On examination the patient appeared to be in moderate to severe respiratory distress. He was anxious, confused, and disoriented. The patient stated that he could not take a deep enough breath. His vital signs were as follows: respiratory rate, 35 breaths per minute; heart rate, 145 beats per minute; blood pressure, 145/90; and temperature, 37° C. The patient was moderately overweight and had a barrel chest. His skin appeared cyanotic. He had a frequent weak cough. He produced a moderate amount of purulent, gray-yellow sputum with each cough. In an upright position, he used accessory muscles of inspiration. He had prolonged exhalations and he was pursed-lip breathing. He had 3+ pitting edema of his legs, ankles, and feet. His neck veins were distended. The patient had clubbing of his fingers and toes.

Palpation revealed decreased chest expansion. Hyperresonant percussion notes were present over both lung fields. Auscultation revealed diminished heart and breath sounds, with bilateral wheezes, rhonchi, and crackles heard over all lung fields. An x-ray film taken in the emergency room with a portable unit showed lung hyperinflation, depressed diaphragms, increased bronchial vascular markings, and an enlarged right side of the heart. Bedside spirometry was attempted, but the patient was too weak and confused to generate a good expiratory maneuver. Arterial blood gas values on a 2 L/min oxygen cannula were pH 7.24, Pa_{CO_2} 110, HCO_3^- 55, Pa_{O_2} 47, Sp_{O_2} 77%. Laboratory results reveal a hemoglobin level of 19 g%. The respiratory therapist working in the emergency room documented the following assessment.

Respiratory Assessment and Plan

S: "I can't take a deep breath."

O: Moderate to severe respiratory distress. Vital signs: RR 35 bpm, HR: 145 bpm, BP: 145/90, T: 37° C. Barrel chest, cyanotic, frequent weak cough, moderate amount of purulent, gray-yellow sputum, using accessory muscles of inspiration, prolonged exhalation, pursed-lip breathing. 3+ pitting edema on legs, ankles, and feet. Distended neck veins, digital clubbing. Decreased chest expansion. Aus: diminished heart and breath sounds. Bilateral wheezes, rhonchi, and crackles could be heard over all lung fields. CXR: hyperinflation, depressed diaphragms, increased bronchial vascular markings, and an enlarged right heart. Arterial blood gas values on a 2 L/min O_2 cannula were pH 7.24, Pa_{CO_2} 110, HCO_3^- 55, Pa_{O_2} 47, Sp_{O_2} 77%. Hemoglobin level of 19 g%.

A: Bronchospasm (wheezing)
Excessive airway secretions (COPD history, rhonchi, crackles, purulent, gray-yellow secretions)
Pulmonary infection (yellow sputum)
Poor ability to mobilize secretions (weak cough effort)
Air trapping (hyperresonant percussion notes, hyperinflation on x-ray film, barrel chest)
Acute ventilatory failure on top of chronic ventilatory failure with moderate to severe hypoxemia (ABGs)
Cor pulmonale (swollen feet, ankles, and legs; enlarged right heart on x-ray film)

P: Notify physician stat regarding acute ventilatory failure superimposed on chronic ventilatory failure. Also inform the physician about the clinical manifestations associated with cor pulmonale. Recommend **Mechanical Ventilation Protocol** and **Oxygen Therapy Protocol**. Start **Bronchopulmonary Hygiene Therapy Protocol** (chest physical therapy qid; suctioning prn). Start **Aerosolized Medication Protocol** (combination short-acting $beta_2$-agonist plus long-acting anticholinergic—e.g., salbutamol/ipratropium). Supplement these agents with an inhaled glucocorticosteroid (beclomethasone tid).

Discussion

This case nicely demonstrates the clinical manifestations associated with both chronic bronchitis and emphysema—that is, COPD. The clinical manifestations of chronic bronchitis seen in this case include chronic productive cough, cor pulmonale (swollen lower extremities and distended neck veins), rhonchi, crackles and wheezing on auscultation, digital clubbing, and polycythemia (elevated hemoglobin level).

That the patient's bronchitis was accompanied by emphysema was indicated by his lung hyperinflation (on inspection and on his chest x-ray film), his hyperresonant percussion note, and the presence of his pursed-lip breathing. The fact that he was in hypoxemic, hypercapnic respiratory failure—and that he required ventilator support—does not help to separate the two diagnoses. These arterial blood gas abnormalities can be seen in either condition. The clinical manifestations (clinical scenarios) in this case are caused by the anatomic alteration of the lungs associated with both chronic bronchitis and emphysema; these clinical scenarios are as follows:

- Chronic bronchitis
    - **Bronchospasm** (see Figure 9-11)
    - **Excessive bronchial secretions** (see Figure 9-12)
- Emphysema
    - **Distal airway and alveolar weakening** (see Figure 9-13)

Treatment in this case was first driven by the selection of a **Ventilator Management Protocol.** With this in place, the **Oxygen Therapy Protocol** and elements of the **Bronchopulmonary Hygiene** and **Aerosolized Medication Protocols** were begun with standard protocol specifics.

Determination of severe via the GOLD standards depend on spirometric demonstrations, which were not possible here. However, "respiratory failure" does qualify the patient as having Stage IV: Very Severe COPD, which raises the requirement for long-term oxygen therapy and consideration of surgical treatments "if applicable." In this case, component 4 of the GOLD guidelines (Manage Exacerbations) was followed once the patient met the arterial blood gas criteria of respiratory acidosis and severe hypoxemia.

Unfortunately, this patient did not do well, and became ventilator-dependent. He died in a skilled nursing facility 3 months later, still "missing his smokes" and listening to rhythm and blues on his radio.

SELF-ASSESSMENT QUESTIONS

evolve Answers to questions can be found on Evolve. To access additional student assessment questions and case studies for application of text material to real-life scenarios, visit **http://evolve.elsevier.com/DesJardins/respiratory**.

1. In chronic bronchitis:
1. The bronchial walls are narrowed because of vasoconstriction
2. The bronchial glands are enlarged
3. The number of goblet cells is decreased
4. The number of cilia lining the tracheobronchial tree is increased
    a. 1 only
    b. 2 only
    c. 3 only
    d. 3 and 4 only

2. Which of the following common bacteria are found in the tracheobronchial tree of patients with chronic bronchitis?
1. *Staphylococcus*
2. *Haemophilus influenzae*
3. *Klebsiella*
4. *Streptococcus pneumonia*
    a. 1 only
    b. 2 only
    c. 3 and 4 only
    d. 2 and 4 only

3. In chronic bronchitis, the patient commonly demonstrates which of the following?
1. Increased FVC
2. Decreased FEV_1/FVC ratio
3. Increased VC
4. Decreased FEV_1
    a. 2 only
    b. 1 and 3 only
    c. 2 and 4 only
    d. 3 and 4 only

4. The patient with severe chronic bronchitis (late stage) commonly has which of the following arterial blood gas values?
1. Normal pH
2. Decreased HCO_3^-
3. Increased $Paco_2$
4. Normal Pao_2
    a. 1 only
    b. 1 and 3 only
    c. 2 and 3 only
    d. 3 and 4 only

5. Patients with severe chronic bronchitis may demonstrate which of the following?
1. Peripheral edema
2. Distended neck veins
3. An elevated hemoglobin concentration
4. An enlarged liver
    a. 3 only
    b. 2 and 4 only
    c. 2, 3, and 4 only
    d. 1, 2, 3, and 4

6. What type of emphysema creates an abnormal enlargement of all structures distal to the terminal bronchioles?
   a. Centrilobular emphysema
   b. Alpha$_1$–protease inhibitor deficiency emphysema
   c. ZZ phenotype emphysema
   d. Panlobular emphysema

7. What is the normal level of alpha$_1$-protease inhibitor?
   a. 0 to 200 mg/dL
   b. 200 to 400 mg/dL
   c. 400 to 600 mg/dL
   d. 600 to 800 mg/dL

8. The DLCO of patients with severe emphysema is:
   a. Increased
   b. Decreased
   c. Normal
   d. The DLCO test is not used to assess emphysema patients.

9. Patients with severe emphysema commonly demonstrate which of the following oxygenation indices?
1. Decreased $S\bar{v}o_2$
2. Increased O_2ER
3. Decreased Do_2
4. Increased $C(a-\bar{v})o_2$
   a. 1 only
   b. 3 only
   c. 4 only
   d. 1, 2, and 3 only

10. Which phenotype is associated with the lowest serum concentration of alpha$_1$-antitrypsin?
   a. MM phenotype
   b. MZ phenotype
   c. ZZ phenotype
   d. M phenotype

11. Which of the following pulmonary function study findings are associated with severe emphysema?
1. Increased FRC
2. Decreased PEFR
3. Increased RV
4. Decreased FVC
   a. 3 and 4 only
   b. 2 and 3 only
   c. 2, 3, and 4 only
   d. 1, 2, 3, and 4

12. The patient with severe COPD commonly demonstrates which of the following hemodynamic indices?
1. Decreased CVP
2. Increased $\overline{PA}$
3. Decreased RVSWI
4. Increased PVR
   a. 1 only
   b. 3 only
   c. 2 and 4 only
   d. 1 and 2 only

13. Because acute ventilatory changes are often seen in patients with chronic ventilatory failure (compensated respiratory acidosis), the respiratory care practitioner must be alert for this problem in patients with severe COPD. Which of the following arterial blood gas values represent(s) acute alveolar hyperventilation superimposed on chronic ventilatory failure?
1. Increased pH
2. Increased $Paco_2$
3. Increased HCO_3^-
4. Increased Pao_2
   a. 2 only
   b. 2 and 4 only
   c. 1 and 3 only
   d. 1, 2, and 3 only

14. The lung parenchyma in the chest radiograph of a patient with emphysema appears:
1. Opaque
2. White
3. More translucent than normal
4. Dark
   a. 2 only
   b. 1 and 3 only
   c. 2 and 3 only
   d. 3 and 4 only

15. What is the single most important etiologic factor in emphysema?
   a. Alpha$_1$-antitrypsin deficiency
   b. Cigarette smoking
   c. Infection
   d. Sulfur dioxide

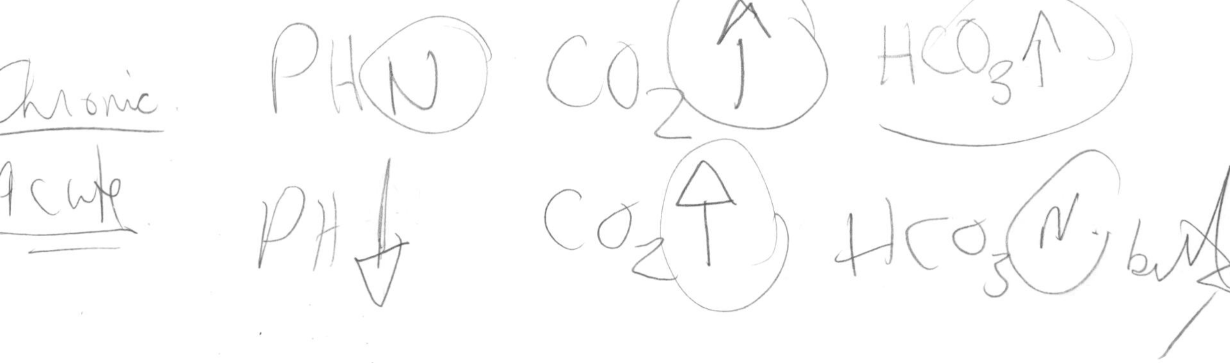

Asthma

12

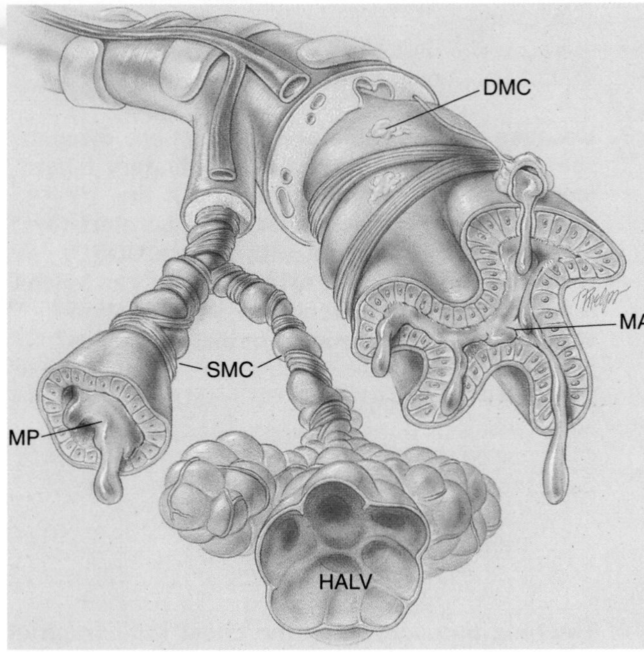

FIGURE 12-1 Asthma. *DMC,* Degranulation of mast cell; *HALV,* hyperinflation of alveoli; *MA,* mucous accumulation; *MP,* mucous plug; *SMC,* smooth muscle constriction (bronchospasm).

Chapter Objectives

After reading this chapter, you will be able to:

- Describe the role of the following organizations in the management of asthma:
  - National Asthma Education and Prevention Program (NAEPP)
  - Global Initiative for Asthma (GINA)
- List the anatomic alterations of the lungs associated with asthma.
- Describe the epidemiology and risk factors associated with asthma, including the following types of asthma:
  - Extrinsic asthma
  - Intrinsic asthma
- Describe the challenges associated with the diagnosis of asthma, and include the tests used to diagnosis and monitor asthma.
- Differentiate the classifications of asthma severity.
- Describe the cardiopulmonary clinical manifestations associated with asthma.
- Describe the general management of asthma.
- Describe the clinical strategies and rationales of the SOAPs presented in the case study.
- Define key terms and complete self-assessment questions at the end of the chapter and on Evolve.

Key Terms

Allergic or Atopic Asthma
Anaphylaxic Hypersensitivity Reaction
Asthma Educator
Controller Medications
Exercise-Induced Asthma
Extrinsic Asthma
Global Initiative for Asthma (GINA)
IgE-Mediated Allergic Reaction
Immunologic Mechanism
Inhaled Corticosteroids (ICSs)
Intrinsic Asthma
Long-Acting Beta$_2$-Agonists (LABA)
National Asthma Education and Prevention Program (NAEPP)
National Heart, Lung, and Blood Institute (NHLBI)
National Institutes of Health (NIH)
Nonallergic or Nonatopic Asthma
Occupational Asthma
Occupational Sensitizers
Pulsus Paradoxus
Reliever (Rescue) Medications
Short-Acting Beta$_2$-Agonists (SABA)
Status Asthmaticus
World Health Organization (WHO)

Chapter Outline

Introduction

The burdens associated with asthma in the United States—and worldwide—are enormous. Although the precise annual numbers are not known, asthma is clearly linked to a multitude of lost school days, countless missed work days, numerous doctor visits, frequent hospital outpatient visits, and recurrent emergency department visits and hospitalizations. According to the Department of Health and Human Services' Centers for Disease Control and Prevention, within the United States in 2005 more than 22 million people were diagnosed with asthma, more than 12 million people had experienced an asthma episode in the previous year, and nearly 4000 Americans died of asthma.* The **World Health Organization (WHO)** estimates that about 180,000 people worldwide die because of asthma each year. Clearly, asthma's impact on health, quality of life, and the economy is substantial.

A relatively new role of the respiratory care practitioner is that of **asthma educator.** In this function, the practitioner's goal is to be sure that the patient and the family are cognizant of their role and functions in the care of this usually chronic and often serious condition. The asthma educator must serve as a "change agent," and his or her effect as a convincing, empathetic communicator will be tested. Toward this end, we have greatly expanded this chapter from previous editions.

Fortunately, over the past two decades several new and important gains have been made by expert panels in the development of evidence-based clinical guidelines directed toward the education, prevention, diagnosis, and management of asthma. These guidelines are based on an extensive scientific foundation that has provided our current understanding of the pathophysiologic mechanisms, clinical manifestations, and treatment recommendations used to control asthma. Updated clinical guidelines are developed and disseminated on a regular basis by the **National Asthma Education and Prevention Program (NAEPP)** and the **Global Initiative for Asthma (GINA).**

National Asthma Education and Prevention Program

The first evidence-based asthma guidelines were published in 1991 by NAEPP, under the coordination of the **National Heart, Lung, and Blood Institute (NHLBI)** of the **National Institutes of Health (NIH).** These guidelines were updated in 1997, 2002, and 2007.† Today the guidelines are structured around the following four components of care: (1) assessment and monitoring of asthma, (2) patient education, (3) control of factors contributing to asthma severity, and (4) the pharmacologic treatments. The NAEPP "stepwise asthma management charts" have been widely used and now specify optimal treatment for specific age groups 0 to 4 years, 5 to 11 years, and 12 years and older.

*www.cdc.gov/asthma/aag07.htm.

†Expert Panel Response 3 (EPR 3): *Guidelines for the diagnosis and management of asthma,* 2007. Available at: www.nhlbi.nih.gov/guidelines/asthma/asthgdln.htm.

Global Initiative for Asthma

GINA* was launched in 1993 in collaboration with the National Heart, Lung, and Blood Institute of NIH and WHO. GINA works with a network of asthma experts and researchers, health-care professionals, professional organizations, and public health-care officials from around the world. GINA gathers and disseminates asthma-related information while also ensuring that a system is in place to incorporate the results of scientific investigations into asthma care. GINA's specific goals are the following:

- Increase awareness of asthma and it public health consequences
- Promote identification of reasons for the increased prevalence of asthma
- Promote study of the association between asthma and the environment
- Reduce asthma morbidity and mortality
- Improve management of asthma
- Improve availability and accessibility of effective asthma therapy

Collectively, by using the evidence-based guidelines provided by NAEPP, along with the extensive information gathered worldwide from asthma experts and researchers, GINA now provides an outstanding—and user-friendly—evidence-based guideline program for the management of asthma. As of this writing, the GINA programs, which are freely available on the internet (www.ginasthma.org), include the following publications:

- *Global Strategy for Asthma Management and Prevention* (2007). Scientific information and recommendations for asthma programs.
- *Pocket Guide for Asthma Management and Prevention* (2006). Summary of patient care information for primary health-care professionals.
- *Pocket Guide for Asthma Management and Prevention in Children* (2006). Summary of patient care information for pediatricians and other health-care professionals.
- *What You and Your Family Can Do About Asthma.* An information booklet for patients and their families.

In this chapter, GINA's five components of asthma care are presented under the general management of asthma section.

Anatomic Alterations of the Lungs

Asthma is described as a lung disorder characterized by (1) reversible bronchial airway smooth muscle constriction, (2) airway inflammation, and (3) increased airway responsiveness to an assortment of stimuli. During an asthma attack, the smooth muscles surrounding the small airways

*Global Initiative for Asthma (GINA): *Global strategy for asthma management and prevention,* updated 2007. The GINA reports are available at www.ginasthma.org.

constrict. Over time the smooth muscle layers hypertrophy and can increase to three times their normal thickness. The airway mucosa becomes infiltrated with eosinophils and other inflammatory cells, which in turn causes airway inflammation and mucosal edema. The goblet cells proliferate, and the bronchial mucous glands enlarge. The airways become filled with thick, whitish, tenacious mucus. Extensive mucous plugging and atelectasis may develop. The cilia are damaged, and the basement membrane of the mucosa is thicker than normal. As a result of smooth muscle constriction, bronchial mucosal edema, and excessive bronchial secretions, air trapping and alveolar hyperinflation develop. If chronic inflammation develops over time, these anatomic alterations become irreversible, resulting in loss of airway caliber. A remarkable feature of bronchial asthma, however, is that many of the pathologic anatomic alterations of the lungs that occur during an asthmatic attack are completely *absent* between asthmatic episodes (Figure 12-1).

The major pathologic or structural changes observed during an asthmatic episode are as follows:

- Smooth muscle constriction of bronchial airways (bronchospasm)
- Bronchial wall inflammation
- Excessive production of thick, whitish bronchial secretions
- Mucous plugging
- Hyperinflation of alveoli (air trapping)
- In severe cases, atelectasis caused by mucous plugging

Etiology and Epidemiology

Asthma was first recognized by Hippocrates more than 2000 years ago. It remains one of the most common diseases encountered in clinical medicine. In fact, over the past decade the incidence of asthma has increased dramatically. Today, it is estimated that more than 25 million Americans have asthma. About 500,000 Americans are hospitalized annually for severe asthma, and about 4000 die as a result of asthma annually. According to WHO, about 180,000 people worldwide die because of asthma each year. In the United States, asthma is found in 3% to 5% of adults and 7% to 10% of children. Approximately 50% of people with asthma develop it before age 10. Asthma is the most common chronic illness of childhood. Among young children, asthma is about two times more prevalent in boys than in girls. After puberty, however, asthma is more common in girls.

Risk Factors

Many asthma experts divide asthma into two major types according to its precipitating risk factors: **extrinsic asthma,** or asthma caused by external or environmental agents, and **intrinsic asthma,** or asthma that occurs in the absence of (or without clear evidence of) an antigen-antibody reaction. Although some authorities believe that the distinction between these terms is of minimal clinical value, the terms are nevertheless widely used.

According to GINA, the risk factors for asthma can be divided into (1) the risk factors with which one is born that cause the development of asthma (e.g., genetic factors or sex), and (2) the risk factors that trigger asthma symptoms (e.g., domestic mites, furred animals, cockroach allergen, fungi, molds, infections, tobacco smoke). The risk factors for asthma with which the individual is born are primarily genetic in nature; the risk factors that trigger asthma symptoms are usually environmental factors. Regardless of the fact that the various asthma authorities are not in full agreement as to how asthma should be categorized, they are—for the most part—in agreement regarding the following causes, or risk factors, of asthma.

Extrinsic Asthma (Allergic or Atopic Asthma)

When an asthmatic episode can clearly be linked to exposure to a specific allergen (antigen), the patient is said to have *extrinsic asthma* (also called **allergic** or **atopic asthma**). Common indoor allergens include house dust, mites, furred animal dander (e.g., dogs, cats, and mice), cockroach allergen, fungi, molds, and yeast. Outdoor allergens include pollens, fungi, molds, and yeast. In addition, there are a number of occupational substances associated with asthma (see next section).

Extrinsic asthma is an immediate (Type I) **anaphylactic hypersensitivity reaction**. It occurs in individuals who have atopy, a hypersensitivity condition associated with genetic predisposition and an excessive amount of immunoglobulin E (IgE) antibody production in response to a variety of antigens. From 10% to 20% of the general population are atopic and therefore have a tendency to develop an **IgE-mediated allergic reaction** such as asthma, hay fever, allergic rhinitis, and eczema. Such individuals develop a wheal-and-flare reaction to a variety of skin test allergens, called a *positive skin test result.* Extrinsic asthma is family-related and usually appears in children and in adults younger than 30 years old. It often disappears after puberty.

Because extrinsic asthma is associated with an antigen-antibody–induced bronchospasm, an **immunologic mechanism** plays an important role. As with other organs, the lungs are protected against injury by certain immunologic mechanisms. Under normal circumstances these mechanisms function without any apparent clinical evidence of their activity. In patients susceptible to extrinsic or allergic asthma, however, the hypersensitive immune response actually creates the disease by causing acute and chronic inflammation.

Immunologic mechanism.

1. When a susceptible individual is exposed to a certain antigen, lymphoid tissue cells form specific IgE (reaginic) antibodies. The IgE antibodies attach themselves to the surface of mast cells in the bronchial walls (Figure 12-2, *A*).
2. Reexposure or continued exposure to the same antigen creates an antigen-antibody reaction on the surface of the mast cell, which in turn causes the mast cell to degranulate and release chemical mediators such as histamine, eosinophil chemotactic factor of anaphylaxis (ECF-A), neutrophil chemotactic factors (NCFs), leukotrienes (formerly known as *slow-reacting substances of*

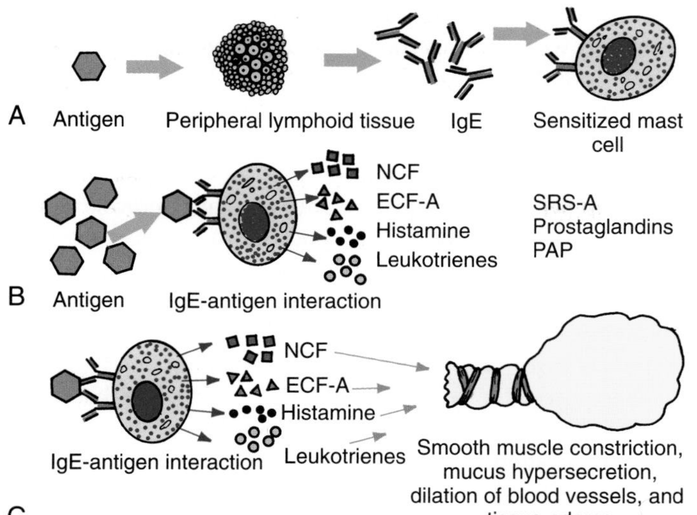

FIGURE 12-2 The immunologic mechanisms in asthma.

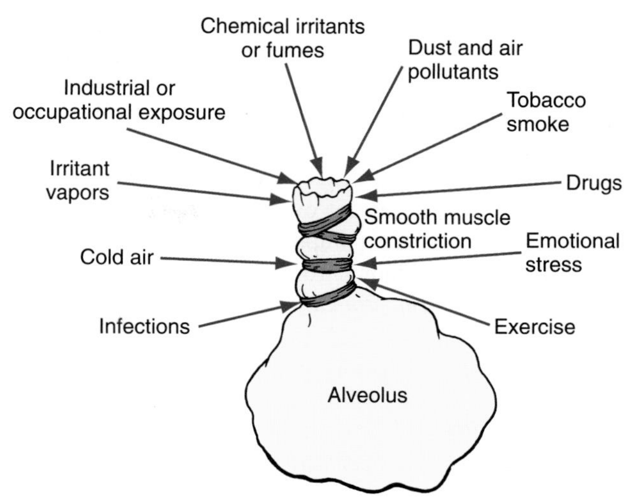

FIGURE 12-3 Some factors known to trigger intrinsic asthma.

Box 12-1 Agents Associated with Occupational Asthma

Animal and Plant Proteins

- Flour, amylase
- Storage mites
- *Bacillus subtilis* enzymes (detergent manufacturing)
- Colophony, such as pine resin (electrical soldering)
- Soybean dust
- Midges, parasites (fish food manufacturing)
- Coffee bean dust, meat tenderizer, tea, shellfish, amylase, egg proteins, pancreatic enzymes, papain
- Storage mites, *Aspergillus*, indoor ragweed, grass (granary workers)
- Psyllium, latex (hospital workers)
- Ispaghula, psyllium (laxative manufacturing)
- Poultry droppings, mites, feathers
- Locusts, dander, urine proteins
- Wood dust, such as western red cedar, oak, mahogany, zebrawood, redwood, Lebanon cedar, African maple, eastern white cedar
- Grain dust, molds, insects, grain
- Silk worm moths and larvae

Inorganic Chemicals

- Persulfate (beauticians)
- Nickel salts
- Platinum salts, vanadium

Organic Chemicals

- Ethanolamine diisocyanate (automobile painting)
- Disinfectants, such as sulfathiazole, chloramines, formaldehyde, and glutaraldehyde; latex (hospital workers)
- Antibiotics, piperazine, methyldopa, salbutamol, cimetidine (manufacturing)
- Ethylene diamine, phthalic anhydride
- Toluene diisocyanate, dephenylene, tetramines, trimellitic anhydride, hexamethyl tetramine, acrylates (plastics industry)

anaphylaxis [SRS-A]), prostaglandins, and platelet-activating factor ([PAP]; Figure 12-2, *B*).

3. The release of these chemical mediators stimulates parasympathetic nerve endings in the bronchial airways, leading to reflex bronchoconstriction and mucous hypersecretion. Moreover, these chemical mediators increase the permeability of capillaries, which results in the dilation of blood vessels and tissue edema (Figure 12-2, *C*).

The patient with extrinsic asthma may demonstrate an early asthmatic (allergic) response, a late asthmatic response, or a biphasic asthmatic response. The early asthmatic response begins within minutes of exposure to an inhaled antigen and resolves in approximately 1 hour. A late asthmatic response begins several hours after exposure to an inhaled antigen but lasts much longer. The late asthmatic response may or may not follow an early asthmatic response. An early asthmatic response followed by a late asthmatic response is called a *biphasic response.*

Occupational sensitizers (occupational asthma). Occupational asthma is defined as asthma caused by exposure to an agent encountered in the work environment. More than 300 different substances have been associated with occupational asthma. Occupational asthma is seen predominantly in adults. It is estimated that **occupational sensitizers** cause about 1 in 10 cases of asthma among adults of working age. High-risk work environments for occupational asthma include farming and agricultural work, painting (including spray painting), cleaning work, and plastic manufacturing. Most occupational asthma is immunologically mediated and has a latency period of months to years after the onset of exposure. Although the cause is not fully understood, it is known that an IgE-mediated allergic reaction and cell-mediated allergic reactions are often involved. Box 12-1 shows additional agents known to cause occupational asthma.

Intrinsic Asthma (Nonallergic or Nonatopic Asthma)

When an asthmatic episode cannot be directly linked to a specific antigen or extrinsic inciting factor, it is referred to as *intrinsic asthma* (also called **nonallergic or nonatopic asthma**) (Figure 12-3). The etiologic factors responsible for intrinsic asthma are elusive. Individuals with intrinsic asthma are not hypersensitive or atopic to environmental antigens and have a normal serum IgE level. The onset of intrinsic asthma usually occurs after the age of 40 years, and typically there is no strong family history of allergy.

In spite of the general distinctions between extrinsic and intrinsic asthma, a significant overlap exists. Distinguishing between the two is often impossible in a clinical setting. Precipitating factors known to cause intrinsic asthma are referred to as *nonspecific stimuli.* Some of the more common nonspecific stimuli associated with intrinsic asthma are discussed in the following paragraphs.

Other Risk Factors

Obesity. Obesity has been shown to be a risk factor for asthma. It is thought that certain mediators, such as leptins, may have an effect on airway function that can lead to the development of asthma.

Sex. Male sex is a risk factor for asthma in children. Up to 14 years of age, the prevalence of asthma is nearly twice as great in boys as in girls. The difference in prevalence of asthma in males and in females progressively narrows through the teenage years. By adulthood, the prevalence of asthma is greater in women than in men. The reason for this sex difference in asthma is unclear. It is suggested that the lung size is smaller in males than in females at birth, but larger in adulthood.

Infections. Although bacterial infections may cause asthma, viral upper airway infections are more likely to contribute to asthma. For example, intrinsic asthma is commonly seen in children after respiratory syncytial virus (RSV), parainfluenza virus, or rhinovirus infection. These conditions often produce a pattern of symptoms that parallel many features of childhood asthma. For example, it is estimated that about 40% of children with RSV infection will continue to wheeze or have asthma into later childhood.

Exercise-induced asthma. Asthma is sometimes associated with vigorous exercise. The asthmatic episode typically occurs 3 to 10 minutes after the exercise. The asthmatic episode usually resolves in about 1 hour. Although the precise mechanism is not understood, it is believed that the heat loss, water loss, and increased osmolarity of the lower airways causes the release of certain mediators from the basophils and tissue mast cells. The release of the mediators, in turn, causes bronchospasm. Exercise in cold, dry air (e.g., jogging, ice skating, cross-country skiing) also may provoke an asthmatic response in susceptible individuals.

Outdoor and indoor air pollution. Outbreaks of asthma exacerbations have been reported in areas of increased levels of air pollution. The role of outdoor air pollution in causing asthma remains controversial. Similar associations have been reported in relation to indoor pollutants, such as smoke and fumes from gas and biomass fuels used for heating and cooling, molds, and cockroach infestation. These conditions are not IgE mediated.

Drugs, food additives, and food preservatives. Asthma is associated with the ingestion of aspirin and other nonsteroidal antiinflammatory drugs (NSAIDs). As much as 20% of the asthmatic population may be sensitive to aspirin and NSAIDs. Various beta-adrenergic blocking agents used to treat hypertension and some cardiac disorders (e.g., propranolol, metoprolol) also may provoke an asthmatic episode. The yellow food-coloring agent tartrazine may provoke an asthmatic episode. The ingestion of tartrazine especially is contraindicated in patients sensitive to aspirin. Bisulfites and metabisulfites, commonly used as preservatives and antioxidants in restaurant food (e.g., salad bars, certain wines, beers, dried fruits), are known to provoke bronchoconstriction. About 5% of the asthmatic population is sensitive to foods and drinks that contain sulfites.

Gastroesophageal reflux. Gastroesophageal reflux disease (GERD), or regurgitation, appears to contribute significantly to bronchoconstriction in some patients. The precise mechanism of this relationship is not known. The patient may complain of burning, substernal pain, belching, and a bitter, acid taste, particularly when lying down.

Sleep (nocturnal asthma). Patients with asthma often have more difficulty late at night or in the early morning. Precipitating factors associated with nocturnal asthma include gastroesophageal reflux, retained airway secretions (caused by a suppressed cough reflex during sleep), exposure to irritants or allergens in the bedroom, and prolonged time between medication doses. Eradication of nocturnal asthma is one measure of good asthma control.

Emotional stress. In some patients the exacerbation of asthma appears to correlate with emotional stress and other psychologic factors.

Perimenstrual asthma (catamenial asthma). The clinical manifestations associated with asthma often worsen in women during the premenstrual and menstrual periods. The peak of worsening symptoms generally occurs 2 to 3 days before menstruation begins. Perimenstrual asthma correlates with the late luteal phase of ovarian activity, the phase during which circulating progesterone and estrogen levels are at their lowest.

Diagnosis of Asthma

The diagnosis of asthma can often be challenging. For example, the diagnosis of asthma in early childhood is based primarily on the assessment of the child's symptoms and physical findings—and good clinical judgment. In the older child and the adult, a complete history and physical examination—along with the demonstration of reversible and variable airflow obstruction—will in most cases confirm the diagnosis of asthma. In the elderly patient, asthma is often undiagnosed because of the presence of comorbid diseases that complicate the diagnosis.

Furthermore, the diagnosis of asthma is often missed in the patient who acquires asthma in the workplace. This form of asthma is called **occupational asthma** (see Box 12-1). Because occupational asthma usually has a slow and insidious onset, the patient's asthma is often misdiagnosed as chronic bronchitis or COPD. As a result, the asthma is either not treated at all or treated inappropriately. Finally, even though asthma can usually be distinguished from COPD, in some patients—those who have chronic respiratory clinical manifestations and fixed airflow limitations—it is often very difficult to differentiate between the two disorders—that is, asthma or COPD.

GINA provides a general guideline to help in the clinical diagnosis of asthma, which is based on the patient's symptoms and medical history. There are many signs and symptoms that should increase the suspicion of asthma. This includes wheezing and a history of any of the following:

- cough
- recurrent wheeze
- recurrent difficult breathing
- recurrent chest tightness

Other indicators are if the symptoms occur or worsen at night or in a seasonal pattern. The presence of eczema, hay fever or a family history of asthma or atopic disease may also be an indicator. Another sign is if an individual has colds that "go to the chest" or that take more than 10 days to clear up. There are also situations in which asthma related symptoms may worsen, such as exposure to:

- animals with fur
- aerosol chemicals
- changes in temperature
- domestic dust mites
- drugs (aspirin, beta-blockers)
- exercise
- pollens
- respiratory (viral) infections
- smoke
- strong emotional expression

These symptoms often respond to appropriate antiasthma therapy.

Diagnostic and Monitoring Test for Asthma

There are several tests used to diagnose and monitor asthma. These tests measure the severity, reversibility, and variability of airflow limitations. Common tests used to for diagnostic and monitoring asthma include the following:

Spirometry measures airflow limitation and its reversibility. An increase in FEV_1 of $\geq 12\%$ (or ≥ 200 ml) after administration of a bronchodilator indicates reversible airflow limitation consistent with asthma.

Peak expiratory flow (PEF) measurements are used to diagnose and monitor asthma. An improvement of 60 L/min (or $\geq 20\%$ of the prebronchodilator [PEF] after inhalation of a bronchodilator), or diurnal variation in PEF of more than 20% (with twice-daily readings, more than 10%), suggests a diagnosis of asthma.

Other tests include measurements of airway responsiveness to methacholine, histamine, mannitol, or exercise in order to diagnose. The presence of allergies (including a positive skin test with allergens or measurement of specific IgE in serum) increases the probability of a diagnosis of asthma, and can help identify risk factors that cause asthma symptoms in individual patients.

Classification of Asthma Severity

GINA provides a general classification of asthma severity based on the clinical features before treatment. The four categories of symptoms include intermittent, mild persistent, moderate persistent, and severe persistent.

- **Intermittent** symptoms are described as those that occur less than once a week and possible brief exacerbations. They may also include nocturnal symptoms not more than twice a month. (Forced expiratory volume in 1 second [FEV_1] or peak expiratory flow [PEF] $\geq$ 80% predicted; PEF or FEV_1 variability $< 20\%$.)
- **Mild persistent** symptoms occur more than once a week, but less than once a day and exacerbations may affect activity and sleep. Nocturnal symptoms also occur more than twice a month. (FEV_1 or PEF $\geq 80\%$ predicted; PEF or FEV_1 variability $< 20\%$ to 30%.)
- **Moderate persistent** symptoms occur daily and exacerbations effect activity and sleep. Nocturnal symptoms occur more than once a week and an individual uses an inhaled short-acting $beta_2$-agonist. (FEV_1 or PEF 60% to 80% predicted; PEF or FEV_1 variability $> 30\%$.)
- **Severe persistent** symptoms occur daily along with frequent nocturnal symptoms. There are also limitations on physical activity. (FEV_1 or PEF $\leq 60\%$ predicted; PEF or FEV_1 variability $> 30\%$.)

Although the classification of asthma based on severity is useful when decisions are being made about treatment plans during the initial assessment of the patient, GINA points out that this classification model has the following limitations:

- It is important to recognize that asthma severity involves both the severity of the underlying disease and its responsiveness to treatment. For example, asthma can cause severe symptoms and airflow obstruction and be classified as "severe persistent" on initial presentation, but respond fully to treatment and then be classified as "moderate persistent" asthma.
- In addition, severity is not an unvarying feature of an individual patient's asthma, but may change over months or years.
- Because of these considerations, the classification of asthma severity provided in Table 12-3, which is based on expert opinion rather than evidence, is no longer recommended as the basis for ongoing treatment decisions.
- Its main limitation is its poor value in predicting what treatment will be required and what a patient's response to that treatment might be.
- For this purpose, a periodic assessment of asthma control is more relevant and useful.

OVERVIEW of the Cardiopulmonary Clinical Manifestations Associated with Asthma

The following clinical manifestations result from the pathophysiologic mechanisms caused (or activated) by **Bronchospasm** (see Figure 9-11) and **Excessive Bronchial Secretions** (see Figure 9-12)—the major anatomic alterations of the lungs associated with an asthmatic episode (see Figure 12-1).

CLINICAL DATA OBTAINED AT THE PATIENT'S BEDSIDE

The Physical Examination

Vital Signs

Increased Respiratory Rate (Tachypnea)

Several pathophysiologic mechanisms operating simultaneously may lead to an increased ventilatory rate:

- Stimulation of peripheral chemoreceptors (hypoxemia)
- Decreased lung compliance and increased ventilatory rate relationship (when lungs are hyperinflated)
- Anxiety

Increased Heart Rate (Pulse), and Blood Pressure

Use of Accessory Muscles during Inspiration

Use of Accessory Muscles during Expiration

Pursed-Lip Breathing

Substernal Intercostal Retractions

Substernal, supraclavicular, and intercostal retractions during inspiration may be seen, particularly in children.

Increased Anteroposterior Chest Diameter (Barrel Chest)

Cyanosis

Cough and Sputum Production

During an asthmatic episode the patient may produce an excessive amount of thick, whitish, tenacious mucus. Because of the presence of large numbers of eosinophils and other white blood cells, the sputum is often purulent.

Pulsus Paradoxus

When an asthmatic episode produces severe alveolar air trapping and hyperinflation, pulsus paradoxus is a classic clinical manifestation. Pulsus paradoxus is defined as systolic blood pressure that is more than 10 mm Hg lower on inspiration than on expiration. This exaggerated waxing and waning of arterial blood pressure can be detected by using a blood pressure cuff or, in severe cases, by palpating the strength of the pulse. Pulsus paradoxus during an asthmatic attack is believed to be caused by the major intrapleural pressure swings that occur during inspiration and expiration.

Decreased Blood Pressure during Inspiration

During inspiration the patient frequently recruits accessory muscles of inspiration. The accessory muscles help produce an extremely negative intrapleural pressure, which in turn enhances intrapulmonary air flow. The increased negative intrapleural pressure, however, also causes blood vessels in the lungs to dilate and blood to pool. Consequently, the volume of blood returning to the left ventricle decreases. This causes a reduction in cardiac output and arterial blood pressure during inspiration.

Increased Blood Pressure during Expiration

During expiration, the patient often activates the accessory muscles of expiration in an effort to overcome the increased airway resistance. The increased power produced by these muscles generates a greater positive intrapleural pressure. Although increased positive intrapleural pressure may help offset the airway resistance, it also works to narrow or squeeze the blood vessels of the lung. This increased pressure on the pulmonary blood vessels enhances left ventricular filling and results in an increased cardiac output and arterial blood pressure during expiration.

Chest Assessment Findings

- Expiratory prolongation (I : E ratio >1 : 3)
- Decreased tactile and vocal fremitus
- Hyperresonant percussion note
- Diminished breath sounds
- Diminished heart sounds
- Wheezing and rhonchi

CLINICAL DATA OBTAINED FROM LABORATORY AND SPECIAL PROCEDURES

Pulmonary Function Test Findings
Moderate to Severe Asthmatic Episode
(Obstructive Lung Pathology)

FORCED EXPIRATORY FLOW RATE FINDINGS

FVC	FEV_T	FEV_1/FVC ratio	$FEF_{25\%-75\%}$
↓	↓	↓	↓

$FEF_{50\%}$	$FEF_{200-1200}$	PEFR	MVV
↓	↓	↓	↓

LUNG VOLUME AND CAPACITY FINDINGS

V_T	IRV	ERV	RV
N or ↑	N or ↓	N or ↓	↑

VC	IC	FRC	TLC	RV/TLC ratio
↓	N or ↓	↑	N or ↑	N or ↑

Arterial Blood Gases

MILD TO MODERATE ASTHMATIC EPISODE
Acute Alveolar Hyperventilation
(Acute Respiratory Alkalosis) with Hypoxemia

pH	$Paco_2$	HCO_3^-	Pao_2
↑	↓	↓(slightly)	↓

SEVERE ASTHMATIC EPISODE (STATUS ASTHMATICUS)
Acute Ventilatory Failure
(Acute Respiratory Acidosis) with Hypoxemia

pH*	$Paco_2$	HCO_3^- *	Pao_2
↓	↑	↑ (Slightly)	↓

*When tissue hypoxia is severe enough to produce lactic acid, the pH and HCO_3 values will be lower than expected for a particular $Paco_2$ level.

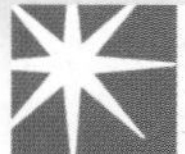

OVERVIEW of the Cardiopulmonary Clinical Manifestations Associated with Asthma—cont'd

Oxygenation Indices*

MODERATE SEVERE STAGES

$\dot{Q}_S/\dot{Q}_T$	Do_2†	$\dot{V}o_2$	$C(a-\bar{v})o_2$	O_2ER	$S\bar{v}o_2$
↑	↓	N	N	↑	↓

†The Do_2 may be normal in patients who have compensated to the decreased oxygenation status with (1) an increased cardiac output, (2) an increased hemoglobin level, or (3) a combination of both. When the Do_2 is normal, the O_2ER is usually normal.

ABNORMAL LABORATORY TESTS AND PROCEDURES

Sputum Examination

- Eosinophils
- Charcot-Leyden crystals
- Casts of mucus from small airways (Kirschman spirals)
- IgE level (elevated in extrinsic asthma)

RADIOLOGIC FINDINGS

Chest Radiograph

- Increased anteroposterior diameter ("barrel chest")
- Translucent (dark) lung fields
- Depressed or flattened diaphragms

*$C(a-\bar{v})o_2$, Arterial-venous oxygen difference; Do_2, total oxygen delivery; O_2ER, oxygen extraction ratio; $\dot{Q}_S/\dot{Q}_T$, pulmonary shunt fraction; $S\bar{v}o_2$, mixed venous oxygen saturation; $\dot{V}o_2$, oxygen consumption.

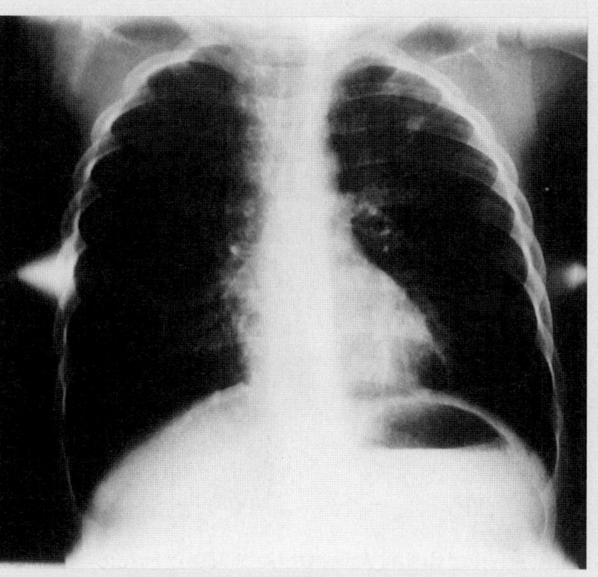

FIGURE 12-4 Chest x-ray film of a 2-year-old patient during an acute asthma attack.

As the alveoli become enlarged during an asthmatic attack, the residual volume and functional residual capacity increase. This condition decreases the radiographic density of the lungs.

Consequently, the chest x-ray film shows lung shadows that are translucent or darker than normal in appearance. Because of the increased residual volume, functional residual capacity, and total lung capacity, the diaphragms are depressed and flattened (Figure 12-4).

General Management of Asthma

Using the scientific evidence-based information developed by the **National Asthma Education and Prevention Program** (NAEPP), and the extensive research and input provided by leading asthma experts from around the world, the **Global Initiative for Asthma (GINA)** now provides an excellent—and user friendly—clinical guideline program for the management and prevention of asthma. The complete GINA documents are available at the following web site: http://www.ginasthma.org. The five major components of asthma care described by GINA are:

Component 1: Develop Patient/Doctor Partnership
Component 2: Identify and Reduce Exposure to Risk Factors
Component 3: Assess, Treat, and Monitor Asthma
Component 4: Manage Asthma Exacerbations
Component 5: Special Considerations in Managing Asthma

Component 1: Develop Patient-Doctor Partnership

If a patient establishes and maintains a good working relationship with their doctor, he or she will learn to avoid risk factors, take medication correctly, understand the differences between the types of asthma medication, monitor symptoms and take action and seek medical help when appropriate.

Component 2: Identify and Reduce Exposure to Risk Factors

Reducing the exposure to risk factors can improve control of asthma and reduce medication needs. It is important to develop strategies to avoid the risk factors such as staying away from tobacco smoke as well as foods, drugs and additives that may trigger symptoms. Also reduce or avoid exposure to occupational sensitizers.

Component 3: Assess, Treat, and Monitor Asthma

Evaluating a patient is necessary before successful treatment can begin. Once a patient has been assessed and the level of control has been established, a patient can be properly treated. Many drugs can be used in the treatment of asthma. The following is a list of inhaled glucocorticosteroids commonly used in the treatment of asthma:

TABLE 12-1 Controller Medications Commonly Used to Treat Asthma

Generic Name	Brand Name	Dose and Administration
Inhaled Corticosteroids (ICSs)		
Beclomethasone dipropionate	QVAR	MDI: 2 puffs, 40 µg/puff or 80 µg/puff, bid
Triamcinolone acetonide	Azmacort	MDI: 2 puffs, 100 µg/puff, tid, qid
Flunisolide	Aerobid, Aerobid-M	MDI: 2 puffs, 250 µg/puff, bid
Flunisolide hemihydrate	Aerospan	MDI: 2 puffs, 80 µg/puff, bid
Fluticasone propionate	Flovent HFA	MDI: 2 puffs, 44 µg/puff, 110 µg/puff, 220 µg/puff, bid
	Flovent Diskus	DPI: 50 µg, 100 µg, 250 µg, 100-1000 µg, bid
Ciclesonide	Alvesco	MDI: 1-2 puffs, 80 µg/puff abd 160 µg/puff, daily
Budesonide	Pulmicort Turbuhaler	DPI: 200 µg/actuation, 200-800 µg, bid
	Pulmicort Respules	SVN: 0.25 mg/2 mL, 0.5 mg/2 mL, once daily or bid
Mometasone furoate	Asmanex Twisthaler	DPI: 220 µg/actuation, 220-880 µg, q day
Systemic Corticosteroids		
Prednisone	Deltasone	Tablets and syrups: For acute attacks 40-60 mg daily in 1 or 2 divided doses for adults or 1-2 mg/kg daily in children
Methylprednisolone	Medrol	
	Solu-Medrol	
Hydrocortisone	Solu-Cortef	
Prednisolone	Orapred	
Long-Acting Beta$_2$ Agents (LABAs)		
Salmeterol	Serevent	DPI: 50 µg/inhalation, bid
Formoterol	Foradil	DPI: 12 µg/inhalation, bid
Arformoterol	Brovana	SVN: 15 µg/2 mL unite dose, bid
Inhaled Corticosteroids and Long-Acting Beta$_2$ Agents		
Fluticasone propionate and salmeterol	Advair Diskus Advair HFA	DPI: 100 µg, 250 µg, or 500 µg fluticasone with 50 µg salmeterol, 1 inhalation bid MDI: 45 µg, 115 µg, or 230 µg, 1-2 inhalations bid
Budesonide and formoterol fumarate	Symbicort	MDI: 80 µg and 160 µg budesonide with 4.5 µg formoterol, 1-2 inhalations bid
Mast Cell–Stabilizing Agents		
Cromolyn sodium	Intal	SVN: 1 ampule, 20 mg/2 mL qid MDI: 2 puffs, 800 µg/puff, qid
Nedocromil sodium	Tilade	MDI: 2 puffs, 1.75 mg/puff, qid
Leukotriene Inhibitors (Antileukotrienes)		
Zafirlukast	Accolate	Tablet: 10 and 20 mg Adults and children ≥12 yr: 20 mg twice daily, without food Children 5-11 yr: 10 mg twice daily
Montelukast	Singulair	Tablets: 10 mg and 4- and 5-mg cherry-flavored chewable; 4-mg packet of granules Adults and children ≥15 yr: one 10 mg tablet daily Children 6-14 yr: one 5-mg chewable tablet daily Children 2-5 yr: one 4-mg chewable tablet or one 4-mg packet of granules daily 6-24 months: one 4-mg packet of granules daily
Zileuton	Zyflo	Tablets: 600 mg Adults and children ≥12 yr: one 600-mg tablet 4 times per day
Monoclonal Anti–Immunoglobulin E (IgE) Antibody		
Omalizumab	Xolair	Adults and children ≥12 yr: Subcutaneous injection every 4 weeks; dose dependent on weight and serum immunoglobulin E (IgE) level

TABLE 12-1 Controller Medications Commonly Used to Treat Asthma—cont'd

Generic Name	Brand Name	Dose and Administration
Xanthine Derivatives		
Theophylline	Slo-phyllin, Theolair, Quibron-T/SR Dividose, Bronkodyl, Elixophyllin, Theo-Dur, Uniphyl	Dose formulations are based on individual metabolism Tablets, capsules, syrup, elixir, extended-release tablets, capsules, injection
Oxtriphylline	Choledyl SA	Dose formulations are based on individual metabolism Tablets, syrup, elixir, sustained-release tablets
Aminophylline	Aminophylline	Dose formulations are based on individual metabolism Tablets, oral liquid, injection, suppositories
Dyphylline	Dylix, Lufyllin	Dose formulations are based on individual metabolism Tablets, elixir

Data from *Global Initiative for Asthma (GINA): Global Strategy for Asthma Management and Prevention*, updated 2008. Available at: www.goldcopd.org; and Gardenshire DS: *Rau's repiratory care pharmacology*, ed 7, St. Louis, 2008, Elsevier.
DPI, Dry powder inhaler; *MDI*, metered dose inhaler; *SVN*, small-volume nebulizer.

TABLE 12-2 Reliever Medications (Rescue Medications) Commonly Used to Treat Asthma

Medication	Trade Name	Adult Dosage
Ultra-Short–Acting Bronchodilator Agents		
Epinephrine	Adrenaline CL, Epinephrine Mist, Primatene Mist	SVN: 1% solution (1:100), 0.25-0.5 mL (2.5-5.0 mg) qid MDI: 0.22 mg/puff, puffs as ordered or needed
Racemic epinephrine	MicroNefrin, Nephron, S2	SVN: 2.25% solution, 0.25-0.5 mL (5.63-11.25 mg) qid
Isoetharine	Isoetharine (HCL)	SVN: 1% solution, 0.5 mL (5.0 mg) q4h
Short-Acting Adrenergic Bronchodilator Agents (SABAs) (Beta$_2$ Agents)		
Metaproterenol	Alupent	SVN: 0.4%, 0.6%, 5% solution, 0.3 mL (15 mg) tid, qid MDI: 650 μg/puff, 2 or 3 puffs tid, qid Tab: 10 mg and 20 mg, tid, qid Syrup: 10 mg/5 mL
Albuterol	Proventil	SVN: 0.5% solution, 0.5 mL (2.5 mg), 0.63 mg, 1.25 mg, and 2.5 mg unit dose, tid, qid
	Ventolin	MDI: 90 μg/puff, 2 puffs tid, qid
	AccuNeb	Tab: 2 mg, 4 mg, and 8 g, bid, tid, qid
	ProAir	Syrup: 2 mg/5 mL, 1-2 tsp tid, qid
Pirbuterol	Maxair Autohaler	MDI: 200 μg/puff, 2 puffs q4-6h
Levalbuterol	Xopenex, Xopenex HFA	SVN: 0.31 mg/3 mL tid, 0.63 mg/3 mL tid, or 1.25 mg/3 mL tid; concentrate 1.25 mg/0.5 mL, tid MDI: 45 μg/puff, 2 puffs q4-6h
Anticholinergics (Chronic Obstructive Pulmonary Disease [COPD])		
Ipratropium bromide	Atrovent Atrovent HFA	MDI: 18 μg/puff, 2 puffs qid HFA MDI: 17 μg/puff, 2 puffs qid SVN: 0.02% solution (0.2 mg/mL) 500 μg tid, qid
Tiotropium	Spiriva	DPI: 18 μg/inhalation, 1 inhalation daily (one capsule)
Beta$_2$ Agents and Anticholinergic Agents		
Ipratropium and albuterol	Combivent	MDI: ipratropium 18 μg/puff and albuterol 90 μg/puff, 2 puffs qid
	DuoNeb	SVN: ipratropium 0.5 mg and albuterol 2.5 mg

Data from *Global Initiative for Asthma (GINA): Global Strategy for Asthma Management and Prevention, updated 2008*. Available at: www.goldcopd.org; and Gardenshire DS: *Rau's repiratory care pharmacology*, ed 7, St. Louis, 2008, Elsevier.
COPD, Chronic obstructive pulmonary disease; *DPI*, dry powder inhaler; *MDI*, metered dose inhaler; *SVN*, small volume nebulizer.

- beclomethasone dipropionate
- budesonide
- ciclesonide
- flunisolide
- fluticasone
- mometasone furoate
- triamcinolone acetonide

Common controller medications used in the treatment of asthma are presented in Table 12-1. Table 12-2 provides an overview of common reliever medications used to manage acute exacerbations of asthma.

TABLE 12-3 Classification of Severity of Acute Asthma Exacerbations

	Mild	Moderate	Severe	Respiratory Arrest Imminent
Symptoms				
Breathlessness	While walking	While talking (infant: softer, shorter cry; difficulty feeding)	While at rest (infant: stops feeding)	
	Can lie down	Prefers sitting	Sits upright	
Talks in	Sentences	Phrases	Words	
Alertness	May be agitated	Usually agitated	Usually agitated	Drowsy or confused
Signs				
Respiratory rate	Increased	Increased	Often >30/min	
		Guide on rates of breathing in awake children:		
		Age	**Normal Rate**	
		<2 mo	<60/min	
		2-12 mo	<50/min	
		1-5 yr	<40/min	
		6-8 yr	<30/min	
Use of accessory muscles; suprasternal retractions	Usually not	Commonly	Usually	Paradoxical thoraco-abdominal movement
Wheeze	Moderate, often only end expiratory	Loud; throughout exhalation	Usually loud; throughout inhalation and exhalation	Absence of wheeze
Pulse/min	<100	100-120	>120	Bradycardia
		Guide to normal pulse rates in children:		
		Age	**Normal Rate**	
		2-12 mo	<160/min	
		1-2 yr	<120/min	
		2-8 yr	<110/min	
Pulsus paradoxus	Absent <10 mm Hg	May be present 10-25 mm Hg	Often present >25 mm Hg (adult) 20-40 mm Hg (child)	Absence suggests respiratory muscle fatigue
Functional Assessment				
PEF (% predicted or % personal best)	80%	~50%-80%	<50% predicted or personal best or response lasts <2 h	
Pa_{O_2} (on air)	Normal (test not usually necessary)	>60 mm Hg (test not usually necessary)	<60 mm Hg: possible cyanosis	
and/or				
P_{CO_2}	<42 mm Hg (test not usually necessary)	<42 mm Hg (test not usually necessary)	≥42 mm Hg: possible respiratory failure	
Sa_{O_2} % (on air) at sea level	>95% (test not usually necessary)	91%-95%	<91%	
	Hypercapnia (hypoventilation) develops more readily in young children than in adults and adolescents.			

From National Asthma Education and Prevention Program, National Heart, Lung, and Blood Institute, Expert Panel Report 2: *Guidelines for the diagnosis and management of asthma*, NIH Pub No. 97, July 1997.

Note: The presence of several parameters, but not necessarily all, indicates the general classification of the exacerbation. Many of these parameters have note been systematically studied, so they serve only as general guides.

Component 4: Manage Asthma Exacerbations

Asthma exacerbation (also called an asthma attack or asthma episode) is defined as a progressive increase in shortness of breath, cough, wheezing, or chest tightness or a combination of these symptoms. A severe asthma exacerbation is life threatening. Table 12-3 provides a clinical scale to classify the severity of asthma exacerbations. The table categorizes the signs, symptoms and assessment into four categories: mild, moderate, severe and respiratory arrest imminent.

Component 5: Special Considerations in Managing Asthma

Special considerations to consider when managing asthma are:

- pregnancy
- surgery

- rhinitis, sinusitism and nasal polyps
- occupational asthma
- respiratory infection
- gastroesophageal reflux
- aspirin-induced asthma
- anaphalaxis

Respiratory Care Treatment Protocols

Oxygen Therapy Protocol

Oxygen therapy is used to treat hypoxemia, decrease the work of breathing, and decrease myocardial work. The hypoxemia that develops in asthma is usually caused by the hypoventilation and shuntlike effect associated with bronchospasm and increased airway secretions. Hypoxemia caused by a shuntlike effect can at least partly be corrected by oxygen therapy (see Oxygen Therapy Protocol, Protocol 9-1).

Bronchopulmonary Hygiene Therapy Protocol

Because of the excessive mucous production and secretion accumulation associated with asthma, a number of bronchial hygiene treatment modalities may be used to enhance the mobilization of bronchial secretions (see Bronchopulmonary Hygiene Therapy Protocol, Protocol 9-2).

Aerosolized Medication Protocol

Both sympathomimetic and parasympatholytic agents commonly are used in the treatment of asthma to induce bronchial smooth muscle relaxation (see Aerosolized Medication Protocol, Protocol 9-4).

Mechanical Ventilation Protocol

Because acute ventilatory failure is associated with **status asthmaticus,** continuous mechanical ventilation may be required to maintain an adequate ventilatory status. Status asthmaticus is defined as a severe asthmatic episode that does not respond to conventional pharmacologic therapy. When the patient becomes fatigued, the ventilatory rate decreases. Clinically, the patient demonstrates a progressive decrease in $Pa{O_2}$ and pH and a steady increase in $Pa{CO_2}$ (acute ventilatory failure). If this trend is not reversed, mechanical ventilation becomes necessary (see Mechanical Ventilation Protocols, Protocols 9-5, 9-6, and 9-7).

CASE STUDY

Asthma

Admitting History and Physical Examination

A 8-year-old girl was admitted to the emergency department (ED) in severe respiratory distress. Her respiratory symptoms dated to age 6 months, when she first developed wheezing. She was hospitalized in different hospitals on a number of occasions and was usually managed satisfactorily with aerosolized albuterol, intravenous (IV) steroids, and aminophylline. She developed a cough and wheezing the night before admission and became progressively worse during the night. Her cough was nonproductive. At 8 AM, she was brought to the ED.

Physical examination revealed an extremely anxious, well-developed female child in acute respiratory distress. She stated, "It is very hard for me to breathe." Her vital signs were as follows: blood pressure 152/115, pulse 220/min, and respiratory rate 62/min. Her temperature was 100° F. Her extremities appeared cyanotic, and her tonsils were enlarged. She was using her accessory muscles of respiration. On auscultation, rhonchi and wheezing could be heard throughout both lung fields. Her PEFR was 70 L/min. (Her personal best was about 200 to 250 L/min.) Arterial blood gases on 2 L/min nasal cannula oxygen were pH 7.17, $Pa{CO_2}$ 71, HCO_3^- 22, and $Pa{O_2}$ 47. A chest x-ray examination was ordered but not performed. The physician ordered a respiratory care consultation and stated that she did not want to commit the patient to a ventilator at this time if possible. The physician asked that aggressive noninvasive pulmonary care be tried first. At this time the respiratory care practitioner documented the following.

Respiratory Assessment and Plan

S Patient stated, "It is very hard for me to breathe"

O Vital signs: BP 152/115, HR 220, RR 62, T 100°. Cyanotic and using accessory muscles. Wheezing and rhonchi over both lungs. PEFR: 70 L/min. ABGs pH 7.17, $Pa{CO_2}$ 71, HCO_3^- 22, and $Pa{O_2}$ 47. No CXR yet.

A
- Severe exacerbation of asthma
- Respiratory distress (increased heart rate, blood pressure, respiratory rate)
- Bronchospasm (wheezing, decreased PEFR, history)
- Excessive airway secretions (rhonchi)
- Acute ventilatory failure (acute respiratory acidosis) with moderate to severe hypoxemia (ABG)
- Metabolic acidosis also likely (both pH and HCO_3^- are both lower than expected for a $Pa{CO_2}$ of 71). Likely caused by lactic acid (low $Pa{O_2}$ of 47)

P **Oxygen Therapy Protocol** ($F{IO_2}$ 80%-100% via oxygen nonrebreather mask). Monitor $Sp{O_2}$ with oximeter. **Aerosolized Medication Therapy Protocol** (med. neb. every 30 minutes with albuterol 0.15 mL in 2.0 mL normal saline via nebulizer). Monitor PEFR and breath sounds. **Bronchopulmonary Hygiene Therapy Protocol** (cough and deep breathe as tolerated). Monitor breath sounds. Place endotracheal tube and mechanical ventilator on standby. Repeat ABG in 30 minutes. Respiratory care practitioner to remain in ED.

In addition to this plan, the patient was treated vigorously with IV aminophylline, steroids, and a beclomethasone inhaler (2 puffs every 30 minutes × 4 per emergency room standing orders for asthma) over the next 2 hours. After 2 hours of therapy, her aminophylline blood level was therapeutic at 12 mg/L. Although the patient seemed to improve slightly, her next arterial blood gas reading showed that her Pa_{CO_2} had increased slightly to 79.

The respiratory therapist notified the doctor immediately. After this, the patient was lightly sedated, paralyzed (with vecuronium [Norcuron]), intubated, and placed on a mechanical ventilator. The ventilator parameters were set per the **Mechanical Ventilation Protocol.** The next morning, on an F_{IO_2} of 0.4 and a mechanical ventilator in SIMV mode at a backup rate of 12 breaths per minute, her arterial blood gases were pH 7.38, Pa_{CO_2} 37, HCO_3^- 23, and Pa_{O_2} 124. Her vital signs were blood pressure 122/87, heart rate 93, temperature 98.8° F. Her wheezes and rhonchi had diminished but were still present. At this point, the following information was recorded.

Respiratory Assessment and Plan

S N/A (patient sedated and paralyzed on ventilator)

O Sedated, paralyzed, fewer wheezes and rhonchi. Vital signs: BP 122/87, HR 93, T 98.8° F. ABG: pH 7.38, Pa_{CO_2} 37, HCO_3^- 23, Pa_{O_2} 124 (on mechanical ventilator in SIMV mode at a ventilatory rate of 12 and an F_{IO_2} of 0.4)

A
- Less bronchospasm (decreased wheezing, normal ABGs)
- Less bronchial secretions (decreased rhonchi)
- Adequately ventilated and oxygenated on present ventilator settings (ABG)

P Discuss with physician: D/C Norcuron. Continue in-line med. nebs. IMV wean and O_2 wean as per **Mechanical Ventilation Protocol**. Continue to monitor O_2 saturation.

The patient remained intubated for another 24 hours, at which time her lungs were clear and when suctioned returned scant but clear secretions. She was weaned from the ventilator with ease and was extubated shortly thereafter. The patient was discharged the following day, after review of the Asthma Action Plan with her parents.

Discussion

Asthma is a potentially fatal disease—largely because its severity is often unrecognized in the home or outpatient setting. The clinical manifestations presented in this case can all be easily traced back through the **Bronchospasm clinical scenario** (see Figure 9-11) and **Excessive Airway Secretions clinical scenario** (see Figure 9-12). For example, the patient's increased blood pressure, heart rate, and respiratory rate can all be followed back to the hypoxemia caused by the decreased $\dot{V}/\dot{Q}$ ratio, pulmonary shunting, and venous admixture activated by bronchospasm and **Excessive Bronchial Secretions** (see Figure 9-11 and 9-12). The patient's anxiety and previous use of beta$_2$-agonists also may have contributed to her abnormal vital signs (tachycardia).

In addition, the decreased PEFR, use of accessory muscles, diminished breath sounds, rhonchi, and wheezing reflect the increased airway resistance and air trapping caused by the **Bronchospasm** (see Figure 9-11) and **Excessive Airway Secretions** (see Figure 9-12). The fact that the patient's arterial blood gas values showed acute ventilatory failure confirmed that the patient was in the severe stages of an asthmatic episode and that mechanical ventilation was justified, although vigorous routine respiratory care was first tried to prevent this.

After the initial assessment, the respiratory care practitioner chose a fairly aggressive approach to both the **Oxygen Therapy Protocol** (Protocol 9-1) and the **Aerosolized Medication Therapy Protocol** (Protocol 9-4). Use of a nonrebreather oxygen therapy mask at initially high F_{IO_2} levels (0.8 to 1.0) allowed him to adjust the F_{IO_2} in small, precise concentration changes while not risking rebreathing of expired air. Frequent monitoring of ABGs and Sp_{O_2} levels was appropriate. Note also the frequency with which he chose to administer inhaled bronchodilators (every 30 minutes) in the **Aerosolized Medication Therapy Protocol.** An alternative approach, often used in pediatric patients, would be to use *continuous* bronchodilator or aerosol therapy.

The manner in which any therapy modality is up-regulated may be (1) a different aerosolized drug or procedure, (2) a larger dose of a drug or therapy, or (3) more frequent use of such drugs or therapy. In this case, he chose the last course, only to see it fail (the patient required intubation).

Among the lessons to be learned here is that some asthmatic episodes worsen despite vigorous therapy. This patient received optimal emergent treatment of her resistant asthma but required intubation and mechanical ventilation nonetheless. Almost continuous assessment by the respiratory care practitioner is necessary if more aggressive therapy (including induced sedation, paralysis, and mechanical ventilation) is to be effective.

The use of IV aminophylline in the emergency treatment of acute asthma in the emergency department is controversial. Care must be taken to avoid theophylline toxicity, and symptoms of toxicity often do not reflect serum concentrations of the drug. The acutely ill asthmatic requires almost continuous monitoring and frequent SOAP notes if the patient care team is to be constantly apprised of the patient's progress. The two such notes recorded here are but a small portion of the more than 14 notes that we found on analysis of the patient's medical record after her ED discharge alone.

SELF-ASSESSMENT QUESTIONS

evolve Answers to questions can be found on Evolve. To access additional student assessment questions and case studies for application of text material to real-life scenarios, visit **http://evolve.elsevier.com/DesJardins/respiratory**.

1. During an asthmatic episode, the smooth muscle of the bronchi may hypertrophy as much as

a. Two times normal thickness
b. Three times normal thickness
c. Four times normal thickness
d. Five times normal thickness

2. Asthma is associated with which of the following?

1. Increase in goblet cells
2. Damage to cilia and deduced mucous clearance
3. Increase in bronchial gland size
4. Decrease in eosinophils

a. 1 and 3 only
b. 2 and 4 only
c. 1, 2, and 3 only
d. 2, 3, and 4 only

3. During an extrinsic-type asthma attack, the lymphoid tissue cells form which antibody?

a. IgA
b. IgM
c. IgG
d. IgE

4. When chemical mediators from mast cells are released:

1. Bronchial dilation occurs
2. Bronchial gland hypersecretion occurs
3. Blood vessels constrict
4. Tissue edema occurs

a. 1 only
b. 2 only
c. 2 and 4 only
d. 1 and 3 only

5. Which of the following are associated with intrinsic asthma?

1. NSAIDs
2. Respiratory syncytial virus
3. Gastroesophageal reflux
4. Bisulfites

a. 2 and 3 only
b. 3 and 4 only
c. 2, 3, and 4 only
d. 1, 2, 3, and 4

6. When pulsus paradoxus appears during an asthma attack:

1. Left ventricle filling is increased during inspiration
2. Cardiac output decreases during expiration
3. Left ventricle filling increases during expiration
4. Cardiac output increases during inspiration

a. 1 only
b. 2 only
c. 3 only
d. 1 and 2 only

7. During an asthmatic episode, which of the following abnormal lung volume and capacity findings are found?

1. Increased FRC
2. Decreased ERV
3. Increased FEV_1
4. Decreased RV

a. 1 only
b. 2 only
c. 1 and 2 only
d. 3 and 4 only

8. During mast cell degranulation, which of the following chemical mediators are released?

1. NCFs
2. ECF-A
3. Histamine
4. Leukotrienes

a. 2 only
b. 3 only
c. 2 and 4 only
d. 1, 2, 3, and 4

9. Patients commonly exhibit which of the following arterial blood gas values early during an acute mild to moderate asthmatic episode?

1. Increased pH
2. Increased $Paco_2$
3. Decreased HCO_3^-
4. Decreased Pao_2

a. 1 and 3 only
b. 2 and 4 only
c. 1, 2, and 3 only
d. 1, 3, and 4 only

10. The onset of intrinsic asthma usually occurs after which age?

a. 20 years
b. 30 years
c. 40 years
d. 50 years

Bronchiectasis

13

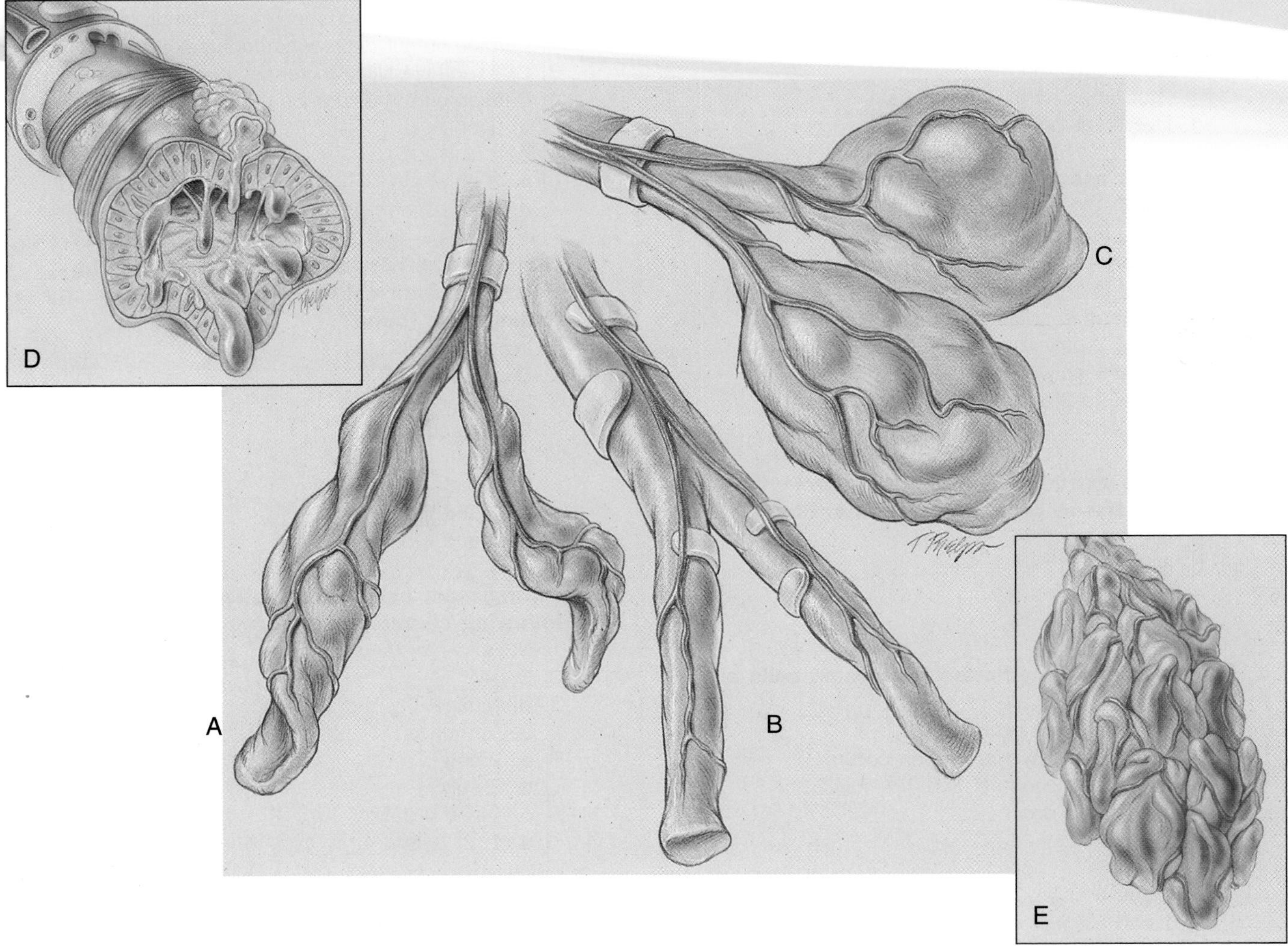

FIGURE 13-1 Bronchiectasis. **A**, Varicose bronchiectasis. **B**, Cylindrical bronchiectasis. **C**, Cystic (saccular) bronchiectasis. Also illustrated are excessive bronchial secretions (**D**) and atelectasis (**E**), which are both common anatomic alterations of the lungs in this disease.

Chapter Objectives

After reading this chapter, you will be able to:

- Describe the anatomic alterations of the lungs associated with bronchiectasis, including the following:
  - Varicose (fusiform) form of bronchiectasis
  - Cylindrical (tubular) form of bronchiectasis
  - Cystic (saccular) form of bronchiectasis
- Differentiate between the following possible types of bronchiectasis:
  - Acquired bronchiectasis
  - Congenital bronchiectasis
- Describe the cardiopulmonary clinical manifestations associated with bronchiectasis.
- Describe the general management of bronchiectasis.
- Describe the clinical strategies and rationales of the SOAPs presented in the case study.
- Define key terms and complete self-assessment questions at the end of the chapter and on Evolve.

Key Terms

Acquired Bronchiectasis
Congenital Bronchiectasis

Cylindrical (Tubular) Bronchiectasis
Cystic (Saccular) Bronchiectasis
Kartagener's Syndrome
Varicose (Fusiform) Bronchiectasis

Chapter Outline

Anatomic Alterations of the Lungs

Bronchiectasis is characterized by chronic dilation and distortion of one or more bronchi as a result of extensive inflammation and destruction of the bronchial wall cartilage, blood vessels, elastic tissue, and smooth muscle components. One or both lungs may be involved. Bronchiectasis is commonly limited to a lobe or segment and is frequently found in the lower lobes. The smaller bronchi, with less supporting cartilage, are predominantly affected.

Because of bronchial wall destruction, the mucociliary clearance mechanism is impaired. This results in the accumulation of copious amounts of bronchial secretions and blood that often become foul-smelling because of secondary colonization with anaerobic organisms. This condition may lead to secondary bronchial smooth muscle constriction and fibrosis. The small bronchi and bronchioles distal to the affected areas become partially or totally obstructed with secretions. This condition leads to one or both of the following anatomic alterations: (1) hyperinflation of the distal alveoli as a result of expiratory check-valve obstruction or (2) atelectasis, consolidation, and fibrosis as a result of complete bronchial obstruction.

Three forms or anatomic varieties of bronchiectasis have been described: cylindrical (tubular), varicose (fusiform), and cystic (saccular).

Cylindrical Bronchiectasis (Tubular Bronchiectasis)

In **cylindrical (tubular) bronchiectasis,** the bronchi are dilated and rigid and have regular outlines similar to a tube. X-ray examination shows that the dilated bronchi fail to taper for 6 to 10 generations and then appear to end abruptly because of mucous obstruction (see Figure 13-1, *B*).

Varicose Bronchiectasis (Fusiform Bronchiectasis)

In **varicose (fusiform) bronchiectasis,** the bronchi are dilated and constricted in an irregular fashion similar to varicose veins, ultimately resulting in a distorted, bulbous shape (see Figure 13-1, *A*).

Cystic Bronchiectasis (Saccular Bronchiectasis)

In **cystic (saccular) bronchiectasis,** the bronchi progressively increase in diameter until they end in large, cystlike sacs in the lung parenchyma. This form of bronchiectasis causes the greatest damage to the tracheobronchial tree. The bronchial walls become composed of fibrous tissue alone—cartilage, elastic tissue, and smooth muscle are all absent (see Figure 13-1, *C*).

The following are the major pathologic or structural changes associated with bronchiectasis:

- Chronic dilation and distortion of bronchial airways
- Excessive production of often foul-smelling sputum (see Figure 13-1, *D*)
- Bronchospasm
- Hyperinflation of alveoli (air trapping)
- Atelectasis (see Figure 13-1, *E*)
- Consolidation and parenchymal fibrosis
- Hemorrhage secondary to bronchial arterial erosion

Etiology and Epidemiology

Bronchiectasis is not as common today as it was a few decades ago because of increased use of antibiotics for lower respiratory infections. The underlying cause of bronchiectasis is not known in more than 60% of the cases. Bronchiectasis is commonly classified by cause as being either **acquired bronchiectasis** or **congenital bronchiectasis.**

Acquired Bronchiectasis

Recurrent Pulmonary Infection

Bronchiectasis is commonly seen in individuals who have recurrent and prolonged episodes of lower respiratory tract infections (e.g., pneumonia, tuberculosis, and fungal infections). For example, children who have frequent bouts of bronchopneumonia—because of the respiratory complications of measles, chickenpox, whooping cough, or influenza—may acquire some form of bronchiectasis later in life.

Bronchial Obstruction

Bronchial obstruction caused by aspiration of a foreign body, mucous plugs, tumors, or enlarged hilar lymph nodes may result in bronchiectasis distal to the obstruction. These conditions impair the mucociliary clearance mechanism, and this impairment in turn favors the development of necrotizing bacterial infections.

Inhalation and Aspiration

Bronchiectasis is sometimes seen in patients who have inhaled large amounts of fumes (e.g., ammonia) or who chronically aspirate gastric fluids.

Congenital Bronchiectasis

Cystic Fibrosis

It is estimated that cystic fibrosis causes approximately 50% of the bronchiectasis cases in the United States today. Because of the impairment of the mucociliary clearance mechanism—and the abundance of stagnant, thick mucus—associated with cystic fibrosis, bronchial obstruction from mucous plugging and bronchial wall infection frequently result. The necrotizing inflammation that develops under these conditions often leads to secondary bronchiectasis.

Kartagener's Syndrome

Kartagener's syndrome (also known as Kartagener's triad, Siewert's syndrome, dextrocardia-bronchiectasis-sinusitis syndrome, primary ciliary dyskinesia [PCD], and immotile ciliary syndrome) is an autosomal recessive genetic disorder. Kartagener's syndrome is described as a triad disorder consisting of bronchiectasis, dextrocardia (having the heart on the right side of the chest), and rhinosinusitis. Patients with Kartagener's syndrome have defective cilia lining throughout the respiratory tract, lower and upper sinuses, Eustachian tubes, middle ears, and fallopian tubes. Because of the defective cilia lining throughout the tracheobronchial tree, the patient is unable to adequately clear airway secretions and pathogenic bacteria. This condition leads to chronic mucous retention, recurrent respiratory tract infections, and damaged airway walls. Kartagener's syndrome accounts for as much as 20% of all congenital bronchiectasis.

Systemic Disorders

Bronchiectasis is associated with several systemic conditions such as rheumatologic disorders, inflammatory bowel disease, and acquired immunodeficiency syndrome (AIDS).

Text continued on p. 208

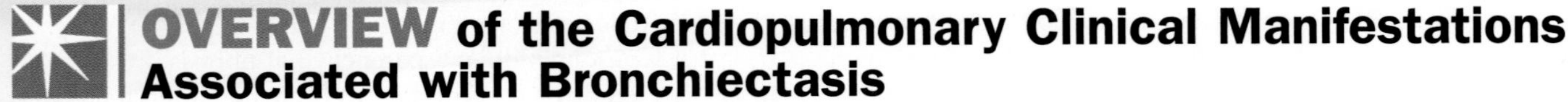

OVERVIEW of the Cardiopulmonary Clinical Manifestations Associated with Bronchiectasis

The following clinical manifestations result from the pathophysiologic mechanisms caused (or activated) by **Excessive Bronchial Secretions** (see Figure 9-12), **Bronchospasm** (see Figure 9-11), **Atelectasis** (see Figure 9-8), **Consolidation** (see Figure 9-9), and **Increased Alveolar-Capillary Membrane Thickness**) (See Figure 9-10)—the major anatomic alterations of the lungs associated with bronchiectasis (see Figure 13-1).

CLINICAL DATA OBTAINED AT THE PATIENT'S BEDSIDE

Depending on the amount of bronchial secretions and the degree of bronchial destruction and fibrosis associated with bronchiectasis, the disease may create an obstructive or a restrictive lung disorder or a combination of both. If the majority of the bronchial airways are only partially obstructed, the bronchiectasis manifests primarily as an obstructive lung disorder. If, on the other hand, the majority of the bronchial airways are completely obstructed, the distal alveoli collapse, atelectasis results, and the bronchiectasis manifests primarily as a restrictive disorder. Finally, if the disease is limited to a relatively small portion of the lung—as it often is—the patient may not have any of the following clinical manifestations.

The Physical Examination

Vital Signs

Increased Respiratory Rate (Tachypnea)

Several pathophysiologic mechanisms operating simultaneously may lead to an increased ventilatory rate:

- Stimulation of peripheral chemoreceptors (hypoxemia)
- Decreased lung compliance and increased ventilatory rate relationship
- Anxiety

Increased Heart Rate (Pulse) and Blood Pressure

Use of Accessory Muscles during Inspiration

Use of Accessory Muscles during Expiration

Pursed-Lip Breathing (When Primarily Obstructive in Nature)

Increased Anteroposterior Chest Diameter (Barrel Chest) (When Primarily Obstructive in Nature)

Cyanosis

Digital Clubbing

Peripheral Edema and Venous Distention

Because polycythemia and cor pulmonale are associated with severe bronchiectasis, the following may be seen:

- Distended neck veins
- Pitting edema
- Enlarged and tender liver

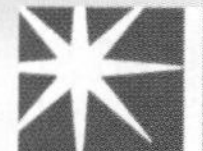

OVERVIEW of the Cardiopulmonary Clinical Manifestations Associated with Bronchiectasis—cont'd

Cough, Sputum Production, and Hemoptysis

Chronic cough with production of large quantities of foul-smelling sputum is a hallmark of bronchiectasis. A 24-hour collection of sputum is usually voluminous and tends to settle into several different layers. Streaks of blood are seen frequently in the sputum, presumably originating from necrosis of the bronchial walls and erosion of bronchial blood vessels. Frank hemoptysis may also occur from time to time, but it is rarely life threatening. Because of the excessive bronchial secretions, secondary bacterial infections are frequent. *Haemophilus influenzae, Streptococcus, Pseudomonas aeruginosa,* and various anaerobic organisms are commonly cultured from the sputum of patients with bronchiectasis.

The productive cough in bronchiectasis is triggered by the large amount of secretions that fill the tracheobronchial tree. The stagnant secretions stimulate the subepithelial mechanoreceptors, which in turn produce a vagal reflex that triggers a cough. The subepithelial mechanoreceptors are found in the trachea, bronchi, and bronchioles, but they are predominantly located in the upper airways.

Chest Assessment Findings

When the bronchiectasis is primarily obstructive in nature:

- Decreased tactile and vocal fremitus
- Hyperresonant percussion note
- Diminished breath sounds
- Wheezing
- Rhonchi and wheezing

When the bronchiectasis is primarily restrictive in nature (over areas of atelectasis and consolidation):

- Increased tactile and vocal fremitus
- Bronchial breath sounds
- Crackles
- Whispered pectoriloquy
- Dull percussion note

CLINICAL DATA OBTAINED FROM LABORATORY TESTS AND SPECIAL PROCEDURES

Pulmonary Function Test Findings
Moderate to Severe Bronchiectasis
(When Primarily Obstructive Lung Pathophysiology)

FORCED EXPIRATORY FLOW RATE FINDINGS

FVC	FEV_T	FEV_1/FVC ratio	$FEF_{25\%-75\%}$
↓	↓	↓	↓

$FEF_{50\%}$	$FEF_{200-1200}$	PEFR	MVV
↓	↓	↓	↓

LUNG VOLUME AND CAPACITY FINDINGS

V_T	IRV	ERV	RV
N or ↑	N or ↓	N or ↓	↑

VC	IC	FRC	TLC	RV/TLC ratio
↓	N or ↓	↑	N or ↑	N or ↑

Pulmonary Function Test Findings
Moderate to Severe Bronchiectasis
(When Primarily Restrictive Lung Pathophysiology)

FORCED EXPIRATORY FLOW RATE FINDINGS

FVC	FEV_T	FEV_1/FVC ratio	$FEF_{25\%-75\%}$
↓	N or ↓	N or ↑	N or ↓

$FEF_{50\%}$	$FEF_{200-1200}$	PEFR	MVV
N or ↓	N or ↓	N or ↓	N or ↓

LUNG VOLUME AND CAPACITY FINDINGS

V_T	IRV	ERV	RV
N or ↓	↓	↓	↓

VC	IC	FRC	TLC	RV/TLC ratio
↓	↓	↓	↓	N

Arterial Blood Gases
Bronchiectasis

MILD TO MODERATE STAGES
Acute Alveolar Hyperventilation with Hypoxemia
(Acute Respiratory Alkalosis)

pH	$Paco_2$	HCO_3^-	Pao_2
↑	↓	↓ (slightly)	↓

SEVERE STAGE
Chronic Ventilatory Failure with Hypoxemia
(Compensated Respiratory Acidosis)

pH	$Paco_2$	HCO_3^-	Pao_2
N	↑	↑ (significantly)	↓

Acute Ventilatory Changes Superimposed on Chronic Ventilatory Failure

Because acute ventilatory changes are frequently seen in patients with chronic ventilatory failure, the respiratory care practitioner must be familiar with and alert for the following:

- Acute alveolar hyperventilation superimposed on chronic ventilatory failure, and/or
- Acute ventilatory failure (acute hypoventilation) superimposed on chronic ventilatory failure

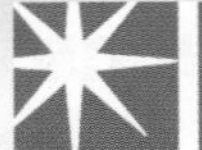

OVERVIEW of the Cardiopulmonary Clinical Manifestations Associated with Bronchiectasis—cont'd

Oxygenation Indices*
Bronchiectasis
Moderate to Severe Stages

$\dot{Q}_S/\dot{Q}_T$	DO_2[†]	$\dot{V}O_2$	$C(a\text{-}\bar{v})O_2$	O_2ER	$S\bar{v}O_2$
↑	↓	N	N	↑	↓

[†]The DO_2 may be normal in patients who have compensated to the decreased oxygenation status with (1) an increased cardiac output, (2) an increased hemoglobin level, or (3) a combination of both. When the DO_2 is normal, the O_2ER is usually normal.

Hemodynamic Indices[†]
Bronchiectasis Moderate to Severe Stages

CVP	RAP	$\overline{PA}$	PCWP	CO	SV
↑	↑	↑	N	N	N
SVI	**CI**	**RVSWI**	**LVSWI**	**PVR**	**SVR**
N	N	↑	N	↑	N

ABNORMAL LABORATORY TESTS AND PROCEDURES

Hematology

- Increased hematocrit and hemoglobin
- Elevated white blood count (WBC) if patient is acutely infected

Sputum Examination

- *Streptococcus pneumoniae*
- *Haemophilus influenzae*
- *Pseudomonas aeruginosa*
- Anaerobic organisms

RADIOLOGIC FINDINGS

Chest Radiograph

When the Bronchiectasis Is Primarily Obstructive in Nature

- Translucent (dark) lung fields
- Depressed or flattened diaphragms
- Long and narrow heart (pulled down by diaphragms)
- Enlarged heart
- Areas of consolidation and/or atelectasis may or may not be seen

When the pathophysiology of bronchiectasis is primarily obstructive in nature, the lungs become hyperinflated, leading to an increased functional residual capacity and depressed diaphragms. Because right and left ventricular enlargement and failure may develop as secondary problems during the advanced stages of bronchiectasis, an enlarged heart may be seen on the chest radiograph.

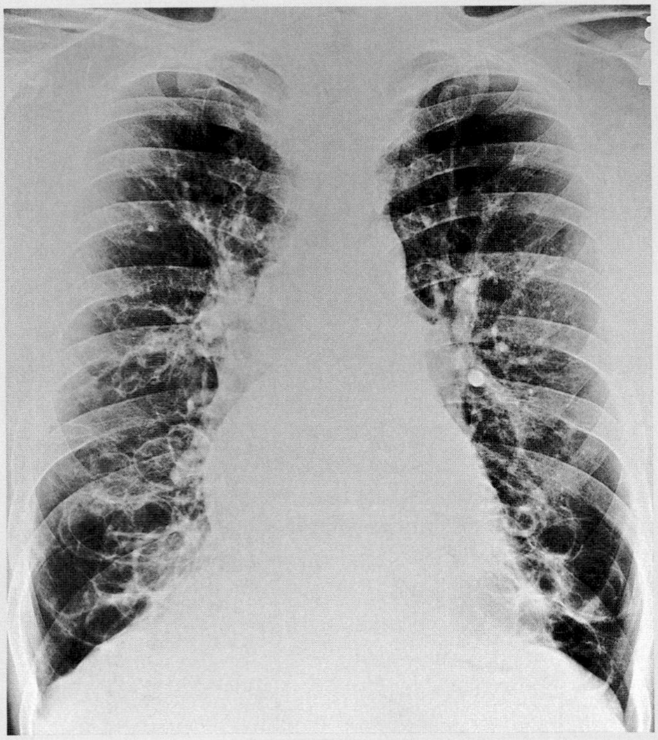

FIGURE 13-2 Gross cystic bronchiectasis. Posteroanterior chest radiograph showing overinflated lungs. There are multiple ring opacities, most obvious at the lung bases, ranging from 3 to 15 mm in diameter. (From Hansell DM, Armstrong P, Lynch DA, McAdams HP, eds: *Imaging of diseases of the chest,* ed 4, Philadelphia, 2005, Elsevier.)

Although the chest radiograph is not be as valuable as the computed tomography (CT) scan in identifying a specific type of bronchiectasis (i.e., cystic, varicose, or cylindrical), a careful analysis of chest radiographs usually reveals abnormalities in the majority of the cases. Figure 13-2, for example, shows a patient with gross cystic bronchiectasis and overinflated lungs.

When the Bronchiectasis Is Primarily Restrictive in Nature

- Atelectasis and consolidation
- Infiltrates (suggesting pneumonia)
- Increased opacity

In generalized bronchiectasis, such as commonly seen in cystic fibrosis, there is usually overinflation of the lungs. However, when the bronchiectasis is localized, the chest radiograph often reveals a restrictive pathology such as atelectasis, consolidation, or infiltrates. When atelectasis and consolidation develop as a result of bronchiectasis, an increased

*$C(a\text{-}\bar{v})O_2$, Arterial-venous oxygen difference; DO_2, total oxygen delivery; O_2ER, oxygen extraction ratio; $\dot{Q}_S/\dot{Q}_T$, pulmonary shunt fraction; $S\bar{v}O_2$, mixed venous oxygen saturation; $\dot{V}O_2$, oxygen consumption.

[†]*CO,* Cardiac output; *CVP,* central venous pressure; *LVSWI,* left ventricular stroke work index; $\overline{PA}$, mean pulmonary artery pressure; *PCWP,* pulmonary capillary wedge pressure; *PVR,* pulmonary vascular resistance; *RAP,* right atrial pressure; *RVSWI,* right ventricular stroke work index; *SV,* stroke volume; *SVI,* stroke volume index; *SVR,* systemic vascular resistance.

OVERVIEW of the Cardiopulmonary Clinical Manifestations Associated with Bronchiectasis—cont'd

opacity and reduced lung volume are seen in these areas on the radiograph. For example, Figure 13-3 illustrates a marked volume loss in a patient with left lower lobe bronchiectasis. Figure 13-4 shows a patient with Kartagener's syndrome with severe volume loss.

Bronchogram

Bronchography (the injection of an opaque contrast material into the tracheobronchial tree) is occasionally performed on patients with bronchiectasis. Bronchograms may be useful in diagnosing bronchiectasis and delineating the extent and type of tracheobronchial involvement. In cylindrical bronchiectasis, the bronchogram shows dilated, cylinder-shaped bronchioles (Figure 13-5). In cystic bronchiectasis, the bronchogram shows large, saclike structures; fibrotic markings; associated atelectasis; and adjacent emphysema (Figure 13-6). In varicose bronchiectasis, the bronchogram may show bronchi that are dilated and constricted in an irregular fashion and terminate

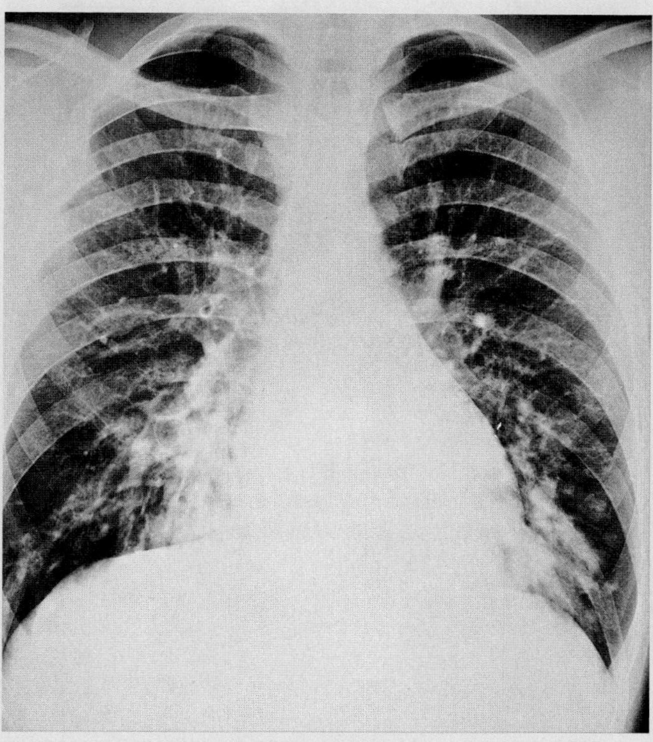

FIGURE 13-3 Left lower lobe bronchiectasis. The marked volume loss of left lower lobe is indicated by a depressed hilum, vertical left mainstem bronchus, mediastinal shift, and left-sided transradiancy. (From Hansell DM, Armstrong P, Lynch DA, McAdams HP, eds: *Imaging of diseases of the chest,* ed 4, Philadelphia, 2005, Elsevier.)

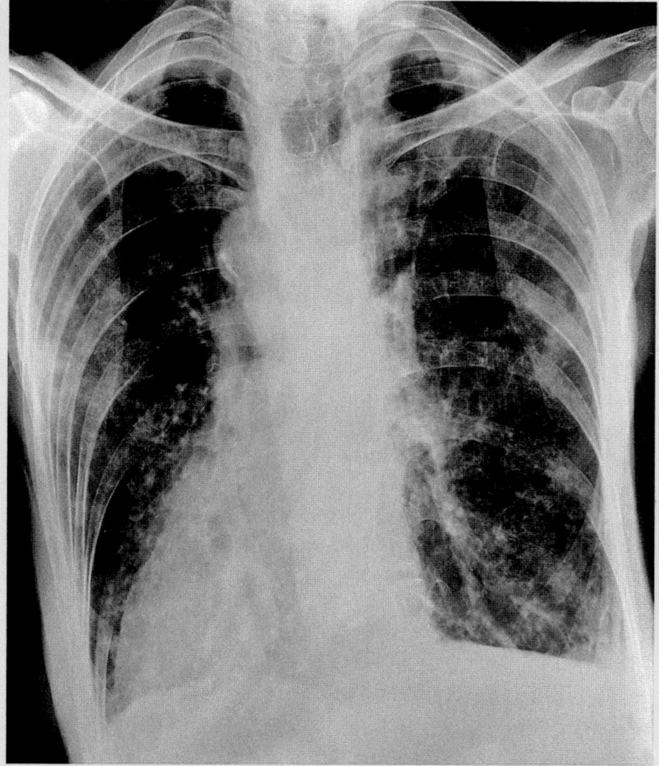

FIGURE 13-4 Ciliary dyskinesia syndrome–Kartagener's syndrome. This 62-year-old woman gave a 40-year history consistent with bronchiectasis. The aortic arch, descending aorta, heart, and gastric air bubble are all on the right. There is diffuse complex pulmonary shadowing with many ring opacities. Broad-branching band shadows can just be seen through the heart and represent dilated fluid-filled airways. (From Hansell DM, Armstrong P, Lynch DA, McAdams HP, eds: *Imaging of diseases of the chest,* ed 4, Philadelphia, 2005, Elsevier.)

OVERVIEW of the Cardiopulmonary Clinical Manifestations Associated with Bronchiectasis—cont'd

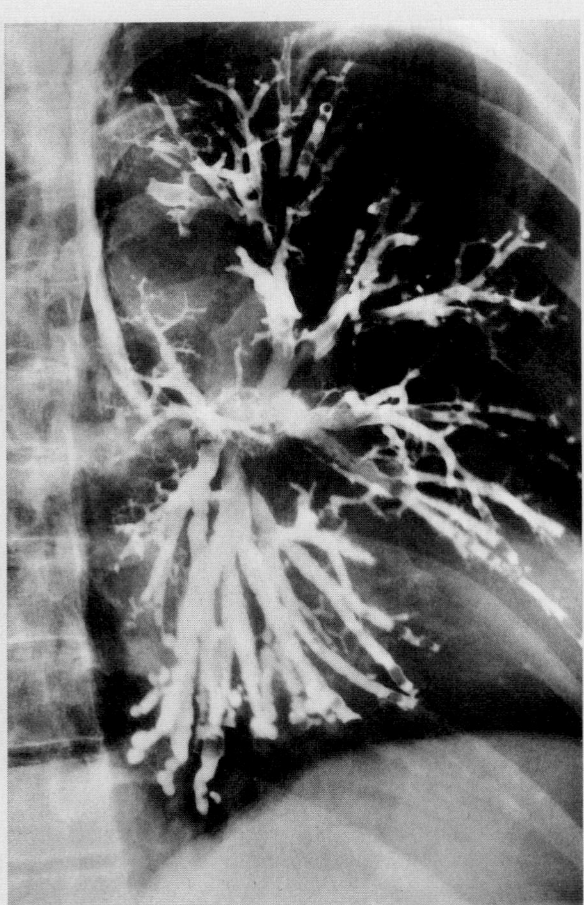

FIGURE 13-5 Cylindrical bronchiectasis. Left posterior oblique projection of a left bronchogram showing cylindrical bronchiectasis affecting the whole of the lower lobe except for the superior segment. Few side branches fill. Basal airways are crowded together, indicating volume loss of the lower lobe, a common finding in bronchiectasis. (From Hansell DM, Armstrong P, Lynch DA, McAdams HP, eds: *Imaging of diseases of the chest,* ed 4, Philadelphia, 2005, Elsevier.)

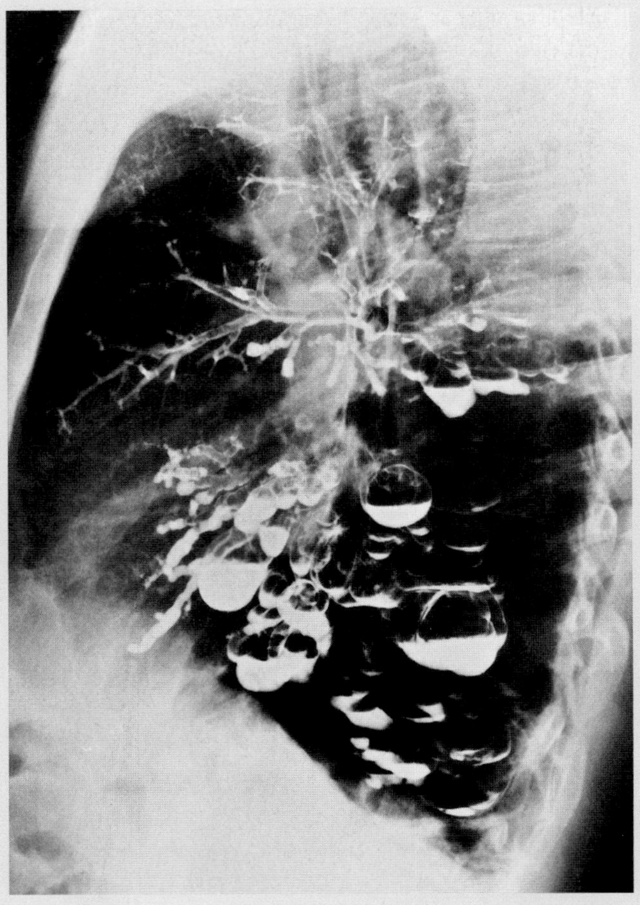

FIGURE 13-6 Cystic (saccular) bronchiectasis. Right lateral bronchogram showing cystic bronchiectasis affecting mainly the lower lobe and posterior segment of the upper lobe. (From Hansell DM, Armstrong P, Lynch DA, McAdams HP, eds: *Imaging of diseases of the chest,* ed 4, Philadelphia, 2005, Elsevier.)

in a distorted, bulbous shape (Figure 13-7). CT of the chest has largely replaced this technique.

Computed Tomography (CT Scan)

Increased bronchial wall opacity is often seen. The bronchial walls may appear as follows:

- Thick
- Dilated
- Characterized by ring lines or clusters
- Signet ring–shaped
- Flame-shaped

The CT scan changes may include many findings that are similar to those seen on the chest radiograph. The bronchial walls may appear thick, dilated, or as rings of opacities arranged in lines or clusters. A characteristic appearance in bronchiectasis is the end-on signet ring opacity produced by the ring shadow of a dilated airway with its accompanying artery (Figure 13-8).

The specific type of bronchiectasis can be confirmed with the CT scan. For example, Figure 13-9 confirms the presence of cylindrical bronchiectasis. Figure 13-10 shows varicose bronchiectasis and Figure 13-11 shows cystic bronchiectasis. Airways that are filled with secretions produce rounded or flame-shaped opacities that can be identified by following them through adjacent sections to unfilled airways. The CT scan also confirms atelectasis, consolidation, fibrosis, scarring, and hyperinflation.

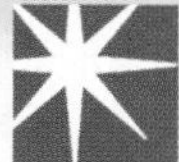

OVERVIEW of the Cardiopulmonary Clinical Manifestations Associated with Bronchiectasis—cont'd

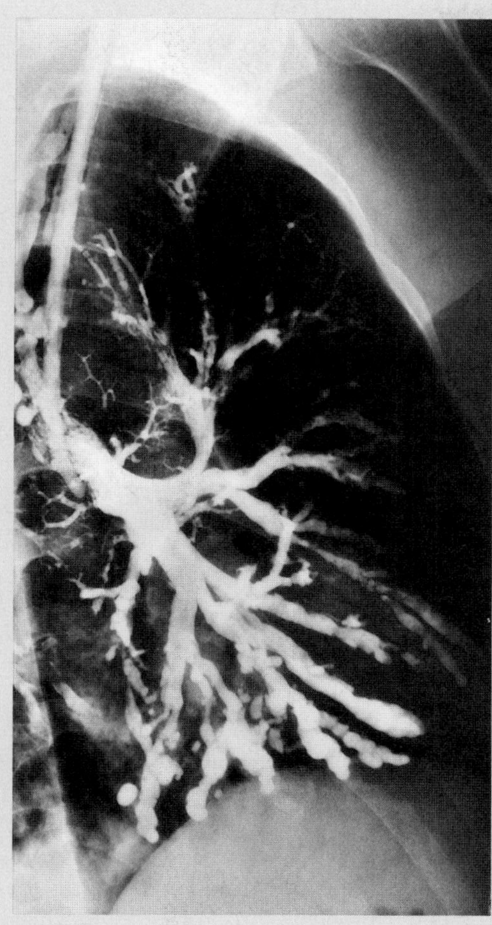

FIGURE 13-7 Varicose bronchiectasis. Left posterior oblique projection of left bronchogram in a patient with the ciliary dyskinesia syndrome. All basal bronchi are affected by varicose bronchiectasis. (From Hansell DM, Armstrong P, Lynch DA, McAdams HP, eds: *Imaging of diseases of the chest,* ed 4, Philadelphia, 2005, Elsevier.)

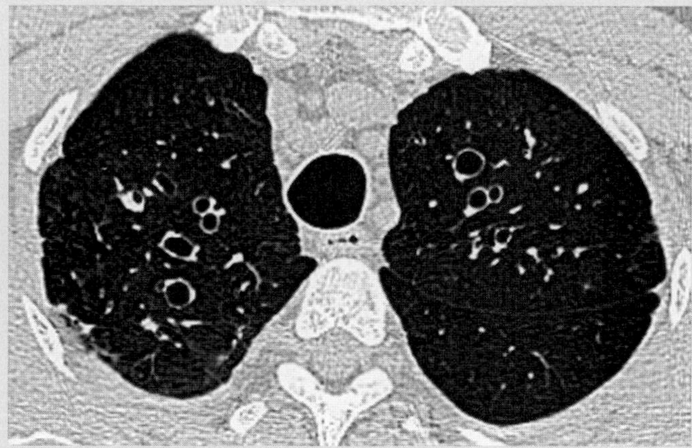

FIGURE 13-8 Signet ring sign in patient with cystic fibrosis. (From Hansell DM, Armstrong P, Lynch DA, McAdams HP, eds: *Imaging of diseases of the chest,* ed 4, Philadelphia, 2005, Elsevier.)

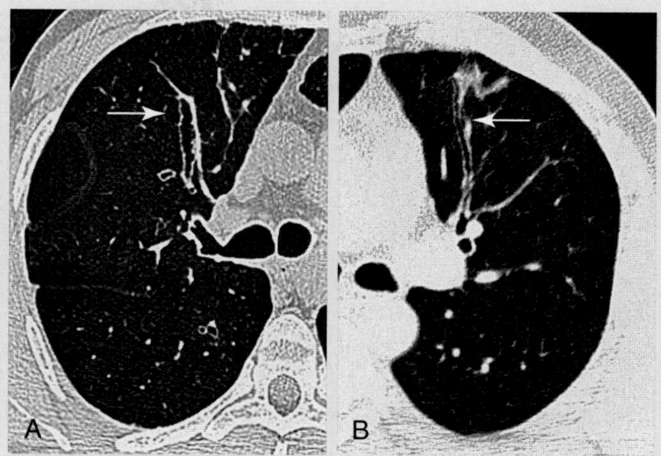

FIGURE 13-9 Cylindrical bronchiectasis. Examples from two patients. Airways parallel to the plane of section in anterior segment of an upper lobe show changes of cylindrical bronchiectasis; bronchi are wider than normal and fail to taper as they proceed toward the lung periphery (arrow). (From Hansell DM, Armstrong P, Lynch DA, McAdams HP, eds: *Imaging of diseases of the chest,* ed 4, Philadelphia, 2005, Elsevier.)

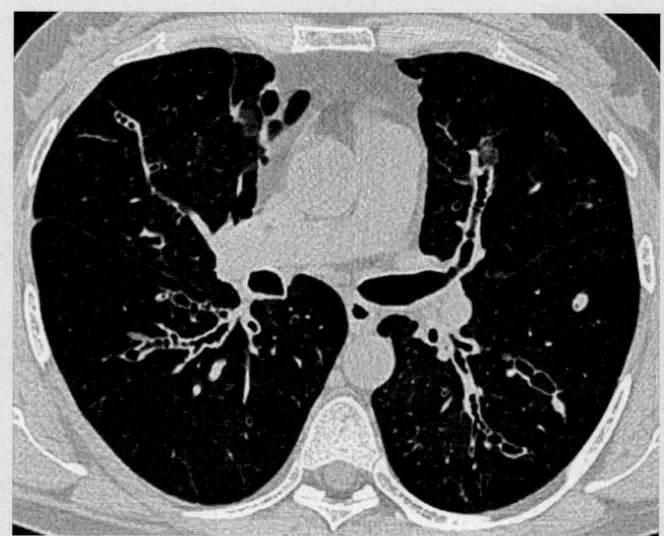

FIGURE 13-10 Varicose bronchiectasis. Patient with allergic bronchopulmonary aspergillosis and cystic fibrosis. The bronchiectatic airways have a corrugated, or beaded, appearance. (From Hansell DM, Armstrong P, Lynch DA, McAdams HP, eds: *Imaging of diseases of the chest,* ed 4, Philadelphia, 2005, Elsevier.)

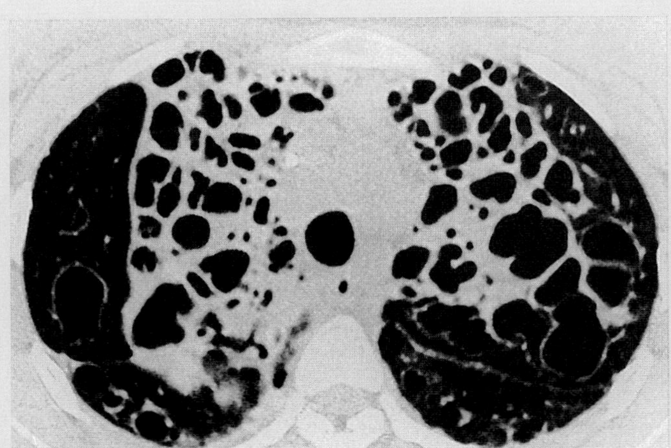

FIGURE 13-11 Cystic bronchiectasis (advanced) in the upper lobes. (From Hansell DM, Armstrong P, Lynch DA, McAdams HP, eds: *Imaging of diseases of the chest*, ed 4, Philadelphia, 2005, Elsevier.)

General Management of Bronchiectasis

The general treatment plan is aimed at controlling pulmonary infections, airway secretions, and airway obstruction and preventing complications. Daily postural drainage and effective coughing exercises to remove bronchial secretions are routine parts of the treatment. Antibiotics, bronchodilators, and expectorants are often prescribed during periods of exacerbation. Childhood vaccinations and yearly influenza vaccinations help reduce the prevalence of some infections. The avoidance of upper respiratory infections, smoking, and polluted environments also helps reduce susceptibility to pneumonia in these patients. Surgical lung resection may be indicated for those patients who respond poorly to therapy or experience massive bleeding.

Respiratory Care Treatment Protocols

Oxygen Therapy Protocol

Oxygen therapy is used to treat hypoxemia, decrease the work of breathing, and decrease myocardial work. The hypoxemia that develops in bronchiectasis is usually caused by the pulmonary shunting associated with the disorder. When the patient demonstrates chronic ventilatory failure during the advanced stages of bronchiectasis, caution must be taken not to overoxygenate the patient (see Oxygen Therapy Protocol, Protocol 9-1).

Bronchopulmonary Hygiene Therapy Protocol

A number of bronchial hygiene treatment modalities may be used to enhance the mobilization of bronchial secretions (see Bronchopulmonary Hygiene Therapy Protocol, Protocol 9-2).

Lung Expansion Therapy Protocol

Attempts to keep distal lung units inflated may involve the use of deep breathing and coughing and incentive spirometry (see Lung Expansion Therapy Protocol, Protocol 9-3).

Aerosolized Medication Therapy Protocol

Both sympathomimetic and parasympatholytic agents are commonly used in bronchiectasis to induce bronchial smooth muscle relaxation (see Aerosolized Medication Therapy Protocol, Protocol 9-4 and Appendix II).

Mechanical Ventilation Protocol

Mechanical ventilation may be necessary to provide and support alveolar gas exchange and eventually return the patient to spontaneous breathing. Because acute ventilatory failure superimposed on chronic ventilatory failure is often seen in patients with severe bronchiectasis, continuous mechanical ventilation is justified when the acute ventilatory failure is thought to be reversible—for example, when acute pneumonia exists as a complicating factor (see Mechanical Ventilation Protocols, Protocol 9-5, Protocol 9-6, and Protocol 9-7).

Medications Commonly Prescribed by the Physician

Expectorants

Expectorants sometimes are ordered when oral liquids and aerosol therapy alone are not sufficient to facilitate expectoration (see Appendix II, Expectorants). Their clinical effectiveness is doubtful.

Antibiotics

Antibiotics commonly are administered to treat associated respiratory tract infections (see Appendix III, Antibiotics).

CASE STUDY

Bronchiectasis

Admitting History and Physical Examination

A 31-year-old male patient consulted his physician regarding an increasingly productive cough. He reported a "bad case" of right lower lobe pneumonia 7 years ago and several episodes of pulmonary infection since that time. On those occasions he usually received an antibiotic, and until 6 months ago the infections responded readily to treatment. However, 6 months ago he noticed that his chronic cough had become increasingly severe, and for the first time his cough became productive. Recently, he had produced as much as a cup of thick, tenacious, yellow-white sputum per day. Within the past 2 to 3 days, he noticed some dark blood mixed with the sputum. He also noticed some dyspnea on exertion, but this had not been particularly troublesome. The past medical history revealed chronic sinusitis since adolescence but was otherwise unremarkable.

Physical examination revealed a well-developed male adult in no apparent distress. Vital signs were within normal limits. His oral temperature was 98.4° F. He coughed frequently during the examination and produced a moderate amount of thick, yellow, blood-streaked sputum. Crackles and rhonchi were heard over the right lower lung fields posteriorly. His Spo_2 on room air while at rest was 85%.

Laboratory results showed a mild leukocytosis but were otherwise normal. Sputum culture indicated the presence of *H. influenzae.* A CT scan of the chest revealed cystic dilations of the right lower lobe bronchus. The respiratory care practitioner assigned to assess and treat the patient at this time recorded the following in the patient's chart.

Respiratory Assessment and Plan

S Productive cough, hemoptysis, worse in past 5 months. Mild dyspnea on exertion.

O Vital signs: normal. Afebrile. Observed moderate amount of mucopurulent, blood-streaked sputum. Crackles and rhonchi over RLL. Sputum culture: *H. influenzae.* CT scan suggests saccular dilation of RLL bronchi.

A
- Postpneumonic bronchiectasis RLL (history and CT scan)
- Excessive airway secretions and sputum production (rhonchi and sputum expectoration)
- Acute bronchial infection and hemoptysis (yellow, blood-streaked sputum)
- Moderate hypoxemia (Spo_2)

P **Oxygen Therapy Protocol** (O_2 via 2 L/min nasal cannula). **Aerosolized Medication** and **Bronchopulmonary Hygiene Protocols** (med neb 2.0 cc 20% acetylcysteine with albuterol 0.5 cc, followed by CPT and PD, q6h).

The patient was treated vigorously with chest physiotherapy and mucolytic therapy. The physician prescribed antibiotics and administered pneumonia vaccine. The patient was discharged from the hospital after 3 days with considerable improvement. He was instructed to seek prompt medical attention for all future pulmonary infections. His wife was instructed in postural drainage techniques.

Approximately 6 months later, the patient arrived at the emergency department complaining of a productive cough, pain on the left side of the chest (made worse by deep breathing), shaking chills and fever for 3 days, and noticeable swelling of both ankles. Since his previous visit, he had been performing CPT and PD only "once or twice a week," had gained 30 pounds, and had taken a new job as a painter's apprentice. He admitted to smoking an occasional cigarette. There had been no known infectious disease exposure.

Physical examination revealed a young man in obvious respiratory distress. His vital signs were blood pressure 160/100, heart rate 110 bpm and regular, respiratory rate 20/min, and oral temperature 101.5° F. His sputum was foul-smelling (a fecal odor), thick, and yellow-green. His cough was strong. Auscultation revealed sibilant rhonchi and crackles over both bases. There was mild clubbing of fingers and toes. The physician wrote "bronchiectasis" in the working diagnosis section of the patient's chart.

Although a chest x-ray film had been taken, it was not yet available. The patient's WBC was 23,500 mm^3, with 80% segmented neutrophils and 10% bands. Room air ABG showed pH 7.51, $Paco_2$ 28 mm Hg, HCO_3^- 21, and Pao_2 45 mm Hg. His Spo_2 at rest on room air was 86%; it fell to 78% when he got out of bed to go to the bathroom. The respiratory care practitioner recorded the following note in the patient's emergency department chart.

Respiratory Assessment and Plan

S Cough, pleuritic left-sided chest pain, chills, fever, leg swelling. Has not been doing CPT and PD on regular basis. 30 lb weight gain. Smoking.

O HR 110; RR 20; BP 160/100; T 101.5° F; Spo_2 (room air, rest) 86%, falls to 78% with mild exertion. Sputum thick, yellow-green, foul-smelling. Rhonchi and crackles both bases. Strong cough. Clubbing of digits. WBC 23,500 (80% neutrophils, 10% bands). Room air ABG; pH 7.51; $Paco_2$ 28 mm Hg; HCO_3^- 21; Pao_2 45 mm Hg.

A
- Bronchiectasis (old chart record)
- Excessive airway secretions (thick sputum, rhonchi)
- Infection likely (fever, yellow-green sputum); good ability to mobilize secretions (strong cough)
- Acute alveolar hyperventilation with moderate hypoxemia (ABG)
- Postural drainage therapy and smoking cessation noncompliance (history)

P Review CXR. **Oxygen Therapy Protocol** (2 L/min per nasal cannula). **Aerosolized Medication Protocol** and **Bronchopulmonary Hygiene Protocols** (med. neb. 2.0 cc 20% acetylcysteine with albuterol 0.5 cc, followed by CPT and PD q4h). Obtain sputum culture. Check

I&O. Repeat ABG in am. Review deep breathe and cough, flutter valve, and pulmonary rehabilitation strategies with patient and his wife. Offer smoking cessation and weight reduction programs.

Discussion

The main challenge facing the respiratory care practitioner caring for the patient with bronchiectasis is one of efficient removal of excessive bronchopulmonary secretions. Over the years, postural drainage and percussion, good systemic hydration, and judicious use of antibiotics have been the hallmarks of therapy. More recently, intermittent use of mucolytics, percussive ventilation, and **Lung Expansion Therapy** (see Protocol 9-3) has become more common. Pneumococcal prophylaxis is, of course, important, as is prompt attention to parenchymal pulmonary infections such as pneumonia. The clinical distinction between chronic bronchiectasis and cystic fibrosis is a subtle one at the bedside, and the latter condition must always be ruled out in patients with bronchiectasis. The goal of long-term therapy in bronchiectasis is prevention of lung parenchyma–destroying pulmonary infections and avoidance of frequent hospitalizations. Hemoptysis is often a sign of more deep-seated infection requiring antibiotic therapy.

The clinical manifestations throughout this case were all based on the clinical scenario associated with **excessive airway secretions**. For example, the thick yellow sputum resulted in decreased $\dot{V}/\dot{Q}$ ratios, venous admixture, and hypoxemia. These pathophysiologic mechanisms caused clinical manifestations of an increase in blood pressure and heart rate, acute alveolar hyperventilation with moderate hypoxemia, and rhonchi.

Digital clubbing associated with hypoxemia is another clinical manifestation of bronchiectasis. After the first assessment, both the **Oxygen Therapy Protocol** and **Bronchopulmonary Hygiene Therapy Protocol** were administered appropriately (see Protocols 9-1 and 9-2). The therapist's review of the chest x-ray allowed him to target the postural drainage therapy. Low-flow oxygen per nasal cannula, aerosolized bronchodilators (albuterol) and mucolytic medication (acetylcysteine), chest percussion, and postural drainage therapy were selected from these protocols and applied with good results.

Finally, during the second admission, patient noncompliance was evident (i.e., weight gain, resumption of smoking, employment in a dusty workplace, failure to continue CPT and PD), which further complicated the patient's respiratory disorder. In response to the patient's condition, the whole respiratory care regimen was upgraded by an increase in frequency of treatments, with a strong emphasis on the patient's responsibility for his own care.

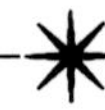

SELF-ASSESSMENT QUESTIONS

evolve Answers to questions can be found on Evolve. To access additional student assessment questions and case studies for application of text material to real-life scenarios, visit **http://evolve.elsevier.com/DesJardins/respiratory.**

1. In which of the following forms of bronchiectasis are the bronchi dilated and constricted in an irregular fashion?

1. Fusiform
2. Saccular
3. Varicose
4. Cylindrical
   - a. 2 only
   - b. 3 only
   - c. 2 and 4 only
   - d. 1 and 3 only

2. Which of the following is or are common causes of acquired bronchiectasis?

1. Hypogammaglobulinemia
2. Pulmonary tuberculosis
3. Kartagener's syndrome
4. Cystic fibrosis
   - a. 1 only
   - b. 2 only
   - c. 3 only
   - d. 3 and 4 only

3. In the primarily obstructive form of bronchiectasis, the patient commonly demonstrates which of the following?

1. Decreased FRC
2. Increased $FEF_{25\%-75\%}$
3. Decreased PEFR
4. Increased $\dot{V}max_{50}$
   - a. 1 only
   - b. 3 only
   - c. 1 and 4 only
   - d. 2 and 4 only

4. Which of the following radiologic findings is or are associated with bronchiectasis that is primarily obstructive in nature?

1. Enlarged heart
2. Depressed or flattened diaphragms
3. Long and narrow heart
4. Translucent lung fields
   - a. 1 and 2 only
   - b. 3 and 4 only
   - c. 2, 3, and 4 only
   - d. 1 , 2, 3, and 4

5. Which of the following is considered *the* hallmark of bronchiectasis?

a. Chronic cough and large quantities of foul-smelling sputum
b. Abnormal bronchogram
c. Acute ventilatory failure superimposed on chronic ventilatory failure
d. Presentation as both a restrictive and obstructive pulmonary disorder

6. Which of the following is or are commonly cultured in the sputum of patients with bronchiectasis?

1. *Streptococcus pneumoniae*
2. *Pseudomonas aeruginosa*
3. *Haemophilus influenzae*
4. *Klebsiella*

a. 3 only
b. 4 only
c. 1, 2, and 3 only
d. 1, 2, 3, and 4

7. When the pathophysiology of bronchiectasis is primarily obstructive in nature, the patient demonstrates which of the following clinical manifestations?

1. Decreased tactile and vocal fremitus
2. Bronchial breath sounds
3. Dull percussion note
4. Rhonchi and wheezing

a. 2 only
b. 3 only
c. 1 and 4 only
d. 2 and 4 only

8. Which of the following diagnostic procedures is or are used to positively diagnose bronchiectasis?

1. Arterial blood gases
2. Bronchography
3. Oxygenation indices
4. Computed tomography

a. 2 only
b. 3 only
c. 1 and 3 only
d. 2 and 4 only

9. Which of the following is or are congenital causes of bronchiectasis?

1. Pertussis
2. Cystic fibrosis
3. Chickenpox
4. Measles

a. 1 only
b. 2 only
c. 3 and 4 only
d. 1 and 3 only

10. Which of the following hemodynamic indices is or are associated with bronchiectasis?

1. Decreased CVP
2. Increased PA
3. Decreased RVSWI
4. Increased RAP

a. 2 only
b. 3 only
c. 2 and 4 only
d. 1 and 3 only

Cystic Fibrosis

14

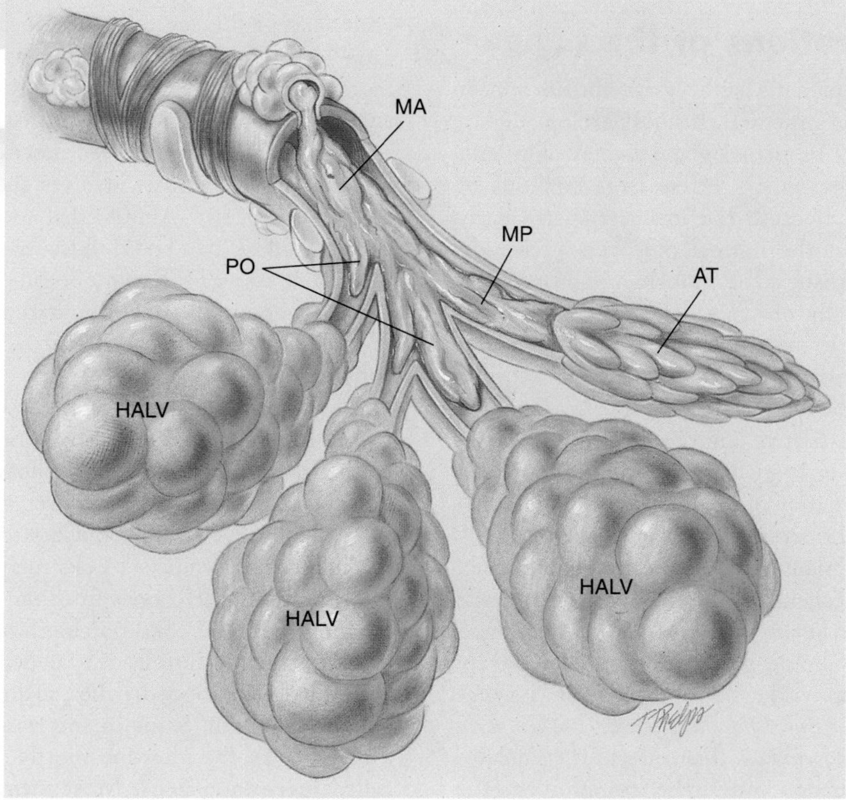

FIGURE 14-1 Cystic fibrosis. *AT,* Atelectasis; *HALV,* hyperinflation of alveoli; *MA,* mucous accumulation; *MP,* mucous plug; *PO,* partial obstruction of the airways.

Chapter Objectives

After reading this chapter, you will be able to:

- List the anatomic alterations of the lungs associated with cystic fibrosis.
- Describe the causes and classifications of cystic fibrosis.
- List the cardiopulmonary clinical manifestations associated with cystic fibrosis.
- Describe the general management of cystic fibrosis.
- Describe the clinical strategies and rationales of the SOAPs presented in the case study.
- Define key terms and complete self-assessment questions at the end of the chapter and on Evolve.

Key Terms

Amniocentesis
Chorionic Villus Biopsy
Cystic Fibrosis Transmembrane Conductance Regulator (CFTR)
Electrical Potential Difference
Genetic Test
Immunoreactive Trypsinogen Test (IRT)
Meconium Ileus
Nasal Potential Difference (NPD)
Pilocarpine
Standard Mendelian Pattern
Sweat Test

Chapter Outline

General Management of Cystic Fibrosis
Respiratory Care Treatment Protocols
Medications and Special Procedures Prescribed by the Physician

Case Study: Cystic Fibrosis
Self Assessment Questions

Anatomic Alterations of the Lungs*

Although the lungs of patients with cystic fibrosis appear normal at birth, abnormal structural changes develop quickly. Initially, the patient has bronchial gland hypertrophy and metaplasia of goblet cells, which secrete large amounts of thick, tenacious mucus. Because the mucus is particularly tenacious, impairment of the normal mucociliary clearing mechanism ensues, and many small bronchi and bronchioles become partially or totally obstructed (mucous plugging). Partial obstruction leads to overdistention of the alveoli, and complete obstruction leads to patchy areas of atelectasis. The anatomic alterations of the lungs associated with cystic fibrosis may result in both restrictive and obstructive lung characteristics, but excessive bronchial secretions, bronchial obstruction, and hyperinflation of the lungs are the predominant features of cystic fibrosis in the advanced stages.

The abundance of stagnant mucus in the tracheobronchial tree also serves as an excellent culture medium for bacteria, particularly *Staphylococcus aureus, Haemophilus influenzae,* and *Pseudomonas aeruginosa.* Some gram-negative bacteria are also commonly associated with cystic fibrosis, such as *Stenotrophomonas maltophilia, Burkholderia cepacia, Burkholderia pickettii,* and *Burkholderia gladioli.* The infection stimulates additional mucous production and further compromises the mucociliary transport system. This condition may lead to secondary bronchial smooth muscle constriction. Finally, as the disease progresses, the patient may develop signs and symptoms of recurrent pneumonia, chronic bronchitis, bronchiectasis, and lung abscesses (Figure 14-1).

The major pathologic or structural changes associated with cystic fibrosis are as follows:

- Excessive production and accumulation of thick, tenacious mucus in the tracheobronchial tree
- Partial bronchial obstruction (mucous plugging)
- Hyperinflation of the alveoli
- Total bronchial obstruction (mucous plugging)
- Atelectasis

Etiology and Epidemiology

Cystic fibrosis is the most common inherited disorder in childhood. Cystic fibrosis is an autosomal recessive gene disorder caused by mutations in a pair of genes located on chromosome 7. Under normal conditions, every cell in the body (except the sex cells) has 46 chromosomes—23 pairs (one half inherited from father and the other half from mother). Over 1000 different mutations in the gene that encodes for the **cystic fibrosis transmembrane conductance regulator (CFTR)** have been described. One genetic defect linked to cystic fibrosis involves the absence of three base pairs in codon 508 (ΔF508) that codes for phenylalanine on chromosome 7 (band q31). Because of the loss of these three base pairs, the CFTR gene becomes dysfunctional. This is the most common genetic mutation associated with cystic fibrosis and accounts for 70% to 75% of the cystic fibrosis patients tested.

The abnormal expression of the CFTR results in abnormal transport of sodium and chloride across many types of epithelial surfaces, including those lining the bronchial airways, intestines, pancreas, liver ducts, sweat glands, and vas deferens. As a result, thick, viscous mucus accumulates in the lungs, and mucus blocks the passageways of the pancreas, preventing enzymes from the pancreas from reaching the intestines. This condition inhibits the digestion of protein and fat, which in turn leads to deficiencies of vitamins A, D, E, and K. In addition, diarrhea, malnutrition, and weight loss are also common. Some infants with cystic fibrosis develop a blockage of the intestine shortly after birth—a condition called **meconium ileus.** Most men with cystic fibrosis are infertile as a result of a missing or an underdeveloped vas deferens. Infertility is not common in women with cystic fibrosis.

How the Cystic Fibrosis Gene Is Inherited

Because cystic fibrosis is a recessive gene disorder, the child must inherit two copies of the defective cystic fibrosis gene—one from each parent (cystic fibrosis carriers)—to have the disease. Even though the carrier of the cystic fibrosis gene may be identified through genetic testing, the carrier (heterozygote) does not demonstrate evidence of the disease. However, if both parents carry the cystic fibrosis gene, the possibility of their children having cystic fibrosis (regardless of gender) follows the **standard Mendelian pattern:** there is a 25% chance that each child will have cystic fibrosis, a 25% chance that each child will be completely normal (and not carry the gene), and a 50% chance that each child will be a carrier. Thus, when both patients have the cystic fibrosis gene, there is a one in four chance that the child will have cystic fibrosis (Figure 14-2). It is estimated that more than 10 million Americans are unknowing, symptomless carriers of the mutant cystic fibrosis gene.

According to the Cystic Fibrosis Foundation, cystic fibrosis affects about 30,000 children and adults in the United

*Cystic fibrosis does not affect the lungs exclusively. It also affects the function of exocrine glands in other parts of the body. In addition to being characterized by abnormally viscid secretions in the lungs, the disease is clinically manifested by pancreatic insufficiency and high sodium concentrations in the sweat.

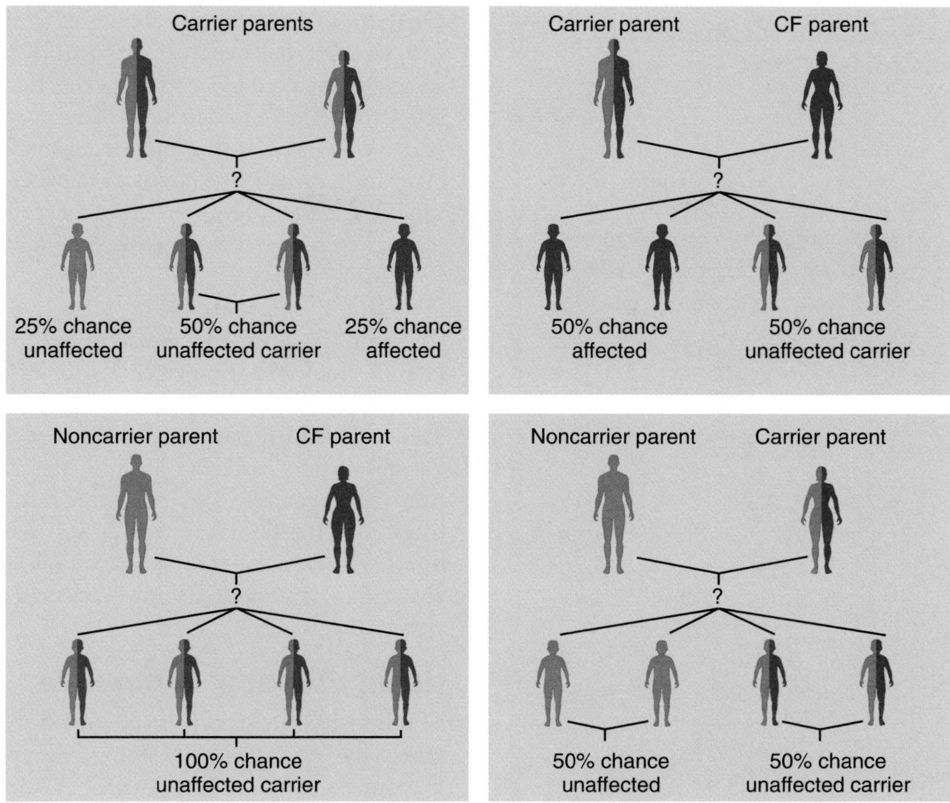

FIGURE 14-2 Standard Mendelian pattern of inheritance of cystic fibrosis.

States. About 1000 new cases of cystic fibrosis are diagnosed each year in the United States (70,000 worldwide). More than 70% of the patients are diagnosed by age 2. More than 40% of the cystic fibrosis patient population is age 18 or older.* Other researchers state that whites are most often affected (1 in 2500 to 3500). Cystic fibrosis is less common in Hispanics (1 in 9500) and African-Americans (1 in 17,000). Cystic fibrosis is rarely seen in Asians (1 in 31,000). The predicted median life expectancy is 37 years. Death usually is caused by pulmonary complications.

Screening and Diagnosis

The diagnosis of cystic fibrosis is based on clinical manifestations associated with cystic fibrosis, family history of cystic fibrosis, and laboratory findings. Box 14-1 provides common clinical indicators that justify evaluation for cystic fibrosis.

The diagnosis of cystic fibrosis is based on results of one or more of the laboratory tests discussed in the following sections.

Sweat Test

The **sweat test** (sometimes called the sweat chlorine test) is the gold standard diagnostic test for cystic fibrosis. The sweat test is a reliable test for the identification of approximately 98% of patients with cystic fibrosis. This test measures the amount of sodium and chloride in the patient's sweat. During the procedure a small amount of a colorless, odorless sweat-producing chemical called **pilocarpine** is applied to the patient's arm or leg—usually the forearm. An electrode is attached to the chemically prepared area, and a mild electric current is applied to stimulate sweat production (Figure 14-3). To collect the sweat, the area is covered with a gauze pad or filter paper and wrapped in plastic. After about 30 minutes the plastic is removed, and the sweat collected in the pad or paper is sent to the laboratory for analysis. The test is usually done twice.

Although the sweat glands of patients with cystic fibrosis are microscopically normal, the glands secrete up to four times the normal amount of sodium and chloride. The actual volume of sweat, however, is no greater than that produced by a normal individual. In children, a sweat chloride concentration greater than 60 mEq/L is considered to be a diagnostic sign of the disease. In adults, a sweat chloride concentration greater than 80 mEq/L usually is required to confirm the diagnosis. The sweat chloride level in the patient with cystic fibrosis may be up to five times greater than normal.

Immunoreactive Trypsinogen Test

An **immunoreactive trypsinogen test (IRT)** (also called *trypsin-like immunoreactivity, serum trypsinogen,* and *serum trypsin*) may be ordered as an initial test for (1) babies who are not creating enough sweat to perform a sweat test, or (2) infants with meconium ileus (no stools in the first 24 to 48 hours of life). The test may be particularly useful for small or malnourished infants in whom the sweat chloride test cannot be performed successfully. An IRT is also ordered for children and adults with signs and symptoms associated with cystic fibrosis and pancreatic dysfunction, such as persistent

*Cystic Fibrosis Foundation (www.cff.org).

Box 14-1 Clinical Indicators Justifying the Initial Evaluation for Cystic Fibrosis

Pulmonary

Wheezing
Chronic cough
Sputum production
Frequent respiratory infections *(Staphylococcus aureus, Pseudomonas aeruginosa, Haemophilus influenzae)*
Abnormal chest radiograph and/or computed tomography (CT) scan
Nasal polyps
Parasinusitis
Digital clubbing

Gastrointestinal

Failure to thrive
Foul-smelling, greasy stools
Voracious appetite
Milk and formula intolerance
Rectal prolapse
Meconium ileus
Meconium peritonitis
Distal intestinal obstruction syndrome
Pancreatic insufficiency
Pancreatitis

Hepatobiliary

Hepatomegaly
Focal biliary cirrhosis
Prolonged neonatal jaundice
Cholelithiasis

Nutritional Deficits

Fat-soluble vitamin deficiency (vitamins A, D, E, K)
Hypoproteinemia
Hypochloremia (metabolic alkalosis)

Infertility (male)

Obstructive azolspermia

diarrhea; foul-smelling, bulky, greasy stools; malnutrition; and vitamin deficiency. During this procedure, a blood sample is analyzed twice for a specific protein called *trypsinogen.* Patients with cystic fibrosis have elevated blood levels of IRT. Two positive test results indicate cystic fibrosis, abnormal pancreatic enzyme production, pancreatitis, or pancreatic cancer. Elevated levels need to be followed with further testing, such as a cystic fibrosis gene mutation test.

Stool Fecal Fat Test

The stool fecal fat test measures the amount of fat in the infant's stool and the percentage of dietary fat that is not absorbed by the body. The test is used to evaluated how the liver, gallbladder, pancreas, and intestines are functioning. Fat absorption requires bile from the gallbladder, enzymes from the pancreas, and normal intestines. Under normal conditions the fat absorption is less than 7 g of fat per 24 hours. An elevated stool fecal fat value (i.e., decreased fat absorption) is associated with a variety of disorders, including cystic fibrosis.

Nasal Potential Difference

The impaired transport of sodium (Na^+) and chloride (Cl^-) across the epithelial cells lining the airways of the cystic fibrosis patient can be measured. As the Na^+ and Cl^- ions move across the epithelial cell membrane they general what is called an **electrical potential difference**—the amount of energy required to move an electrical charge from one point to another. In the nasal passages this electrical potential difference is called the **nasal potential difference (NPD).** The NPD can be measured with a surface electrode over the nasal epithelial cells lining the inferior turbinate. An increased (i.e., more negative) nasal potential difference strongly suggests cystic fibrosis. The NPD is recommended for patients with clinical features of cystic fibrosis who have borderline or normal sweat test values and nondiagnostic cystic fibrosis genotyping.

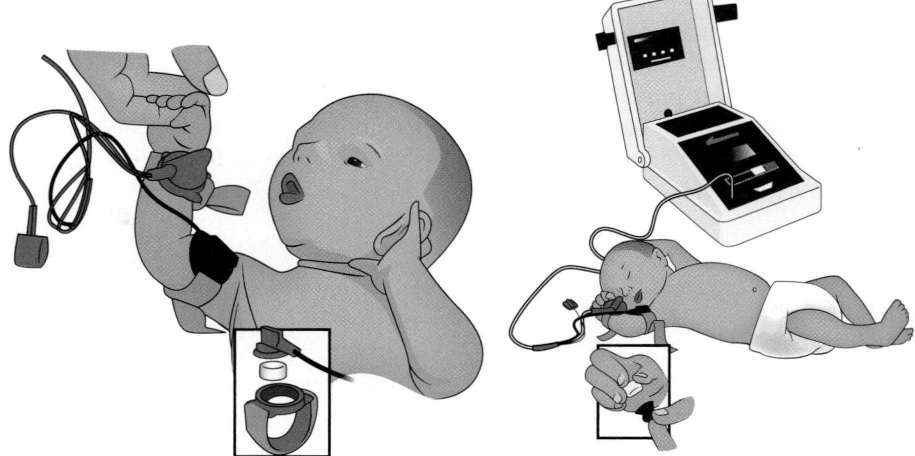

FIGURE 14-3 Sweat test. During the procedure a small amount of a colorless, odorless sweat-producing chemical called **pilocarpine** is applied to the patient's arm or leg—usually the forearm. An electrode is attached to the chemically prepared area, and a mild electric current is applied to stimulate sweat production. Used with permission Wescor, Inc—an ELITech Group Company.

Genetic Testing

With a sample of the patient's blood, a **genetic test** (also called a *genotype test, gene mutation test,* or *mutation analysis*) can be performed to analyze deoxyribonucleic acid (DNA) for the presence of CFTR gene mutations. From over 1000 different CFTR gene mutations, the most common gene alteration in cystic fibrosis is ΔF508. Although genetic testing for cystic fibrosis is considered a valuable diagnostic tool, it does have its limitations. For example, some individuals have CFTR mutations but demonstrate no typical clinical manifestations of cystic fibrosis. In addition, some patients may have CFTR mutations, but the mutations cannot be identified with our current gene analysis methods. It is estimated that genetic testing can confirm cystic fibrosis in about 80% to 85% of the patients tested. As a general rule, genetic testing is performed in patients who have negative sweat test results but still demonstrate a variety of clinical manifestations associated with cystic fibrosis (see following section).

Prenatal Testing

In women who are pregnant and who wish to make informed reproductive decisions, prenatal diagnosis may be performed by **chorionic villus biopsy** in the first trimester or by **amniocentesis** in the second or third trimester. Such testing is usually carried out in a family that has previously had a child with cystic fibrosis.

- Amniocentesis—the amniotic fluid is obtained and tested to determine if both of the CFTR genes from the fetus are normal. Amniocentesis can be used to diagnose a large number of genetic and chromosomal abnormalities, including cystic fibrosis.
- Chorionic villus biopsy—with the aid of an ultrasound examination, a thin tube is inserted into the uterus to obtain a piece of the placenta to biopsy. The cells of the placenta are then tested for a variety of genetic defects, including cystic fibrosis.

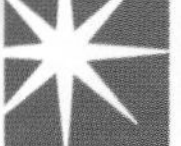

OVERVIEW of the Cardiopulmonary Clinical Manifestations Associated with Cystic Fibrosis

The following clinical manifestations result from the pathophysiologic mechanisms caused (or activated) by **Atelectasis** (see Figure 9-8), **Bronchospasm** (see Figure 9-11), and **Excessive Bronchial Secretions** (see Figure 9-12)—the major anatomic alterations of the lungs associated with cystic fibrosis (CF) (see Figure 14-1).

CLINICAL DATA OBTAINED AT THE PATIENT'S BEDSIDE

The Physical Examination

Vital Signs

Increased Respiratory Rate (Tachypnea)

Several pathophysiologic mechanisms operating simultaneously may lead to an increased ventilatory rate:

- Stimulation of peripheral chemoreceptors (hypoxemia)
- Decreased lung compliance–increased ventilatory rate relationship
- Anxiety

Increased Heart Rate (Pulse), and Blood Pressure

Use of Accessory Muscles during Inspiration

Use of Accessory Muscles during Expiration

Pursed-Lip Breathing

Increased Anteroposterior Chest Diameter (Barrel Chest)

Cyanosis

Digital Clubbing

Peripheral Edema and Venous Distention

Because polycythemia and cor pulmonale are associated with CF, the following may be seen:

- Distended neck veins
- Pitting edema
- Enlarged and tender liver

Cough, Sputum Production, and Hemoptysis

Chest Assessment Findings

- Decreased or increased tactile and vocal fremitus
- Hyperresonant percussion note
- Diminished breath sounds
- Diminished heart sounds
- Bronchial breath sounds (over atelectasis)
- Crackles, rhonchi, and wheezing

Spontaneous Pneumothorax

Spontaneous pneumothorax commonly is seen in patients with CF. The incidence is greater than 20% in adults with CF. When a patient with CF has a pneumothorax, there is about a 50% chance that it will recur. The respiratory care practitioner must be alert for the signs and symptoms of this complication (e.g., pleuritic pain, shoulder pain, sudden shortness of breath). Precipitating factors include excessive exertion, high altitude, and positive-pressure breathing (see Pneumothorax, Chapter 22.)

OVERVIEW of the Cardiopulmonary Clinical Manifestations Associated with Cystic Fibrosis—cont'd

CLINICAL DATA OBTAINED FROM LABORATORY TESTS AND SPECIAL PROCEDURES

Pulmonary Function Test Findings
Moderate to Severe Cystic Fibrosis (Obstructive Lung Pathophysiology)*

FORCED EXPIRATORY FLOW RATE FINDINGS

FVC	FEV_T	FEV_1/FVC ratio	$FEF_{25\%-75\%}$
↓	↓	↓	↓

$FEF_{50\%}$	$FEF_{200-1200}$	PEFR	MVV
↓	↓	↓	↓

LUNG VOLUME AND CAPACITY FINDINGS

V_T	IRV	ERV	RV
N or ↑	N or ↓	N or ↓	↑

VC	IC	FRC	TLC	RV/TLC ratio
↓	N or ↓	↑	N or ↑	N or ↑

*Cystic fibrosis is primarily an obstructive lung disorder. However, when extensive total lung obstruction (from mucous plugging) and atelectasis is present throughout the lungs, restrictive pulmonary function testing values will likely appear.

Arterial Blood Gases

MILD TO MODERATE STAGES OF CYSTIC FIBROSIS
Acute Alveolar Hyperventilation with Hypoxemia
(Acute Respiratory Alkalosis)

pH	Pa_{CO_2}	HCO_3^-	Pa_{O_2}
↑	↓	↓ (slightly)	↓

SEVERE STAGE OF CYSTIC FIBROSIS
Chronic Ventilatory Failure with Hypoxemia
(Compensated Respiratory Acidosis)

pH	Pa_{CO_2}	HCO_3^-	Pa_{O_2}
N	↑	↑ (significantly)	↓

ACUTE VENTILATORY CHANGES SUPERIMPOSED ON CHRONIC VENTILATORY FAILURE

Because acute ventilatory changes are frequently seen in patients with chronic ventilatory failure, the respiratory care practitioner must be familiar with and alert for the following:

- Acute alveolar hyperventilation superimposed on chronic ventilatory failure, and/or
- Acute ventilatory failure (acute hypoventilation) superimposed on chronic ventilatory failure

Oxygenation Indices*
Moderate to Severe Stages

$\dot{Q}_S/\dot{Q}_T$	D_{O_2}[†]	$\dot{V}_{O_2}$	$C(a-\bar{v})_{O_2}$	O_2ER	$S\bar{v}_{O_2}$
↑	↓	N	N	↑	↓

[†]The D_{O_2} may be normal in patients who have compensated to the decreased oxygenation status with (1) an increased cardiac output, (2) an increased hemoglobin level, or (3) a combination of both. When the D_{O_2} is normal, the O_2ER is usually normal.

Hemodynamic Indices[†]
Moderate to Severe Stages

CVP	RAP	$\overline{PA}$	PCWP	CO	SV
↑	↑	↑	N	N	N

SVI	CI	RVSWI	LVSWI	PVR	SVR
N	N	↑	N	↑	N

ABNORMAL LABORATORY TESTS AND PROCEDURES

Hematology
- Increased hematocrit and hemoglobin
- Increased white blood cell count

Electrolytes
- Hypochloremia (chronic ventilatory failure)
- Increased serum bicarbonate (chronic ventilatory failure)

Sputum examination
- Increased white blood cells
- Gram-positive bacteria
  - *Staphylococcus aureus*
  - *Haemophilus influenzae*
- Gram-negative bacteria
  - *Stenotrophomonas maltophilia*
  - *Burkholderia cepacia*
  - *Burkholderia pickettii*
  - *Burkholderia gladioli*
  - *Pseudomonas aeruginosa*

RADIOLOGIC FINDINGS

Chest Radiograph
- Translucent (dark) lung fields
- Depressed or flattened diaphragms
- Right ventricular enlargement
- Areas of atelectasis and fibrosis

*$C(a-\bar{v})_{O_2}$, Arterial-venous oxygen difference; D_{O_2}, total oxygen delivery; O_2ER, oxygen extraction ratio; $\dot{Q}_S/\dot{Q}_T$, pulmonary shunt fraction; $S\bar{v}_{O_2}$, mixed venous oxygen saturation; $\dot{V}_{O_2}$, oxygen consumption.

[†]*CO*, Cardiac output; *CVP*, central venous pressure; *LVSWI*, left ventricular stroke work index; *$\overline{PA}$*, mean pulmonary artery pressure; *PCWP*, pulmonary capillary wedge pressure; *PVR*, pulmonary vascular resistance; *RAP*, right atrial pressure; *RVSWI*, right ventricular stroke work index; *SV*, stroke volume; *SVI*, stroke volume index; *SVR*, systemic vascular resistance.

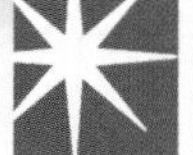

OVERVIEW of the Cardiopulmonary Clinical Manifestations Associated with Cystic Fibrosis—cont'd

- Bronchiectasis (often a secondary complication)
- Pneumothorax (spontaneous)
- Abscess formation (occasionally)

During the late stages of CF, the alveoli become hyperinflated, which causes the residual volume and functional residual capacity to increase. Because this condition decreases the density of the lungs and therefore reduces the resistance to x-ray penetration, the chest radiograph appears darker. As the patient's residual volume and functional residual capacity increase, the diaphragm moves downward and appears flattened or depressed on the radiograph (Figure 14-4).

Figure 14-5 presents four serial chest radiographs of the progression of CF over 26 years. Because right ventricular enlargement and failure often develop as secondary problems during the advanced stages of CF, an enlarged heart may be identified on the radiograph. In some patients, areas of atelectasis, abscess formation, or a pneumothorax may be seen. Finally, computed tomography (CT) and positron emission tomography (PET) scans may be helpful when borderline radiographic findings are present.

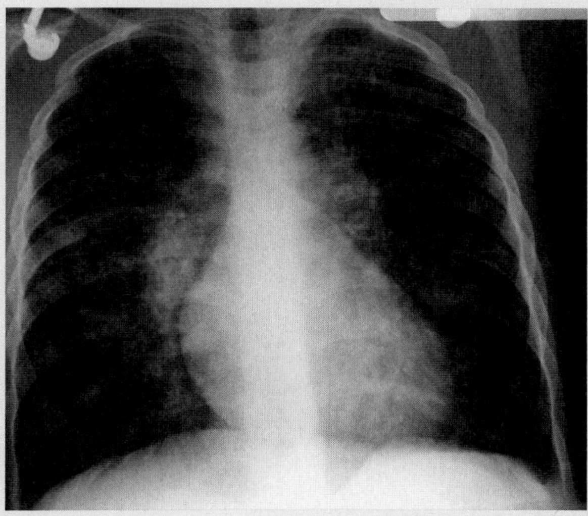

FIGURE 14-4 Chest x-ray of a patient with cystic fibrosis. Note the lung overinflation, the diffuse infiltrates, and the large main pulmonary artery segment.

COMMON NONRESPIRATORY CLINICAL MANIFESTATIONS

Meconium Ileus

Meconium ileus is an obstruction of the small intestine of the newborn that is caused by the impaction of thick, dry, tenacious meconium, usually at or near the ileocecal valve. This results from a deficiency in pancreatic enzymes and is the earliest manifestation of CF. The disease is suspected in newborns who demonstrate abdominal distention and fail to pass meconium within 12 hours after birth. Meconium ileus may occur in as many as 25% of infants with CF.

Meconium Ileus Equivalent

Meconium ileus equivalent is an intestinal obstruction (similar to meconium ileus in neonates) that occurs in older children and young adults with CF.

Malnutrition and Poor Body Development

In CF, the pancreatic ducts become plugged with mucus, which leads to fibrosis of the pancreas. The pancreatic insufficiency that ensues inhibits the digestion of protein and fat. This condition leads to a deficiency of vitamins A, D, E, and K. Vitamin K deficiency may be the cause of easy bruising and bleeding. Approximately 80% of all patients with CF have vitamin deficiencies and therefore show signs of malnutrition and poor body development throughout life.

Nasal Polyps and Sinusitis

About 20% of patients with CF have nasal polyps and sinusitis. The polyps are usually multiple and may cause nasal obstruction; in some cases, they cause distortion of the normal facial features.

Infertility

Approximately 99% of men with CF are sterile. Women with CF who become pregnant are not likely to carry the infant to term. An infant who is carried to term will either have CF or be a carrier (see Figure 14-2).

OVERVIEW of the Cardiopulmonary Clinical Manifestations Associated with Cystic Fibrosis—cont'd

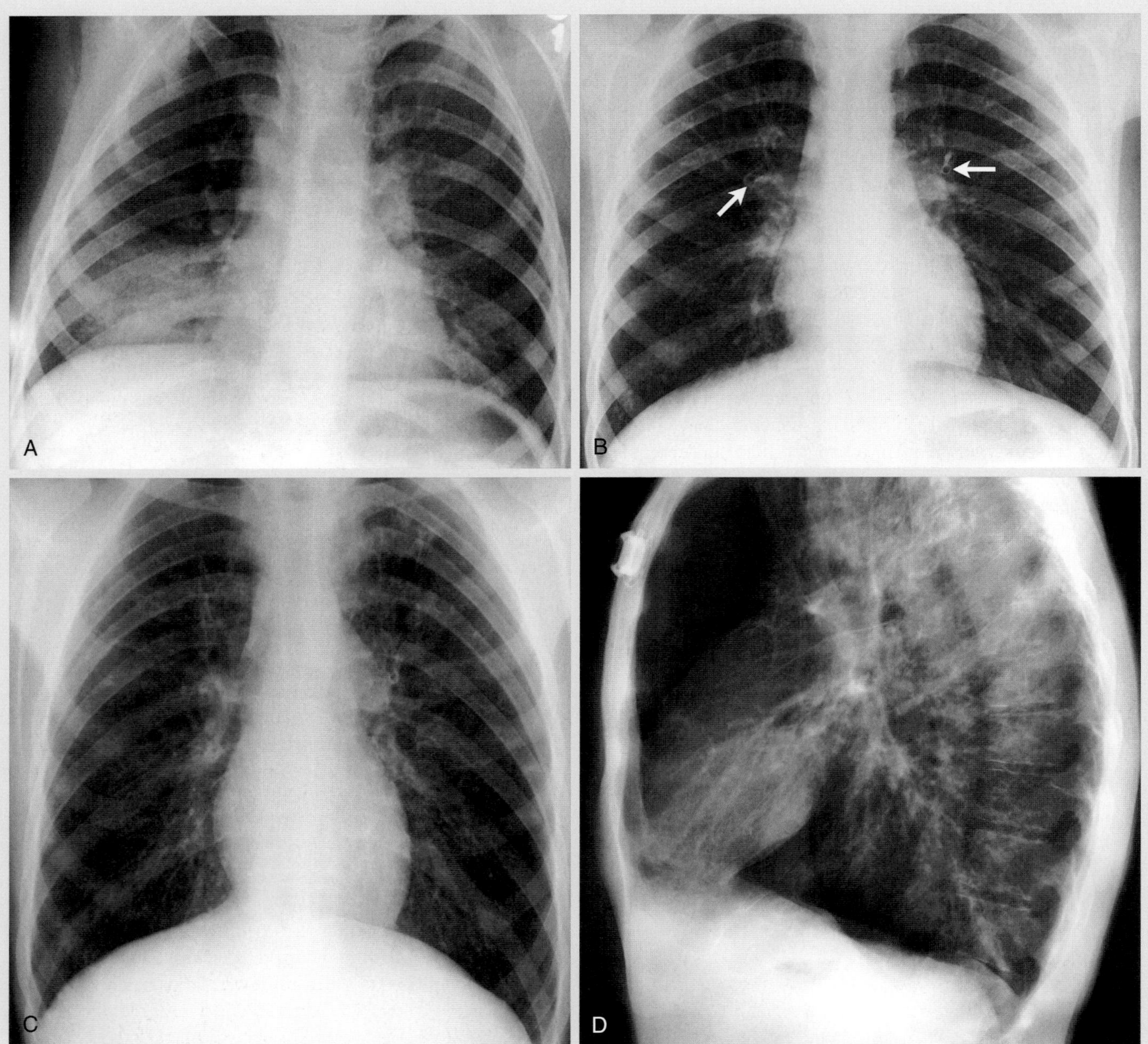

FIGURE 14-5 Cystic fibrosis. Serial chest imaging over a 26-year period showing the progressive changes of cystic fibrosis. **A**, At 3 years of age, the patient had right middle lobe pneumonia. **B**, Mild hyperinflation and bronchial wall thickening *(arrow)* present at age 7 years. **C**, At age 15 years, the patient demonstrates progressive hyperinflation, bronchiectasis, and enlargement of the hila on the chest radiograph. **D**, Lateral chest radiograph at 29 years shows typical findings of end-stage cystic fibrosis. Note marked hyperinflation and "barrel chest" deformity, severe bronchiectasis, and tubular opacities consistent with mucous plugs. (From Hansell DM, Armstrong P, Lynch DA, McAdams HP: *Imaging of diseases of the chest,* ed 4, Philadelphia, 2005, Elsevier.)

General Management of Cystic Fibrosis

The management of cystic fibrosis entails an interdisciplinary approach. The primary goals are to prevent pulmonary infections, reduce the amount of thick bronchial secretions, improve air flow, and provide adequate nutrition. The patient and the patient's family should be instructed regarding the disease and the way it affects bodily functions. They should be taught home care therapies, the goals of these therapies, and the way to administer medications. Patients with severe cystic fibrosis commonly are best managed by a pulmonary rehabilitation team. Such teams include a respiratory care practitioner, a physical therapist, a respiratory nurse specialist, an occupational therapist, a dietitian, a social worker, and a psychologist. A pediatrician or an internist trained in respiratory rehabilitation outlines and orchestrates the patient's therapeutic program.

Patients with cystic fibrosis should have regular medical checkups for comparative purposes to determine their general health, weight, height, pulmonary function abilities, and sputum culture results. In addition, oral time-released pancreatic enzymes, such as pancreatic lipase, are prescribed for patients with cystic fibrosis to aid food digestion. Patients also are encouraged to replace body salts either by heavily salting their food or by taking sodium supplements. Supplemental multivitamins and minerals also are important. To accomplish these objectives, the management of cystic fibrosis includes the protocols discussed in the following sections.

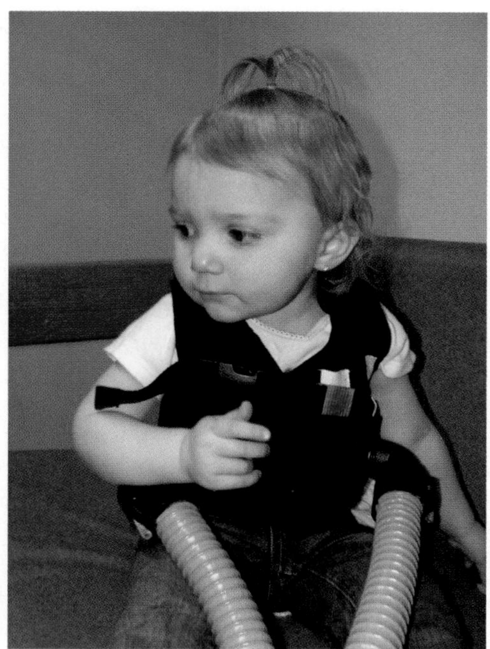

FIGURE 14-6 An 18-month-old female cystic fibrosis patient wearing a high-frequency chest compression (HFCC) vest (the inCourage System). Today, HFCC is a commonly used bronchopulmonary hygiene treatment for airway clearance in patients with cystic fibrosis.

Respiratory Care Treatment Protocols

Oxygen Therapy Protocol

Oxygen therapy is used to treat hypoxemia, decrease the work of breathing, and decrease myocardial work. The hypoxemia that develops in cystic fibrosis is caused by the pulmonary shunting associated with the disorder. When the patient demonstrates chronic ventilatory failure during the advanced stages of cystic fibrosis, caution must be taken not to overoxygenate the patient (see Oxygen Therapy Protocol, Protocol 9-1).

Bronchopulmonary Hygiene Therapy Protocol

Because of the excessive mucous production and accumulation associated with cystic fibrosis, a number of respiratory therapy modalities are used to enhance the mobilization of bronchial secretions. Aggressive and vigorous bronchial hygiene—especially chest physical therapy and postural drainage—should be performed regularly on patients both in the hospital and at home. Because many patients with cystic fibrosis require bronchial hygiene therapy at least twice a day for 20 to 30 minutes, a mechanical percussor or a high-frequency chest compression vest can be especially helpful in moving thick bronchial secretions (Figure 14-6) (see Bronchopulmonary Hygiene Therapy Protocol, Protocol 9-2).

Lung Expansion Therapy Protocol

Lung expansion therapy may be administered to help offset the alveolar atelectasis associated with cystic fibrosis (see Lung Expansion Therapy Protocol, Protocol 9-3).

Aerosolized Medication Protocol

Various sympathomimetic, parasympatholytic, and mucolytic agents are commonly used to induce bronchial smooth muscle relaxation and mucous thinning. **Dornase alpha** (Pulmozyme—also known as *rhDNase* or *DNase*) has been shown to be especially helpful in the management of cystic fibrosis. This aerosolized agent is an enzyme that breaks down the DNA of the thick bronchial mucus associated with cystic fibrosis. Dornase alpha has shown good results in improving the lung function of patients with cystic fibrosis while reducing the frequency and severity of respiratory infections (see Aerosolized Medication Protocol, Protocol 9-4 and Appendix II).

Mechanical Ventilation Protocol

Because acute ventilatory failure superimposed on chronic ventilatory failure often is seen in patients with severe cystic fibrosis, mechanical ventilation may be required to maintain an adequate ventilatory status. Continuous mechanical ventilation is justified when the acute ventilatory failure is thought to be reversible—for example, when pneumonia complicates the condition (see Mechanical Ventilation Protocols, Protocol 9-5, Protocol 9-6, and Protocol 9-7).

Medications and Special Procedures Prescribed by the Physician

Xanthines

Xanthines are occasionally used to enhance bronchial smooth muscle relaxation (see Appendix II, Xanthine Bronchodilators).

Expectorants

Expectorants often are used when water alone or aerosolized mucolytics are not sufficient to facilitate expectoration (see Appendix II, Expectorants).

Antibiotics

Antibiotics are commonly administered to prevent or combat secondary respiratory tract infections. For example, an antibiotic treatment widely used to treat *P. aeruginosa* in the cystic fibrosis patient is inhaled tobramycin (TOBI). Unfortunately, a major drawback of long-term use of antibiotics is the development of bacteria that become resistant to drug therapy. In addition, the long-term use of antibiotics often leads to fungal infections of the mouth, oral pharynx, and tracheobronchial tree (see Appendix II, Antibiotic Agents).

Lung or Heart-Lung Transplantation

Several large organ transplant centers currently are performing lung or heart-lung transplantations in selected patients with cystic fibrosis whose general body condition is good. According to the Cystic Fibrosis Foundation, approximately 900 lung transplants are performed each year in the United States. Since 1991, about 1600 cystic fibrosis patients have received lung transplants—120 to 150 patients per year. In 2003, 368 patients were accepted for the lung transplant procedure. The success of lung transplantation in patients with cystic fibrosis is as good as or better than in patients with other lung diseases (e.g., emphysema). As many as 90% of the patients with cystic fibrosis are alive 1 year after transplantation, and 50% are alive after 5 years.*

Future Treatments

Since the identification of the mutant gene that disrupts the CFTR, some advances have been made in gene therapy for patients with cystic fibrosis. For example, researchers have had some success with the tracheal instillation of copies of normal genes over the surface of the epithelial cells of the respiratory tract. However, because of the myriad complex challenges associated with this DNA research, effective gene therapy for cystic fibrosis is not close at hand.

---

*Cystic Fibrosis Foundation (www.cff.org).

CASE STUDY

Cystic Fibrosis

Admitting History

A 27-year-old man has a long history of respiratory problems caused by cystic fibrosis. Even though his medical records are incomplete, he reported on admission that his parents told him that he had experienced several episodes of pneumonia during his early years. He is an adopted child and therefore does not know his biologic family history. His parents are actively involved in his general care, which entails the home care suggestions and therapeutic procedures presented by the pulmonary rehabilitation team. He takes supplemental multivitamins and timed-release oral pancreatic enzymes regularly, as prescribed by his doctor.

During his teens he had fewer respiratory symptoms than he has today and was able to lead a relatively normal life. During that time, he took up water-skiing and became proficient in the slalom event. He is known to most of his associates as a "wonder." Although he qualifies for disability income because of his continual shortness of breath, he is able to do various small jobs, which always relate to water-skiing. He is well known throughout the water-skiing circuit as an excellent chief judge at national and regional tournaments. In addition, he is a certified driver for jump-trick and slalom events and recently has become involved in selling water-ski tournament ropes and handles, which provides him with a small additional income.

Over the past 3 years, his cough has become more persistent and increasingly productive, with about a cupful of sputum noted daily. Over the same period, he has noted intermittent hemoptysis and has become short of breath when climbing stairs. Even though the man has a normal appetite, he has lost a great deal of weight over the past 2 years. On admission, he reported a history of severe shortness of breath. He denied experiencing any recent changes in bowel habits, despite his weight loss, but said that he has noticed a tendency to pass rather pale stools. Much to the chagrin of his doctor, 3 years ago he began smoking about 10 cigarettes a day, his reason being that the cigarettes help him cough up the sputum.

Physical Examination

On examination the patient appeared pale, cyanotic, and thin. He had a barrel chest and was using his accessory muscles of respiration. Clubbing of the fingers was present. He demonstrated a frequent, productive cough. His sputum was sweet-smelling, thick, and yellow-green. His neck veins were distended, and he showed mild-to-moderate peripheral edema. He stated that he had not been this short of breath in a long time.

He had a blood pressure of 142/90, a heart rate of 108 bpm, and a respiratory rate of 28/min. He was afebrile. Palpation of the chest was unremarkable. Expiration was prolonged. Hyperresonant notes were elicited bilaterally during percussion. Auscultation revealed diminished breath sounds and heart sounds. Crackles and rhonchi were heard throughout both lung fields.

His chart showed that during his last medical checkup (about 10 months before this admission) a pulmonary function test (PFT) was conducted. Results revealed moderate-to-severe airway obstruction. No blood gases were analyzed.

His chest x-ray examination on this admission revealed hyperlucent lung fields, depressed hemidiaphragms, and mild cardiac enlargement (Figure 14-7). His arterial blood gas values (ABGs) on 1.5 L/min oxygen by nasal cannula were as follows: pH 7.51, $Pa{CO_2}$ 58 mm Hg, HCO_3^- 43, and $Pa{O_2}$ 66 mm Hg. His hemoglobin oxygen saturation measured by pulse oximetry ($Sp{O_2}$) was 94%. On the basis of these clinical data, the following SOAP was documented.

Respiratory Assessment and Plan

S "I've not been this short of breath in a long time."

O Skin: pale, cyanotic; barrel chest and use of accessory muscles of respiration; digital clubbing; cough frequent and productive; sputum: sweet-smelling, thick, yellow-green; distended neck veins and peripheral edema; vital signs: BP 142/90, HR 108, RR 28, T normal; bilateral hyperresonant percussion notes; diminished breath sounds; crackles and rhonchi; CXR: hyperlucency, flattened diaphragms, and mild cardiac enlargement; ABGs (1.5 L/min O_2 by nasal cannula): pH 7.51, $Pa{CO_2}$ 58, HCO_3^- 43, $Pa{O_2}$ 66; $Sp{O_2}$ 94%

A
- Respiratory distress (general appearance, vital signs)
- Excessive tracheobronchial tree secretions (productive cough)

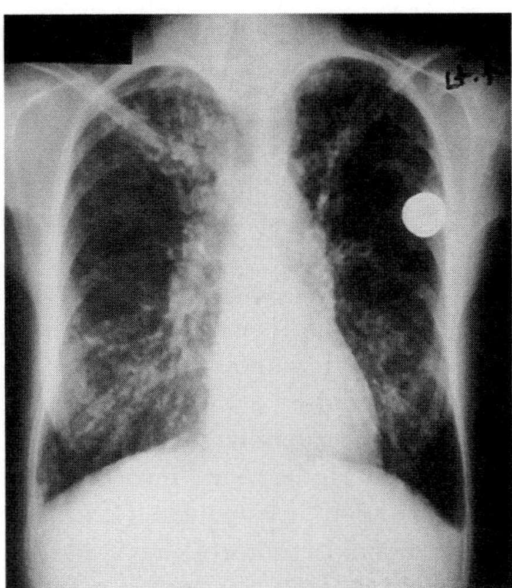

FIGURE 14-7 Chest x-ray film from a 27-year-old man with cystic fibrosis.

- Infection likely (yellow-green sputum)
- Hyperinflated alveoli (barrel chest, use of accessory muscles, CXR)
- Acute alveolar hyperventilation superimposed on chronic ventilatory failure with mild hypoxemia (history, ABGs)
- Possible impending acute ventilatory failure
- Cor pulmonale (distended neck veins, peripheral edema, CXR)

P **Bronchopulmonary Hygiene Therapy Protocol** (cough and deep breathe Tx q4h), sputum culture). **Oxygen Therapy Protocol** (2 L/min by nasal cannula). Monitor possible impending ventilatory failure closely (pulse oximetry, vital signs, ABGs).

48 Hours after Admission

The respiratory therapist from the Consult Service noted that the patient was again in respiratory distress. The man stated that he could not get enough air to sleep even 10 minutes. He appeared cyanotic and was using his accessory muscles of respiration. His vital signs were as follows: blood pressure 147/95, heart rate 117 bpm, respiratory rate 32/min, and temperature 37° C (98.6° F).

He coughed frequently, and although his cough was weak, he produced large amounts of thick, green sputum. Hyperresonant notes were produced during percussion over both lung fields. On auscultation, breath sounds and heart sounds were diminished. Crackles, rhonchi, and wheezing were heard throughout both lung fields. No recent chest x-ray film was available. A sputum culture confirmed the presence of *Pseudomonas aeruginosa.* His Spo_2 was 92% and his ABGs were as follows: pH 7.55, $Paco_2$ 54 mm Hg, HCO_3^- 45, and Pao_2 57 mm Hg. On the basis of these clinical data, the following SOAP was documented.

Respiratory Assessment and Plan

S "I can't get enough air to sleep 10 minutes!"

O Cyanosis and use of accessory muscles of respiration; vital signs: BP 147/95, HR 117, RR 32, T 37° C (98.6° F); cough: frequent, weak, and productive of large amounts of thick, green sputum; *Pseudomonas aeruginosa* cultured; bilateral hyperresonant notes and diminished breath sounds; crackles, rhonchi, and wheezes; Spo_2 92%; ABGs: pH 7.55, $Paco_2$ 54, HCO_3^- 45, Pao_2 57

A
- Continued respiratory distress (general appearance, vital signs, use of accessory muscles)
- Excessive bronchial secretions (cough, sputum, breath sounds)
- Poor ability to mobilize secretions (weak cough)
- Acute alveolar hyperventilation superimposed on chronic ventilatory failure with mild- to-moderate hypoxemia (ABGs)
- Possible impending ventilatory failure

P Start **Aerosolized Medication Protocol** (0.5 cc albuterol in 2 cc rhDNase q4h). Up-regulate **Bronchopulmonary Hygiene Therapy** per protocol (CPT and PEP therapy q2h). Up-regulate **Oxygen Therapy Protocol** (HAFOE mask at Fio_2 0.35). Continue to monitor possible impending ventilatory failure closely.

64 Hours after Admission

The respiratory care practitioner noted that the patient was in obvious respiratory distress. The patient said he could not find a position that allowed him to breathe comfortably. He appeared cyanotic and was using pursed-lip breathing, using his accessory muscles of respiration. His vital signs were as follows: blood pressure 145/90, heart rate 120 bpm, respiratory rate 22/min, and oral temperature 38° C (100.5° F). Palpation was normal, but bilateral hyperresonant percussion notes were elicited. Auscultation revealed crackles, rhonchi, and wheezing bilaterally. No recent chest x-ray film was available. His Spo_2 was 65%, and his ABGs were as follows: pH 7.33, $Paco_2$ 79 mm Hg, HCO_3^- 41, and Pao_2 37 mm Hg. On the basis of these clinical data, the following SOAP was entered in the patient's chart.

Respiratory Assessment and Plan

S "I can't get into a comfortable position to breathe."

O Cyanosis; pursed-lip breathing and use of accessory muscles of respiration; vital signs: BP 145/90, HR 120, RR 22, T 38° C (100.5° F); bilateral hyperresonant percussion notes, crackles, rhonchi, and wheezing; Spo_2 65%; ABGs: pH 7.33, $Paco_2$ 79, HCO_3^- 41, PaO_2 37

A
- Continued respiratory distress (general appearance, vital signs, use of accessory muscles, pursed-lip breathing)
- Excessive bronchial secretions (cough, sputum, breath sounds)
- Acute ventilatory failure superimposed on chronic ventilatory failure with severe hypoxemia (ABGs, vital signs)

P Contact physician stat. Consider intubation and implementation of the **Mechanical Ventilation Protocol.** Continue **Aerosolized Medication and Bronchial Hygiene Therapy Protocol** (after patient has been placed on ventilator). Up-regulate **Oxygen Therapy Protocol** (initially, Fio_2 0.50 on ventilator). Monitor closely.

Discussion

The science of respiratory care has advanced over the years, and the prognosis for patients with this multisystem genetic disorder has improved. In this patient's lifetime, the following four therapeutic landmarks can be noted:

1. Vigorous use of chest physical therapy (percussion and postural drainage)
2. Intermittent treatment of secretions with antibiotics and mucolytics, such as Pulmozyme
3. Positive expiratory pressure (PEP) therapy
4. Lung transplantation (when all else fails)

This patient had received at least three of these treatments and was in the hands of caring parents. His own stubborn nature and interest in athletics were clearly helpful in his prolonged survival. Important to note are the circumstances surrounding his admission, especially the fact that he had experienced hemoptysis, dyspnea, and weight loss during the several years preceding his admission. Note also that he had started smoking cigarettes.

In this case study, the patient's chief complaints purposely have been buried in the admitting history. The reader should have discerned that the patient was coughing productively and had hemoptysis, dyspnea, and weight loss. The recommended therapeutic strategy arises from recognition of these four presenting complaints. Note also that on admission the patient had neck vein distention and peripheral edema, suggesting cor pulmonale. If the experience with chronic obstructive pulmonary disease can be translated to patients with cystic fibrosis, this is a bad prognostic sign and one that clearly calls for intensification of the therapeutic regimen.

Note that on the initial physical examination, the patient demonstrated **excessive bronchial secretions** and a productive cough; no baseline arterial blood gases existed with which to compare his current values (see **Bronchospasm**, Figure 9-11). Thus the observation of an elevated Pa_{CO_2} should be taken very, very seriously, because (at least initially) whether this value is a "chronic" arterial blood gas value is unclear.

At the time of the second evaluation the patient clearly was not improving. The up-regulation of **Bronchopulmonary Hygiene Therapy** (see Protocol 9-2) and addition of the **Aerosolized Medication Protocol** at this point was appropriate—the increased chest physical therapy (along with PEP therapy) q2h, and Pulmozyme therapy. A repeat chest x-ray study would not be out of order at this time. We could argue that the Aerosolized Medication Protocol should have been started earlier.

The third assessment suggests that the patient clearly was deteriorating despite vigorous noninvasive therapy. At this point, the patient was placed on an F_{IO_2} of 0.5, and the stat call to the physician regarding the acute ventilatory failure was clearly justified. The addition of intubation and mechanical ventilation at this time would prevent fatigue, allow deep nasal tracheal suctioning, and facilitate repeat therapeutic bronchoscopy if it were to become necessary.

Despite this initial downhill course, the patient was placed on a ventilator and slowly improved. Over the next 7 days, the patient was extubated. The therapist should note that despite all the "good" things the patient and family did to treat his illness, the patient's initiation of smoking clearly could be a "last-straw" phenomenon. The patient should be placed on a smoking-cessation program. This step is as important for the long-term prognosis as is the skill of the practitioner caring for him during this bout of acute ventilatory failure.

SELF-ASSESSMENT QUESTIONS

evolve Answers to questions can be found on Evolve. To access additional student assessment questions and case studies for application of text material to real-life scenarios, visit **http://evolve.elsevier.com/DesJardins/respiratory.**

1. Which of the following organisms is or are commonly found in the tracheobronchial tree secretions of patients with cystic fibrosis?
1. Staphylococcus
2. Haemophilus influenzae
3. Streptococcus
4. Pseudomonas aeruginosa
    a. 1 only
    b. 2 only
    c. 1 and 4 only
    d. 1, 2, and 4 only

2. When two carriers of cystic fibrosis produce children, there is a:
1. 75% chance that the baby will be a carrier
2. 25% chance that the baby will be completely normal
3. 50% chance that the baby will have cystic fibrosis
4. 25% chance that the baby will have cystic fibrosis
    a. 1 only
    b. 3 only
    c. 2 and 4 only
    d. 1 and 2 only

3. The cystic fibrosis gene is located on which chromosome?
    a. 5
    b. 6
    c. 7
    d. 8

4. In cystic fibrosis the patient commonly demonstrates which of the following?
1. Increased FEV_T
2. Decreased MVV
3. Increased RV
4. Decreased FEV_1/FVC ratio
    a. 1 only
    b. 3 only
    c. 3 and 4 only
    d. 2, 3, and 4 only

5. During the advanced stages of cystic fibrosis, the patient generally demonstrates which of the following?
1. Bronchial breath sounds
2. Dull percussion notes
3. Diminished breath sounds
4. Hyperresonant percussion notes
    a. 1 and 3 only
    b. 2 and 4 only
    c. 1 and 4 only
    d. 1, 3, and 4 only

6. Approximately 80% of all patients with cystic fibrosis demonstrate a deficiency in which of the following vitamins?

1. A
2. B
3. D
4. E
5. K

a. 3 and 4 only
b. 1, 4, and 5 only
c. 2, 3, and 4 only
d. 1, 3, 4, and 5 only

7. In children, which of the following sweat chloride concentration values is diagnostic of cystic fibrosis?

a. 50 mEq/L
b. 60 mEq/L
c. 70 mEq/L
d. 80 mEq/L

8. Which of the following is or are mucolytic agents?

1. DNase
2. Pulmozyme
3. Tobramycin
4. Dornase alpha

a. 1 only
b. 2 only
c. 3 and 4 only
d. 1, 2, and 4 only

9. With regard to the secretion of sodium and chloride, the sweat glands of patients with cystic fibrosis secrete up to:

a. 3 times the normal amount
b. 5 times the normal amount
c. 7 times the normal amount
d. 10 times the normal amount

10. Which of the following clinical manifestations are associated with severe cystic fibrosis?

1. Decreased hemoglobin concentration
2. Increased central venous pressure
3. Decreased breath sounds
4. Increased pulmonary vascular resistance

a. 1 and 3 only
b. 2 and 3 only
c. 3 and 4 only
d. 2, 3, and 4 only

PART III

Infectious Pulmonary Diseases

Pneumonia

15

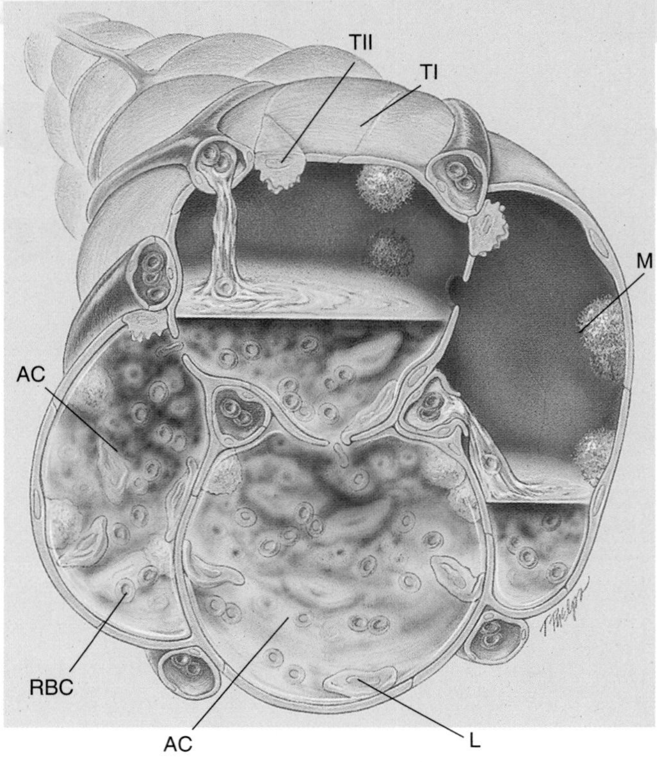

FIGURE 15-1 Cross-sectional view of alveolar consolidation in pneumonia. *AC,* Alveolar consolidation; *L,* leukocyte; *M,* macrophage; *RBC,* red blood cell; *TI,* type I cell.

Chapter Objectives

After reading this chapter, you will be able to:

- List the anatomic alterations of the lungs associated with pneumonia.
- Describe the causes and classifications of pneumonia.
- List the cardiopulmonary clinical manifestations associated with pneumonia.
- Describe the general management of pneumonia.
- Describe the clinical strategies and rationales of the SOAPs presented in the case study.
- Define key terms and complete self-assessment questions at the end of the chapter and on Evolve.

Key Terms

Acquired Pneumonia Classifications
Adenovirus
Anaerobic Organisms
Aspiration
Aspiration Pneumonia
Aspiration Pneumonitis
Atypical Organisms
Avian Influenza A
Bacteroides asaccharolyticus
Bacteroides melaninogenicus
Chlamydia pneumoniae
Chlamydia psittaci
Community-Acquired Pneumonia (CAP)
Consolidated
Coronavirus
Croup
Cytomegalovirus
"Double Pneumonia"
Dysphagia
***Enterobacter* species**
Escherichia coli
Fungal Infections
Fusobacterium necrophorum
Gastroesophageal Reflux Disease (GERD)
Gram-Negative Organisms
Gram-Positive Organisms
Haemophilus influenzae
Hospital-Acquired Pneumonia
Influenza Virus
Klebsiella
Legionella pneumophila
Lipoid Pneumonitis

Lobar Pneumonia
Multiple Drug-Resistant *Staphyloccus aureus* (MDRSA)
Mendelson's Syndrome
Moraxella catarrhalis
Mycoplasma pneumoniae
Nursing Home-Acquired Pneumonia
Parainfluenza Viruses
Peptostreptococcus Species
Pneumocystis carinii
Porphyromonas endodontalis
Porphyromonas gingivalis
Pseudomonas aeruginosa
Respiratory Syncytial Virus (RSV)
Rickettsial Infections
Rubella
Serratia Species
Severe Acute Respiratory Syndrome (SARS)
Silent Aspiration
Staphylococcus
Streptococcus
Swallowing Mechanics
Tuberculosis
Varicella
Ventilator-Associated Pneumonia
Walking Pneumonia

Chapter Outline

Anatomic Alterations of the Lungs

Pneumonia, or pneumonitis with consolidation, is the result of an inflammatory process that primarily affects the gas exchange area of the lung. In response to the inflammation, fluid (serum) and some red blood cells (RBCs) from adjacent pulmonary capillaries pour into the alveoli. This process of fluid transfer is called *effusion.* Polymorphonuclear leukocytes move into the infected area to engulf and kill invading bacteria on the alveolar walls. This process has been termed *surface phagocytosis.* Increased numbers of macrophages also appear in the infected area to remove cellular and bacterial debris. If the infection is overwhelming, the alveoli become filled with fluid, RBCs, polymorphonuclear leukocytes, and macrophages. When this occurs, the lungs are said to be **consolidated** (Figure 15-1). Atelectasis is often associated with patients who have **aspiration pneumonia.**

The major pathologic or structural changes associated with pneumonia are as follows:

- Inflammation of the alveoli
- Alveolar consolidation
- Atelectasis (e.g., aspiration pneumonia)

Etiology and Epidemidogy

Pneumonia and influenza combined are the eighth leading cause of death among all Americans and the sixth leading cause of death among all Americans over the age of 65. It is estimated that more than 60,000 Americans die of pneumonia each year. Pneumonia and influenza are especially life threatening in individuals whose lungs are already damaged by chronic obstructive pulmonary disease (COPD), asthma, or smoking. The risk of death from pneumonia or influenza is also higher among people with heart disease, diabetes, or a weakened immune system. As discussed in further detail later, causes of pneumonia include bacteria, viruses, fungi, **tuberculosis,** anaerobic organisms, **aspiration,** and the inhalation of irritating chemicals such as chlorine.

Pneumonia involving an entire lobe of the lung is called **lobar pneumonia.** When both lungs are involved, the condition is called **double pneumonia.** Although the term "**walking pneumonia**" has no clinical significance, it is often used to describe a mild case of pneumonia. For example, patients infected with ***Mycoplasma pneumoniae,*** who generally have mild symptoms and remain ambulatory, are sometimes told that they have "walking pneumonia". Initially, pneumonia often mimics a common cold or the flu (e.g., the signs and symptoms develop quickly). For example, the patient suddenly experiences chills, shivering, high fever, sweating, chest pain (pleurisy), and a dry and nonproductive cough.

Pneumonia is an insidious disease because its symptoms vary greatly depending on the patient's specific underlying condition and the type of organism causing the pneumonia. Often what is initially thought to be a cold or the flu can in fact be a much more serious pulmonary infection. The early recognition and treatment of pneumonia provide the best chance for a full recovery. There are over 30 causes of pneumonia. The major ones are listed in Box 15-1 and are discussed in the following paragraphs.

Bacterial Causes

Several types of bacteria can cause pneumonia. Bacterial pneumonia often occurs after an individual has had an upper respiratory infection such as a cold or the flu. Early signs and symptoms include shaking chills, shaking, a high fever, sweating, chest pain, an increased respiratory rate, and cough that produces yellow and green sputum. The patient may be confused or delirious. Bacterial pneumonia is often confined to just one lobe of the lung. This is called *lobar pneumonia.* Bacterial causes are divided into **gram-positive organisms, gram-negative organisms,** and **anaerobic organisms.** The most common are discussed in the following paragraphs.

Box 15-1 Causes of Pneumonia and Classifications

Bacterial Causes

Gram-Positive Organisms

Streptococcus
Staphylococcus

Gram-Negative Organisms

Haemophilus influenzae
Klebsiella
Pseudomonas aeruginosa
Moraxella catarrhalis
Escherichia coli
Serratia species
Enterobacter species

Atypical Organisms

Mycoplasma pneumoniae
Legionella pneumophila
Chlamydia psittaci
Chlamydia pneumoniae

Anaerobic Organisms

Peptostreptococcus species
Bacteroides melaninogenicus
Fusobacterium necrophorum
Bacteroides asaccharolyticus
Porphyromonas endodontalis
Porphyromonas gingivalis

Viral Causes

Influenza virus, including H1N1
Respiratory syncytial virus
Parainfluenza virus
Adenovirus
Coronavirus (severe acute respiratory syndrome [SARS])

Other Causes

Rickettsial infections
Varicella
Rubella
Aspiration pneumonitis
Lipoid pneumonitis
Pneumocystis carinii
Cytomegalovirus
Tuberculosis (see Chapter 17)
Fungal infections (see Chapter 18)
Avian influenza A

Acquired Pneumonia Classification

Community-acquired pneumonia
Nursing home–acquired pneumonia
Hospital-acquired pneumonia
Ventilator-associated pneumonia

Gram-Positive Organisms

Streptococcal pneumonia. *Streptococcus pneumoniae* accounts for more than 80% of all the bacterial pneumonias. The organism is a gram-positive, nonmotile coccus that is found singly, in pairs (called *diplococci*), and in short chains (Figure 15-2). The cocci are enclosed in a smooth, thick polysaccharide capsule that is essential for virulence. There are more than 80 different types of *S. pneumoniae.* Serotype 3 organisms are the most virulent. Streptococci are generally transmitted by aerosol from a cough or sneeze of an infected individual. Most strains of *S. pneumoniae* are sensitive to penicillin and its derivatives. *S. pneumoniae* also is commonly cultured from the sputum of patients having an acute exacerbation of chronic bronchitis.

Staphylococcal pneumonia. There are two major groups of ***Staphylococcus:*** (1) *Staphylococcus aureus,* which is responsible for most "staph" infections in humans, and (2) *Staphylococcus albus* and *Staphylococcus epidermidis,* which are part of the normal skin flora. The staphylococci are gram-positive cocci found singly, in pairs (called *diplococci*), and in irregular clusters (Figure 15-3). Staphylococcal pneumonia often follows a predisposing virus infection and is seen most often in children and immunosuppressed adults. *S. aureus* is commonly transmitted by aerosol from a cough or sneeze of an infected individual and indirectly via contact with contaminated

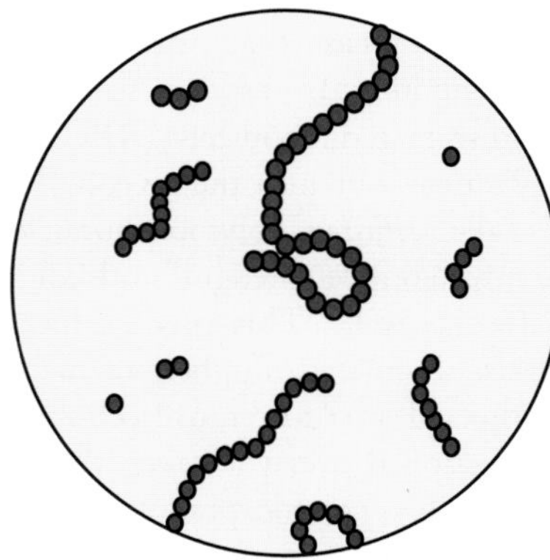

FIGURE 15-2 The *Streptococcus* organism is a gram-positive, nonmotile bacterium that occurs singly, in pairs, and in short chains.

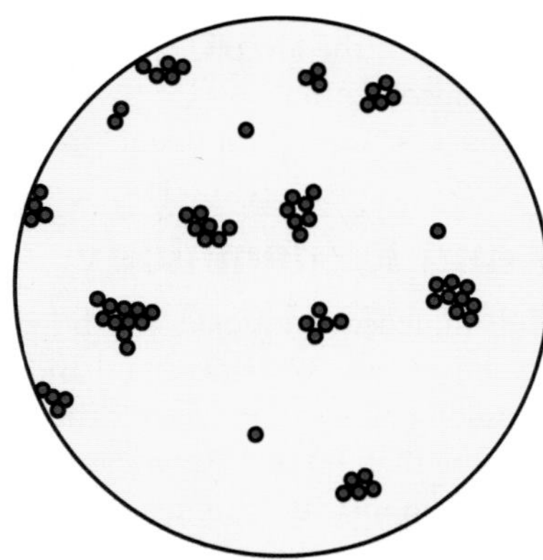

FIGURE 15-3 The *Staphylococcus* organism is a gram-positive, nonmotile coccus that is found singly, in pairs, and in irregular clusters.

floors, bedding, clothes, and the like. Staphylococci are a common cause of **hospital-acquired pneumonia** and are becoming increasingly antibiotic resistant—thus the term **multiple drug–resistant *S. aureus* (MDRSA)** organisms (some centers shorten this acronym to *MRSA*).

Gram-Negative Organisms

The major gram-negative organisms responsible for pneumonia are rod-shaped microorganisms called *bacilli* (Figure 15-4). The bacilli described in the following sections are frequently seen in the clinical setting.

Haemophilus influenzae. ***Haemophilus influenzae*** is a common inhabitant of human pharyngeal flora. *H. influenzae* is one of the smallest gram-negative bacilli, measuring about 1.5 mm in length and 0.3 mm in width. It appears as coccobacilli on Gram stain. There are six types of *H. influenzae,* designated A to F, but only type B is commonly pathogenic. Pneumonia caused by *H. influenzae* type B is seen most often in children aged 1 month to 6 years old. *H. influenzae* type B is almost always the cause of acute epiglottitis. The organism is transmitted via aerosol or contact with contaminated objects. It is sensitive to cold and does not survive long after expectoration. *H. influenzae* is commonly cultured from the sputum of patients having an acute exacerbation of chronic bronchitis. Additional risk factors for *H. influenzae* infection include COPD, defects in B-cell function, functional and anatomic asplenia, and human immunodeficiency virus (HIV) infection.

Klebsiella pneumoniae* (Friedländer's Bacillus).** *K. pneumoniae* organisms have long been associated with lobar pneumonia, particularly in men older than 40 years and in chronic alcoholics of both genders. ***Klebsiella is a gram-negative bacillus that is found singly, in pairs, and in chains of varying lengths. It is a normal inhabitant of the human gastrointestinal tract. The organism can be transmitted directly by aerosol or indirectly by contact with freshly contaminated articles. *K. pneumoniae* is a common nosocomial, or hospital-acquired, disease. It is typically transmitted by routes such as clothing, intravenous solutions, foods, and the hands of health-care workers. The mortality of patients with *K. pneumoniae* is quite high because septicemia is a frequent complication.

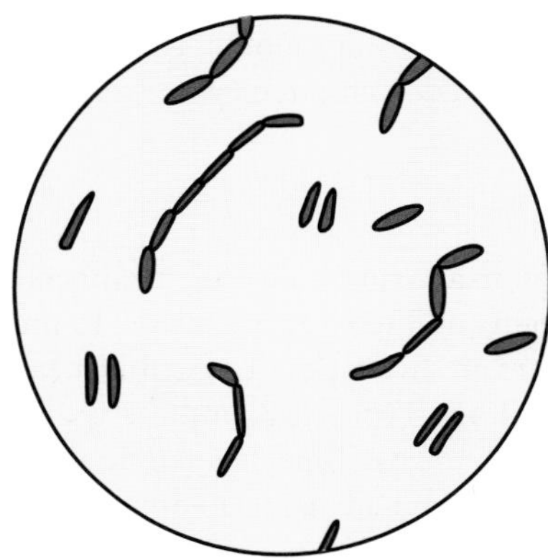

FIGURE 15-4 Bacilli are rod-shaped microorganisms and are the major gram-negative organisms responsible for pneumonia.

***Pseudomonas aeruginosa* (Bacillus Pyocyaneus).** *P. aeruginosa* is a highly motile, gram-negative bacillus. It colonizes the gastrointestinal tract, burns, and catheterized urinary tract and is a contaminant in many aqueous solutions. Risk factors include neutropenia, HIV infection, preexisting lung disease, endotracheal intubation, and prior antibiotic use. *P. aeruginosa* frequently is cultured from the respiratory tract of chronically ill, tracheostomized patients and is a leading cause of hospital-acquired pneumonia. This makes *P. aeruginosa* a particular problem for the respiratory care practitioner. Because the *Pseudomonas* organism thrives in dampness, it is frequently cultured from contaminated respiratory therapy equipment. The organism is commonly transmitted by aerosol or by direct contact with freshly contaminated articles. The sputum from patients with *Pseudomonas* infection is frequently green and sweet-smelling.

Moraxella catarrhalis. *M. catarrhalis* is a natural inhabitant of the human pharynx. After *S. pneumoniae* and *H. influenzae, M. catarrhalis* is the third most common cause of acute exacerbation of chronic bronchitis.

Escherichia coli. *E. coli* is a normal inhabitant of the intestinal tract. It is sometimes the cause of nosocomial pneumonia (see the discussion of hospital-acquired pneumonia, page 230).

Serratia species. ***Serratia* species** cause about 7% of the cases of nosocomial pneumonia (see discussion of hospital-acquired pneumonia, page 230).

Enterobacter species. ***Enterobacter* species** *(Enterobacter cloacae* and *Enterobacter aerogenes)* are sometimes the cause of pneumonia.

Atypical Organisms

Mycoplasma pneumoniae. *M. pneumoniae* is a common cause of mild pneumonia. These organisms cause symptoms similar to both bacterial and viral pneumonia, although the symptoms develop more gradually and are often milder. A common symptom of mycoplasma pneumonia is a cough that tends to come in violent attacks, producing only a small amount of white mucus. Chills and fever are early symptoms. Some patients experience nausea or vomiting. Some patients may experience a profound weakness that lasts for a long time.

The mycoplasma are tiny, cell wall–deficient organisms. They are smaller than bacteria but larger than viruses. The pneumonia caused by the mycoplasmal organism is described as *primary atypical pneumonia*—atypical because the organism escapes identification by standard bacteriologic tests. *M. pneumoniae* is most frequently seen in people younger than 40 years of age during the late summer and early fall months. This type of pneumonia spreads easily in areas where people congregate, such as child-care centers, schools, and homeless shelters. Patients with *M. pneumoniae* often are said to have "*walking pneumonia*" because the condition is mild (i.e., slight fever, fatigue, and a characteristic dry, hacking cough) and the patient is usually ambulatory.

Legionella pneumophila. In July 1976, a severe pneumonia-like disease outbreak occurred at an American Legion convention in Philadelphia. The causative agent eluded identification for many months, despite the concerted efforts of the nation's top epidemiologic experts. When the organism finally was recovered from a patient, it was found to be an unusual and fastidious gram-negative bacillus with atypical concentrations of certain branched-chain lipids. The initial isolate was designated as *Legionella pneumophila.* More than 20 *Legionella* species have now been identified.

Most of the species are free-living in soil and water, where they act as decomposer organisms. The organism also multiplies in standing water such as contaminated mud puddles, large air-conditioning systems, and water tanks. The organism is transmitted when it becomes airborne and enters the patient's lungs as an aerosol. No convincing evidence suggests that the organism is transmitted from person to person. The organism can be detected in pleural fluid, sputum, or lung tissue by direct fluorescent antibody microscopy. Although it is rarely found outside the lungs, the organism may be found in other tissues. The disease is most commonly seen in middle-aged men who smoke.

***Chlamydia psittaci* (Psittacosis).** *C. psittaci* is a small gram-negative bacterium in the respiratory tract and feces of a variety of birds (e.g., parrots, parakeets, lorikeets, cockatoos, chickens, pigeons, ducks, pheasants, turkeys). *C. psittaci* is transmitted from birds to humans by aerosol or direct contact. The clinical manifestations of *C. psittaci* closely resemble those caused by *M. pneumoniae.*

Chlamydia pneumoniae. *C. pneumoniae* recently has been identified as a cause of pneumonia in adults. It has been detected in schools, military institutions, and families. It is associated with meningoencephalitis, myocarditis, endocarditis, coronary artery disease, and Guillain-Barré syndrome.

Anaerobic Bacterial Infections

The major anaerobic organisms associated with pneumonia are ***Peptostreptococcus* species,** *Bacteroides melaninogenicus, Fusobacterium necrophorum, Bacteroides asaccharolyticus, Porphyromonas endodontalis,* and *Porphyromonas gingivalis.* Aspiration of oropharyngeal secretions and gastric fluids are the major causes of anaerobic lung infections. Predisposing risk factors of aspiration include a decreased level of consciousness, impaired swallowing, poor dental hygiene, and gastrointestinal abnormalities. Aspiration pneumonia is often multimicrobial.

Viral Causes

Approximately half of all pneumonias are caused by viruses. More and more viruses are being identified as the cause of respiratory infections. Although most viruses attack the upper airways, some can produce pneumonia. Most of these pneumonias are not life threatening and last only a short time. Viral pneumonia tends to start with flulike signs and symptoms. The early symptoms are a dry (nonproductive) cough, headache, fever, muscle pain, and fatigue. As the disease progresses, the patient may become short of breath, cough, and produce a small amount of clear or white sputum. Viral pneumonia always carries the risk of development of a secondary bacterial pneumonia.

Viruses are minute organisms not visible by ordinary light microscopy. They are parasitic and depend on nutrients inside cells for their metabolic and reproductive needs. Approximately 90% of acute upper respiratory tract infections and 50% of lower respiratory tract infections are caused by viruses. Respiratory viruses are the most common cause of pneumonia in young children, peaking between the ages of 2 and 3. By school age, *M. pneumoniae* become more prevalent (see previous section). The most common viruses that cause respiratory infections are described in the following paragraphs.

Influenza Virus

Although the **influenza virus** has several subtypes, influenza A and B are the most common causes of viral respiratory tract infections. In the United States, influenza A and B commonly occur in epidemics during the winter months. Children, young adults, and older individuals are most at risk. Influenza is transmitted from person to person by aerosol droplets. Often the first sign of an epidemic is an increase in school absenteeism. The virus survives well in conditions of low temperatures and low humidity. It also has been found in horses, swine, and birds. Influenza viruses have an incubation period of 1 to 3 days and usually cause upper respiratory tract infections. Epidemiologists fear a pandemic of influenza, stating it is an issue of "when" and "where" rather than "if." The recent epidemic of H1N1 ("swine flu") is a case in point.

Respiratory Syncytial Virus

The **respiratory syncytial virus (RSV)** (see Chapter 36) is a member of the paramyxovirus group. Parainfluenza, mumps, and **rubella** viruses also belong to this group. RSV is most often seen in children less than 12 months of age and in older adults with underlying heart or pulmonary disease. Almost all children will be infected with RSV by their second birthday. The infection is rarely fatal in infants. RSV often goes unrecognized but may play an important role as a forerunner to bacterial infections. Early attempts to develop an RSV vaccine have been unsuccessful. The virus is transmitted by aerosol and by direct contact with infected individuals. RSV infections are most commonly seen in patients during the late fall, winter, or early spring months. Many times the virus is misdiagnosed in older children, who are given antibiotics that do not work.

Parainfluenza Virus

The **parainfluenza viruses** also are members of the paramyxovirus group and therefore are related to mumps, rubella, and RSV. There are five types of parainfluenza viruses: types 1, 2, 3, 4A, and 4B. Types 1, 2, and 3 are the major causes of infections in humans. Type 1 is considered a **croup** type of virus. Types 2 and 3 are associated with severe infections. Although type 3 is seen in persons of all ages, it usually is seen in infants younger than 2 months of age; types 1 and 2 are seen most often in children between the ages of 6 months and 5 years. Types 1 and 2 typically occur in the fall, whereas type 3 infection most often is seen in the late spring and summer. Parainfluenza viruses are transmitted by aerosol droplets and by direct person-to-person contact. The parainfluenza viruses are known for their ability to spread rapidly among members of the same family.

Adenoviruses

There are more than 30 **adenovirus** subgroups. Serotypes 4, 7, 14, and 21 cause viral infections and pneumonia in all age groups. Serotype 7 has been related to fatal cases of pneumonia in children. Adenoviruses are transmitted by aerosol. Pneumonia caused by adenoviruses generally occurs during the fall, winter, and spring.

Severe Acute Respiratory Syndrome

In 2002 China reported the first case of **severe acute respiratory syndrome (SARS)**. Shortly after this report, the disease was documented in numerous countries, including Vietnam, Singapore, and Indonesia. Both the United States and Canada have reported imported cases. Health officials believe that the cause of SARS is a newly recognized virus strain called a **coronavirus.** Other viruses, however, are still under investigation as potential causes. Coronaviruses are a group of viruses that have a halo or corona-like appearance when observed under an electron microscope. Known forms of coronavirus cause common colds and upper respiratory tract infections. SARS is highly contagious on close personal contact with infected individuals. It spreads through droplet transmission by coughing and sneezing. SARS might be transmitted through the air or from objects that have become contaminated.

The incubation period for SARS typically is 2 to 7 days. Initially, the patient usually develops a fever (>100.4° F or >38.0° C), followed by chills, headaches, general feeling of discomfort, and body aches. Toward the end of the incubation period, the SARS patient usually develops a dry, nonproductive cough, shortness of breath, and malaise. In severe causes, hypoxemia develops. According to the Centers for Disease Control and Prevention (CDC), 10% to 20% of SARS patients require mechanical ventilation. In spite of this fact, death from SARS is rare. No specific treatment recommendations exist at this time. The CDC, however, recommends that SARS patients receive the same treatment used for any patient with serious community-acquired atypical pneumonia of unknown cause.

Other Causes

Rickettsiae

Rickettsiae are small, pleomorphic coccobacilli. Most rickettsiae are intracellular parasites possessing both ribonucleic acid (RNA) and deoxyribonucleic acid (DNA). There are several pathogenic members of the *Rickettsia* family: *Rickettsia rickettsii* (Rocky Mountain spotted fever), *Rickettsia akari* (rickettsialpox), *Rickettsia prowazekii* (typhus), and *Rickettsia burnetii*, also called *Coxiella burnetii* (Q fever).

All species of the genus *Rickettsia* are unstable outside of cells except for *R. burnetii* (Q fever), which is extremely resistant to heat and light. Q fever can cause pneumonia as well as a prolonged febrile illness, an influenza-like illness, and endocarditis. The organism is commonly transmitted by arthropods (lice, fleas, ticks, mites). It also may be transmitted by cattle, sheep, and goats and possibly in raw milk.

Varicella (Chickenpox)

The **varicella** virus usually causes a benign disease in children aged 2 to 8 years, and complications of varicella are not common. In some cases, however, varicella has been noted to spread to the lungs and cause a serious secondary pneumonitis. The mortality rate of varicella pneumonia is about 20%.

Rubella (Measles)

Measles virus spreads from person to person by the respiratory route. Respiratory complications often are encountered in measles because of the widespread involvement of the mucosa of the respiratory tract (e.g., excessive bronchial secretions and infection).

Aspiration Pneumonitis

Aspiration of gastric fluid with a pH of 2.5 or less causes a serious and often fatal form of pneumonia. Aspiration of oropharyngeal secretions and gastric fluids are the major causes of anaerobic lung infections (see discussion of anaerobic bacterial infections, earlier). **Aspiration pneumonitis** is commonly missed because acute inflammatory reactions may not begin until several hours after aspiration of the gastric fluid. The inflammatory reaction generally increases in severity for 12 to 26 hours and may progress to acute respiratory distress syndrome (ARDS), which includes interstitial and intraalveolar edema, intraalveolar hyaline membrane formation, and atelectasis. In the absence of a secondary bacterial infection, the inflammation usually becomes clinically insignificant in approximately 72 hours. In 1946 Mendelson first described the clinical manifestations of tachycardia, dyspnea, and cyanosis associated with the aspiration of acid stomach contents. The clinical picture he described is now known as **Mendelson's syndrome** and is usually confined to aspiration pneumonitis in pregnant women.

Aspiration pneumonia is broadly defined as the pulmonary result of the entry of material from the stomach or upper respiratory tract into the lower airways. There are at least three distinctive forms of aspiration pneumonia, classified according to the nature of the aspirate, the clinical presentation, and management guidelines, as follows:

1. Toxic injury to the lung (such as that caused by gastric acid)
2. Obstruction (by foreign body or fluids)
3. Infection

Aspiration is the presumed cause of nearly all cases of anaerobic pulmonary infections. Studies suggest that anaerobic bacteria are the most common causative agents of lung abscesses; they are also commonly isolated in cases of empyema.

There is a difference between the aspiration of gastric contents and the aspiration of food. Aspiration of gastric contents causes initial hypoxemia regardless of the aspirate's pH level. Consequently, oximetry is a good measurement if aspiration is suspected. If the aspirate's pH is relatively high (greater than 5.9), the initial injury is rapidly reversible. Such aspiration occurs in patients who receive antacids or proton pump inhibitors (PPIs). If the pH is low (pH of unbuffered gastric contents normally ranges from 1 to 1.5), parenchymal damage may occur, with inflammation, edema, and hemorrhage. When food is aspirated, obliterative bronchiolitis with subsequent granuloma formation occurs.

Gastroesophageal reflux disease (GERD) is the regurgitation of stomach contents into the esophagus. GERD causes disruption in nerve-mediated reflexes in the distal esophagus, resulting in alteration of the primary and secondary peristaltic wave and reflux. Therefore "to-and-fro" peristalsis can result from spasticity at the distal esophageal sphincter and retropulsion of middle and upper esophageal contents. This may result in aspiration, although not necessarily.

GERD is three times more prevalent in patients with asthma than in other patients. In other words, GERD is a frequently unrecognized cause of asthma. Presumably, acid reflux into the esophagus causes vagal stimulation, resulting in a reflexive increase in bronchial tone in patients with asthma. Recent literature suggests that asymptomatic reflux does not contribute to worsening lung function. Nevertheless, GERD does cause chronic cough in 10% to 20% of patients.

Normal **swallowing mechanics** has four phases, as follows:

1. Oral preparatory
2. Oral
3. Pharyngeal
4. Esophageal

The first two phases are considered voluntary stages (cerebral). These phases occur as the food or liquid is prepared for entry to the pharynx and esophagus. The airway is open while food is prepared in the oral cavity. Adequate tongue function is important for the manipulation and propulsion of the prepared food or liquid (called a *bolus*) into the pharynx. Spillage of liquid into the pharynx during the chewing of food is usually not a problem in patients with good airway protection.

The pharyngeal phase (involuntary brain stem function) of swallowing involves numerous physiologic actions that direct the bolus into the esophagus:

- Elevation and retraction of the velopharyngeal port (velum closure)
- Pharyngeal muscle contraction
- Elevation and forward excursion of the larynx (epiglottic closure)
- Closure of the laryngeal vestibule, false vocal folds, and true vocal folds (laryngeal closure)
- Relaxation of the upper esophageal sphincter (UES)

Airway closure progresses inferiorly to superiorly in the larynx as the food bolus is directed laterally around the airway and into the esophagus.

Respiration is halted during the pharyngeal phase for an approximately 1-second apneic period, although duration varies with bolus volume and viscosity. Bolus transit in the esophageal phase (under both brain stem and intrinsic neural control) lasts 8 to 20 seconds. In this phase the UES relaxes to receive the bolus with a peristaltic wave from the pharyngeal superior constrictor muscles, forcing the bolus through the relaxed UES. The primary peristalsis propels the bolus through the esophagus and lower esophageal sphincter and into the stomach.

Six cranial nerves carry motor signals generated by cerebral and brain stem swallowing centers:

- V (trigeminal)
- VII (facial)
- IX (glossopharyngeal)
- X (vagus)
- XI (spinal accessory [minor involvement])
- XII (hypoglossal)

The relationship between respiration and swallowing is not random. Expiration before and after the pharyngeal phase in normal swallowing is believed to serve as an inherent closure and clearance mechanism against penetration of food or liquids into the airway entrance.

Dysphagia is the result of an abnormal swallow that can involve the oral, pharyngeal, and esophageal phases. Penetration into the laryngeal vestibule occurs when food or liquid (or both) enters the larynx but does not pass through the vocal cords into the trachea. Aspiration is the passage of food or liquid into the trachea via the vocal cords.

Diagnostic tests for dysphagia include the modified barium swallow (MBS), videofluoroscopy, videofiberoptic endoscopy, and the modified Evan's blue dye test. Evan's blue dye test involves instilling a deep blue dye into the gastrointestinal tract and seeing if it can be suctioned from the trachea. If it can, it suggests a communication between the two structures, such as a fistula. The MBS and videofluoroscopy tests are most definitive for identification of the particular phase of the swallow that is dysfunctional. The modified Evan's blue dye test can be unreliable (as much as 40% of the time) as a test suggesting aspiration in a tracheostomized patient. Both false-positive and false-negative test results occur.

A compromised respiratory system can cause dysphagia, and conversely, dysphagia may cause respiratory complications. COPD can result in a slowed oral and pharyngeal transit time, reduced coordination and strength of the oral and pharyngeal musculature, and reduced airway clearance by coughing.

Treatment of dysphagia is specific to the nature of the disorder. Varied methods of presentation of foods and liquids, bolus volumes and consistency, postural movements, and food temperature can affect the dynamics of the relation between respiration and swallowing. Large volumes of liquid requiring uninterrupted swallowing result in longer apneic periods and can be difficult for patients with shortness of breath and dyspnea. Small-volume bites and swallows make sense in this setting.

Unilateral cerebrovascular accidents (strokes) and hemorrhage tend to cause hypopharyngeal hemiparesis. Difficulty in swallowing (with impairment of the oral phase) and aspiration of thin fluids therefore may follow. The facial and tongue weakness can result in poor bolus control in the oral cavity.

Silent aspiration is defined as aspiration that does not evoke clinically observable adverse symptoms such as coughing, choking, and immediate respiratory distress. Some patients have silent aspiration after a stroke. Evidence also suggests that some sequelae of stroke include laryngopharyngeal sensory deficits with no subjective or objective evidence of dysphagia, such as choking, gagging, or cough.

Some patients with severe and bilateral sensory deficits develop aspiration pneumonia. The clinical findings of dysphonia, dysarthria, abnormal gag reflex, abnormal volitional cough, cough after swallow, and voice change after swallow all significantly relate to aspiration and are predictors of silent aspiration. Conversely, a normal reflex cough after a stroke indicates an intact laryngeal cough reflex, a protected airway, and low risk for developing aspiration pneumonia with oral feeding. The cough reflex is significantly reduced in older patients.

Tracheostomized patients are at high risk for silent aspiration. Perhaps 55% to 70% of intubated or tracheostomized patients aspirate. A tracheostomy tube has a direct effect on the pharyngeal phase of a swallow because of the alteration of normal respiratory function (exhalation timing) as well as the anatomic alteration and the physical resistance imposed by the tracheostomy tube itself. Laryngeal elevation is reduced, particularly with the cuff inflated, which leads to inadequate airway closure and increased pharyngeal residue.

Poor sensory response to material entering the larynx contributes to the slowing of an uncoordinated laryngeal closure. The protective cough may be lessened because of the impaired laryngeal sensation. Subglottic air pressure (coordinated exhalation with swallow) helps prevent entry of material into the trachea and is reduced in patients with a tracheostomy. An inflated cuffed tracheostomy can cause complications that can anchor the larynx to the anterior wall of the neck and desensitize the pharynx. Delayed triggering of the swallowing response and increased pharyngeal residue are prevalent.

Recommendations for oral feeding include considerations of dietary consistency, specifically defined for solids and liquids; skilled supervision with oral intake; safe swallowing strategies; positioning requirements; cuff deflation; and tracheal occlusion issues. It may be necessary to coordinate mealtime with ventilator weaning attempts to optimize more positive pressure generation to aid in expelling laryngeal residue and creating subglottic pressure.

Partial or complete endotracheal cuff deflation during meals promotes laryngeal elevation, allows expectoration of secretions, reduces the effect of friction on the tracheoesophageal wall, and enhances the senses of taste and smell. If an uncuffed tracheostomy is in place, possible placement of a Passey-Muir valve or capping of a fenestrated tracheostomy tube will aid in subglottic negative pressure and assist in an effective swallow.

The dynamic changes a patient may experience clinically necessitate a coordinated team approach, including physical, occupational, and respiratory therapists; a speech-language pathologist; registered dietitian; and nurse. This approach allows for effective management of tracheostomized and nontracheostomized patients and avoidance of aspiration.

Lipoid Pneumonitis

The aspiration of mineral oil, used medically as a lubricant, also has been known to cause pneumonitis–**lipoid pneumonitis.** The severity of the pneumonia depends on the type of oil aspirated. Oils from animal fats cause the most serious reaction, whereas oils of vegetable origin are relatively inert. When mineral oil is inhaled in an aerosolized form, an intense pulmonary tissue reaction occurs.

Pneumocystis carinii Pneumonia

P. jiroveci is an opportunistic, often fatal, form of pneumonia seen in profoundly immunosuppressed patients. Although the *Pneumocystis* organism has been identified as a protozoan, recent information suggests that it is more closely related to fungi. *Pneumocystis* normally can be found in the lungs of humans, but it does not cause disease in healthy hosts, only in individuals whose immune systems are critically impaired. Currently, *Pneumocystis pneumonia is the major pulmonary infection seen in patients with acquired immunodeficiency syndrome (AIDS) and HIV infection.*

In vulnerable hosts the disease spreads rapidly throughout the lungs. Before AIDS, *P. carinii* pneumonia was seen primarily in patients with malignancy, in organ transplant recipients, and in patients with diseases requiring treatment with large doses of immunosuppressive agents. Today, most cases of *P. carinii* pneumonia are seen in patients with AIDS. The early clinical manifestations of *Pneumocystis* in patients with AIDS are indistinguishable from those of any other pneumonia. Typical signs and symptoms include progressive exertional dyspnea, a dry cough that may or may not produce mucoid sputum, difficulty in taking a deep breath (not caused by pleurisy), and fever with or without sweats. The therapist may hear normal breath sounds on auscultation or end-inspiratory crackles. The chest x-ray film may be normal at first; later it will show bilateral interstitial infiltrates, which may progress to alveolar filling and "white out" of the chest x-ray film.

Cytomegalovirus

Cytomegalovirus (CMV), a member of the herpesvirus family, is the most common viral pulmonary complication of AIDS. CMV infection commonly coexists with *P. carinii* infection.

Tuberculosis

Tuberculosis (see Chapter 17) is an infectious disease caused by *Mycobacterium tuberculosis. M. tuberculosis* is a slender, rod-shaped aerobic organism. Predisposing factors of tuberculosis include homelessness, drug abuse, and AIDS. The initial response of the lung is an inflammatory reaction that is similar to any acute pneumonia (see Chapter 17).

Fungal Infections

Because most fungi are aerobes, the lung is a prime site for **fungal infections** (see Chapter 18). Primary fungal pathogens include *Histoplasma capsulatum, Coccidioides immitis,* and *Blastomyces dermatitidis.* In addition, the opportunistic yeast pathogens *Candida albicans, Cryptococcus neoformans,* and *Aspergillus* also may cause pneumonia in certain patients. For example, *C. albicans,* which occurs as normal flora in the oral cavity, genitalia, and large intestine, is rarely seen in the tracheobronchial tree or lung parenchyma. In patients with AIDS, however, *C. albicans* commonly causes an infection of the mouth, pharynx, esophagus, vagina, skin, and lungs. A *C. albicans* infection of the mouth is called *thrush;* it is characterized by a white, adherent, patchy infection of the membranes of the mouth, gums, cheeks, and throat.

C. neoformans proliferates in pigeon droppings, which have a high nitrogen content, and readily scatters into the air and dust. Today, the highest rate of cryptococcosis occurs among patients with AIDS and persons undergoing steroid therapy. The molds of the genus *Aspergillus* may be the most pervasive of all fungi—especially *Aspergillus fumigatus. Aspergillus* is found in soil, vegetation, leaf detritus, food, and compost heaps. Persons who breathe the air of granaries, barns, and silos are at the greatest risk. Aspergillus infection usually occurs in the lungs. *Aspergillus* is almost always an opportunistic infection and lately has posed a serious threat to patients with AIDS. When fungal organisms are inhaled, the initial response of the lung is an inflammatory reaction similar to that produced by any acute pneumonia (see Chapter 18).

Avian Influenza A

Avian influenza A (also called *bird flu* and *H5N1*) is a subype of the A strain virus and is highly contagious in birds. Historically, bird flu has not been known to infect humans. However, in Hong Kong in 1997 the first avian influenza virus to infect humans directly was reported. This outbreak was linked to chickens and classified as avian influenza A (H5N1). Since the Hong Kong outbreak, the bird flu virus has been reported in parts of Europe, Turkey, Romania, the Near East, and Africa. Many of the infected people have died. Experts are concerned that if the avian flu virus continues to spread, a worldwide pandemic outbreak could occur. People with bird flu may develop life-threatening complications, such as viral pneumonia and ARDS (the most common cause of bird flu–related deaths).

Acquired Pneumonia Classifications

Pneumonia is often classified according to the location or method of exposure. Common **acquired pneumonia classifications** are **community-acquired pneumonia (CAP), hospital-acquired pneumonia, ventilator-associated pneumonia (VAP),** and **nursing home–acquired pneumonia.**

Community-Acquired Pneumonia

Community-acquired pneumonia is defined as a lower respiratory tract infection that is acquired outside of the hospital or during the first 48 hours of hospitalization. More than 4 million adults are diagnosed with CAP each year in the United States. The most common cause of CAP is ***Streptococcus.*** Other organisms associated with CAP include *M. pneumoniae, H. influenzae, C. pneumoniae, L. pneumophila, S. aureus,* and *M. tuberculosis.*

Hospital-Acquired Pneumonia

Hospital-acquired pneumonia (also called *nosocomial pneumonia*) is defined as a pneumonia that develops 48 hours or longer after admission to the hospital. Nosocomial pneumonia is estimated to account for more than 15% of all respiratory infections. Nosocomial infections include *P. aeruginosa; S. aureus,* including MDRSA; *S. pneumoniae; Enterobacter; E. coli; Klebsiella;* and oral anaerobes (aspiration).

Ventilator-Acquired Pneumonia

Ventilator-acquired pneumonia (also called *ventilator-associated pneumonia*) is defined as a pneumonia that develops more than 48 to 72 hours after endotracheal intubation. Common ventilator-associated infections include *P. aeruginosa, Enterobacter, Klebsiella, Stenotrophomonas maltophilia,* and *S. aureus.* Concern that the occurrence of VAP is preventable lies as the root of possible reimbursement penalties for hospitals in which it occurs.

Nursing Home–Acquired Pneumonia

Nursing home–acquired pneumonia is defined as a respiratory tract infection that develops in a long-term care facility. Common nursing home–acquired infections include mixed aerobic and anaerobic mouth flora, *S. aureus,* enteric gram-negative bacilli, influenza, and *M. tuberculosis.*

OVERVIEW of the Cardiopulmonary Clinical Manifestations Associated with Pneumonia

The following clinical manifestations result from the pathologic mechanisms caused (or activated) by **Alveolar Consolidation** (see Figure 9-9), **Increased Alveolar-Capillary Membrane Thickness** (see Figure 9-10), and **Atelectasis** (see Figure 9-8)—the major anatomic alterations of the lungs associated with pneumonia (see Figure 15-1).

During the resolution stage of pneumonia, **Excessive Bronchial Secretions** (see Figure 9-12) also may play a part in the clinical presentation.

CLINICAL DATA OBTAINED AT THE PATIENT'S BEDSIDE

The Physical Examination

Vital Signs

Increased Respiratory Rate (Tachypnea)

Several pathophysiologic mechanisms operating simultaneously may lead to an increased ventilatory rate:

- Stimulation of peripheral chemoreceptors (hypoxemia)
- Decreased lung compliance–increased ventilatory rate relationship

OVERVIEW of the Cardiopulmonary Clinical Manifestations Associated with Pneumonia—cont'd

- Stimulation of J receptors
- Pain, anxiety, fever

Increased Heart Rate (Pulse) and Blood Pressure

Chest Pain and Decreased Chest Expansion

Cyanosis

Cough, Sputum Production, and Hemoptysis

Initially the patient with pneumonia usually has a nonproductive barking or hacking cough. As the disease progresses, however, the cough becomes productive. When the disease progresses to this point, the patient often expectorates small amounts of purulent, blood-streaked, or rusty sputum. This is caused by fluid moving from the pulmonary capillaries into the alveoli in response to the inflammatory process. As fluid crosses into the alveoli, some red blood cells (RBCs) also move into the alveoli and produce the blood-streaked or rusty appearance of the fluid (see Figure 15-1). Some of the fluid that moves in the alveoli also may work its way into the bronchioles and bronchi. As the fluid accumulates in the bronchial tree, the subepithelial receptors in the trachea, bronchi, and bronchioles are stimulated and initiate a cough reflex. Because the bronchioles and the smaller bronchi are deep in the lung parenchyma, the patient with pneumonia initially has a dry, hacking cough, and fluid cannot be easily expectorated until secretions reach the larger bronchi.

Chest Assessment Findings

- Increased tactile and vocal fremitus
- Dull percussion note
- Bronchial breath sounds
- Crackles and rhonchi
- Pleural friction rub (if process extends to pleural surface)
- Whispered pectoriloquy

CLINICAL DATA OBTAINED FROM LABORATORY TESTS AND SPECIAL PROCEDURES

Pulmonary Function Test Findings (Restrictive Lung Pathophysiology)

FORCED EXPIRATORY FLOW RATE FINDINGS

FVC	FEV_T	FEV_1/FVC ratio	$FEF_{25\%-75\%}$
↓	N or ↓	N or ↑	N or ↓

$FEF_{50\%}$	$FEF_{200-1200}$	PEFR	MVV
N or ↓	N or ↓	N or ↓	N or ↓

LUNG VOLUME AND CAPACITY FINDINGS

V_T	IRV	ERV	RV
N or ↓	↓	↓	↓

VC	IC	FRC	TLC	RV/TLC ratio
↓	↓	↓	↓	N

Arterial Blood Gases

MILD TO MODERATE STAGES

Acute Alveolar Hyperventilation with Hypoxemia (Acute Respiratory Alkalosis)

pH	Pa_{CO_2}	HCO_3^-	Pa_{O_2}
↑	↓	↓ (slightly)	↓

SEVERE STAGE

Acute Ventilatory Failure with Hypoxemia (Acute Respiratory Acidosis)

pH*	Pa_{CO_2}	HCO_3^- *	Pa_{O_2}
↓	↑	↑ (slightly)	↓

*When tissue hypoxia is severe enough to produce lactic acid, the pH and HCO_3^- values will be lower than expected for a particular Pa_{CO_2} level.

Oxygenation Indices*

$\dot{Q}_S/\dot{Q}_T$	D_{O_2}†	$\dot{V}_{O_2}$	$C(a-\bar{v})_{O_2}$	O_2ER	$S\bar{v}_{O_2}$
↑	↓	N	N	↑	↓

†The D_{O_2} may be normal in patients who have compensated to the decreased oxygenation status with (1) an increased cardiac output, (2) an increased hemoglobin level, or (3) a combination of both. When the D_{O_2} is normal, the O_2ER is usually normal.

ABNORMAL LABORATORY TEST AND PROCEDURE RESULTS

Abnormal sputum examination findings (see discussion of etiology in this chapter, Box 15-1)

RADIOLOGIC FINDINGS

Chest Radiograph

- Increased density (from consolidation and atelectasis)
- Air bronchograms
- Pleural effusions

The radiographic signs vary considerably depending on the causative agent. In general, pneumonia (alveolar consolidation) appears as an area of increased density that may involve a small lung segment, a lobe, or one or both lungs (Figure 15-5). The process may appear patchy or uniform throughout the area. As the alveolar consolidation intensifies, alveolar density increases and air bronchograms may be seen (Figure 15-6). A pleural effusion may be identified on the chest radiograph (see Chapter 23).

Computed Tomography Scan

Alveolar consolidation and air bronchograms also can be seen on the computed tomography (CT) scan (Figure 15-7).

*$C(a-\bar{v})_{O_2}$, Arterial-venous oxygen difference; D_{O_2}, total oxygen delivery; O_2ER, oxygen extraction ratio; $\dot{Q}_S/\dot{Q}_T$, pulmonary shunt fraction; $S\bar{v}_{O_2}$, mixed venous oxygen saturation; $\dot{V}_{O_2}$, oxygen consumption.

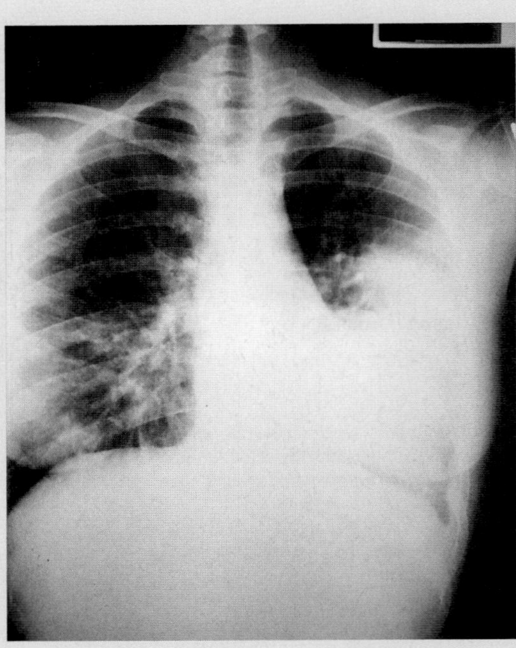

FIGURE 15-5 Chest x-ray film of a 20-year-old woman with severe pneumonia of the left lung and patchy pneumonia in the right middle and lower lobes.

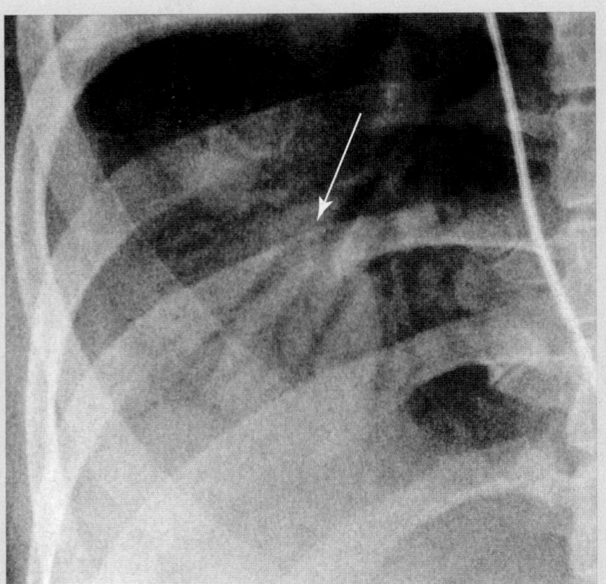

FIGURE 15-6 Air bronchogram. The branching linear lucencies within the consolidation in the right lower lobe are particularly well demonstrated in this example of staphylococcal pneumonia. (From Hansell DM, Armstrong P, Lynch DA, McAdams HP, eds: *Imaging of diseases of the chest,* ed 4, Philadelphia, 2005, Elsevier.)

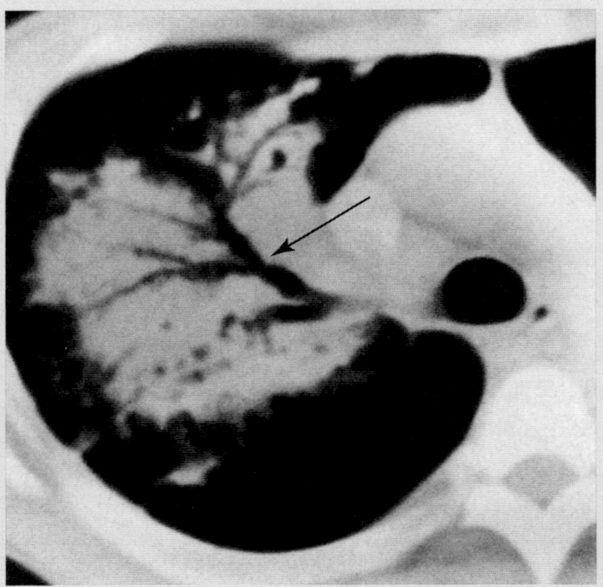

FIGURE 15-7 Air bronchograms shown by computed tomography in a patient with pneumonia. (From Hansell DM, Armstrong P, Lynch DA, McAdams HP, eds: *Imaging of diseases of the chest,* ed 4, Philadelphia, 2005, Elsevier.)

TABLE 15-1 Commonly Encountered Organisms Responsible for Pneumonia and the Therapeutic Agents Used to Treat Them

Organism Responsible for Pneumonia	Common Treatment Choices
Gram-Positive Organisms	
Staphylococcus aureus	Methicillin-susceptible strains: nafcillin or oxacillin with or without rifampin Methicillin-resistant strains: vancomycin with or without rifampin Alternative choice: cephalosporins, clindamycin
Streptococcus	Penicillins: procaine penicillin G or aqueous penicillin G, amoxicillin Alternative choice: macrolides, cephalosporins, doxycycline, quinolones Cefotaxime or ceftriaxone; antipseudomonal fluoroquinolones (levofloxacin, gatifloxacin, moxifloxacin)
Gram-Negative Organisms	
Haemophilus influenzae	Ampicillin, third- or fourth-generation cephalosporin, macrolides (azithromycin, clarithromycin), fluoroquinolones
Klebsiella pneumoniae	Third- and/or fourth-generation cephalosporins (cefotaxime, ceftriaxone) plus aminoglycoside, antipseudomonal penicillin, monobactam (aztreonam), or quinolone
Pseudomonas aeruginosa	Tobramycin (TOBI), aminoglycoside, and antipseudomonal agents (ticarcillin, piperacillin, mezlocillin, ceftazidime)
Atypical Organisms	
Mycoplasma pneumoniae	Doxycycline, macrolides or fluoroquinolones
Legionella pneumophila	Erythromycin ± rifampin (in severely compromised patient) or clarithromycin, or a macrolide (azithromycin), or a fluoroquinolone (ofloxacin, levofloxacin, sparfloxacin)
Chlamydia pneumoniae	Tetracycline, erythromycin, macrolide, quinolone
Anaerobic bacterial infections *Peptostreptococcus species* *Bacteroides melaninogenica* *Fusobacterium necrophorum* *Bacteroides asaccharolyticus* *Porphyromonas endodontalis* *Porphyromonas gingivalis*	Most of these organisms are oral contaminants. For anaerobic coverage use metronidazole (Flagyl) or clindamycin; or metronidazole + ceftriaxone; or penicillin + amoxicillin. Infections respond slowly; 4-6 weeks of therapy is generally recommended. Most of the problem with aspiration pneumonia is secondary to the acid present in stomach contents, causing a chemical pneumonia. Quinolones, penicillins are also useful. Aspiration fluid should be cultured immediately (even with bronchoscopy and special culture), then the patient started on coverage medication while culture results are awaited. If the culture is negative, stop the antibiotics, then reculture if chest x-ray findings or patient's condition gets worse. Monitor closely for superinfections such as candida, other yeasts. May add vancomycin and Diflucan to cover nosocomial suprainfections.
Viral Causes	
Influenza virus	Type A: amantadine and rimantadine Type A/B: zanamivir, oseltamivir phosphate
Respiratory syncytial virus	Ribavirin (Virazole)
Other Common Causes	
Pneumocystis jiroveci	Pentamidine (NebuPent) Trimethoprim-sulfamethoxazole (TMP-SMZ), dapsone-trimethoprim, primaquine plus clindamycin
Fungal infections	Amphotericin B, itraconazole, fluconazole, ketoconazole
Tuberculosis *(Mycobacterium tuberculosis)*	Isoniazid (INH), rifampin, pyrazinamide, ethambutol, streptomycin

General Management of Pneumonia

The treatment of pneumonia is based on (1) the specific cause of the pneumonia, and (2) the severity of symptoms demonstrated by the patient. For bacterial pneumonia, the first line of defense is usually an antibiotic. Although there are a few viral pneumonias that may be treated with antiviral medications, the recommended treatment is usually the same as for the flu—bed rest and plenty of fluids. In addition, over-the-counter medications are often helpful to reduce fever, treat aches and pains, and depress the dry cough associated with pneumonia. In severe pneumonia, hospitalization may be required. The following is an overview of the treatments used for pneumonia.

Medications and Procedures Commonly Prescribed by the Physician

Antibiotics

Antibiotics are commonly administered to combat the infective agents that cause bacterial pneumonia. Table 15-1 provides an overview of the commonly encountered organisms responsible for pneumonia and the therapeutic agents currently used to treat them.

Respiratory Care Treatment Protocols

Oxygen Therapy Protocol

Oxygen therapy is used to treat hypoxemia, decrease the work of breathing, and decrease myocardial work. Because of the hypoxemia associated with pneumonia, supplemental oxygen may be required. The hypoxemia that develops in pneumonia is most commonly caused by alveolar consolidation and capillary shunting associated with the disorder. Hypoxemia caused by capillary shunting is at least partially refractory to oxygen therapy (see Oxygen Therapy Protocol, Protocol 9-1).

Bronchopulmonary Hygiene Therapy Protocol

Because of the airway secretions associated with the resolution stage of pneumonia, a number of bronchopulmonary hygiene treatment modalities may be used to enhance the mobilization of bronchial secretions. In addition, because of food particles in the aspirate, the bronchopulmonary hygiene protocol is useful in the treatment of aspiration pneumonia (see Bronchopulmonary Hygiene Therapy Protocol, Protocol 9-2).

Lung Expansion Therapy Protocol

Lung expansion therapy may be administered to attempt to offset the atelectasis associated with some pneumonias (see Lung Expansion Therapy Protocol, Protocol 9-3).

Thoracentesis

Therapeutically, thoracentesis may be used to treat pleural effusion (see Chapter 23). Fluid samples may be examined for the following:

- Color
- Odor
- RBC count
- Protein
- Glucose
- Lactic dehydrogenase (LDH)
- Amylase
- pH
- Wright's, Gram, and acid-fast bacillus (AFB) stains
- Aerobic, anaerobic, tuberculosis, and fungal cultures
- Cytology

CASE STUDY

Pneumonia

Admitting History and Physical Examination

A 47-year-old man was deer hunting in northern Michigan with some friends. They spent considerable time outdoors in inclement weather and indulged freely in alcoholic beverages during the afternoons and evenings. Previously the man had been essentially healthy. He smoked one pack of cigarettes a day.

Returning home, he felt listless and thought that he was "coming down with a cold." That night, he noticed a mild, nonproductive cough. He had a headache and some pain in the right side of his chest on deep inspiration and noticed that he was somewhat short of breath when he climbed one flight of stairs. During the night, he woke up and felt very chilled, then very warm. His wife put her hand on his forehead and was certain that he had a "high fever." Because he felt miserable, they went to the emergency room of the nearest hospital.

On physical examination, his vital signs were as follows: blood pressure 150/88, pulse 116/min, respiratory rate 28/min, and temperature (oral) 39.9° C. He was in moderate distress. Percussion of the chest revealed dullness on the right lower side, and on inspiration there were fine crackles heard in that area. The breath sounds were described as "bronchial." The chest radiograph showed pneumonic consolidation of the right lower lung field. On room air, his arterial blood gas values were pH 7.53, $Pa{CO_2}$ 27, HCO_3^- 21, and $Pa{O_2}$ 62. The respiratory therapist assigned to assess and treat the patient charted the following SOAP note.

Respiratory Assessment and Plan

S "I feel miserable." Mild dyspnea.

O Alert, cooperative, acutely ill. Mild nonproductive cough. Vital signs: T 39.9° C, BP 150/88, P 116, RR 28. Dull to percussion over RLL, along with crackles and bronchial breath sounds. CXR: Pneumonic consolidation RLL. ABG on room air: pH 7.53, $Pa{CO_2}$ 27, HCO_3^- 21, and $Pa{O_2}$ 62.

A
- RLL consolidation (pneumonia presumed)
- Acute alveolar hyperventilation with mild hypoxemia (ABG)

P **Oxygen Therapy Protocol:** Monitor $Sp{O_2}$. (Titrate O_2 per NC as needed to keep $Sp{O_2}$ >90%.)

The patient was started on oxygen (2 L/min) via a nasal cannula. The physician prescribed intravenous antibiotic therapy.

Over the next 72 hours, the patient steadily improved, although he felt nauseated and vomited three times. On the fourth hospital day, however, the patient complained of increased shortness of breath. He started to cough up large amounts (3 to 4 tablespoons every 2 hours) of foul-smelling, greenish-yellow sputum. He also complained of choking on his secretions (aspiration likely), a bitter taste in his mouth, belching, mild substernal discomfort, and chills.

On physical examination, the patient appeared anxious. His vital signs were blood pressure 120/82, pulse 140 bpm, respiratory rate 20/min, and oral temperature 40° C. His sputum was thick, yellow-green, and foul-smelling. His cough was strong. He had bronchial breath sounds, rhonchi, and nonclearing crackles in the right middle of the anterior chest and over both lower lobes posteriorly. There was mild cyanosis of the nail beds. The abdominal examination was unremarkable. There was no peripheral edema. A chest x-ray examination showed a new infiltrate in the right middle lung field and left lower lobe. The opaque infiltrate obstructed the view of the heart and was described by the radiologist as consolidation. On 2 L/min O_2 nasal cannula, his ABGs were as follows: pH 7.50, $Pa{CO_2}$ 29, HCO_3^- 20, $Pa{O_2}$ 36, and $Sa{O_2}$ 69%. At this time the respiratory therapist charted the following SOAP progress note.

Respiratory Assessment and Plan

S Increased dyspnea. Symptoms of belching and substernal chest pain.

O Anxious appearance. BP 120/82, HR 140, RR 20, T 40° C. Cyanotic. Strong productive cough (sputum foul-smelling, yellow-green). Bronchial breath sounds, rhonchi, persistent crackles in right middle anterior chest and both bases. CXR: RML and LLL infiltrate and consolidation. ABG (on 2 L/min): pH 7.50, $Pa{CO_2}$ 29, HCO_3^- 20, $Pa{O_2}$ 36, and $Sa{O_2}$ 69%.

A
- Aspiration complicating community-acquired pneumonia, involving RML and LLL (history, CXR)
- Alveolar consolidation (CXR)
- Excessive airway secretions (thick, yellow-green sputum)
- Good ability to mobilize secretions (strong cough)
- Acute alveolar hyperventilation with severe hypoxemia (ABG)

P **Oxygen Therapy Protocol:** Increase $F{I}{O_2}$ to 0.60 via HAFOE mask. **Bronchopulmonary Hygiene Protocol:** DB&C instruction, prn oropharyngeal suctioning. Trial P&D to lower lobes and RML q shift as tolerated). **Aerosolized Medication Protocol:** 2.0 mL 10% acetylcysteine with 0.5 mL albuterol q4h. ABG in 1 hour.

Discussion

A history of cold exposure in conjunction with the use of alcoholic beverages before the onset of pneumonia is not uncommon. The first part of this case begins with a classic presentation for community-acquired pneumonia with alveolar consolidation (see **Alveolar Consolidation**, Figure 9-9). For example, the fever and tachycardia represent a normal functioning immune response, and the tachycardia and tachypnea reflect the body's response to shunt-induced hypoxemia. The auscultation of crackles and bronchial breath sounds also reflects the patient's pulmonary consolidation. An attempt at improving his oxygenation, though not successful, was certainly in order. It was hoped that by providing an oxygen-enriched gas to both normal and partially consolidated alveoli, the effects of pulmonary shunting would be at least partially offset.

The second SOAP presents the complication of the patient's community-acquired pneumonia with aspiration pneumonitis. Alcoholics frequently have gastritis or esophagitis, and the patient's eructation (belching) and pyrosis (heartburn) were clues to the development of that complication. At this time there were new clinical manifestations associated with **Excessive Bronchial Secretions** (see Figure 9-12). For example, the patient demonstrated a cough, sputum, rhonchi, and crackles. The **Bronchopulmonary Hygiene Therapy Protocol** (e.g., mucolytic with a bronchodilator, DB&C, suctioning, and P&D) was appropriate. A trial of **Lung Expansion Therapy** (see Protocol 9-3) was not given in this case. However, **Atelectasis** (see Figure 9-8) often complicates aspiration pneumonia, and such a trial would not have been inappropriate.

In cases of pneumonia, the respiratory care practitioner is often tempted to do too much. Typically, volume expansion therapy, bronchodilator aerosol therapy, and bland aerosol therapy have all been ordered for affected patients, even in the acute, consolidative stage of their pneumonia. Often, however, all that is needed is the appropriate selection of antibiotics, rest, fluids, and supplementary oxygen. When the pneumonia "breaks up" (resolution stage) or is complicated by aspiration (as in this case), **Excessive Bronchial Secretions** (Figure 9-12) and even **Bronchospasm** (Figure 9-11) may appear. When this happens, use of other protocol modalities is necessary.

SELF-ASSESSMENT QUESTIONS

evolve Answers to questions can be found on Evolve. To access additional student assessment questions and case studies for application of text material to real-life scenarios, visit **http://evolve.elsevier.com/DesJardins/respiratory.**

1. Which of the following is also known as Friedländer's bacillus?
- a. *Haemophilus influenzae*
- b. *Pseudomonas aeruginosa*
- c. *Legionella pneumophila*
- d. *Klebsiella*

2. Of the six types of *Haemophilus influenzae*, which type is most frequently pathogenic?
- a. Type A
- b. Type B
- c. Type C
- d. Type D

3. Which of the following is associated with Q fever?
- a. *Mycoplasma pneumoniae*
- b. *Rickettsia*
- c. Ornithosis
- d. Varicella

4. Mendelson's syndrome is associated with which of the following?
- a. Lipoid pneumonitis
- b. Rubella
- c. Varicella
- d. Aspiration pneumonia

5. Which of the following is the most common *viral* pulmonary complication of AIDS?
- a. *Aspergillus*
- b. *Cryptococcus*
- c. *Pneumocystis carinii*
- d. Cytomegalovirus

6. Ribavirin aerosol has been shown to be effective in treating children with which of the following?
- a. *Klebsiella*
- b. *Haemophilus influenzae* type B
- c. Respiratory syncytial virus
- d. *Pseudomonas aeruginosa*

7. Which of the following is almost always the cause of acute epiglottitis?
- a. *Haemophilus influenzae* type B
- b. *Klebsiella*
- c. *Streptococcus*
- d. *Mycoplasma pneumoniae*

8. Which of the following is most associated with croup?
- a. *Streptococcus*
- b. Parainfluenza virus
- c. *Mycoplasma pneumoniae*
- d. Adenovirus

9. In the absence of a secondary bacterial infection, lung inflammation caused by the aspiration of gastric fluids usually becomes insignificant in approximately how many days?

a. 2
b. 3
c. 5
d. 7

10. Which of the following is or are associated with pneumonia?

1. Decreased tactile and vocal fremitus
2. Increased $C(a-\bar{v})O_2$
3. Decreased PEFR
4. Increased VC

a. 1 only
b. 3 only
c. 2 and 4 only
d. 1 and 3 only

Lung Abscess

16

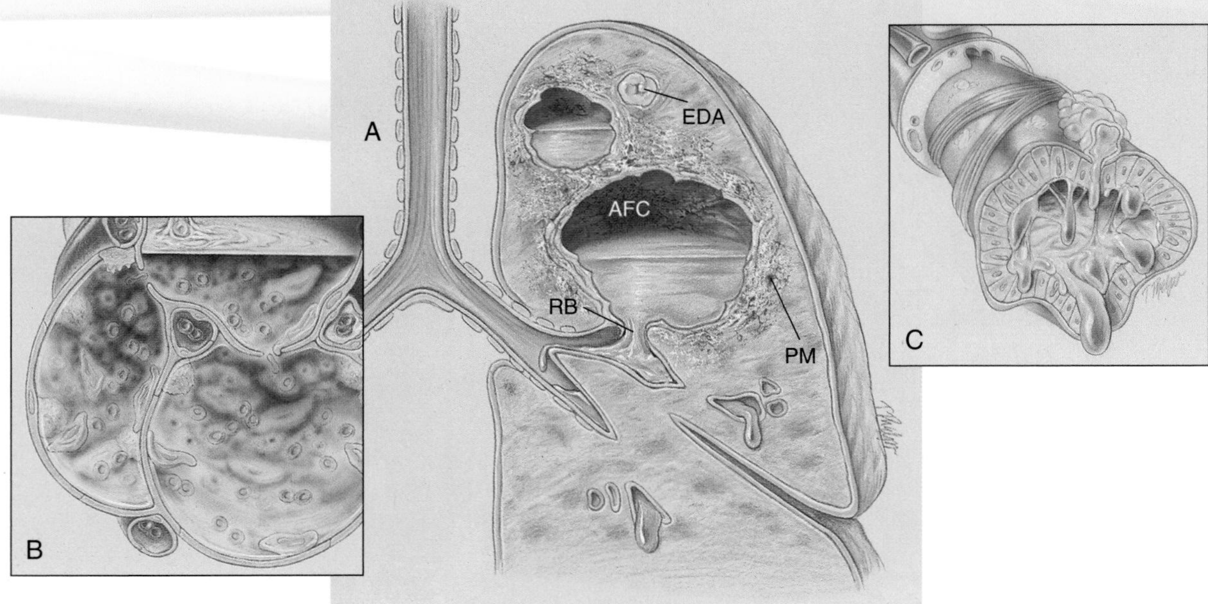

FIGURE 16-1 Lung abscess. **A,** Cross-sectional view of lung abscess. **B,** Consolidation and (**C**) excessive bronchial secretions are common secondary anatomic alterations of the lungs. *AFC,* Air-fluid cavity; *EDA,* early development of abscess; *PM,* pyogenic membrane; *RB,* ruptured bronchus (and drainage of the liquefied contents of the cavity).

Chapter Objectives

After reading this chapter, you will be able to:

- List the anatomic alterations of the lungs associated with lung abscess.
- Describe the causes of lung abscess.
- List the cardiopulmonary clinical manifestations associated with lung abscess.
- Describe the general management of lung abscess.
- Describe the clinical strategies and rationales of the SOAPs presented in the case study.
- Define key terms and complete self-assessment questions at the end of the chapter and on Evolve.

Key Terms

Anaerobic Gram-Negative Bacilli
Anaerobic Gram-Positive Cocci
Bacteroides fragilis
Flash Burn
Fusobacterium
Peptococci
Peptostreptococci
Prevotella melaninogenica
Staphylococcus

Chapter Outline

Anatomic Alterations of the Lungs
Etiology and Epidemiology
Overview of Cardiopulmonary Clinical Manifestations Associated with Lung Abscess
General Management of Lung Abscess
Medications and Procedures Commonly Prescribed by the Physician
Respiratory Care Treatment Protocols
Case Study: Lung Abscess
Self Assessment Questions

Anatomic Alterations of the Lungs

A *lung abscess* is defined as a necrosis of lung tissue that in severe cases leads to a localized air- and fluid-filled cavity. The fluid in the cavity is a collection of purulent exudate that is composed of liquefied white blood cell remains, proteins, and tissue debris. The air- and fluid-filled cavity is encapsulated in a so-called *pyogenic membrane* that consists of a layer of fibrin, inflammatory cells, and granulation tissue.

During the early stages of a lung abscess, the pathology is indistinguishable from that of any acute pneumonia. Polymorphonuclear leukocytes and macrophages move into the infected area to engulf any invading organisms. This action causes the pulmonary capillaries to dilate, the interstitium to fill with fluid, and the alveolar epithelium to swell from the edema fluid. In response to this inflammatory reaction, the alveoli in the infected area become consolidated (see Figure 15-1).

As the inflammatory process progresses, tissue necrosis involving all the lung structures occurs. In severe cases the tissue necrosis ruptures into a bronchus and allows a partial or total drainage of the liquefied contents into the cavity. An air- and fluid-filled cavity also may rupture into the intrapleural space via a bronchopleural fistula and cause pleural effusion and empyema (see Chapter 23, Pleural Diseases). This may lead to inflammation of the parietal pleura, chest pain, atelectasis, and decreased chest expansion. After a period of time, fibrosis and calcification of the tissues around the cavity encapsulate the abscess (see Figure 16-1).

The major pathologic or structural changes associated with a lung abscess are as follows:

- Alveolar consolidation
- Alveolar-capillary and bronchial wall destruction
- Tissue necrosis
- Cavity formation
- Fibrosis and calcification of the lung parenchyma
- Bronchopleural fistulas and empyema
- Atelectasis
- Excessive airway secretions

Etiology and Epidemiology

A lung abscess is commonly associated with the aspiration of gastric and oral fluids. Aspiration can cause either (1) chemical pneumonia, (2) anaerobic bacterial pneumonia, or (3) a combination of both (see Chapter 15). The aspiration of acidic gastric fluids is associated with immediate injury to the tracheobronchial tree and lung parenchyma—often likened to a **flash burn.** Common anaerobic organisms found in the normal flora of the mouth, upper respiratory tract, and gastrointestinal tract include the following:

- **Anaerobic gram-positive cocci**
  - **Peptococci**
  - **Peptostreptococci**
- **Anaerobic gram-negative bacilli**
  - ***Bacteroides fragilis***
  - ***Prevotella melaninogenica***
  - ***Fusobacterium*** species

Anaerobic organisms often colonize in the small grooves and spaces between the teeth and gums in patients with poor oral hygiene; anaerobic organisms are frequently associated with gingivitis and dead or abscessed teeth. Aspiration often occurs in the patient with a decreased level of consciousness. Predisposing factors include (1) alcohol abuse, (2) seizure disorders, (3) general anesthesia, (4) head trauma, (5) cerebrovascular accidents, and (6) swallowing disorders. The incidence of lung abscesses caused by anaerobic organisms is also high in patients with poor oral hygiene. Anaerobic organisms are cultured in 62% to 87% of cases of aspiration pneumonia, in 85% to 93% of lung abscess cases, in 62% to 76% of patients with empyema, and as many as 94% of patients with exacerbations of bronchiectasis.

Other organisms known to cause a lung abscess are *Klebsiella,* ***Staphylococcus,*** *Mycobacterium tuberculosis* (including the atypical organisms *Mycobacterium kansasii* and *Mycobacterium avium*), *Histoplasma capsulatum, Coccidioides immitis, Blastomyces,* and *Aspergillus fumigatus.* Some parasites such as *Paragonimus westermani, Echinococcus,* and *Entamoeba histolytica* may also cause lung abscess formation. On rare occasions a lung abscess may also be caused by *Streptococcus pneumoniae, Pseudomonas aeruginosa,* or *Legionella pneumophila.* Typically, more than one type of bacterium is involved, as in an infection with anaerobic organisms mixed with aerobic ones.

Finally, a lung abscess may develop as a result of (1) bronchial obstruction with secondary cavitating infection (e.g., distal to bronchogenic carcinoma or an aspirated foreign body), (2) vascular obstruction with tissue infarction (e.g., septic embolism, vasculitis), (3) interstitial lung disease with cavity formation (e.g., pneumoconiosis [silicosis], Wegener's granulomatosis, and rheumatoid nodules), (4) bullae or cysts that become infected (e.g., congenital or bronchogenic cysts), or (5) penetrating chest wounds that lead to an infection (e.g., bullet wound).

Anatomically, a lung abscess most commonly forms in the superior segments of the lower lobes and the posterior segments of the upper lobes. The tendency for an abscess to form in these areas is because of the effect of gravity and the dependent position of the tracheobronchial tree at the time of aspiration, which commonly occurs while the patient is in the supine position. The right lung is more commonly involved than the left.

Box 16-1 on p. 247 summarizes organisms known to cause lung abscess.

OVERVIEW of the Cardiopulmonary Clinical Manifestations Associated with Lung Abscess

The following clinical manifestations result from the pathologic mechanisms caused (or activated) by **Alveolar Consolidation** (see Figure 9-9) and, when the abscess is draining, by **Excessive Bronchial Secretions** (see Figure 9-12)—the major anatomic alterations of the lungs associated with lung abscess (see Figure 16-1).

CLINICAL DATA OBTAINED AT THE PATIENT'S BESIDE

The Physical Examination

Vital Signs

Increased Respiratory Rate (Tachypnea)

Several pathophysiologic mechanisms operating simultaneously may lead to an increased ventilatory rate:

- Stimulation of peripheral chemoreceptors (hypoxemia)
- Decreased lung compliance–increased ventilatory rate relationship
- Stimulation of J receptors
- Pain, anxiety, fever

Increased Heart Rate (Pulse) and Blood Pressure

Chest Pain, Decreased Chest Expansion

Cyanosis

Cough, Sputum Production, and Hemoptysis

During the early stages, when the lung abscess is in the inflammatory pneumonia-like phase, the patient generally has a nonproductive barking or hacking cough. If the abscess progresses into an air- and fluid-filled cavity and ruptures through a bronchus, the patient may suddenly cough up large amounts of sputum. Foul-smelling brown or gray sputum indicates a putrid infection that is caused by numerous organisms, including anaerobes. An odorless green or yellow sputum indicates a nonputrid infection caused by a single aerobic organism. Blood-streaked sputum is common in patients with a lung abscess. Occasionally, frank hemoptysis is seen.

Chest Assessment Findings

- Increased tactile and vocal fremitus
- Crackles and rhonchi

The following may be noted directly over the abscess:

- Dull percussion note
- Bronchial breath sounds
- Diminished breath sounds
- Whispered pectoriloquy
- Pleural friction rub (if abscess is near pleural surface)

CLINICAL DATA OBTAINED FROM LABORATORY TESTS AND SPECIAL PROCEDURES

Pulmonary Function Test Findings
Severe and Extensive Cases
(Restrictive Lung Pathophysiology)

FORCED EXPIRATORY FLOW RATE FINDINGS

FVC	FEV_T	FEV_1/FVC ratio	$FEF_{25\%-75\%}$
↓	N or ↓	N or ↑*	N or ↓
$FEF_{50\%}$	$FEF_{200-1200}$	PEFR	MVV
N or ↓	N or ↓	N or ↓	N or ↓

*May be down in when airway obstruction is present.

Lung Volume and Capacity Findings

V_T	IRV	ERV	RV	
N or ↓	↓	↓	↓	
VC	IC	FRC	TLC	RV/TLC ratio
↓	↓	↓	↓	N

Arterial Blood Gases

MILD TO MODERATE LUNG ABSCESS
Acute Alveolar Hyperventilation with Hypoxemia
(Acute Respiratory Alkalosis)

pH	Pa_{CO_2}	HCO_3^-	Pa_{O_2}
↑	↓	↓ (slightly)	↓

SEVERE LUNG ABSCESS
Acute Ventilatory Failure with Hypoxemia
(Acute Respiratory Acidosis)

pH*	Pa_{CO_2}	HCO_3^-*	Pa_{O_2}
↓	↑	↑ (slightly)	↓

*When tissue hypoxia is severe enough to produce lactic acid, the pH and HCO_3^- values will be lower than expected for a particular Pa_{CO_2} level.

Oxygenation Indices*

$\dot{Q}_S/\dot{Q}_T$	D_{O_2}†	$\dot{V}_{O_2}$	$C(a-\bar{v})_{O_2}$	O_2ER	$S\bar{v}_{O_2}$
↑	↓	N	N	↑	↓

†The D_{O_2} may be normal in patients who have compensated to the decreased oxygenation status with (1) an increased cardiac output, (2) an increased hemoglobin level, or (3) a combination of both. When the D_{O_2} is normal, the O_2ER is usually normal.

*$C(a-\bar{v})_{O_2}$, Arterial-venous oxygen difference; D_{O_2}, total oxygen delivery; O_2ER, oxygen extraction ratio; $\dot{Q}_S/\dot{Q}_T$, pulmonary shunt fraction; $S\bar{v}_{O_2}$ mixed venous oxygen saturation; $\dot{V}_{O_2}$ oxygen consumption.

OVERVIEW of the Cardiopulmonary Clinical Manifestations Associated with Lung Abscess—cont'd

ABNORMAL LABORATORY TEST AND PROCEDURE RESULTS

Sputum Examination—Most Common Organisms (See Discussion of Etiology)

Anaerobic Organisms

Anaerobic Gram-Positive Cocci

- Peptococci
- Peptostreptococci

Anaerobic Gram-Negative Bacilli

- *Bacteroides fragilis*
- *Prevotella melaninogenica*
- *Fusobacterium* species

RADIOLOGIC FINDINGS

Chest Radiograph

- Increased opacity
- Cavity formation
- Cavities with air-fluid levels
- Fibrosis and calcification
- Pleural effusion

The chest radiograph typically reveals localized consolidation during the early stages of lung abscess formation. Later, the characteristic radiographic appearance of a lung abscess appears after (1) the infection ruptures into a bronchus, (2) tissue destruction and necrosis have occurred, and (3) partial evacuation of the purulent contents has occurred. The abscess usually appears on the radiograph as a circular radiolucency that contains an air-fluid level surrounded by a dense wall of lung parenchyma (Figure 16-2).

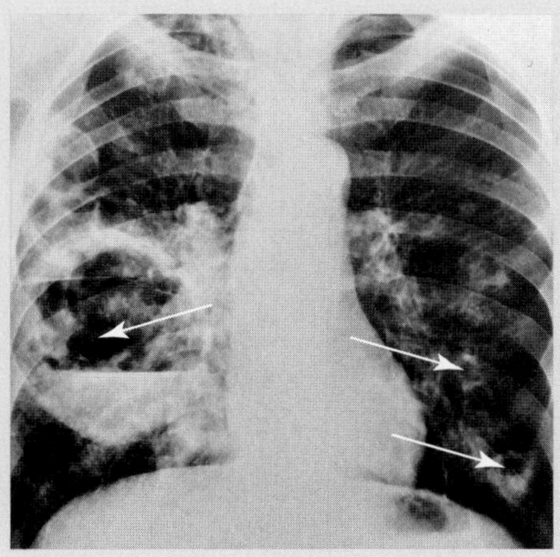

FIGURE 16-2 Reactivation tuberculosis with a large cavitary lesion containing an air-fluid level in the right lower lobe. Smaller cavitary lesions are also seen in other lobes. (From Hansell DM, Armstrong P, Lynch DA, McAdams HP, eds: *Imaging of diseases of the chest,* ed 4, Philadelphia, 2005, Elsevier.)

Box 16-1 Organisms Known to Cause Lung Abscess

Common Organisms Associated with Aspiration

Anaerobic Gram-positive Cocci

Peptococci
Peptostreptococci

Anaerobic Gram-Negative Bacilli

Bacteroides fragilis
Prevotella melaninogenica
Fusobacterium species

Less Common Organisms

Klebsiella
Staphylococcus
Mycobacterium tuberculosis (plus atypical organisms *Mycobacterium kansasii* and *Mycobacterium avium*)
Histoplasma capsulatum
Coccidioides immitis
Blastomyces
Aspergillus fumigatus

Some Parasites

Paragonimus westermani
Echinococcus
Entamoeba histolytica

Rare Occurrences

Streptococcus pneumonia
Pseudomonas aeruginosa
Legionella pneumophila

General Management of Lung Abscess

Treatment varies based on the severity of the pneumonia and lung abscess. Treatment includes appropriate antimicrobial therapy coupled with prompt drainage and surgical debridement. When treated properly, most patients with a lung abscess show improvement. In acute cases the size of the abscess quickly decreases and eventually closes altogether. In severe or chronic cases, the patient's improvement may be slow or insignificant, even with appropriate therapy.

Medications and Procedures Commonly Prescribed by the Physician

Antibiotics

Antibiotics are the primary treatment for a lung abscess. For example, oropharyngeal anaerobic infections are treated with penicillin G. For anaerobic coverage, metronidazole (Flagyl) or clindamycin may be used. Because most of the problems associated with aspiration pneumonia are secondary to the inhaled acidic gastric contents—which in turn cause a chemical pneumonia—quinolones and penicillins are also used. When *Klebsiella* is the causative agent, the following may be administered: third- and/or fourth-generation cephalosporins (cefotaxime, ceftriaxone) plus aminoglycosides, antipseudomonal penicillins, monobactam (aztreonam), or quinolones.

When lung abscesses are caused by methicillin-susceptible strains of *Staphylococcus aureus,* nafcillin or oxacillin (with or without rifampin) may be used. In the case of methicillin-resistant strains of *S. aureus,* vancomycin (with or without rifampin) is commonly administered. Good alternative choices are cephalosporins and clindamycin. (See Appendix III, Antibiotics.)

Respiratory Care Treatment Protocols

Oxygen Therapy Protocol

Oxygen therapy is used to treat hypoxemia, decrease the work of breathing, and decrease myocardial work. The hypoxemia that develops in lung abscess is usually caused by pulmonary capillary shunting. Hypoxemia caused by capillary shunting is often refractory to oxygen therapy (see Oxygen Therapy Protocol, Protocol 9-1).

Bronchopulmonary Hygiene Therapy Protocol

Because of the excessive mucous production and accumulation associated with a ruptured lung abscess, a number of bronchial hygiene treatment modalities may be used to enhance the mobilization of bronchial secretions (see Bronchopulmonary Hygiene Therapy Protocol, Protocol 9-2).

Lung Expansion Therapy Protocol

Because of the alveolar consolidation and atelectasis associated with a lung abscess, lung expansion may be tried to offset these anatomic alterations of the lungs (see Lung Expansion Therapy Protocol, Protocol 9-3).

CASE STUDY

Lung Abscess

Admitting History and Physical Examination

This 64-year-old unemployed man sought medical attention because of an increasingly severe cough that produced moderate amounts of foul-smelling sputum. He had undergone splenectomy for removal of a ruptured spleen 1 year ago. He reported that on several occasions recently he had a slight fever and that his appetite was poor; he had lost about 6 pounds. For the past 3 days he had noticed some right-sided chest pain, and his cough had become very productive. The patient denied cigarette smoking.

Physical examination showed a small and poorly nourished male in moderate distress, coughing throughout the interview. The patient's vital signs were blood pressure 160/90, heart rate 120/min, respiratory rate 22/min, and oral temperature 100.6° F. There was brawny discoloration of the legs below the knees. His teeth were in deplorable condition, and he had marked halitosis. Examination of the chest revealed dullness to percussion, crackles, rhonchi, and bronchial breath sounds in the right lower lobe.

His frequent cough produced large amounts of foul-smelling brown and gray sputum. His cough was strong. The chest x-ray film showed a 4-cm diameter cavity in the right lower lobe with a clear air-fluid level. Patches of alveolar consolidation surrounded the cavity. There was no evidence of air trapping. Sputum for a culture and sensitivity study was obtained, but the results were still pending. His arterial blood gas values were as follows: pH 7.51, $Pa{CO_2}$ 29, HCO_3^- 22, and $Pa{O_2}$ 61 on room air. Intravenous antibiotic therapy was begun. The respiratory care practitioner assigned to his case recorded the following.

Respiratory Assessment and Plan

S "I can't stop coughing." Complains of low-grade fever, loss of appetite, weight loss (6 lb).

O Cachectic. BP 160/90, HR 120, RR 22, T 100.6° F orally. Teeth carious. Flat to percussion over RLL. Crackles, rhonchi, and bronchial breath sounds over RLL. CXR: 4-cm diameter cavity with fluid level and consolidation RLL. ABGs: pH 7.51, $Pa{CO_2}$ 29, HCO_3^- 22, and $Pa{O_2}$ 61. Excessive amount of foul-smelling, thick brown and gray sputum.

A
- Acute infection (fever)
- Malnourished (inspection)
- Lung abscess and consolidation, RLL (CXR)
- Acute alveolar hyperventilation with mild hypoxemia (ABG)
- Excessive and thick airway secretions (sputum, rhonchi)
- Good ability to mobilize secretions (strong cough)

P **Oxygen Therapy Protocol**: 2 L/min per nasal cannula. $Sp{O_2}$ spot check to verify appropriateness of O_2 therapy. O_2 titration if necessary. **Bronchopulmonary Hygiene Therapy Protocol**: Deep breathe and cough, with postural drainage to right lower lobe q6h. **Aerosolized Medication Protocol**: Trial period of med nebs: 2.0 cc acetylcysteine with 0.5 mL albuterol ½ hour before postural drainage q6h × 3 days, then reevaluate.

After reviewing the results of sputum culture sensitivity studies, the physician adjusted the patient's antibiotic therapy. Over the next 5 days, the patient's general condition improved. His cough and sputum production decreased remarkably but not completely. The sputum produced was no longer thick. His $Pa{O_2}$ increased to 86 mm Hg, and he no longer had acute alveolar hyperventilation. A chest radiograph revealed that his lung abscess was slightly reduced in size compared with the chest radiograph taken on the day of his admission, and his pneumonia had improved significantly. A complete pulmonary function test (PFT) study revealed a mild reduction in lung volumes, capacities, and expiratory flow rates. Social Service worked with him on two occasions during his hospitalization and scheduled a follow-up appointment at his home 4 weeks after discharge. An oral surgery consultation was obtained and extraction of the patient's carious teeth was scheduled. The patient was instructed on deep-breathing and coughing techniques and general bronchial hygiene and was discharged on the morning of the sixth day. He was discharged on a month-long course of oral antibiotics.

Discussion

This case illustrates some of the classic clinical manifestations of a lung abscess. For example, the **Alveolar Consolidation** (see Figure 9-9), which was identified on the chest x-ray film, surrounding the abscess likely played a role in producing the patient's fever and increased heart rate, blood pressure, and respiratory rate. In addition, the pneumonic consolidation also contributed to the patient's alveolar hyperventilation and hypoxemia, the bronchial breath sounds, and the reduced lung volumes and capacities and flow rates identified on his PFT.

In addition, the clinical manifestations associated with **Excessive Bronchial Secretions** (see Figure 9-12) also were seen in this case. Not only did the excessive airway secretions contribute to the patient's hypoxemia, secondary to the decreased $\dot{V}/\dot{Q}$ ratio and pulmonary shunting, but they also contributed to the increased airway resistance (caused by the secretions) that resulted in the rhonchi, sputum production, and reduced air-flow rates seen in the PFT.

The primary treatments started by the respiratory care practitioner were directed to the patient's excessive secretions. **Lung Expansion Therapy** (see Protocol 9-3) was not employed in this case. One could argue that it should have been, given the chest x-ray film infiltrates, which could have represented atelectasis just as well as pneumonia. The appropriate respiratory care of patients with lung abscesses closely resembles that of those with bronchiectasis (see Chapter 13). Identification of this patient's lung abscess in the right lower lobe allowed targeted chest physical therapy to be practiced. The suggestion that a Social Service representative see the patient to instruct him regarding his personal hygiene was entirely appropriate. Finally, extraction of his carious teeth was suggested by the Dental Service, hopefully, to eradicate this source of infection once and for all.

SELF-ASSESSMENT QUESTIONS

evolve Answers to questions can be found on Evolve. To access additional student assessment questions and case studies for application of text material to real-life scenarios, visit **http://evolve.elsevier.com/DesJardins/respiratory.**

1. Which of the following is or are anaerobic organisms?

1. *Blastomyces*
2. *Peptococcus*
3. *Coccidioides immitis*
4. *Bacteroides*
   a. 1 and 2 only
   b. 2 and 4 only
   c. 3 and 4 only
   d. 2, 3, and 4 only

2. Which of the following is or are predisposing factors to the aspiration of gastrointestinal fluids (and anaerobes)?

1. Seizure disorders
2. Head trauma
3. Alcoholic binges
4. General anesthesia
   a. 2 and 4 only
   b. 2 and 3 only
   c. 2, 3, and 4 only
   d. 1, 2, 3, and 4

3. Which of the following is or are associated with the formation of a lung abscess?

1. Bullae or cysts that become infected
2. Interstitial lung disease with cavity formation
3. Bronchial obstruction with secondary cavitating infection
4. Penetrating chest wounds that lead to an infection
   a. 1 only
   b. 3 only
   c. 2 and 4 only
   d. 1, 2, 3, and 4

4. Anatomically, a lung abscess most commonly forms in which part(s) of the lung?

1. Posterior segment of the upper lobe
2. Lateral basal segment of the lower lobe
3. Anterior segment of the upper lobe
4. Superior segment of the lower lobe
   a. 1 only
   b. 3 only
   c. 1 and 4 only
   d. 2 and 3 only

5. Which of the following pulmonary function findings may be associated with a severe and extensive lung abscess?

1. Decreased FVC
2. Increased PEFR
3. Decreased RV
4. Increased FRC
   a. 3 only
   b. 2 and 4 only
   c. 3 and 4 only
   d. 1 and 3 only

Tuberculosis

17

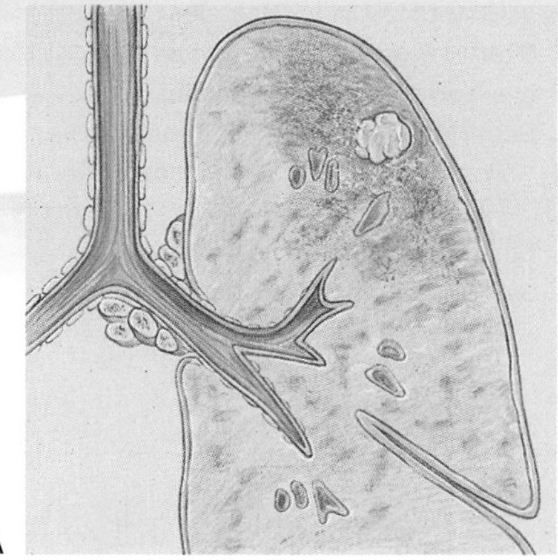

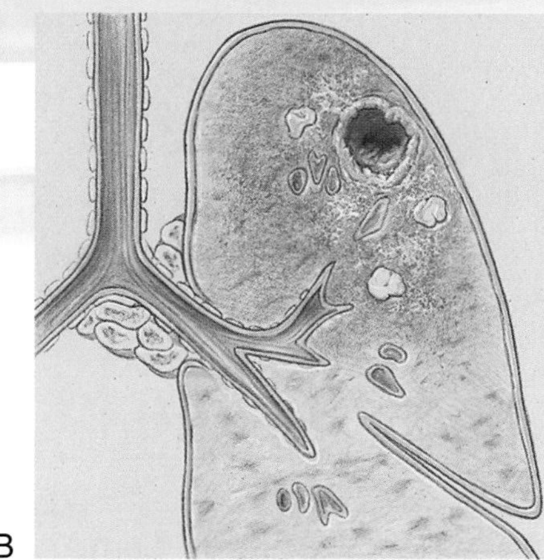

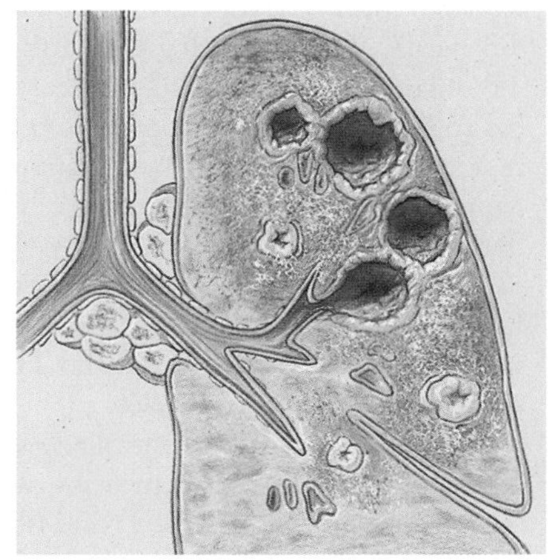

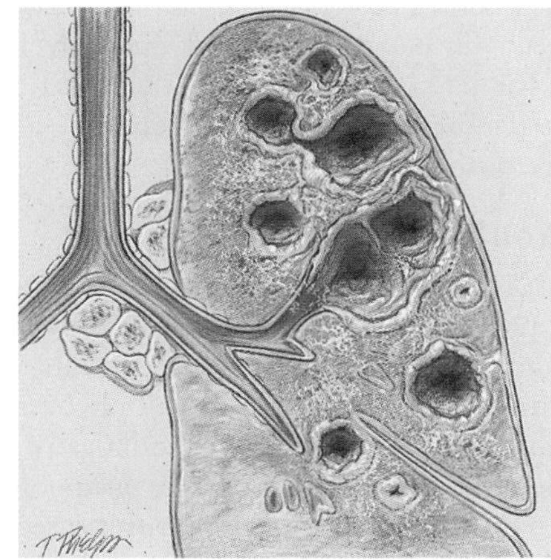

FIGURE 17-1 Tuberculosis. **A,** Early primary infection. **B,** Cavitation of a caseous tubercle and new primary lesions developing. **C,** Further progression and development of cavitations and new primary infections. Note the subpleural location of some of these lesions. **D,** Severe lung destruction caused by tuberculosis.

Chapter Objectives

After reading this chapter, you will be able to:

- List the anatomic alterations of the lungs associated with tuberculosis.
- Describe the causes of tuberculosis.
- List the cardiopulmonary clinical manifestations associated with tuberculosis.
- Describe the general management of tuberculosis.
- Describe the clinical strategies and rationales of the SOAP presented in the case study.
- Define key terms and complete self-assessment questions at the end of the chapter and on Evolve.

Key Terms

Acid-Fast Bacilli
Acid-Fast Bacteria
Caseous Granuloma
Caseous Lesion
Directly Observed Therapy (DOT)
Disseminated Tuberculosis
Dormant TB
Ethambutol
Fluorescent Acid-Fast Stain
Ghon Complex
Ghon Nodules
Granuloma
Induration
Isolation Procedure
Isoniazid (INH)
Latent TB
Mantoux Tuberculin Skin Test
Miliary TB

Mycobacterium avium
Mycobacterium kansasii
Mycobacterium tuberculosis
Nontuberculous Acid-Fast Mycobacteria
Postprimary Tuberculosis
Primary Tuberculosis
Prophylactic use of INH
Pyrazinamide
Rifampin
Sputum Smear
Streptomycin
Tubercle
Ziehl-Neelsen Stain

Chapter Outline

Anatomic Alterations of the Lungs

Tuberculosis (TB) is a contagious chronic bacterial infection that primarily affects the lungs, although it may involve almost any part of the body. Clinically, TB is classified as either **primary tuberculosis, postprimary tuberculosis,** or **disseminated tuberculosis.**

Primary Tuberculosis

Primary TB (also called the *primary infection stage*) follows the patient's first exposure to the TB pathogen, ***Mycobacterium tuberculosis.*** Primary TB begins when the inhaled bacilli implant in the alveoli. As the bacilli multiply over a 3- to 4-week period, the initial response of the lungs is an inflammatory reaction that is similar to any acute pneumonia (see Figure 15-1). In other words, a large influx of polymorphonuclear leukocytes and macrophages moves into the infected area to engulf—but not fully kill—the bacilli. This action also causes the pulmonary capillaries to dilate, the interstitium to fill with fluid, and the alveolar epithelium to swell from the edema fluid. Eventually the alveoli become consolidated (i.e., filled with fluid, polymorphonuclear leukocytes, and macrophages). Clinically, this phase of TB coincides with a positive tuberculin reaction—a positive purified protein derivative (PPD) skin test result (see discussion of diagnosis later in this chapter).

Unlike pneumonia, however, the lung tissue that surrounds the infected area slowly produces a protective cell wall called a **tubercle,** or **granuloma.** In essence, the tubercles work to encapsulate—that is, put in a nutshell-like structure—the TB bacilli (see Figure 17-1, *A*). Although the initial lung lesions may be difficult to identify on a chest radiograph, the lesions may be seen as small, sharply defined opacities. When detected on a chest radiograph, these initial lung lesions are called **Ghon nodules.** As the disease progresses, the combination of tubercles and the involvement of the lymph nodes in the hilar region is known as the **Ghon complex.**

Structurally, a tubercle consists of a central core containing TB bacilli. The central core also has enlarged macrophages with an outer wall composed of fibroblasts, lymphocytes, and neutrophils. A tubercle takes about 2 to 10 weeks to form. The function of the tubercle is to contain the TB bacilli, thus preventing the further spread of infectious TB organisms. Unfortunately, the central core of the tubercle has the potential to break down from time to time, especially in a patient with a depressed immune system. When this happens, the center of the tubercle fills with necrotic tissue that resembles dry cottage cheese. During this stage the tubercle is called a **caseous lesion** or **caseous granuloma** (see Figure 17-1, *B*). The patient is potentially contagious at this stage. In most cases, however, the TB bacilli are effectively contained within the tubercles.

Once the bacilli are controlled—either by the patient's immunologic defense system or by antituberculous drugs—the healing process begins. Tissue fibrosis and calcification of the lung parenchyma slowly replace the tubercle. This tissue fibrosis and calcification cause lung tissue retraction and scarring. In some cases the calcification and fibrosis cause the bronchi to distort and dilate—that is, to develop bronchiectasis.

Finally, when the bacilli are isolated within tubercles and immunity develops, the TB bacilli may remain dormant for months, years, or life. Individuals with **dormant TB** (also called **latent TB**) do not feel sick or have any TB-related symptoms. They are still infected with TB but do not have clinically active TB. The only indication of a TB infection is a positive reaction to the tuberculin skin test, or TB blood test, and the finding of possible residual scarring on the chest radiograph. Individuals with dormant (latent) TB are not infectious and cannot spread the TB bacilli to others.

Postprimary Tuberculosis

Postprimary TB (also called *reactivation TB, reinfection TB,* or *secondary TB*) is a term used to describe the reactivation of TB months or even years after the initial infection has been controlled. Even though most patients with primary TB recover completely from a clinical standpoint, it is important to note that live tubercle bacilli can remain dormant for decades. A positive tuberculin reaction generally persists even after the primary infection stage has been controlled. At any time, TB may become reactivated, especially in patients with depressed immune systems. Most new TB cases are associated with the following risk factors:

- Malnourished individuals
- People in institutional housing (e.g., nursing homes, prisons, homeless shelters)
- People living in overcrowded conditions
- Immunosuppressed patients (e.g., organ transplant patients, cancer patients)
- Human immunodeficiency virus (HIV)–infected patients (TB is a leading cause of death in HIV patients)
- Alcoholism

If the TB infection is uncontrolled, cavitation of the caseous granuloma tubercle develops. The patient progressively experiences more severe symptoms, including violent cough episodes, greenish or bloody sputum, low-grade fever, anorexia, weight loss, extreme fatigue, night sweats, and chest pain. It is this gradual wasting of the body that provided the basis for the earlier name for TB—*consumption.* The patient is highly contagious at this stage. In severe cases a deep tubercle cavity may rupture and allow air and infected material to flow into the pleural space or the tracheobronchial tree. Pleural complications are common in TB (see Figure 17-1, *C*).

Disseminated Tuberculosis

Disseminated TB (also called *extrapulmonary TB,* **miliary TB,** and *tuberculosis—disseminated*) refers to infection from TB bacilli that escape from a tubercle and travel to sites other throughout the body by means of the bloodstream or lymphatic system. In general, the TB bacilli that gain entrance to the bloodstream usually gather and multiply in portions of the body that have a high tissue oxygen tension. The most common location is the apex of the lungs. Other oxygen-rich areas in the body include the regional lymph nodes, kidneys, long bones, genital tract, brain, and meninges.

Genital TB in males damages the prostate gland, epididymis, seminal vesicle, and testes; and in females, the fallopian tubes, ovaries, and uterus. The spine is a frequent site of TB infection, although the hip, knee, wrist, and elbow can also be involved. Tubercular meningitis is caused by an active brain lesion seeding TB bacilli into the meninges. Over time, the infection may cause mental deterioration, permanent retardation, blindness, and deafness. When a large number of bacilli are freed into the bloodstream, the result can be the presence of numerous small tubercles—about the size of a pinhead—scattered throughout the body. This condition is commonly called *miliary TB.*

TB is primarily a chronic restrictive pulmonary disorder. The major pathologic or structural changes of the lungs associated with TB (mainly postprimary TB) are as follows:

- Alveolar consolidation
- Alveolar-capillary membrane destruction
- Caseous tubercles or granulomas
- Cavity formation
- Fibrosis and secondary calcification of the lung parenchyma
- Distortion and dilation of the bronchi
- Increased bronchial secretions

Etiology and Epidemiology

TB is one of the oldest diseases known to man and remains one of the most widespread diseases in the world. Unmistakable evidence has been provided from mummies from the Stone Age, ancient Egypt, and Peru that TB is an ancient human disease. In early writings, the disease was called "consumption," "Captain of the Men of Death," and "white plague." In the nineteenth century, the disease was named *tuberculosis,* a term that derives mainly from the tubercle formations found during postmortem examinations of victims of the disease.

According to the Centers for Disease Control and Prevention (CDC), there were 13,299 new cases of TB reported in the United States in 2007—the lowest since the reporting of TB began in 1953. The number of TB cases reported annually in the United States dropped 74% between 1953 and 1985 (84,304 to 22,201). Starting in 1986, however, the incidence of TB trended upward each year in the United States, with a peak of 26,673 reported cases in 1992. The resurgence of TB during this period is well correlated with (1) increased immigration from endemic areas, (2) the sudden rise of the HIV infection epidemic, and (3) the increased use of immunosuppressive drugs. From 1994 to 2007 the yearly incidence of TB again trended downward to its lowest level of 13,299. The decline of TB in the United States is believed to be the result of a number of factors, including new TB medications, a better understanding of the disease, and better public health education. The mortality rate from TB in the United States is currently 0.6 deaths per 100,000, which represents approximately 1700 deaths per year. In 1953 the mortality rate was 12.5 deaths per 100,000 per year.

Globally, TB is still very prevalent. According the World Health Organization (WHO) 2008 report, a third of the world's population is infected by TB. In 2006, WHO estimated that 9.2 million new cases of TB occurred, and about 709,000 (7.7%) were among HIV-positive individuals. WHO reported that the following counties account for nearly 75% of all TB cases: India, China, Pakistan, the Philippines, Thailand, Indonesia, Bangladesh, and the Democratic Republic of Congo. In the European region, it is estimated that 49 new TB cases and seven TB-related deaths occur every hour. According to WHO, the global incidence of TB per capita peaked around 2003 and appears to have stabilized or begun to decline. However, the fall in the TB incidence per capita will likely be more than offset by the expected global population growth. In other words, the overall absolute number of new TB cases each year can be expected to increase (e.g., new TB cases increased from 9.1 to 9.2 million from 2005 to 2006.

In humans, TB is primarily caused by *M. tuberculosis.* The mycobacteria are long, slender, straight or curved rods. The *M. tuberculosis* organism enters humans via the following three routes: the respiratory tract, the gastrointestinal tract, and an open wound in the skin. Most TB infections are contracted via the airborne route (e.g., inhalation of aerosol droplets containing organisms of the tubercle bacillus from an infected individual).

The TB bacilli are highly aerobic organisms and thrive best in areas of the body with high oxygen tension—especially in the apex of the lung. When stained, the hard outer layer of the tubercle bacilli resists decolorization by acid or alcohol; therefore the bacilli are called **acid-fast bacilli.** In addition, the hard outer coat of the tubercle bacillus also protects the organism against killing and digestion by phagocytes and renders the bacilli more resistant to antituberculous drugs.

The TB bacilli are almost exclusively transmitted within aerosol droplets produced by the coughing, sneezing, or laughing of an individual with active TB. This accounts for the use of strict **isolation procedures** in patients acutely hospitalized and suspected of having active tuberculosis. In fact, in fine dried aerosol droplets, the TB bacilli can remain suspended in air for several hours after a cough or sneeze. When inhaled, some of the bacilli may be trapped in the mucus of the nasal passages and removed. The smaller bacilli, however, can easily be inhaled as an aerosol into the bronchioles and alveoli. People living in closed, small rooms with limited access to sunlight and fresh air are especially at risk. The aerosol is composed of organisms contained in small particles known as droplet nuclei. Other possible ways of contracting TB include the ingestion of unpasteurized milk from cattle infected with the TB pathogen (usually *Mycobacterium bovis*) or, in rare cases, direct inoculation through the skin (e.g., a laboratory accident during a postmortem examination).

Diagnosis

The most frequently used diagnostic methods for TB are the **Mantoux tuberculin skin test,** acid-fast staining, sputum cultures, and chest radiographs. Recently a new blood test for TB, called the QuantiFERON-TB Gold (QFT-G) test, has been approved.

Mantoux Tuberculin Skin Test

The most widely used tuberculin test is the Mantoux test, which consists of an intradermal injection of a small amount of a PPD of the tuberculin bacillus (Figure 17-2). The skin is then observed for **induration** (a wheal) after 48 hours and 72 hours, with results interpreted as follows:

- An induration less than 5 mm is a negative result.
- An induration of 5 to 9 mm is considered suspicious, and retesting is required.
- An induration of 10 mm or greater is considered a positive result. A positive reaction is fairly sound evidence of recent or past infection or disease.

It should be stressed, however, that a positive reaction does not necessarily confirm that a patient has active TB, only that the patient has been exposed to the bacillus and has developed cell-mediated immunity to it.

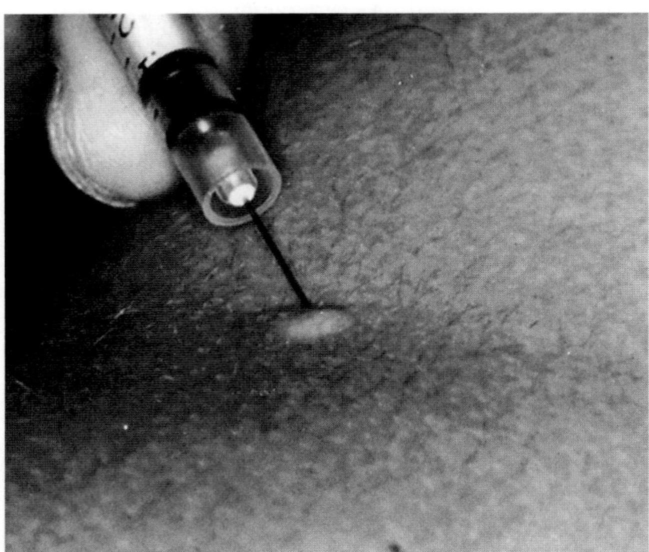

FIGURE 17-2 The Mantoux test, which consists of an intradermal injection of a small amount of a purified protein derivative (PPD) of the tuberculin bacillus. An induration of 10 mm or greater is considered positive. A positive reaction is fairly sound evidence of recent or past infection or disease. From Price SA, Wilson LM: *Pathophysiology: Clinical concepts of disease processes*, 6e. St Louis, 2002, Elsevier.

Acid-Fast Staining

Because the *M. tuberculosis* organism has an unusual, waxy coating on the cell surface, which makes the cells impervious to staining, an **acid-fast bacteria** (AFB) test (also called a **sputum smear**) is performed instead. Several variations of the acid-fast stain are currently in use. The frequently used **Ziehl-Neelsen stain** reveals bright red acid-fast bacilli against a blue background (Figure 17-3, *A*). Another popular technique involves a **fluorescent acid-fast stain** that reveals luminescent yellow-green bacilli against a dark brown background. The fluorescent acid-fast stain is becoming the acid-fast test of choice because it is easier to read and provides a striking contrast (Figure 17-3, *B*).

Sputum Culture

Because a variety of nontuberculous strains of *Mycobacterium* can show up on an AFB smear, a sputum culture is often necessary to differentiate *M. tuberculosis* from other acid-fast organisms. For example, common **nontuberculous acid-fast mycobacteria** associated with chronic obstructive pulmonary disease (COPD) are ***Mycobacterium avium*** and ***Mycobacterium kansasii.*** Sputum cultures can also identify drug-resistant bacilli and their sensitivity to antibiotic therapy. *M. tuberculosis* grows very slowly. It takes up to 6 weeks for colonies to appear in culture. When the TB bacterium was first studied, it was given the misleading prefix *Myco,* which gave the impression that the TB pathogen was fungal in nature. This was because the bacterium growing in agars appeared as colonies, similar to fugal colonies (Figure 17-4). They are unrelated; TB is caused by a bacterium and not a fungus.

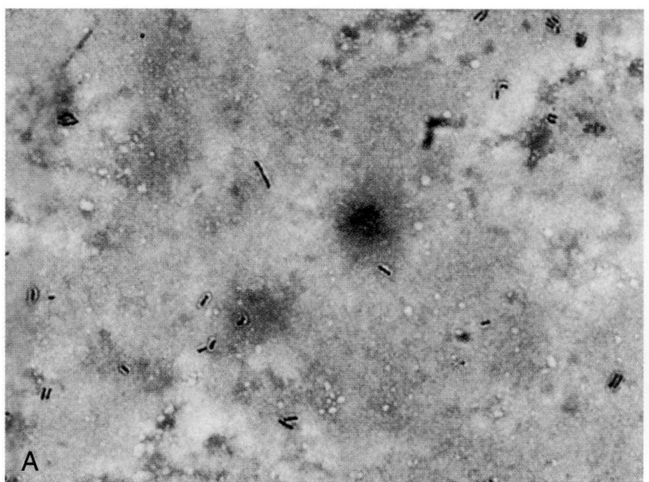

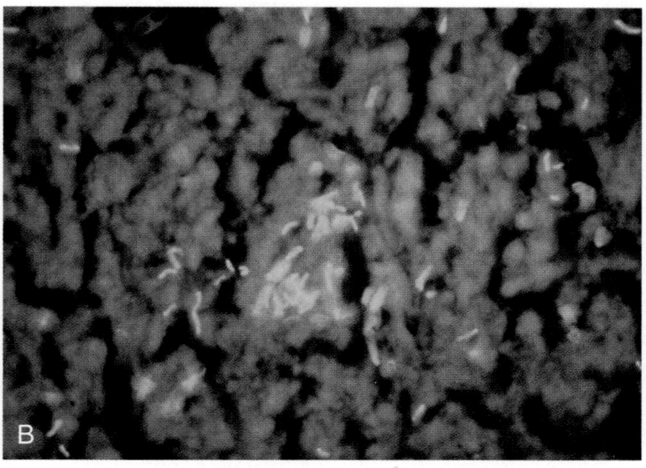

FIGURE 17-3 Acid-fast staining techniques. **A,** Ziehl-Neelsen staining of *Mycobacterium tuberculosis* from sputum. The red rods are *M. tuberculosis.* **B,** A fluorescent acid-fast stain of *M. tuberculosis* from sputum. (From Cowan, MK: *Microbiology: A systems approach,* ed 2, copyright 2009. Reproduced with permission of The McGraw-Hill Companies, New York.)

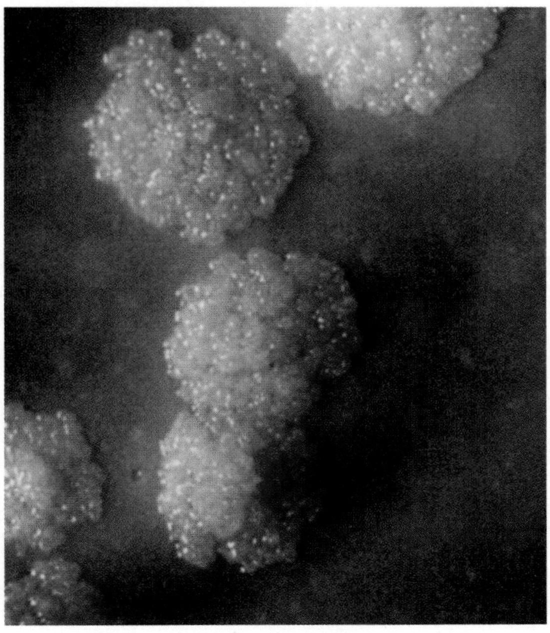

FIGURE 17-4 Cultural appearance of *Mycobacterium tuberculosis.* (From Cowan, MK: *Microbiology: A systems approach,* ed 2, copyright 2009. Reproduced with permission of The McGraw-Hill Companies, New York.)

QuantiFERON-TB Gold Test

In 2005 the U.S. Food and Drug Administration (FDA) approved the QFT-G test. The QFT-G test is a whole-blood test used for diagnosing *M. tuberculosis* infection, including latent TB infection. Samples of the patient's blood are mixed with antigens (substances that can generate an immune response) and controls. The QFT-G test contains synthetic antigens that represent two *M. tuberculosis* proteins (ESAT-6 and CFP-10). The mixture is then allowed to incubate for 16 to 24 hours. After this period the mixture is measured for the presence of interferon-gamma (IFN-gamma). In patients infected with *M. tuberculosis,* the white blood cells will release IFN-gamma when in contact with the TB antigens. An elevated IFN-gamma level is diagnostic of TB. Additional clinical evaluations, such as AFB stain of the sputum smear and chest radiograph, are recommended to further support a positive QFT-G finding.

OVERVIEW of the Cardiopulmonary Clinical Manifestations Associated with Tuberculosis

The following clinical manifestations result from the pathophysiologic mechanisms caused (or activated) by **Alveolar Consolidation** (see Figure 9-9) and **Increased Alveolar-Capillary Membrane Thickness** (see Figure 9-10)—the major anatomic alterations of the lungs associated with tuberculosis (see Figure 17-1).

CLINICAL DATA OBTAINED AT THE PATIENT'S BEDSIDE

The Physical Examination

Vital Signs

Increased Respiratory Rate (Tachypnea)

Several pathophysiologic mechanisms operating simultaneously may lead to an increased ventilatory rate:

OVERVIEW of the Cardiopulmonary Clinical Manifestations Associated with Tuberculosis—cont'd

- Stimulation of peripheral chemoreceptors
- Decreased lung compliance–increased ventilatory rate relationship
- Pain, anxiety, fever

Increased Heart Rate (Pulse) and Blood Pressure

Chest Pain, Decreased Chest Expansion

Cyanosis

Digital Clubbing

Peripheral Edema and Venous Distention

Because polycythemia and cor pulmonale are associated with severe tuberculosis (TB), the following may be seen:

- Distended neck veins
- Pitting edema
- Enlarged and tender liver

Cough, Sputum Production, and Hemoptysis

Chest Assessment Findings

- Increased tactile and vocal fremitus
- Dull percussion note
- Bronchial breath sounds
- Crackles, rhonchi, and wheezing
- Pleural friction rub (if process extends to pleural surface)
- Whispered pectoriloquy

CLINICAL DATA OBTAINED FROM LABORATORY TESTS AND SPECIAL PROCEDURES

Pulmonary Function Test Findings (Severe and Extensive Cases)* (Restrictive Lung Pathology)

FORCED EXPIRATORY FLOW RATE FINDINGS

FVC	FEV_T	FEV_1/FVC ratio	$FEF_{25\%-75\%}$
↓	N or ↓	N or ↑	N or ↓

$FEF_{50\%}$	$FEF_{200-1200}$	PEFR	MVV
N or ↓	N or ↓	N or ↓	N or ↓

*Pulmonary function test (PFT) findings are usually normal in most cases of TB.

LUNG VOLUME AND CAPACITY FINDINGS

V_T	IRV	ERV	RV
N or ↓	↓	↓	↓

VC	IC	FRC	TLC	RV/TLC ratio
↓	↓	↓	↓	N

Arterial Blood Gases

MODERATE TUBERCULOSIS

Acute Alveolar Hyperventilation with Hypoxemia (Acute Respiratory Alkalosis)

pH	$Paco_2$	HCO_3^-	Pao_2
↑	↓	↓ (slightly)	↓

EXTENSIVE TUBERCULOSIS WITH PULMONARY FIBROSIS

Chronic Ventilatory Failure with Hypoxemia (Compensated Respiratory Acidosis)

pH	$Paco_2$	HCO_3^-	Pao_2
N	↑	↑ (significantly)	↓

ACUTE VENTILATORY CHANGES SUPERIMPOSED ON CHRONIC VENTILATORY FAILURE

Because acute ventilatory changes are frequently seen in patients with chronic ventilatory failure, the respiratory care practitioner must be familiar with and alert for the following:

- Acute alveolar hyperventilation superimposed on chronic ventilatory failure, and/or
- Acute ventilatory failure (acute hypoventilation) superimposed on chronic ventilatory failure

Oxygenation Indices* Moderate to Severe Stages

$\dot{Q}_S/\dot{Q}_T$	Do_2†	$\dot{V}o_2$	$C(a-\bar{v})o_2$	O_2ER	$S\bar{v}o_2$
↑	↓	N	N	↑	↓

†The Do_2 may be normal in patients who have compensated to the decreased oxygenation status with (1) an increased cardiac output, (2) an increased hemoglobin level, or (3) a combination of both. When the Do_2 is normal, the O_2ER is usually normal.

Hemodynamic Indices‡ Severe Tuberculosis

CVP	RAP	$\overline{PA}$	PCWP	CO	SV
↑	↑	↑	N	N	N

SVI	CI	RVSWI	LVSWI	PVR	SVR
N	N	↑	N	↑	N

ABNORMAL LABORATORY TEST AND PROCEDURE RESULTS

- Positive tuberculosis skin test (PPD)
- Positive sputum acid-fast bacillus (AFB) stain test
- Positive sputum culture

*$C(a-\bar{v})o_2$, Arterial-venous oxygen difference; Do_2, total oxygen delivery; O_2ER, oxygen extraction ratio; $\dot{Q}_S/\dot{Q}_T$, pulmonary shunt fraction; $S\bar{v}o_2$, mixed venous oxygen saturation; $\dot{V}o_2$, oxygen consumption.

‡CO, Cardiac output; CVP, central venous pressure; LVSWI, left ventricular stroke work index; $\overline{PA}$, mean pulmonary artery pressure; PCWP, pulmonary capillary wedge pressure; PVR, pulmonary vascular resistance; RAP, right atrial pressure; RVSWI, right ventricular stroke work index; SV, stroke volume; SVI, stroke volume index; SVR, systemic vascular resistance.

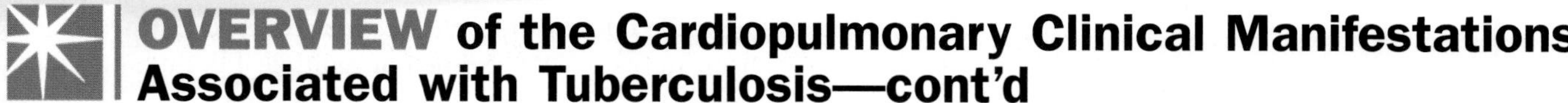

OVERVIEW of the Cardiopulmonary Clinical Manifestations Associated with Tuberculosis—cont'd

RADIOLOGIC FINDINGS

Chest Radiograph

- Increased opacity
- Ghon nodule
- Ghon complex
- Cavity formation
- Cavity lesion containing an air-fluid level (see Figure 16-2)
- Pleural effusion
- Calcification and fibrosis
- Retraction of lung segments or lobe
- Right ventricular enlargement

Chest radiography is most valuable in the diagnosis of pulmonary TB. During the initial primary infection stage, peripheral pneumonic infiltrates (Ghon nodules) can be identified. As the disease progresses, the combination of tubercles and involvement of the lymph nodes in the hilar region (the Ghon complex) can be seen. In severe cases, cavity formation and pleural effusion are seen (Figure 17-5). Healed lesions appear fibrotic or calcified. Retraction of the healed lesions or segments also is revealed on chest radiographs. In patients with postprimary TB of the lungs, lesions involving the apical and posterior segments of the upper lobes are often seen. In disseminated miliary tuberculosis, the lungs may show myriad 2- to 3-mm granulomatous foci. The radiographic result is widespread fine nodules, which are uniformly distributed and equal in size (Figure 17-6). Finally, because right-sided heart failure (cor pulmonale) may develop as a secondary problem during the advanced stages of TB, an enlarged heart may be seen on the chest radiograph.

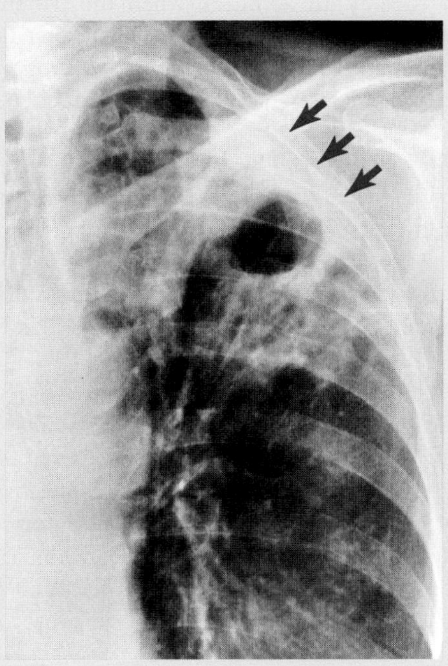

FIGURE 17-5 Cavitary reactivation tuberculosis showing a left upper lobe cavity and localized pleural thickening *(arrows).* (From Hansell DM, Armstrong P, Lynch DA, McAdams HP, eds: *Imaging of diseases of the chest,* ed 4, Philadelphia, 2005, Elsevier.)

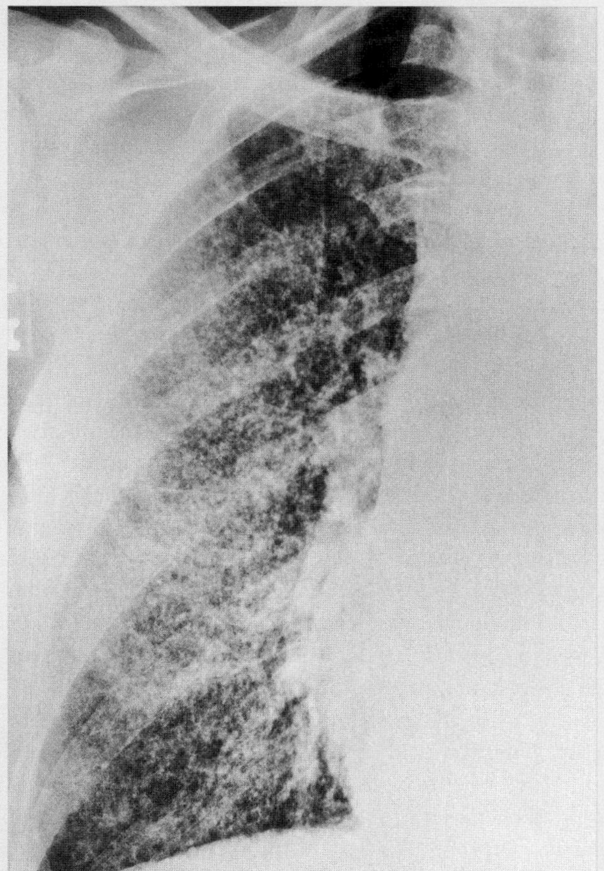

FIGURE 17-6 Miliary tuberculosis showing widespread uniformly distributed fine nodulation of the lung. (From Hansell DM, Armstrong P, Lynch DA, McAdams HP, eds: *Imaging of diseases of the chest,* ed 4, Philadelphia, 2005, Elsevier.)

General Management of Tuberculosis

Because the tubercle bacillus can exist in open cavitary lesions, in closed lesions, and within the cytoplasm of macrophages, a drug that may be effective in one of these environments may be ineffective in another. In addition, some of the TB bacilli are drug resistant. Because of this problem, several drugs usually are prescribed *concurrently* for individuals with TB. Because toxicity is associated with some of the antituberculosis drugs, frequent examinations are performed to identify toxicity manifested in the kidneys, liver, eyes, and ears. In noncompliant patients the drug may need to be administered under the direct supervision of a health-care worker.

Pharmacologic Agents Used to Treat Tuberculosis

The standard pharmacologic agents used to treat *M. tuberculosis* consist of two to four drugs for 6 to 9 months. Examples of these protocols are as follows:

- **6-month treatment protocol:** For the first 2 months (called the *induction phase*) the patient takes a daily dose of **isoniazid (INH), rifampin, pyrazinamide,** and either **ethambutol** or **streptomycin.** For the next 4 months the patient takes isoniazid and rifampin daily or twice weekly.
- **9-month treatment protocol:** For the first 1 to 2 months the patient takes a daily dose of isoniazid and rifampin, followed by twice-weekly isoniazid and rifampin until the full 9-month period has been completed.

Isoniazid (INH) and rifampin (Rifadin) are first-line agents prescribed for the entire 9 months. Isoniazid is considered to be the most effective first-line antituberculosis agent. Rifampin is bactericidal and is most commonly used with isoniazid. Although patients with TB usually are not contagious after a few weeks of treatment, a full course of treatment is necessary to kill all the bacteria. The **prophylactic *use of isoniazid*** is often prescribed as a daily dose for 1 year in individuals who have been exposed to the TB bacilli or who demonstrate a positive tuberculin reaction (even when the acid-fast sputum stain is negative).

When the TB bacterium is resistant to one or more of these agents, at least three or more antibiotics must be added to the treatment regimen and the duration should be extended. A major problem with TB therapy is noncompliance on the part of the patient to take the TB medication as prescribed. Even under the best circumstances, it is very difficult to maintain a regimen of multiple TB antibiotics on a daily basis for months. Unfortunately, most TB patients are not living under the best circumstances. In addition, failure to adhere to an antibiotic regimen often leads to antibiotic resistance in the slow-growing microorganism. In fact, many *M. tuberculosis* isolates are now found to be multiple drug–resistant TB (MDRTB).

In response to the problem of noncompliance, it is recommended that all patients with TB be treated by **directly observed therapy (DOT)**—that is, the ingestion of medication is directly observed by a responsible individual. In communities where DOT has been used, the rate of drug-resistant TB and the rate of TB relapse have been shown to decrease.

A new strain of drug-resistant *M. tuberculosis* was identified in Africa in 2006. It is especially lethal for HIV-infected individuals and has been named *extensively drug-resistant TB* (XDRTB).

Respiratory Care Treatment Protocols

Oxygen Therapy Protocol

Oxygen therapy is used to treat hypoxemia, decrease the work of breathing, and decrease myocardial work. Because of the hypoxemia associated with TB, supplemental oxygen may be required. The hypoxemia that develops in patients with lung abscess is usually caused by pulmonary capillary shunting. Hypoxemia caused by capillary shunting is often refractory to oxygen therapy. In addition, when the patient demonstrates chronic ventilatory failure during the advanced stages of TB, caution must be taken not to overoxygenate the patient (see Oxygen Therapy Protocol, Protocol 9-1).

Bronchopulmonary Hygiene Therapy Protocol

Because of the excessive mucous production and accumulation sometimes associated with severe TB, a number of bronchial hygiene treatment modalities may be used to enhance the mobilization of bronchial secretions (see Bronchopulmonary Hygiene Therapy Protocol, Protocol 9-2).

Mechanical Ventilation Protocol

Because acute ventilatory failure is occasionally associated with TB, mechanical ventilation may be required to maintain an adequate ventilatory status. Continuous mechanical ventilation is justified when the acute ventilatory failure is thought to be reversible—for example, when pneumonia complicates the condition (see Mechanical Ventilation Protocols, Protocol 9-5, Protocol 9-6, and Protocol 9-7).

CASE STUDY

Tuberculosis

Admitting History and Physical Examination

This 60-year-old male patient had been in good health until about 4 months before admission, when he first noted the onset of night sweats, occasionally accompanied by chills. About 3 months ago he noted that his appetite was decreasing, and he lost about 25 pounds after that time.

Approximately 3 weeks before his admission, he noted that his long-standing "smoker's cough" had become more productive. For the 2 weeks prior to admission, his daily sputum production had increased to about a cup of thick yellow sputum with an occasional fleck or two of blood. There was a concomitant increase in dyspnea. About 10 days before admission, he had a gradual onset of moderately sharp left-sided chest pain. It was aggravated by deep breathing but did not radiate.

The past history gave little useful information. About 35 years ago, he was told during a routine medical exam that he had a positive TB skin test, but that he had no pulmonary problems. Subsequently he had had several chest x-ray examinations in mobile chest x-ray units, once for an insurance application. The last x-ray examination was performed 5 years ago.

For the previous 35 years, he had been employed in a foundry as a "cone maker" and "shaker." He volunteered the information that he worked in a "dusty" environment and that he had worn a protective mask only for the previous few months. His family history was noncontributory. He and his wife lived in the same house with his married daughter and two young granddaughters.

Physical examination revealed a thin man who appeared to be both chronically and acutely ill. His vital signs were blood pressure 132/90, heart rate 116/min, respiratory rate 32/min, and oral temperature 102.4° F. His room air Spo_2 was 90%. He was coughing up large amounts of yellow, blood-streaked sputum. There was marked dullness to percussion in both apical areas, and diffuse inspiratory crackles and expiratory rhonchi were present in the right upper and middle lobes. A chest x-ray film demonstrated extensive bilateral apical calcification, cavity formation in the right upper lobe, and diffuse infiltrate and consolidation in the right middle lobe. He was admitted to the hospital and placed in respiratory isolation. The following initial respiratory assessment was entered into the patient's chart.

Respiratory Assessment and Plan

S Productive cough, slight hemoptysis; moderate dyspnea. History of left-sided chest pain for 10 days.

O Febrile to 102.4° F. RR 32, HR 116, BP 132/90. Room air Spo_2 90%. Productive cough: large amounts yellow, blood-streaked sputum. Crackles and rhonchi in right upper and middle lobes. CXR: Apical calcification; RUL cavity; RML infiltrate/consolidation.

A
- Probable tuberculosis (patient possibly infectious)
- Excessive airway secretions (yellow sputum, cough)
- Mild hypoxemia (Spo_2 90%)

P Flag chart: Continue respiratory isolation pending AFB smear results. Obtain sputum for routine, anaerobic, and acid-fast cultures and cytology—induce if necessary. Obtain baseline ABG on room air. **Bronchopulmonary Hygiene Therapy Protocol:** C&DB q2h. Based on ABG results, titrate oxygen therapy per **Oxygen Therapy Protocol.** Discuss need for bedside spirogram with physician.

Discussion

Two primary clinical scenarios were activated in this case. First, the **Alveolar Consolidation** (see Figure 9-9) identified on the chest x-ray film reflected the patient's challenged immune response. This was further manifested by the objective data noted at the patient's bedside—fever, dull percussion notes, and increased heart rate, blood pressure, and respiratory rate. In addition, the alveolar consolidation undoubtedly contributed to the patient's pulmonary shunting and mild hypoxemia (see Figure 9-9).

Secondly, clinical manifestations associated with **Excessive Bronchial Secretions** (see Figure 9-12) also were present in this patient: daily cough, yellow sputum production, crackles, and rhonchi. His oxygen desaturation was mild (Spo_2 = 90%), and a room air ABG and subsequent oxygen titration (presumably with low-flow oxygen by nasal cannula) were appropriate.

As expected, the patient produced sputum containing acid-fast organisms. The attending physician prescribed isoniazid, rifampin, and streptomycin for 2 months, followed by an outpatient course of isoniazid and rifampin for 4 months. The patient also was instructed regarding several different **Bronchopulmonary Hygiene Therapy** (see Protocol 9-2) to perform at home. The patient did well through 1 year of follow-up.

SELF-ASSESSMENT QUESTIONS

evolve Answers to questions can be found on Evolve. To access additional student assessment questions and case studies for application of text material to real-life scenarios, visit **http://evolve.elsevier.com/DesJardins/respiratory.**

1. What is the first stage of tuberculosis known as?

1. Reinfection tuberculosis
2. Primary tuberculosis
3. Secondary tuberculosis
4. Primary infection stage
   - a. 2 only
   - b. 3 only
   - c. 1 and 3 only
   - d. 2 and 4 only

2. What is the name of the protective wall that surrounds and encases lung tissue infected with tuberculosis?

1. Miliary tuberculosis
2. Reinfection tuberculosis
3. Granuloma
4. Tubercle
   - a. 1 only
   - b. 3 only
   - c. 4 only
   - d. 3 and 4 only

3. The tubercle bacillus is:

1. Highly aerobic
2. Acid-fast
3. Capable of surviving for months outside of the body
4. Rod-shaped
   - a. 2 only
   - b. 4 only
   - c. 2 and 3 only
   - d. 1, 2, 3, and 4

4. At which size wheal is a tuberculin skin test considered to be positive?

- a. Greater than 4 mm
- b. Greater than 6 mm
- c. Greater than 8 mm
- d. Greater than 10 mm

5. Which of the following is often prescribed as a prophylactic daily dose for 1 year in individuals who have been exposed to tuberculosis bacilli?

- a. Streptomycin
- b. Ethambutol
- c. Isoniazid
- d. Rifampin

Fungal Diseases of the Lung

18

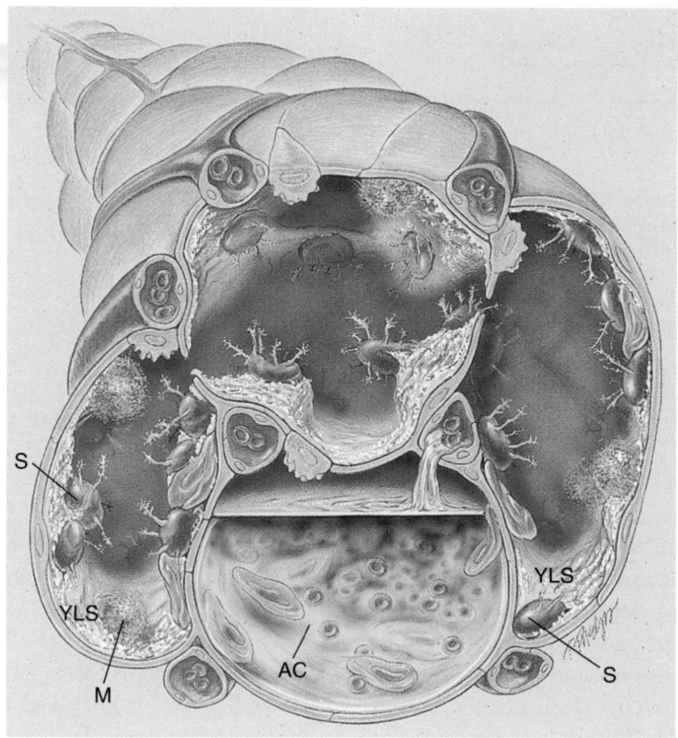

FIGURE 18-1 Fungal disease of the lung. Cross-sectional view of alveoli infected with *Histoplasma capsulatum*. *AC,* Alveolar consolidation; *M,* alveolar macrophage; *S,* Fungal spore; *YLS,* yeastlike substance.

Chapter Objectives

After reading this chapter, you will be able to:

- List the anatomic alterations of the lungs associated with fungal disease.
- Describe the causes of fungal disease.
- List the cardiopulmonary clinical manifestations associated with fungal disease.
- Describe the general management of fungal disease.
- Describe the clinical strategies and rationales of the SOAPs presented in the case study.
- Define key terms and complete self-assessment questions at the end of the chapter and on Evolve.

Key Terms

Acute Symptomatic Pulmonary Histoplasmosis
Amphotericin B (Fungizone)
Anidulafungin
Aspergillus
Asymptomatic Primary Histoplasmosis
Azoles
Blastomyces dermatitidis
Blastomycosis
California Disease
Candida albicans
Caseous Tubercles
Caspofungin
Cavity Formation
Chicago Disease
Chronic Histoplasmosis
Coccidioides immitis
Coccidioidomycosis
Cryptococcus neoformans
Desert Arthritis
Desert Bumps
Desert Fever
Desert Rheumatism
Disseminated Histoplasmosis
Echinocandins
Fluconazole
Gilchrist's Disease
Granulomas
Histoplasma capsulatum

Histoplasmosis
Itraconazole
Ketoconazole
Micafungin
North American Blastomycosis
Ohio Valley Fever
San Joaquin Valley Disease
Valley Fever

Chapter Outline

Anatomic Alterations of the Lungs

When fungal spores are inhaled, they may reach the lungs and germinate. When this happens, the spores produce a frothy, yeastlike substance that leads to an inflammatory response. Polymorphonuclear leukocytes and macrophages move into the infected area and engulf the fungal spores. The pulmonary capillaries dilate, the interstitium fills with fluid, and the alveolar epithelium swells with edema fluid. Regional lymph node involvement commonly occurs during this period. Because of the inflammatory reaction, the alveoli in the infected area eventually become consolidated (Figure 18-1). Airway secretions may also develop at this time.

In severe cases, tissue necrosis, **granulomas,** and cavity formation may be seen. During the healing process, fibrosis and calcification of the lung parenchyma ultimately replace the granulomas. In response to the fibrosis and occasionally calcification, the lung tissue retracts and becomes firm. The apical and posterior segments of the upper lobes are most commonly involved. The anatomic changes of the lungs caused by fungal diseases are similar to those seen in tuberculosis.

Fungal diseases of the lung cause a chronic restrictive pulmonary disorder. The major pathologic or structural changes of the lungs associated with fungal diseases of the lungs are as follows:

- Alveolar consolidation
- Alveolar-capillary destruction
- **Caseous tubercles** or granulomas
- **Cavity formation**
- Fibrosis and secondary calcification of the lung parenchyma
- Bronchial airway secretions

Etiology and Epidemiology

Fungal spores are widely distributed throughout the air, soil, fomites, and animals, and even exist in the normal flora of humans. As many as 300 fungal species may be linked to disease in animals. In plants, fungal disease is the most common cause of death and destruction. In humans, most exposures to fungal pathogens do not lead to overt infection because humans have a relatively high resistance to them. Human fungal disease (also called *mycotic disease* or *mycosis*) can be caused, however, by primary or "true" fungal pathogens that exhibit some degree of virulence or by opportunistic or secondary pathogens that take advantage of a weakened immune defense system (e.g., in acquired immunodeficiency syndrome [AIDS] and human immunodeficiency virus [HIV] infection).

Primary Pathogens

Histoplasmosis

Histoplasmosis is the most common fungal infection in the United States. It is caused by the dimorphic fungus ***Histoplasma capsulatum.*** In the United States, the prevalence of histoplasmosis is especially high along the major river valleys of the Midwest (e.g., Ohio, Michigan, Illinois, Mississippi, Missouri, Kentucky, Tennessee, Georgia, and Arkansas). In fact, on the basis of skin test surveys it is estimated that 80% to 90% of the population throughout these areas shows signs of previous infection. Histoplasmosis is often called **Ohio Valley Fever.**

H. capsulatum is commonly found in soils enriched with bird excreta, such as the soil near chicken houses, pigeon lofts, barns, and trees where starlings and blackbirds roost. The birds themselves, however, do not carry the organism, although the *H. capsulatum* spore may be carried by bats. Generally, an individual acquires the infection by inhaling the fungal spores that are released when the soil from an infected area is disturbed (e.g., children playing in dirt).

When the *H. capsulatum* organism reaches the alveoli, at body temperature it converts from its mycelial form (mold) to a parasitic yeast form. The clinical manifestations of histoplasmosis are strikingly similar to those of tuberculosis. The incubation period for the infection is approximately 17 days. Only about 40% of those infected demonstrate symptoms, and only about 10% of these patients are ill enough to consult a physician. Depending on the individual's immune system, the disease may take on one of the following forms: **asymptomatic primary histoplasmosis, acute symptomatic**

pulmonary histoplasmosis, chronic histoplasmosis, and **disseminated histoplasmosis.**

Asymptomatic histoplasmosis is the most common form of histoplasmosis. Normally it produces no signs or symptoms in otherwise healthy individuals who become infected. The only residual sign of infection may be a small, healed lesion of the lung parenchyma or calcified hilar lymph nodes. The patient has a positive histoplasmin skin test result.

Acute symptomatic pulmonary histoplasmosis tends to occur in otherwise healthy individuals who have had an intense exposure to *H. capsulatum.* Depending on the number of spores inhaled, the individual signs and symptoms may range from a mild to serious illness. Mild signs and symptoms include fever, muscle and joint pain, headache, dry hacking cough, chills, chest pain, weight loss, and sweats. People who have inhaled a large number of spores may develop a severe acute pulmonary syndrome, a potentially life-threatening condition in which the individual becomes extremely short of breath. The acute pulmonary syndrome is often referred to as *spelunker's lung* because it frequently develops after excessive exposure to bat excrement stirred up by individuals exploring caves. During this phase of the disease, the patient's chest radiograph generally shows single or multiple infection sites resembling those associated with pneumonia.

Chronic pulmonary histoplasmosis is characterized by infiltration and cavity formation in the upper lobes of one or both lungs. This type of histoplasmosis often affects people with an underlying lung disease such as emphysema. It is most commonly seen in middle-aged white men who smoke. Signs and symptoms include fatigue, fever, night sweats, weight loss, a productive cough, and hemoptysis—similar to signs and symptoms of tuberculosis. Often the infection is self-limiting. In some patients, however, progressive destruction of lung tissue and dissemination of the infection may occur.

Disseminated histoplasmosis may follow either self-limited histoplasmosis or chronic histoplasmosis. It is most often seen in very young or very old patients with compromised immune systems (e.g., patients with HIV infection). Even though the macrophages can remove the fungi from the bloodstream, they are unable to kill the fungal organisms. As a result, disseminated histoplasmosis can affect nearly any part of the body, including eyes, liver, bone marrow, skin, adrenal glands, and intestinal tract. Depending on which body organs are affected, the patient may develop anemia; pneumonia; pericarditis; meningitis; adrenal insufficiency; and ulcers of the mouth, tongue, or intestinal tract. If untreated, disseminated histoplasmosis is usually fatal.

Screening and Diagnosis

Fungal culture. The fungal culture test is considered the gold standard for detecting histoplasmosis. A small amount of blood, sputum, or tissue from a lymph node, lung, or bone marrow is cultured. The disadvantage of this test is that it takes time for the fungus to grow—4 weeks or longer. For this reason, it is not the test of choice for cases of disseminated histoplasmosis. Treatment delays in these patients may prove fatal.

Fungal stain. In the fungal stain test, a tissue sample, which may be obtained from sputum, bone marrow, lungs, or a skin lesion, is stained with dye and examined under a microscope for *H. capsulatum.* A positive test result is 100% accurate. The disadvantage of this test is that obtaining a sputum sample can be difficult, and obtaining a sample from other sites requires invasive procedures.

Serology. A blood serology test checks blood serum for antigens and antibodies. When an individual is exposed to histoplasmosis spores (antigens), the body's immune system produces antibodies (proteins) to react to the histoplasmosis antigens. Tests that check for histoplasmosis antigen and antibody reactions are relatively fast and fairly accurate. False-negative results, however, may occur in people who have compromised immune systems or who are infected with other types of fungi.

Coccidioidomycosis

Coccidioidomycosis is caused by inhalation of the spores of ***Coccidioides immitis,*** which are spheric fungi carried by wind-borne dust particles. The disease is endemic in hot, dry regions. In the United States, coccidioidomycosis is especially prevalent in California, Arizona, Nevada, New Mexico, Texas, and Utah. About 80% of the people in the San Joaquin Valley are coccidioidin skin test positive. Because the prevalence of coccidioidomycosis is high in these regions, the disease is also known as **California Disease, Desert Fever, San Joaquin Valley Disease,** and **Valley Fever.** The fungus has been isolated in these regions from soils, plants, and a large number of vertebrates (e.g., mammals, birds, reptiles, amphibians).

When *C. immitis* spores are inhaled, they settle in the lungs, begin to germinate, and form round, thin-walled cells called *spherules.* The spherules, in turn, produce endospores that make more spherules (the spherule-endospore phase). The disease usually takes the form of an acute, primary, self-limiting pulmonary infection with or without systemic involvement. Some cases, however, progress to disseminated disease.

Clinical manifestations are absent in about 60% of the people who have a positive skin test result. In the remaining 40%, most of the patients demonstrate coldlike symptoms such as fever, chest pain, cough, headaches, and malaise. In uncomplicated cases, patients generally recover completely and enjoy lifelong immunity. In approximately 1 in 200 cases, however, the primary infection does not resolve and progresses with varied clinical manifestations. Chronic progressive pulmonary disease is characterized by nodular growths called *fungomas* and cavity formation in the lungs. Disseminated coccidioidomycosis occurs in about 1 in 6000 exposed persons. When this condition exists, the lymph nodes, meninges, spleen, liver, kidney, skin, and adrenals may be involved. The skin lesions (e.g., bumps on the face and chest) are commonly accompanied by arthralgia or arthritis, especially in the ankles and knees. This condition is commonly called **desert bumps, desert arthritis,** or **desert rheumatism.** Death is most commonly caused by meningitis.

Screening and Diagnosis

The diagnosis of coccidioidomycosis can be made by the direct visualization of distinctive spherules in microscopy of the patient's sputum, tissue exudates, biopsies, or spinal fluid. The diagnosis can be further supported by blood tests that detect antibodies to the fungus or a culture of the organism from infected fluid or tissue.

Blastomycosis

Blastomycosis (also called **Chicago disease, Gilchrist's disease,** and **North American blastomycosis**) is caused by ***Blastomyces dermatitidis.*** Blastomycosis occurs in people living in the south-central and midwestern United States and Canada. The infection occurs in 1 to 2 out of every 100,000 people in these areas. Cases also have been reported in Central America, South America, Africa, and the Middle East. *B. dermatitidis* inhabits areas high in organic matter, such as forest soil, decaying wood, animal manure, and abandoned buildings. Blastomycosis is most common among pregnant women and middle-aged African-American men. The disease also is found in dogs, cats, and horses.

The primary portal of entry of *B. dermatitidis* is the lungs. The acute clinical manifestations resemble those of acute histoplasmosis, including fever, cough, hoarseness, aching of the joints and muscles, and, in some cases, pleuritic pain. Unlike histoplasmosis, however, the cough is frequently productive, and the sputum is purulent. Acute pulmonary infections may be self-limiting or progressive. When the condition is progressive, nodules and abscesses develop in the lungs. Extrapulmonary lesions commonly involve the skin, bones, reproductive tract, spleen, liver, kidney, or prostate gland. The skin lesions may, in fact, be the first signs of the disease. It often begins on the face, hands, wrists, or legs as subcutaneous nodules that erode to the skin surface. Dissemination of the yeast also may cause arthritis and osteomyelitis, and involvement of the central nervous system causes headache, convulsions, coma, and mental confusion. Standardized testing procedures for blastomycosis are not available. The diagnosis of blastomycosis can be made from direct visualization of the yeast in sputum smears. Culture of the fungus also can be performed. An accurate blastomycin skin test is not available.

Opportunistic Pathogens

Opportunistic yeast pathogens such as ***Candida albicans, Cryptococcus neoformans,*** and ***Aspergillus*** also are associated with lung infections in certain patients.

C. albicans occurs as normal flora in the oral cavity, genitalia, and large intestine. *C. albicans* infection of the mouth is characterized by a white, adherent, patchy infection of the mouth, gums, cheeks, and throat. In patients with HIV infection, *C. albicans* often causes infection of the mouth, pharynx, vagina, skin, and lungs.

C. neoformans proliferates in the high nitrogen content of pigeon droppings and is readily scattered into the air and dust. Today, *Cryptococcus* is most often seen in patients with HIV infection and persons undergoing steroid therapy.

Aspergillus may be the most pervasive of all fungi—especially *Aspergillus fumigatus. Aspergillus* is found in soil, vegetation, leaf detritus, food, and compost heaps. Persons breathing the air of granaries, barns, and silos are at greatest risk. *Aspergillus* infection usually occurs in the lungs. It is almost always an opportunistic infection and poses a serious threat to patients with HIV infection.

OVERVIEW of the Cardiopulmonary Clinical Manifestations Associated with Fungal Diseases of the Lungs

The following clinical manifestations result from the pathophysiologic mechanisms caused (or activated) by **Alveolar Consolidation** (see Figure 9-9) and, in severe cases, with fibrosis, **Increased Alveolar-Capillary Membrane Thickness** (see Figure 9-10)—the major anatomic alterations of the lungs associated with fungal diseases of the lungs (see Figure 18-1).

CLINICAL DATA OBTAINED AT THE PATIENT'S BEDSIDE

The Physical Examination

Vital Signs

Increased Respiratory Rate (Tachypnea)

Several pathophysiologic mechanisms operating simultaneously may lead to an increased ventilatory rate:

- Stimulation of peripheral chemoreceptors
- Decreased lung compliance–increased ventilatory rate relationship
- Pain, anxiety, fever

Increased Heart Rate (Pulse) and Blood Pressure

Chest Pain, Decreased Chest Expansion

Cyanosis

Digital Clubbing

Peripheral Edema and Venous Distention

Because polycythemia and cor pulmonale are associated with severe tuberculosis (TB), the following may be seen:

- Distended neck veins
- Pitting edema
- Enlarged and tender liver

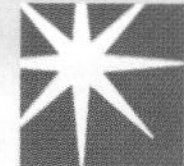

OVERVIEW of the Cardiopulmonary Clinical Manifestations Associated with Fungal Diseases of the Lungs—cont'd

Cough, Sputum Production, and Hemoptysis

Chest Assessment Findings

- Increased tactile and vocal fremitus
- Dull percussion note
- Bronchial breath sounds
- Crackles, rhonchi, and wheezing
- Pleural friction rub (if process extends to pleural surface)
- Whispered pectoriloquy

CLINICAL DATA OBTAINED FROM LABORATORY TESTS AND SPECIAL PROCEDURES

Pulmonary Function Test Findings (Moderate to Severe) (Restrictive Lung Pathology)

FORCED EXPIRATORY FLOW RATE FINDINGS

FVC	FEV_T	FEV_1/FVC ratio	$FEF_{25\%-75\%}$
↓	N or ↓	N or ↑	N or ↓

$FEF_{50\%}$	$FEF_{200-1200}$	PEFR	MVV
N or ↓	N or ↓	N or ↓	N or ↓

LUNG VOLUME AND CAPACITY FINDINGS

V_T	IRV	ERV	RV	
N or ↓	↓	↓	↓	

VC	IC	FRC	TLC	RV/TLC ratio
↓	↓	↓	↓	N

Arterial Blood Gases

MODERATE FUNGAL DISEASE

Acute Alveolar Hyperventilation with Hypoxemia

(Acute Respiratory Alkalosis)

pH	$Paco_2$	HCO_3^-	Pao_2
↑	↓	↓ (slightly)	↓

SEVERE FUNGAL DISEASE WITH PULMONARY FIBROSIS

Chronic Ventilatory Failure with Hypoxemia

(Compensated Respiratory Acidosis)

pH	$Paco_2$	HCO_3^-	Pao_2
N	↑	↑ (significantly)	↓

ACUTE VENTILATORY CHANGES SUPERIMPOSED ON CHRONIC VENTILATORY FAILURE

Because acute ventilatory changes are frequently seen in patients with chronic ventilatory failure, the respiratory care practitioner must be familiar with and alert for the following:

- Acute alveolar hyperventilation superimposed on chronic ventilatory failure, and/or
- Acute ventilatory failure (acute hypoventilation) superimposed on chronic ventilatory failure

Oxygenation Indices*

Moderate to Severe Stages

$\dot{Q}_S/\dot{Q}_T$	Do_2†	$\dot{V}o_2$	$C(a-\bar{v})o_2$	O_2ER	$S\bar{v}o_2$
↑	↓	N	N	↑	↓

†The Do_2 may be normal in patients who have compensated to the decreased oxygenation status with (1) an increased cardiac output, (2) an increased hemoglobin level, or (3) a combination of both. When the Do_2 is normal, the O_2ER is usually normal.

Hemodynamic Indices‡

Severe Fungal Disease

CVP	RAP	$\overline{PA}$	PCWP	CO	SV
↑	↑	↑	N	N	N

SVI	CI	RVSWI	LVSWI	PVR	SVR
N	N	↑	N	↑	N

ABNORMAL LABORATORY TEST AND PROCEDURE RESULTS

Radiologic Findings

Chest Radiograph

- Increased opacity
- Cavity formation
- Pleural effusion
- Calcification and fibrosis
- Right ventricular enlargement

During the early stages of many pulmonary fungal infections, localized infiltration and consolidation with or without lymph node involvement are commonly seen (Figure 18-2). Single or numerous spheric nodules may be seen (Figure 18-3). During the advanced stages, bilateral cavities in the apical and posterior segments of the upper lobes are often seen (Figure 18-4). In disseminated disease a diffuse bilateral micronodular pattern and pleural effusion may be seen. Fibrosis and calcification of healed lesions can be identified. Finally, because right-sided heart failure may develop as a secondary problem during the advanced stages of fungal disease, an enlarged heart may be seen on the chest radiograph. These radiologic findings are very similar to those seen in pulmonary TB.

**$C(a-\bar{v})o_2$*, Arterial-venous oxygen difference; *Do_2*, total oxygen delivery; *O_2ER*, oxygen extraction ratio; *$\dot{Q}_S/\dot{Q}_T$*, pulmonary shunt fraction; *$S\bar{v}o_2$*, mixed venous oxygen saturation; *$\dot{V}o_2$*, oxygen consumption.

‡*CO*, Cardiac output; *CVP*, central venous pressure; *LVSWI*, left ventricular stroke work index; *$\overline{PA}$*, mean pulmonary artery pressure; *PCWP*, pulmonary capillary wedge pressure; *PVR*, pulmonary vascular resistance; *RAP*, right atrial pressure; *RVSWI*, right ventricular stroke work index; *SV*, stroke volume; *SVI*, stroke volume index; *SVR*, systemic vascular resistance.

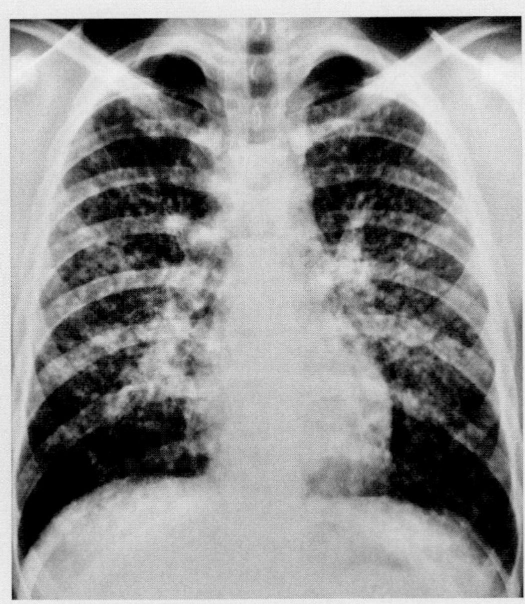

FIGURE 18-2 Acute inhalational histoplasmosis in an otherwise healthy patient. This young man developed fever and cough after tearing down an old barn. The study shows bilateral hilar adenopathy and diffuse nodular opacities. (From Hansell DM, Armstrong P, Lynch DA, McAdams HP, eds: *Imaging of diseases of the chest,* ed 4, Philadelphia, 2005, Elsevier.)

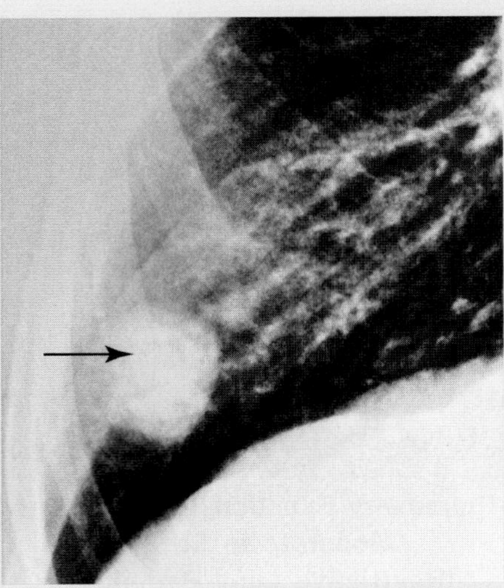

FIGURE 18-3 Histoplasmoma, showing a well-defined spheric nodule. The central portion of the nodule shows calcification. (From Hansell DM, Armstrong P, Lynch DA, McAdams HP, eds: *Imaging of diseases of the chest,* ed 4, Philadelphia, 2005, Elsevier.)

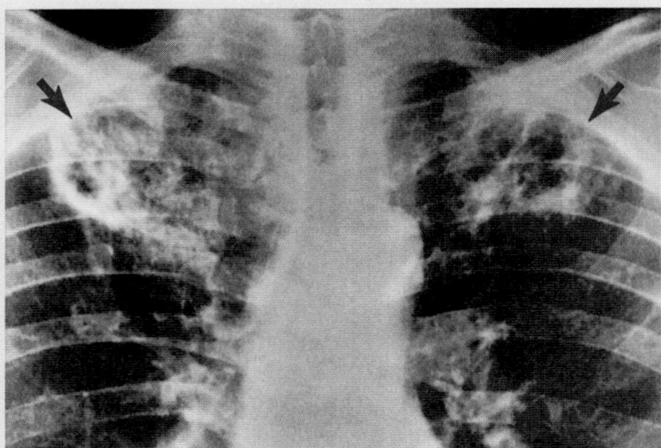

FIGURE 18-4 Chronic cavitary histoplasmosis. Note the striking upper zone predominance of the shadows. Numerous large cavities. (From Hansell DM, Armstrong P, Lynch DA, McAdams HP, eds: *Imaging of diseases of the chest,* ed 4, Philadelphia, 2005, Elsevier.)

General Management of Fungal Disease

The antifungal agents are the first line of defense in treating fungal lung infections. In general, the drug of choice for most fungal infections is intravenously administered polyene **amphotericin B (Fungizone).** Although **ketoconazole** was used as a first-line agent against common fungal organisms, it has largely been replaced by the trizoles, **fluconazole** and **itraconazole.** The **echinocandins,** a relatively new class of antifungal agents, are now available (Table 18-1).

Respiratory Care Treatment Protocols

Oxygen Therapy Protocol

Oxygen therapy is used to treat hypoxemia, decrease the work of breathing, and decrease myocardial work. Because of the hypoxemia associated with the fungal pulmonary condition, supplemental oxygen may be required. Because of the alveolar consolidation produced by a fungal disorder, capillary shunting may be present. Hypoxemia caused by capillary shunting is often refractory to oxygen therapy. In addition, when the patient demonstrates chronic ventilatory failure during the advanced stages of fungal disease, caution must be taken not to overoxygenate the patient (see Oxygen Therapy Protocol, Protocol 9-1).

Bronchopulmonary Hygiene Therapy Protocol

Because of the excessive mucous production and accumulation sometimes associated with fungal disease, a number of bronchial hygiene treatment modalities may be used to enhance the mobilization of bronchial secretions (see Bronchopulmonary Hygiene Therapy Protocol, Protocol 9-2).

Mechanical Ventilation Protocol

Mechanical ventilation may be necessary to provide and support alveolar gas exchange and eventually return the patient to spontaneous breathing. Because acute ventilatory failure is occasionally seen in patients with severe fungal disease, continuous mechanical ventilation may be required. Continuous mechanical ventilation is justified when the acute ventilatory failure is thought to be reversible (see Mechanical Ventilation Protocols, Protocol 9-5, Protocol 9-6, and Protocol 9-7).

TABLE 18-1 Antifungal Agents

Agents	Common Uses (Microorganisms)
Polyenes	
Amphotericin B (Fungizone)	*Cryptococcus neoformans, Histoplasma capsulatum, Blastomyces dermatitidis, Coccidioides immitis, Candida* species, *Aspergillus* species
Amphotericin B colloidal dispersion (Amphotec)	*Candida* species, *Aspergillus* species, mucormycosis, *C. neoformans*
Azoles	
Ketoconazole (Nizoral)	*Candida* species, *C. neoformans, H. capsulatum, B. dermatitidis*
Fluconazole (Diflucan)	*Candida* species, *Aspergillus* species, *C. neoformans, H. capsulatum*
Itraconazole (Sporanox)	*B. dermatitidis, C. immitis, Sporothrix schenckii*
Echinocandins	
Caspofungin (Cancidas)	*Aspergillus* species, *Candida* species
Micafungin (Mycamine)	
Anidulafungin (Eraxis)	
Other Antifungals	
Flucytosine (Ancobon)	*Aspergillus* species, *Candida* species, *C. neoformans*
Griseofulvin (Fulvicin)	Tinea corporis, tinea cruris, tinea barbae
Terbinafine (Lamisil)	Tinea corporis, tinea pedis, tinea manuum

Modified from Gardenhire DS: *Rau's respiratory care pharmacology,* ed 7, St Louis, 2008, Elsevier.

CASE STUDY

Fungal Diseases of the Lungs

Admitting History

A 56-year-old cattle driver was admitted to the arthritis clinic of a small hospital just outside Phoenix because of joint pain. The man stated that the tenderness in his joints prevented him from riding his horse for any extended period. He was born on a cattle ranch in New Mexico and spent most of his adult life working as a cattle driver in Arizona, New Mexico, and Colorado. He had always considered himself an "outdoors" kind of man. He loved the range, wide open spaces, clear air, and beauty of the desert.

In his early 20s he traveled to the East Coast to attend college. While there, he became withdrawn and depressed and felt confined. After 1 year he dropped out of college and returned to New Mexico. Shortly after returning home, his symptoms of depression disappeared. He worked on a large cattle ranch, made several new friends, and was content with the fact that he "belonged on the open range." He never married or settled down in one place he could call home. He often said that the great outdoors was his home. He never owned an automobile. In fact, he often said that the only things of real value he owned were a roan quarter horse and a saddle.

The hospital had no past medical record on the patient. The man reported, however, that although he was rarely ill, he had gone to see a doctor while in Colorado about a year ago for severe "cold" symptoms, which included fever, cough, chest pain, headaches, and a general feeling of fatigue. He was a nonsmoker, although he did chew tobacco for a short time in his teens. The patient verified that he consumed alcohol regularly on Friday and Saturday nights. The man estimated that on average he consumed between 6 and 10 beers per outing and sometimes more. Despite the patient's somewhat rugged living conditions and alcohol consumption, he was not overweight and was in reasonably good physical condition.

Physical Examination

The patient appeared to be a well-developed, well-nourished white man in moderate respiratory distress. He complained of soreness and stiffness in all his joints. He also stated that he thought he had a "bad cold" and that he was short of breath.

The patient's knees and ankle joints were warm, swollen, and tender to the touch. Although his skin appeared weathered and tan, his lips and nail beds were cyanotic. He demonstrated a frequent cough productive of a moderate amount of thick, yellow sputum. Although the cough was strong, he experienced difficulty raising sputum during each coughing episode. His vital signs were as follows: blood pressure 160/90, heart rate 90 bpm, respiratory rate 18/min, and oral temperature 37.8° C (100° F). Palpation revealed a few erythematous lesions on his anterior chest, of which he was unaware. In addition, a walnut-sized erythematous lesion was present on the patient's left cheek. Percussion of the chest was not remarkable. Auscultation revealed bilateral crackles and rhonchi in the lung apices.

The patient's chest x-ray film showed scattered infiltrates consistent with fibrosis and calcification and multiple spheric nodules throughout both lungs. In the upper lobes of both lungs, two to three small, 1- to 3-cm cavities were visible. On room air the patient's arterial blood gas values (ABGs) were as follows: pH 7.51, $Pa{CO_2}$ 29, HCO_3^- 22, and $Pa{O_2}$ 64 mm Hg. The patient was admitted to the hospital. Concerned about the patient's respiratory status, the physician requested a respiratory care consultation. On the basis of these clinical data, the following SOAP was documented.

Respiratory Assessment and Plan

S "I feel short of breath, and my joints are swollen and painful."

O Cyanosis; cough: frequent and strong, producing moderate amounts of thick, yellow sputum; vital signs: BP 160/90, HR 90, RR 18, T 37.8° C (100° F); palpation: red lesions on anterior chest and left cheek; auscultation: bilateral crackles and rhonchi in lung apices; CXR: bilateral fibrosis and calcification and spheric nodules; two to three 1- to 3-cm cavities in both upper lobes; ABGs (room air): pH 7.51, $Pa{CO_2}$ 29, HCO_3^- 22, $Pa{O_2}$ 64

A
- Moderate respiratory distress (cyanosis, vital signs)
- Large amounts of thick, yellow secretions (sputum, rhonchi)
- Infection likely (yellow sputum)
- Pulmonary fibrosis, calcification, and cavities (CXR)
- Acute alveolar hyperventilation with mild hypoxemia (ABGs)

P Initiate **Oxygen Therapy Protocol** (2 L/min per nasal cannula) and **Bronchopulmonary Hygiene Therapy Protocol** (C&DB instruction, PD to both upper lobes q shift × 3 days). Order sputum culture (routine, AFB, and fungal). Encourage fluid intake. Monitor (oximeter, I&O).

5 Days after Admission

After microscopy of the patient's sputum and a spherulin skin test, the diagnosis of coccidioidomycosis was written in the patient's chart. The patient had been receiving amphotericin B intravenously for 2 days. A complete pulmonary function study revealed a moderate-to-severe restrictive disorder, with a moderate obstructive component as well.

When the respiratory practitioner entered the patient's room, the man was sitting up in bed, appearing cyanotic, short of breath, and fatigued. He stated that he was becoming tired of people in white outfits coming in and out of his room, day and night, with "needles, pills, and bills." He further stated that he still could not get a good breath of air.

In fact, he said it was more difficult for him to breathe today than it had been on the day he entered the hospital.

The patient still had a frequent, strong cough productive of moderate amounts of thick, opaque sputum. His vital signs were as follows: blood pressure 165/95, heart rate 96 bpm, respiratory rate 24/min, and temperature 37° C (98.6° F). Auscultation revealed persistent bilateral tight wheezes, and bilateral crackles and rhonchi in the apices of both lungs. A current chest x-ray film was not available. His hemoglobin oxygen saturation measured by pulse oximetry (Spo_2) was 88%. His ABGs were as follows: pH 7.54, $Paco_2$ 27, HCO_3^- 21, and Pao_2 55. At this time, the following SOAP was charted.

Respiratory Assessment and Plan

S "I still can't get a good breath of air."

O Respiratory distress: cyanotic, short of breath; positive spherulin skin test; coccidioidomycosis organisms seen in sputum smear; frequent strong cough: moderate amount of thick, opaque sputum; vital signs: BP 165/95, HR 96, RR 24, T normal; bilateral crackles and rhonchi in the lung apices; Spo_2 88%; ABGs: pH 7.54, $Paco_2$ 27, HCO_3^- 21, Pao_2 55

A
- Coccidioidomycosis (positive spherulin skin test, sputum smear)
- Continued respiratory distress (cyanosis, vital signs)
- Excessive amounts of thick bronchial secretions (sputum, rhonchi)
- Acute alveolar hyperventilation with moderate hypoxemia (worsening ABGs)

P Up-regulate **Oxygen Therapy Protocol** (3 L/min nasal cannula). Add **Aerosolized Medication Protocol;** up-regulate **Bronchopulmonary Hygiene Therapy Protocol** (2 mL 10% acetylcysteine with 0.2 mL albuterol q6h followed by C&DB and PD to both upper lobes). Add supervised use of flutter valve 2 times per shift. Request repeat CXR. Continue to monitor and reevaluate.

10 Days after Admission

On this day, the respiratory therapist found the patient walking up and down the corridor talking to various staff members and patients. The man appeared to be in no respiratory distress. He stated that he was breathing much better and was ready to ride his horse a long distance in any direction away from the hospital.

No spontaneous cough was noted. When asked to generate a cough, the patient produced a strong, nonproductive cough. His vital signs were as follows: blood pressure 135/88, heart rate 80 bpm, respiratory rate 14/min, and normal temperature. Auscultation revealed persistent bilateral crackles in the apices of both lungs. A recent chest x-ray film was not available. His pulse oximetry on room air showed an Spo_2 of 91%. His ABGs were as follows: pH 7.44, $Paco_2$ 34, HCO_3^- 23, and Pao_2 71. On the basis of these clinical data, the following SOAP note was written.

Respiratory Assessment and Plan

S "I'm breathing much better."

O No obvious respiratory distress; no spontaneous cough; strong, nonproductive cough on request; vital signs: BP 135/88, HR 80, RR 14, T normal; bilateral crackles in the lung apices; Spo_2 91%; ABGs: pH 7.44, $Paco_2$ 34, HCO_3^- 23, Pao_2 71

A
- Adequate bronchial hygiene status (nonproductive cough, absence of rhonchi, crackles expected in lung fibrosis)
- Normal acid-base status with mild hypoxemia (ABGs)

P Discontinue **Oxygen Therapy Protocol.** Recheck Spo_2 on room air ("spot check") in 1 hour. Discontinue **Bronchopulmonary Hygiene Therapy Protocol.** Instruct patient in trial use of Combivent (albuterol/ipratropium) MDI. Reevaluate the patient when he is off all therapy modalities but on self-administered MDI in AM; then sign off.

Discussion

Respiratory care practitioners (RCPs) who work in the Southwest, where coccidioidomycosis is endemic, would probably anticipate this diagnosis in the patient with bilateral pulmonary infiltrates, swollen tender joints, and the skin rash typical of this lesion. Others could not be blamed if they missed this potential diagnosis until the coccidioidal skin test came back positive and the sputum fungal smear demonstrated the presence of the coccidioidomycosis organism. In this case, the patient demonstrated the clinical manifestations associated with the following two anatomic alterations of the lungs: **Increased Alveolar-Capillary Membrane Thickness** (e.g., bilateral fibrosis and calcification; see Figure 9-10) and **Excessive Bronchial Secretions** (e.g., cough, sputum, and rhonchi; see Figure 9-12).

The first assessment—that the patient is hypoxemic despite alveolar hyperventilation and that he has alveolar fibrosis and cavity formation—is correct. For the hypoxemia, oxygen therapy is appropriate and should be started with a nasal oxygen cannula at 1 to 2 L/min and then regulated with a pulse oximeter. In treating this patient, as with any other pneumonia, the assessing RCP should quickly obtain sputum, Gram stain, and acid-fast bacillus and fungal preparations; this step was appropriately done in this case. The treating RCP would do well to understand the use of tuberculin and fungal testing in such patients and to understand that, as with other pneumonic infiltrates, the therapist's impact once such testing was done would probably be minimal.

In the second assessment, the offending organism has been isolated and appropriate therapy with intravenous amphotericin B started. The patient is still hypoxemic, and up-regulation of his **Oxygen Therapy Protocal** (perhaps to 3 or 4 L/min, or with a nonrebreathing mask if the former is unsuccessful) is indicated. Because the patient is still wheezing and coughing up thick, opaque sputum and because his dyspnea is not relieved so far, up-regulation of the **Bronchopulmonary Hygiene Therapy Protocol** and addition of the **Aerosolized Medication Protocol** with a trial of bronchodilator therapy and mucolytic therapy are in order. Because the patient is not improving, a repeat chest x-ray examination appears to be indicated.

At the last assessment 10 days after the patient's admission to the hospital, clear improvement is noted. Oximetry reveals good peripheral oxygen saturation, and the blood gases are much improved. Now is the time for the treating therapist to reduce the intensity of the patient's respiratory care, and this step is illustrated in the appropriate response for this section of the case study. Follow-up pulmonary function testing 6 to 12 months after the abatement of acute illness would be worthwhile.

SELF-ASSESSMENT QUESTIONS

evolve Answers to questions can be found on Evolve. To access additional student assessment questions and case studies for application of text material to real-life scenarios, visit **http://evolve.elsevier.com/DesJardins/respiratory.**

1. Which of the following is the most common fungal infection in the United States?
   a. Coccidioidomycosis
   b. Histoplasmosis
   c. San Joaquin Valley disease
   d. Blastomycosis

2. Incidence of histoplasmosis is especially high in which of the following area(s)?
   1. Arizona
   2. Mississippi
   3. Nevada
   4. Texas
      a. 2 only
      b. 4 only
      c. 2 and 4 only
      d. 2 and 3 only

3. The condition called *desert bumps, desert arthritis,* or *desert rheumatism* is associated with which fungal disorder?
   a. Ohio Valley fever
   b. Blastomycosis
   c. Coccidioidomycosis
   d. Aspergillosis

4. Which of the following is or are used to treat fungal diseases?
   1. Streptomycin
   2. Amphotericin B
   3. Penicillin G
   4. Itraconazole
      a. 1 only
      b. 2 only
      c. 4 only
      d. 2 and 4 only

5. Which of the following forms of histoplasmosis is characterized by healed lesions in the hilar lymph nodes as well as a positive histoplasmin skin test response?
   a. Disseminated infection
   b. Latent asymptomatic disease
   c. Chronic histoplasmosis
   d. Self-limiting primary disease

PART IV

Pulmonary Vascular Diseases

Pulmonary Edema 19

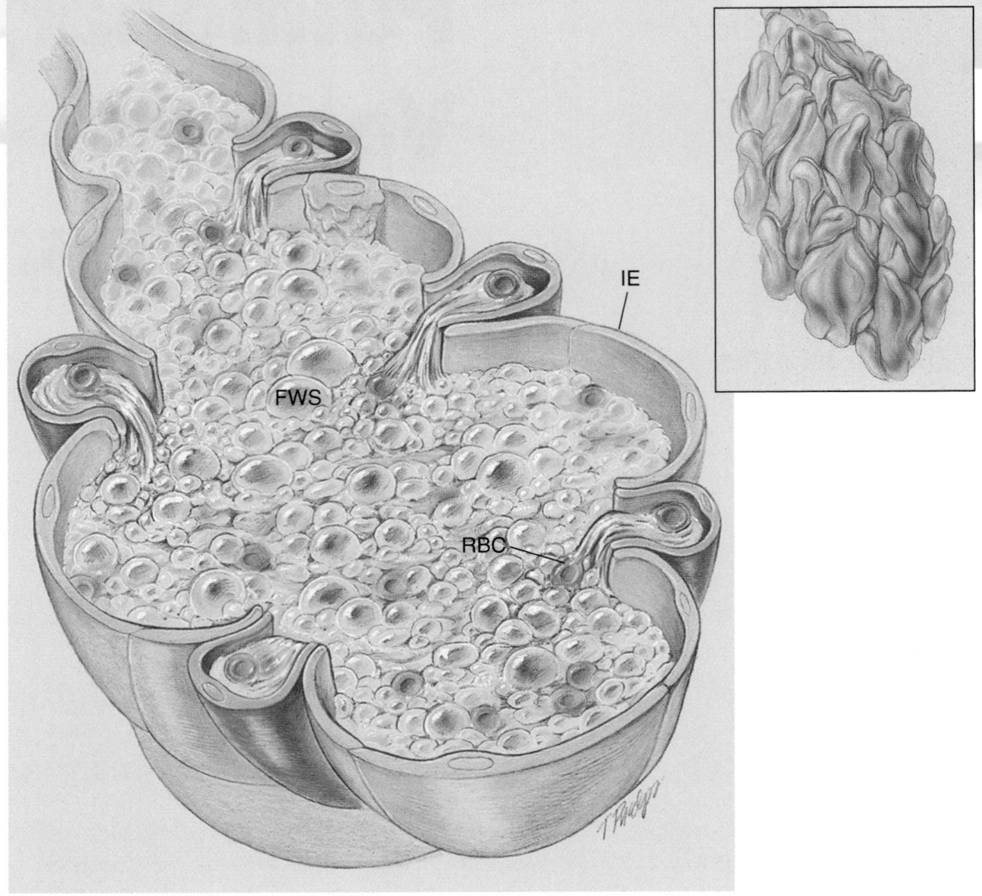

FIGURE 19-1 Pulmonary edema. Cross-sectional view of alveoli and alveolar duct in pulmonary edema. *FWS,* Frothy white secretions; *IE,* interstitial edema; *RBC,* red blood cell. *Inset,* Atelectasis, a common secondary anatomic alteration of the lungs.

Chapter Objectives

After reading this chapter, you will be able to:

- List the anatomic alterations of the lungs associated with pulmonary edema.
- Describe the causes of pulmonary edema.
- List the cardiopulmonary clinical manifestations associated with pulmonary edema.
- Describe the general management of pulmonary edema.
- Describe the clinical strategies and rationales of the SOAPs presented in the case study.
- Define key terms and complete self-assessment questions at the end of the chapter and on Evolve.

Key Terms

Afterload Reduction
Albumin
Amiodarone
Angiotension-Converting Enzyme (ACE) Inhibitors
Antidysrhythmic Agents
Bat's Wing x-ray Appearance
Bretylium
Butterfly Pattern
Calcium Channel Blockers
Captopril
Cardiogenic Pulmonary Edema
Congestive Heart Failure (CHF)
Decompression Pulmonary Edema
Digitalis
Direct-Acting Vasodilators
Dobutamine
Dopamine
Hydralazine
Increased Capillary Permeability
Indirect-Acting Vasodilators
Isosorbide
Kerley A and B Lines

Lisinopril
Mannitol
Mask CPAP
Metoprolol
Minoxidil
Morphine Sulfate
Nifedipine
Nitroglycerin
Nitroprusside
Noncardiogenic Pulmonary Edema
Oncotic Pressure
Orthopnea
Paroxysmal Nocturnal Dyspnea (PND)
Positive Inotropic Agents
Prazosin
Procainamide
Starling's Equation
Transudate
Trimazosin
Verapamil

Chapter Outline

Anatomic Alterations of the Lungs

Pulmonary edema results from excessive movement of fluid from the pulmonary vascular system to the extravascular system and air spaces of the lungs. Fluid first seeps into the perivascular and peribronchial interstitial spaces; depending on the degree of severity, fluid may progressively move into the alveoli, bronchioles, and bronchi (see Figure 19-1).

As a consequence of this fluid movement, the alveolar walls and interstitial spaces swell. As the swelling intensifies, the alveolar surface tension increases and causes alveolar shrinkage and atelectasis. Moreover, much of the fluid that accumulates in the tracheobronchial tree is churned into a frothy white (sometimes blood-tinged or pink) sputum as a result of air moving in and out of the lungs. The abundance of fluid in the interstitial spaces causes the lymphatic vessels to widen and the lymph flow to increase.

Pulmonary edema is a restrictive pulmonary disorder. The major pathologic or structural changes of the lungs associated with pulmonary edema are as follows:

- Interstitial edema, including fluid engorgement of the perivascular and peribronchial spaces and the alveolar wall interstitium
- Alveolar flooding
- Increased surface tension of alveolar fluids
- Alveolar shrinkage and atelectasis
- Frothy white (or pink) secretions throughout the tracheobronchial tree

Etiology and Epidemiology

The causes of pulmonary edema can be divided into two major categories: cardiogenic and noncardiogenic.

Cardiogenic Pulmonary Edema

The most common cause of cardiac pulmonary edema is left-sided heart failure—commonly called **congestive heart failure (CHF).** According to the Centers for Disease Control and Prevention (CDC), about 5 million people in the United States have CHF—or about 1.7% of the overall population. Approximately 550,000 new cases of CHF are diagnosed annually. Heart failure is most common in people over age 65 and is more common in African-Americans. CHF is a leading cause of hospitalization in people over the age of 65 and is estimated to be a contributing factor to nearly 300,000 deaths annually. In 2008 the estimated annual direct and indirect costs associated with heart failure totaled nearly 35 billion dollars. As the median age of the U.S. population of "baby boomers" continues to grow older—between the present and 2040—the number of patients diagnosed with CHF, along with the direct and indirect costs associated with CHF, will undoubtedly continue to rise.

Cardiac pulmonary edema occurs when the left ventricle is not able to pump out all of the blood that it receives from the lungs. As a result, the blood pressure inside the pulmonary veins and capillaries increases. This action literally causes fluid to be pushed through the capillary walls and into the alveoli in the form of a **transudate.** The basic pathophysiologic mechanism for this action is described in the following sections.

Ordinarily, hydrostatic pressure of about 10 to 15 mm Hg tends to move fluid *out* of the pulmonary capillaries into the interstitial space. This force is normally offset by colloid osmotic forces of about 25 to 30 mm Hg that tend to keep fluid *in* the pulmonary capillaries. The colloid osmotic pressure is referred to as **oncotic pressure** and is produced by the **albumin** and globulin in the blood. The stability of fluid within the pulmonary capillaries is determined by the balance between hydrostatic and oncotic pressure. This relationship also maintains fluid stability in the interstitial compartments of the lung.

Movement of fluid in and out of the capillaries is expressed by **Starling's equation:**

$$J = K\,(Pc - Pi) - (\pi c - \pi i)$$

where J is the net fluid movement out of the capillary, K is the capillary permeability factor, Pc and Pi are the hydrostatic pressures in the capillary and interstitial space, and πc and πi are the oncotic pressures in the capillary and interstitial space.

Although conceptually valuable, this equation has limited practical use. Of the four pressures, only the oncotic and hydrostatic pressures of blood in the pulmonary capillaries can be measured with any certainty. The oncotic and hydrostatic pressures within the interstitial compartments cannot be readily determined.

When the hydrostatic pressure within the pulmonary vascular system rises to more than 25 to 30 mm Hg, the oncotic pressure loses its holding force over the fluid within the pulmonary capillaries. Consequently fluid starts to spill into the interstitial and air spaces of the lungs (see Figure 19-1).

Clinically, the patient with left ventricular failure often has anxiety, delirium, dyspnea, orthopnea, paroxysmal nocturnal dyspnea, cough, fatigue, and adventitious breath sounds. Because of poor peripheral circulation, such patients often have cool skin, diaphoresis, cyanosis of the digits, and peripheral pallor. Increased pulmonary capillary hydrostatic pressure is the most common cause of pulmonary edema. Box 19-1 provides common causes of **cardiogenic pulmonary edema.** Box 19-2 provides common risk factors for coronary heart disease (CHD).

Box 19-1 Common Causes of Cardiogenic Pulmonary Edema

- Arrhythmias (e.g., premature ventricular contractions or bradycardia producing low cardiac output)
- Systemic hypertension
- Congenital heart defects
- Excessive fluid administration
- Left ventricular failure
- Mitral or aortic valve disease
- Myocardial infarction
- Cardiac Tamponade
- Pulmonary embolus
- Renal failure
- Rheumatic heart disease (myocarditis)
- Cardiomyopathies (e.g., viral)

Box 19-2 Risk Factors for Coronary Heart Disease (CHD)

- Age
  Male >45 years old
  Female >55 years old
- Family history of CHD
  Male relative: <55 years old
  Female relative: <65 years old
- Cigarette smoker
- Overweight
- Hypertension: (blood pressure >140/90 mm Hg or on antihypertensive agents)
- High level of low-density–lipoprotein cholesterol (LDL-C): >130 mg/dL ("bad cholesterol")
- Low level of high-density–lipoprotein cholesterol (HDL-C): <35 mg/dL ("good cholesterol")
- High level of homocysteine: >10 mg/dL
- High total cholesterol level (>150-200 mg/dL) and high triglyceride level (>200-300 mg/dL)
- Diabetes mellitus (type 1 and type 2)

Noncardiogenic Pulmonary Edema

There are numerous noncardiogenic causes of pulmonary edema. In these conditions, fluid can readily flow from the pulmonary capillaries into the alveoli—even in the absence of the back pressure caused by an abnormal heart. The more common conditions include those discussed in the following paragraphs.

Increased Capillary Permeability

Pulmonary edema may develop as a result of **increased capillary permeability** stemming from infectious, inflammatory, and other processes. The following are some causes of increased capillary permeability:

- Alveolar hypoxia
- Acute respiratory distress syndrome (ARDS)
- Inhalation of toxic agents such as chlorine, sulfur dioxide, nitrogen dioxides, ammonia, and phosgene
- Pulmonary infections (e.g., pneumonia)
- Therapeutic radiation of the lungs
- Acute head injury (also known as *cephalogenic pulmonary edema*)

Lymphatic Insufficiency

Should the lungs' normal lymphatic drainage be decreased, intravascular and extravascular fluid begins to pool, and pulmonary edema ensues. Lymphatic drainage may be slowed because of obliteration or distortion of lymphatic vessels. The lymphatic vessels may be obstructed by tumor cells in lymphangitic carcinomatosis. Because the lymphatic vessels empty into systemic veins, increased systemic venous pressure may slow lymphatic drainage. Lymphatic insufficiency also has been observed after lung transplantation.

Decreased Intrapleural Pressure

Reduced intrapleural pressure may cause pulmonary edema. With severe airway obstruction, for example, the negative pressure exerted by the patient during inspiration may create a suction effect on the pulmonary capillaries and cause fluid to move into the alveoli. Furthermore, the increased negative intrapleural pressure promotes filling of the right side of the heart and hinders blood flow in the left side of the heart. This condition may cause pooling of the blood in the lungs and subsequently an elevated hydrostatic pressure and pulmonary edema. A related kind of pulmonary edema is caused by the sudden removal of a pleural effusion. Clinically this condition is called **decompression pulmonary edema.**

Decreased Oncotic Pressure

Although this condition is rare, if the oncotic pressure is reduced from its normal 25 to 30 mm Hg and falls below the patient's normal hydrostatic pressure of 10 to 15 mm Hg, fluid may begin to seep into the interstitial and air spaces of the lungs. Decreased oncotic pressure may be caused by the following:

Box 19-3 Other Causes of Noncardiogenic Pulmonary Edema

- Allergic reaction to drugs
- Excessive sodium consumption
- Drug overdose (e.g., heroin, aspirin, amphetamines, cocaine, antituberculosis agents, cancer chemotherapy agents)
- Metal poisoning (e.g., cobalt, iron, lead)
- Chronic alcohol ingestion
- Aspiration (e.g., near drowning)
- Central nervous system stimulation
- Encephalitis
- High altitudes (greater than 8,000 to 10,000 feet)

- Overtransfusion and/or rapid transfusion of intravenous fluids
- Uremia
- Hypoproteinemia (e.g., severe malnutrition)
- Acute nephritis
- Polyarteritis nodosa

Although the exact mechanisms are not known, Box 19-3 provides other causes of conditions associated with **noncardiogenic pulmonary edema.**

OVERVIEW of the Cardiopulmonary Clinical Manifestations Associated with Pulmonary Edema

The following clinical manifestations result from the pathologic mechanisms caused (or activated) by **Atelectasis** (see Figure 9-8), **Increased Alveolar-Capillary Membrane Thickness** (see Figure 9-10), and, in severe cases, **Excessive Bronchial Secretions** (see Figure 9-12)—the major anatomic alterations of the lungs associated with pulmonary edema (see Figure 19-1).

CLINICAL DATA OBTAINED AT THE PATIENT'S BEDSIDE

The Physical Examination

Vital Signs

Increased Respiratory Rate (Tachypnea)

Several pathophysiologic mechanisms operating simultaneously may lead to an increased ventilatory rate:

- Stimulation of peripheral chemoreceptors (hypoxemia)
- Decreased lung compliance–increased ventilatory rate relationship
- Stimulation of J receptors
- Anxiety

Increased Heart Rate (Pulse) and Blood Pressure

Cheyne-Stokes Respiration

Cheyne-Stokes respiration may be seen in patients with severe left-sided heart failure and pulmonary edema. Some authorities have suggested that the cause of Cheyne-Stokes respiration in these patients may be related to the prolonged circulation time between the lungs and the central chemoreceptors. Cheyne-Stokes respiration is a classic clinical manifestation in central sleep apnea (see Chapter 30).

Paroxysmal Nocturnal Dyspnea (PND) and Orthopnea

Patients with pulmonary edema often awaken with severe dyspnea after several hours of sleep. This condition is called paroxysmal nocturnal dyspnea. This condition is particularly prevalent in patients with cardiogenic pulmonary edema. While the patient is awake, more time is spent in the erect position and, as a result, excess fluids tend to accumulate in the dependent portions of the body. When the patient lies down, however, the excess fluids from the dependent parts of the body move into the bloodstream and cause an increase in venous return to the lungs. This action raises the pulmonary hydrostatic pressure and promotes pulmonary edema. The pulmonary edema in turn produces pulmonary shunting, venous admixture, and hypoxemia. When the hypoxemia becomes severe, the peripheral chemoreceptors are stimulated and initiate an increased ventilatory rate (see Figure 4-4). The decreased lung compliance, J receptor stimulation, and anxiety also may contribute to the paroxysmal nocturnal dyspnea commonly seen in this disorder at night. A patient is said to have **orthopnea** when dyspnea increases while the patient is in a recumbent position.

Cyanosis

Cough and Sputum (Frothy and Pink in Appearance)

Chest Assessment Findings

- Increased tactile and vocal fremitus
- Crackles, rhonchi, and wheezing

CLINICAL DATA OBTAINED FROM LABORATORY TESTS AND SPECIAL PROCEDURES

Pulmonary Function Test Findings (Moderate to Severe) (Restrictive Lung Pathology)

FORCED EXPIRATORY FLOW RATE FINDINGS

FVC	FEV_T	FEV_1/FVC ratio	$FEF_{25\%-75\%}$
↓	N or ↓	N or ↑	N or ↓
$FEF_{50\%}$	$FEF_{200-1200}$	PEFR	MVV
N or ↓	N or ↓	N or ↓	N or ↓

OVERVIEW of the Cardiopulmonary Clinical Manifestations Associated with Pulmonary Edema—cont'd

LUNG VOLUME AND CAPACITY FINDINGS

V_T	IRV	ERV	RV	
N or ↓	↓	↓	↓	
VC	IC	FRC	TLC	RV/TLC ratio
↓	↓	↓	↓	N

Arterial Blood Gases

MILD TO MODERATE PULMONARY EDEMA

Acute Alveolar Hyperventilation with Hypoxemia

(Acute Respiratory Alkalosis)

pH	Pa_{CO_2}	HCO_3^-	Pa_{O_2}
↑	↓	↓ (slightly)	↓

SEVERE STAGE PULMONARY EDEMA

Acute Ventilatory Failure with Hypoxemia

(Acute Respiratory Acidosis)

pH*	Pa_{CO_2}	HCO_3^- *	Pa_{O_2}
↓	↑	↑ (slightly)	↓

*When tissue hypoxia is severe enough to produce lactic acid, the pH and HCO_3^- values will be lower than expected for a particular Pa_{CO_2} level.

Oxygenation Indices*

$\dot{Q}_S/\dot{Q}_T$	D_{O_2}†	$\dot{V}_{O_2}$	$C(a-\bar{v})_{O_2}$	O_2ER	$S\bar{v}_{O_2}$
↑	↓	N	N	↑	↓

†The D_{O_2} may be normal in patients who have compensated to the decreased oxygenation status with (1) an increased cardiac output, (2) an increased hemoglobin level, or (3) a combination of both. When the D_{O_2} is normal, the O_2ER is usually normal.

Hemodynamic Indices‡

Cardiogenic Pulmonary Edema Moderate to Severe Stages

CVP	RAP	$\overline{PA}$	PCWP	CO	SV
↑	↑	↑	↑	↓	↓
SVI	CI	RVSWI	LVSWI	PVR	SVR
↓	↓	↑	↓	↑	↑

ABNORMAL LABORATORY TEST AND PROCEDURE RESULTS

- Serum chloride: low
- Serum potassium: low
- Serum sodium: low

Hypokalemia, hyponatremia and hypochloremia are often seen in patients with left-sided heart failure and may result from diuretic therapy or excessive fluid retention.

*$C(a-\bar{v})_{O_2}$, Arterial-venous oxygen difference; D_{O_2}, total oxygen delivery; O_2ER, oxygen extraction ratio; $\dot{Q}_S/\dot{Q}_T$, pulmonary shunt fraction; $S\bar{v}_{O_2}$, mixed venous oxygen saturation; $\dot{V}_{O_2}$, oxygen consumption.

‡*CO,* Cardiac output; *CVP,* central venous pressure; *LVSWI,* left ventricular stroke work index; *$\overline{PA}$,* mean pulmonary artery pressure; *PCWP,* pulmonary capillary wedge pressure; *PVR,* pulmonary vascular resistance; *RAP,* right atrial pressure; *RVSWI,* right ventricular stroke work index; *SV,* stroke volume; *SVI,* stroke volume index; *SVR,* systemic vascular resistance.

RADIOLOGIC FINDINGS

Chest Radiograph

- Bilateral fluffy opacities
- Dilated pulmonary arteries
- Left ventricular hypertrophy (cardiomegaly)
- Kerley A and B lines
- Bat's wing or butterfly pattern
- Pleural effusion

Cardiogenic Pulmonary Edema

The radiographic findings associated with left heart failure are commonly described as follows:

- Mild left-sided heart failure: Pulmonary venous congestion with dilated pulmonary arteries is present.
- Moderate left-sided heart failure: Cardiomegaly, engorgement of the pulmonary arteries, and **Kerley A** and **Kerley B** lines are present. When cardiomegaly is present, the heart is greater than half the diameter of the thorax in a posterior-anterior chest radiograph (Figure 19-2). Because radiographic densities primarily reflect alveolar filling and not early interstitial edema, by the time abnormal findings are encountered, the pathologic changes associated with pulmonary edema are advanced. Chest x-ray films typically reveal dense, fluffy opacities that spread outward from the hilar areas to the peripheral borders of the lungs (Figure 19-2).

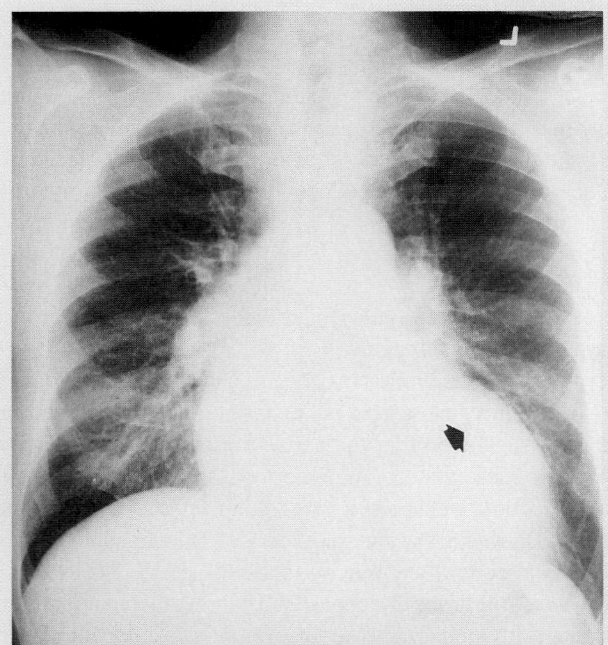

FIGURE 19-2 Cardiomegaly *(arrow)*, hilar prominence, and pulmonary edema in congestive heart failure. Note that the heart diameter is greater than half the diameter of the thorax.

OVERVIEW of the Cardiopulmonary Clinical Manifestations Associated with Pulmonary Edema—cont'd

Kerley A lines, which represent deep interstitial edema, radiate out from the hilum into the central portions of the lungs. Kerley A lines do not reach the pleura and are most prevalent in the middle and upper lung regions. **Kerley B lines** are short, thin, horizontal lines of interstitial edema, usually less than 1 cm in length, that extend inward from the pleural surface. They appear peripherally in contact with the pleura and are parallel to one another at right angles to the pleura. Although they may be seen in any lung region, they are most commonly seen in the lung bases (Figure 19-3).

- Severe left-sided heart failure: During this stage, the patient's chest radiograph shows cardiomegaly; pulmonary artery engorgement; interstitial pulmonary edema; fluffy, patchy areas of alveolar edema; and often the appearance of the **bat's wing pattern** (also called the butterfly pattern)—the peripheral portion of the lungs often remains clear, and this produces what is described as a "butterfly" or "bat's wing" distribution (Figure 19-4). Pleural effusion may also be seen.

Noncardiogenic Pulmonary Edema

In noncardiogenic pulmonary edema the chest radiograph commonly shows areas of fluffy densities that are usually more dense near the hilum. The density may be unilateral or bilateral. Pleural effusion is usually not present, and (most important) the cardiac silhouette is not enlarged.

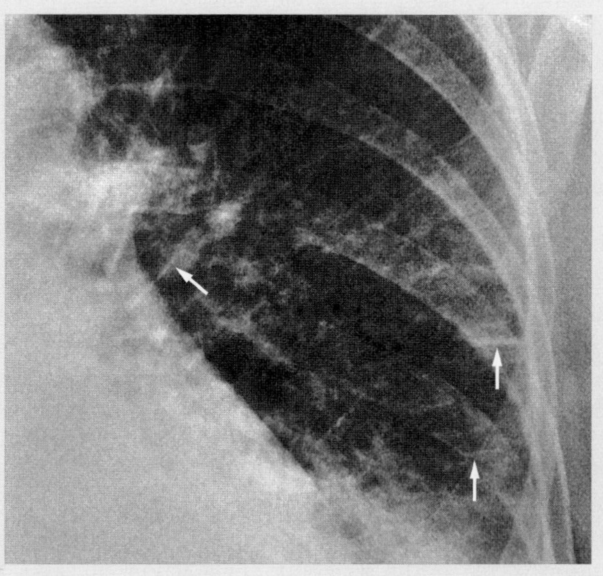

FIGURE 19-3 Kerley lines. Septal lines caused by pulmonary edema. Kerley B lines are short horizontal lines at the lung periphery *(vertical arrows)*. Kerley A lines are lines radiating from the hila *(oblique arrow)*. (From Hansell DM, Armstrong P, Lynch DA, McAdams HP, eds: *Imaging of diseases of the chest,* ed 4, Philadelphia, 2005, Elsevier.)

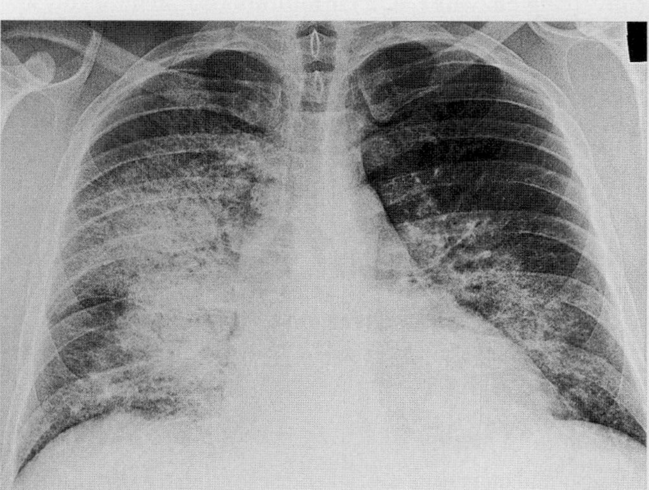

FIGURE 19-4 Bat's wing or butterfly pattern caused by pulmonary edema. This example is typical in that it is bilateral but not symmetrical. The shadowing is maximal in the central (perihilar) portions of the lung, and the outer portions of the lungs are relatively clear. (From Hansell DM, Armstrong P, Lynch DA, McAdams HP, eds: *Imaging of diseases of the chest,* ed 4, Philadelphia, 2005, Elsevier.)

General Management of Pulmonary Edema

The treatment of pulmonary edema is based on knowledge of the underlying cause. Common therapeutic interventions are discussed in the following sections.

Medications and Procedures Commonly Prescribed by the Physician

Antidysrhythmic Agents

Because cardiac dysrhythmias can cause or exacerbate left ventricular heart failure, drugs to control bradycardia (e.g., atropine) or tachycardia (e.g., **procainamide, metoprolol,** or **bretylium**) **(antidysrhythmic agents)** may be administered.

Positive Inotropic Agents (Improve Cardiac Output)

When left-sided heart failure is present, **positive inotropic agents** (e.g., **digitalis, dopamine, dobutamine,** and **amiodarone**) are commonly administered to increase cardiac output. Digitalis is the most frequently prescribed inotropic agent for heart failure and is the drug of choice (see Appendix II, Positive Inotropic Agents).

Cardiac Workload Reduction (Afterload Reduction)

The most effective way to decrease the cardiac workload is to reduce the cardiac afterload **(afterload reduction).** This is primarily achieved by patient lifestyle changes and use of medications. In general, important lifestyle changes include getting exercise, lowering stress, losing weight if necessary, and consuming a low-salt diet. In some cases, bed rest and sedation may be helpful in reducing anxiety and agitation. Medications used to reduce systemic hypertension—and therefore to reduce the cardiac afterload—include **direct-acting vasodilators** (e.g., **nitroglycerin, nitroprusside, isosorbide, hydralazine,** and **minoxidil**).

Indirect-acting vasodilators are also be used to reduce the left ventricular afterload. Such agents include the alpha-adrenergic receptor–blocking agents (e.g., **prazosin, trimazosin**), which block the vasoconstrictive effects of norepinephrine. Vasodilation and afterload reduction are also achieved with the administration of **angiotension-converting enzyme (ACE) inhibitors** (e.g., **lisinopril, captopril**) or **calcium channel blockers** (e.g., **verapamil, nifedipine**). **Morphine sulfate** is used to reduce afterload by inducing venodilation and venous pooling. It also is used for sedation and relief of anxiety.

Sodium and Fluid Retention Therapy

Common methods used to reduce sodium and fluid retention include the following: (1) bed rest in the supine position, which enhances natural diuresis by the kidneys (sitting in the upright position reduces sodium and water excretion and therefore should be avoided), (2) restriction of sodium and water intake, and (3) high-dose diuretic therapy.

Albumin and Mannitol

Albumin or **mannitol** is sometimes administered to increase the patient's oncotic pressure in an effort to offset the increased hydrostatic forces of cardiogenic pulmonary edema, if the patient's osmotic pressure is low.

Respiratory Care Treatment Protocols

Oxygen Therapy Protocol

Oxygen therapy is used to treat hypoxemia, decrease the work of breathing, and decrease myocardial work. The hypoxemia that develops in pulmonary edema is most commonly caused by the interstitial and alveolar fluid, atelectasis, and capillary shunting associated with the disorder. Hypoxemia caused by capillary shunting is at least partially refractory to oxygen therapy (see Oxygen Therapy Protocol, Protocol 9-1).

Bronchopulmonary Hygiene Therapy Protocol

Because of the excessive frothy white secretions associated with pulmonary edema, bronchial hygiene treatment modalities may be used to enhance the mobilization of bronchial secretions (see Bronchopulmonary Hygiene Therapy Protocol, Protocol 9-2).

Lung Expansion Therapy Protocol

Lung expansion therapy is commonly prescribed to offset the fluid accumulation and alveolar shrinkage associated with pulmonary edema. For example, high-flow mask continuous positive airway pressure (CPAP) has been shown to produce a significant and rapid improvement in oxygenation and ventilatory status in patients with pulmonary edema. **Mask CPAP** improves decreased lung compliance, decreases the work of breathing, enhances gas exchange, and decreases vascular congestion in patients with pulmonary edema. In fact, mask CPAP is prescribed (at least for a trial period) for patients with pulmonary edema who have arterial blood gas values that reveal impending or acute ventilatory failure—the hallmark clinical manifestation for mechanical ventilation. Often, mask CPAP dramatically improves oxygenation and ventilatory status in these patients and eliminates the need for mechanical ventilation (see Lung Expansion Therapy Protocol, Protocol 9-3).

Aerosolized Medication Protocol

Both sympathomimetic and parasympatholytic agents are commonly used to induce bronchial smooth muscle relaxation (see Aerosolized Medication Protocol, Protocol 9-4 and Appendix II). They often are not effective in this disorder, however.

Alcohol (Ethanol, Ethyl Alcohol)

Because alcohol is a specific surface-active agent, it may be aerosolized into the patient's lungs to lower the surface tension of the frothy secretions. This action enhances the mobilization of secretions. Generally, 5 to 15 mL of 30% to 50% alcohol solution is administered. Such therapy is rarely used today.

Decreasing Hydrostatic Pressure

In an effort to lower hydrostatic pressure, the physician may order the following:

- Positioning the patient in Fowler's position (sitting up)
- Rotating tourniquets (rarely used)
- Phlebotomy (rarely used)

CASE STUDY

Pulmonary Edema

Admitting History and Physical Examination

This 76-year-old man was admitted to the emergency room in obvious respiratory distress. His wife reported that her husband had gone to bed feeling well. He woke up with chest pain at about 2:30 AM, very short of breath. She became concerned and called an ambulance. Neither the patient nor the wife were good historians, but they did report that the patient had been under a physician's care for some time for "heart trouble" and that he was taking "little white pills" on a daily basis. For the previous 3 days, he had not taken any medication.

On admission to the emergency room, the patient was mildly disoriented and slightly cyanotic. He repeatedly tried to take the oxygen mask from his face. He complained of a feeling of suffocation. His neck veins were distended, and the skin of his extremities was mottled. On auscultation, there were coarse rhonchi and crackles in both lower lung fields and some crackles in the middle and upper lung fields.

His cough was productive of pinkish, frothy sputum. His vital signs were as follows: blood pressure 105/50, heart rate 124/min, and respiratory rate 28/min. He was afebrile. ECG showed evidence of an old infarct, sinus tachycardia, and an occasional premature ventricular contraction. X-ray films taken in the emergency room with the patient in a sitting position revealed bilateral fluffy infiltrates, more marked in the lower lung fields. The heart was enlarged. All other laboratory findings were within normal limits. Blood gases on an F_{IO_2} of 0.30 were pH 7.11, Pa_{CO_2} 72, HCO_3^- 27, and Pa_{O_2} 56. His oxygen saturation by oximetry (Sp_{O_2}) was 87%. The respiratory therapist working in the emergency room during the night shift recorded the following SOAP note.

Respiratory Assessment and Plan

S Patient states "a feeling of suffocation."

O Cyanosis, disorientation. Distended neck veins and mottled extremities. BP 105/50, HR 124, RR 28. ECG: sinus tach and occasional PVCs. Distended neck veins, mottled extremities, coarse rhonchi and crackles bilaterally. Frothy pink sputum. CXR: Bilateral fluffy infiltrates and an enlarged heart. ABG: pH 7.11, Pa_{CO_2} 72, HCO_3^- 25, and Pa_{O_2} 56 (F_{IO_2} 0.30). Sp_{O_2} 87%.

A
- Acute pulmonary edema (CXR)
- Acute ventilatory failure with moderate hypoxemia (ABG)
- Large and small airway secretions (rhonchi and crackles)

P **Oxygen Therapy Protocol:** Increase F_{IO_2} to 0.60 via continuous CPAP mask at 25 cm H_2O per **Lung Expansion Therapy Protocol.** Remain on standby for emergency endotracheal intubation and ventilator support. Continue ECG and oximetry monitoring, and repeat ABG in 30 minutes.

The patient was admitted on the cardiology service with a diagnosis of pulmonary edema–CHF. ECG monitoring and continuous oximetry were followed. Treatment consisted of intravenous furosemide, dopamine, and nitroprusside, as well as mask CPAP at 25 cm H_2O pressure with an F_{IO_2} of 0.6. A Foley catheter was placed.

Two hours later, the patient's condition was very much improved, and he was no longer cyanotic. Vital signs were as follows: blood pressure 126/70, heart rate 96/min, and respiratory rate 18/min. ECG revealed mild sinus tachycardia and no ectopic beats. Auscultation showed considerable improvement. There were still some basilar crackles, but the upper lung fields were clear. Cough was much reduced and no longer productive. Repeat chest x-ray examination at the bedside showed considerable improvement. Urine output was in excess of 600 mL/hr. The patient was calm and rational, stating that he was less short of breath and had no pain. Repeat arterial blood gases revealed pH 7.35, Pa_{CO_2} 46, HCO_3^- 24, and Pa_{O_2} 120 on an F_{IO_2} of 0.50. The following respiratory therapy SOAP note was made at the time.

Respiratory Assessment and Plan

S Patient states, "I'm less short of breath. No pain."

O Not cyanotic. BP 126/70, HR 96, RR 18. ECG: Mild sinus tachycardia without ectopic beats. Fewer crackles; no sputum production; CXR: Improved. ABG: pH 7.35, Pa_{CO_2} 46, HCO_3^- 24, Pa_{O_2} 120 (F_{IO_2} 0.50).

A
- Decreased pulmonary edema (overall impression from the data)
- No longer in ventilatory failure (ABG)
- Acceptable acid-base status with excessively corrected hypoxemia (ABG)
- Secretions controlled (no sputum and fewer crackles)

P Reduce O_2 per **Oxygen Therapy Protocol** to 2 L/min by nasal cannula. Discontinue CPAP per **Lung Expansion Therapy Protocol.** Continue ECG and oximetric monitoring. Repeat ABG in 60 minutes.

Discussion

Acute pulmonary edema is a classic finding in CHF. Several clinical manifestations associated with **Increased Alveolar-Capillary Membrane Thickness** (see Figure 9-10) were present in this case. For example, the patient's decreased lung compliance was manifested in his tachycardia and tachypnea, whereas his hypoxemia reflected diffusion blockade associated with classic pulmonary edema. His lung compliance was so reduced that he had progressed to acute ventilatory failure—the severe stage of pulmonary edema. Some **Atelectasis** (see Figure 9-8) was doubtless also present and was the rationale for CPAP therapy. In addition, the clinical scenario associated with **Excessive Bronchial Secretions** (see Figure

9-12) also was evident initially with frothy blood-tinged sputum and coarse rhonchi and crackles in both lower lung fields. The patient was too ill to allow valid pulmonary function testing, but the suspicion is that a combined obstructive and restrictive pattern may have been present at the time of the first assessment.

The **Aerosolized Medication Protocol** and **Bronchopulmonary Hygiene Therapy Protocol** were not used in this case. Often, the first-line management of pulmonary edema consists only of improving myocardial efficiency, decreasing the cardiovascular afterload, decreasing the hypervolemia, providing CPAP, and improving oxygenation. Furosemide (Lasix) is a potent loop diuretic, dopamine has direct inotropic effects, and nitroprusside is a potent peripheral vasodilator. The combination of these drugs, along with CPAP and oxygen therapy, resulted in marked improvement of the patient's myocardial activity and a rapid change in the clinical picture.

In short, this patient had an acute respiratory problem, but the basic cause was cardiac. After the cardiac condition was treated, the respiratory symptoms rapidly disappeared. CPAP and an increased F_{IO_2} were adequate, and this patient was spared the trauma and risk associated with intubation and mechanical ventilation. No evidence of acute myocardial infarction was found. He was discharged after 48 hours, his condition much improved. He was instructed to take his cardiac medication and diuretics without fail and to return to his family physician in 3 days.

SELF-ASSESSMENT QUESTIONS

evolve Answers to questions can be found on Evolve. To access additional student assessment questions and case studies for application of text material to real-life scenarios, visit **http://evolve.elsevier.com/DesJardins/respiratory.**

1. In pulmonary edema, fluid first moves into the:
1. Alveoli
2. Perivascular interstitial space
3. Bronchioles
4. Peribronchial interstitial space
   a. 2 only
   b. 3 only
   c. 1 and 3 only
   d. 2 and 4 only

2. What is the normal hydrostatic pressure in the pulmonary capillaries?
   a. 5 to 10 mm Hg
   b. 10 to 15 mm Hg
   c. 15 to 20 mm Hg
   d. 20 to 25 mm Hg

3. What is the normal oncotic pressure of the blood?
   a. 10 to 15 mm Hg
   b. 15 to 20 mm Hg
   c. 20 to 25 mm Hg
   d. 25 to 30 mm Hg

4. Which of the following are causes of cardiogenic pulmonary edema?
1. Excessive fluid administration
2. Right ventricular failure
3. Mitral valve disease
4. Pulmonary embolus
   a. 1 and 2 only
   b. 1, 2, and 3 only
   c. 2, 3, and 4 only
   d. 1, 3, and 4 only

5. As a result of pulmonary edema, the patient's:
1. RV is decreased
2. FRC is increased
3. VC is increased
4. TLC is increased
   a. 1 only
   b. 1 and 4 only
   c. 2 and 3 only
   d. 3 and 4 only

Pulmonary Embolism

20

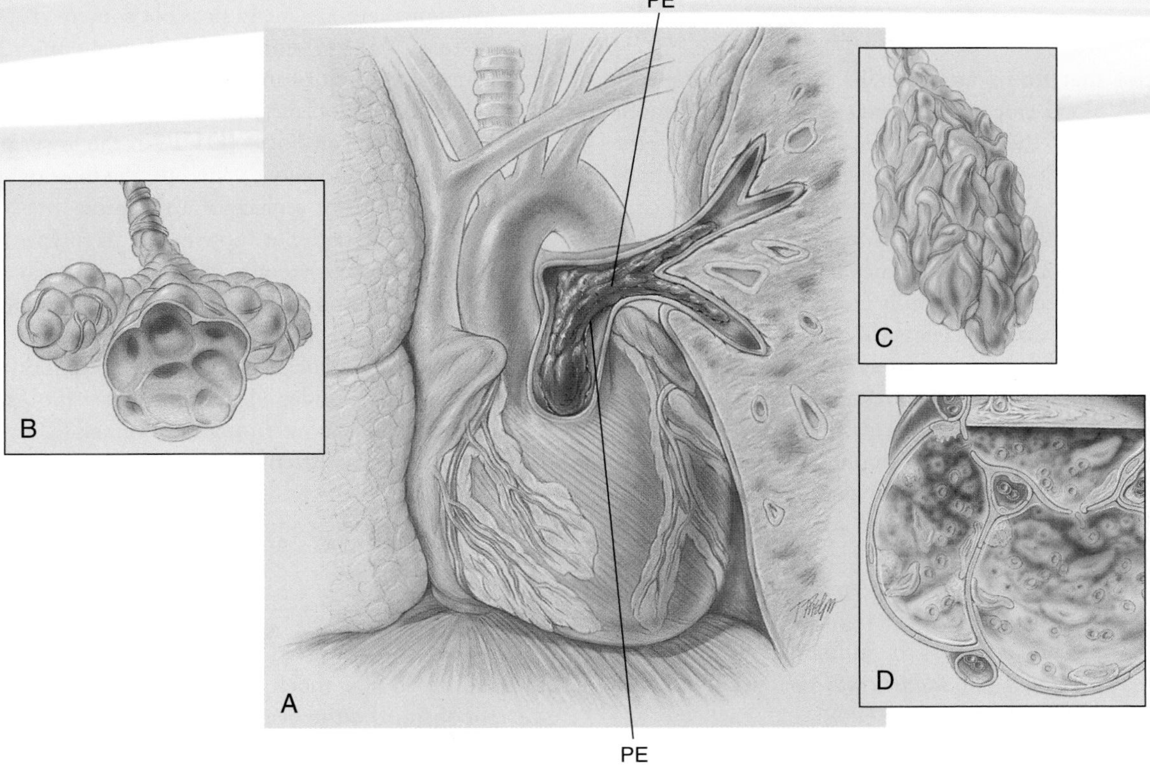

FIGURE 20-1 **A**, Pulmonary embolism *(PE)*. Bronchial smooth muscle constriction (**B**), atelectasis (**C**), and alveolar consolidation (**D**) are common secondary anatomic alterations of the lungs.

Chapter Objectives

After reading this chapter, you will be able to:

- List the anatomic alterations of the lungs associated with pulmonary embolism.
- Describe the causes of pulmonary embolism.
- List the cardiopulmonary clinical manifestations associated with pulmonary embolism.
- Describe the general management of pulmonary embolism.
- Describe the clinical strategies and rationales of the SOAPs presented in the case study.
- Define key terms and complete self-assessment questions at the end of the chapter and on Evolve.

Key Terms

Alteplase
Coumadin
D-dimer Blood Test
Deep Venous Thrombosus (DVT)
Duplex Venous Ultrasonography
Embolus
Extremity Venography
High–Molecular-Weight Heparin
Inferior Vena Cava Vein Filter
Low–Molecular-Weight Heparins
Panwarfarin
Pulmonary Angiogram
Pulmonary Embolectomy
Pulmonary Embolism CT Scan
Reteplase
Saddle Embolus
Streptokinase
Thrombolytic Agents
Thrombus
Urokinase
Ventilation-Perfusion Scan ($\dot{V}/\dot{Q}$ Scan)
Virchow's Triad
Warfarin

Chapter Outline

Anatomic Alterations of the Lungs

A blood clot that forms and remains in a vein is called a **thrombus.** A blood clot that becomes dislodged and travels to another part of the body is called an **embolus.** If the embolus significantly disrupts pulmonary blood flow, pulmonary infarction develops and causes alveolar atelectasis, consolidation, and tissue necrosis. Bronchial smooth muscle constriction occasionally accompanies pulmonary embolism. Although the precise mechanism is not known, it is believed that the embolism causes the release of cellular mediators such as serotonin, histamine, and prostaglandins from platelets, which in turn leads to bronchoconstriction. Local areas of alveolar hypocapnia and hypoxemia also may contribute to the bronchoconstriction associated with pulmonary embolism.

An embolus may originate from one large thrombus or occur as a shower of small thrombi and may or may not interfere with the right side of the heart's ability to perfuse the lungs adequately. When a large embolus detaches from a thrombus and passes through the right side of the heart, it may lodge in the bifurcation of the pulmonary artery, where it forms what is known as a ***saddle embolus*** (partially shown in Figure 20-1). This is often fatal.

The major pathologic or structural changes of the lungs associated with pulmonary embolism are as follows:

- Blockage of the pulmonary vascular system
- Pulmonary infarction
- Alveolar atelectasis
- Alveolar consolidation
- Bronchial smooth muscle constriction (bronchospasm)

Etiology and Epidemiology

A pulmonary embolus is a clinically insidious disorder. If the pulmonary embolus is relative small, the early signs and symptoms of its presence are often vague and nonspecific. On the other hand, a large pulmonary embolus can cause sudden death. A massive pulmonary embolism is one of the most common causes of sudden and unexpected death in all age groups. Many pulmonary emboli are undiagnosed and therefore untreated. In fact, because of the subtle and misleading clinical manifestations associated with a pulmonary embolus, the possibility of a blood clot lodged in the lung is often not considered until autopsy in about 70% to 80% of cases. There are approximately 650,000 cases of pulmonary embolism reported each year in the United States. About 50,000 Americans die annually from the condition. The experienced health care practitioner actively works to confirm the diagnosis of a pulmonary embolism as soon the suspicion arises. This is especially true when the origin of the signs and symptoms cannot be identified.

Although there are many possible sources of pulmonary emboli (e.g., fat, air, amniotic fluid, bone marrow, tumor fragments), blood clots are by far the most common. Most pulmonary blood clots originate—or break away from—**sites of deep venous thrombosus (DVT)** in the lower part of the body (i.e., the leg and pelvic veins and the inferior vena cava). When a thrombus or a piece of a thrombus breaks loose in a deep vein, the blood clot (now called an *embolus*) is carried through the venous system to the right atrium and ventricle of the heart and ultimately lodges in the pulmonary arteries or arterioles. There are three primary factors, known as **Virchow's triad,** associated with the formation of DVT. Virchow's triad includes (1) venous stasis (i.e., slowing or stagnation of blood flow through the veins), (2) hypercoagulability (i.e., the increased tendency of blood to form clots), and (3) injury to the endothelial cells that line the vessels. Box 20-1 provides common risk factors for pulmonary embolism.

Diagnosis and Screening

Depending on how much of the lung is involved, the size of the embolism, and the overall health of the patient, the signs and symptoms of a pulmonary embolism can vary greatly. Box 20-2 provides common signs and symptoms that often justify additional—and sometimes urgently needed—diagnostic procedures used to diagnose a suspected pulmonary embolism. Prompt diagnosis and treatment can dramatically reduce the mortality and morbidity of the disease.

Chest X-Ray Film

Although the chest x-ray film is often normal in the patient with a pulmonary embolism, it can be used to rule out conditions that mimic a pulmonary embolism, such as pneumonia and pneumothorax. In addition, infiltrate or atelectasis will be seen in about 50% of the pulmonary embolism cases, and an elevated hemidiaphragm occurs in about 40% of the cases.

Spiral (Helical) Computed Tomography Scan

The spiral or helical computed tomography (CT) scan (**pulmonary embolism CT scan**) is fast becoming the first-line test for diagnosing suspected pulmonary embolism Figure 20-2). Because the spiral CT scanner rotates continuously around the body, it can provide a three-dimensional image of any abnormalities with a higher degree of accuracy. A dye (contrast medium) is usually used to help visualize the structures of the lungs. It only takes about 20 seconds as opposed to 20 minutes for the standard CT scan. Because the spiral CT scan is fast, it is easier to capture the dye while it is still in the pulmonary arteries. The spiral CT scan exposes the patient to more radiation than the standard x-ray

Box 20-1 Risk Factors Associated with Pulmonary Embolism

Venous Stasis
- Inactivity
  - Prolonged bed rest and/or immobilization
  - Prolonged sitting (e.g., car or plane travel)
- Congestive heart failure
- Varicose veins
- Thrombophlebitis

Surgical Procedures
- Hip surgery
- Pelvic surgery
- Knee surgery
- Certain obstetric or gynecologic procedures

Trauma
- Bone fractures (especially of the pelvis and the long bones of the lower extremities)
- Extensive injury to soft tissue
- Postoperative or postpartum states
- Extensive hip or abdominal operations
- Phlegmasia alba dolens puerperarum ("milk-leg" of pregnancy)

Hypercoagulation Disorders
- Oral contraceptives
- Polycythemia
- Multiple myeloma

Others
- Obesity
- Pacemakers or venous catheters
- Pregnancy and childbirth
- Supplemental estrogen (estrogen in birth control formulations can increase clotting factors)
- Family history of venous thromboembolism
- Smoking
- Malignant neoplasms
- Burns

examination but increases the risk of an allergic reaction to the contrast medium (rare). The spiral CT scan is considered to be more sensitive than the **ventilation-perfusion scan ($\dot{V}/\dot{Q}$ scan)** and **pulmonary angiogram,** discussed later.

Electrocardiogram

The most common electrocardiographic abnormality in pulmonary embolism is nonspecific ST-T wave changes. Sinus tachycardia is the most commonly seen rhythm disturbance. Atrial fibrillation and flutter may also occur. The electrocardiogram (ECG) is an excellent test for ruling out disorders such as pericarditis and myocardial infarction.

Ventilation-Perfusion Scan

A $\dot{V}/\dot{Q}$ scan is reliable only at the extremes of interpretation (i.e., the test confirms that the lungs are normal or that there is a high probability of a pulmonary embolism). The $\dot{V}/\dot{Q}$ scan often raises more questions than it answers. This test is slowly being replaced by more sensitive and rapid tests, such as spiral CT scans.

Box 20-2 Signs and Symptoms Commonly Associated with Pulmonary Embolism

- Sudden shortness of breath
- Tachycardia
- Weak pulse
- Lightheadedness or fainting
- Anxiety
- Excessive sweating
- Cyanosis
- Cool or clammy skin to the touch
- Chest pain that resembles a heart attack—that is, chest pain that may radiate to the shoulder, arm, neck or jaw. The pain is often described as sharp, stabbing, aching, or dull. The pain often intensifies when the patient inhales deeply, coughs, eats, or bends over. The pain often intensifies during exertion but will not go away during rest.
- Cough
- Blood-streaked sputum
- Wheezing
- Leg swelling

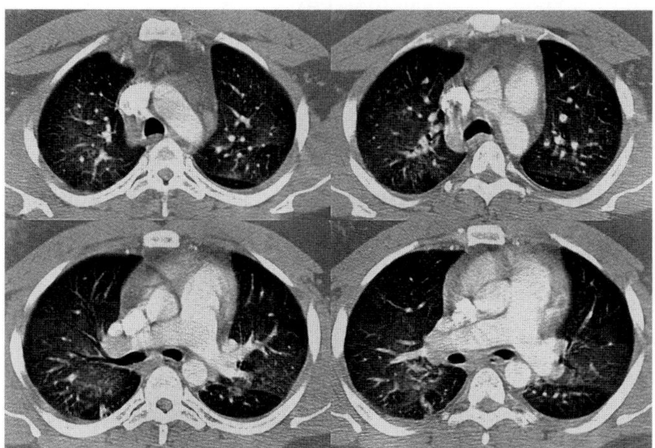

FIGURE 20-2 Fat embolism in a young man with dyspnea and hypoxemia after repair of a femur fracture with an intramedullary nail. Computed tomography (CT) shows scattered nondependent ground-glass opacities, likely resulting from fat embolism. The patient did not develop further stigmata of fat embolism syndrome, and his symptoms improved gradually over the next few days. (From Hansell DM, Armstrong P, Lynch DA, McAdams HP, eds: *Imaging of diseases of the chest,* ed 4, Philadelphia, 2005, Elsevier.)

Pulmonary Angiogram

A pulmonary angiogram provides a clear image of the blood flow in the lung's arteries. It is an extremely accurate test for diagnosis of pulmonary embolism. However, because it is invasive (catheter insertion and dye injection) and time-consuming (about 1 hour) and requires a high degree of skill to administer, it is usually performed when other tests have failed to provide a definitive diagnosis. More contrast dye is used in this study than in the pulmonary embolism CT scan.

Additional Tests Used to Detect Blood Clots in Veins

In addition to the previously described tests that are used to detect a pulmonary embolism, several tests can be performed to detect a blood clot in the vein—called a *venous thromboembolism* (VTE).

D-dimer Blood Test

The **D-dimer blood test** (also called the *fibrinogen test*) is used to check for an increased level of the protein fibrinogen—an integral component of the blood-clotting process. The test is relatively simple and fast; it entails drawing a blood sample, and the results can be available in less than 1 hour. D-dimer values higher than 500 ng/mL are considered positive—which may suggest the possibility of blood clots. However, it should be emphasized that there are many conditions that can increase an individual's D-dimer level, including recent surgery. Thus, an elevated D-dimer value is usually used to supplement other clinical information. A normal D-dimer level essentially rules out the possibility of blood clots.

Duplex Venous Ultrasonography

A **duplex venous ultrasonography** test uses high-frequency sound waves to detect blood clots in the thigh veins. The test is noninvasive and takes only 30 minutes or less to perform. A wand-shaped transducer is used to direct the sound waves to the thigh veins being tested. The sound waves are then reflected back to the transducer and converted to a moving image on a computer screen. The test is very accurate for the diagnosis of blood clots behind the knee or thigh. Although it is relatively sensitive in detecting DVT above the knee, it is insensitive in detecting DVT below the knee.

Extremity Venography

The **extremity venography** test is a more complex and invasive procedure. It entails the insertion of a catheter into a vein of the patient's arm or leg. A contrast dye is injected into the vein to make it visible on x-ray examination. Although venography can accurately detect DVT, it has largely been replaced by duplex venous ultrasonography.

Magnetic Resonance Imaging

A magnetic resonance imaging (MRI) scan of the chest may be used for individuals whose kidneys may be harmed by dyes used in x-ray tests and for women who are pregnant.

Magnetic Resonance Angiography

Magnetic resonance angiography (MRA) may be used to differentiate between blood (usual), thromboemboli, and tumor emboli in patients with malignancy.

Blood Tests

In individuals who (1) have a family history of blood clots, (2) have had more than one episode of blood clots, or (3) have experienced blood clots for no known reason, the doctor may prescribe a series of blood tests to determine if there are any inherited abnormalities in the blood-clotting system. When genetic abnormalities (e.g., Factor V [Leyden] Deficiency) are found or there is a history of blood clots, the physician may recommend a lifelong therapy of anticoagulants. The doctor may also recommend that other members of the family receive a series of blood tests.

OVERVIEW of the Cardiopulmonary Clinical Manifestations Associated with Pulmonary Embolism*

The following clinical manifestations result from the pathologic mechanisms caused (or activated) by **Atelectasis** (see Figure 9-8)—the major anatomic alteration of the lungs associated with a pulmonary embolism (see Figure 20-1). **Bronchospasm** (see Figure 9-11) also may explain some of the following findings. It occurs rarely and is of little clinical significance compared with the atelectasis and increased physiologic dead space caused by the embolism.

CLINICAL DATA OBTAINED AT THE PATIENT'S BEDSIDE

The Physical Examination

*In an uncomplicated pulmonary embolism, none of the clinical scenarios presented in Figures 9-8 through 9-13 are activated. In these patients, "wasted" or increased alveolar dead space ventilation is the primary pathophysiologic mechanism (i.e., the ventilation of embolized [nonperfused] pulmonary subsegments, segments, or lobes).

Vital Signs

Increased Respiratory Rate (Tachypnea)

Several unique mechanisms probably work simultaneously to increase the rate of breathing in patients with pulmonary embolism.

Stimulation of Peripheral Chemoreceptors (Hypoxemia)

When an embolus lodges in the pulmonary vascular system, blood flow is reduced or completely absent distal to the obstruction. Consequently the alveolar ventilation beyond the obstruction is wasted, or dead space, ventilation. In other words, no carbon dioxide–oxygen exchange occurs. The ventilation-perfusion ($\dot{V}/\dot{Q}$) ratio distal to the pulmonary embolus is high and may even be infinite if there is no perfusion at all (Figure 20-3). In chronic cases, pulmonary embolism or wasted or dead space ventilation can be identified in cardiopulmonary exercise testing.

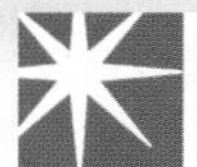

OVERVIEW of the Cardiopulmonary Clinical Manifestations Associated with Pulmonary Embolism—cont'd

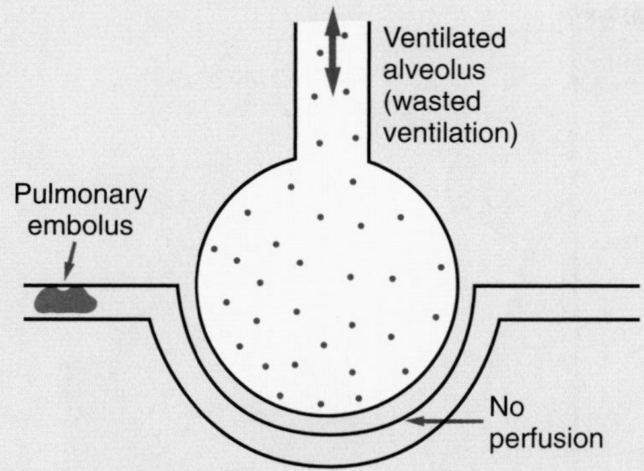

FIGURE 20-3 Dead-space ventilation in pulmonary embolism.

Although portions of the lungs have a high $\dot{V}/\dot{Q}$ ratio at the onset of a pulmonary embolism, this condition is quickly reversed, and a decrease in the $\dot{V}/\dot{Q}$ ratio occurs. The pathophysiologic mechanisms responsible for the decreased $\dot{V}/\dot{Q}$ ratio are as follows: In response to the pulmonary embolus, pulmonary infarction develops and causes alveolar atelectasis, consolidation, and parenchymal necrosis. In addition, the embolus is believed to activate the release of humoral agents such as serotonin, histamine, and prostaglandins into the pulmonary circulation, causing bronchial constriction. Collectively, the alveolar atelectasis, consolidation, tissue necrosis, and bronchial constriction lead to decreased alveolar ventilation relative to the alveolar perfusion (decreased $\dot{V}/\dot{Q}$ ratio). As a result of the decreased $\dot{V}/\dot{Q}$ ratio, pulmonary shunting and venous admixture ensue.

The result of the venous admixture is a decrease in the patient's Pa_{O_2} and Ca_{O_2} (Figure 20-4). It should be emphasized that it is not the pulmonary embolism but rather the decreased $\dot{V}/\dot{Q}$ ratio that develops from the pulmonary infarction (atelectasis and consolidation) and bronchial constriction (release of cellular mediators) that actually causes the reduction of the patient's arterial oxygen level. As this condition intensifies, the patient's oxygen level may decline to a point low enough to stimulate the peripheral chemoreceptors, which in turn initiates an increased ventilatory rate.

Reflexes from the Aortic and Carotid Sinus Baroreceptors

If obstruction of the pulmonary vascular system is severe, left ventricular output will diminish and cause the systemic blood pressure to drop. The decreased systemic blood pressure reduces the tension of the walls of the aorta and carotid artery, which activates the baroreceptors. Activation of the baroreceptors in turn initiates an increased heart rate and an increased ventilatory rate.

Other pathophysiologic mechanisms that may increase the patient's ventilatory rate include the following:

- Stimulation of the J receptors
- Anxiety, pain, fever

Increased Heart Rate

The two major mechanisms responsible for the increased heart rate associated with pulmonary embolism are (1) reflexes

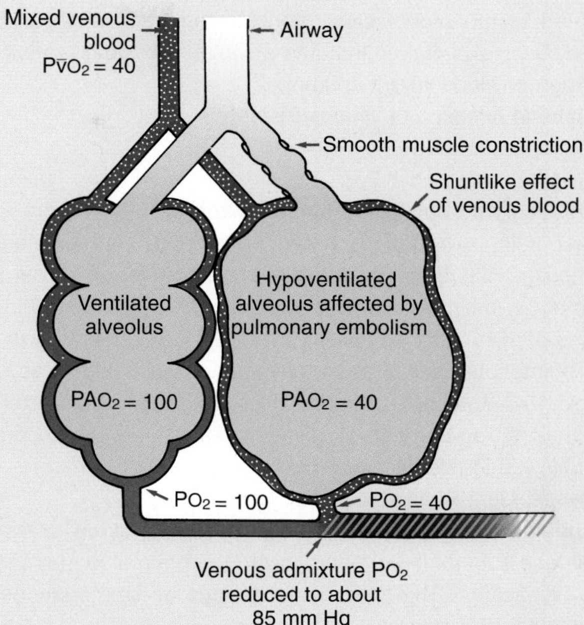

FIGURE 20-4 Venous admixture may develop in pulmonary embolism as a result of bronchial smooth muscle constriction (shuntlike effect). Venous admixture also may occur when an embolus leads to pulmonary infarction and causes alveolar atelectasis and consolidation (true capillary shunt). Alveolar atelectasis and consolidation are not shown in this illustration.

from the aortic and carotid sinus baroreceptors and (2) stimulation of the pulmonary reflex mechanism.

For a discussion of reflexes from the aortic and carotid sinus baroreceptors, see the previous section on increased respiratory rate. The increased heart rate also may reflect an indirect response to hypoxic stimulation of the peripheral chemoreceptors, mainly the carotid bodies. When the carotid bodies are stimulated in this manner, the patient's ventilatory rate increases. As a result of the increased rate of lung inflation, the pulmonary reflex mechanism is activated; this mechanism triggers tachycardia.

Systemic Hypotension (Decreased Blood Pressure)

When significant pulmonary hypertension develops in pulmonary embolic disease, it is nearly always present because of the decrease in the cross-sectional area of the pulmonary vascular system, which reduces cardiac return and causes a decrease in left ventricular output and systemic hypotension.

Cyanosis

Cough and Hemoptysis

As a result of the pulmonary hypertension, the pulmonary hydrostatic pressure, normally about 15 mm Hg, often becomes higher than the pulmonary oncotic pressure (normally about 25 mm Hg). This increase in the hydrostatic pressure permits plasma and red blood cells to move across the alveolar-capillary membrane and into alveolar spaces. If this process continues, the subepithelial mechanoreceptors

OVERVIEW of the Cardiopulmonary Clinical Manifestations Associated with Pulmonary Embolism—cont'd

located in the bronchioles, bronchi, and trachea are stimulated. Such stimulation initiates a cough reflex and the expectoration of blood-tinged sputum.

Peripheral Edema and Venous Distention

- Distended neck veins
- Swollen and tender liver

Chest Pain and Decreased Chest Expansion

Chest pain is frequently noted in patients with pulmonary embolism. The origin of the pain is obscure. It may be cardiac or pleural, but it is one of the common early findings in all forms of pulmonary embolism, even in the absence of obvious cor pulmonale or pleural involvement. If the patient has systemic hypotension, perfusion of the coronary arteries decreases, and angina-like chest pain (and electrocardiographic [ECG] findings) may result.

Syncope, Light-Headedness, and Confusion

If the left ventricular output and systemic blood pressure decrease substantially, blood flow to the brain also may diminish significantly. This may cause periods of lightheadedness, confusion, and even syncope.

Abnormal Heart Sounds

- Increased second heart sound (S_2)
- Increased splitting of the second heart sound (S_2)
- Third heart sound (or ventricular gallop)

Increased Second Heart Sound (S_2)

As a result of pulmonary embolization, abnormally high blood pressure develops in the pulmonary artery. This condition causes the pulmonic valve to close more forcefully. As a result the sound produced by the pulmonic valve (P_2) is often louder than the aortic sound (A_2), which causes a louder second heart sound, or S_2.

Increased Splitting of the Second Heart Sound (S_2)

Two major mechanisms either individually or together may contribute to the increased splitting of S_2 sometimes noted in pulmonary embolism: (1) increased pulmonary hypertension and (2) incomplete right bundle branch block.

The incomplete right bundle branch block that sometimes accompanies pulmonary embolism also may contribute to the increased splitting of S_2. In an incomplete block the electrical activity through the right side of the heart is delayed; this delayed activity in turn slows right ventricular contraction. The blood pressure in the pulmonic valve area remains higher than normal for a longer time during right ventricular contraction. As a result, the closure of the pulmonic valve is delayed, which may further widen the S_2 split.

Third Heart Sound (Ventricular Gallop)

A third heart sound (S_3), or ventricular gallop, is sometimes heard in patients with pulmonary embolism. It occurs early in diastole, about 0.12 to 0.16 seconds after S_2. Although its precise origin is unknown, S_3 is thought to be created by cardiac wall vibrations during diastole, when the rush of blood into the ventricles is abruptly stopped by ventricular walls that have lost some of their elasticity because of hypertrophy. An S_3 generated in the right ventricle usually is best heard to the right of the apex, close to the lower sternal border during inspiration.

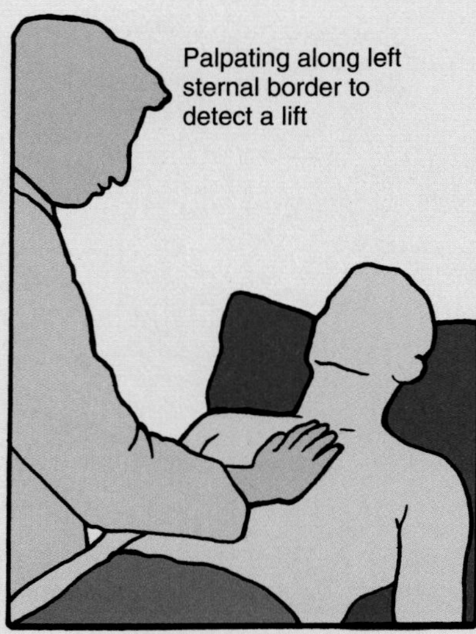

FIGURE 20-5 A right ventricular lift can be detected in patients with a pulmonary embolism if significant pulmonary hypertension is present.

Other Cardiac Manifestations

Right Ventricular Heave or Lift

As a consequence of the elevated pulmonary blood pressure, right ventricular strain or right ventricular hypertrophy (or both) often develops. When this occurs, a sustained lift of the chest wall can be felt at the lower left side of the sternum during systole (Figure 20-5), because the right ventricle lies directly beneath the sternum.

Chest Assessment Findings

- Crackles
- Wheezes
- Pleural friction rub (especially when pulmonary infarction involves the pleura)

CLINICAL DATA OBTAINED FROM LABORATORY TESTS AND SPECIAL PROCEDURES

Arterial Blood Gases

MILD TO MODERATE STAGES
Acute Alveolar Hyperventilation with Hypoxemia
(Acute Respiratory Alkalosis)

pH	Pa_{CO_2}	HCO_3^-	Pa_{O_2}
↑	↓	↓ (slightly)	↓

SEVERE STAGE
Acute Ventilatory Failure with Hypoxemia
(Acute Respiratory Acidosis)

pH*	Pa_{CO_2}	HCO_3^- *	Pa_{O_2}
↓	↑	↑ (slightly)	↓

*When tissue hypoxia is severe enough to produce lactic acid, the pH and HCO_3^- values will be lower than expected for a particular Pa_{CO_2} level.

OVERVIEW of the Cardiopulmonary Clinical Manifestations Associated with Pulmonary Embolism—cont'd

Oxygenation Indices*

$\dot{Q}_S/\dot{Q}_T$	Do_2[†]	$\dot{V}o_2$	$C(a-\bar{v})o_2$	O_2ER	$S\bar{v}o_2$
↑	↓	N	N	↑	↓

[†]The Do_2 may be normal in patients who have compensated to the decreased oxygenation status with (1) an increased cardiac output, (2) an increased hemoglobin level, or (3) a combination of both. When the Do_2 is normal, the O_2ER is usually normal.

Hemodynamic Indices[‡]

EXTENSIVE PULMONARY EMBOLISM

CVP	RAP	$\overline{PA}$	PCWP	CO	SV
↑	↑	↑	↓ or N	↓	↓
SVI	**CI**	**RVSWI**	**LVSWI**	**PVR**	**SVR**
↓	↓	↑	↓	↑	N

Normally the pulmonary artery pressure is no greater than 25/10 mm Hg, with a mean pulmonary artery pressure of approximately 15 mm Hg. Most patients with a pulmonary embolism, however, have a mean pulmonary artery pressure in excess of 20 mm Hg. Three major mechanisms may contribute to the pulmonary hypertension: (1) decreased cross-sectional area of the pulmonary vascular system because of the embolism, (2) vasoconstriction induced by humoral agents, and (3) vasoconstriction induced by alveolar hypoxia.

Decreased Cross-Sectional Area of the Pulmonary Vascular System because of the Embolus

The cross-sectional area of the pulmonary vascular system will decrease significantly if a large embolus becomes lodged in a major artery or if many small emboli become lodged in numerous small pulmonary vessels.

Vasoconstriction Induced by Humoral Agents

One of the consequences of pulmonary embolism is the release of certain humoral agents, primarily serotonin and prostaglandin. These agents induce smooth muscle constriction of both the tracheobronchial tree and the pulmonary vascular system. Such smooth muscle vasoconstriction may further reduce the total cross-sectional area of the pulmonary vascular system and cause the pulmonary artery pressure to rise further.

Vasoconstriction Induced by Alveolar Hypoxia

In response to the humoral agents liberated in pulmonary embolism, the smooth muscles of the tracheobronchial tree constrict and cause the $\dot{V}/\dot{Q}$ ratio to decrease and the Pao_2 to decline. Although the precise mechanism is unclear, when the Pao_2 and $Paco_2$ decrease, pulmonary vasoconstriction routinely ensues. This action appears to be a normal compensatory mechanism that offsets the shunt produced by underventilated alveoli. When the number of hypoxic areas becomes significant, however, generalized pulmonary vasoconstriction may develop and further contribute to the increase in pulmonary blood pressure. When the pulmonary embolism is severe, right-sided heart strain and cor pulmonale may ensue. Cor pulmonale leads to an increased CVP, distended neck veins, and a swollen and tender liver.

ABNORMAL ELECTROCARDIOGRAPHIC PATTERNS

- Sinus tachycardia
- Atrial arrhythmias
  - Atrial tachycardia
  - Atrial flutter
  - Atrial fibrillation
- Acute right ventricular strain pattern and right bundle branch block
- P pulmonale (peaked P waves)

In some cases the obstruction of pulmonary blood flow produced by pulmonary emboli leads to abnormal ECG patterns. However, there is no single ECG pattern diagnostic of pulmonary embolism. Abnormal patterns merely suggest the possibility of pulmonary embolic disease. Sinus tachycardia is the most common arrhythmia seen. The sinus tachycardia and atrial arrhythmias sometimes noted also are thought to be related to the increased right-sided heart strain and cor pulmonale.

RADIOLOGIC FINDINGS

Chest Radiograph

- Increased density (in infarcted areas)
- Hyperradiolucency distal to the embolus (in noninfarcted areas)
- Dilation of the pulmonary arteries
- Pulmonary edema
- Right ventricular cardiomegaly (cor pulmonale)
- Pleural effusion (usually small)

Patients with a pulmonary embolus often demonstrate no radiographic signs. However, a density with an appearance similar to that of pneumonia may be seen if infarction has occurred. Hyperradiolucency also may be apparent distal to the embolus; it is caused by decreased vascularity (Westermark's sign). Dilation of the pulmonary artery on the affected side, pulmonary edema (common after a fat embolus), right ventricular cardiomegaly, and pleural effusions also may be seen.

Ventilation-Perfusion Lung Scan Findings

Ventilation-perfusion lung scanning provides important information in this disease. The patient first breathes a gas mixture containing a small amount of radioactive gas, usually xenon-

*$C(a-\bar{v})o_2$, Arterial-venous oxygen difference; Do_2, total oxygen delivery; O_2ER, oxygen extraction ratio; $\dot{Q}_S/\dot{Q}_T$, pulmonary shunt fraction; $S\bar{v}o_2$, mixed venous oxygen saturation; $\dot{V}o_2$, oxygen consumption.

[‡]*CO*, Cardiac output; *CVP*, central venous pressure; *LVSWI*, left ventricular stroke work index; *$\overline{PA}$*, mean pulmonary artery pressure; *PCWP*, pulmonary capillary wedge pressure; *PVR*, pulmonary vascular resistance; *RAP*, right atrial pressure; *RVSWI*, right ventricular stroke work index; *SV*, stroke volume; *SVI*, stroke volume index; *SVR*, systemic vascular resistance.

OVERVIEW of the Cardiopulmonary Clinical Manifestations Associated with Pulmonary Embolism—cont'd

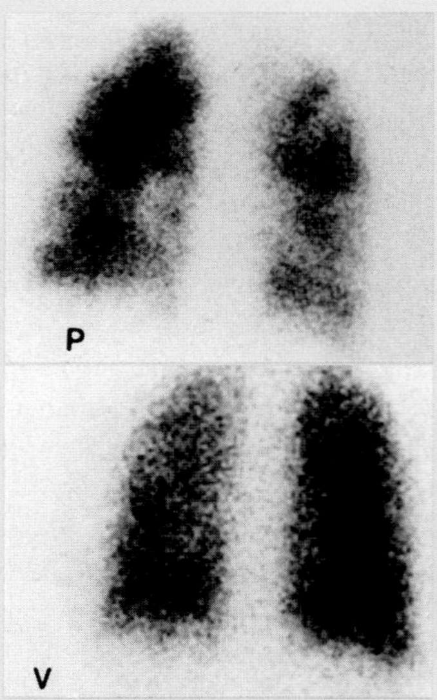

FIGURE 20-6 Fat embolism in a patient with dyspnea and hypoxemia after a recent orthopedic procedure. Perfusion *(P)* and ventilation *(V)* radionuclide scans show multiple peripheral subsegmental perfusion defects suggestive of fat embolism. (From Hansell DM, Armstrong P, Lynch DA, McAdams HP, eds: *Imaging of diseases of the chest,* ed 4, Philadelphia, 2005, Elsevier.)

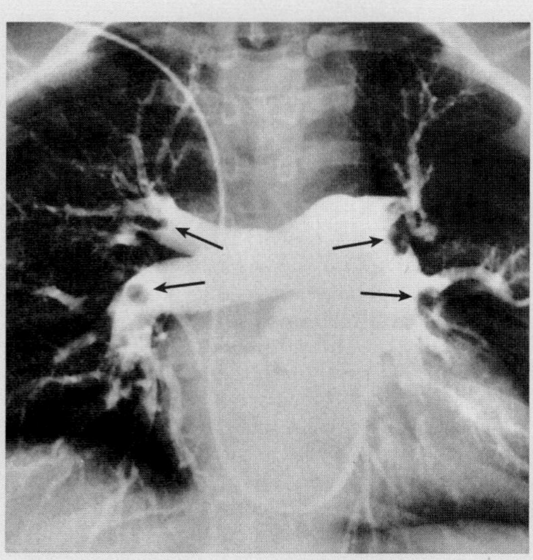

FIGURE 20-7 Pulmonary emboli. Pulmonary angiogram shows numerous filling defects. Trailing ends of the occluding thromboemboli are particularly well shown *(arrows).* (From Hansell DM, Armstrong P, Lynch DA, McAdams HP, eds: *Imaging of diseases of the chest,* ed 4, Philadelphia, 2005, Elsevier.)

133. The presence of the xenon is detected by an external scintillation camera during a wash-in or wash-out breathing maneuver. Patients with pulmonary embolism usually demonstrate normal ventilation in the region of their perfusion defect (Figure 20-6, *V*).

Next, intravenous injection of radiolabeled particles 20 to 50 µm in diameter is performed. Particles labeled with a gamma-emitting isotope, usually iodine or technetium, are injected into venous blood. The isotope accompanies the venous blood through the chambers of the right side of the heart and into the pulmonary vascular system. Because blood flow is decreased or absent distal to a pulmonary embolus, fewer radioactive particles are present in that area of the thorax. This is also recorded by an external scintillation camera (Figure 20-6, *P*). Areas of lung with normal ventilation and absent or reduced perfusion should be suspected of having pulmonary emboli.

Pulmonary Angiographic Findings

Pulmonary angiography is the gold standard used to confirm the presence of pulmonary embolism in patients with borderline or indeterminate ventilation-perfusion lung scans. A catheter is advanced through the right side of the heart and into the pulmonary artery. A radiopaque dye is then rapidly injected into the pulmonary artery while serial roentgenograms are taken. Pulmonary embolism is confirmed by abnormal filling within the artery or a cutoff of the artery. A dark area appears on the angiogram distal to the embolization because the radiopaque material is prevented from flowing past the obstruction (Figure 20-7). The procedure generally poses no risk to the patient unless there is severe pulmonary hypertension (mean pulmonary artery pressure >45 mm Hg) or the patient is in shock or allergic to the contrast medium. The pulmonary angiogram is rarely positive if the ventilation-perfusion lung scan is normal.

General Management of Pulmonary Embolism

The treatment of pulmonary embolism usually begins with treating the symptoms. Oxygen is administered per the Oxygen Therapy Protocol. The physician provides analgesics for pain, and fluids and cardiovascular agents to correct blood pressure.

Fast-acting anticoagulants, such as heparin, are given (1) to prevent existing blood clots from growing, and (2) to prevent the formation of new ones. Heparin is administered intravenously to achieve a rapid effect. **High–molecular-weight heparin** (unfractionated heparin) has, until recently, been the mainstay of treatment for patients with acute pulmonary embolism. The unfractionated heparin dosing must be governed by frequent monitoring of the activated partial thromboplastin time (APTT). This is because bleeding from unfractionated heparin can develop. Recently, **low–molecular-weight heparins** have become available (e.g., enoxaparin, dalteparin, and tinzaparin) and have been shown to be safer and more effective than unfractionated heparin for prophylaxis of DVT or pulmonary emboli. They are also more cost-effective and do not necessitate APTT monitoring. Doctors strive to achieve a full anticoagulant effect within the first 24 hours of treatment.

This is typically followed by the slow-acting, oral anticoagulant **warfarin (Coumadin, Panwarfarin).** Heparin and warfarin are given together for 5 to 7 days, until blood tests show that the warfarin is effectively preventing clotting. Then the heparin is discontinued. How long anticoagulants are given varies, based on each patient's condition. For example, if the pulmonary embolism is caused by a temporary risk factor, such as surgery, treatment is given for 2 to 3 months. If the cause is from some long-term condition, such as prolonged bed rest, the treatment is usually given for 3 to 6 months. Some patients may need to take anticoagulants indefinitely. For example, patients who have recurrent pulmonary embolism because of a hereditary clotting disorder may need to take anticoagulants for life. Patients taking warfarin need to have their blood tested periodically to determine if the dose needs to be adjusted.

Because many drugs can adversely interact with warfarin, the patient needs to be careful—that is, check with the physician—before taking any other drugs. Drugs that alter the blood's ability to clot include the over-the-counter acetaminophens, ibuprofens, herbal preparations, and dietary supplements. In addition, foods that are high in vitamin K (which affects blood clotting), such as broccoli, spinach, and other leafy green vegetables, liver, grapefruit and grapefruit juice, and green tea, may also need to be avoided.

Thrombolytic Agents

The use of the fibrinolytic agents such as **streptokinase** (Streptase), **urokinase** (Abbokinase), **alteplase** (Activase), and **reteplase** (Retavase) actually dissolves blood clots. These agents (commonly referred to as "clot-busters") have proved beneficial in treating acute pulmonary embolism. These **thrombolytic agents** are sometimes used in conjunction with heparin. Their effect in patients with hemodynamic instability may be dramatic. Because of the excessive risk of bleeding, however, the use of fibrinolytic agents in treating pulmonary embolism has been limited.

Preventive Measures

Directions to patients at high risk for thromboembolic disease include the following:

- Walking—If possible, walk frequently. When riding in a car, stop often to walk around or perform a few deep knee bends. When flying in an airplane, move around the cabin every hour or so.
- Exercise while seated—When sitting, flex, extend, and rotate your ankles or press your feet against the seat in front of you. Try rising up and down on your toes. Avoid sitting with your legs crossed.
- Drink fluids—Drink plenty of water to avoid dehydration, which can contribute to the formation of blood clots. Avoid alcohol, which also contributes to fluid loss.
- Graduated compression stockings—Tight-fitting elastic stockings squeeze the patient's legs, helping the veins and leg muscles move blood more efficiently. They provide a safe, simple, and inexpensive way to keep blood from stagnating. Research has shown that compression stockings used in combination with heparin are much more effective than heparin alone.

Vein Filter

An **inferior vena cava vein filter** (e.g., a Greenfield filter) may be surgically placed in the inferior vena cava to prevent clots from being carried into the pulmonary artery.

Pneumatic Compression

This treatment uses thigh-high cuffs that automatically inflate every few minutes to massage and compress the veins in a patient's legs. Studies show that this procedure can significantly decrease the risk of blood clots, especially in patients who undergo hip replacement surgery.

Pulmonary Embolectomy

Surgical removal of blood clots from the pulmonary circulation **(pulmonary embolectomy)** is generally a last resort in treating pulmonary embolism because of the mortality rate associated with the procedure and because of the availability of fibrinolytic agents to treat pulmonary embolism.

Respiratory Care Treatment Protocols

Oxygen Therapy Protocol

Oxygen therapy is used to treat hypoxemia, decrease the work of breathing, and decrease myocardial work. The hypoxemia that develops with pulmonary emboli usually is caused by wasted (dead space) ventilation. Hypoxemia caused by dead space ventilation is generally refractory to oxygen therapy (see Oxygen Therapy Protocol, Protocol 9-1).

Aerosolized Medication Protocol

Both sympathomimetic and parasympatholytic agents may be used to induce bronchial smooth muscle relaxation when wheezing is present (see Aerosolized Medication Protocol, Protocol 9-4 and Appendix II).

CASE STUDY

Pulmonary Embolism

Admitting History

A 32-year-old motorcycle enthusiast who smoked one pack of cigarettes per day fell asleep and fell from his bike while riding with a group of Harley "hogs" to the annual Sturgis Rally in North Dakota. Although his motorcycle sustained extensive damage, the man was conscious when the ambulance arrived. Before he was transported to the local hospital, he was treated in the field; splints and an immobilizer were applied. His injuries were thought to include a fractured pelvis, left tibia, and left knee.

En route to the hospital, a partial rebreathing oxygen mask was placed over the man's face. An intravenous infusion was started with 5% glucose solution. The patient was alert and able to answer questions. His vital signs were as follows: blood pressure 150/90, heart rate 105 bpm, and respiratory rate 20/min. Various small lacerations and scrapes on his face and left shoulder were treated. Each time the man was moved slightly or when the ambulance suddenly bounced or turned sharply as it moved over the highway, he complained of abdominal and bilateral chest pain. The emergency medical technician (EMT) crew all believed that his helmet and his youth had saved his life.

In the emergency room, a laboratory technician drew the patient's blood; several x-ray films were taken, and the man was given morphine for the pain. Within an hour the patient was taken to surgery to have the broken bones in his left leg repaired. He was transferred 4 hours later to the intensive care unit (ICU) with his left leg in a cast. Thrombosis and embolism prophylaxis had been started with low-dose heparin. Busy with another surgery, the physician ordered a respiratory care consultation for the patient.

Physical Examination

The respiratory care practitioner found the patient lying in bed with his left leg suspended about 25 cm (10 inches) above the bed surface. He had a partial rebreathing oxygen mask on his face and was alert. His wife and twin boys, who were 10 years of age and wearing black motorcycle jackets, were at the man's bedside. The patient stated that he was feeling much better and that his breathing was OK.

His vital signs were as follows: blood pressure 115/75, heart rate 75 bpm, and respiratory rate 12/min. He was afebrile, and his skin color appeared good. No remarkable breathing problems were noted. Palpation revealed mild tenderness over the left shoulder and left anterior chest area. Percussion was unremarkable, and auscultation revealed normal vesicular breath sounds. The chest x-ray film taken earlier that morning in the emergency room was normal. His arterial blood gas values (ABGs) on a partial rebreathing mask were as follows: pH 7.40, $Pa{CO_2}$ 41, HCO_3^- 24, and $Pa{O_2}$ 504. His oxygen saturation measured by pulse oximetry ($Sp{O_2}$) was 97%. On the basis of these clinical data, the following SOAP was documented.

Respiratory Assessment and Plan

S "My breathing is OK."

O No remarkable respiratory distress noted. Vital signs: BP 115/75, HR 75, RR 12; afebrile; tenderness over left shoulder and left anterior chest area; normal vesicular breath sounds; CXR: normal; ABGs (partial rebreathing mask): pH 7.40, $Pa{CO_2}$ 41, HCO_3^- 24, $Pa{O_2}$ 504 mm Hg; $Sp{O_2}$ 97%.

A
- No remarkable respiratory problems
- Normal acid-base status with overoxygenation

P Reduce oxygen therapy per protocol (2 L/min by nasal cannula). Recheck $Sp{O_2}$.

3 Days after Admission

The man's general course of recovery was uneventful until the third day after his admission, when the nurses noticed swelling of the left calf while giving him a bath. A Doppler venogram revealed a left femoral vein deep venous thrombosis (DVT). The physician was informed. Anticoagulant therapy was started. Five hours later, the patient became short of breath and agitated. A spontaneous cough was noted, with productive of a small amount of blood-tinged sputum. Concerned, the nurse called the physician and respiratory care.

When the respiratory care practitioner walked into the patient's room, the man appeared cyanotic, was extremely short of breath, and stated that he felt awful. The patient also said that he had precordial chest pain, felt lightheaded, and had a feeling of impending doom. His vital signs were as follows: blood pressure 90/45, heart rate 125 bpm, respiratory rate 30/min, and oral temperature 37.2° C (99° F). Palpation and percussion of the chest were unremarkable. Auscultation revealed faint wheezing throughout both lung fields. A pleural friction rub was audible anteriorly over the right middle lobe. A pulmonary artery catheter had been inserted.

The patient's electrocardiogram (ECG) pattern alternated between a normal sinus rhythm, sinus tachycardia, and atrial flutter. His hemodynamic indices showed an increased central venous pressure (CVP), right atrial pressure (RAP), mean pulmonary artery pressure ($\overline{PA}$), right ventricular stroke work index (RVSWI), and pulmonary vascular resistance (PVR), as well as a decreased pulmonary capillary wedge pressure (PCWP), cardiac output (CO), stroke volume (SV), stroke volume index (SVI), and cardiac index (CI). The chest x-ray showed increased density in the right middle lobe consistent with atelectasis and consolidation. On an F_{IO_2} of 0.50, the ABGs were as follows: pH 7.53, $Pa{CO_2}$ 26, HCO_3^- 21, and $Pa{O_2}$ 53. His $Sp{O_2}$ was 89%. The physician started the patient on intravenous streptokinase, ordered a ventilation-perfusion lung scan, and requested that respiratory care see the patient again. On the basis of these clinical data, the following SOAP was documented.

Respiratory Assessment and Plan

S "I feel awful. I'm short of breath and lightheaded."

O Cyanosis; agitation; dyspnea; cough productive of small amount of blood-tinged sputum; vital signs: BP 90/45, HR 125, RR 30, T 37.2° C (99° F), slight wheezing throughout both lung fields; pleural friction rub, right midlung; ECG: varies among normal sinus rhythm, sinus tachycardia, atrial flutter. Hemodynamic indices: increased CVP, RAP, $\overline{PA}$, RVSWI, and PVR and decreased PCWP, CO, SV, SVI, and CI. CXR: atelectasis and consolidation in the right middle lobe. On F_{IO_2} = 0.5, ABGs: pH 7.53, Pa_{CO_2} 26, HCO_3^- 21, Pa_{O_2} 53; Sp_{O_2} 89%.

A
- Hypotension (BP)
- Respiratory distress (cyanosis, heart rate, respiratory rate, ABGs)
- Pulmonary embolism and infarction likely (history, vital signs, CXR, ECG, blood-tinged sputum, wheezing, pleural friction rub)
- Bronchospasm, probably secondary to pulmonary embolism or infarction (wheezing)
- Alveolar atelectasis and consolidation (CXR)
- Acute alveolar hyperventilation with moderate hypoxemia (ABGs)
- Pulmonary artery hypertension and low cardiac output probably secondary to pulmonary embolism (clinical presentation and hemodynamic data)

P Contact physician to request transfer to ICU. Increase **oxygen therapy** per **Protocol.** Begin **Aerosolized Medication Protocol** (med. neb. with 2 mL albuterol premix qid). Monitor and reevaluate in 30 minutes (e.g., ABG). Remain on standby with mechanical ventilator available.

2 Hours Later

The ventilation-perfusion scan showed no blood flow to the right middle lobe. The patient's eyes were closed, and he no longer was responsive to questions. His skin appeared cyanotic, and his cough was productive of a small amount of blood-tinged sputum. His vital signs were as follows: blood pressure 70/35, heart rate 160 bpm, respiratory rate 25/min and shallow, and rectal temperature 37.5° C (99.2° F). Findings on palpation of the chest were normal. Dull percussion notes were elicited over the right midlung. Wheezing was heard throughout both lung fields, and a pleural friction rub was audible over the right middle lobe.

The patient demonstrated an ECG pattern that alternated among a normal sinus rhythm, sinus tachycardia, and atrial flutter. His hemodynamic indices continued to show increased CVP, RAP, $\overline{PA}$, RVSWI, and PVR and decreased PCWP, CO, SV, SVI, and CI. The patient's ABGs on 100% oxygen were as follows: pH 7.25, Pa_{CO_2} 69, HCO_3^- 27, and Pa_{O_2} 37. His Sp_{O_2} was 64%. On the basis of these clinical data, the following SOAP was documented.

Respiratory Assessment and Plan

S N/A (patient not responsive)

O Ventilation-perfusion scan: no blood flow to right middle lobe; cyanosis; cough: small amount of blood-tinged sputum; vital signs: BP 70/35, HR 160, RR 25 and shallow, T 37.5° C (99.2° F); palpation negative; dull percussion notes over right middle lobe; wheezing over both lung fields; pleural friction rub over right middle lobe; ECG: alternating among normal sinus rhythm, sinus tachycardia, and atrial flutter; hemodynamic indices: increased CVP, RAP, $\overline{PA}$, RVSWI, and PVR and decreased PCWP, CO, SV, SVI, and CI; ABGs on 100% O_2: pH 7.25, Pa_{CO_2} 69, HCO_3^- 27, Pa_{O_2} 37; Sp_{O_2} 64%

A
- Pulmonary embolism and infarction (history, vital signs, hemodynamics, CXR, ECG, blood-tinged sputum, wheezing, pleural friction rub)
- Bronchospasm (wheezing)
- Acute ventilatory failure with severe hypoxemia (ABGs)

P Contact physician stat. Discuss acute ventilatory failure and need for intubation and **Mechanical Ventilation Protocol.** Manually ventilate until physician arrives. Continue **Oxygen Therapy Protocol** via manual resuscitation at an F_{IO_2} of 1.0. Increase **Aerosolized Medication Protocol** (changing med. nebs. to IPPB to assist patient's work of breathing q4h).

Discussion

Risk factors for development of a fatal pulmonary embolism include immobilization, malignant disease, and a history of thrombotic disease (including venous thrombosis), congestive heart failure, and chronic lung disease. Only about 10% of patients with pulmonary emboli do not have at least one of these risk factors. The symptoms of ultimately fatal pulmonary embolism include dyspnea (in about 60% of patients), syncope (in about 25%), altered mental status, apprehension, nonpleuritic chest pain, sweating, cough, and hemoptysis (in a smaller percentage of patients).

The signs of acute pulmonary embolism and infarction include tachypnea, tachycardia, crackles, low-grade fever, lower extremity edema, hypotension, cyanosis, gallop rhythm, diaphoresis, and clinically evident phlebitis (in a small percentage of patients).

Today, the spiral or helical CT scan is fast becoming the first-line test for diagnosing suspected pulmonary embolism. The D-dimer blood test, duplex venous ultrasonography, and extremity venography may also be helpful in confirming the diagnosis of a suspected pulmonary embolism.

It is interesting to note that in surgical patients at least half of the deaths caused by pulmonary embolism occur within the first week after the surgical procedure, most commonly on the third to seventh day after the operation. The remainder of the deaths, however, divide equally among the second, third, and fourth postoperative weeks. The current patient certainly had one of the obvious causes for pulmonary embolism—namely, immobilization of the left leg, which was put in a cast after surgery.

At the time of the first assessment the patient was not in any respiratory distress. His chest physical examination was basically unremarkable, as were the chest x-ray film and arterial blood gas values. The patient might well have been placed on hyperexpansion therapy, as with incentive spirometry, because his known fractures were expected to be surgically reduced. This fact was particularly important for this patient, who was on morphine and might have been prone to hypoventilate because of his left shoulder and left anterior chest pain and tenderness.

By the time of the second assessment, however, things had changed, and the patient demonstrated many of the signs and symptoms listed previously. The assessing therapist should have recognized the seriousness of the situation from the patient's complaints, physical findings, hemodynamic parameters, and arterial blood gas values. The patient's wheezing most likely was a result of pulmonary embolism and infarction, as was the atelectasis. However, a trial of aerosolized bronchodilation was not inappropriate. The data were abnormal enough to prompt the therapist to suggest that the patient be transferred to the intensive care unit and to prepare for ventilator standby because acute ventilatory failure might not have been far off.

Indeed, in the last assessment, things had progressed to the point at which the patient was in severe respiratory acidemia with severe hypoxemia, and mechanical ventilation became necessary. The treating therapist should recognize that the therapeutic options in such cases are limited by the amount of ventilation "wasted" in these patients because of their embolic disease. High minute volume ventilation may be necessary to improve (even slightly) the arterial blood gas values in such patients.

One final note: The outlook for this patient was extremely poor. Indeed, he died during the fifth week of his hospitalization. He remained on ventilatory support until the time of his death.

SELF ASSESSMENT QUESTIONS

evolve Answers to questions can be found on Evolve. To access additional student assessment questions and case studies for application of text material to real-life scenarios, visit **http://evolve.elsevier.com/DesJardins/respiratory.**

1. Most pulmonary emboli originate from thrombi in the:
   a. Lungs
   b. Right side of the heart
   c. Leg and pelvic veins
   d. Pulmonary veins

2. The aortic and carotid sinus baroreceptors initiate which of the following in response to a decreased systemic blood pressure?
   1. Increased heart rate
   2. Increased ventilatory rate
   3. Decreased heart rate
   4. Decreased ventilatory rate
   5. Ventilatory rate is not affected by the aortic and carotid sinus baroreceptors.
      a. 1 and 5 only
      b. 2 and 3 only
      c. 3 and 4 only
      d. 1 and 2 only

3. What is the upper limit of the normal mean pulmonary artery pressure?
   a. 5 mm Hg
   b. 10 mm Hg
   c. 15 mm Hg
   d. 20 mm Hg

4. Pulmonary hypertension develops in pulmonary embolism because of which of the following?
   1. Increased cross-sectional area of the pulmonary vascular system
   2. Vasoconstriction caused by humoral agent release
   3. Vasoconstriction induced by decreased arterial oxygen pressure (P_{AO_2})
   4. Vasoconstriction induced by decreased alveolar oxygen pressure (Pa_{O_2})
      a. 1 and 3 only
      b. 2 and 4 only
      c. 1, 2, and 3 only
      d. 2, 3, and 4 only

5. In severe pulmonary embolism, which of the following hemodynamic indices is or are commonly seen?
   1. Decreased PVR
   2. Increased $\overline{PA}$
   3. Decreased CVP
   4. Increased PCWP
      a. 2 only
      b. 3 only
      c. 4 only
      d. 1 and 2 only

6. When humoral agents such as serotonin are released into the pulmonary circulation, which of the following occur?
   1. The bronchial smooth muscles dilate.
   2. The $\dot{V}/\dot{Q}$ ratio decreases.
   3. The bronchial smooth muscles constrict.
   4. The $\dot{V}/\dot{Q}$ ratio increases.
      a. 1 only
      b. 2 only
      c. 4 only
      d. 2 and 3 only

7. Which of the following is or are thrombolytic agents?

1. Urokinase
2. Heparin
3. Warfarin
4. Streptokinase
   a. 1 only
   b. 4 only
   c. 2 and 3 only
   d. 1 and 4 only

8. Which of the following is the most prominent source of pulmonary emboli?

a. Fat
b. Blood clots
c. Bone marrow
d. Air

PART V

Chest and Pleural Trauma

Flail Chest

21

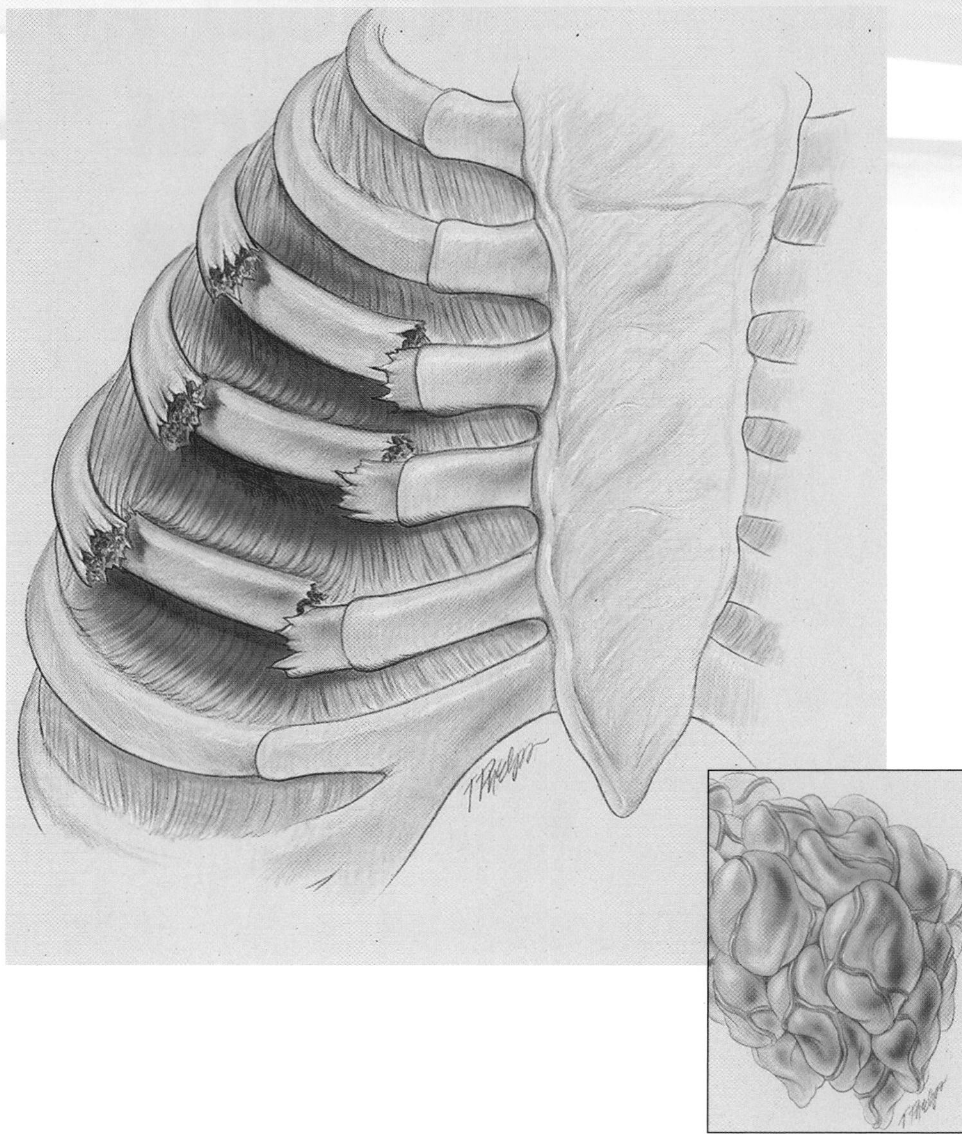

FIGURE 21-1 Flail chest. Double fractures of three or more adjacent ribs produce instability of the chest wall and paradoxic motion of the thorax. *Inset,* Atelectasis, a common secondary anatomic alteration of the lungs.

Chapter Objectives

After reading this chapter, you will be able to:

- List the anatomic alterations of the lungs associated with a flail chest.
- Describe the causes of a flail chest.
- List the cardiopulmonary clinical manifestations associated with a flail chest.
- Describe the general management of a flail chest.
- Describe the clinical strategies and rationales of the SOAPs presented in the case study.
- Define key terms and complete self-assessment questions at the end of the chapter and on Evolve.

Key Terms

Flail
Fractured Ribs
Paradoxic Movement of the Chest Wall
Pendelluft
PEEP
Venous Admixture

Chapter Outline

Anatomic Alterations of the Lungs

A flail chest is the result of double fractures of at least three or more adjacent ribs, which causes the thoracic cage to become unstable—to flail (see Figure 21-1). The affected ribs cave in (flail) during inspiration as a result of the subatmospheric intrapleural pressure. This compresses and restricts the underlying lung area and promotes a number of pathologies, including atelectasis and lung collapse. In addition, the lung also may be contused under the fractured ribs.

A flail chest causes a restrictive lung disorder. The major pathologic or structural changes of the lungs associated with flail chest are as follows:

- Double fracture of numerous adjacent ribs
- Rib instability
- Lung volume restriction
- Atelectasis
- Lung collapse (pneumothorax)
- Lung contusion
- Secondary pneumonia

Etiology and Epidemiology

A blunt or crushing injury to the chest is usually the cause of flail chest. Such trauma may result from the following:

- Motor vehicle accidents
- Falls
- Blast injury
- Direct compression by a heavy object
- Industrial accidents

OVERVIEW of the Cardiopulmonary Clinical Manifestations Associated with Flail Chest

The following clinical manifestations result from the pathologic mechanisms caused (or activated) by **Atelectasis** (see Figure 9-8) and **Consolidation** (see Figure 9-9)—the major anatomic alterations of the lungs associated with flail chest (see Figure 21-1).

CLINICAL DATA OBTAINED AT THE PATIENT'S BEDSIDE

The Physical Examination

Vital Signs

Increased Respiratory Rate (Tachypnea)

Several pathophysiologic mechanisms operating simultaneously may lead to an increased ventilatory rate. These include the following:

- Stimulation of peripheral chemoreceptors (hypoxemia)
- Paradoxic movement of the chest wall
- Other mechanisms

Paradoxic Movement of the Chest Wall

When double fractures exist in at least three or more adjacent ribs, a paradoxic movement of the chest wall is seen. During inspiration the **fractured ribs** are pushed inward by the atmospheric pressure surrounding the chest and negative intrapleural pressure. During expiration (and particularly during forced exhalation), the flail area bulges outward when the intrapleural pressure becomes greater than the atmospheric pressure.

As a result of the paradoxic movement of the chest wall, the lung area directly beneath the broken ribs is compressed during inspiration and is pushed outward through the flail area during expiration. This abnormal chest and lung movement causes air to be shunted from one lung to another during a ventilatory cycle.

When the lung on the affected side is compressed during inspiration, gas moves into the lung on the unaffected side. During expiration, however, air from the unaffected lung moves into the affected lung. The shunting of air from one lung to another is known as **pendelluft** (Figure 21-2). As a consequence of the pendelluft, the patient rebreathes dead-space gas and hypoventilates. In addition to the hypoventilation produced by the pendelluft, alveolar ventilation also may be

OVERVIEW of the Cardiopulmonary Clinical Manifestations Associated with Flail Chest—cont'd

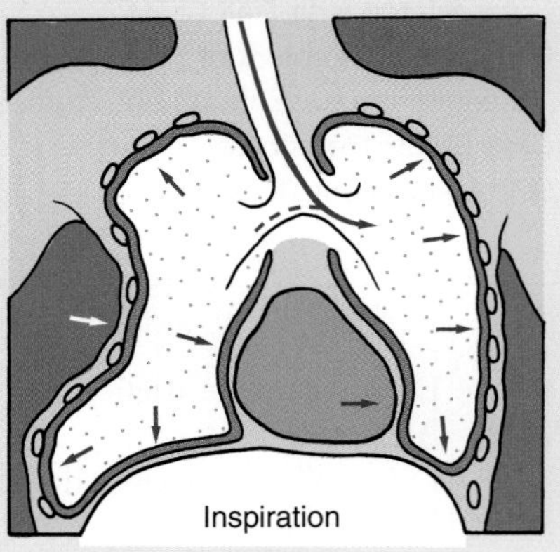

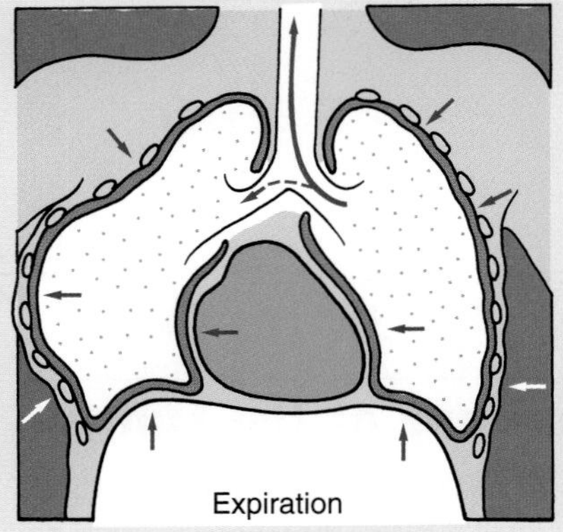

FIGURE 21-2 Lateral flail chest with accompanying pendelluft.

decreased by the lung compression and atelectasis associated with the unstable chest wall.

As a result of the pendelluft, lung compression, and atelectasis, the $\dot{V}/\dot{Q}$ ratio decreases. This leads to intrapulmonary shunting and **venous admixture** (Figure 21-3). Because of the venous admixture, the patient's Pa_{O_2} and Ca_{O_2} decrease. As this condition intensifies, the patient's oxygen level may decline to a point low enough to stimulate the peripheral chemoreceptors, which in turn initiate an increased ventilatory rate.

Other Possible Mechanisms

- Decreased lung compliance–increased ventilatory rate relationship
- Activation of the deflation receptors
- Activation of the irritant receptors
- Stimulation of the J receptors
- Pain, anxiety

Increased Heart Rate (Pulse) and Blood Pressure

Cyanosis

Chest Assessment Findings

- Diminished breath sounds, on both the affected and the unaffected sides

Mixed venous blood $P\bar{v}_{O_2} = 40$
Airway
Shuntlike effect of venous blood
(In equilibrium with $P\bar{v}_{O_2}$)
Ventilated alveolus
Hypoventilated alveolus affected by flail chest
Flail chest compressing alveoli
$PA_{O_2} = 100$
$PA_{O_2} = 40$
$P_{O_2} = 100$
$P_{O_2} = 40$
Venous admixture P_{O_2} reduced to about 85 mm Hg

FIGURE 21-3 Venous admixture in flail chest.

CLINICAL DATA OBTAINED FROM LABORATORY TESTS AND SPECIAL PROCEDURES

Pulmonary Function Test Findings
(Restrictive Lung Pathology)

LUNG VOLUME AND CAPACITY FINDINGS

V_T	IRV	ERV	RV	
N or ↓	↓	↓	↓	
VC	IC	FRC	TLC	RV/TLC ratio
↓	↓	↓	↓	N

Arterial Blood Gases

MILD TO MODERATE FLAIL CHEST
Acute Alveolar Hyperventilation with Hypoxemia
(Acute Respiratory Alkalosis)

pH	Pa_{CO_2}	HCO_3^-	Pa_{O_2}
↑	↓	↓ (slightly)	↓

SEVERE FLAIL CHEST
Acute Ventilatory Failure with Hypoxemia
(Acute Respiratory Acidosis)

pH*	Pa_{CO_2}	HCO_3^- *	Pa_{O_2}
↓	↑	↑ (slightly)	↓

*When tissue hypoxia is severe enough to produce lactic acid, the pH and HCO_3^- values will be lower than expected for a particular Pa_{CO_2} level.

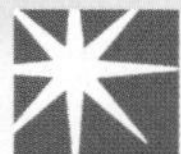

OVERVIEW of the Cardiopulmonary Clinical Manifestations Associated with Flail Chest—cont'd

Oxygenation Indices*					
$\dot{Q}_S/\dot{Q}_T$	Do_2[†]	$\dot{V}o_2$	$C(a-\bar{v})o_2$	O_2ER	$S\bar{v}o_2$
↑	↓	N	↑ (severe)	↑	↓

[†]The Do_2 may be normal in patients who have compensated to the decreased oxygenation status with (1) an increased cardiac output, (2) an increased hemoglobin level, or (3) a combination of both. When the Do_2 is normal, the O_2ER is usually normal.

Hemodynamic Indices[‡] Severe Flail Chest Disorder					
CVP	RAP	$\overline{PA}$	PCWP	CO	SV
↑	↑	↑	↓	↓	↓
SVI	CI	RVSWI	LVSWI	PVR	SVR
↓	↓	↑	↓	↑	↓

*$C(a-\bar{v})o_2$, Arterial-venous oxygen difference; Do_2, total oxygen delivery; O_2ER, oxygen extraction ratio; $\dot{Q}_S/\dot{Q}_T$, pulmonary shunt fraction; $S\bar{v}o_2$, mixed venous oxygen saturation; $\dot{V}o_2$, oxygen consumption.

[‡]*CO,* Cardiac output; *CVP,* central venous pressure; *LVSWI,* left ventricular stroke work index; *$\overline{PA}$,* mean pulmonary artery pressure; *PCWP,* pulmonary capillary wedge pressure; *PVR,* pulmonary vascular resistance; *RAP,* right atrial pressure; *RVSWI,* right ventricular stroke work index; *SV,* stroke volume; *SVI,* stroke volume index; *SVR,* systemic vascular resistance.

RADIOLOGIC FINDINGS

Chest Radiograph

- Increased opacity (in atelectatic areas or areas with postflail pneumonia).
- Rib fractures (may need special films—rib series—to demonstrate).
- Because of the lung compression and atelectasis associated with flail chest, the density of the lung on the affected side increases. The increase in lung density is revealed on the chest radiograph as increased opacity (i.e., whiter in appearance). The chest radiograph may also shows the rib fractures (Figure 21-4).

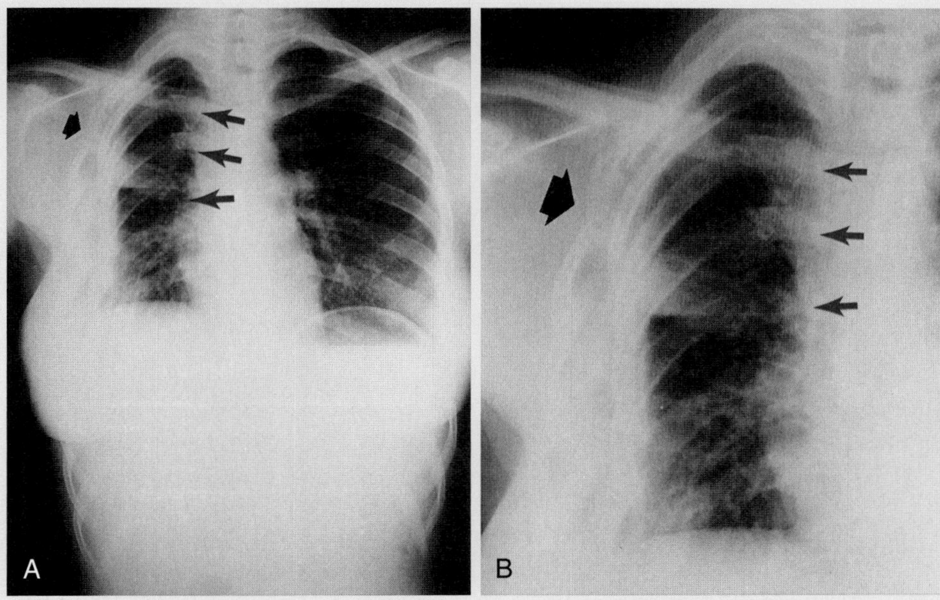

FIGURE 21-4 **A,** Chest x-ray film of a 20-year-old woman with a severe right-sided flail chest. **B,** Close-up of the same x-ray film, demonstrating rib fractures *(arrows).*

General Management of Flail Chest

In mild cases, medication for pain and routine bronchial hygiene may be the only treatments needed. In more severe cases, however, stabilization of the chest is usually required to allow bone healing and prevent atelectasis. Today, volume-controlled ventilation, accompanied by **positive end-expiratory pressure** (PEEP), is commonly used to stabilize a flail chest. Generally, mechanical ventilation for 5 to 10 days is adequate for sufficient bone healing to occur.

Respiratory Care Treatment Protocols

Oxygen Therapy Protocol

Oxygen therapy is used to treat hypoxia, decrease the work of breathing, and decrease myocardial work. It should be noted, however, that the hypoxemia that develops in flail chest is most commonly caused by the alveolar atelectasis and capillary shunting associated with the disorder. Hypoxemia caused by capillary shunting is often refractory to oxygen therapy (see Oxygen Therapy Protocol, Protocol 9-1).

Lung Expansion Therapy Protocol

Lung expansion techniques are commonly administered to offset and prevent the alveolar consolidation and atelectasis associated with flail chest (see Lung Expansion Therapy Protocol, Protocol 9-3).

Mechanical Ventilation Protocol

Because acute ventilatory failure is associated with flail chest, continuous mechanical ventilation is often required to maintain an adequate ventilatory status (see Mechanical Ventilation Protocols, Protocol 9-5, Protocol 9-6, and Protocol 9-7).

CASE STUDY

Flail Chest

Admitting History and Physical Examination

A 40-year-old obese male truck driver was involved in a serious four-vehicle accident and was taken to the emergency department of a nearby medical center, where he was found to be markedly agitated and uncooperative. He was conscious and in obvious respiratory distress. His vital signs were as follows: blood pressure 80/62, pulse 90/min, respiration rate 42/min and shallow. Bilateral **paradoxic movement of the chest wall** was evident.

He had a laceration of the right eyelid and deep lacerations of the right thigh with rupture of the patellar tendon. Pain and tenderness were present on palpation of the right posterior chest wall. The ribs moved inward with inspiration. The anteroposterior (AP) diameter of the chest was increased. Breath sounds were decreased bilaterally, and expiration was prolonged.

X-ray examination revealed posterolateral fractures of ribs 2 through 10 on the right and fractures of the necks of ribs 11 and 12 on the left. He had a 4+ hematuria, but his other laboratory findings were within normal limits.

The patient was intubated in the emergency department and placed on a mechanical ventilator with 3 cm H_2O PEEP, a V_T of 15 mL/kg and ventilatory rate of 12. An arterial line was placed, and the patient was taken to the operating room, where surgical repair of the eyelid and thigh was performed. In the operating room, with an F_{IO_2} of 1.0, the patient's blood gas values were pH 7.48, Pa_{CO_2} 30, HCO_3^- 23, and Pa_{O_2} 360. The patient was transferred to the surgical intensive care unit, where the respiratory care practitioner on duty made the following assessment.

Respiratory Assessment and Plan

S N/A—patient is intubated, put on mechanical ventilator, sedated, and paralyzed (Norcuron).

O No spontaneous respirations. No paradoxic movement of chest wall on ventilator. BP 110/70, HR 100 regular, RR 12 on vent. On 100% O_2, pH 7.48, Pa_{CO_2} 30, HCO_3^- 23, and Pa_{O_2} 360. CXR: Bilateral rib fractures, left lung contused, no pneumothorax, no hemothorax.

A
- Bilateral flail chest (history, paradoxic chest movement, CXR)
- Acute alveolar hyperventilation with overoxygenation (ABG)

P **Mechanical Ventilation Protocol:** Decrease V_T to correct acute alveolar hyperventilation and maintain patient on controlled ventilation per protocol until chest wall is stable. Wean oxygen per **Ventilator Protocol** (decreased to F_{IO_2} 0.4). Alert charge nurse (to request increased sedation and muscle paralysis) if the patient begins to inhale above preset mechanical ventilation rate. Routine ABG monitoring and continuous Sa_{O_2} monitoring. Careful chest assessment and auscultation to monitor for secondary pneumothorax and pneumonia.

Over the next 72 hours, the patient was kept intubated and ventilated with an F_{IO_2} of 0.4 and a mechanical ventilation rate of 12/min. However, his hospital course was stormy. Aggressive fluid volume resuscitation with intravenous fluids at the rate of 10 mL/hour was given. His sputum rapidly became thick and yellow. **Lung Expansion Therapy Protocol** was increased to a PEEP of 5 cm H_2O. On the second day, a right pneumothorax was demonstrated and a chest tube was inserted. A persistent air leak was present.

The next day, his pulse rose to 160/min and the pulmonary artery catheter showed evidence of left ventricular failure. His blood pressure was 142/82. His rectal temperature was 99.2° F. His ventilator rate was 12 breaths/min, with a PEEP of 10 cm H_2O. Auscultation revealed bilateral crackles. On an F_{IO_2} of 0.7, his ABGs were as follows: pH 7.37, Pa_{CO_2} 38, HCO_3^- 23, and Pa_{O_2} 58. He was rapidly diuresed, and his cardiac function improved dramatically. His Swan-Ganz catheter failed to "wedge." Over the next few days, the chest x-ray film showed dense infiltrates in both lungs, and it was difficult to maintain adequate oxygenation, even with high inspired oxygen concentrations. His sputum was yellow and thick. Whenever his Sa_{O_2} dropped below 90%, he became restless and agitated. At this time, the respiratory assessment was as follows:

Respiratory Assessment and Plan

S N/A—intubated, sedated, and paralyzed.

O Afebrile. HR 160 regular, BP 142/82, RR 12 (on vent). Right chest tube shows air leak. Crackles bilaterally. CXR: Fractures appear in line; bilateral dense infiltrates. ABG on an F_{IO_2} of 0.7: pH 7.37, Pa_{CO_2} 38, HCO_3^- 23, and Pa_{O_2} 58. Sputum thick, yellow.

A
- Persistent bilateral flail chest (CXR)
- Bilateral dense infiltrates suggest atelectasis vs pulmonary edema vs ARDS vs pneumonia (CXR)
- Adequate alveolar ventilation with moderate hypoxemia on present ventilator settings; oxygenation continues to worsen (ABG)
- Thick, yellow bronchial secretions (sputum)
- Pneumonia possible (despite normal temperature)
- Bronchopleural fistula on right side (chest tube bubbles)

P **Mechanical Ventilation Protocol** and **Lung Expansion Therapy Protocol.** Increase PEEP to 12 cm H_2O. Oxygen therapy per protocol (increase F_{IO_2} to 0.8). Institute Bronchopulmonary **Hygiene Therapy Protocol** and **Aerosolized Medication Protocol** (in-line med. neb. with 2.0 mL premixed albuterol, followed by direct instillation of acetylcysteine q4h, and suction prn. Obtain sputum for Gram stain and culture). Assist physician in the replacement of the Swan-Ganz catheter to optimize fluid therapy. Continue Sa_{O_2} monitoring.

During the patient's first week of hospitalization, his BUN increased to 60 mg% and his creatinine to 1.9 mg%. Liver function values remained within normal limits. The abnormal BUN and creatinine gradually returned to normal during the second week. The patient was slowly but successfully weaned off the ventilator over the next 2 weeks.

Discussion

This complicated case demonstrates the care of the traumatized patient with multiorgan failure. In this case the second organ system affected was the cardiovascular system, probably secondary to fluid overload. Initial therapy included chest wall rest and internal fixation with mechanical ventilation. By the time of the second assessment, the more classic clinical manifestations of pulmonary parenchymal change secondary to flail chest had developed. The clinical scenarios of **Atelectasis** (see Figure 9-8) and/or **Alveolar Consolidation** (see Figure 9-9) were well established, with oxygen-refractory pulmonary capillary shunting clearly in evidence.

Later, when what appeared to be acute respiratory distress syndrome (ARDS) supervened, PEEP was added, both for its effect on the ARDS and to stabilize the chest wall. Although these problems were dramatic enough, the therapist alertly noted the thick yellow bronchial secretions and added acetylcysteine and vigorous suctioning to deal with this problem. **Aerosolized Bronchodilator Therapy** (in this case albuterol) must always be given before or concurrently with acetylcysteine because the latter agent may cause bronchospasm if given alone. The ordering of a sputum Gram stain and culture was appropriate.

Clearly, a patient this ill should be assessed at least once—possibly more—per shift. Because this patient was hospitalized for 40 days, more than 120 such assessments were found in his chart! As we reviewed his case, this certainly did not seem to be excessive.

SELF-ASSESSMENT QUESTIONS

evolve Answers to questions can be found on Evolve. To access additional student assessment questions and case studies for application of text material to real-life scenarios, visit **http://evolve.elsevier.com/DesJardins/respiratory.**

1. In flail chest, which of the following occur?
1. V_T increases
2. Atelectasis often occurs
3. Intrapulmonary shunting occurs
4. Pneumothorax is rare
   a. 1, 2, and 4 only
   b. 1 and 3 only
   c. 2 and 3 only
   d. 2 and 4 only

2. When a patient has a severe flail chest, which of the following occurs?
1. Venous return increases.
2. Cardiac output decreases.
3. Systemic blood pressure increases.
4. Central venous pressure increases.
   a. 1 only
   b. 3 only
   c. 3 and 4 only
   d. 2 and 4 only

3. A flail chest consists of a double fracture of at least:
   a. Two adjacent ribs
   b. Three adjacent ribs
   c. Four adjacent ribs
   d. Five adjacent ribs

4. As a consequence of a severe flail chest, which of the following occurs?
1. RV increases.
2. V_T decreases.
3. VC increases.
4. FRC decreases.
   a. 4 only
   b. 1 and 3 only
   c. 2 and 4 only
   d. 2, 3, and 4 only

5. When mechanical ventilation is used to stabilize a flail chest, how much time generally is needed for adequate bone healing to occur?
   a. 5 to 10 days
   b. 10 to 15 days
   c. 15 to 20 days
   d. 20 to 25 days

Pneumothorax

22

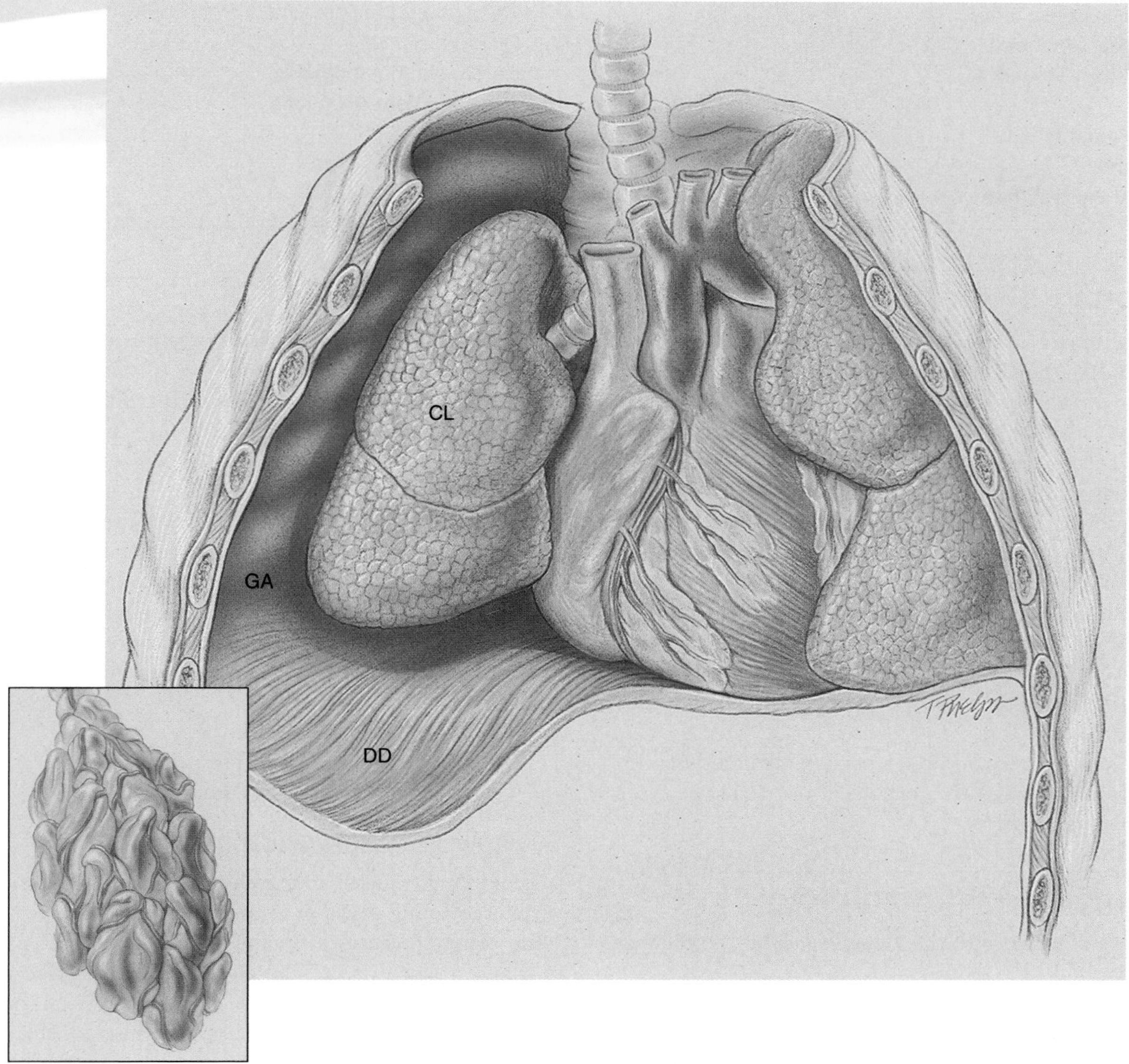

FIGURE 22-1 A right tension pneumothorax. *CL,* Collapsed lung; *DD,* depressed diaphragm; *GA,* gas accumulation in the pleura cavity; *Inset,* Atelectasis, a common secondary anatomic alteration of the lungs.

Chapter Objectives

After reading this chapter, you will be able to:

- List the anatomic alterations of the lungs associated with a pneumothorax.
- Describe the causes of a pneumothorax.
- List the cardiopulmonary clinical manifestations associated with a pneumothorax.
- Describe the general management of a pneumothorax.
- Describe the clinical strategies and rationales of the SOAPs presented in the case study.
- Define key terms and complete self-assessment questions at the end of the chapter and on Evolve.

Key Terms

Bleomycin Sulfate
Chest (Thoracostomy) Tube
Closed Pneumothorax
Iatrogenic Pneumothorax
Open Pneumothorax
Pendelluft
Pleurisy
Pleurodesis
Prophylactic Chest Tubes
Spontaneous Pneumothorax
Sucking Chest Wound
Talc
Tension Pneumothorax
Tetracycline
Traumatic Pneumothorax

Chapter Outline

Anatomic Alterations of the Lungs

A pneumothorax exists when gas (sometimes called *free air*) accumulates in the pleural space (see Figure 22-1). When gas enters the pleural space, the visceral and parietal pleura separate. This enhances the natural tendency of the lungs to recoil, or collapse, and the natural tendency of the chest wall to move outward, or expand. As the lung collapses, the alveoli are compressed and atelectasis ensues. In severe cases, the great veins may be compressed and cause the venous return to the heart to diminish.

A pneumothorax is a restrictive lung disorder. The major pathologic or structural changes associated with a pneumothorax are as follows:

- Lung collapse
- Atelectasis
- Chest wall expansion (in tension pneumothorax)
- Compression of the great veins and decreased cardiac venous return

Etiology and Epidemiology

Gas can gain entrance to the pleural space in the following three ways:

1. From the lungs through a perforation of the visceral pleura
2. From the surrounding atmosphere through a perforation of the chest wall and parietal pleura or, rarely, through an esophageal fistula or a perforated abdominal viscus
3. From gas-forming microorganisms in an empyema in the pleural space (rare)

A pneumothorax may be classified as either closed or open according to the way gas gains entrance to the pleural space. In a **closed pneumothorax,** gas in the pleural space is not in direct contact with the atmosphere. An **open pneumothorax,** on the other hand, is a condition in which the pleural space is in direct contact with the atmosphere such that gas can move freely in and out. A pneumothorax in which the intrapleural pressure exceeds the intraalveolar (or atmospheric) pressure is known as a **tension pneumothorax.** Some forms of pneumothorax are identified on the basis of origin, as follows:

- **Traumatic pneumothorax**
- **Spontaneous pneumothorax**
- **Iatrogenic pneumothorax**

Traumatic Pneumothorax

Penetrating wounds to the chest wall from a knife, a bullet, or an impaling object in an automobile or industrial accident are common causes of traumatic pneumothorax. When this type of trauma occurs, the pleural space is in direct contact with the atmosphere, and gas can move into and out of the pleural cavity. This condition is known as a **sucking chest wound** and is classified as an open pneumothorax (Figure 22-2).

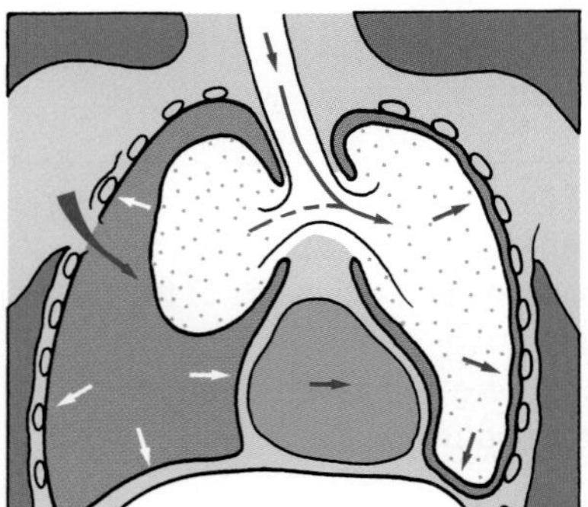

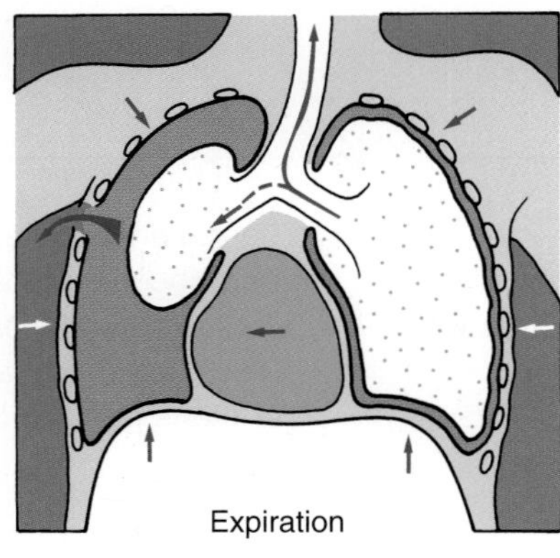

FIGURE 22-2 Sucking chest wound with accompanying pendelluft in an open pneumothorax. The large arrow illustrates the chest wall injury.

A piercing chest wound also may result in a **closed** (valvular) or **tension pneumothorax** through a one-way valvelike action of the ruptured parietal pleura. In this form of pneumothorax, gas enters the pleural space during inspiration but cannot leave during expiration because the parietal pleura (or, more infrequently, the chest wall itself) acts as a check valve. This condition may cause the intrapleural pressure to exceed the atmospheric pressure in the affected area. Technically this form of pneumothorax is classified as a tension pneumothorax (Figure 22-3). This form of pneumothorax is the most serious of all.

When a crushing chest injury occurs, the pleural space may not be in direct contact with the atmosphere, but the sharp end of a fractured rib may pierce or tear the visceral pleura. This may permit gas to leak into the pleural space from the lungs. Technically, this form of pneumothorax is classified as a closed pneumothorax.

Spontaneous Pneumothorax

When a pneumothorax occurs suddenly and without any obvious underlying cause, it is referred to as a *spontaneous pneumothorax.* A spontaneous pneumothorax is secondary to certain underlying pathologic processes such as pneumonia, tuberculosis, and chronic obstructive pulmonary disease (COPD). A spontaneous pneumothorax is sometimes caused by the rupture of a small bleb or bulla on the surface of the lung. This type of pneumothorax often occurs in tall, thin persons aged 15 to 35 years. It may result from the high negative intrathoracic pressure and mechanical stresses that take place in the upper zone of the upright lung (Figure 22-4).

A spontaneous pneumothorax also may behave as a tension pneumothorax. Air from the lung parenchyma may enter the pleural space via a tear in the visceral pleura during inspiration but is unable to leave during expiration because the visceral tear functions as a check valve (see Figure 22-4). This condition may cause the intrapleural pressure to exceed the intraalveolar pressure. This form of pneumothorax is classified as both a closed pneumothorax and a tension pneumothorax.

Iatrogenic Pneumothorax

An iatrogenic pneumothorax sometimes occurs during specific diagnostic or therapeutic procedures. For example, a pleural or liver biopsy may cause a pneumothorax. Thoracentesis, intercostal nerve block, cannulation of a subclavian vein, and tracheostomy are other possible causes of an iatrogenic pneumothorax.

An iatrogenic pneumothorax is always a hazard during positive-pressure mechanical ventilation—particularly when high tidal volumes or high system pressures are used. This is particularly common in COPD and in human immunodeficiency virus (HIV)–related acute respiratory distress syndrome (ARDS). Indeed, when very high mean airway pressures are required to ventilate such patients, **prophylactic** bilateral tube thoracostomies are often mandatory.

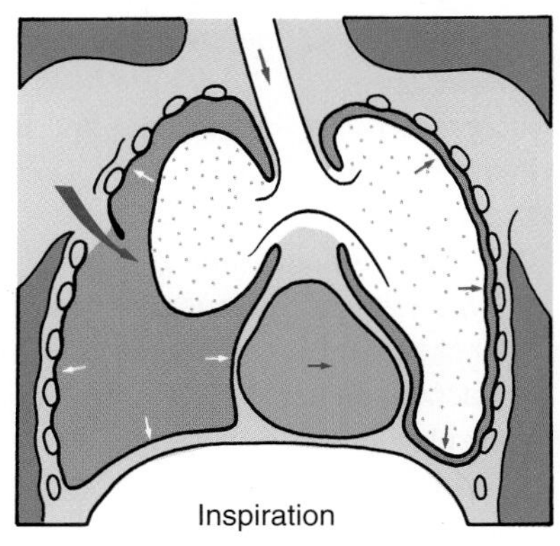

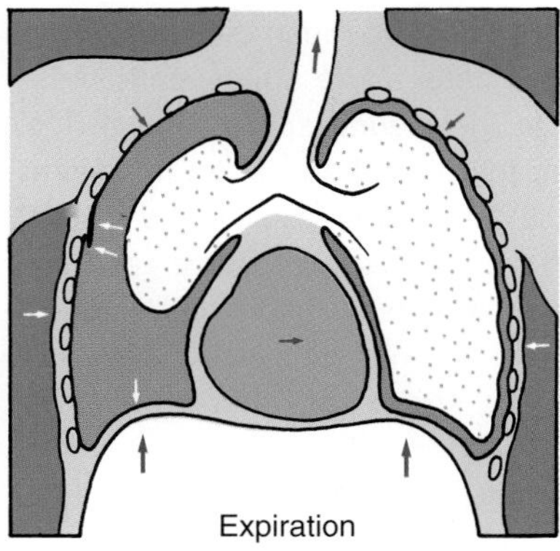

FIGURE 22-3 Closed (tension) pneumothorax produced by a chest wall wound. The large arrow illustrates the chest wall injury. The small arrows indicate the parietal pleural "value."

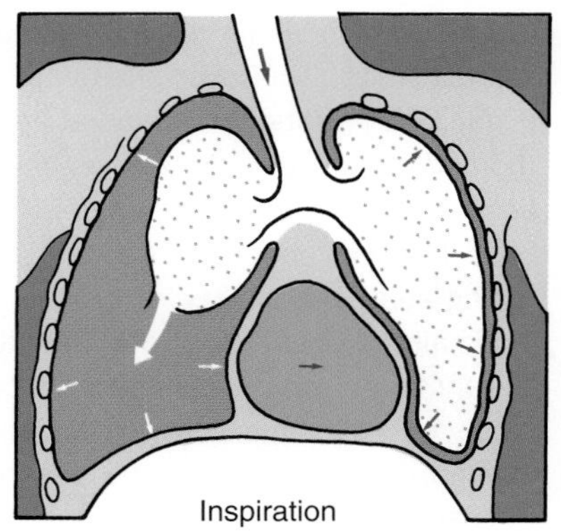

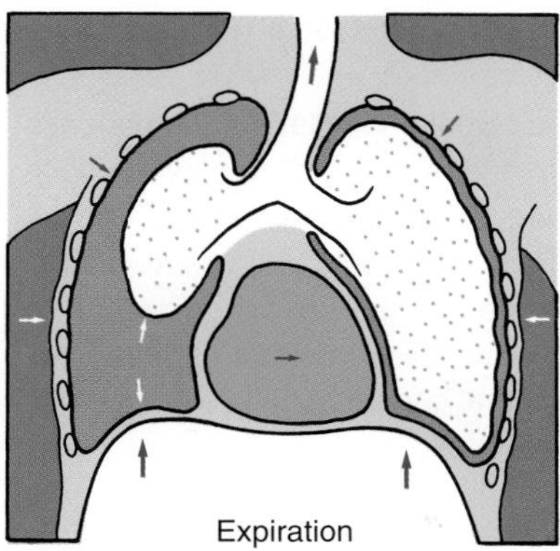

FIGURE 22-4 Right pneumothorax produced by a rupture in the visceral pleura that functions as a check valve. Progressive enlargement of the pneumothorax occurs, producing atelectasis on the affected side.

OVERVIEW of the Cardiopulmonary Clinical Manifestations Associated with Pneumothorax

The following clinical manifestations result from the pathologic mechanisms caused (or activated) by **Atelectasis** (see Figure 9-8)—the major anatomic alteration of the lungs associated with pneumothorax (see Figure 22-1).

CLINICAL DATA OBTAINED AT THE PATIENT'S BEDSIDE

The Physical Examination

Vital Signs

Increased Respiratory Rate (Tachypnea)

Several pathophysiologic mechanisms operating simultaneously may lead to an increased ventilatory rate.

Stimulation of Peripheral Chemoreceptors (Hypoxemia)

As gas moves into the pleural space, the visceral and parietal pleura separate and the lung on the affected side begins to collapse. As the lung collapses, atelectasis develops, and alveolar ventilation decreases.

If the patient has a pneumothorax as a result of a sucking chest wound, an additional mechanism also may promote hypoventilation. In other words, when a patient with this type of pneumothorax inhales, the intrapleural pressure on the unaffected side decreases. As a result the mediastinum often moves to the unaffected side, where the pressure is lower, and compresses the normal lung. The intrapleural pressure on the affected side also may decrease, and some air may enter through the chest wound and further shift the mediastinum toward the normal lung. During expiration the intrapleural pressure on the affected side rises above atmospheric pressure, and gas escapes from the pleural space through the chest wound. As gas leaves the pleural space, the mediastinum moves back toward the affected side. Because of this back-and-forth movement of the mediastinum, some gas from the normal lung may enter the collapsed lung during expiration and cause it to expand slightly. During inspiration, however, some of this "rebreathed dead space gas" may move back into the normal lung. This paradoxic movement of gas within the lungs is known as **pendelluft.** As a result of the pendelluft, the patient hypoventilates (see Figure 22-2).

Therefore when a patient has a pneumothorax, alveolar ventilation is reduced because of lung collapse and atelectasis. If the pneumothorax is accompanied by a sucking chest wound, alveolar ventilation may be further decreased by pendelluft.

As a result of the reduced alveolar ventilation, the patient's $\dot{V}/\dot{Q}$ ratio decreases. This leads to intrapulmonary shunting and venous admixture (Figure 22-5). Because of the venous admixture, the Pa_{O_2} and Ca_{O_2} decrease. As this condition intensifies, the patient's arterial oxygen level may decline to a point low enough to stimulate the peripheral chemoreceptors. Stimulation of the peripheral chemoreceptors in turn initiates an increased ventilatory rate.

Other Possible Mechanisms

- Decreased lung compliance–increased ventilatory rate relationship

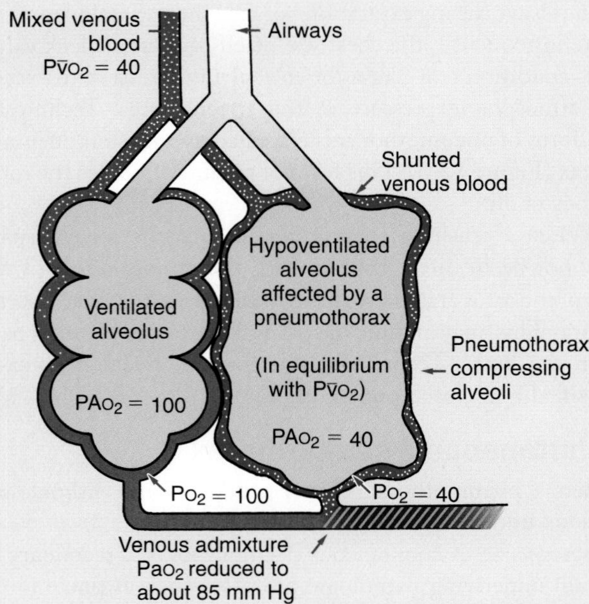

FIGURE 22-5 Venous admixture in pneumothorax.

- Activation of the deflation receptors
- Activation of the irritant receptors
- Stimulation of the J receptors
- Pain, anxiety

Increased Heart Rate (Pulse) and Blood Pressure (Small Pneumothorax)

Cyanosis

Chest Assessment Findings

- Hyperresonant percussion note over the pneumothorax
- Diminished breath sounds over the pneumothorax
- Tracheal shift
- Displaced heart sounds
- Increased thoracic volume on the affected side (particularly in tension pneumothorax)

As gas accumulates in the pleural space, the ratio of air to solid tissue increases. Percussion notes resonate more freely throughout the gas in the pleural space as well as in the air spaces within the lung (Figure 22-6). When this area is auscultated, however, the breath sounds are diminished (Figure 22-7). When intrapleural gas accumulates, and intrathoracic pressure is excessively high, the mediastinum may be forced to the unaffected side. If this is the case, there will be a tracheal shift and the heart sounds will be displaced during auscultation.

Finally, the gas that accumulates in the pleural space enhances not only the natural tendency of the lungs to collapse but also the natural tendency of the chest wall to expand. Therefore in a large pneumothorax the chest often appears larger on the affected side. This is especially true in patients with a severe tension pneumothorax (Figure 22-8).

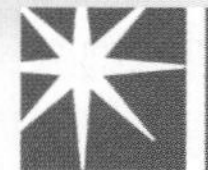

OVERVIEW of the Cardiopulmonary Clinical Manifestations Associated with Pneumothorax—cont'd

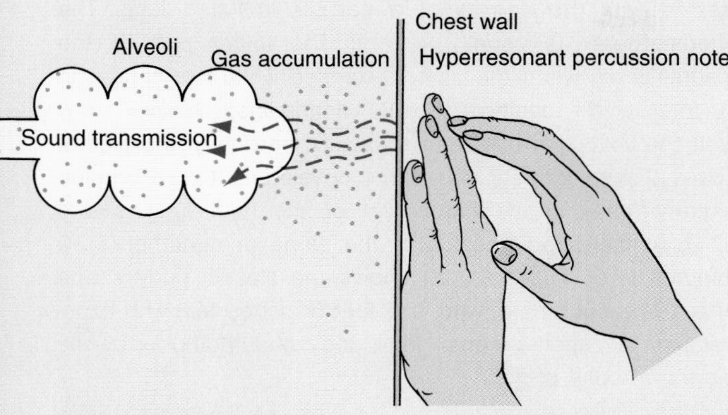

FIGURE 22-6 Because the ratio of extrapulmonary gas to solid tissue increases in a pneumothorax, hyperresonant percussion notes are produced over the affected area.

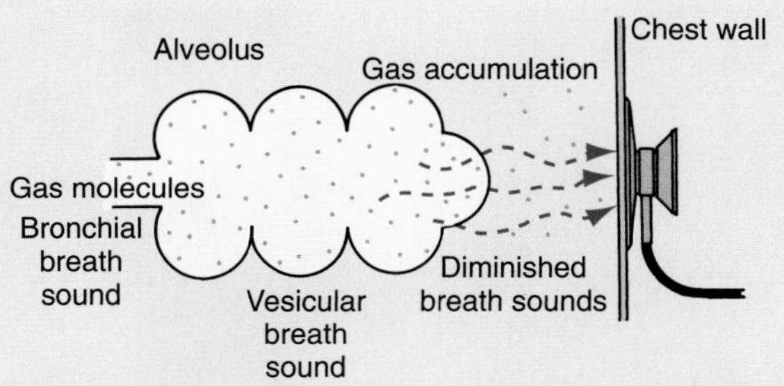

FIGURE 22-7 Breath sounds diminish as gas accumulates in the intrapleural space.

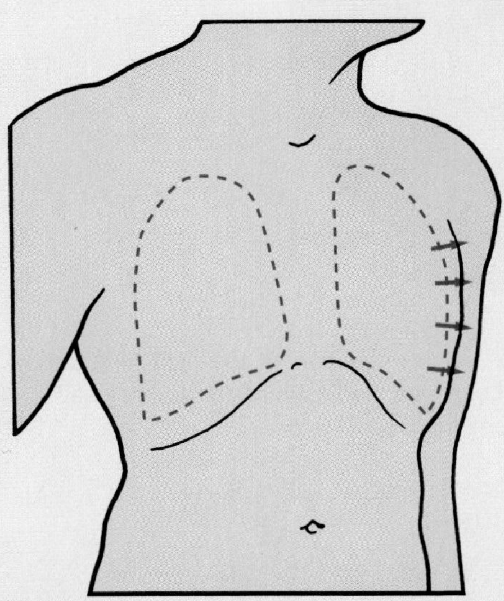

FIGURE 22-8 As gas accumulates in the intrapleural space, the chest diameter increases on the affected side in a tension pneumothorax.

CLINICAL DATA OBTAINED FROM LABORATORY TESTS AND SPECIAL PROCEDURES

Pulmonary Function Test Findings (Restrictive Lung Pathology)

LUNG VOLUME AND CAPACITY FINDINGS

V_T	IRV	ERV	RV	
N or ↓	↓	↓	↓	
VC	**IC**	**FRC**	**TLC**	**RV/TLC ratio**
↓	↓	↓	↓	N

Arterial Blood Gases

SMALL PNEUMOTHORAX

Acute Alveolar Hyperventilation with Hypoxemia

(Acute Respiratory Alkalosis)

pH	$Paco_2$	HCO_3^-	Pao_2
↑	↓	↓ (slightly)	↓

LARGE PNEUMOTHORAX

Acute Ventilatory Failure with Hypoxemia

(Acute Respiratory Acidosis)

pH*	$Paco_2$	HCO_3^- *	Pao_2
↓	↑	↑ (slightly)	↓

*When tissue hypoxia is severe enough to produce lactic acid, the pH and HCO_3^- values will be lower than expected for a particular $Paco_2$ level.

Oxygenation Indices*

$\dot{Q}_S/\dot{Q}_T$	Do_2†	$\dot{V}o_2$	$C(a-\bar{v})o_2$	O_2ER	$S\bar{v}o_2$
↑	↓	N	↑ (severe)	↑	↓

†The Do_2 may be normal in patients who have compensated to the decreased oxygenation status with (1) an increased cardiac output, (2) an increased hemoglobin level, or (3) a combination of both. When the Do_2 is normal, the O_2ER is usually normal.

Hemodynamic Indices‡ (Large Pneumothorax)

CVP	RAP	$\overline{PA}$	PCWP	CO	SV
↑	↑	↑	↓	↓	↓
SVI	**CI**	**RVSWI**	**LVSWI**	**PVR**	**SVR**
↓	↓	↑	↓	↑	↓

*$C(a-\bar{v})o_2$, Arterial-venous oxygen difference; DO_2, total oxygen delivery; O_2ER, oxygen extraction ratio; $\dot{Q}_S/\dot{Q}_T$, pulmonary shunt fraction; $S\bar{v}o_2$, mixed venous oxygen saturation; $\dot{V}o_2$, oxygen consumption.

†*CO,* Cardiac output; *CVP,* central venous pressure; *LVSWI,* left ventricular stroke work index; $\overline{PA}$, mean pulmonary artery pressure; *PCWP,* pulmonary capillary wedge pressure; *PVR,* pulmonary vascular resistance; *RAP,* right atrial pressure; *RVSWI,* right ventricular stroke work index; *SV,* stroke volume; *SVI,* stroke volume index; *SVR,* systemic vascular resistance.

OVERVIEW of the Cardiopulmonary Clinical Manifestations Associated with Pneumothorax—cont'd

RADIOLOGIC FINDINGS

Chest Radiograph

- Increased translucency (darker lung fields) on the side of pneumothorax
- Mediastinal shift to unaffected side in tension pneumothorax
- Depressed diaphragm
- Lung collapse
- Atelectasis

Ordinarily, the presence of a pneumothorax is easily identified on the chest radiograph in the upright posteroanterior view. A small collection of air is often visible if the exposure is made at the end of maximal expiration because the translucency of the pneumothorax is more obvious when contrasted with the density of a partially deflated lung. The pneumothorax is usually seen in the upper part of the pleural cavity when the film is exposed while the patient is in the upright position. Severe adhesions, however, may limit the collection of gas to a specific portion of the pleural space. Figure 22-9, *A* shows the development of a tension pneumothorax in the lower part of the right lung. Figure 22-9, *B* shows progression of the same pneumothorax 30 minutes later. Figure 22-10 shows the classic body shape of a 19-year-old male, who is 6 feet 5 inches tall, who experienced a spontaneous left-sided pneumothorax while playing a round of golf.

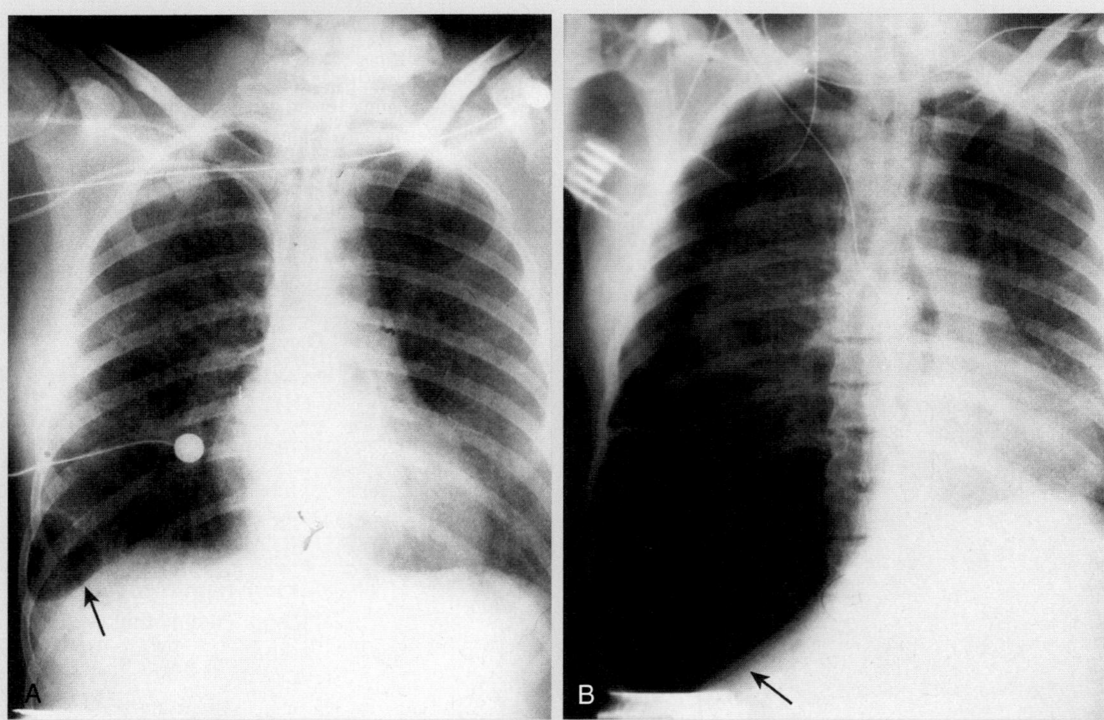

FIGURE 22-9 **A**, Development of a small tension pneumothorax in the lower part of the right lung *(arrow)*. **B**, The same pneumothorax 30 minutes later. Note the shift of the heart and mediastinum to the left away from the tension pneumothorax. Also note the depression of the right hemidiaphragm *(arrow)*.

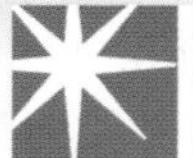

OVERVIEW of the Cardiopulmonary Clinical Manifestations Associated with Pneumothorax—cont'd

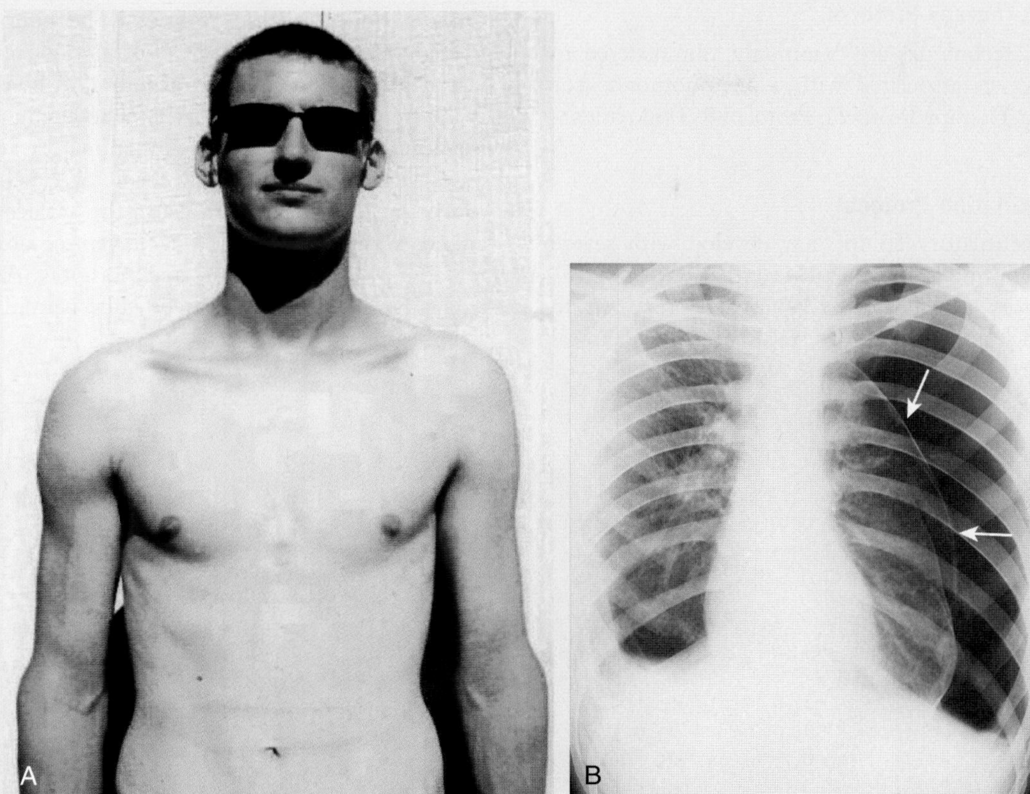

FIGURE 22-10 **A**, A 19-year-old male patient, 6 feet 5 inches tall, who experienced a sudden spontaneous left-sided pneumothorax while playing a round of golf. A spontaneous pneumothorax is not uncommon in people who are tall and thin. **B**, Chest radiograph of the same patient 45 minutes later in the emergency room. Note the shift of the heart and mediastinum to the right (toward the unaffected side), away from the tension pneumothorax, and the depressed diaphragm on the patient's left side.

General Management of Pneumothorax

The management of pneumothorax depends on the degree of lung collapse. When the pneumothorax is relatively small (15% to 20%), the patient may need only bed rest or limited physical activity. In such cases, resorption of intrapleural gas usually occurs within 30 days.

When the pneumothorax is larger than 20%, it should be evacuated. In less severe cases, air may simply be withdrawn from the pleural cavity by needle aspiration. In more serious cases, a **thoracostomy chest tube** attached to an underwater seal is inserted into the patient's pleural cavity. Because air rises, the tube is usually placed anteriorly near the lung's apex. Typically, a No. 28 to No. 36 French gauge thoracostomy tube is used for adults, with smaller sizes used for children. The tube permits evacuation of air and enhances the reexpansion and pleural adherence of the affected lung. The chest tube may or may not be attached to gentle suction. When suction is used, the negative pressure need not exceed −12 cm H_2O; −5 cm H_2O is generally all that is needed. After the lung has reexpanded and bubbling from the chest tube has ceased, the tube is clamped and left in place without suction for another 24 to 48 hours.

Respiratory Care Treatment Protocols

Oxygen Therapy Protocol

Oxygen therapy is used to treat hypoxemia, decrease the work of breathing, and decrease myocardial work. It should be noted, however, that the hypoxemia that develops in a pneumothorax is most commonly caused by the alveolar atelectasis and capillary shunting associated with the disorder. Hypoxemia caused by capillary shunting is often refractory to oxygen therapy (see Oxygen Therapy Protocol, Protocol 9-1).

Lung Expansion Therapy Protocol

Lung expansion techniques are commonly administered to offset the atelectasis associated with a pneumothorax (see Lung Expansion Therapy Protocol, Protocol 9-3) in patients with chest tubes.

Mechanical Ventilation Protocol

Because acute ventilatory failure may develop with severe pneumothorax, continuous mechanical ventilation with positive end-expiratory pressure (PEEP) may be required to maintain an adequate ventilatory status (see Mechanical Ventilation Protocols, Protocol 9-5, Protocol 9-6, and Protocol 9-7).

Pleurodesis

On occasion, a thoracentesis may be performed before a procedure called **pleurodesis.** During this procedure a chemical or medication (**talc, tetracycline,** or **bleomycin sulfate**) is injected into the chest cavity. The chemical substance or medication causes an intense inflammatory reaction over the outer surface of the lung and inside of the chest cavity. This procedure is performed to cause the surface of the lung to adhere to the chest cavity, thus preventing or reducing recurrent fluid accumulation or pneumothorax. An intense pleuritis is produced, which may be quite painful (**pleurisy**).

CASE STUDY

Spontaneous Pneumothorax

Admitting History and Physical Examination

This patient was a 20-year-old male university student who was in excellent health until 5 hours before admission. He was sitting quietly in his dorm room studying for an examination when he suddenly developed a sharp pain in his left lower thoracic region. It was most acute in the anterior axillary line. The pain was exacerbated by deep inspiration and radiated anteriorly, almost to the midline. It did not radiate into the shoulder or neck. The patient became mildly dyspneic and had episodes of nonproductive cough that seemed to increase the chest pain. These symptoms worsened, and at 1 AM his roommate drove him to the university hospital emergency department.

On examination the patient was a well-nourished, well-developed young man in moderately acute distress. His trachea was shifted to the right of the midline. His blood pressure was 150/82, pulse 96, and respirations 28 and shallow. The left side of the chest was tympanitic to percussion, and the breath sounds were described as "distant." The patient was not cyanotic. The emergency department physician was momentarily busy with another patient and asked the respiratory therapist on duty to assess the patient's respiratory status. The respiratory care practitioner assigned to the emergency room during the night shift made the following assessments and plans.

Respiratory Assessment and Plan

S Left chest pain worsened by cough; shortness of breath

O Normal vital signs. Left chest hyperresonant. Trachea shifted to the right. Breath sounds on left "distant."

A Probable left tension pneumothorax (history and objective indicators)

P Notify physician (who is in the next room). Request stat CXR and ABG. **Oxygen Therapy Protocol** (partial rebreathing mask with F_{IO_2} between 0.6 to 0.8). Oxygen therapy via partial rebreathing mask (F_{IO_2} 0.6 to 0.8). Obtain supplies for tube thoracostomy and place at patient's bedside.

The patient stated that he was more comfortable on the oxygen mask, but that some left-sided chest pain was still present. His physical findings were unchanged from his initial evaluation. The chest radiograph confirmed the diagnosis of a 50% left-sided pneumothorax, lung collapse, and mediastinal shift to the right. The arterial blood gas values on a partial rebreathing mask were pH 7.53, Pa_{CO_2} 29, HCO_3^- 21, and Pa_{O_2} 56. The physician was still busy with the patient in the next room. With this new information, the respiratory therapist charted the following.

Respiratory Assessment and Plan

S "This oxygen mask helps a little."

O Persistent symptoms and physical findings as in SOAP-1 above. CXR: 50% left tension pneumothorax. Mediastinum shifted to right. ABGs: pH 7.53, Pa_{CO_2} 29, HCO_3^- 21, and Pa_{O_2} 56 (on partial rebreathing mask).

A
- 50% left pneumothorax with mediastinal shift—lung collapse and atelectasis (CXR)
- Acute alveolar hyperventilation with mild hypoxemia (ABG)

P Inform physician of previous and current assessment. Up-regulate **Oxygen Therapy Protocol** (Increase F_{IO_2} to 0.8 to 1.0 via a nonrebreathing mask). Stay at patient's bedside until physician arrives. Assist in placement of chest tube.

Approximately 15 minutes later, the attending physician entered the room and quickly reviewed the clinical data and assessments. Moments later, he inserted a thoracostomy tube and began underwater drainage. The respiratory therapist placed a CPAP mask on the patient's face at 5 cm H_2O. The F_{IO_2} on the mask was adjusted to 0.8. Over the next 30 minutes, the lung expanded well and the patient's ventilatory and oxygenation status quickly improved. The chest tube was removed after 48 hours. Follow-up examination after 2 weeks revealed full expansion of the left lung. There was no evidence of blebs or bullae. A tuberculin skin test result was negative, and the cause of the pneumothorax was never found.

Discussion

Few respiratory conditions persist with a "crisis" onset, and this is one of them. Other instances include foreign body aspiration, pulmonary embolism, anaphylactic shock, and some cases of asthma.

This case nicely demonstrates the signs and symptoms of **Atelectasis** and intrapulmonary shunting (see Figure 9-8). The physician and respiratory therapist could not hear crackles, however, presumably because the atelectatic segments were separated (distant) from the chest wall and the examiner's stethoscope.

Although the respiratory care administered in this case (oxygen therapy) was fairly pedestrian, the therapist's assistance in the assessment of this patient and his presence at bedside made a great difference in the speed and ease with which the patient was treated. The value of an assessing and treating therapist in this situation cannot be overestimated.

SELF-ASSESSMENT QUESTIONS

evolve Answers to questions can be found on Evolve. To access additional student assessment questions and case studies for application of text material to real-life scenarios, visit **http://evolve.elsevier.com/DesJardins/respiratory.**

1. When gas moves between the pleural space and the atmosphere during a ventilatory cycle, the patient is said to have a(n):
1. Closed pneumothorax
2. Open pneumothorax
3. Valvular pneumothorax
4. Sucking chest wound
   a. 2 only
   b. 3 only
   c. 1 and 3 only
   d. 2 and 4 only

2. When gas enters the pleural space during inspiration but is unable to leave during expiration, the patient is said to have a(n):
1. Iatrogenic pneumothorax
2. Valvular pneumothorax
3. Tension pneumothorax
4. Open pneumothorax
   a. 1 only
   b. 3 only
   c. 2 and 3 only
   d. 3 and 4 only

3. Which of the following may cause a pneumothorax?
1. Pneumonia
2. Tuberculosis
3. Chronic obstructive pulmonary disease
4. Blebs
   a. 1 and 2 only
   b. 2 and 3 only
   c. 2, 3, and 4 only
   d. 1, 2, 3, and 4

4. When a patient has a pneumothorax because of a sucking chest wound, which of the following occurs?
1. Intrapleural pressure on the unaffected side increases during inspiration.
2. The mediastinum often moves to the unaffected side during inspiration.
3. Intrapleural pressure on the affected side often rises above the atmospheric pressure during expiration.
4. The mediastinum often moves to the affected side during expiration.
   a. 1 and 4 only
   b. 1 and 3 only
   c. 2 and 3 only
   d. 2, 3, and 4 only

5. The increased ventilatory rate commonly manifested in patients with pneumothorax may result from which of the following?
1. Stimulation of the J receptors
2. Increased lung compliance
3. Increased stimulation of the Hering-Breuer reflex
4. Stimulation of the irritant reflex
   a. 1 and 4 only
   b. 2 and 3 only
   c. 3 and 4 only
   d. 2, 3, and 4 only

6. The physician usually elects to evacuate the intrathoracic gas when the pneumothorax is greater than:
   a. 5%
   b. 10%
   c. 15%
   d. 20%

7. During treatment of a pneumothorax with a chest tube and suction, the negative (suction) pressure usually need not exceed:
   a. −6 cm H_2O
   b. −8 cm H_2O
   c. −10 cm H_2O
   d. −12 cm H_2O

8. A patient with a severe tension pneumothorax demonstrates which of the following on the affected side?
1. Diminished breath sounds
2. Hyperresonant percussion note
3. Dull percussion notes
4. Whispered pectoriloquy
   a. 2 only
   b. 1 and 2 only
   c. 3 and 4 only
   d. 1, 2, and 4 only

9. When a patient has a large tension pneumothorax, which of the following occur(s)?
1. $Paco_2$ decreases.
2. pH increases.
3. HCO_3^- decreases.
4. $Paco_2$ increases.
   a. 1 only
   b. 4 only
   c. 3 and 4 only
   d. 2 and 3 only

10. When a patient has a large tension pneumothorax, which of the following occur(s)?
1. PVR decreases.
2. $\overline{PA}$ increases.
3. CVP decreases.
4. CO increases.
   a. 1 only
   b. 2 only
   c. 3 only
   d. 1 and 3 only

PART VI

Disorders of the Pleura and of the Chest Wall

Pleural Effusion and Empyema

23

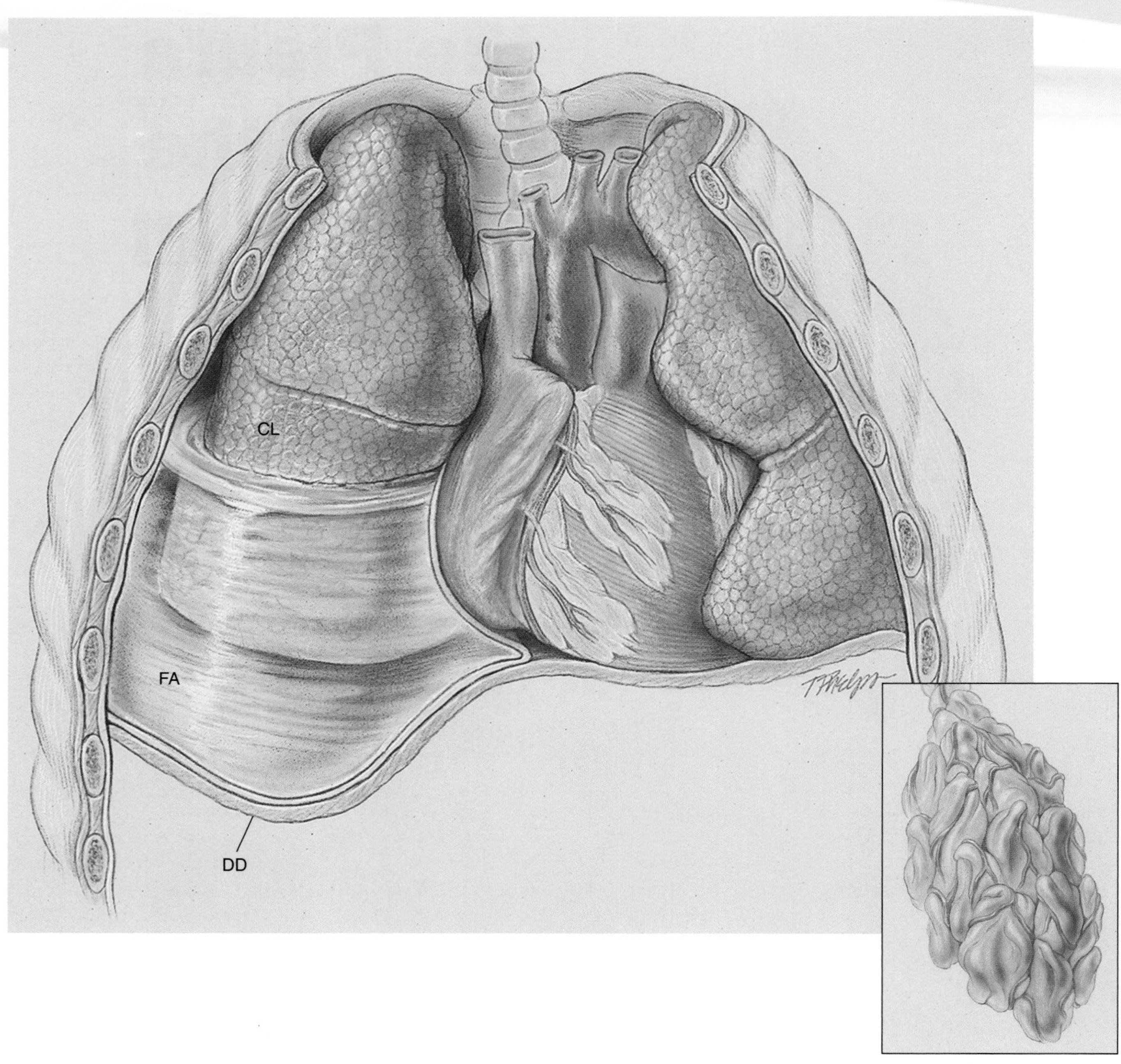

FIGURE 23-1 Right-sided pleural effusion. *CL,* Collapsed lung (partially collapsed); *DD,* depressed diaphragm; *FA,* fluid accumulation. *Inset,* Atelectasis, a common secondary anatomic alteration of the lungs.

Chapter Objectives

After reading this chapter, you will be able to:

- List the anatomic alterations of the lungs associated with pleural diseases.
- Describe the causes of pleural diseases.
- List the cardiopulmonary clinical manifestations associated with pleural diseases.
- Describe the general management of pleural diseases.

- Describe the clinical strategies and rationales of the SOAPs presented in the case study.
- Define key terms and complete self-assessment questions at the end of the chapter and on Evolve.

Key Terms

Chylothorax
Congestive Heart Failure
Empyema
Exudative Pleural Effusions
Hemothorax
Hepatic Hydrothorax
Left-Sided Heart Failure
Malignant Mesothelioma
Meniscus Sign
Nephrotic Syndrome
Peritoneal Dialysis
Pleurodesis
Postpneumonic Pleural Effusion
Pulmonary Embolism or Infarction
Right-Sided Heart Failure
Transudative Pleural Effusions

Chapter Outline

Anatomic Alterations of the Lungs

A number of pleural diseases can cause fluid to accumulate in the pleural space; this fluid is called a **pleural effusion**, or if infected, an **empyema** (see Figure 23-1). Similar to free air in the pleural space, fluid accumulation separates the visceral and parietal pleura and compresses the lungs. In severe cases, atelectasis will develop, the great veins may be compressed, and cardiac venous return may be diminished. Pleural effusion and empyema produce a restrictive lung disorder.

The major pathologic or structural changes associated with significant pleural effusion are as follows:

- Lung compression
- Atelectasis
- Compression of the great veins and decreased cardiac venous return

Etiology and Epidemiology

Pleural effusion affects approximately 1.3 million people each year in the United States. Early signs and symptoms include pleuritic chest pain, "chest pressure," dyspnea, and cough. Chest *pain* can occur early when there is intense inflammation of the pleural surfaces. "Chest pressure" usually develops until the effusion is in the moderate (500 to 1500 mL) to large (>1500 mL) category. Dyspnea rarely occurs in small effusions unless significant pleurisy is present. A cough is usually directly related to the degree of atelectasis caused by the effusion.

A pleural effusion may be transudative or exudative. A transudate develops when fluid from the pulmonary capillaries moves into the pleural space. The fluid is thin and watery, containing a few blood cells and little protein. The pleural surfaces are not involved in producing the transudate. In contrast, an exudate develops when the pleural surfaces are diseased. The fluid has a high protein content and a great deal of cellular debris. Exudate is usually caused by inflammation, infection, or malignancy. **Transudative pleural effusions** and **exudative pleural effusions** are differentiated by comparing the chemistries of the pleural fluid with those of the blood. The pleural effusion is classified as exudative when one or more of the following is found in the pleural fluid:

- Pleural fluid protein >2.9 g/dL (29 g/L)
- Pleural fluid cholesterol >45 mg/dL (1.16 mmol/L)
- Pleural fluid lactate dehydrogenase (LDH) >60% of upper limit for serum

Common Causes of Transudative Pleural Effusion

Congestive Heart Failure

Congestive heart failure is the most common cause of pleural effusion. Both right- and left-sided heart failure can result in pleural effusion. In general, left-sided heart failure is more likely to produce pleural effusion than right-sided heart failure. In **right-sided heart failure** (cor pulmonale), an increase in the hydrostatic pressure in the systemic circulation can (1) increase the rate of pleural fluid formation and (2) decrease lymphatic drainage from the pleural space because of the elevated systemic venous pressure. In **left-sided heart failure**, an increase in hydrostatic pressure in the pulmonary circulation can (1) decrease the rate of pleural fluid absorption through the visceral pleura and (2) cause fluid movement through the visceral pleura into the pleural space.

Hepatic Hydrothorax

Occasionally, pleural effusions can develop as a complication of hepatic cirrhosis, particularly when ascitic fluid is present in the abdomen. The pleural effusion in these patients is generally right-sided.

Peritoneal Dialysis

As in the pleural effusion that occurs as a result of abdominal ascites, pleural fluid also may develop as a complication of

peritoneal dialysis. When the peritoneal dialysis is stopped, the pleural effusion usually disappears rapidly.

Nephrotic Syndrome

Pleural effusion is commonly seen in patients with **nephrotic syndrome.** It is generally bilateral. The effusion is a result of the decreased plasma oncotic pressure that develops in patients with this disorder.

Pulmonary Embolism or Infarction

Thirty percent to 50% of patients with pulmonary arterial emboli develop pleural effusion. Two distinct mechanisms are responsible. First, obstruction of the pulmonary vasculature can lead to right-sided heart failure, which in turn can lead to pleural effusion. The second mechanism involves the increased permeability of the capillaries in the visceral pleura that develops in response to the ischemic infarction caused by the pulmonary emboli.

Common Causes of Exudative Pleural Effusion

Malignant Pleural Effusions

About two thirds of malignant pleural effusions occur in women. Malignant pleural effusions are highly associated with breast and gynecologic malignancies.

Malignant Mesotheliomas

Malignant mesotheliomas arise from the mesothelial cells that line the pleural cavities. Individuals with chronic asbestos exposure have a much greater risk for developing mesothelioma. The pleural fluid is exudative and generally contains a mixture of normal mesothelial cells, differentiated and undifferentiated malignant mesothelial cells, and a varying number of lymphocytes and polymorphonuclear leukocytes.

Bacterial Pneumonias

As many as 40% of patients with bacterial pneumonia have an accompanying pleural effusion. Most pleural effusions associated with pneumonia resolve without any specific therapy. Approximately 10%, however, require some sort of therapeutic intervention. If appropriate antibiotic therapy is not instituted, bacteria invade the pleural fluid from the lung parenchyma. Eventually, pus will accumulate in the pleural cavity **(empyema)**. Pleural effusion also can be produced by viruses, *Mycoplasma pneumoniae,* and *Rickettsia,* although the pleural effusions are usually small.

Tuberculosis

Pleural effusion may develop from extension of a caseous tubercle into the pleural cavity. It also is possible that the inflammatory reaction that develops in tuberculosis obstructs the lymphatic pores in the parietal pleura. This in turn leads to an accumulation of protein and fluid in the pleural space. Pleural effusion caused by tuberculosis is generally unilateral and small to moderate in size (see Chapter 17).

Fungal Diseases

Patients with fungal diseases occasionally have secondary pleural effusions. Common fungal diseases that may produce pleural effusions are histoplasmosis, coccidioidomycosis, and blastomycosis (see Chapter 18).

Pleural Effusion Resulting from Diseases of the Gastrointestinal Tract

Pleural effusion is sometimes associated with diseases of the gastrointestinal tract such as pancreatitis, subphrenic abscess, intrahepatic abscess, esophageal perforation, abdominal operations, and diaphragmatic hernia.

Pleural Effusion Resulting from Collagen Vascular Diseases

Pleural effusion occasionally develops as a complication of collagen vascular diseases. Such diseases include rheumatoid pleuritis, systemic lupus erythematosus, Sjögren's syndrome, familial Mediterranean fever, and Wegener's granulomatosis.

Other Pathologic Fluids That Separate the Parietal from the Visceral Pleura

In addition to transudate and exudate, other pathologic fluids can separate the parietal pleura from the visceral pleura.

Empyema

The accumulation of pus in the pleural cavity is called *empyema.* Empyema commonly develops as a result of inflammation. Thoracentesis may confirm the diagnosis and determine the specific causative organism. The pus is usually removed by chest tube drainage. Open thoracotomy drainage may occasionally be necessary.

Chylothorax

Chylothorax is the presence of chyle in the pleural cavity. Chyle is a milky liquid produced from the food in the small intestine during digestion. It consists mainly of fat particles in a stable emulsion. Chyle is taken up by fingerlike intestinal lymphatics called *lacteals* and transported by the thoracic duct to the neck. From the thoracic duct the chyle moves into the venous circulation and mixes with blood. The presence of chyle in the pleural cavity is usually caused by trauma to the neck or thorax or by cancer occluding the thoracic duct.

Hemothorax

The presence of blood in the pleural space is known as a **hemothorax.** Most of these are caused by penetrating or blunt chest trauma. An iatrogenic hemothorax may develop from trauma caused by the insertion of a central venous or pulmonary artery catheter.

Blood can gain entrance into the pleural space from trauma to the chest wall, diaphragm, lung, or mediastinum. A hematocrit of the pleural fluid should always be obtained if the pleural fluid looks like blood. A hemothorax is said to be present only when the hematocrit of the pleural fluid is at least 50%.

OVERVIEW of the Cardiopulmonary Clinical Manifestations Associated with Pleural Effusion and Empyema

The following clinical manifestations result from the pathologic mechanisms caused (or activated) by **Atelectasis** (see Figure 9-7)—the major anatomic alteration of the lungs associated with pleural effusion (see Figure 24-1).

CLINICAL DATA OBTAINED AT THE PATIENT'S BEDSIDE

The Physical Examination

Vital Signs

Increased Respiratory Rate (Tachypnea)

Several pathophysiologic mechanisms operating simultaneously may lead to an increased ventilatory rate:

- Stimulation of peripheral chemoreceptors (hypoxemia)
- Decreased lung compliance–increased ventilatory rate relationship
- Activation of the deflation receptors
- Activation of the irritant receptors
- Stimulation of J receptors
- Pain, anxiety

Increased Heart Rate (Pulse) and Blood Pressure

Chest Pain, Decreased Chest Expansion

Cyanosis

Cough (Dry, Nonproductive)

Chest Assessment Findings

- Tracheal shift
- Decreased tactile and vocal fremitus
- Dull percussion note
- Diminished breath sounds
- Displaced heart sounds
- Pleural friction rub (occasionally)

CLINICAL DATA OBTAINED FROM LABORATORY TESTS AND SPECIAL PROCEDURES

Pulmonary Function Test Findings (Restrictive Lung Pathology)

LUNG VOLUME AND CAPACITY FINDINGS

V_T	IRV	ERV	RV	
N or ↓	↓	↓	↓	
VC	IC	FRC	TLC	RV/TLC ratio
↓	↓	↓	↓	N

Arterial Blood Gases

SMALL PLEURAL EFFUSION

Acute Alveolar Hyperventilation with Hypoxemia (Acute Respiratory Alkalosis)

pH	Pa_{CO_2}	HCO_3^-	Pa_{O_2}
↑	↓	↓ (slightly)	↓

LARGE PLEURAL EFFUSION

Acute Ventilatory Failure with Hypoxemia (Acute Respiratory Acidosis)

pH*	Pa_{CO_2}	HCO_3^- *	Pa_{O_2}
↓	↑	↑ (slightly)	↓

*When tissue hypoxia is severe enough to produce lactic acid, the pH and HCO_3^- values will be lower than expected for a particular Pa_{CO_2} level.

Oxygenation Indices* (Large Pleural Effusion)

$\dot{Q}_S/\dot{Q}_T$	D_{O_2}†	$\dot{V}_{O_2}$	$C(a-\bar{v})_{O_2}$	O_2ER	$S\bar{v}_{O_2}$
↑	↓	N	↑ (severe)	↑	↓

†The D_{O_2} may be normal in patients who have compensated to the decreased oxygenation status with (1) an increased cardiac output, (2) an increased hemoglobin level, or (3) a combination of both. When the D_{O_2} is normal, the O_2ER is usually normal.

Hemodynamic Indices‡ (Large Pleural Effusion)

CVP	RAP	$\overline{PA}$	PCWP	CO	SV
↑	↑	↑	↓	↓	↓
SVI	CI	RVSWI	LVSWI	PVR	SVR
↓	↓	↑	↓	↑	↓

RADIOLOGIC FINDINGS

Chest Radiograph

- Blunting of the costophrenic angle
- Fluid level on the affected side (see Figure 23-2)
- Depressed diaphragm
- Mediastinal shift (possibly) to unaffected side
- Atelectasis
- "Meniscus sign"

The diagnosis of a pleural effusion is generally based on the chest x-ray film. A pleural effusion of less than 300 mL usually cannot be seen on an upright chest x-ray film. In moderate pleural effusion (>1000 mL) in the upright position, an increased density usually appears at the costophrenic angle. The fluid first accumulates posteriorly in the most dependent part of the thoracic cavity between the inferior surface of the lower lobe and the diaphragm. As the fluid volume increases, it extends upward around the anterior, lateral, and posterior thoracic walls in the so-called "**meniscus sign**" (see Figure 23-3). Interlobar fissures are sometimes highlighted as a result of fluid filling.

As nicely illustrated in the chest radiograph of a pleural effusion shown in Figure 23-2, the lateral costophrenic angle is usually obliterated, and the outline of the diaphragm on the

*$C(a-\bar{v})_{O_2}$, Arterial-venous oxygen difference; D_{O_2}, total oxygen delivery; O_2ER, oxygen extraction ratio; $\dot{Q}_S/\dot{Q}_T$, pulmonary shunt fraction; $S\bar{v}_{O_2}$, mixed venous oxygen saturation; $\dot{V}_{O_2}$, oxygen consumption.

†*CO*, Cardiac output; *CVP*, central venous pressure; *LVSWI*, left ventricular stroke work index; *$\overline{PA}$*, mean pulmonary artery pressure; *PCWP*, pulmonary capillary wedge pressure; *PVR*, pulmonary vascular resistance; *RAP*, right atrial pressure; *RVSWI*, right ventricular stroke work index; *SV*, stroke volume; *SVI*, stroke volume index; *SVR*, systemic vascular resistance.

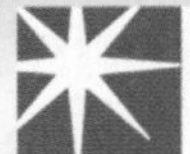

OVERVIEW of the Cardiopulmonary Clinical Manifestations Associated with Pleural Effusion and Empyema—cont'd

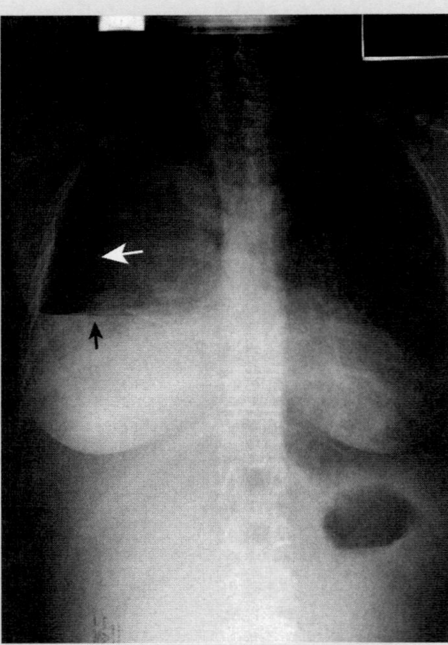

FIGURE 23-2 Right-sided pleural effusion *(small black arrow)* complicated by a pneumothorax *(large white arrow)*. Note that the lateral costophrenic angle on the right side is obliterated, and the outline of the diaphragm on the affected side is lost.

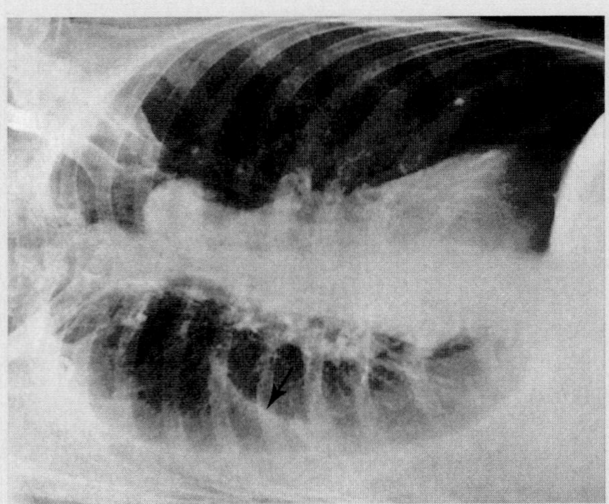

FIGURE 23-3 Subpulmonic pleural effusion. Right lateral decubitus view. Subdiaphragmatic fluid has run up the lateral chest wall, producing a band of soft tissue or water density (meniscus sign). The medial curvilinear shadow *(arrow)* indicates fluid in the major fissure.

affected side is lost. In severe cases the weight of the fluid may cause the diaphragm to become inverted (concave). Clinically this inversion is seen only in left-sided pleural effusions; the gastric air bubble is pushed downward, and the superior border of the left diaphragmatic leaf is concave. In addition, the mediastinum may be shifted to the unaffected side, and the intercostal spaces may appear widened.

Pleural effusion, atelectasis, and parenchymal infiltrates can obliterate one or both diaphragms. Therefore when a posteroanterior or lateral chest radiograph suggests pleural effusion, additional radiographic studies are generally necessary to document the presence of pleural fluid or other pathology. The lateral decubitus radiograph is recommended because free fluid gravitates to the most dependent part of the pleural space and layers out there (Figure 23-3).

General Management of Pleural Effusion

The management of each patient with a pleural effusion must be individualized. Questions to be asked include the following: Should a thoracentesis be performed? Can the underlying cause be treated? What is the appropriate antibiotic? Should a chest tube be inserted? When it is determined that a chest tube should be inserted, it is normally placed in the fourth or fifth intercostal space at the midaxillary line. Typically, a No. 28 to No. 36 French gauge thoracostomy tube is used for adults, with a smaller size used for children.

The best way to resolve a pleural effusion is to direct the treatment at what is causing it, rather than treating the effusion itself. For example, if the heart failure is reversed or the lung infection is cured by antibiotics, the effusion usually resolves. When the cause of the pleural effusion is not readily evident, microscopic and chemical examination of pleural fluid may determine whether the effusion is a transudate or an exudate. If the fluid is a transudate, treatment is directed to the underlying problem (e.g., congestive heart failure, cirrhosis, nephrosis).

When an exudate is present, a cytologic examination may identify a malignancy. The fluid also may be examined for its biochemical makeup (e.g., protein, sugar, various enzymes) and for the presence of bacteria. Examination of the effusion may reveal blood after trauma or surgery, pus in empyema, or milky fluid in chylothorax. The presence of blood in the pleural fluid in the absence of trauma or surgery suggests malignant disease or pulmonary embolization or infarction.

Respiratory Care Treatment Protocols

Oxygen Therapy Protocol

Oxygen therapy is used to treat hypoxemia, decrease the work of breathing, and decrease myocardial work. The hypoxemia that develops in pleural effusion is mostly caused by the **atelectasis** and pulmonary shunting associated with the disorder. Hypoxemia caused by capillary shunting is often refractory to oxygen therapy (see Oxygen Therapy Protocol, Protocol 9-1).

Lung Expansion Therapy Protocol

Lung expansion techniques are often administered to offset the alveolar atelectasis associated with pleural effusions (see Lung Expansion Therapy Protocol, Protocol 9-3).

Mechanical Ventilation Protocol

Because acute ventilatory failure and hypoxemia may be seen in severe pleural effusions, continuous mechanical ventilation may be required to maintain an adequate ventilatory status. Continuous mechanical ventilation is justified when the acute ventilatory failure is thought to be reversible (see Mechanical Ventilation Protocols, Protocol 9-5, Protocol 9-6, and Protocol 9-7).

Pleurodesis

A **pleurodesis** may be performed to cause irritation and inflammation (pleuritis) between the parietal and visceral layers of the pleural. This action causes the pleurae to stick together and thereby prevents subsequent fluid accumulation of the pleura.

CASE STUDY

Pleural Effusion and Empyema

Admitting History

Against her doctor's advice, a 38-year-old white woman had discharged herself from the hospital about 2 months before the admission discussed here. She had originally been admitted for severe right lower lobe pneumonia. After 5 days of treatment, she became angry because she was not allowed to smoke. She was a longtime, three-pack-per-day smoker. When a nurse found her smoking in her hospital bed while on a 2 L/min oxygen nasal cannula, the nurse quickly confiscated her cigarettes and matches.

The woman became upset. She told her doctor that this was the last straw and that she was going to leave the hospital on her own. Her doctor wanted her to remain so that a thorough follow-up could be performed for what was described as a "spot" on her lower right lung. The woman promised that she would make an appointment at the doctor's office the next week. She then got dressed and left. However, 2 days after she left the hospital, she felt so much better that she decided the spot on her lung was not an issue for concern. The woman told her friends that smoking one pack of cigarettes made her feel better than 5 days' worth of nurses, doctors, and hospitals.

On the day of the admission discussed here, the woman appeared at the doctor's office without an appointment. She told the receptionist that something was very wrong. She thought that she had the flu and that it had been getting progressively worse over the previous 4 days. At the time of the office visit, she could speak in short sentences only and was unable to inhale deeply. Seeing that the woman was in obvious respiratory distress, the nurse interrupted the doctor. Within 5 minutes, the doctor had the woman transported and admitted to the hospital a few blocks away.

Physical Examination

The woman appeared malnourished, exhibited poor personal hygiene, and had yellow tobacco stains around her fingers. She appeared to be in moderate to severe respiratory distress. Her nails and mucous membranes were cyanotic, and her shirt was wet from perspiration. She demonstrated an occasional hacking, nonproductive cough. She stated that she could not take a deep breath and that maybe the problem stemmed from "that spot" on her lung.

Her vital signs were as follows: blood pressure 130/60, heart rate 112 bpm, and respiratory rate 36/min with shallow respirations. She was slightly febrile, with an oral temperature of 37.7° C (99.8° F). Palpation showed that the trachea was shifted slightly to the left. Dull percussion notes were found over the right middle and right lower lobes. Auscultation revealed normal vesicular breath sounds over the left lung fields and upper right lobe. No breath sounds could be heard over the right middle and right lower lobes.

The patient's chest x-ray film showed a large, right-sided pleural effusion. The right costophrenic angle demonstrated blunting, the right hemidiaphragm was depressed, and the right middle and lower lung lobes were partially collapsed and showed changes consistent with pneumonia. The arterial blood gas values (ABGs) on a 3 L/min oxygen nasal cannula were as follows: pH 7.48, $Pa{CO_2}$ 24, HCO_3^- 17, and $Pa{O_2}$ 37. The oxygen saturation measured by pulse oximetry ($Sp{O_2}$) was 72%. The doctor, assisted by the respiratory therapist, performed a thoracentesis on the patient at the bedside. Slightly more than 2 L of yellow fluid was withdrawn. The patient then was started on intravenous antibiotics. A portable chest x-ray examination was ordered, and a respiratory care consultation was requested. On the basis of these clinical data, the following SOAP was documented.

Respiratory Assessment and Plan

S "I can't take a deep breath."

O Malnourished appearance with poor personal hygiene; cyanosis with an occasional hacking, nonproductive cough; vital signs: BP 130/60, HR 112, RR 36 and shallow, T 37.7° C (99.8° F); trachea slightly shifted to the left; dull percussion notes over the right middle and right lower lobes; normal vesicular breath sounds over the left lung fields and right upper lobe; no breath sounds over the right middle and right lower lobes; CXR: large, right-sided pleural effusion, right middle and right lower lobes partially collapsed and consolidated; about 2 L of yellow fluid obtained via thoracentesis; ABGs (on 3 L/min O_2 by nasal cannula): pH 7.48 , $Pa{CO_2}$ 24, HCO_3^- 17, $Pa{O_2}$ 37, $Sp{O_2}$ 72%

A
- Right-sided pneumonia and pleural effusion (CXR)
- Partially collapsed right middle and lower lobes; atelectasis versus pneumonia (CXR)
- Respiratory distress (vital signs, ABGs)
- Acute alveolar hyperventilation with severe hypoxemia (ABGs)
- Metabolic (lactic) acidosis likely (ABGs compared with $P{CO_2}$/HCO_3^-/pH relationship nomogram)

P Begin **Lung Expansion Therapy Protocol** (incentive spirometry q2h) and **Oxygen Therapy Protocol** ($F{IO_2}$ = 0.50 per HAFOE mask). Monitor vital signs carefully and reevaluate.

3 Hours after Admission

At this time the patient was sitting up in bed. She stated that although she was feeling better, she did not feel great. She still had an occasional dry-sounding, nonproductive cough. Her skin appeared pale. She was still cyanotic. She was no longer perspiring, as she was when she was first admitted. Her vital signs were as follows: blood pressure 135/85, heart rate 100 bpm, respiratory rate 24/min, and temperature normal. Her respiratory efforts, however, no longer appeared shallow. Palpation of the chest was not remarkable. Dull percussion notes were found over the right middle and right lower lobes. Normal vesicular breath sounds were heard over the left lung and upper right lung. Loud bronchial breath sounds were audible over the right middle and right lower lobes.

The patient's chest x-ray showed a small, right-sided pleural effusion. Increased opacity was still present in the right middle and lower lung, consistent with pneumonia. The patient's trachea and mediastinum were in their normal positions. On an F_{IO_2} of 0.50, her ABGs were as follows: pH 7.52, Pa_{CO_2} 29, HCO_3^- 22, and Pa_{O_2} 57. Her Sp_{O_2} was 92%. At this time, the following SOAP was charted.

Respiratory Assessment and Plan

S "I'm feeling better but not great yet."

O Cyanotic and pale appearance; occasional dry, nonproductive cough; vital signs: BP 135/85, HR 100, RR 24, T normal; dull percussion notes over right middle and right lower lobes; normal vesicular breath sounds over left lung and over right upper lobe; bronchial breath sounds over right middle and lower lobes; CXR: small right-sided pleural effusion; right middle and right lower lobe consolidation; ABGs: pH 7.52, Pa_{CO_2} 29, HCO_3^- 22, Pa_{O_2} 57; Sp_{O_2} 92% on an F_{IO_2} of 0.50.

A
- Small right-sided pneumonia and pleural effusion, greatly improved (CXR)
- Atelectasis and consolidation in right middle and lower lung lobes (CXR)
- Continued respiratory distress, but improving (vital signs, ABGs)
- Acute alveolar hyperventilation with moderate hypoxemia, improved (ABGs)

P Up-regulate **Lung Expansion Therapy Protocol** (CPAP mask at 10 cm H_2O q2h for 15 minutes). Up-regulate **Oxygen Therapy Protocol** (F_{IO_2} = 0.60 per HAFOE mask). Monitor and reevaluate.

5 Hours after Admission

The patient was sitting in a semi-Fowler's position. She appeared relaxed and alert. She stated that she had finally caught her breath. Although she still appeared pale, she did not look cyanotic. No spontaneous cough was observed at this time.

Her vital signs were as follows: blood pressure 128/79, heart rate 88 bpm, respiratory rate 16/min, and temperature normal. Palpation of the chest was unremarkable. Dull percussion notes were found over the right middle and right lower lobes. Normal vesicular breath sounds were heard over the left lung and right upper lobe. Bronchial breath sounds were audible over the right middle and right lower lobes. No current chest x-ray was available. The patient's ABG values on an F_{IO_2} of 0.60 were as follows: pH 7.45, Pa_{CO_2} 36, HCO_3^- 24, and Pa_{O_2} 77. Her Sp_{O_2} was 95%. On the basis of these clinical data, the following SOAP was documented.

Respiratory Assessment and Plan

S "I've finally caught my breath."

O Relaxed, alert appearance, in semi-Fowler's position; paleness but no cyanosis; no spontaneous cough; vital signs: BP 128/79, HR 88, RR 16, T normal; dull percussion notes in right middle and right lower lung lobes; normal vesicular breath sounds over left lung and right upper lobe; bronchial breath sounds over right middle and right lower lobes; ABGs: pH 7.45, Pa_{CO_2} 36, HCO_3^- 24, Pa_{O_2} 77; Sp_{O_2} 95%

A
- Small, right-sided pneumonia and pleural effusion, greatly improved (previous CXR)
- Atelectasis and consolidation in right middle and right lower lung lobes (previous CXR)
- Normal acid-base status with mild hypoxemia (ABGs)

P Maintain present level of **Lung Expansion Therapy Protocol** and **Oxygen Therapy Protocols.** Monitor and reevaluate each shift.

Discussion

This case illustrates a patient with postpneumonic pleural effusion, one of the pleural diseases that generally can be improved with appropriate therapy (in this case a 2-L thoracentesis).

During the first assessment, the respiratory care practitioner recognizes that the patient has significant respiratory morbidity. Indeed, the patient has an extensive right-sided pneumonia and pleural effusion and partially collapsed right middle and lower lobes. Clearly the patient is in respiratory distress. The patient's acute alveolar hyperventilation and severe hypoxemia are a direct result of the partial collapse of the lung lobes. Because of the extremely low Pa_{O_2} noted on the initial arterial blood gas, the presence of lactic acid is very likely. In fact, this was confirmed by the respiratory practitioner with the P_{CO_2}/HCO_3^-/pH nomogram. Understanding that **Atelectasis** is the main pathophysiologic mechanism operating in this case (see Figure 9-8), the practitioner correctly assesses the situation as one that requires careful monitoring and begins the **Lung Expansion Therapy Protocol** (Protocol 9-3) (with incentive spirometry) and the **Oxygen Therapy Protocol** (Protocol 9-1) (with a high concentration of oxygen).

A trial of **bronchopulmonary hygiene therapy** would not be unwarranted in this case, given the patient's cigarette smoking history alone or the degree of severity of the condition. Admittedly, the physical findings in this patient (no sputum production) did not indicate such therapy. Given the patient's history, the respiratory care practitioner also would be interested in the results of the cytologic studies for malignancy in both the sputum and thoracentesis fluid. Frequently, blood gases do not improve immediately after a thoracentesis, despite the fluid removal, because the atelectasis under the pleural effusion takes some time (hours or days) to dissipate. For this reason, the **Lung Expansion Therapy Protocol,** after thoracentesis, is appropriate.

At the time of the second assessment, the patient was beginning to improve, although she still had signs of right middle and lower lobe **Consolidation** (Figure 9-9). Good breath sounds were heard over the left lung and upper right lung, although bronchial breath sounds reflecting consolidation were still noted on the right. The respiratory care practitioner was appropriately concerned that atelectasis was still present, and in such a case he or she should increase the **Lung Expansion Therapy Protocol** (Protocol 9-3). In this case, the practitioner selected a continuous positive airway pressure (CPAP) mask at 10 cm H_2O every 2 hours for 15 minutes. The practitioner could have also intensified use of incentive spirometry, carefully used intermittent positive-pressure breathing (IPPB) or extended the amount of time the patient was using the CPAP mask.

In the last assessment the patient continued to do fairly well, although she was far from returning to baseline values. The pneumonitis, atelectasis, and mild hypoxemia, which persisted despite supplemental oxygen therapy, suggested the need for continued significant (though unchanged) therapy. This case demonstrates that in-place therapy often does not need to be changed at each assessment. Indeed, this guide may apply to as many as 50% to 60% of accurately performed seriatim assessments. For pedagogic reasons, this option has not been exercised often in this text. However, this third assessment (in a patient with pleural effusion and underlying atelectasis and pneumonia) is a good case in point.

SELF-ASSESSMENT QUESTIONS

evolve Answers to questions can be found on Evolve. To access additional student assessment questions and case studies for application of text material to real-life scenarios, visit **http://evolve.elsevier.com/DesJardins/respiratory.**

1. Which of the following is or are associated with exudative effusion?

1. Few blood cells
2. Inflammation
3. Thin and watery fluid
4. Disease of the pleural surfaces

   a. 2 only
   b. 4 only
   c. 1 and 3 only
   d. 2 and 4 only

2. Which of the following is probably the most common cause of a transudative pleural effusion?

a. Pulmonary embolus
b. Congestive heart failure
c. Hepatic hydrothorax
d. Nephrotic syndrome

3. A hemothorax is said to be present when the hematocrit of the pleural fluid is at least what?

a. 20%
b. 30%
c. 40%
d. 50%

4. Approximately what percentage of patients with pulmonary emboli develop pleural effusion?

a. 0% to 20%
b. 20% to 30%
c. 30% to 50%
d. 50% to 60%

5. Which of the following is or are associated with pleural effusion?

1. Increased RV
2. Decreased FRC
3. Increased V_T
4. Decreased VC

   a. 1 only
   b. 3 only
   c. 1 and 3 only
   d. 2 and 4 only

Kyphoscoliosis

24

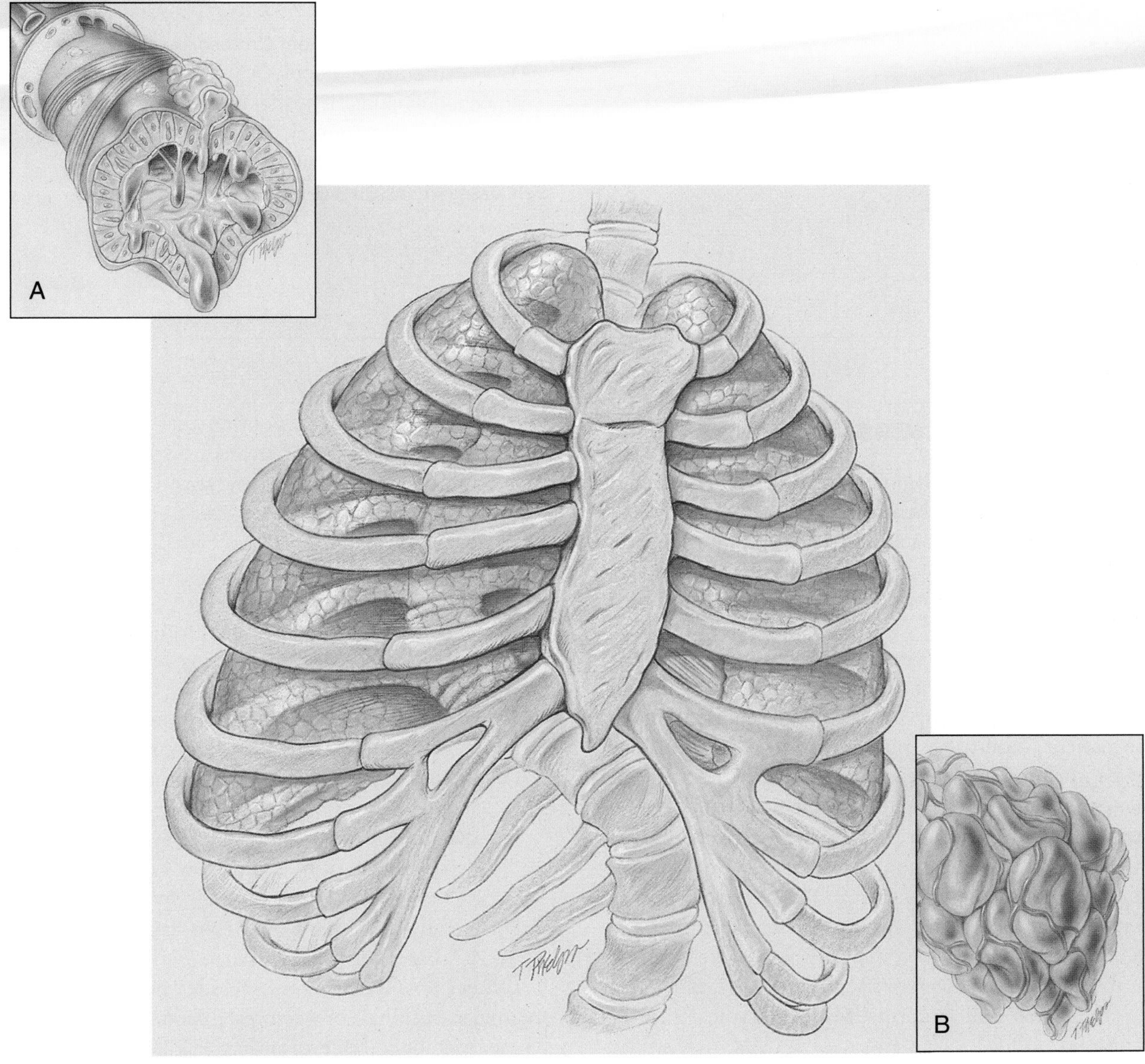

FIGURE 24-1 Kyphoscoliosis. Posterior and lateral curvature of the spine causing lung compression. Excessive bronchial secretions (**A**) and atelectasis (**B**) are common secondary anatomic alterations of the lungs.

Chapter Objectives

After reading this chapter, you will be able to:

- List the anatomic alterations of the lungs associated with kyphoscoliosis.
- Describe the causes of kyphoscoliosis.
- List the cardiopulmonary clinical manifestations associated with kyphoscoliosis.
- Describe the general management of kyphoscoliosis.
- Describe the clinical strategies and rationales of the SOAPs presented in the case study.
- Define key terms and complete self-assessment questions at the end of the chapter and on Evolve.

Key Terms

Adolescent Scoliosis
Boston Brace
Charleston Bending Brace
Cobb Angle
Congenital Scoliosis
Harrington Rod
Idiopathic Scoliosis
Infantile Scoliosis
Juvenile Scoliosis
Kyphoscoliosis
Kyphosis
Milwaukee Brace
Neuromuscular Scoliosis
Nonstructural Scoliosis
Rod Instrumentation
Scoliosis
Spinal Fusion
Structural Scoliosis

Chapter Outline

Anatomic Alterations of the Lungs

Kyphoscoliosis is a combination of two thoracic deformities that commonly appear together. **Kyphosis** is a posterior curvature of the spine (humpback). In **scoliosis** the spine is curved to one side, typically appearing as an S or C shape. Its appearance is most obvious in the anterior-posterior plane.

In severe kyphoscoliosis the deformity of the thorax compresses the lungs and restricts alveolar expansion, which in turn causes alveolar hypoventilation and atelectasis. In addition, the patient's ability to cough and mobilize secretions also may be impaired, further causing atelectasis as secretions accumulate throughout the tracheobronchial tree. Because kyphoscoliosis involves both a posterior and a lateral curvature of the spine, the thoracic contents generally twist in such a way as to cause a mediastinal shift in the same direction as the lateral curvature of the spine. Severe kyphoscoliosis causes a chronic restrictive lung disorder that makes it more difficult to clear airway secretions. Figure 24-1 illustrates the lung and chest wall abnormalities in a typical case of kyphoscoliosis.

The major pathologic or structural changes of the lungs associated with kyphoscoliosis are as follows:

- Lung restriction and compression as a result of the thoracic deformity
- Mediastinal shift
- Mucous accumulation throughout the tracheobronchial tree
- Atelectasis

Etiology and Epidemiology

Kyphoscoliosis affects approximately 2% of the people in the United States—mostly young children who are going through a growing spurt. Kyphoscoliosis rarely develops in the adult—unless it is a worsening condition that started in childhood and was not diagnosed or treated. Kyphoscoliosis may also develop in adults from a degenerative joint condition in the spine. Although the precise cause of kyphoscoliosis is unknown, it is commonly associated with the following general conditions:

- **Congenital scoliosis**
  - A condition resulting from a formation of the spine or fused ribs during fetal development.
- **Neuromuscular scoliosis**
  - A condition caused by poor muscle control, muscle weakness, or paralysis because of diseases such as cerebral palsy, muscular dystrophy, spina bifida, or poliomyelitis.
- **Idiopathic scoliosis**
  - Scoliosis from an unknown cause. It appears in a previously straight spine. When kyphoscoliosis arises without a known cause (80% to 85% of cases), it is called *idiopathic kyphoscoliosis.*

Other possible causes include hormonal imbalance, trauma, extraspinal contractures, infections involving the vertebrae, metabolic bone disorders (e.g., rickets, osteoporosis, osteogenesis imperfecta), joint disease, and tumors.

Depending on the child's age at the time of onset, idiopathic scoliosis is classified as infantile, juvenile, or adolescent. In **infantile scoliosis** the curvature of the spine develops during the first 3 years of life. In **juvenile scoliosis** the curvature occurs at 4 years of age to the onset of adolescence. In **adolescent scoliosis** the spinal curvature develops after the age of 10. Adolescent scoliosis is the most common. Early signs (i.e., appearing when a child is approximately 8 years of age) of scoliosis include uneven shoulder height, prominent shoulder blade(s), uneven waist height, elevated hips, and leaning to one side. Risk factors include the following:

- Sex—Girls are more likely to develop curvature of the spine than boys.

- Age—The younger the child is when the diagnosis is first made, the greater the chance of curve progression.
- Angle of the curve—The greater the curvature of the spine, the greater the risk that the curve progression will worsen.
- Location—Curves in the middle to lower spine are less likely to progress than those in the upper spine.
- Height—Taller people have a greater chance of curve progression.
- Spinal problems at birth—Children with scoliosis at birth (congenital scoliosis) have a greater risk for worsening of the curve.

Diagnosis

Scoliosis is diagnosed by means of the patient's medical history, physical examination, x-ray evaluation, and curve measurement. Clinically, scoliosis is commonly defined according to the following factors related to the curvature of the spine:

- Shape (**nonstructural scoliosis** and **structural scoliosis**)—A nonstructural scoliosis is a curve that develops side-to-side as a C- or S-shaped curve. This form of scoliosis results from a cause other than the spine itself (e.g., poor posture, leg length discrepancy, pain). A structural scoliosis is a curvature of the spine associated with vertebral rotation. A structural scoliosis involves the twisting of the spine and appears in three dimensions.
- Location—The curve of the spine may develop in the upper back area where the ribs are located (thoracic), the lower back area (lumbar), or in both areas (thoracolumbar).
- Direction—Scoliosis can bend the spine left or right.
- Angle—A normal spine viewed from the back is zero degrees—a straight line. Scoliosis is defined as a spinal curvature of greater than 10 degrees (i.e., bending toward the ground when in the upright position). The degree of the lateral curvature is expressed by the **Cobb angle,** which is calculated from a radiograph as shown in Figure 24-2.

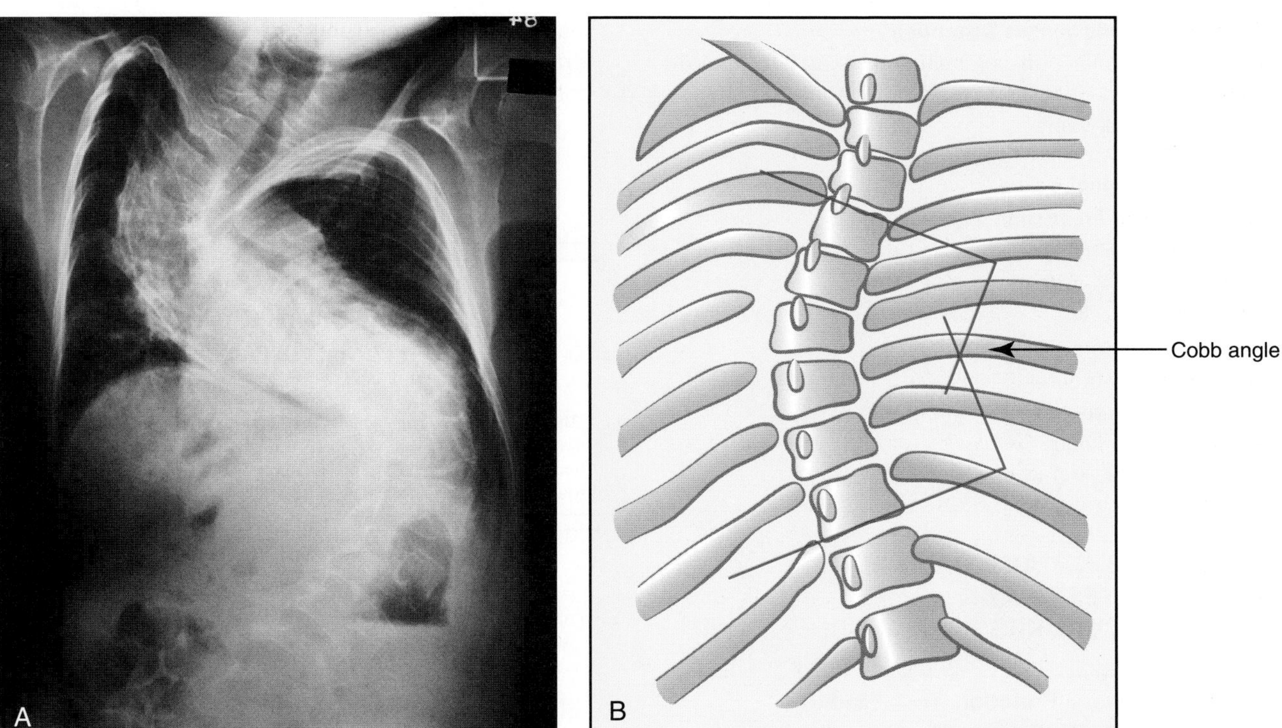

FIGURE 24-2 **A**, Chest x-ray on patient with kyphoscoliosis. **B**, Method of calculating the Cobb angle. *Scoliosis* is defined as a spinal curvature of 10 degrees or greater. Because the Cobb angle reflects curvature only in a single plane, it may fail to fully identify the severity of the scoliosis—especially when the patient has vertebral rotation and three-dimensional spinal deformity.

OVERVIEW of the Cardiopulmonary Clinical Manifestations Associated with Kyphoscoliosis

The following clinical manifestations result from the pathophysiologic mechanisms caused (or activated) by **Atelectasis** (see Figure 9-8) and **Excessive Airway Secretions** (see Figure 9-12)—the major anatomic alterations of the lungs associated with kyphoscoliosis (see Figure 24-1).

CLINICAL DATA OBTAINED AT THE PATIENT'S BEDSIDE

The Physical Examination

Vital Signs

Increased Respiratory Rate (Tachypnea)

Several pathophysiologic mechanisms operating simultaneously may lead to an increased ventilatory rate:

- Stimulation of peripheral chemoreceptors (hypoxemia)
- Decreased lung compliance–increased ventilatory rate relationship
- Activation of the deflation receptors
- Activation of the irritant receptors
- Stimulation of the J receptors
- Pain, anxiety

Increased Heart Rate (pulse) and Blood Pressure

Cyanosis

Digital Clubbing

Peripheral Edema and Venous Distention

Because polycythemia and cor pulmonale are late findings associated with kyphoscoliosis, the following may be seen:

- Distended neck veins
- Pitting edema
- Enlarged and tender liver

Cough and Sputum Production

Chest Assessment Findings

- Obvious thoracic deformity
- Tracheal shift
- Increased tactile and vocal fremitus
- Dull percussion note
- Bronchial breath sounds
- Whispered pectoriloquy
- Crackles, rhonchi, and wheezing

CLINICAL DATA OBTAINED FROM LABORATORY TESTS AND SPECIAL PROCEDURES

Pulmonary Function Test Findings
Moderate to Severe Kyphoscoliosis
(Restrictive Lung Pathology)

FORCED EXPIRATORY FLOW RATE FINDINGS

FVC	FEV_T	FEV_1/FVC ratio	$FEF_{25\%-75\%}$
↓	N or ↓	N or ↑	N or ↓

$FEF_{50\%}$	$FEF_{200-1200}$	PEFR	MVV
N or ↓	N or ↓	N or ↓	N or ↓

LUNG VOLUME AND CAPACITY FINDINGS

V_T	IRV	ERV	RV
N or ↓	↓	↓	↓

VC	IC	FRC	TLC	RV/TLC ratio
↓	↓	↓	↓	N

Arterial Blood Gases

MILD TO MODERATE KYPHOSCOLIOSIS

Acute Alveolar Hyperventilation with Hypoxemia
(Acute Respiratory Alkalosis)

pH	Pa_{CO_2}	HCO_3^-	Pa_{O_2}
↑	↓	↓ (slightly)	↓

SEVERE KYPHOSCOLIOSIS

Chronic Ventilatory Failure with Hypoxemia
(Compensated Respiratory Acidosis)

pH	Pa_{CO_2}	HCO_3^-	Pa_{O_2}
N	↑	↑ (significantly)	↓

ACUTE VENTILATORY CHANGES SUPERIMPOSED ON CHRONIC VENTILATORY FAILURE

Because acute ventilatory changes are frequently seen in patients with chronic ventilatory failure, the respiratory care practitioner must be familiar with and alert for the following:

- Acute alveolar hyperventilation superimposed on chronic ventilatory failure, and/or
- Acute ventilatory failure (acute hypoventilation) superimposed on chronic ventilatory failure

Oxygen Indices*
Moderate to Severe Kyphoscoliosis

$\dot{Q}_S/\dot{Q}_T$	Do_2†	$\dot{V}o_2$	$C(a-\bar{v})o_2$	O_2ER	$S\bar{v}o_2$
↑	↓	N	N	↑	↓

†The Do_2 may be normal in patients who have compensated to the decreased oxygenation status with (1) an increased cardiac output, (2) an increased hemoglobin level, or (3) a combination of both. When the Do_2 is normal, the O_2ER is usually normal.

Hemodynamic Indices‡
Moderate to Severe Kyphoscoliosis

CVP	RAP	$\overline{PA}$	PCWP	CO	SV
↑	↑	↑	N	N	N

SVI	CI	RVSWI	LVSWI	PVR	SVR
N	N	↑	N	↑	N

**$C(a-\bar{v})o_2$*, Arterial-venous oxygen difference; *Do_2*, total oxygen delivery; *O_2ER*, oxygen extraction ratio; *$\dot{Q}_S/\dot{Q}_T$*, pulmonary shunt fraction; *$S\bar{v}o_2$*, mixed venous oxygen saturation; *$\dot{V}o_2$*, oxygen consumption.

‡*CO*, Cardiac output; *CVP*, central venous pressure; *LVSWI*, left ventricular stroke work index; *$\overline{PA}$*, mean pulmonary artery pressure; *PCWP*, pulmonary capillary wedge pressure; *PVR*, pulmonary vascular resistance; *RAP*, right atrial pressure; *RVSWI*, right ventricular stroke work index; *SV*, stroke volume; *SVI*, stroke volume index; *SVR*, systemic vascular resistance.

OVERVIEW of the Cardiopulmonary Clinical Manifestations Associated with Kyphoscoliosis—cont'd

LABORATORY FINDINGS

Severe and/or Late Stage Kyphoscoliosis (if the Patient Is Chronically Hypoxemic)

- Increased hematocrit and hemoglobin (polycythemia)
- Hypochloremia (Cl^-)
- Hypernatremia (Na^+)

RADIOLOGIC FINDINGS

Chest Radiograph

- Thoracic deformity
- Mediastinal shift
- Increased lung opacity
- Atelectasis in areas of compressed (atelectatic) lungs
- Enlarged heart (cor pulmonale)

The extent of the thoracic deformity in kyphoscoliosis is demonstrated in anteroposterior and lateral radiographs. When present, a mediastinal shift is best shown on an anteroposterior chest radiograph. As the alveoli collapse, the density of the lung increases and is revealed on the chest radiograph as increased opacity (Figure 24-3). In severe cases, cor pulmonale may be seen.

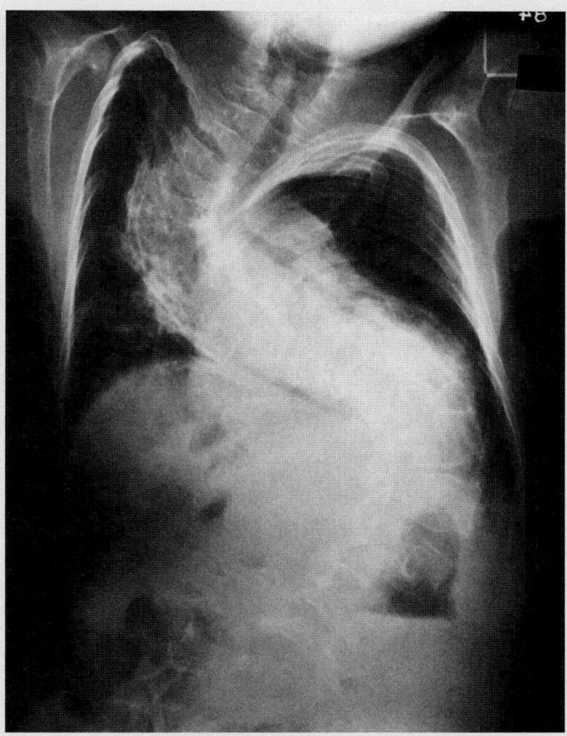

FIGURE 24-3 Severe kyphoscoliosis in a 14-year-old male patient.

General Management of Scoliosis

The treatment of scoliosis largely depends on the cause of the scoliosis, the size and location of the curve, and how much more growing the patient is expected to do. In most cases of scoliosis (less than 20 degrees), the degree of abnormal spine curvature is relatively small and requires only observation to ensure that the curve does not worsen. Observation is usually recommended in patients with a spine curvature of less than 20 degrees. In young children who are still growing, observation checkups are usually scheduled at 3- to 6-month intervals. When the curve is determined to be progressing to a more serious degree (more than 25 to 30 degrees in a child who is still growing), the following treatments options are available:

Braces

A brace device is usually recommended as the first line of defense for growing children who have a spinal curvature of 25 to 45 degrees. The mechanical objective of the brace is to hyperextend the spine and to limit forward flexion. It does not reverse the curve. Although a brace does not cure scoliosis (or even improve the condition), it has been shown to prevent the curve progression in more than 90% of patients who wear it. Bracing is not effective in congenital or neuromuscular scoliosis. The therapeutic effects of bracing are also less helpful in infantile and juvenile idiopathic scoliosis. Today a number of braces are available, including the **Boston brace, Charleston bending brace,** and **Milwaukee brace** (Figure 24-4). The type of brace is selected according to a the patient's age, the specific characteristics of the curve, and the willingness of the patient to tolerate a specific brace.

The Boston brace (also called a *thoracolumbosacral orthosis* [TLSO], a *low-profile brace,* or an *underarm brace*) is composed of plastic that is custom-molded to fit the patient's body. The Boston brace extends from below the breast to the top of the pelvic area in front, and from below the scapula to the coccyx in the back. The Boston brace is typically used for curves in the lumbar (low-back) or thoracolumbar sections of the spine. The Boston brace is worn about 23 hours a day but can be taken off to shower, swim, or engage in sports.

The Charleston bending brace (also known as a *part-time brace*) is worn only for 8 to 10 hours at night, when the human growth hormone (HGH) level is at its highest. The Charleston bending brace is molded to conform to the patient's body when the patient bends toward the convexity—or outward bulge—of the curve. This brace works to overcorrect the curve while the patient is asleep. In order for the Charleston brace to be effective, the patient's curve must be in the 20- to 40-degree range and the apex of the curve needs to be below the level of the scapula. The Charleston bending brace works on the principle that the spine should be bent to grow in the correct direction during the time of

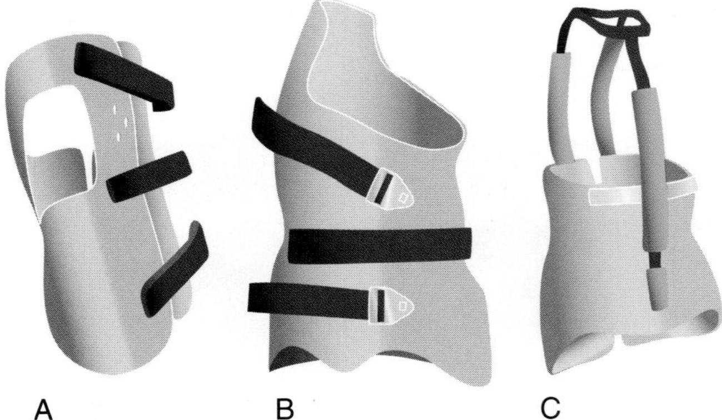

FIGURE 24-4 Common types of braces for scoliosis. **A,** Boston back brace (also called a *thoracolumbosacral orthosis* [TLSO], a *low-profile brace,* or an *underarm brace*). Typically used for curves in the lumbar (low-back) or thoracolumbar sections of the spine. **B,** Charleston bending brace (also known as a *part-time brace*). Commonly used for spinal curves of 20 to 35 degrees, with the apex of the curve below the level of the shoulder blade. **C,** Milwaukee brace (also called cervicothoracolumbosacral orthosis [CTLSO]) is used for high thoracic (mid-back) curves.

day that most growing occurs. Many studies have shown that the Charleston nighttime brace is as effective as the braces that need to be worn for 23 hours.

The Milwaukee brace (also known as a *cervicothoracolumbosacral orthosis* [CTLSO]) is used for high thoracic (mid-back) curves. The Milwaukee brace is a full-torso brace with a neck ring that serves as a rest for the chin and for the back of the head. It extends from the neck to the pelvis. It consists of a specially contoured plastic pelvic girdle and a neck ring that is connected by metal bars in the front and back of the brace. The metal bars work to extend the length of the torso, and the neck ring keeps the head centered over the pelvis. The Milwaukee brace is used less frequently now that more form-fitting plastic braces are available.

Surgery

In general, surgery is performed to correct unacceptable deformity and prevent further curvature. Surgery is usually recommended in patients who have curvatures of the spine greater than 40 to 50 degrees. As a general rule, even the best surgical techniques do not completely straighten the patient's spine. Also, surgery often does not improve ventilatory function. Surgical procedures include the following.

Spinal Fusion

A **spinal fusion,** followed by casting, involves placing pieces of bone between two or more vertebrae. The bone sections are taken from the patient's pelvis or rib. Eventually the bone pieces and the vertebrae fuse together. This procedure has now been largely replaced by **rod instrumentation.**

Rod Instrumentation

Rod instrumentation involves the insertion of metal rods (e.g., **Harrington rod**), hooks, screws, and wires to prevent the curve from moving for 3 to 12 months and to allow the fusion to become solid (Figure 24-5). The system provides disruption to the concave side of the spine and compression to the convex side. This action enhances stabilization, reduces any rotational tendency, and applies force to the spine to correct the curvature. Up to 50% improvement of the curvature may occur in patients who elect to have this procedure.

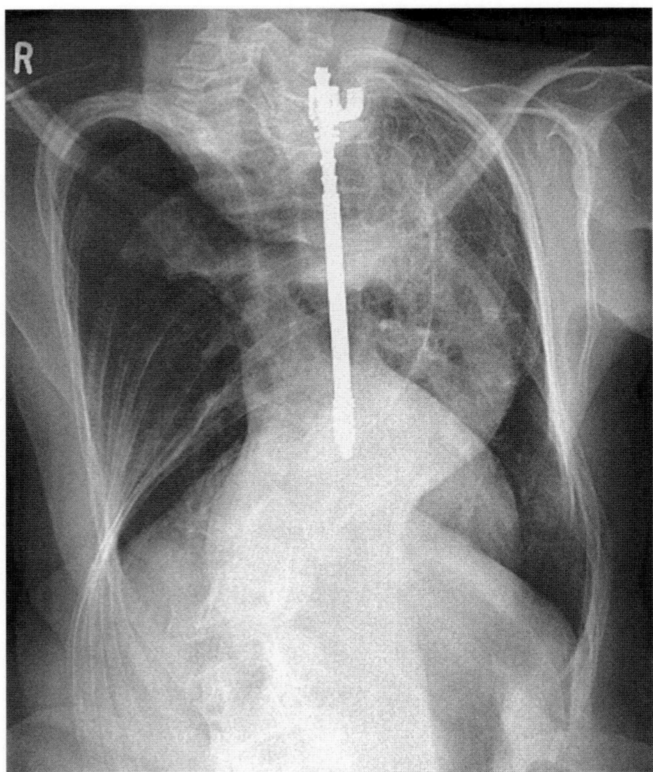

FIGURE 24-5 Radiograph of patient with scoliosis treated with a Harrington rod. (From Albert RK, Spiro SG, Jett JR: *Clinical respiratory medicine,* ed 3, St Louis, 2008, Elsevier.)

Other Approaches

Some physicians may try electrical stimulation of muscles, chiropractic manipulation, and exercise to treat scoliosis. There is no evidence that any of these procedures will stop the progression of spine curvature. Exercise, however, may improve the patient's overall health and well-being. Prophylactic deep breathing and coughing (DB&C) exercises are also taught. Their long-term effect is debatable.

Respiratory Care Treatment Protocols

Oxygen Therapy Protocol

Oxygen therapy is used to treat hypoxemia, decrease the work of breathing, and decrease myocardial work. The hypoxemia that develops in kyphoscoliosis is commonly caused by **atelectasis** and pulmonary shunting. Hypoxemia caused by capillary shunting is often refractory to oxygen therapy. In addition, when the patient demonstrates chronic ventilatory failure during the advanced stages of kyphoscoliosis, caution must be taken not to overoxygenate the patient (see Oxygen Therapy Protocol, Protocol 9-1).

Bronchopulmonary Hygiene Therapy Protocol

A number of bronchial hygiene treatment modalities may be used to enhance the mobilization of the excessive bronchial secretions associated with kyphoscoliosis (see Bronchopulmonary Hygiene Therapy Protocol, Protocol 9-2).

Lung Expansion Therapy Protocol

Lung expansion therapy is ordered to offset atelectasis (see Lung Expansion Therapy Protocol, Protocol 9-3).

CASE STUDY

Kyphoscoliosis

Admitting History

A 62-year-old woman began to develop kyphoscoliosis when she was 6 years old. She lived in the mountains of Virginia all her life, first with her parents and later with her two older sisters. Although she wore various types of body braces until she was 17 years old, her disorder was classified as severe by the time she was 15 years old. Her doctors, who were few and far between, always told her that she would have to learn to live with her condition the best she could, and as a general rule she did.

She finished high school with no other remarkable physical or personal problems. She was well liked by her classmates and was actively involved in the school newspaper and art club. After graduation she continued to live with her parents for a few more years. At 21 years of age, she moved in with her two older sisters, who were buying a large farmhouse near a small but popular tourist town. All three sisters made various arts and crafts, which they sold at local tourist shops. The woman's physical disability and general health were relatively stable until she was about 40 years old. At that time, she started to experience frequent episodes of dyspnea, coughing, and sputum production. As the years progressed, her baseline condition was marked by increasingly severe dyspnea.

Because the sisters rarely ventured into the city, the woman's medical resources were poor until she was introduced to a social worker at a nearby church. The church had just become part of an outreach program based in a large city nearby. The social worker was charmed by the woman and fascinated by the beauty of the colorful quilts she made.

The social worker, however, also was concerned by the woman's limited ability to move because of her severe chest deformity. In addition, the social worker thought that the woman's cough sounded serious. She noted that the woman appeared grayish-blue, weak, and ill. The sisters told the social worker that their sibling had had a bad "cold" for about 6 months. After much urging, the social worker persuaded the woman to travel, accompanied by her sisters, to the city to see a doctor at a large hospital associated with the church outreach program. The woman was immediately admitted to the hospital. The sisters stayed in a nearby hotel room provided by the hospital.

Physical Examination

Although the patient appeared to be well nourished, the lateral curvature of her spine was twisted significantly to the left. She also demonstrated anterior bending of the thoracic spine. She appeared older than her stated age, and she was in obvious respiratory distress. The patient stated that she was having trouble breathing. Her skin was cyanotic. She had digital clubbing, and her neck veins were distended, especially on the right side. The woman demonstrated a frequent but adequate cough. During each coughing episode she expectorated a moderate amount of thick, yellow sputum.

When the patient generated a strong cough, a large unilateral bulge appeared at the right anterolateral base of her neck, directly posterior to the clavicle. The patient referred to the bulge as her "Dizzy Gillespie pouch." The doctor thought that the bulge was a result of the severe kyphoscoliosis, which had in turn stretched and weakened the suprapleural membrane that normally restricts and contains the parietal pleura at the apex of the lung. Because of the weakening of the suprapleural membrane, any time the woman performed Valsalva's maneuver for any reason (e.g., for coughing), the increased intrapleural pressure herniated the suprapleural membrane outward. Despite the odd appearance of the bulge, the doctor did not consider it a serious concern.

The patient's vital signs were as follows: blood pressure 160/100, heart rate 90 bpm, respiratory rate 18/min, and oral temperature 36.3° C (97.4° F). Palpation revealed a trachea deviated to the right. Dull percussion notes were produced over both lungs; crackles and rhonchi were heard over them as well. There was 2+ pitting edema below both knees. A pulmonary function test (PFT) conducted that morning showed vital capacity (VC), functional residual capacity (FRC), and residual volume (RV) of 45% to 50% of predicted values.

Although the patient's electrolyte levels were all normal, her hematocrit was 58%, and her hemoglobin level was 18 g%. A chest x-ray examination revealed a severe thoracic and spinal deformity, a mediastinal shift, an enlarged heart with prominent pulmonary artery segments bilaterally, and bilateral infiltrates in the lung bases consistent with pneumonia and atelectasis. The patient's arterial blood gas values (ABGs) on room air were as follows: pH 7.52, Pa_{CO_2} 58, HCO_3^- 46, and Pa_{O_2} 49. Her oxygen saturation measured by pulse oximetry (Sp_{O_2}) was 88%. The physician requested a respiratory care consultation and stated that mechanical ventilation was not an option at this time per the patient's request and his knowledge of the case. On the basis of these clinical data, the following SOAP was documented.

Respiratory Assessment and Plan

S "I'm having trouble breathing."

O Well-nourished appearance; severe anterior and left lateral curvature of the spine; cyanosis, digital clubbing, and distended neck veins—especially on the right side; cough: frequent, adequate, and productive of moderate amounts of thick yellow sputum; 2+ pitting edema below both knees; vital signs: BP 160/100, HR 90, RR 18, T 36.3° C (97.4° F); trachea deviated to the right; both lungs: dull percussion notes, crackles, and rhonchi; PFT: VC, FRC, and RV 45% to 50% of predicted; Hct 58%, Hb 18 g%; CXR: severe thoracic and spinous deformity, mediastinal shift, cardiomegaly, and bilateral infiltrates in the lung bases consistent with pneumonia or atelectasis; ABGs (room air): pH 7.52, $Pa{CO_2}$ 58, HCO_3^- 46, $Pa{O_2}$ 49; $Sp{O_2}$ 88%

A
- Severe kyphoscoliosis (history, CXR, physical examination)
- Increased work of breathing (elevated blood pressure, heart rate, and respiratory rate)
- Excessive bronchial secretions (sputum, rhonchi)
- Infection likely (thick, yellow sputum)
- Good ability to mobilize secretions (strong cough)
- Atelectasis and consolidation (CXR)
- Acute alveolar hyperventilation superimposed on chronic ventilatory failure with moderate hypoxemia (ABGs)
- Cor pulmonale (CXR and physical examination)

P Initiate **Oxygen Therapy Protocol** (HAFOE at $F{IO_2}$ 0.28; be careful not to overoxygenate the patient). **Bronchopulmonary Hygiene Therapy Protocol** (obtain sputum for culture; C&DB instructions and oral suction prn). **Lung Expansion Therapy Protocol** (incentive spirometry qid and prn). **Aerosolized Medication Protocol** (aerosolized Xopenex 0.5 mL in 1.5 mL 10% acetylcysteine q4h). Notify physician of admitting ABGs and impending ventilatory failure. Place mechanical ventilator on standby. Monitor closely.

10 Hours after Admission

The patient's condition had not improved, and she was transferred to an intensive care unit. The physician had trouble titrating the cardiac drugs and decided to insert a pulmonary artery catheter, a central venous catheter, and an arterial line. Because of the woman's cardiac problems, several medical students, respiratory therapists, nurses, and doctors were constantly in and out of her room, performing and assisting in various procedures. As a result, working with the patient for any length of time was difficult, and the intensity of respiratory care was less than desirable. Eventually, the patient's cardiac status stabilized, and the physician requested an update on the woman's pulmonary condition.

The respiratory therapist working on the pulmonary consultation team found the patient in extreme respiratory distress. She was sitting up in bed, appeared frightened, and stated that she was extremely short of breath. Both of her sisters were in the room; one sister was putting cold towels on the patient's face while the other sister was holding the patient's hands. Both sisters were crying softly. The woman's skin appeared cyanotic, and perspiration was visible on her face. Her neck veins were still distended. She demonstrated a weak, spontaneous cough. Although no sputum was noted, she sounded congested when she coughed. Dull percussion notes, crackles, and rhonchi were still present throughout both lungs. Her vital signs were as follows: blood pressure 180/120, heart rate 130 bpm, respiratory rate 26/min, and rectal temperature 37.8° C (100° F).

Several of the patient's hemodynamic indices were elevated: CVP, RAP, PA, RVSWI, and PVR.* Her oxygenation indices were as follows: increased $\dot{Q}_S/\dot{Q}_T$ and O_2ER and decreased $D{O_2}$ and $S\bar{v}{O_2}$. Her $\dot{V}{O_2}$ and $C(a\text{-}\bar{v})O_2$ were normal.[†] No recent chest x-ray film was available. Her ABGs on an $F{IO_2}$ of 0.28 were as follows: pH 7.57, $Pa{CO_2}$ 49, HCO_3^- 44, and $Pa{O_2}$ 43. Her $Sp{O_2}$ was 87%. On the basis of these clinical data, the following SOAP was documented.

Respiratory Assessment and Plan

S Severe dyspnea; "I'm extremely short of breath."

O Extreme respiratory distress; cyanosis and perspiration; distended neck veins; weak, spontaneous cough; sounds of congestion but no sputum produced; bilateral dull percussion notes, crackles, and rhonchi; vital signs: BP 180/120, HR 130, RR 26, T 37.8° C (100° F); hemodynamics: increased CVP, RAP, PA, RVSWI, and PVR; oxygenation indices: increased $\dot{Q}_S/\dot{Q}_T$, and O_2ER and decreased $D{O_2}$ and $S\bar{v}{O_2}$; $\dot{V}{O_2}$ and $C(a\text{-}\bar{v})O_2$ normal; ABGs; pH 7.57, $Pa{CO_2}$ 49, HCO_3^- 44, $Pa{O_2}$ 43; $Sp{O_2}$ 87%

A
- Severe kyphoscoliosis (history, physical exam, CXR)
- Increased work of breathing, worsening (increased blood pressure, heart rate, and respiratory rate)
- Excessive bronchial secretions (rhonchi, congested cough)
- Atelectasis and consolidation (previous CXR)
- Acute alveolar hyperventilation superimposed on chronic ventilatory failure with moderate-to-severe hypoxemia (ABGs and history)
  - Impending ventilatory failure
- Continued critically ill status, but chances of avoiding ventilatory failure improving

P Up-regulate **Oxygen Therapy Protocol** (HAFOE at 0.35). Up-regulate **Bronchopulmonary Hygiene Therapy Protocol** (add CPT and PD qid). Up-regulate **Aerosolized Medication Protocol** (increase med. nebs. to q2h). Contact physician regarding possible ventilatory failure. Discuss therapeutic bronchoscopy with physician. Continue to keep mechanical ventilator on standby. Monitor and reevaluate in 30 minutes.

24 Hours after Admission

At this time the respiratory care practitioner found the patient watching the morning news on television with her two sisters. The woman was situated in a semi-Fowler's position eating the last few bites of her breakfast. The patient stated that she felt "so much better" and that "finally I have enough wind to eat some food."

Although her skin still appeared cyanotic, she did not look as ill as she had the day before. On request, she produced a strong cough and expectorated a small amount of white sputum. Her vital signs were as follows: blood pressure 140/85, heart rate 83 bpm, respiratory rate 14/min, and temperature normal. Chest assessment findings demonstrated

**CVP,* Central venous pressure; *PA,* mean pulmonary artery pressure; *PVR,* pulmonary vascular resistance; *RAP,* right atrial pressure; *RVSWI,* right ventricular stroke work index.

† $C(a\text{-}\bar{v})O_2$, Arterial-venous oxygen difference; $D{O_2}$, total oxygen delivery; O_2ER, oxygen extraction ratio; $\dot{Q}_S/\dot{Q}_T$, pulmonary shunt fraction; $S\bar{v}{O_2}$, mixed venous oxygen saturation; $\dot{V}{O_2}$, oxygen consumption.

crackles, rhonchi, and dull percussion notes over both lung fields. The rhonchi were less intense, however, than they had been the day before.

Although the patient's hemodynamic and oxygenation indices were better than they had been the day before, she still had room for improvement. Her hemodynamic parameters, still abnormal, revealed an elevated CVP, RAP, PA, RVSWI, and PVR. All other hemodynamic indices were normal. Her oxygenation indices still showed an increased $\dot{Q}_S/\dot{Q}_T$ and O_2ER and a decreased Do_2 and $S\bar{v}o_2$. Her $\dot{V}o_2$ and $C(a\text{-}\bar{v})o_2$ were normal. The patient's chest x-ray film, taken earlier that morning, showed some clearing of the pneumonia and atelectasis described on admission. Her ABGs on an Fio_2 of 0.35 were as follows: pH 7.45, $Paco_2$ 73, HCO_3^- 49, and Pao_2 68. Her Spo_2 was 94%. On the basis of these clinical data, the following SOAP was recorded.

Respiratory Assessment and Plan

S "I feel so much better. I finally have enough wind to eat some food."

O Cyanotic appearance; cough: strong, small amount of white sputum; vital signs: BP 140/85, HR 83, RR 14, T normal; crackles, rhonchi, and dull percussion notes over both lung fields; rhonchi improving; hemodynamic and oxygenation indices improving, but still an elevated CVP, RAP, PA, RVSWI, and PVR and still an increased $\dot{Q}_S/\dot{Q}_T$ and O_2ER and a decreased Do_2 and $S\bar{v}o_2$; CXR: improvement of the bilateral pneumonia and atelectasis; ABGs: pH 7.45, $Paco_2$ 73, HCO_3^- 49, Pao_2 68; Spo_2 94%

A
- Generally improved respiratory status (history, CXR, hemodynamic and oxygenation indices, ABGs)
- Significant improvement in problem with excessive bronchial secretions (rhonchi, cough)
- Improvement in atelectasis and consolidation (CXR)
- Chronic ventilatory failure with mild hypoxemia (ABGs)
- Current ABGs are likely close to patient's normal (baseline) ABGs

P Down-regulate **Oxygen Therapy Protocol, Bronchopulmonary Hygiene Therapy Protocol,** and **Aerosolized Medication Protocols.** Continue to monitor and reevaluate (ABGs on reduced Fio_2). Recommend pulmonary rehabilitation and patient and family education (cuirass respiratory ventilation, possibly rocking bed, BIPAP, or positive expiratory pressure [PEP]).

Discussion

This case provides an excessive amount of extraneous historical and personal material. This was done to demonstrate, in part, how the respiratory care worker must cut through to the core of the case in the SOAP notes. Care of the patient with symptomatic advanced kyphoscoliosis consists of (1) treatment of the conditions that can complicate it (e.g., bronchitis, pneumonia, atelectasis, pleural effusion) and (2) treatment of the underlying condition itself.

In the first assessment, the SOAP documented excessive bronchial secretions and a likely infection because of the thick yellow sputum and recent history. The patient had a good ability to mobilize the secretions as charted by a strong cough. The chest radiograph confirmed atelectasis and consolidation. Although acute alveolar hyperventilation on top of chronic ventilatory failure was present, the possibility of impending ventilatory failure was real. The therapist's decision to oxygenate the patient with a low Fio_2 (0.28), administer bronchial hygiene and mucolytic aerosols, and be prepared for ventilator support were all appropriate. The patient's secondary polycythemia and cor pulmonale would have been expected to improve as overall oxygenation improved, although this improvement could take some time. The digital clubbing and cor pulmonale itself suggested that the hypoxemia was long-standing.

At the time of the second assessment, the intensity of the patient's respiratory distress was increasing. This was verified by the continued observation of the high pulse and respiratory rate, excessive bronchial secretions, dull percussion notes, acute alveolar hyperventilation on top of chronic ventilatory failure with moderate to severe hypoxemia, atelectasis on the chest x-ray film, and poor response to oxygen therapy. Undoubtedly, impending ventilatory failure was more likely. Atelectasis is often refractory to oxygen therapy, suggesting that therapeutic bronchoscopy might have been worthwhile. At that point in time, the up-regulation of the **Oxygen Therapy Protocol** (Protocol 9-1), **Bronchopulmonary Hygiene Therapy Protocol** (Protocol 9-2), and **Aerosolized Medication Protocol** (Protocol 9-4) were all justified by the clinical indicators.

In the last assessment, the clinical manifestations associated with the patient's disorder had all decreased substantially. The down-regulation of the **Oxygen Therapy Protocol, Bronchopulmonary Hygiene Therapy Protocol,** and **Aerosolized Medication Protocol** was appropriate. The recommendation of pulmonary rehabilitation and family education was appropriately considered. The ABGs were most likely at the patient's baseline level, because the pH was in the normal range. In fact, according to the pH (normal but on the alkalotic side of normal) the patient's usual $Paco_2$ was most likely somewhat higher than the last assessment value.

Comparison with baseline values (if available) would be appropriate at such a time, and consideration of cuirass ventilation, a rocking bed, or positive expiratory pressure (PEP) to assist nocturnal ventilation might be in order. Oxygenation easily can be assessed by oximetry at home. This case is an excellent example of the value of hemodynamic monitoring (specifically the normal PCWP) in differentiating left-sided from right-sided cardiac failure.

SELF-ASSESSMENT QUESTIONS

evolve Answers to questions can be found on Evolve. To access additional student assessment questions and case studies for application of text material to real-life scenarios, visit **http://evolve.elsevier.com/DesJardins/respiratory.**

1. What kind of curvature of the spine is manifested in kyphosis?
- a. Posterior
- b. Anterior
- c. Lateral
- d. Medial

2. Kyphoscoliosis affects approximately what percentage of the U.S. population?
- a. 2
- b. 5
- c. 10
- d. 15

3. Which of the following is or are associated with kyphoscoliosis?
1. Increased FRC
2. Decreased V_T
3. Increased TLC
4. Decreased RV
- a. 1 only
- b. 4 only
- c. 2 and 4 only
- d. 3 and 4 only

4. Which of the following are associated with kyphoscoliosis?
1. Bronchial breath sounds
2. Hyperresonant percussion note
3. Whispered pectoriloquy
4. Diminished breath sounds
- a. 1 and 3 only
- b. 2 and 4 only
- c. 3 and 4 only
- d. 2, 3, and 4 only

5. During the advanced stages of kyphoscoliosis, the patient commonly demonstrates which of the following arterial blood gas values?
1. Increased HCO_3^-
2. Decreased pH
3. Increased $Paco_2$
4. Normal pH
5. Decreased HCO_3^-
- a. 2 only
- b. 3 and 4 only
- c. 2 and 5 only
- d. 1, 3, and 4 only

PART VII

Environmental Lung Diseases

Interstitial Lung Diseases

25

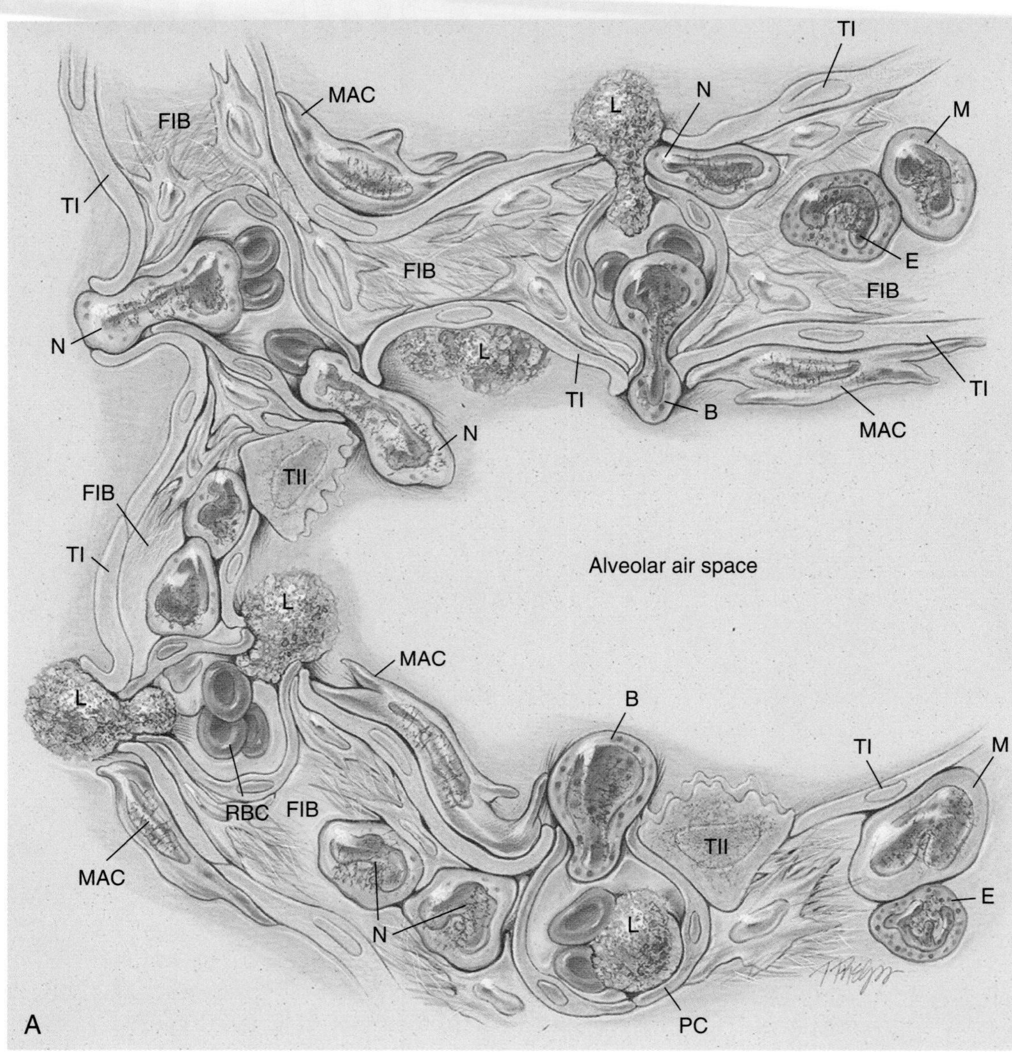

FIGURE 25-1 **A**, Interstitial lung disease. Cross-sectional microscopic view of alveolar-capillary unit. *B,* Basophil; *E,* eosinophil; *FIB,* fibroblast (fibrosis); *L,* lymphocyte; *M,* monocyte; *MAC,* macrophage; *N,* neutrophil; *PC,* pulmonary capillary; *RBC,* red blood cell; *TI,* type I alveolar cell; *TII,* type II alveolar cell.

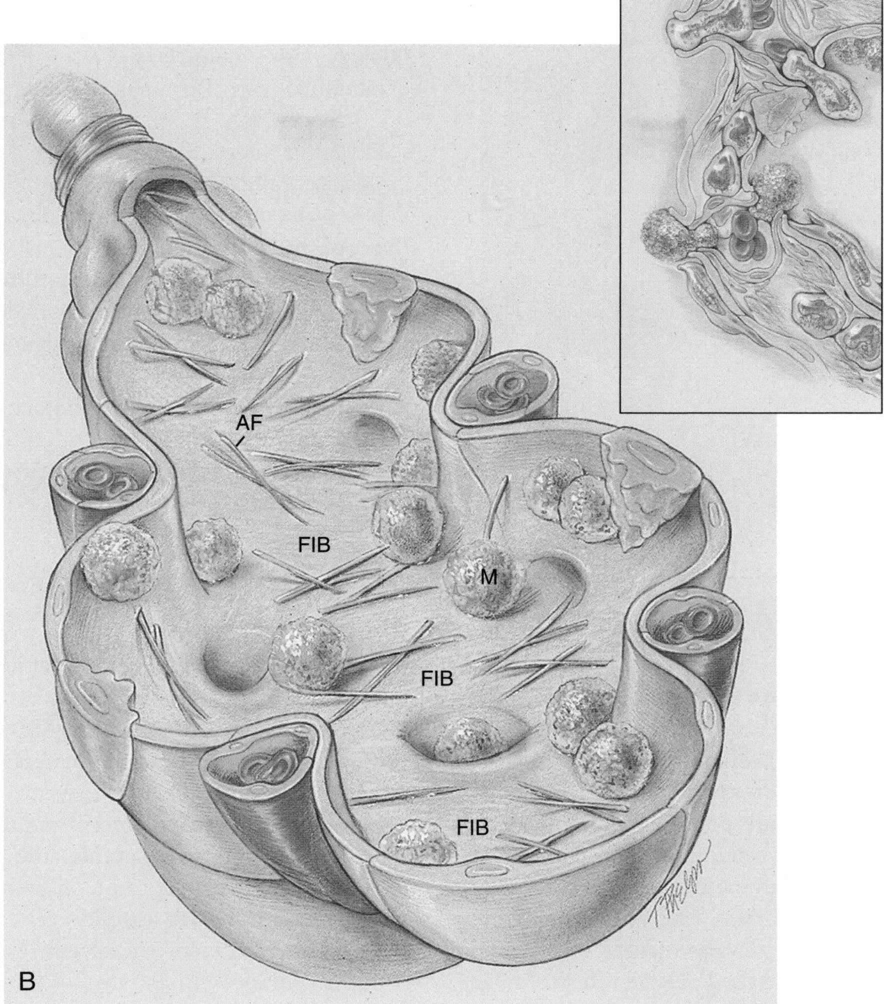

FIGURE 25-1, cont'd B, Asbestosis (close-up of one alveolar unit). *AF,* Asbestos fiber; *FIB,* fibrosis; *M,* macrophage.

Chapter Objectives

After reading this chapter, you will be able to:

- List the anatomic alterations of the lungs associated with chronic interstitial lung disease.
- Describe the causes of chronic interstitial lung disease.
- List the cardiopulmonary clinical manifestations associated with chronic interstitial lung disease.
- Describe the general management of chronic interstitial lung disease.
- Describe the clinical strategies and rationales of the SOAPs presented in the case study.
- Define key terms and complete self-assessment questions at the end of the chapter and on Evolve.

Key Terms

Allergic Alveolitis
Acute Pneumonitic Phase
Asbestos/Asbestosis
Beryllium/Berylliosis
Black Lung
Bronchiolitis Obliterans Organizing Pneumonia (BOOP)
Chronic Eosinophilic Pneumonia
Churg-Strauss Syndrome
Coal Miner's Lung
Coal Worker's Pneumoconiosis (CWP)
Connective Tissue (Collagen Vascular) Diseases
Cryptogenic Organizing Pneumonia (COP)
Desquamative Interstitial Pneumonia (DIP)
Extrinsic Allergic Alveolitis
Focal Emphysema
Grinder's Disease
Goodpasture's Syndrome
Honeycombing
Hypersensitivity Pneumonitis
Idiopathic Pulmonary Fibrosis (IPF)
Idiopathic Pulmonary Hemosiderosis
Interstitial Lung Disease (ILD)
Late Fibrotic Phase
Lymphangioleiomyomatosis (LAM)
Lymphocytic Interstitial Pneumonia (LIP)
Lymphomatoid Granulomatosis
Organic Exposure

Plasmapheresis
Polymyositis-Dermatomyositis
Progressive Massive Fibrosis (PMF)
Progressive Systemic Sclerosis (PSS)
Pulmonary Alveolar Proteinosis
Pulmonary Langerhans Cell Histiocytosis (PLCH)
Pulmonary Vasculitides
Quartz Silicosis (Grinder's Disease)
Rheumatoid Pneumoconiosis
Sarcoidosis
Scleroderma
Silica
Silicosis
Sjögren's Syndrome
Systemic Lupus Erythematosus (SLE)
Usual Interstitial Pneumonia (UIP)
Wegener's Granulomatosis

Chapter Outline

Introduction

The term **interstitial lung disease (ILD)** (also called *diffuse interstitial lung disease, fibrotic interstitial lung disease, pulmonary fibrosis,* and *pneumoconiosis*) refers to a broad group of inflammatory lung disorders. More than 180 disease entities are characterized by acute, subacute, or chronic inflammatory infiltration of alveolar walls by cells, fluid, and connective tissue. If left untreated, the inflammatory process can progress to irreversible pulmonary fibrosis. The ILD group consists of a wide range of illnesses with varied causes, treatments, and prognoses. However, because the ILDs all reflect similar anatomic alterations of the lungs and therefore cardiopulmonary clinical manifestations, they are presented as a group in this chapter.

Anatomic Alterations of the Lungs

The anatomic alterations of ILD may involve the bronchi, alveolar walls, and adjacent alveolar spaces. In severe cases the extensive inflammation leads to pulmonary fibrosis, granulomas, **honeycombing,** and cavitation. During the acute stage of any ILD, the general inflammatory condition is characterized by edema and the infiltration of a variety of white blood cells (e.g., neutrophils, eosinophils, basophils, monocytes, macrophages, and lymphocytes) in the alveolar walls and interstitial spaces (see Figure 25-1,*A*). Bronchial inflammation and thickening and increasing airway secretions may be also present.

During the chronic stage the general inflammatory response is characterized by the infiltration of numerous white blood cells (especially monocytes, macrophages, and lymphocytes), and some fibroblasts may also be present in the alveolar walls and interstitial spaces. This stage may be followed by further interstitial thickening, fibrosis, granulomas, and, in some cases, honeycombing and cavity formation. Pleural effusion also may be present. In the chronic stages the basic pathologic features of interstitial fibrosis are identical in any interstitial lung disorder (so-called *end-stage pulmonary fibrosis*).

As a general rule, the interstitial lung disorders produce a restrictive lung disease. However, because bronchial inflammation and excessive airway secretions also can develop in the small airways, the clinical manifestations associated with an obstructive lung disorder may also be seen. Therefore the patient with ILD may demonstrate a restrictive disorder, an obstructive disorder, or a combination of both.

The major pathologic or structural changes associated with chronic ILDs are as follows:

- Destruction of the alveoli and adjacent pulmonary capillaries
- Fibrotic thickening of the respiratory bronchioles, alveolar ducts, and alveoli
- Granulomas
- Honeycombing and cavity formation
- Fibrocalcific pleural plaques (particularly in asbestosis)
- Bronchospasm
- Excessive bronchial secretions (caused by inflammation of airways)

Etiology and Epidemiology

Because there are over 180 different pulmonary disorders classified as ILD, it is helpful to group them according to their occupational or environmental exposure, disease associations, and specific pathology. Table 25-1 provides an overview of common ILD groups. A discussion of the more common ILDs follows.

Interstitial Lung Diseases of Known Causes or Associations

Occupational, Environmental and Therapeutic Exposures

Inorganic particulate (dust) exposure.

Asbestos. Exposure to **asbestos** may cause **asbestosis**—a common form of ILD. Asbestos fibers are a mixture of fibrous minerals composed of hydrous silicates of magne-

TABLE 25-1 Overview of Interstitial Lung Diseases

Occupational, Environmental, and Therapeutic Exposures	Systemic Disease	Idiopathic Interstitial Pneumonia	Specific Pathology	Miscellaneous Interstitial Lung Diseases
Occupational or Environmental	Connective tissue disease	Idiopathic pulmonary fibrosis	Lymphangioleiomyomatosis	Goodpasture's syndrome
Inorganic exposure	Scleroderma	Nonspecific	Pulmonary Langerhans cell histiocytosis	Idiopathic pulmonary hemosiderosis
Asbestosis	Rheumatoid arthritis	Cryptogenic-organizing pneumonia	Pulmonary alveolar proteinosis	Chronic eosinophilic pneumonia
Coal dust	Sjögren's syndrome	Lymphocytic interstitial pneumonia	Pulmonary vasculitides	
Silica	Polymyositis or dermatomyositis		Wegener's granulomatosis	
Beryllium	Systemic lupus erythematosus		Churg-Strauss syndrome	
Aluminum	Sarcoidosis		Lymphomatoid granulomatosis	
Barium				
Clay				
Iron				
Certain talcs				
Organic Exposure				
Hypersensitivity pneumonitis				
Moldy hay				
Silage				
Moldy sugar cane				
Mushroom compost				
Barley				
Cheese				
Wood pulp, bark, dust				
Cork dust				
Bird droppings				
Paints				
Medications and Illicit Drugs				
Antibiotics				
Antiinflammatory agents				
Cardiovascular agents				
Chemotherapeutic agents				
Drug-induced systemic lupus erythematosus				
Illicit drugs				
Miscellaneous agents				
Radiation Therapy				
Irritant Gases				

sium, sodium, and iron in various proportions. There are two primary types: the amphiboles (crocidolite, amosite, and anthophyllite) and chrysotile (most commonly used in industry). Asbestos fibers typically range from 50 to 100 μm in length and are about 0.5 μm in diameter. The chrysotiles have the longest and strongest fibers. Box 25-1 lists common sources associated with asbestos fibers.

As shown in Figure 25-1, *B,* asbestos fibers can be seen by microscope within the thickened septa as brown or orange baton-like structures. The fibers characteristically stain for iron with Perls' stain. The pathologic process may affect only one lung, a lobe, or a segment of a lobe. The lower lobes are most commonly affected. Pleural calcification is common and diagnostic in patients with an asbestos exposure history.

Coal dust. The pulmonary deposition and accumulation of large amounts of coal dust causes what is known as **coal worker's pneumoconiosis (CWP).** CWP also is known as **coal miner's lung and black lung**. Miners who use cutting machines at the coal face have the greatest exposure, but even relatively minor exposures may result in the disease. Indeed, cases have been reported in which coal miners' wives developed the disease, presumably from shaking the dust from their husbands' work clothes.

Simple CWP is characterized by the presence of pinpoint nodules called *coal macules (black spots)* throughout the lungs. The coal macules often develop around the first- and second-generation respiratory bronchioles and cause the adjacent alveoli to retract. This condition is called **focal emphysema.**

Complicated CWP or **progressive massive fibrosis** (PMF) is characterized by areas of fibrotic nodules greater than 1 cm in diameter. The fibrotic nodules generally appear in the peripheral regions of upper lobes and extend toward the hilum with growth. The nodules are composed of dense collagenous tissue with black pigmentation. Coal dust by itself is chemically inert. The fibrotic changes in CWP are usually caused by **silica.**

Silica. Silicosis (also called **grinder's disease** or **quartz silicosis**) is caused by the chronic inhalation of crystalline, free silica, or silicon dioxide particles. Silica is the main component of more than 95% of the rocks of the earth. It is found in sandstone, quartz (beach sand is mostly quartz), flint, granite, many hard rocks, and some clays.

Simple silicosis is characterized by small rounded nodules scattered throughout the lungs. No single nodule is greater than 9 mm in diameter. Patients with simple silicosis are usually symptom-free.

Complicated silicosis is characterized by nodules that coalesce and form large masses of fibrous tissue, usually in the upper lobes and perihilar regions. In severe cases the fibrotic regions may undergo tissue necrosis and cavitate. Box 25-2 lists common occupations associated with silica exposure.

Beryllium. Beryllium is a steel-gray, lightweight metal found in certain plastics and ceramics, rocket fuels, and x-ray tubes. As a raw ore, beryllium is not hazardous. When it is processed into the pure metal or one of its salts, however, it may cause a tissue reaction when inhaled or implanted into the skin. The acute inhalation of beryllium fumes or particles may cause a toxic or allergic pneumonitis sometimes accompanied by rhinitis, pharyngitis, and tracheobronchitis. The more complex form of **berylliosis** is characterized by the development of granulomas and a diffuse interstitial inflammatory reaction.

Other inorganic causes. Box 25-3 lists other inorganic causes of ILD.

Organic materials exposure. Hypersensitivity pneumonitis. Hypersensitivity pneumonitis (also called **allergic alveolitis** or **extrinsic allergic alveolitis**) is a cell-mediated immune response of the lungs caused by the inhalation of a variety of offending agents or antigens. Such antigens include grains, silage, bird droppings or feathers, wood dust (especially redwood and maple), cork dust, animal pelts, coffee beans, fish meal, mushroom compost, and molds that grow on sugar cane, barley, and straw. The immune response to these allergens causes production of antibody and an inflammatory response. The lung inflammation, or pneumonitis, develops after repeated and prolonged exposure to the allergen. The term *hypersensitivity pneumonitis* (or *allergic alveolitis*) is often

Box 25-1 Common Sources Associated with Asbestos Fibers

- Acoustic products
- Automobile undercoating
- Brake lining
- Cements
- Clutch casings
- Floor tiles
- Firefighting suits
- Fireproof paints
- Insulation
- Roofing materials
- Ropes
- Steam pipe material

Box 25-2 Common Occupations Associated with Silica Exposure

- Tunneling
- Hard-rock mining
- Sandblasting
- Quarrying
- Stonecutting
- Foundry work
- Ceramics work
- Abrasives work
- Brick making
- Paint making
- Polishing
- Stone drilling
- Well drilling

Box 25-3 Additional Inorganic Causes of Interstitial Lung Disease

Aluminum
- Ammunition workers

Baritosis (barium)
- Barite millers and miners
- Ceramics workers

Kaolinosis (clay)
- Brick makers and potters
- Ceramics workers

Siderosis (iron)
- Welders

Talcosis (certain talcs)
- Ceramics workers
- Papermakers
- Plastics and rubber workers

renamed according to the type of exposure that caused the lung disorder. For example, the hypersensitivity pneumonitis caused by the inhalation of moldy hay is called *farmer's lung.* Table 25-2 provides common causes, exposure sources, and disease syndromes associated with hypersensitivity pneumonitis.

Medications and illicit drugs. As the list of medications and illicit drugs continues to grow, so does the list of possible side effects (Box 25-4). Unfortunately, the lungs are major target organs affected by these side effects. Although it is impossible to discuss in detail the various lung-related side effects of every drug, it is possible to describe some of the general concerns related to drug-induced lung disease and to list some of the pharmacologic agents that may be responsible.

The chemotherapeutic (anticancer agents) are by far the largest group of agents associated with ILD. Bleomycin, mitomycin, busulfan, cyclophosphamide, methotrexate, and carmustine (BCNU) are the major offenders. Nitrofurantoin (an antibacterial drug used in the treatment of urinary tract infections) is also associated with ILD. Gold and penicillamine for the treatment of **rheumatoid arthritis** also have been shown to cause ILD. The excessive long-term administration of oxygen (oxygen toxicity) also is known to cause diffuse pulmonary injury and fibrosis (see Chapter 27). As a general rule, the risk of these drugs causing an interstitial lung disorder is directly related to the cumulative dosage. However, drug-induced interstitial disease may be seen as early as 1 month to as late as several years after exposure to these agents.

The precise cause of drug-induced ILD is not known. Diagnosis is confirmed by an open lung biopsy. When interstitial fibrosis is found with no infectious organisms, a drug-induced interstitial process must be suspected.

Radiation therapy. Radiation therapy in the management of cancer may cause ILD. Radiation-induced lung disease is commonly divided into the following two major phases: the **acute pneumonitic phase** and the **late fibrotic phase**. Acute pneumonitis rarely is seen in patients who receive a total radiation dose of less than 3500 rad. On the other hand, doses in excess of 6000 rad over 6 weeks almost always cause ILD in and near the radiated areas. The acute pneumonitic phase develops approximately 2 to 3 months

Box 25-4 Medications and Illicit Drugs Associated with the Development of Interstitial Lung Disease

Antibiotics
- Nitrofurantoin
- Sulfasalazine

Antiinflammatory agents
- Aspirin
- Gold
- Penicillamine
- Methotrexate
- Etanercept
- Infliximab

Cardiovascular agents
- Amiodarone
- Tocainide

Chemotherapeutic agents
- Bleomycin
- Mitomycin-C
- Busulfan
- Cyclophosphamide
- Chlorambucil
- Melphalan
- Azathioprine
- Cytosine arabinoside
- Methotrexate
- Procarbazine
- Zinostatin
- Etoposide
- Vinblastine
- Imatinib

Drugs associated with drug-induced systemic lupus erythematosus
- Procainamide
- Isoniazid
- Hydralazine
- Hydantoins
- Penicillamine

Illicit drugs
- Heroin
- Methadone
- Propoxyphene
- Talc as an intravenous contaminant

Miscellaneous agents
- Oxygen
- Drugs inducing pulmonary infiltrate and eosinophilia: L-tryptophan
- Hydrochlorothiazide
- Radiation therapy

From Camus P: Drug induced infiltrative lung diseases. In Schwarz MI, Kin TE, eds: *Interstitial lung disease,* ed 4, Hamilton, 2003, BC Decker.

TABLE 25-2 Causes of Hypersensitivity Pneumonitis

Antigen	Exposure Source	Disease (Syndrome)
Bacteria, Thermophilic		
Saccharopolyspora rectivirgula	Moldy hay, silage	Farmer's lung
Thermoactinomyces vulgaris	Moldy sugarcane	Bagassosis
Thermoactinomyces sacchari	Mushroom compost	Mushroom worker's lung
Thermoactinomyces candidus	Heated water reservoirs	Air conditioner lung
Bacteria, Nonthermophilic		
Bacillus subtilis, Bacillus cereus	Water, detergent	Humidifier lung, washing powder lung
Fungi		
Aspergillus species	Moldy hay	Farmer's lung
	Water	Ventilation pneumonitis
Aspergillus clavatus	Barley	Malt worker's lung
Penicillium casei, Penicillium roqueforti	Cheese	Cheese washer's lung
Alternaria species	Wood pulp	Woodworker's lung
Cryptostroma corticale	Wood bark	Maple bark stripper's lung
Graphium, Aureobasidium pullulans	Wood dust	Sequoiosis
Merulius lacrymans	Rotten wood	Dry root lung
Penicillium frequentans	Cork dust	Suberosis
Aureobasidium pullulans	Water	Humidifier lung
Cladosporium species	Hot tub mist	Hot tub HP*
Trichosporon cutaneum	Damp wood and mats	Japanese summer-type HP*
Amebae		
Naegleria gruberi	Contaminated water	Humidifier lung
Acanthamoeba polyphaga	Contaminated water	Humidifier lung
Acanthamoeba castellani	Contaminated water	Humidifier lung
Animal Protein		
Avian proteins	Bird droppings, feathers	Bird-breeder's lung
Urine, serum, pelts	Rates, gerbils	Animal handler's lung
Chemicals		
Isocyanates, trimellitic anhydride	Paints, resins, plastics	Chemical worker's lung
Copper sulfate	Bordeaux mixture	Vineyard sprayer's lung
Phthalic anhydride	Heated epoxy resin	Epoxy resin lung
Sodium diazobenzene sulfate	Chromatography reagent	Pauli's reagent alveolitis
Pyrethrum	Pesticide	Pyrethrum HP*

From Selman M: Hypersensitivity pneumonitis. In Schwarz MI, Kin TE, eds: *Interstitial lung disease,* ed 4, Hamilton, 2003, BC Decker.
*HP, Hypersensitivity pneumonitis.

after exposure. Chronic radiation fibrosis is seen in all patients who develop acute pneumonitis.

The late phase of fibrosis may develop (1) immediately after the development of acute pneumonitis, (2) without an acute pneumonitic period, or (3) after a symptom-free latent period. When fibrosis does develop, it generally does so 6 to 12 months after radiation exposure. Pleural effusion often is associated with the late fibrotic phase.

The precise cause of radiation-induced lung disease is not known. The establishment of a diagnosis is similar to that for drug-induced interstitial disease (i.e., by obtaining a history of recent radiation therapy and confirming the diagnosis with an open lung biopsy).

Irritant gases. The inhalation of irritant gases may cause an acute chemical pneumonitis and, in severe cases, ILD. Most exposures occur in an industrial setting. Table 25-3 lists some of the more common irritant gases and the industrial settings where they may be found.

Systemic Diseases

Connective Tissue (Collagen Vascular) Diseases

Scleroderma. Scleroderma is characterized by chronic hardening and thickening of the skin caused by new collagen formation. It may occur in a localized form or as a systemic disorder (called *systemic sclerosis*). **Progressive systemic sclerosis (PSS)** is a relatively rare autoimmune disorder that affects the blood vessels and connective tissue. It causes fibrous degeneration of the connective tissue of the skin, lungs, and internal organs, especially the esophagus, digestive tract, and kidney.

Scleroderma of the lung appears in the form of ILD and fibrosis. Of all the collagen vascular disorders, scleroderma is

TABLE 25-3 Common Irritant Gases Associated with Interstitial Lung Disease

Gas	Industrial Setting
Chlorine	Chemical and plastic industries; water disinfection
Ammonia	Commercial refrigeration; smelting of sulfide ores
Ozone	Welding
Nitrogen dioxide	May be liberated after exposure of nitric acid to air
Phosgene	Used in the production of aniline dyes

the one in which pulmonary involvement is most severe and most likely to cause significant scarring of the lung parenchyma. The pulmonary complications include diffuse interstitial fibrosis, severe pulmonary hypertension, pleural disease, and aspiration pneumonitis (secondary to esophageal involvement). Scleroderma also may involve the small pulmonary blood vessels and appears to be independent of the fibrotic process involving the alveolar walls. The disease most commonly is seen in women 30 to 50 years of age.

Rheumatoid arthritis. Rheumatoid arthritis primarily is an inflammatory joint disease. It may, however, involve the lungs in the form of (1) pleurisy, with or without effusion; (2) interstitial pneumonitis; (3) necrobiotic nodules, with or without cavities; (4) Caplan's syndrome; and (5) pulmonary hypertension secondary to pulmonary vasculitis.

Pleurisy with or without effusion is the most common pulmonary complication associated with rheumatoid arthritis. When present, the effusion is generally unilateral (often on the right side). Men appear to develop rheumatoid pleural complications more often than women. Rheumatoid interstitial pneumonitis is characterized by alveolar wall fibrosis, interstitial and intraalveolar mononuclear cell infiltration, and lymphoid nodules. In severe cases, extensive fibrosing alveolitis and honeycombing may develop. Rheumatoid interstitial pneumonitis is also more common in male patients. Necrobiotic nodules are characterized by the gradual degeneration and swelling of lung tissue.

The pulmonary nodules generally appear as well-circumscribed masses that often progress to cavitation. The nodules usually develop in the periphery of the lungs and are more common in men. Histologically, the pulmonary nodules are identical to the subcutaneous nodules that develop in rheumatoid arthritis.

Caplan's syndrome (also called **rheumatoid pneumoconiosis**) is a progressive pulmonary fibrosis of the lung commonly seen in coal miners. Caplan's syndrome is characterized by rounded densities in the lung periphery that often undergo cavity formation and, in some cases, calcification. Pulmonary hypertension is a common secondary complication caused by the progression of fibrosing alveolitis and pulmonary vasculitis.

Sjögren's syndrome. Sjögren's syndrome is a lymphocytic infiltration that primarily involves the salivary and lacrimal glands and is manifested by dry mucous membranes, usually of the mouth and eyes. Pulmonary involvement also frequently occurs in Sjögren's syndrome and includes (1) pleurisy with or without effusion, (2) interstitial fibrosis that is indistinguishable from that of other collagen vascular disorders, and (3) infiltration of lymphocytes of the tracheobronchial mucous glands, which in turn causes atrophy of the mucous glands, mucous plugging, atelectasis, and secondary infections. Sjögren's syndrome occurs most often in women (90%) and is commonly associated with rheumatoid arthritis (50% of patients with Sjögren's syndrome).

Polymyositis-dermatomyositis. Polymyositis is a diffuse inflammatory disorder of the striated muscles that primarily weakens the limbs, neck, and pharynx. *Dermatomyositis* is the term used when an erythematous skin rash accompanies the muscle weakness. Pulmonary involvement develops in response to (1) recurrent episodes of aspiration pneumonia caused by esophageal weakness and atrophy, (2) hypostatic pneumonia secondary to a weakened diaphragm, and (3) drug-induced interstitial pneumonitis.

Polymyositis-dermatomyositis is seen more often in women than men, at about a 2 : 1 ratio. The disease occurs primarily in two age groups: before the age of 10 and from 40 to 50 years of age. In about 40% of the patients, the pulmonary manifestations are seen 1 to 24 months before the striated muscle or skin shows signs or symptoms.

Systemic lupus erythematosus. Systemic lupus erythematosus (SLE) is a multisystem disorder that mainly involves the joints and skin. It also may cause serious problems in numerous other organs, including the kidneys, lungs, nervous system, and heart. Involvement of the lungs appears in about 50% to 70% of the cases. Pulmonary manifestations are characterized by (1) pleurisy with or without effusion, (2) atelectasis, (3) diffuse infiltrates and pneumonitis, (4) diffuse ILD, (5) uremic pulmonary edema, (6) diaphragmatic dysfunction, and (7) infections.

Pleurisy with or without effusion is the most common pulmonary complication of SLE. The effusions usually are exudates with high protein concentration and are frequently bilateral. Atelectasis commonly develops in response to the pleurisy, effusion, and diaphragmatic elevation associated with SLE. Diffuse noninfectious pulmonary infiltrates and pneumonitis are common. In severe cases, chronic interstitial pneumonitis may develop. Because SLE frequently impairs the renal system, uremic pulmonary edema may occur. SLE has also been found to be associated with diaphragmatic dysfunction and reduced lung volumes. Some research suggests that a diffuse myopathy affecting the diaphragm is the source of this problem. Approximately 50% of the cases have a complicating pulmonary infection.

Sarcoidosis. Sarcoidosis is a chronic disorder of unknown origin characterized by the formation of tubercles of nonnecrotizing epithelioid tissue (noncaseating granulomas). Common sites are the lungs, spleen, liver, skin, mucous membranes, and lacrimal and salivary glands, usually with the involvement of the lymph glands. The lung is the most frequently affected organ, with manifestations generally including ILD, enlargement of the mediastinal lymph nodes, or a combination of both. One of the clinical hallmarks of sarcoidosis is an increase in all three major immunoglobulins (IgM, IgG, and IgA). The disease is more common among African-Americans and appears most frequently in patients 10 to 40 years of age, with the highest incidence at 20 to 30 years of age. Women are affected more often than men, especially among African-Americans.

Idiopathic Interstitial Pneumonias

Many patients with ILD do not have a readily identified specific exposure, a systemic disorder, or an underlying genetic cause. Such instances of ILD are commonly placed in the idiopathic interstitial pneumonia (IIP) group or the group with specific pathology.

Idiopathic Pulmonary Fibrosis

Idiopathic pulmonary fibrosis (IPF) is a progressive inflammatory disease with varying degrees of fibrosis and, in severe cases, honeycombing. The precise cause is unknown. Although *idiopathic pulmonary fibrosis* is the term most frequently used for this disorder, numerous other names appear in the literature, such as *acute interstitial fibrosis of the lung, cryptogenic fibrosing alveolitis, Hamman-Rich syndrome, honeycomb lung, interstitial fibrosis,* and *interstitial pneumonitis.*

IPF commonly is separated into the following two major disease entities according to the predominant histologic appearance: **desquamative interstitial pneumonia (DIP)** and **usual interstitial pneumonia (UIP)**. In DIP the most prominent features are hyperplasia and desquamation of the alveolar type II cells. The alveolar spaces are packed with macrophages, and there is an even distribution of the interstitial mononuclear infiltrate.

In UIP the most prominent features are interstitial and alveolar wall thickening caused by chronic inflammatory cells and fibrosis. In severe cases, fibrotic connective tissue replaces the alveolar walls, the alveolar architecture becomes distorted, and eventually honeycombing develops. When honeycombing is present, the inflammatory infiltrate is significantly reduced. The prognosis for patients with DIP is significantly better than that for patients with UIP.

Some experts believe that DIP and UIP are two distinct ILD entities. Others, however, believe that DIP and UIP are different stages of the same disease process. IPF most commonly seen is seen in men 40 to 70 years of age. Diagnosis generally is confirmed by an open lung biopsy. Most patients diagnosed with IPF have a more chronic progressive course, and death usually occurs in 4 to 10 years. Death usually is the result of progressive acute ventilatory failure, complicated by pulmonary infection.

Cryptogenic Organizing Pneumonia

Cryptogenic organizing pneumonia (COP) (also known as **bronchiolitis obliterans organizing pneumonia [BOOP]**) is characterized by connective tissue plugs in the small airways (hence the term *bronchiolitis obliterans*) and mononuclear cell infiltration of the surrounding parenchyma (hence the term *organizing pneumonia*). Although the most of the cases have no identifiable cause and therefore are considered idiopathic, COP has been associated with connective tissue disease, toxic gas inhalation, and infection. The chest radiograph commonly shows patchy infiltrates of alveolar rather than interstitial involvement. Diagnosis may require a surgical biopsy when the clinical and radiographic data are uncertain. COP is one of the ILDs in which both restrictive and obstructive pathologic lesions are present.

Lymphocytic Interstitial Pneumonia

Lymphocytic interstitial pneumonia (LIP) is a diffuse pulmonary disorder characterized by fibrosis and accumulation of lymphocytes in the lungs. It is commonly associated with lymphoma and may progress to lymphoma. The diagnosis usually requires a surgical lung biopsy.

Specific Pathology

Lymphangioleiomyomatosis

Lymphangioleiomyomatosis (LAM) is a rare lung disease involving the smooth muscles of the airways and affects women of childbearing age. It is characterized by the proliferation of disorderly smooth muscle proliferation throughout the bronchioles, alveolar septa, perivascular spaces, and lymphatics. LAM causes the obstruction of small airways and lymphatics. Common clinical features associated with LAM are recurrent pneumothorax and chylous pleural effusion. The diagnosis of LAM is confirmed with an open lung biopsy. The prognosis is poor; the disease slowly progresses over 2 to 10 years, ending in death resulting from ventilatory failure.

Pulmonary Langerhans Cell Histiocytosis

Pulmonary Langerhans cell histiocytosis (PLCH) is a smoking-related ILD characterized by midlung-zone star-shaped nodules with adjacent thin-walled cysts. It was once considered a benign condition in adults, but long-term complications such as pulmonary hypertension are becoming increasingly recognized. Diagnosis is confirmed histologically by tissue biopsy.

Pulmonary Alveolar Proteinosis

Pulmonary alveolar proteinosis is a condition of unknown cause in which the alveoli become filled with protein and lipids. The lipoprotein material is similar to the pulmonary surfactant produced by the type II cells. In addition, the alveolar macrophages generally are dysfunctional in this disorder. The disease most commonly is seen in adults 20 to 50 years of age. Men are affected twice as often as women. The chest radiograph typically reveals bilateral infiltrates that are most prominent in the perihilar regions (butterfly pattern). It is often indistinguishable from pulmonary edema. Air bronchograms commonly are seen. The diagnosis is confirmed by transbronchial or open lung biopsy, or by analysis of fluid removed during bronchial lavage.

Pulmonary Vasculitides

The **pulmonary vasculitides** (also called *granulomatous vasculitides*) consist of a heterogeneous group of pulmonary disorders characterized by inflammation and destruction of the pulmonary vessels. The major disorders in this category include **Wegener's granulomatosis, Churg-Strauss syndrome,** and **lymphomatoid granulomatosis.**

Wegener's granulomatosis. Wegener's granulomatosis is a multisystem disorder characterized by (1) a necrotizing, granulomatous vasculitis; (2) focal and segmental glomerulonephritis; and (3) variable degrees of systemic vasculitis of the small veins and arteries. In the lungs, numerous 1- to 9-cm-diameter nodules are commonly seen in the upper lobes, and cavity formation is often associated with the larger lesions.

Wegener's granulomatosis is considered an aggressive and fatal disorder, although the prognosis has significantly improved with the use of cytotoxic agents (e.g., cyclophosphamide). This disorder most commonly is seen in men older than 50 years of age. Diagnosis is confirmed by an open lung biopsy. Histologic examination reveals lesions with marked central necrosis. The area surrounding the necrotizing lesion consists of inflammatory white blood cells (WBCs) with some fibroblasts. Inflammatory cell infiltrate and necrotizing vasculitis are seen in the adjacent blood vessels.

Churg-Strauss syndrome. Churg-Strauss syndrome is a necrotizing vasculitis that predominantly involves the small vessels of the lungs. The granulomatous lesions are characterized by a heavy infiltrate of eosinophils, central necrosis, and peripheral eosinophilia. Cavity formation is rare in this disorder. Clinically, symptoms of asthma usually precede the onset of vasculitis. In recent years, rapid tapering of oral steroids with substitution of leukotriene inhibitors such as montelukast (Singulair) and zafirlukast (Accolate) has been associated with deaths from fulminant Churg-Strauss syndrome reactions. Neurologic disorders such as mononeuritis multiplex, a simultaneous disease of several peripheral nerves, are frequently associated with this disorder. Diagnosis is usually confirmed with an open lung biopsy, and the disease is often rapidly fatal.

Lymphomatoid granulomatosis. Lymphomatoid granulomatosis is a rare necrotizing vasculitis that primarily involves the lungs, although neurologic and cutaneous lesions sometimes are seen. The lesions are usually in the lower lobes, and cavities develop in more than one third of the cases. Pleural effusion is common.

Although the clinical presentation is similar to that of Wegener's granulomatosis, there are some distinct differences. For example, more mature lymphoreticular cells are involved in the formation of the granulomatous lesions and no glomerulonephritis is seen. Histologically, the lesions simulate malignant lymphoma. This disorder most commonly is seen in men 50 to 70 years of age. Diagnosis is confirmed by open lung biopsy.

Miscellaneous Diffuse Interstitial Lung Diseases

Goodpasture's Syndrome

Goodpasture's syndrome is a disease of unknown cause that involves two organ systems—the lungs and the kidneys. In the lungs there are recurrent episodes of pulmonary hemorrhage and in some cases pulmonary fibrosis, presumably as a consequence of the bleeding episodes. In the kidneys there is a glomerulonephritis characterized by the infiltration of antibodies within the glomerular basement membrane (GBM). These circulating antibodies function against the patient's own GBM. They are commonly abbreviated as *anti-GBM antibodies.* It is believed that the anti-GBM antibodies cross-react with the basement membrane of the alveolar wall and that their deposition in the kidneys and lungs is responsible for producing the pathophysiologic processes of the disease.

Goodpasture's syndrome usually is seen in young adults. The average survival period after diagnosis is about 15 weeks. About 50% of the patients die from massive pulmonary hemorrhage, and about 50% die from chronic renal failure. An interesting feature of Goodpasture's syndrome is that the patient frequently demonstrates an increased DLCO, which is in direct contrast to most interstitial lung disorders. The increased carbon monoxide uptake commonly seen in this disorder is thought to be caused by the increased amount of retained blood in the pulmonary tissue.

Idiopathic Pulmonary Hemosiderosis

Idiopathic pulmonary hemosiderosis is a disease entity of unknown cause that is characterized by recurrent episodes of pulmonary hemorrhage similar to that seen in Goodpasture's syndrome. Histologic examination reveals an alveolar hemorrhage with hemosiderin-laden macrophages and hyperplasia of the alveolar epithelium. Unlike in Goodpasture's syndrome, however, there is no evidence of circulating anti-GBM antibodies attacking the alveoli or GBMs, and this disorder is not associated with renal disease.

Idiopathic pulmonary hemosiderosis most often is seen in children. As in Goodpasture's syndrome, patients commonly demonstrate an increased DLCO, which is in direct contrast to most interstitial lung disorders. Again, the increased uptake of carbon monoxide is thought to be caused by the increased amount of blood retained in the lungs.

Chronic Eosinophilic Pneumonia

Chronic eosinophilic pneumonia is characterized by infiltration of eosinophils and, to a lesser extent, macrophages into the alveolar and interstitial spaces. Clinically, a unique feature of this disorder often is seen on the chest radiograph, consisting of a peripheral distribution of pulmonary infiltrates. This radiographic pattern is commonly referred to as a *photographic negative of pulmonary edema.* This is because of the dense peripheral infiltration, with the sparing of the perihilar areas, seen in chronic eosinophilic pneumonia, compared with the central pulmonary infiltration with the sparing of the lung periphery seen in pulmonary edema. An increased number of eosinophils also is commonly seen in the peripheral blood. Histologic diagnosis is made by means of an open lung biopsy.

OVERVIEW of the Cardiopulmonary Clinical Manifestations Associated with Chronic Interstitial Lung Diseases

The following clinical manifestations result from the pathophysiologic mechanisms caused (or activated) by an **Increased Alveolar-Capillary Membrane Thickness** (see Figure 9-10) and **Excessive Bronchial Secretions** (see Figure 9-12)—the major anatomic alterations of the lungs associated with chronic interstitial lung disease (see Figure 28-1).

CLINICAL DATA OBTAINED AT THE PATIENT'S BEDSIDE

The Physical Examination

Vital Signs

Increased Respiratory Rate (Tachypnea)

Several pathophysiologic mechanisms operating simultaneously may lead to an increased ventilatory rate:

- Stimulation of peripheral chemoreceptors (hypoxemia)
- Decreased lung compliance–increased ventilatory rate relationship
- Stimulation of the J receptors
- Pain, anxiety

Increased Heart Rate (Pulse) and Blood Pressure

Cyanosis

Digital Clubbing

Peripheral Edema and Venous Distention

Because polycythemia and cor pulmonale are associated with chronic interstitial lung disease, the following may be seen:

- Distended neck veins
- Pitting edema
- Enlarged and tender liver

Nonproductive Cough

Chest Assessment Findings

- Increased tactile and vocal fremitus
- Dull percussion note
- Bronchial breath sounds
- Crackles, rhonchi
- Pleural friction rub
- Whispered pectoriloquy

CLINICAL DATA OBTAINED FROM LABORATORY TESTS AND SPECIAL PROCEDURES

Pulmonary Function Test Findings
Moderate to Severe Interstitial Lung Disease
(Restrictive Lung Pathology)

FORCED EXPIRATORY FLOW RATE FINDINGS

FVC	FEV_T	FEV_1/FVC ratio	$FEF_{25\%-75\%}$
↓	N or ↓	N or ↑	N or ↓

$FEF_{50\%}$	$FEF_{200-1200}$	PEFR	MVV
N or ↓	N or ↓	N or ↓	N or ↓

LUNG VOLUME AND CAPACITY FINDINGS

V_T	IRV	ERV	RV
N or ↓	↓	↓	↓

VC	IC	FRC	TLC	RV/TLC ratio
↓	↓	↓	↓	N

DECREASED DIFFUSION CAPACITY

There is an exception to the expected decreased diffusion capacity in the following two interstitial lung diseases: Goodpasture's syndrome and idiopathic pulmonary hemosiderosis. The Dlco is often elevated in response to the increased amount of blood retained in the alveolar spaces that is associated with these two disorders.

Arterial Blood Gases

MILD TO MODERATE INTERSTITIAL LUNG DISEASE

Acute Alveolar Hyperventilation with Hypoxemia
(Acute Respiratory Alkalosis)

pH	$Paco_2$	HCO_3^-	Pao_2
↑	↓	↓ (slightly)	↓

SEVERE CHRONIC INTERSTITIAL LUNG DISEASE

Chronic Ventilatory Failure with Hypoxemia
(Compensated Respiratory Acidosis)

pH	$Paco_2$	HCO_3^-	Pao_2
N	↑	↑ (significantly)	↓

Acute Ventilatory Changes Superimposed on Chronic Ventilatory Failure

Because acute ventilatory changes are frequently seen in patients with chronic ventilatory failure, the respiratory care practitioner must be familiar with and alert for the following:

- Acute alveolar hyperventilation superimposed on chronic ventilatory failure, and/or
- Acute ventilatory failure (acute hypoventilation) superimposed on chronic ventilatory failure

Oxygenation Indices*
Moderate to Severe Stage Interstitial Lung Disease

$\dot{Q}_S/\dot{Q}_T$	Do_2†	$\dot{V}o_2$	$C(a-\bar{v})o_2$	O_2ER	$S\bar{v}o_2$
↑	↓	N	N	↑	↓

†The Do_2 may be normal in patients who have compensated to the decreased oxygenation status with (1) an increased cardiac output, (2) an increased hemoglobin level, or (3) a combination of both. When the Do_2 is normal, the O_2ER is usually normal.

* $C(a-\bar{v})o_2$, Arterial-venous oxygen difference; Do_2, total oxygen delivery; O_2ER, oxygen extraction ratio; $\dot{Q}_S/\dot{Q}_T$, pulmonary shunt fraction; $S\bar{v}o_2$, mixed venous oxygen saturation; $\dot{V}o_2$, oxygen consumption.

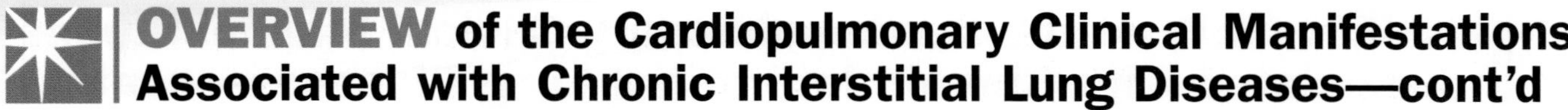

OVERVIEW of the Cardiopulmonary Clinical Manifestations Associated with Chronic Interstitial Lung Diseases—cont'd

Hemodynamic Indices*
Severe Interstitial Lung Disease

CVP	RAP	$\overline{PA}$	PCWP	CO	SV
↑	↑	↑	N	N	N
SVI	**CI**	**RVSWI**	**LVSWI**	**PVR**	**SVR**
N	N	↑	N	↑	N

LABORATORY FINDINGS

- Increased hematocrit and hemoglobin (polycythemia)

RADIOLOGIC FINDINGS

Radiologic findings vary according to the cause.

Chest Radiograph

- Bilateral reticulonodular pattern
- Irregularly shaped opacities
- Granulomas
- Cavity formation

*CO, Cardiac output; CVP, central venous pressure; LVSWI, left ventricular stroke work index; $\overline{PA}$, mean pulmonary artery pressure; PCWP, pulmonary capillary wedge pressure; PVR, pulmonary vascular resistance; RAP, right atrial pressure; RVSWI, right ventricular stroke work index; SV, stroke volume; SVI, stroke volume index; SVR, systemic vascular resistance.

- Honeycombing
- Pleural effusion (see Chapter 23)

As shown in Figure 25-2, a patient with severe scleroderma, a bilateral reticulonodular pattern is commonly seen on the radiographs. In patients with asbestosis the opacity is often described as cloudy in appearance or as having a "ground-glass" appearance and is especially apparent in the lower lobes (Figure 25-3). Calcified pleural plaques may be seen on the superior border of the diaphragm or along the chest wall (Figure 25-4). The inflammatory response elicited by the asbestos fibers also may produce a fuzziness and irregularity of the cardiac and diaphragmatic borders.

Figure 25-5 shows a diffuse parenchymal ground-glass pattern with some areas of consolidation in a patient with acute farmer's lung. The severity of parenchymal opacification in this case is rare.

In Figure 25-6, the honeycomb appearance is nicely illustrated in a computed tomography (CT) scan of a patient with sarcoidosis. Figure 25-7 shows a patient with Wegener's granulomatosis with numerous nodules with a large cavity lesion adjacent to the right hilus. Figure 25-8 shows a pleural effusion in a patient with rheumatoid disease.

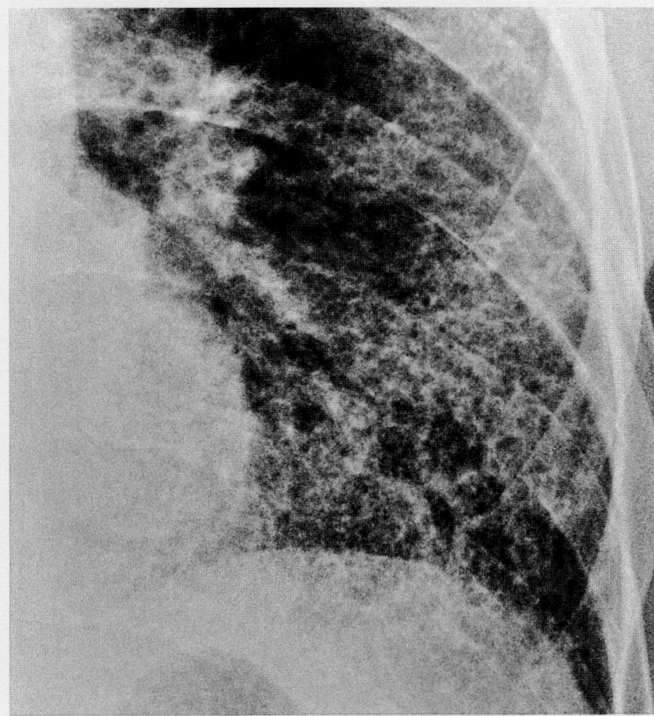

FIGURE 25-2 Reticulonodular pattern of interstitial pulmonary fibrosis in a patient with scleroderma. (From Hansell DM, Armstrong P, Lynch DA, McAdams HP, eds: *Imaging of diseases of the chest,* ed 4, Philadelphia, 2005, Elsevier.)

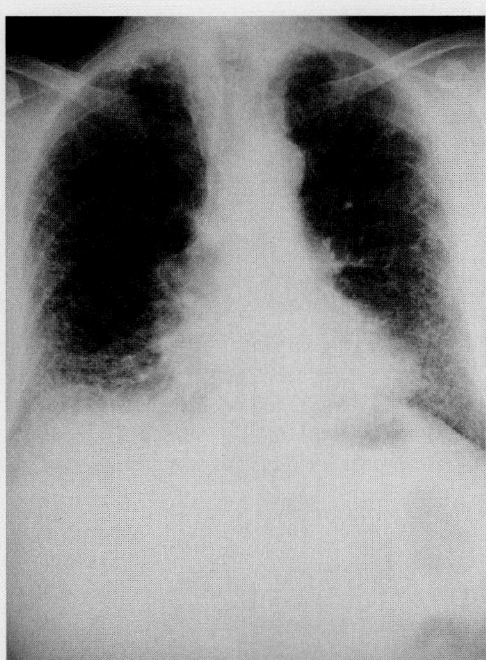

FIGURE 25-3 Chest x-ray film of a patient with asbestosis.

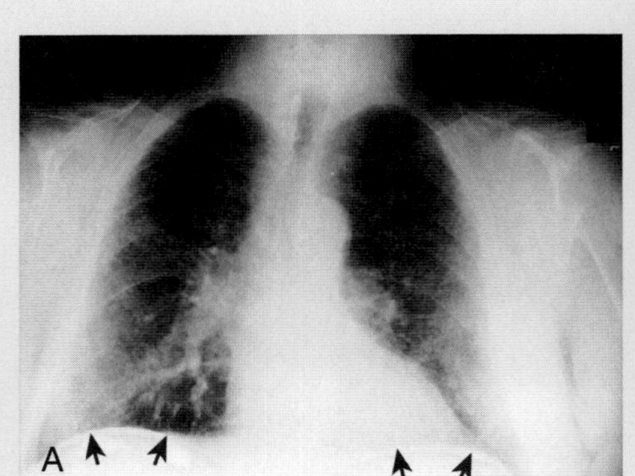

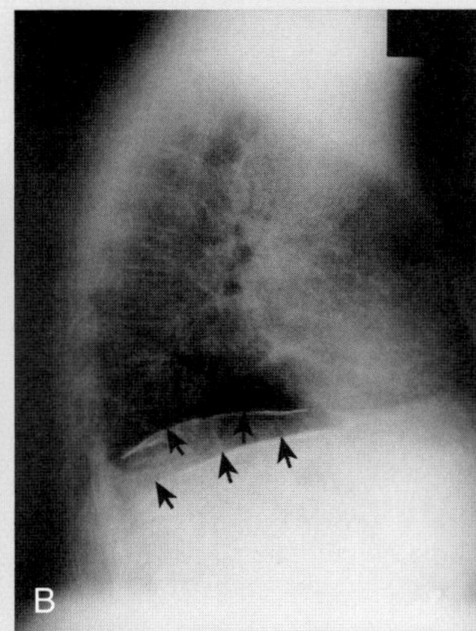

FIGURE 25-4 Calcified pleural plaques on the superior border of the diaphragm *(arrows)* in a patient with asbestosis. Thickening of the pleural margins also is seen along the lower lateral borders of the chest. **A**, Anteroposterior view. **B**, Lateral view.

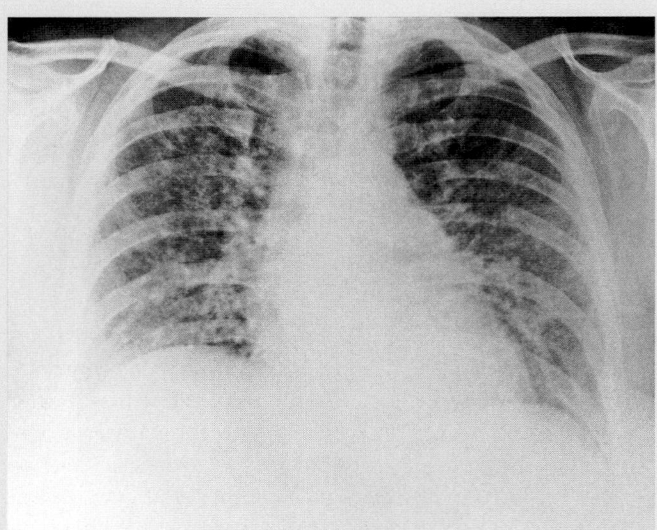

FIGURE 25-5 Acute farmer's lung. Chest radiograph shows diffuse parenchymal ground-glass pattern with some areas of consolidation. The severity of parenchymal opacification in this case is unusual. (From Hansell DM, Armstrong P, Lynch DA, McAdams HP, eds: *Imaging of diseases of the chest,* ed 4, Philadelphia, 2005, Elsevier.)

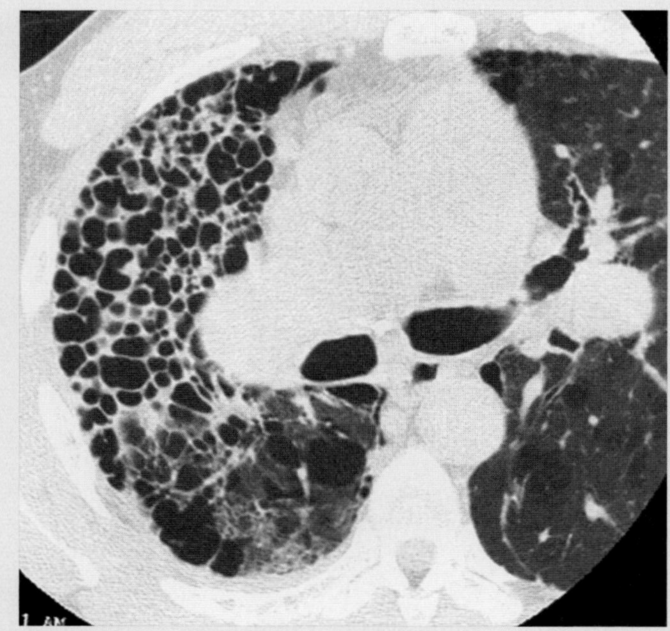

FIGURE 25-6 Honeycomb cysts in sarcoidosis. HRCT through the right midlung shows perfuse clustered honeycomb cysts. The cysts are larger than the typical honeycomb cysts seen in usual interstitial pneumonia. Cysts are much less extensive in the left lung. (From Hansell DM, Armstrong P, Lynch DA, McAdams HP, eds: *Imaging of diseases of the chest,* ed 4, Philadelphia, 2005, Elsevier.)

OVERVIEW of the Cardiopulmonary Clinical Manifestations Associated with Chronic Interstitial Lung Diseases—cont'd

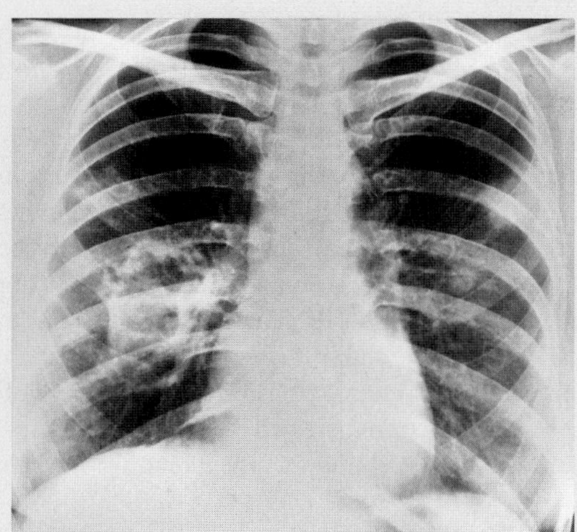

FIGURE 25-7 Wegener's granulomatosis. Numerous nodules with a large (6-cm) cavitary lesion adjacent to the right hilus. Its walls are thick and irregular. (From Hansell DM, Armstrong P, Lynch DA, McAdams HP, eds: *Imaging of diseases of the chest,* ed 4, Philadelphia, 2005, Elsevier.)

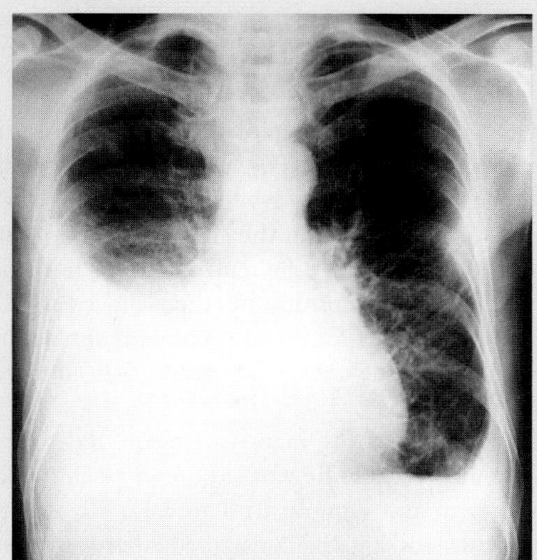

FIGURE 25-8 Pleural effusion in rheumatoid disease. Bilateral pleural effusions are present with mild changes of fibrosing alveolitis. The effusions were painless, and the one on the right had been present, more or less unchanged, for 5 months. Note the bilateral "meniscus signs." (From Hansell DM, Armstrong P, Lynch DA, McAdams HP, eds: *Imaging of diseases of the chest,* ed 4, Philadelphia, 2005, Elsevier.)

General Management of Interstitial Lung Disease

Medications and Procedures Commonly Prescribed by the Physician

The management of interstitial lung disorders is directed at the inflammation associated with the various disorders.

Corticosteroids

Corticosteroids are commonly administered with reasonably good results, but the benefit varies remarkably from one patient to another (see Appendix II).

Respiratory Care Treatment Protocols

Oxygen Therapy Protocol

Oxygen therapy is used to treat hypoxemia, decrease the work of breathing, and decrease myocardial work. Because of the hypoxemia associated with ILDs, supplemental oxygen often is required. The hypoxemia that develops in an interstitial lung disorder most commonly is caused by the **alveolar thickening**, fibrosis, and capillary shunting associated with the disorder. In addition, because the patient may demonstrate chronic ventilatory failure during the advanced stages of an ILD, caution must be taken not to overoxygenate the patient (see Oxygen Therapy Protocol, Protocol 9-1).

Mechanical Ventilation Protocol

Mechanical ventilation may be needed to provide and support alveolar gas exchange and eventually return the patient to spontaneous breathing. Because acute ventilatory failure superimposed on chronic ventilatory failure often is seen in patients with severe ILD, continuous mechanical ventilation may be required. Continuous mechanical ventilation is justified when the acute ventilatory failure is thought to be reversible (see Mechanical Ventilation Protocols, Protocol 9-5, Protocol 9-6, and Protocol 9-7).

Other Treatments

Plasmapheresis

Treatment for Goodpasture's syndrome is directed at reducing the circulating anti-GBM antibodies that attack the patient's GBM. **Plasmapheresis,** which directly removes the anti-GBM antibodies from the circulation, has been of some benefit.

CASE STUDY

Interstitial Lung Disease

Admitting History

A 72-year-old man is well known to the treating-hospital staff members, having received care there for more than 12 years. While in the U.S. Navy during World War II, he worked on the East Coast in the ship construction industry. After his discharge in 1945, he returned to his home in Mississippi for about 6 months; he then moved to Detroit, Michigan, and worked for an automobile manufacturer. His primary job for the next 20 years was undercoating automobiles.

In the early 1970s the man was transferred to a nearby automotive plant, where he worked on an assembly line fastening bumpers and chrome trim to cars. He was popular with his fellow workers and considered a hard worker by the management. When he retired in 1980, he was one of four supervisors in charge of the chrome trim assembly line.

Although the man smoked two packs a day for more than 40 years, his health was essentially unremarkable until about 4 years before he retired. At that time he started to experience periods of coughing, dyspnea, and weakness. A complete examination provided by the company concluded that the man had moderate interstitial lung disease (ILD).

On the basis of the man's work history, the doctor speculated that the ILD was caused by asbestos fibers. This theory was confirmed later with the finding of asbestos fibers in a Perls' stain of sputum, and the diagnosis of asbestosis was noted in the patient's chart. Just before the man retired, his pulmonary function test results (PFTs) showed a mild-to-moderate combined restrictive and obstructive disorder.

Although the man was able to enjoy a couple of relatively good years of retirement with his wife, his health declined rapidly. His cough and dyspnea quickly became a daily problem. Despite his deteriorating health, the man continued to smoke. When he was 68 years old, he was hospitalized for 8 days for treatment of pneumonia and severe respiratory distress. When he was discharged at that time, his PFTs still showed a moderate-to-severe restrictive disorder. He started using oxygen at home regularly.

Approximately 10 months before the current admission, the man was hospitalized because of congestive heart failure. He was treated aggressively and sent home within 5 days. At the time of discharge, his PFTs showed that he had a worsening restrictive respiratory disorder. His arterial blood gas values (ABGs) on 2 L/min oxygen by nasal cannula were as follows: pH 7.38, Pa_{CO_2} 86, HCO_3^- 46, and Pa_{O_2} 63.

Approximately 3 hours before the current admission, the man awoke from an afternoon nap extremely short of breath. His wife stated that he coughed almost continuously and had difficulty speaking. She measured his oral temperature, which read 38° C (100° F). Concerned, she drove her husband to the hospital emergency room.

Physical Examination

As the man was wheeled into the emergency room, he appeared nervous, weak, and in obvious respiratory distress. He was on 1.5 L/min oxygen by nasal cannula, which was connected to an E-tank that was attached to the wheelchair. His skin felt damp and clammy to the touch. He appeared pale and cyanotic. His neck veins were distended, and his fingers and toes were clubbed. He demonstrated a frequent but weak cough productive of a moderate amount of thick, whitish-yellow secretions. He had 3+ peripheral edema of the ankles and feet. He said this was the worst his breathing had ever been.

The patient's vital signs were as follows: blood pressure 180/96, heart rate 108 bpm, respiratory rate 32/min, and oral temperature 38.3° C (100.8° F). Palpation of the chest was negative. Percussion produced bilateral dull notes in the lung bases. Rhonchi and crackles were auscultated throughout both lungs. A pleural friction rub could be heard over the right middle lobe between the sixth and seventh ribs, between the anterior axillary line and midaxillary line.

The patient's lower lobes had a diffuse, "ground-glass" appearance on the chest x-ray film. Irregularly shaped opacities in the right and left lower pleural spaces were identified by the radiologist as calcified pleural plaques. A possible infiltrate consistent with pneumonia also was visible in the right middle lobe. In addition, the chest x-ray suggested that the right side of the heart was moderately enlarged. His ABGs on a 1.5 L/min oxygen nasal cannula were as follows: pH 7.56, Pa_{CO_2} 51, HCO_3^- 42, and Pa_{O_2} 47.

The physician started the patient on intravenous furosemide (Lasix) to treat the man's cor pulmonale and began administering an antibiotic to treat suspected pneumonia. A respiratory care practitioner was called to obtain a sputum culture, perform a respiratory care evaluation, and outline further respiratory therapy. The physician said that she did not want to commit the patient to a ventilator unless absolutely necessary. On the basis of this information, the following SOAP was recorded.

Respiratory Assessment and Plan

S "This is the worst my breathing has ever been."

O Vital signs: BP 180/96, HR 108, RR 32, T 38.3° C (100.8° F); weak appearance; skin: cyanotic, damp, and clammy; distended neck veins and digital clubbing; cough: frequent, weak, moderate amount of thick, whitish yellow secretions; peripheral edema 3+ of ankles and feet. Bilateral dull percussion notes in lung bases. Over both lungs: rhonchi and crackles; pleural friction rub over right middle lobe between sixth and seventh ribs, between anterior axillary line and midaxillary line; CXR: ground-glass appearance in lower lobes; calcified pleural plaques in right and left lower pleural spaces; consolidation in right middle lung lobe; right heart enlargement; ABGs

(1.5 L/min O_2 by nasal cannula): pH 7.56, $Paco_2$ 51, HCO_3^- 42, Pao_2 47.

A
- Respiratory distress (general appearance, vital signs, ABGs)
- Pulmonary fibrosis (history, diagnosis of asbestosis, CXR)
- Alveolar consolidation in right middle lobe (CXR)
- Pleurisy (asbestosis or pneumonitis) in area of right middle lobe (pleural friction rub)
- Excessive bronchial secretions (rhonchi, sputum production)
- Chest infection likely (yellow sputum)
- Acute alveolar hyperventilation superimposed on chronic ventilatory failure with moderate-to-severe hypoxemia (history, ABGs)
- Impending ventilatory failure (ABGs)

P Begin **Oxygen Therapy Protocol** (HAFOE at Fio_2 0.28). **Bronchopulmonary Hygiene Therapy Protocol** (C&DB q4h; obtaining sputum for Gram stain and culture). Initiate **Lung Expansion Therapy Protocol** (incentive spirometry followed by C&DB). Monitor with alarming pulse oximeter set at 85% Spo_2.

The Next Morning

Throughout the night the patient's condition remained unstable. He continued to cough frequently but could not expectorate secretions adequately on his own. When the therapist assisted the patient during coughing episodes, a moderate amount of thick, white and yellow sputum was produced. Even though he was conscious, alert, and able to follow simple directions, he did not answer any of the respiratory care practitioner's specific questions about his breathing.

His skin was cold and damp to the touch, and he appeared short of breath. His color was improved, but he still appeared pale and cyanotic. His neck veins were still distended, although not so severely as they had been on admission, and edema of his ankles and feet could still be seen. The patient's vital signs were as follows: blood pressure 192/108, heart rate 113 bpm, respiratory rate 34/min, and oral temperature 38° C (100.4° F). Palpation of the chest was negative.

Dull percussion notes were elicited over the lung bases. Rhonchi and crackles continued to be auscultated throughout both lungs. A pleural friction rub could still be heard over the right middle lung between the sixth and seventh ribs, between the anterior axillary line and midaxillary line. No recent chest x-ray was available. His ABGs (Fio_2 = 0.28) were as follows: pH 7.57, $Paco_2$ 47, HCO_3^- 36, and Pao_2 40. His oxygen saturation measured by pulse oximetry (Spo_2) was 77%. On the basis of these clinical data, the following SOAP was documented.

Respiratory Assessment and Plan

S N/A (patient too dyspneic to reply)

O Condition unstable; cough: frequent, weak, productive of thick, white and yellow secretions; skin: cyanotic, pale, cool, and damp; distended neck veins and peripheral edema, but improving; vital signs: BP 192/108, HR 113, RR 34, T 38° C (100.4° F); dull percussion notes over both lung bases; rhonchi and crackles throughout both lungs; pleural friction rub over right middle lobe between sixth and seventh ribs, between anterior axillary line and midaxillary line; ABGs (Fio_2 = 0.28): pH 7.57, $Paco_2$ 47, HCO_3^- 36, Pao_2 40; Spo_2 77%

A
- Continued respiratory distress (general appearance, vital signs, ABGs)
- Pulmonary fibrosis in lower lobes (history, diagnosis of asbestosis, recent CXR)
- Alveolar consolidation in right middle lobe (CXR, pneumonia)
- Pleurisy or pneumonia that has extended into pleural space over right middle lobe (pleural friction rub)
- Excessive bronchial secretions (rhonchi, sputum production)
- Infection likely (yellow sputum)
- Acute alveolar hyperventilation superimposed on chronic ventilatory failure with severe hypoxemia, worsening (history, ABGs)
- Impending ventilatory failure (ABGs: increased alveolar hyperventilation and worsening Pao_2)

P Up-regulate **Oxygen Therapy Protocol** (HAFOE to Fio_2 0.40). **Bronchopulmonary Hygiene Therapy Protocol** (adding intensive nasotracheal suctioning q2h). Start **Aerosolized Medication Protocal** (nebulize 2 mL acetylcysteine to the premix albuterol). Continue **Lung Expansion Therapy Protocol** (continuing to coach and monitor incentive spirometry; if FVC falls below 15 mL/kg, administer CPAP mask at +10 cm H_2O for 20 minutes qid while patient is awake). Continue to monitor closely.

20 Hours Later

At 6:15 AM the alarm on the patient's cardiac monitor sounded. The electrocardiogram (ECG) strip showed frequent premature ventricular contractions followed by ventricular flutter and fibrillation. The head nurse called for a Code Blue. Cardiopulmonary resuscitation was started immediately. Because of the severe hypotension (blood pressure 80/50), epinephrine and dopamine were administered through the patient's intravenous line. Approximately 12 minutes into the code, the patient exhibited a normal sinus rhythm and spontaneous respirations.

The patient was intubated, transferred to the intensive care unit (ICU), and placed on a mechanical ventilator. The initial ventilator settings were in assist control mode as follows: 12 breaths per minute, Fio_2 1.0, pressure support 14 cm H_2O, and 10 cm H_2O positive end-expiratory pressure (PEEP). His cardiopulmonary status remained unstable. Premature ventricular contractions were frequently seen on the electrocardiographic monitor. A pulmonary artery catheter and arterial line were inserted.

The patient's skin was pale, cyanotic, and clammy. His neck veins were still distended, and his ankles and feet were swollen. Vital signs were as follows: blood pressure 135/90, heart rate 84 bpm, and rectal temperature 38.3° C (100.8° F). Palpation of the chest wall was negative. Dull percussion notes were noted over the lung bases. Rhonchi and crackles continued to be auscultated throughout both lungs. Thick, greenish-yellow sputum was frequently suctioned from the patient's endotracheal tube.

A pleural friction rub still could be heard over the right middle lung lobe between the sixth and seventh ribs, between the anterior axillary line and midaxillary line. A chest x-ray had been taken but had not yet been interpreted by the radiologist. The patient's hemodynamic indices were as follows: elevated central venous pressure (CVP), right atrial pressure (RAP), mean pulmonary artery pressure (PA), right ventricular stroke work index (RVSWI), and pulmonary vascular resistance (PVR). All other hemodynamic values were normal. His ABGs on 1.0 oxygen were as follows: pH 7.53, $Pa{CO_2}$ 56, HCO_3^- 38, and $Pa{O_2}$ 246. His $Sp{O_2}$ was 98%. At this time, the following SOAP note was charted.

Respiratory Assessment and Plan

S N/A (patient intubated on ventilator)

O Vital signs: BP 135/90 on vasopressors, HR 84, T 38.3° C (100.8° F); frequent premature ventricular contractions; skin: pale, cyanotic, and clammy; distended neck veins; peripheral edema of ankles and feet; dull percussion notes over lung bases; rhonchi and crackles throughout both lungs; thick, greenish-yellow sputum frequently suctioned; pleural friction rub over right middle lung lobe between sixth and seventh ribs and between anterior axillary line and midaxillary line; hemodynamic indices: elevated CVP, RAP, PA, RVSWI, and PVR; ABGs ($FI{O_2}$ = 1.0): pH 7.53, $Pa{CO_2}$ 56, HCO_3^- 38, $Pa{O_2}$ 246, $Sp{O_2}$ 98%

A
- Pulmonary fibrosis, lower lung lobes (history, diagnosis of asbestosis, recent CXR)
- Alveolar consolidation, right middle lobe (recent CXR showing pneumonia)
- Pneumonia possibly extended into pleural space over right middle lobe (pleural friction rub)
- Excessive bronchial secretions (rhonchi, sputum production)
- Infection likely (fever, greenish-yellow sputum, possible new organism)
- Acute alveolar hyperventilation superimposed on chronic ventilatory failure and overly corrected hypoxemia (ABGs)
- Overventilation and overoxygenation caused by mechanical ventilator

P Down-regulate **Oxygen Therapy Protocol** (reduction of $FI{O_2}$ to 0.50). Down-regulate **Mechanical Ventilation Protocol** (decreasing tidal volume to increase $Pa{CO_2}$ to patient's baseline—80 to 90 mm Hg). Continue **Bronchopulmonary Hygiene Therapy Protocol** and **Aerosolized Medication Protocol**. Continue **Lung Expansion Therapy Protocol** (depending on mean airway pressure). Continue to closely monitor and reevaluate.

Discussion

The admitting history revealed that the patient had been diagnosed with moderate pneumoconiosis (probable asbestosis) and that he had been a heavy smoker for more than 40 years. Not surprisingly, pulmonary function tests in the past had shown mild-to-moderate restrictive pulmonary disorders.

Significant new findings were the recent history suggesting congestive heart failure and the arterial blood gas values on his discharge from the hospital 10 months before the admission under discussion, which demonstrated chronic ventilatory failure. The patient's recent fever and cough before his emergency room admission suggested an infectious cause for his symptoms. His cyanosis, neck-vein distention, and digital clubbing suggested chronic hypoxemia. The sputum purulence confirmed that infection may indeed have been present and that the assessing therapist's desire to obtain a sputum culture was appropriate. The pleural rub demonstrated by this patient could have been related to his asbestosis or to a pneumonic infiltrate extending to the pleural surface.

In the initial assessment the patient's severe hypertension and his fever were noted. Both deserved vigorous therapy if his pulmonary function were to improve at all. The patient's severe hypoxemia reflected common clinical indicators caused by **Alveolar-Capillary Membrane Thickening** (see Figure 9-10) and **Excessive Bronchial Secretions** (see Figure 9-12). Although there is no therapy to reverse the increased alveolar membrane thickening, the excessive bronchial secretions can be effectively treated in most cases.

Note that the pulmonary capillary wedge pressure (PCWP) was not measured in the first assessment. Such measurements may have identified an element of left ventricular failure in this hypertensive patient as well. The patient was hyperventilating with respect to his earlier outpatient blood gases. During such an assessment the patient's underlying pulmonary conditions (chronic pulmonary fibrosis, bronchitis, and congestive heart failure) should be recorded, but the assessment should really zero in on the treatable issues, specifically in this case the pulmonary infection, as suggested by the patient's fever, sputum purulence, and chest x-ray film.

At the time of the second evaluation, the patient's hypoxemia had worsened despite oxygen therapy. If not already being used, Venturi oxygen mask (HAFOE) therapy was indicated there, and additional mucolytics and endobronchial suctioning also could be indicated. The trial of **Lung Expansion Therapy Protocol** (Protocol 9-3) was appropriate to attempt to offset the pathologic effects of the alveolar consolidation and, possibly, atelectasis. The physician may have ordered a trial of diuretic therapy to reduce the fluid retention and a course of antibiotic therapy as well.

The last assessment revealed ventricular arrhythmias. The change in the patient's sputum from thick and white to greenish-yellow suggests superinfection with another organism, and reculture of the sputum was appropriate. The respiratory practitioner responded quickly, and appropriately, to readjust the mechanical ventilator. The $FI{O_2}$ was decreased to 0.5 to correct the patient's overoxygenation ($Pa{O_2}$: 246), and the tidal volume was reduced to increase the $Pa{CO_2}$ to the baseline—80 to 90 mm Hg according to the ABG history. Ventilator parameters should be adjusted to provide good pulmonary expansion while avoiding high mean airway pressures. A cautious trial of PEEP would have been in order.

Despite all that was done for this patient, he died 4 days later as a result of left-sided congestive heart failure and pneumonia complicating his pulmonary asbestosis.

SELF-ASSESSMENT QUESTIONS

evolve Answers to questions can be found on Evolve. To access additional student assessment questions and case studies for application of text material to real-life scenarios, visit **http://evolve.elsevier.com/DesJardins/respiratory.**

1. Which of the following is another name for hypersensitivity pneumonitis?
   a. Sarcoidosis
   b. Extrinsic allergic alveolitis
   c. Alveolar proteinosis
   d. Idiopathic pulmonary hemosiderosis

2. Which of the following is or are considered pulmonary vasculitides?
   1. Rheumatoid arthritis
   2. Wegener's granulomatosis
   3. Lymphomatoid granulomatosis
   4. Churg-Strauss syndrome
   a. 1 only
   b. 3 only
   c. 2, 3, and 4 only
   d. 1, 2, and 3 only

3. Which of the following disorders is associated with desquamative interstitial pneumonia and usual interstitial pneumonia?
   a. Idiopathic pulmonary fibrosis
   b. Eosinophilic granuloma
   c. Rheumatoid arthritis
   d. Sarcoidosis

4. Which of the following is/are systemic connective tissue diseases?
   1. Pulmonary Langerhans' cell histiocytosis
   2. Rheumatoid arthritis
   3. Sjögren's syndrome
   4. Alveolar proteinosis
   a. 3 only
   b. 2 and 4 only
   c. 1 and 4 only
   d. 2 and 3 only

5. Which of the following pulmonary function study findings is or are associated with chronic interstitial lung disease?
   1. Increased FRC
   2. Decreased FEV_T
   3. Increased RV
   4. Decreased FVC
   a. 1 only
   b. 3 only
   c. 2 and 4 only
   d. 3 and 4 only

6. Which of the following hemodynamic indices is or are associated with advanced or severe interstitial lung disease?
   1. Increased CVP
   2. Decreased PCWP
   3. Increased $\overline{PA}$
   4. Decreased RAP
   a. 1 only
   b. 4 only
   c. 1 and 3 only
   d. 2 and 4 only

7. The length of asbestos fibers is commonly which of the following?
   a. 10 to 20 μm
   b. 15 to 25 μm
   c. 25 to 50 μm
   d. 50 to 100 μm

8. Which of the following oxygenation indices is or are associated with the pneumoconioses?
   1. Decreased $C(a-\bar{v})O_2$
   2. Increased O_2ER
   3. Decreased $S\bar{v}O_2$
   4. Increased $\dot{V}O_2$
   a. 1 only
   b. 3 only
   c. 2 and 3 only
   d. 1 and 4 only

9. The fibrotic changes that develop in coal worker's pneumoconiosis usually result from which of the following?
   a. Barium
   b. Silica
   c. Iron
   d. Coal dust

10. Which of the following are associated with the ILD?
   1. Pleural friction rub
   2. Dull percussion note
   3. Cor pulmonale
   4. Elevated $\overline{PA}$
   a. 2 and 4 only
   b. 3 and 4 only
   c. 2, 3, and 4 only
   d. 1, 2, 3, and 4

PART VIII

Neoplastic Disease

Cancer of the Lung

26

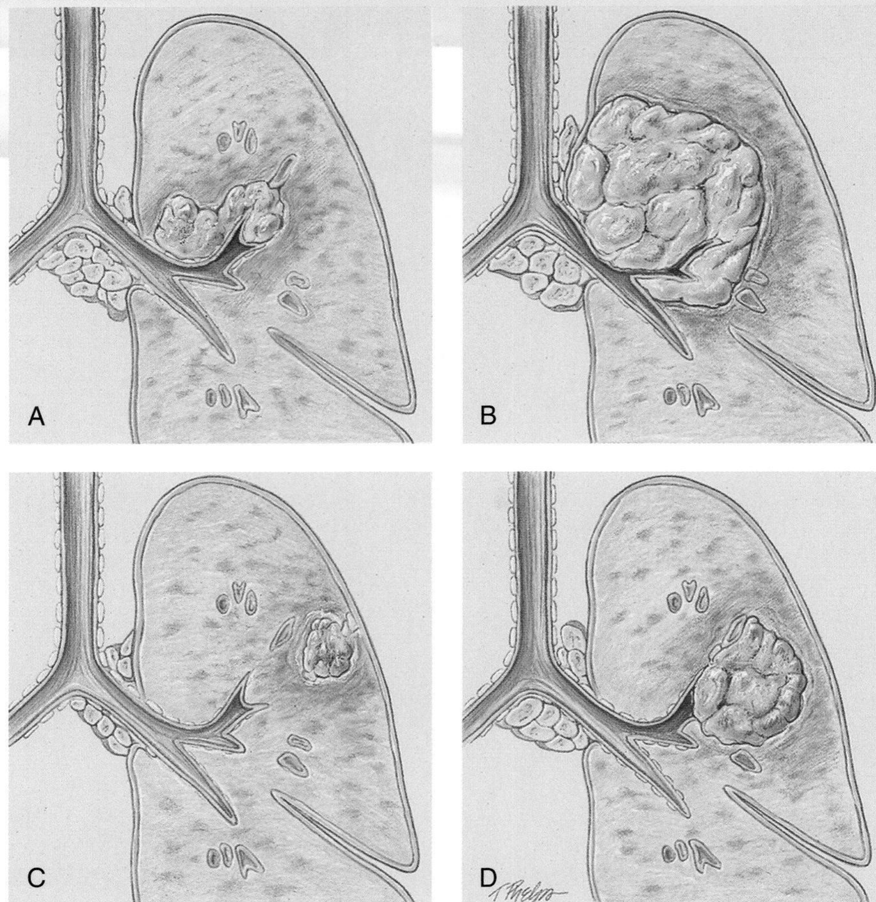

FIGURE 26-1 Cancer of the lung. **A**, Squamous cell carcinoma. **B**, Adenocarcinoma. **C**, Large cell carcinoma. **D**, Small cell (oat cell) carcinoma.

Chapter Objectives

After reading this chapter, you will be able to:

- List the anatomic alterations of the lungs associated with cancer of the lung.
- Describe the causes of cancer of the lung.
- List the cardiopulmonary clinical manifestations associated with cancer of the lung.
- Describe the general management of cancer of the lung.
- Describe the clinical strategies and rationales of the SOAPs presented in the case study.
- Define key terms and complete self-assessment questions at the end of the chapter and on Evolve.

Key Terms

Adenocarcinoma
Benign Tumors
Bilobectomy
Brachytherapy
Bronchogenic Carcinoma
Chemotherapy
Cigarette Smoking
Coin Lesion
Large Cell Carcinoma (Undifferentiated)
Lobectomy
Malignant Tumors
Neoplasm
Non-Small Cell Lung Carcinoma (NSCLC)
Palliative (Comfort) Care
PET/CT Image
Pneumonectomy
Positron Emission Tomography (PET) Scans
Prophylactic Cranial Irradiation (PCI)
Radiation Therapy
Radical Radiotherapy
Segmentectomy
Small Cell (Oat Cell) Carcinoma

Small Cell Lung Carcinoma (SCLC)
Squamous Cell Carcinoma
Staging of Lung Cancer
Stereotactic Radiation Therapy
Superior Vena Cava Syndrome
Wedge Resection

Chapter Outline

Anatomic Alterations of the Lungs

Cancer is a general term that refers to abnormal new tissue growth characterized by the progressive, uncontrolled multiplication of cells. This abnormal growth of new cells is called a **neoplasm** or *tumor.* A tumor may be localized or invasive, benign or malignant.

Benign tumors do not endanger life unless they interfere with the normal functions of other organs or affect a vital organ. They grow slowly and push aside normal tissue but do not invade it. They are usually encapsulated, well-demarcated growths. They are not invasive or metastatic; that is, tumor cells do not travel by way of the bloodstream or lymphatics and invade or form secondary tumors in other organs.

Malignant tumors are composed of embryonic, primitive, or poorly differentiated cells. They grow in a disorganized manner and so rapidly that nutrition of the cells becomes a problem. For this reason, necrosis, ulceration, and cavity formation are commonly associated with malignant tumors. They also invade surrounding tissues and may be metastatic. Although malignant changes may develop in any portion of the lung, they most commonly originate in the mucosa of the tracheobronchial tree.

Lung cancer arises from the epithelium of the tracheobronchial tree. Thus a tumor that originates in the bronchial mucosa is called **bronchogenic carcinoma.** The terms *lung cancer* and *bronchogenic carcinoma* are used interchangeably. As a tumor enlarges, the surrounding bronchial airways and alveoli become irritated, inflamed, and swollen. The adjacent alveoli may fill with fluid or become consolidated or collapse. In addition, as the tumor protrudes into the tracheobronchial tree, excessive mucous production and airway obstruction develop. As the surrounding blood vessels erode, blood enters the tracheobronchial tree. Peripheral tumors also may invade the pleural space and impinge on the mediastinum, chest wall, ribs, or diaphragm. A secondary pleural effusion is often seen in lung cancer. A pleural effusion further compresses the lung and causes atelectasis.

The major pathologic or structural changes associated with bronchogenic carcinoma are as follows:

- Inflammation, swelling, and destruction of the bronchial airways and alveoli
- Excessive mucous production
- Tracheobronchial mucous accumulation and plugging
- Airway obstruction (either from blood, from mucous accumulation, or from a tumor projecting into a bronchus)
- Atelectasis
- Alveolar consolidation
- Cavity formation
- Pleural effusion (when a tumor invades the parietal pleura and mediastinum)

Etiology and Epidemiology

Lung cancer is the leading cause of cancer deaths in the United States. According to the American Cancer Society 2008 surveillance report, it is estimated that more than 214,000 new cases of lung cancer are reported in the United States annually—about 114,000 in males and about 100,000 in females. Although lung cancer accounts for about 15% of all cancers in both men and women, it is responsible for about 31% of all cancer deaths in men and about 26% of all cancers in women. Among women, the lung cancer death rate is now higher than the death rate of any other cancer, including breast cancer (15% for breast cancer versus 26% for lung cancer). The higher incidence of lung cancer in women is primarily because of their increased rate of cigarette smoking. Death from lung cancer generally begins when patients are 35 to 44 years of age. A sharp increase in lung cancer deaths is seen among patients 45 to 55 years of age. The incidence of lung cancer death progressively increases to 74 years of age and then levels off and decreases in extremely old individuals.

Cigarette smoking is the most common cause of lung cancer. Although various studies and professional organizations report slightly different numbers, all the figures are grim. For example, according to the Centers for Disease Control and Prevention (CDC) and the Surgeon General's report, male smokers are 22 times more likely to develop lung cancer than nonsmokers, whereas female smokers are 12 times more likely than female nonsmokers to develop lung cancer. Heavy smokers are 64 times more likely to develop lung cancer. It is estimated that cigarette smoke contains more than 4000 different chemicals, many of which have proved to be carcinogens. Passive, or second-hand, smoking is associated with as much as a 30% increase in the risk for lung cancer. A genetic predisposition toward developing lung cancer also plays a role in the incidence of lung cancer.

Environmental or occupational risk factors for lung cancer include the following:

- Benzopyrene and radon particles associated with uranium mining
- Radiation and nuclear fallout
- Polycyclic aromatic hydrocarbons and arsenicals
- Asbestos fibers
- Diesel exhaust
- Nitrogen mustard gases
- Nickel
- Silica
- Vinyl chloride
- Chlormethyl methyl ether
- Air pollution
- Coal and iron mining

Types of Cancers

There are four major types of bronchogenic tumors: (1) **squamous (epidermoid) cell carcinoma,** (2) **adenocarcinoma** (including bronchial alveolar cell carcinoma), (3) **large cell carcinoma,** and (4) **small cell (oat cell) carcinoma** (see Figure 26-1). For therapeutic reasons, these bronchogenic tumors are commonly divided into the following two groups:

- Non–small cell lung carcinoma (NSCLC)
  - **Squamous cell carcinoma**
  - **Adenocarcinoma**
  - **Large cell carcinoma (Undifferentiated)**
- Small cell lung carcinoma (SCLC)
  - **Small cell (or oat cell carcinoma)**

Each group grows and spreads in different way. For example, SCLC spreads aggressively and responds best to **chemotherapy** and **radiation therapy.** It occurs almost exclusively in smokers and accounts for over 20% of all lung cancers in the United States. NSCLC is more common and accounts for about 80% of all lung cancers in America. When confined to a small area and identified early, this type of cancer often can be removed surgically. Table 26-1 provides general characteristics of these cancer cell types, including growth rates, metastasis, and means of diagnosis. A more in-depth description of each cancer cell type follows.

Non–Small Cell Lung Carcinoma

Squamous cell carcinoma. Squamous cell carcinoma constitutes approximately 30% of the bronchogenic carcinomas. The incidence of this type of cancer has sharply declined over the past two decades. This type of tumor is commonly located near a central bronchus or hilus and projects into the large bronchi. Squamous cell tumors are often seen projecting into the bronchi during bronchoscopy. The tumor originates from the basal cells of the bronchial epithelium and grows through the epithelium before invading the surrounding tissues.

The tumor has a slow growth rate and a late metastatic tendency (mostly to hilar lymph nodes). These tumors generally remain fairly well localized and tend not to metastasize until late in the course of the lung cancer. Cavitation and necrosis within the center of the cancer is a common finding. Surgical resection is the preferred treatment if metastasis has not taken place. In about one third of the cases, squamous cell carcinoma originates in the periphery. Because of the location in the central bronchi, obstructive manifestations are generally nonspecific and include a nonproductive cough and hemoptysis. Pneumonia and atelectasis are often secondary complications of squamous cell carcinoma. Cavity formation with or without an air-fluid interface is seen in 10% to 20% of the cases (see Figure 26-1, *A*).

Adenocarcinoma. Adenocarcinoma arises from the mucous glands of the tracheobronchial tree. In fact, the glandular configuration and the mucous production caused by this type of cancer are the pathologic features that distinguish adenocarcinoma from the other types of bronchogenic carcinoma. It accounts for 35% to 40% of all bronchogenic carcinomas. Adenocarcinoma has the weakest association with smoking. However, among people who have never smoked, adenocarcinoma is the most common form of lung cancer. Adenocarcinoma tumors are usually smaller than 4 cm and are most commonly found in the peripheral regions of the lung parenchyma. The growth rate is moderate and the metastatic tendency is early. Secondary cavity formation and pleural effusion are common (see Figure 26-1, *B*). When the cancer is

TABLE 26-1 Characteristics of Lung Cancers

Tumor Type	Growth Rate	Metastasis	Means of Diagnosis
Squamous cell carcinoma	Slow	Late; mostly to hilar lymph nodes	Biopsy, sputum analysis, bronchoscopy, electron microscopy, immunohistochemistry
Adenocarcinoma	Moderate	Early	Radiography, fiberoptic bronchoscopy, electron microscopy
Large cell carcinoma	Rapid	Early and widespread	Sputum analysis, bronchoscopy, electron microscopy (by exclusion of other cell types)
Small cell (oat cell) carcinoma	Very rapid	Very early; to mediastinum or distally in lung	Radiography, sputum analysis, bronchoscopy, electron microscopy, immunohistochemistry, and clinical manifestations (cough, chest pain, dyspnea, hemoptysis, localized wheezing)

Modified from McCance KL, Huether SE: *Pathophysiology: the biologic basis for disease in adults and children,* ed 5, St Louis, 2006, Mosby.

discovered early, surgical resection is possible in a high percentage of cases.

Bronchial alveolar cell carcinoma is included under the category of adenocarcinoma. These tumors typically arise from the terminal bronchioles and alveoli. They have a slow growth rate, and their metastasis pattern is unpredictable.

Large cell carcinoma (undifferentiated). Large cell carcinoma accounts for about 10% to 15% of all bronchogenic carcinoma cases. Because this tumor has lost all evidence of differentiation, it is commonly referred to as *undifferentiated large cell anaplastic cancer.* Although these tumors commonly arise peripherally, they may also be found centrally—often distorting the trachea and large airways. Large cell carcinoma has a rapid growth rate and early and widespread metastasis. Common secondary complications include chest wall pain, pleural effusion, pneumonia, hemoptysis, and cavity formation (see Figure 26-1, *C*).

Small Cell Lung Carcinoma

Small cell carcinoma accounts for about 14% of all bronchogenic carcinomas. Most of these tumors arise centrally near the hilar region. They tend to arise in the larger airways (primary and secondary bronchi). Cell size ranges from 6 to 8 μm. The tumor grows very rapidly, becoming quite large, and metastasizes early. Because the tumor cells often are compressed into an oval shape, this form of cancer is commonly referred to as oat cell carcinoma. Staging for small cell carcinoma is divided into only two categories: limited disease (20% to 30%) or extensive disease (70% to 80%). Small cell carcinoma has the poorest prognosis. The average survival time for untreated small cell carcinoma is about 1 to 3 months. Small cell carcinoma has the strongest correlation with cigarette smoking and is associated with the worst prognosis (see Figure 26-1, *A*).

Screening and Diagnosis

A routine chest x-ray is the most common screening test used to identify an abnormal mass or nodule in a patient's lung. Computed tomography (CT) and **positron emission tomography (PET) scans** are also frequently used to reveal extremely small lesions and determine whether the cancer has spread to other areas. A definitive diagnosis, however, can be made only by viewing a tissue sample (biopsy) under a microscope. Common procedures used to obtain a tissue biopsy include bronchoscopy, thoracoscopy, mediastinoscopy, transbronchial needle biopsy or open-lung biopsy, sputum cytology, thoracentesis, and videothoracoscopy (see Chapter 8).

Staging of Lung Cancer

Staging is the process of classifying information about cancer. The staging system describes the cancer cell type, the size of the tumor, the level of lymph node involvement, and the extent to which the cancer has spread. The patient's prognosis and treatment depend, to a large extent, on the staging results. The system most often used for the **staging of lung cancer** is the TNM classification (Table 26-2). *T* represents the extent of the primary tumor, *N* denotes the lymph node involvement, and *M* indicates the extent of metastasis. On the basis of the TNM findings, roman numerals are used to identify stages I through IV, with 0 being the least advanced and IV the most advanced. Figure 26-2 provides five representative illustrations of the staging of lung cancer by the TNM classification system. A general overview and description of the staging process for non–small cell lung cancer and small cell lung cancer follows*:

Non–Small Cell Lung Carcinoma

NSCLC is staged according to the size of the tumor, the level of lymph node involvement, and the extent to which the cancer has spread. The stages for non–small cell lung cancer include the following:

- *Stage 0:* The cancer is limited to the lining of the bronchial airways. There is no involvement of the lung tissue or distant metastasis. Stage 0 cancers usually are found during bronchoscopy. When found and treated early, cancers at this stage can often be cured. (TisN0M0)
- *Stage I:* The tumor is less than 3 cm and is located in lobar or distal airways. There is no lung tissue involvement or distant metastasis. (T1N0M0)
- *Stage II:* In this stage the cancer has invaded neighboring lymph nodes or spread to the chest wall. There is no distant metastasis. (T1N1M0)
- *Stage IIIA:* The tumor is any size. The tumor is in the main bronchus, or the tumor is accompanied by atelectasis or obstructive pneumonitis of the entire lung. Local invasion involves chest wall, diaphragm, mediastinal, pleural, or parietal pericardium. There is the presence of metastasis to ipsilateral peribronchial or ipsilateral hilar lymph nodes or both. There is no distant metastasis. (T3N1M0)
- *Stage IIIB:* The cancer has spread locally to areas such as the mediastinum, heart, great vessels, trachea, esophagus, vertebral body, or carina, or malignant pleural or pericardial effusion is present—all within the chest. There may be involvement of any of the lymph node groups. There is no distant metastasis. (T4, any N, M0)
- *Stage IV:* The cancer is of any size, involves any of the lymph node groups, and has spread to other parts of the body, such as the liver, bones, or brain. (any T; any N; M1)

Small Cell Lung Carcinoma

SCLC is staged differently than non–small cell cancer. Roman numerals are not used to identify the stages. Small cell lung cancer is usually classified as either limited or extensive:

- Limited: The cancer is confined to only one lung and to its neighboring lymph nodes.
- Extensive: The cancer has spread beyond one lung and nearby lymph nodes. It may have invaded both lungs, more remote lymph nodes, or other organs.

---

*Not all the subcategories for each stage are provided in this overview. See Table 26-2 for all the stages and their respective definitions.

TABLE 26-2 1997 Revised International System for Staging Lung Cancer

Symbol	Definition
Primary Tumor (T)	
T0	No evidence of tumor
Tx	Tumor that cannot be assessed or is not apparently radiologically or bronchoscopically (malignant cells in bronchopulmonary secretions)
Tis	Carcinoma in situ
T1	Tumor with the following characteristics:
a	Size: ≤3 cm
b	Airway location: in lobar bronchus or distal airways
c	Local invasion: none, surrounded by lung or visceral pleura
T2	Tumor with any of the following characteristics:
a	Size: >3 cm
b	Airway location: tumor in the main bronchus (within 2 cm of the carina) or tumor with atelectasis involvement of the main bronchus (distance to the carina is 2 cm or more) or presence of atelectasis or obstructive pneumonitis that extends to hilar region but does not involve the entire lung
c	Local invasion: involvement of the visceral pleura
T3	Tumor with the following location or invasion:
a	Size: any
b	Airway location: tumor in the main bronchus (within 2 cm of the carina) or tumor with atelectasis or obstructive pneumonitis of the entire lung
c	Local invasion: invasion of chest wall (including superior sulcus tumors), diaphragm,mediastinal pleura, or parietal pericardium
T4	Tumor with the following location or invasion:
a	Size: any
b	Airway location: satellite tumor nodule(s) within the ipsilateral primary-tumor lobe of the lung
c	Local invasion: invasion of the mediastinum, heart, great vessels, trachea, esophagus, vertebral body, or carina; or presence of malignant pleural/pericardial effusion
Lymph Nodes (N)	
Nx	Regional lymph nodes cannot be assessed
N0	Absence of regional lymph node involvement
N1	Presence of metastasis to ipsilateral peribronchial or ipsilateral hilar lymph nodes or both (including direct extension to intrapulmonary nodes)
N2	Presence of metastasis to ipsilateral mediastinal or subcarinal lymph nodes or both
N3	Presence of metastasis to any of the following lymph node groups: contralateral mediastinal, contralateral hilar, ipsilateral or contralateral scalene, or supraclavicular
Distant Metastasis (M)	
Mx	Metastasis cannot be assessed
M0	Absence of distant metastasis
M1	Presence of distant metastasis (separate metastatic tumor nodule[s] in the ipsilateral nonprimary-tumor lobe[s] of the lung also are grouped as M1)
Stage Grouping—TNM Subsets	
Stage 0	TisN0M0
Stage IA	T1N0M0
Stage IB	T2N0M0
Stage IIA	T1N1M0
Stage IIB	T2N1N0; T3N0M0
Stage IIIA	T3N1M0; T(1-3)N2M0
Stage IIIB	T4, any N, M0; any T, N3M0
Stage IV	Any T; any N; M1

From Mountain CF: Revisions in the international system for staging lung cancer. *Chest* 111(6):1710, 1997.

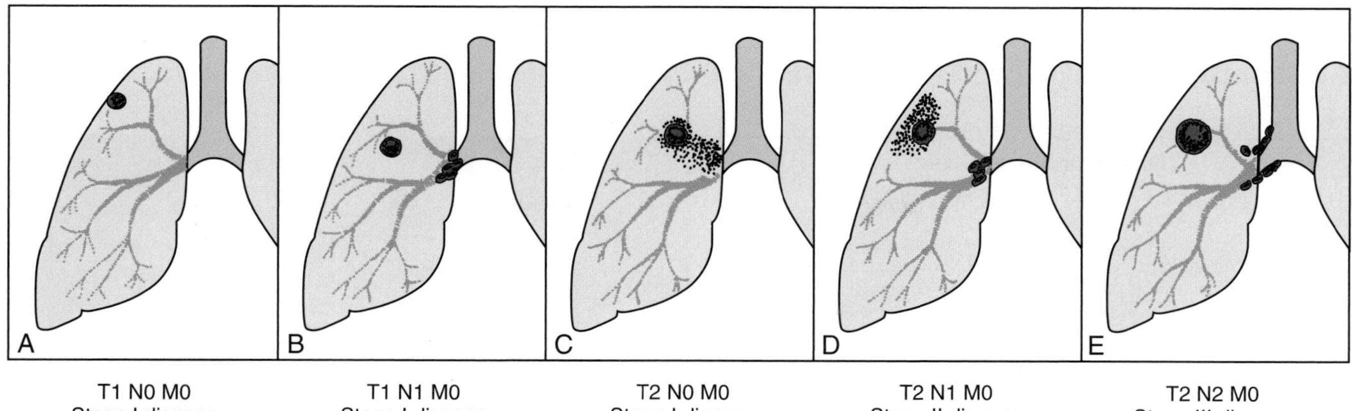

FIGURE 26-2 Staging of lung cancer by the TNM classification system. **A**, **B**, Stage I disease includes tumors classified as T1, with or without metastasis to the lymph nodes in the ipsilateral hilar region. **C**, Also included in stage I are tumors classified as T2 but having no nodal or distant metastases. **D**, Stage II disease includes those tumors classified as T2, with metastasis only to the ipsilateral hilar lymph nodes. **E**, Stage III includes all tumors more extensive than T2 or any tumor with metastasis to the lymph nodes in the mediastinum or with distant metastasis. (Modified from McCance KL, Huether SE: *Pathophysiology: the biologic basis for disease in adults and children,* ed 5, St Louis, 2006, Mosby.)

OVERVIEW of the Cardiopulmonary Clinical Manifestations Associated with Cancer of the Lung

The following clinical manifestations result from the pathologic mechanisms caused (or activated) by **Atelectasis** (see Figure 9-8), **Alveolar Consolidation** (see Figure 9-9), and **Excessive Bronchial Secretions** (see Figure 9-12)—the major anatomic alterations of the lungs associated with cancer of the lung (see Figure 26-1).

CLINICAL DATA OBTAINED AT THE PATIENT'S BEDSIDE

The Physical Examination

Vital Signs

Increased Respiratory Rate (Tachypnea)

Several pathophysiologic mechanisms operating simultaneously may lead to an increased ventilatory rate:

- Stimulation of peripheral chemoreceptors (hypoxemia)
- Decreased lung compliance–increased ventilatory rate relationship
- Stimulation of the J receptors
- Pain, anxiety

Increased Heart Rate (Pulse) and Blood Pressure

Cyanosis

Cough, Sputum Production, and Hemoptysis

Chest Assessment Findings

- Crackles, rhonchi, and wheezing

CLINICAL DATA OBTAINED FROM LABORATORY TESTS AND SPECIAL PROCEDURES

Pulmonary Function Test (PFT) Findings

Relative to where the malignancy originates, the PFT results may show either obstructive or restrictive values. For example, when the malignancy obstructs major airways, the PFT values may show obstructive pathology—especially when chronic obstructive pulmonary disease (COPD) is present. However, when large amounts of pulmonary tissue, chest wall, and/or diaphragm are involved (extensive bronchioalveolar carcinoma), then the pathology may show restrictive PFT values.

Arterial Blood Gases

LOCALIZED (e.g., LOBAR) LUNG CANCER

Acute Alveolar Hyperventilation with Hypoxemia (Acute Respiratory Alkalosis)

pH	Pa_{CO_2}	HCO_3^-	Pa_{O_2}
↑	↓	↓ (slightly)	↓

EXTENSIVE OR WIDESPREAD LUNG CANCER

Acute Ventilatory Failure with Hypoxemia (Acute Respiratory Acidosis)

pH*	Pa_{CO_2}	HCO_3^- *	Pa_{O_2}
↓	↑	↑ (slightly)	↓

*When tissue hypoxia is severe enough to produce lactic acid, the pH and HCO_3^- values will be lower than expected for a particular Pa_{CO_2} level.

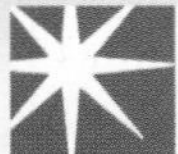

OVERVIEW of the Cardiopulmonary Clinical Manifestations Associated with Cancer of the Lung—cont'd

Oxygenation Indices*

$\dot{Q}_S/\dot{Q}_T$	Do_2[†]	$\dot{V}o_2$	$C(a-\bar{v})o_2$	O_2ER	$S\bar{v}o_2$
↑	↓	N	N	↑	↓

[†]The Do_2 may be normal in patients who have compensated to the decreased oxygenation status with (1) an increased cardiac output, (2) an increased hemoglobin level, or (3) a combination of both. When the Do_2 is normal, the O_2ER is usually normal.

Hemodynamic Indices[‡]

When hypoxemia and acidemia are present, or when a tumor invades the mediastinum and compresses the superior vena cava, the following may be expected.

CVP	RAP	$\overline{PA}$	PCWP	CO	SV
↑	↑	↓	↓ or N	↓ or N	↓ or N

SVI	CI	RVSWI	LVSWI	PVR	SVR
↓ or N	↓ or N	↑	↓ or N	↑	N

RADIOLOGIC FINDINGS

Chest Radiograph

- Small oval or coin lesion
- Large irregular mass
- Alveolar consolidation
- Atelectasis
- Pleural effusion (see Chapter 23)
- Involvement of the mediastinum or diaphragm

A routine chest x-ray examination often provides the first indication or suspicion of lung cancer. Depending on how long the tumor has been growing, the chest x-ray film may show a small radiodense nodule (called a ***coin lesion***) or a large irregular radiodense mass. Unfortunately, by the time a tumor is identified radiographically, regardless of its size, it is usually in the invasive stage and thus difficult to treat. Another common x-ray presentation of lung cancer is that of volume loss involving a single lobe or an individual segment within a lobe.

Because there are four major forms of lung cancer, chest x-ray findings are variable. In general, squamous cell and small cell carcinoma usually appear as a white mass near the hilar region; adenocarcinoma appears in the peripheral portions of the lung; and large cell carcinoma may appear in either the peripheral or the central portion of the lung. Figure 26-3 is a representative example of a large bronchogenic carcinoma in the right lung. Common secondary chest x-ray findings caused by bronchial obstruction include alveolar consolidation, atelectasis, pleural effusion, and mediastinal or diaphragmatic involvement. The x-ray appearance of cavity formation within a bronchogenic carcinoma is similar regardless of the type of cancer.

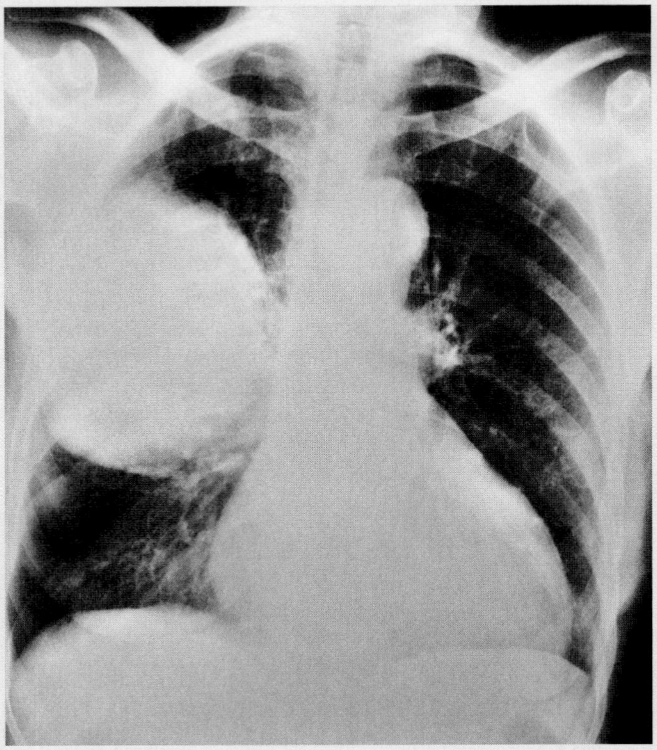

FIGURE 26-3 Right lung squamous cell carcinoma of the bronchus illustrating the huge size these tumors may attain before discovery. (From Hansell DM, Armstrong P, Lynch DA, McAdams HP, eds: *Imaging of diseases of the chest,* ed 4, Philadelphia, 2005, Elsevier.)

Clinically, a positron emission tomography (PET) scan is an excellent test to rule out a possible cancerous area identified on either a chest x-ray film or a computed tomography (CT) scan. For example, Figure 26-4 shows a chest radiograph that identifies two suspicious findings—one small nodule in the right upper lung lobe and a larger density in the left lower lung lobe, just behind the heart. Figure 26-5 shows two CT scans that also identify the two suspicious findings and their precise location. Figures 26-6, 26-7, and 26-8 show PET scans that all confirm a "hot spot" (likely cancer) in the lower left lobe. However, the PET scan shown in Figure 26-9 confirms that the nodule in the right upper lobe is benign (i.e., no hot spot is noted).

Finally, the PET/CT image provides an image of excellent quality and high sensitivity and specificity in detecting malignant lesions in the chest. Figure 26-10 shows a CT/PET scan alongside a CT scan and a PET scan; all the images show the same malignant nodule in the right upper lobe.

*$C(a-\bar{v})o_2$, Arterial-venous oxygen difference; Do_2, total oxygen delivery; O_2ER, oxygen extraction ratio; $\dot{Q}_S/\dot{Q}_T$, pulmonary shunt fraction; $S\bar{v}o_2$, mixed venous oxygen saturation; $\dot{V}o_2$, oxygen consumption.

[‡]*CO,* Cardiac output; *CVP,* central venous pressure; *LVSWI,* left ventricular stroke work index; *$\overline{PA}$,* mean pulmonary artery pressure; *PCWP,* pulmonary capillary wedge pressure; *PVR,* pulmonary vascular resistance; *RAP,* right atrial pressure; *RVSWI,* right ventricular stroke work index; *SV,* stroke volume; *SVI,* stroke volume index; *SVR,* systemic vascular resistance.

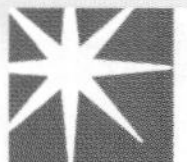

OVERVIEW of the Cardiopulmonary Clinical Manifestations Associated with Cancer of the Lung—cont'd

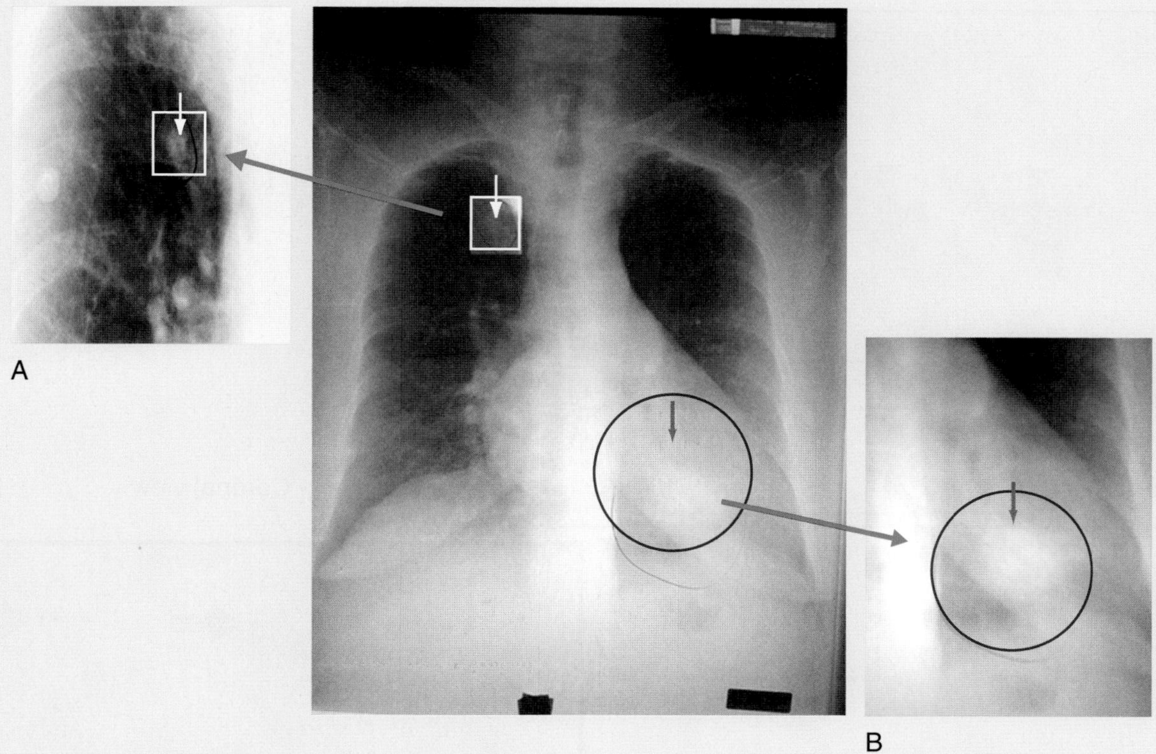

FIGURE 26-4 Chest radiograph identifying two suspicious findings: in the right upper lobe (**A**) and in the left lower lobe (**B**), just behind the heart (*white arrows*).

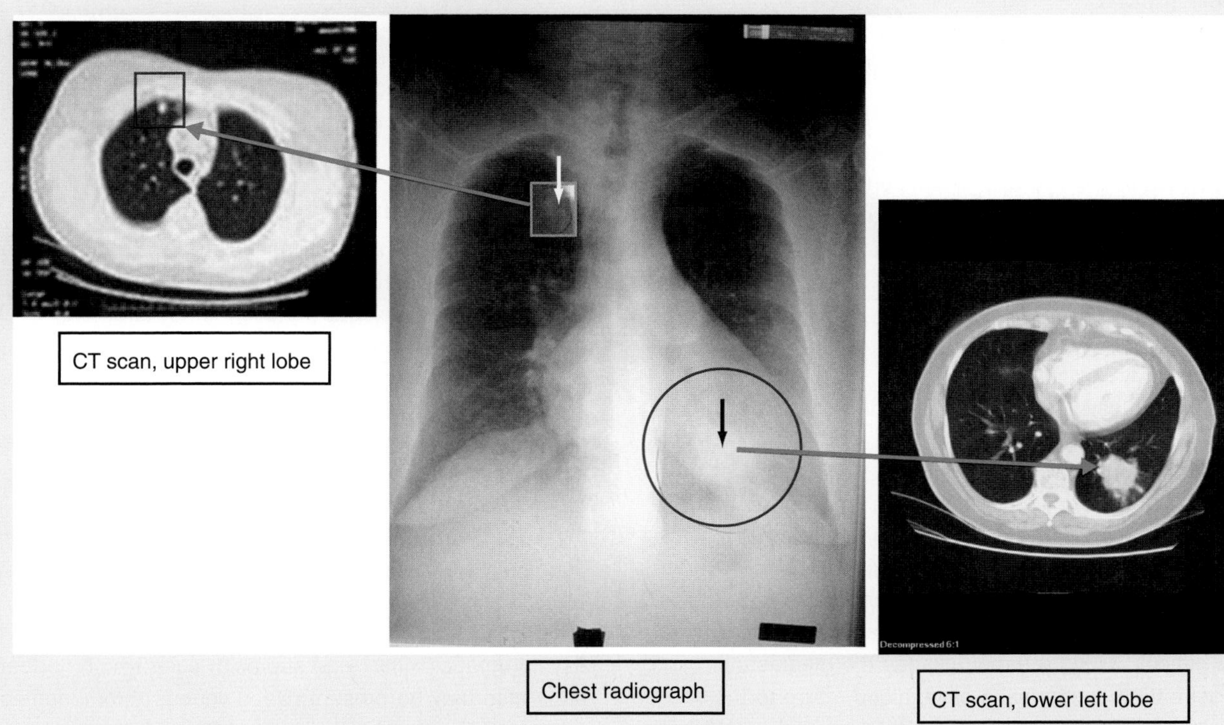

FIGURE 26-5 Same chest radiograph as shown in Figure 26-4. Note that the computed tomography (CT) scan also identifies the suspicious nodules and their precise location.

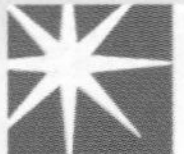

OVERVIEW of the Cardiopulmonary Clinical Manifestations Associated with Cancer of the Lung—cont'd

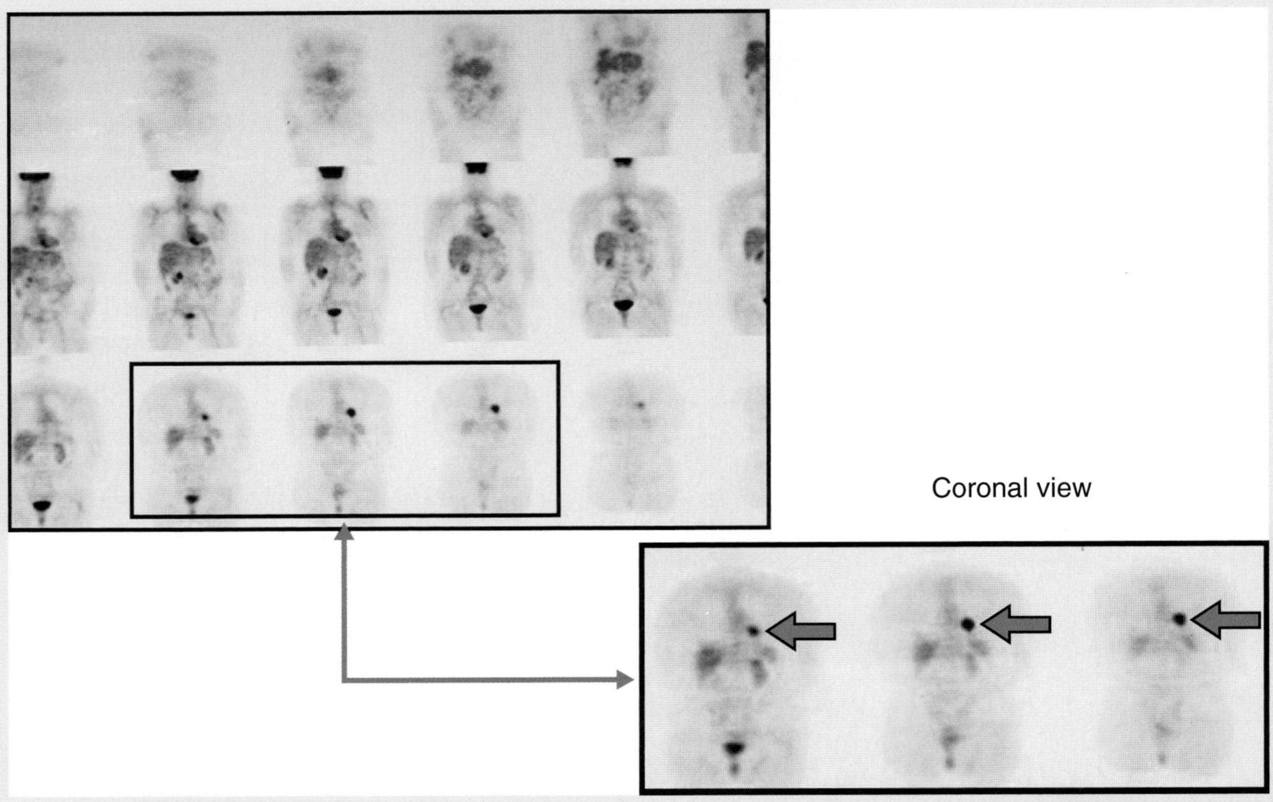

FIGURE 26-6 Positron emission tomography (PET) scan: coronal views. Scans show a "hot spot" in the left lower lobe.

BRONCHOSCOPY FINDINGS

- Bronchial tumor or mass lesion

The fiberoptic bronchoscope may permit direct visualization of a bronchial tumor for further inspection, biopsy, and assessment of the extent of the disease (Figure 26-11).

COMMON NONRESPIRATORY CLINICAL MANIFESTATIONS

- Hoarseness
- Difficulty in swallowing
- Superior vena cava syndrome (distention of the neck veins and neck and facial edema)
- Weakness and weight loss

When a bronchogenic tumor invades the mediastinum, it may involve the left recurrent laryngeal nerve, the esophagus, or the superior vena cava. When the tumor involves the left recurrent laryngeal nerve, the patient's voice becomes hoarse. When the tumor compresses the esophagus, swallowing may become difficult. When a tumor invades the mediastinum and compresses the superior vena cava, blood return to the heart from the head and upper part of the body may be interrupted. When obstruction occurs, the symptoms include an increased ventilatory rate and cough, which is greatly aggravated by recumbency. Clinically, this condition is called *superior vena cava syndrome.*

GENERAL COMMENTS

The clinical manifestations associated with lung cancer may be caused by local effects, tumor extensions into the mediastinum, paraneoplastic endocrine syndromes, or tumor metastases. The most common local signs and symptoms are cough, chest pain, dyspnea, and hemoptysis. Less common signs and symptoms include superior vena cava syndrome, hoarseness resulting from vocal cord paralysis, wheezing, shoulder and upper back pain, and Horner's syndrome (constriction of the pupil and enophthalmos) related to an apical (Pancoast) tumor. Symptoms of metastatic lung cancer include bone pain, weakness, weight loss, and central nervous system signs and symptoms such as headache, seizures, or symptoms mimicking those of a cerebrovascular accident (CVA). Asymptomatic axillary and supraclavicular lymph node metastasis also may be present. Deep venous thrombophlebitis is present at the time of diagnosis in 5% to 10% of patients with lung cancer.

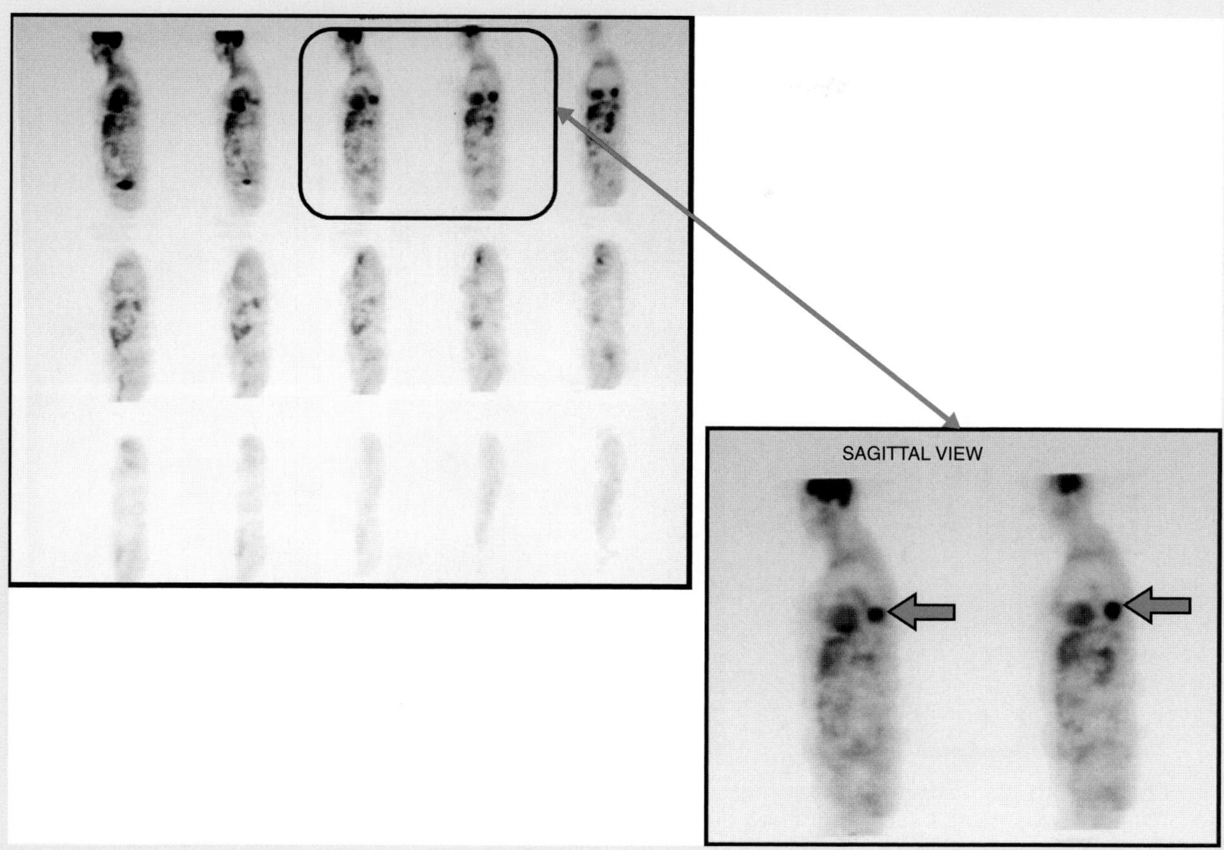

FIGURE 26-7 Positron emission tomography (PET) scan: sagittal views. The encircled images show a "hot spot" in the lower left lobe.

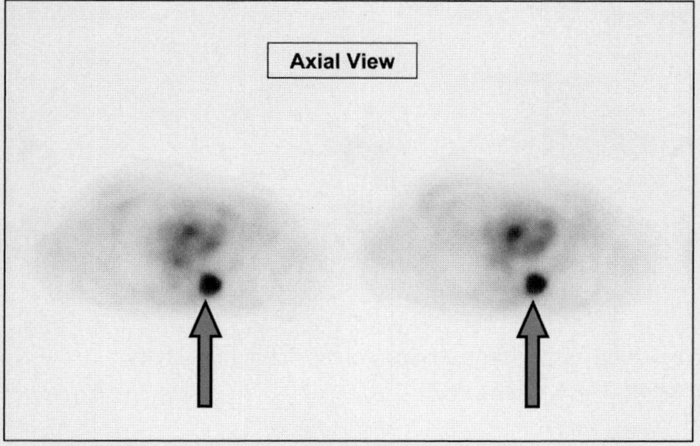

FIGURE 26-8 Positron emission tomography (PET) scan: axial view. A "hot spot" is further confirmed in left lower lobe.

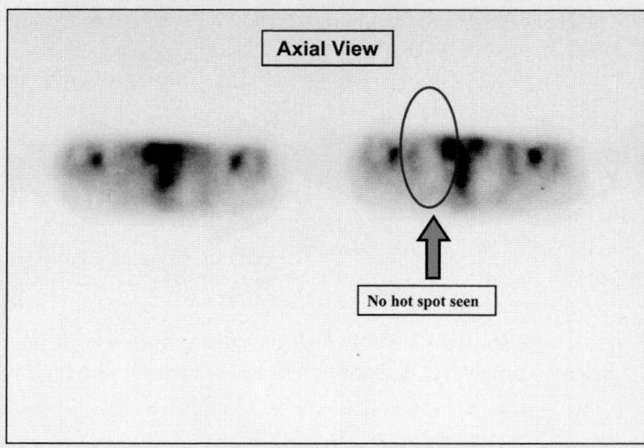

FIGURE 26-9 Positron emission tomography (PET) scan: axial view. This image confirms that the small nodule identified in the upper right lobe in the chest radiograph and computed tomography (CT) scan is benign (i.e., no "hot spot" is evident).

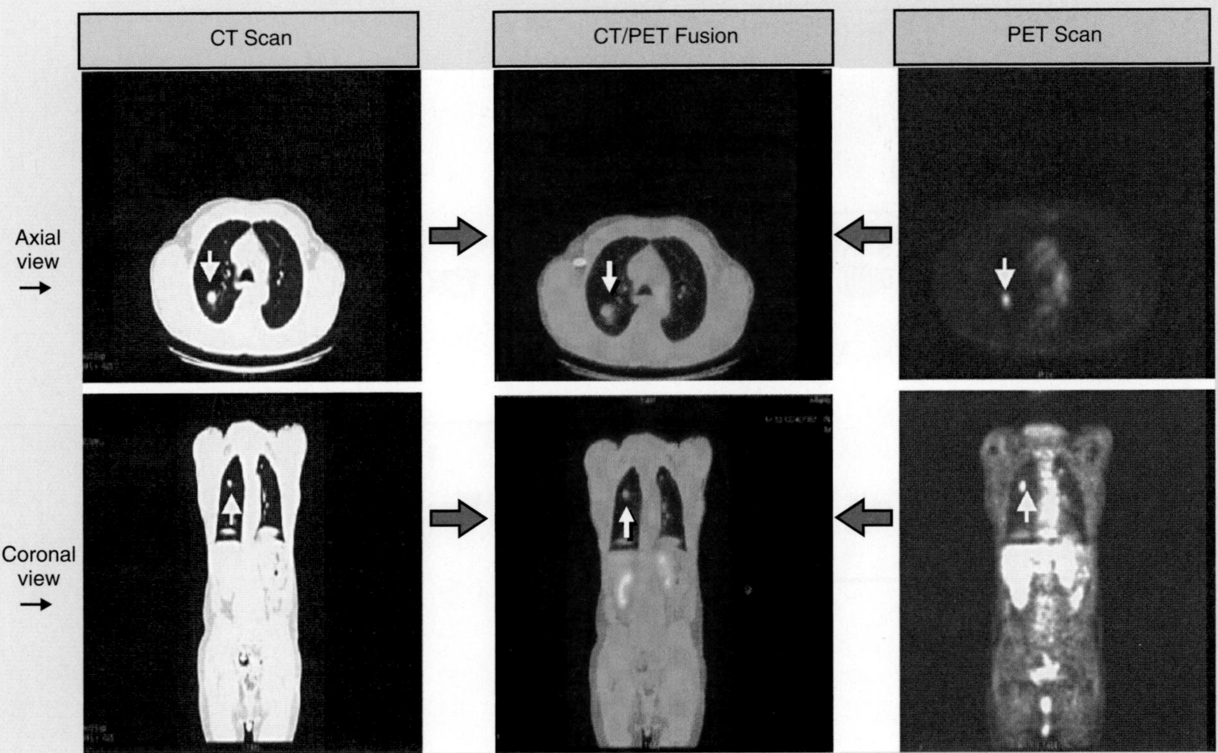

FIGURE 26-10 Computed tomography/positron emission tomography (CT/PET) scan *(center).* CT scan, CT/PET fusion, and PET scan, all showing the same malignant nodule in right upper lobe (*white arrow*). Note: CT/PET fusion is normally presented in color (e.g., red, blue, yellow).

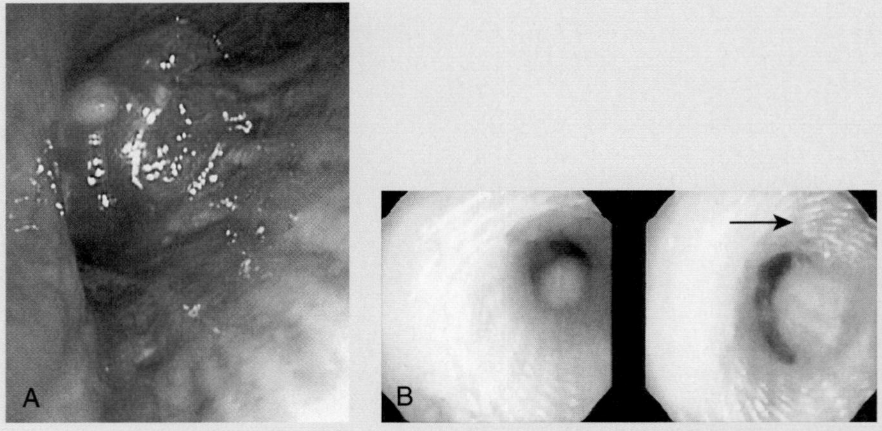

FIGURE 26-11 **A**, Bronchoscopic view of a small cell carcinoma tumor protruding into the right mainstem bronchus. **B**, A wire stent is in place to help hold the airway open *(black arrow).*

General Management of Cancer of the Lung

The treatment of lung cancer depends on the patient's overall health, the type of cancer, the size of the tumor, and the location. Common treatments include surgery, chemotherapy, and radiation therapy.

Surgery

Surgery is usually an option only for patients who have NSCLC that is limited to only one lung, up to stage IIIA. This is usually confirmed with a CT scan and PET scan. In addition, an adequate respiratory reserve must be present to allow good lung function after the lung tissue has been removed. Common surgical procedures include the following:

- **Wedge resection** (partial removal of a lung lobe)
- **Segmentectomy** (removal of a lung segment or segments of the lung)
- **Lobectomy** (removal of one lung lobe)
- **Bilobectomy** (removal of two lung lobes)
- **Pneumonectomy** (removal of whole right or left lung)

In the patient with adequate preoperative respiratory reserve (i.e., a predicted after-surgery forced expiratory volume in 1 second [FEV_1] of 0.8 to 1 L), a lobectomy is the preferred option. A lobectomy reduces the chances of local recurrence. In the patient with an inadequate respiratory reserve, a wedge resection may be performed. The application of radioactive iodine **brachytherapy** at the margins of the wedge resection may minimize the need to perform a lobectomy.

Chemotherapy

Chemotherapy is the general term for any treatment involving the use of chemical agents or drugs that are selectively destructive to malignant cancer cells. Because chemotherapy can eliminate cancer cells at sites away from the original cancer, it is considered a systemic treatment. Unfortunately, because the drugs used in chemotherapy can damage healthy cells along with the cancer cells, serious side effects are common. Fast-growing cells are especially likely to be affected (e.g., cells in the digestive tract, bone marrow, and hair). In addition, the patient may experience nausea and vomiting, dizziness, fatigue, and increased risk of infection.

The primary treatment for SCLC is chemotherapy and radiation; surgery is usually not an option. Chemotherapy is also administered to patients with metastatic NSCLC. The type of chemotherapy is based on the tumor category. SCLC is commonly treated with cisplatin and etoposide. Combinations of carboplatin, gemcitabine, paclitaxel, vinorelbine, topotecan, and irinotecan are also commonly used. NSCLC is commonly treated with cisplatin or carboplatin, in combination with gemcitabine, docetaxel, etoposide, or vinorelbine.

Radiation Therapy

Radiation therapy (external radiation) is often given with chemotherapy. It may be used with curative intent in patients with NSCLC who are not eligible for surgery. This type of high-intensity radiation therapy is called **radical radiotherapy.** In the patient with potentially curable SCLC, radiation therapy and chemotherapy are commonly recommended. In both NSCLC and SCLC, a smaller dose of radiation therapy is often used for symptom control (called *palliative radiotherapy*). Brachytherapy (localized radiotherapy) may also be used when the tumor can be visualized with a bronchoscopy. Brachytherapy entails the use of small radioactive rods (called *seeds*) that are implanted near or directly into the tumor.

In the patient with limited-stage SCLC, **prophylactic cranial irradiation (PCI)** to the brain is often given. PCI is used to minimize the risk of cancer cell metastasis to the brain. Recent advances in targeting and imaging have led to the development of **stereotactic radiation therapy** (also called *stereotactic external-beam radiation therapy* and *stereotaxic radiation therapy*). This type of therapy uses special equipment to position the patient and precisely deliver radiation to a tumor. The total radiation dose is delivered in a small number of doses over several days. It is primarily used in patients who are not surgical candidates.

The goal of radiation therapy is to kill cancer cells without hurting normal tissue cells. Side effects of radiation therapy include redness, swelling, sloughing of skin at the point at which the radiation enters the patient's body, an increased risk of infection, and radiation fibrosis of adjacent lung tissue. In addition, the patient may experience nausea, vomiting, change of taste, fatigue, and malaise.

Comfort (Supportive) Care

Radiation therapy and chemotherapy may not be tolerated when the patient has extensive small cell lung cancer and is in poor health. The patient may choose to receive only comfort or **palliative care**, which means treating the symptoms of the cancer rather than the cancer itself.

Respiratory Care Treatment Protocols

Oxygen Therapy Protocol

Oxygen therapy is used to treat hypoxemia, decrease the work of breathing, and decrease myocardial work. Because hypoxemia is associated with lung cancer, supplemental oxygen may be required. However, capillary shunting is common because of the alveolar compression and consolidation often produced by lung cancer. Hypoxemia caused by capillary shunting often is refractory to oxygen therapy (see Oxygen Therapy Protocol, Protocol 9-1).

Bronchopulmonary Hygiene Therapy Protocol

Because of the excessive mucous production and accumulation associated with lung cancer, a number of bronchial hygiene treatment modalities may be used to enhance the mobilization of bronchial secretions (see Bronchopulmonary Hygiene Therapy Protocol, Protocol 9-2).

Lung Expansion Therapy Protocol

Lung expansion techniques are used to offset (at least temporarily) the alveolar compression and consolidation associated with lung cancer (see Lung Expansion Therapy Protocol, Protocol 9-3).

Aerosolized Medication Protocol

Aerosolized bronchodilators and mucolytics often are indicated, particularly when chronic obstructive pulmonary disease (COPD) coexists, as it does in more than 75% of all cases of lung cancer (see Aerosolized Medication Protocol, Protocol 9-4).

CASE STUDY

Cancer of the Lung

Admitting History

A 66-year-old retired man lives with his wife in a small, two-bedroom ranch house in Peoria, Illinois, during the summer months. During the rest of the year, they live in a 22-foot trailer in a retirement park just outside Las Vegas, Nevada. The trailer park is located conveniently on the casinos' shuttle-bus route; a bus comes by at the top of every hour.

Both the man and his wife are described by their children as addicted gamblers. They gamble almost every day of the year. During the summer months, they play keno and blackjack on the Par-A-Dice Riverboat Casino, which is docked along the shores of the Illinois River in downtown East Peoria. While in Las Vegas, they play bingo, blackjack, and the slot machines at several different casinos. They dress in matching warm-up suits, ride the bus to one of the casinos, and gamble until 10 or 11 PM every day.

Their children, adults with their own families, homes, and jobs in the Peoria area, have been very concerned about their parents' gambling. They have tried to no avail to get their parents to see a compulsive-gambling therapist, who actually is provided by the Par-A-Dice Riverboat Casino. Their children's concern is justified. Their parents are always gambling on a shoestring budget. Although they still own their trailer and small home in Peoria, within the last 2 years they have gambled away most of their life savings, which included stocks, bonds, and mutual funds. Because they let their health insurance premium lapse, their policy recently was cancelled. They still receive a small monthly pension check, and some Social Security income.

Before he retired, the man worked for 17 years as a boiler tender for Methodist Hospital in Peoria. He also was a part-time firefighter. For more than 52 years, he smoked two and a half to three packs of unfiltered cigarettes daily. While in Las Vegas, the man began experiencing periods of dyspnea, coughing, and weakness. His cough was productive of small amounts of clear secretions. Also around this time, his wife first noticed that his voice sounded hoarse.

Although he missed several days of gambling and remained in bed because of weakness, he did not seek medical attention. He hated doctors and thought that he merely had a bad cold and the flu. When he returned to Peoria for the summer, however, the children became concerned and insisted that he see a doctor. Despite the man's lack of health insurance, two medical students from the University of Illinois, who were working as a team, ordered a full diagnostic workup.

A pulmonary function test showed that the man had a restrictive and obstructive pulmonary disorder. CT scanning revealed several masses, ranging from 2 to 5 cm in diameter, in the right and left mediastinum in the hilar regions. The masses, especially on the right side, also could be seen clearly on the posteroanterior chest radiograph. Both the CT scan and the chest x-ray film showed an increased opacity consistent with atelectasis of the medial basal segments of the left lower lobe as well.

A bronchoscopic examination was conducted by the pulmonary physician, with the assistance of a respiratory care practitioner trained in special procedures. It showed several large, protruding bronchial masses in the second- and third-generation bronchi of the right lung; and in the second-, third-, and fourth-generation bronchi of the left lung. During the bronchoscopy, several mucous plugs were suctioned. Biopsy of three of the larger tumors was positive for squamous cell bronchogenic carcinoma, and the man was admitted to the hospital.

The physician told the patient that he had cancer and that his prognosis was poor. Treatment, at best, would be palliative. The patient asked what the odds were on his life expectancy. The physician stated that the patient had only about a 50% chance of living longer than 6 to 8 weeks. Surgery was out of the question. In the interim, however, the physician promised to do what was possible to make the man comfortable. The physician outlined a treatment plan of radiation therapy and chemotherapy and requested a respiratory care consultation.

Physical Examination

The respiratory care practitioner reviewed the admitting history information in the patient's chart and found the man sitting up in bed in obvious respiratory distress. He appeared weak. His skin was cyanotic, and his face, arms, and chest were damp with perspiration. Wheezing was audible without the aid of a stethoscope. He stated in a hoarse voice that he had coughed up a cup of sputum since breakfast 2 hours earlier. He demonstrated a weak cough every few minutes or so. His cough was productive of large amounts of blood-streaked sputum. The viscosity of the sputum was thin. After each coughing episode, he stated that he wanted a cigarette and then laughed.

His vital signs were as follows: blood pressure 155/85, heart rate 90 bpm, respiratory rate 22/min, and temperature normal. Palpation was unremarkable. Percussion produced dull notes over the left lower lobe. On auscultation, rhonchi, wheezing, and crackles could be heard throughout both lung fields. His arterial blood gas values on a 2 L/min oxygen nasal cannula were as follows: pH 7.51, $Pa{CO_2}$ 29, HCO_3^- 24, and $Pa{O_2}$ 66. His oxygen saturation measured by pulse oximetry ($Sp{O_2}$) was 94%. On the basis of these clinical data, the following SOAP was documented.

Respiratory Assessment and Plan

S "I've coughed up a cup of sputum since breakfast."

O Vital signs: BP 155/85, HR 90, RR 22, T normal; perspiring and weak and cyanotic appearance; voice hoarse-sounding; weak cough; large amounts of blood-streaked sputum; dull percussion notes over left lower lobe;

rhonchi, wheezing, and crackles throughout both lung fields; recent PFTs: restrictive and obstructive pulmonary disorder; CT scan and CXR: 2- to 5-cm masses in right and left mediastinum in hilar regions and atelectasis of left lower lobe. Bronchoscopy: protruding tumors in both left and right large airways, mucous plugging. Biopsy: squamous cell bronchogenic carcinoma. ABGs (2 L/min O_2 by nasal cannula): pH 7.51, Pa_{CO_2} 29, HCO_3^- 24, Pa_{O_2} 66; Sp_{O_2} 94%.

A
- Bronchogenic carcinoma (CT scan and biopsy)
- Respiratory distress (vital signs, ABGs)
- Excessive bloody bronchial secretions (sputum, rhonchi)
- Mucous plugging (bronchoscopy)
- Poor ability to mobilize secretions (weak cough)
- Atelectasis of left lower lobe (CXR)
- Acute alveolar hyperventilation with mild hypoxemia (ABGs)

P Initiate **Oxygen Therapy Protocol** (4 L nasal cannula and titration by oximetry). Also begin **Aerosolized Medication Protocol** (0.5 mL albuterol in 2 mL 10% acetylcysteine q6h), followed by **Bronchopulmonary Hygiene Therapy Protocol** (C&DB). Begin **Lung Expansion Therapy Protocol** (incentive spirometry q2h and prn). Closely monitor and reevaluate.

3 Days after Admission

A respiratory care practitioner evaluated the patient during morning rounds. After reviewing the patient's chart, the practitioner went to the patient's bedside and discovered that the man was not tolerating the chemotherapy well. He had been vomiting intermittently for the past 10 hours and was still in obvious respiratory distress. He appeared cyanotic and tired, and his hospital gown was wet from perspiration. His cough was still weak and productive of large amounts of moderately thick, clear, and white sputum. He stated in a hoarse voice that he still was not breathing very well.

His vital signs were as follows: blood pressure 166/90, heart rate 95 bpm, respiratory rate 28/min, and temperature normal. Dull percussion notes were elicited over both the right and left lower lobes. Rhonchi, wheezing, and crackles were auscultated throughout both lung fields. His ABG values were as follows: pH 7.55, Pa_{CO_2} 25, HCO_3^- 23, and Pa_{O_2} 53. His Sp_{O_2} was 92%. On the basis of these clinical data, the following SOAP was documented.

Respiratory Assessment and Plan

S "I'm still not breathing very well."

O Vital signs: BP 166/90, HR 95, RR 28, T normal; vomiting over past 10 hours; cyanosis, tiredness, and dampness from perspiration; cough: weak and productive of moderately thick, clear, and white sputum; dull percussion notes over both right and left lower lobes; rhonchi, wheezing, and crackles over both lung fields; ABGs: pH 7.55, Pa_{CO_2} 25, HCO_3^- 23, Pa_{O_2} 53, Sp_{O_2} 92%

A
- Bronchogenic carcinoma (previous CT scan and biopsy)
- Trouble tolerating chemotherapy well (excessive vomiting)
- Continued respiratory distress
- Excessive bronchial secretions (sputum, rhonchi)
- Mucous plugging still likely (previous bronchoscopy, secretions becoming thicker)
- Poor ability to mobilize secretions (weak cough)
- Atelectasis of left lower lobes; atelectasis likely in right lower lobe now (CXR, dull percussion notes)
- Acute alveolar hyperventilation with moderate hypoxemia, worsening (ABGs)
- Possible impending ventilatory failure

P Up-regulate **Oxygen Therapy Protocol** (oxygen mask). Up-regulate **Aerosolized Medication Protocol** (increasing treatment frequency to q3h). Up-regulate **Bronchopulmonary Hygiene Therapy Protocol** (CPT and PD q3h). Up-regulate **Lung Expansion Therapy Protocol** (changing incentive spirometry to CPAP mask). Contact physician about possible ventilatory failure. Discuss therapeutic bronchoscopy. Closely monitor and reevaluate.

16 Days after Admission

Although the physician's original intention and hope were to discharge the patient soon, stabilizing the man for any length of time proved difficult. Over the next 2 weeks, the patient had continued to be nauseated on a daily basis. He did, however, have occasional periods of relief during which he could breathe, but he generally was in respiratory distress. On day 16 the respiratory therapist observed and collected the following clinical data.

The patient was lying in bed in the supine position. His eyes were closed, and he was unresponsive to the therapist's questions. The patient was in obvious respiratory distress. He appeared pale, cyanotic, and diaphoretic. No cough was observed at this time, but rhonchi easily could be heard from across the patient's room. The nurse in the patient's room stated that the doctor had called the rhonchi a "death rattle." The patient's vital signs were as follows: blood pressure 170/105, heart rate 110 bpm, respiratory rate 12/min and shallow, and rectal temperature normal. Percussion was not performed. Rhonchi, wheezing, and crackles were heard throughout both lung fields. His ABG values were as follows: pH 7.28, Pa_{CO_2} 63, HCO_3^- 28, and Pa_{O_2} 66. His Sp_{O_2} was 89%. At that time, the following SOAP was recorded.

Respiratory Assessment and Plan

S N/A (patient comatose)

O Unresponsive; pale, cyanotic, and perspiring appearance; no cough noted; rhonchi heard without stethoscope; vital signs: BP 170/105, HR 110, RR 12 and shallow, T normal; rhonchi, wheezing, and crackles over both lung fields; ABGs: pH 7.28, Pa_{CO_2} 63, HCO_3^- 28, Pa_{O_2} 66; Sp_{O_2} 89%

A
- Bronchogenic carcinoma (previous CT scan and biopsy)
- Excessive bronchial secretions (rhonchi)
- Mucous plugging still likely (previous bronchoscopy, rhonchi)
- Poor ability to mobilize secretions (no cough)
- Atelectasis (CXR)
- Acute ventilatory failure with moderate hypoxemia (ABGs)

P Contact physician about acute ventilatory failure, and discuss code status. Up-regulate **Oxygen Therapy Protocol, Bronchopulmonary Hygiene Therapy Protocol,** and **Aerosolized Medication Therapy Protocol.** Monitor and reevaluate.

Discussion

This case demonstrates the few specific treatments that a respiratory care practitioner can bring to the care of patients with lung cancer. Specifically, it illustrates that most of the patients have concomitant obstructive pulmonary disease with a need for good **Bronchopulmonary Hygiene Therapy** (see Protocol 9-2). The patient's comfort must be kept in mind at all times.

The first assessment was performed soon after bronchoscopy and diagnosis. The patient's blood-stained sputum could have reflected the primary tumor or, as likely, bleeding from the bronchoscopy sites. In such cases the practitioner must monitor this sputum as the days go along. No improvement in the patient's wheezing can be expected if a bronchial tumor is the cause, but it may improve if bronchospasm (from cigarette smoking) is the causative factor.

The rhonchi, wheezing, and crackles indicated the need for vigorous bronchial hygiene therapy. The atelectasis in the left lower lobe suggested that a trial of careful **Lung Expansion Therapy Protocol** (Protocol 9-3) was in order (see Figure 9-8). The ABG values assessed with the patient on 2 L/min O_2 showed acute alveolar hyperventilation with moderate hypoxemia. A trial of oxygen by Venturi mask (or nonrebreathing mask) would be helpful. Patient anxiety may be alleviated with appropriate treatment of the hypoxemia.

The second assessment revealed that the patient may have developed atelectasis in both the right and left lower lobes (where the tumor masses had been noted previously). This case may present a setting in which therapeutic bronchoscopy or laser-assisted endobronchial resection of the tumor masses may be helpful. The patient continued to be hypoxemic, despite alveolar hyperventilation. A higher F_{IO_2} (for example, through a Venturi oxygen mask) was indicated. Vigorous suctioning was appropriate. Because of the impending ventilatory failure, ordering at least one cycle of ventilator support for such a patient would not be surprising, given that the patient had just recently received radiation and chemotherapy. The patient's wishes in this respect should have been checked against his living will or durable power of attorney for health care, if such a document existed.

The last assessment indicates that the patient did not elect aggressive therapy and that he had slipped into acute ventilatory failure. All health-care personnel had agreed that the patient was close to death. The practitioner may be excused for not suggesting the use of chest physical therapy and postural drainage at this time, because of the patient's wishes. Aerosolized morphine is now being used to relieve dyspnea in terminally ill cancer patients. If, however, aggressive therapy were still in order, formal evaluation and treatment of superimposed atelectasis or pneumonia, or both, would be in order.

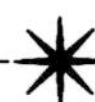

SELF-ASSESSMENT QUESTIONS

evolve Answers to questions can be found on Evolve. To access additional student assessment questions and case studies for application of text material to real-life scenarios, visit **http://evolve.elsevier.com/DesJardins/respiratory.**

1. Which of the following is the most common form of bronchogenic carcinoma?
   a. Squamous cell carcinoma
   b. Oat cell carcinoma
   c. Large cell carcinoma
   d. Adenocarcinoma

2. Which of the following arises from the mucous glands of the tracheobronchial tree?
   a. Small cell carcinoma
   b. Adenocarcinoma
   c. Squamous cell carcinoma
   d. Oat cell carcinoma

3. Which of the following carcinomas has the strongest correlation with cigarette smoking?
   a. Adenocarcinoma
   b. Small cell carcinoma
   c. Large cell carcinoma
   d. Squamous cell carcinoma

4. Which of the following has the fastest growth (doubling) rate?
   a. Large cell carcinoma
   b. Small cell carcinoma
   c. Adenocarcinoma
   d. Squamous cell carcinoma

5. Which of the following is or are associated with bronchogenic carcinoma?
   1. Alveolar consolidation
   2. Pleural effusion
   3. Alveolar hyperinflation
   4. Atelectasis
      a. 2 and 3 only
      b. 1 and 4 only
      c. 2 and 3 only
      d. 1, 2, and 4 only

PART IX

Diffuse Alveolar Disease

Acute Respiratory Distress Syndrome

27

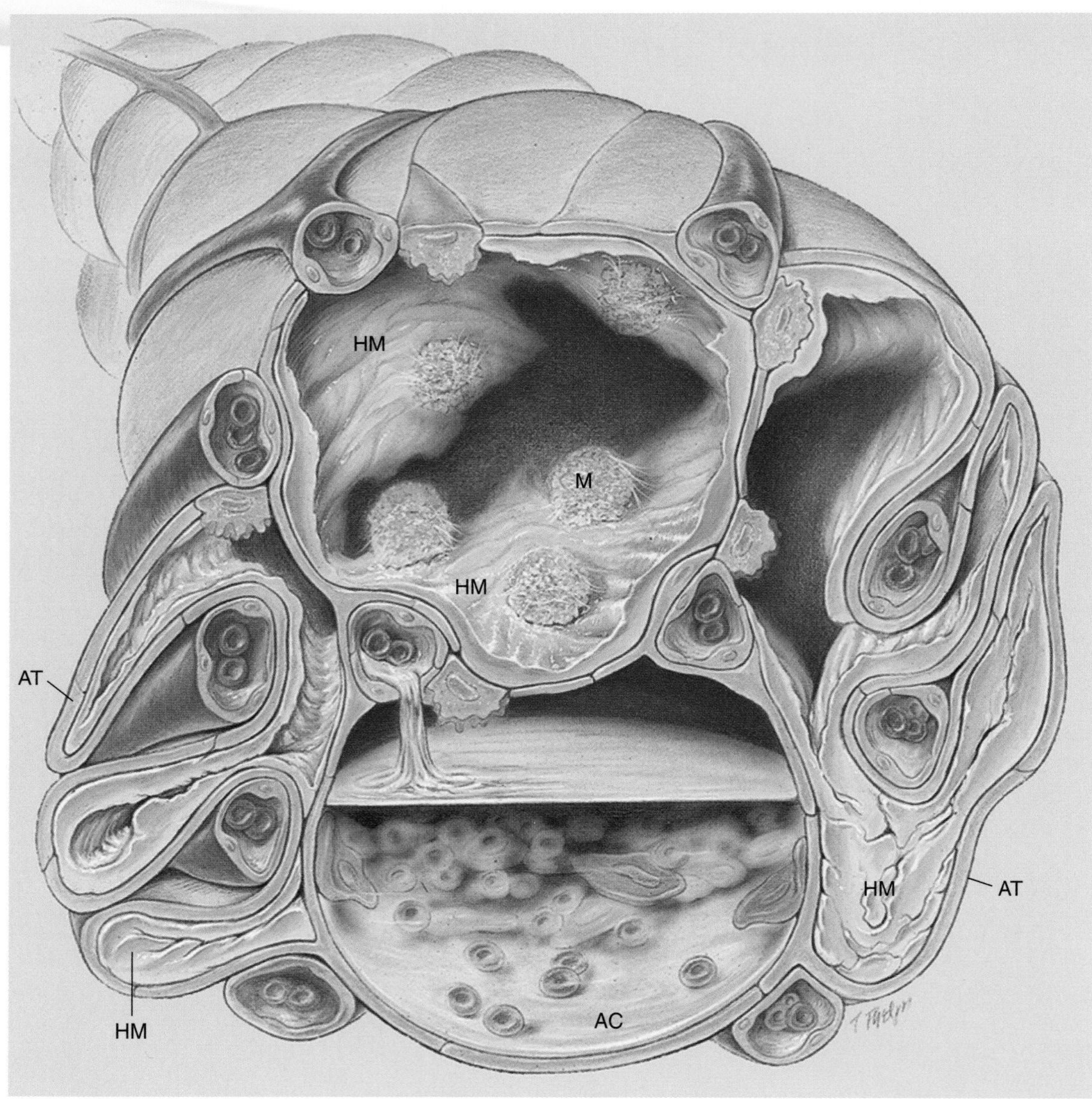

FIGURE 27-1 Cross-sectional view of alveoli in acute respiratory distress syndrome. *AC,* Alveolar consolidation; *AT,* atelectasis; *HM,* hyaline membrane; *M,* macrophage.

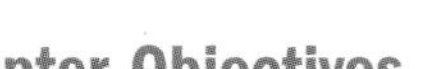
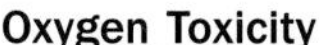

Chapter Objectives

After reading this chapter, you will be able to:

- List the anatomic alterations of the lungs associated with acute respiratory distress syndrome.
- Describe the causes of acute respiratory distress syndrome.
- List the cardiopulmonary clinical manifestations associated with acute respiratory distress syndrome.
- Describe the general management of acute respiratory distress syndrome.
- Describe the clinical strategies and rationales of the SOAPs presented in the case study.
- Define key terms and complete self-assessment questions at the end of the chapter and on Evolve.

Key Terms

Barotrauma
Continuous Positive Airway Pressure (CPAP)
Ground Glass Appearance
Hyaline Membrane
Low Tidal Volume and High Respiratory Rate Ventilation
Oxygen Toxicity
Permissive Hypercapnia
Positive End-Expiratory Pressure (PEEP)
Plateau Pressure
Pulmonary Capillary Wedge Pressure (PWCP)
Transpulmonary Pressures

Chapter Outline

Anatomic Alterations of the Lungs

The lungs of patients affected by acute respiratory distress syndrome (ARDS) undergo similar anatomic changes, regardless of the cause of the disease. In response to injury the pulmonary capillaries become engorged, and the permeability of the alveolar-capillary membrane increases. Interstitial and intraalveolar edema and hemorrhage ensue, as well as scattered areas of hemorrhagic alveolar consolidation. These processes result in a decrease in alveolar surfactant and in alveolar collapse, or atelectasis.

As the disease progresses, the intraalveolar walls become lined with a thick, rippled **hyaline membrane** identical to the hyaline membrane seen in newborns with infant respiratory distress syndrome (hyaline membrane disease). The membrane contains fibrin and cellular debris. In prolonged cases there is hyperplasia and swelling of the type II cells. Fibrin and exudate develop and lead to intraalveolar fibrosis.

In gross appearance the lungs of patients with ARDS are heavy and "red," "beefy," or "liver-like." The anatomic alterations that develop in ARDS create a restrictive lung disorder (see Figure 27-1).

The major pathologic or structural changes associated with ARDS are as follows:

- Interstitial and intra-alveolar edema and hemorrhage
- Alveolar consolidation
- Intraalveolar hyaline membrane formation
- Pulmonary surfactant deficiency or abnormality
- Atelectasis

Historically, ARDS was first referred to as the "shock lung syndrome" when the disease was first identified in combat casualties during World War II. Since that time, the disease has appeared in the medical literature under many different names, all based on the conditions believed to be responsible for the disease. In 1967 the disease was first described as a specific entity, and the term *acute respiratory distress syndrome* was suggested. This term is predominantly used today. Box 27-1 provides some of the other names that have appeared in the medical journals to identify ARDS.

Box 27-1 Other Names Used in the Past to Identify Acute Respiratory Distress Syndrome (ARDS)

- Adult hyaline membrane disease
- Adult respiratory distress syndrome
- Capillary leak syndrome
- Congestion atelectasis
- Da Nang lung (because of the high incidence of ARDS in the Vietnam War)
- Hemorrhagic pulmonary edema
- Noncardiac pulmonary edema
- Oxygen pneumonitis
- Oxygen toxicity
- Postnontraumatic pulmonary insufficiency
- Postperfusion lung
- Postpump lung
- Posttraumatic pulmonary insufficiency
- Shock lung syndrome
- Stiff lung syndrome
- Wet lung
- White lung syndrome

Etiology and Epidemiology

A multitude of causative factors may produce ARDS. Box 27-2 provides some of the better-known causes.

Box 27-2 Common Causes of Acute Respiratory Distress Syndrome

- Aspiration (e.g., of gastric contents, or water in near-drowning episodes)
- Central nervous system (CNS) disease (particularly when complicated by increased intracranial pressure)
- Cardiopulmonary bypass (especially when the bypass is prolonged)
- Disseminated intravascular coagulation (seen in patients with shock; it is a condition of paradoxic simultaneous clotting and bleeding that produces microthrombi in the lungs)
- Drug overdose (e.g., heroin, barbiturates, morphine, methadone)
- Fat or air emboli (the fat emboli act as a source of harmful vasoactive material, including fatty acids and serotonin)
- Infections (bacterial, viral, fungal, parasitic, mycoplasma)
- Inhalation of toxins and irritants (e.g., chlorine gas, nitrogen dioxide, smoke, ozone; oxygen also may be included in this category of irritants)
- Immunologic reaction (e.g., allergic alveolar reaction to inhaled material or Goodpasture's syndrome)
- Massive blood transfusion (in stored blood the quantity of aggregated white blood cells [WBCs], red blood cells [RBCs], platelets, and fibrin increases; these blood components may in turn occlude or damage small blood vessels)
- Nonthoracic trauma
- **Oxygen toxicity** (e.g., when patients are treated with an excessive oxygen concentration—usually greater than 60%—for a prolonged period)
- Pulmonary ischemia (resulting from shock and hypoperfusion; may cause tissue necrosis, vascular damage, and capillary leakage)
- Radiation-induced lung injury
- Shock (e.g., hypovolemia)
- Systemic reactions to processes initiated outside the lungs (e.g., reactions caused by hemorrhagic pancreatitis, burns, complicated abdominal surgery, septicemia)
- Thoracic trauma (direct contusion to the lungs)

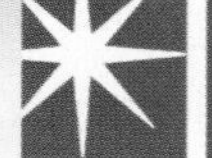

OVERVIEW of the Cardiopulmonary Clinical Manifestations Associated with Acute Respiratory Distress Syndrome

The following clinical manifestations result from the pathologic mechanisms caused (or activated) by **Atelectasis** (see Figure 9-9), **Alveolar Consolidation** (see Figure 9-9), and **Increased Alveolar-Capillary Membrane Thickness** (see Figure 9-10)—the major anatomic alterations of the lungs associated with ARDS (see Figure 27-1).

CLINICAL DATA OBTAINED AT THE PATIENT'S BEDSIDE

The Physical Examination

Vital Signs

Increased Respiratory Rate (Tachypnea)

Several pathophysiologic mechanisms operating simultaneously may lead to an increased ventilatory rate:

- Stimulation of peripheral chemoreceptors (hypoxemia)
- Decreased lung compliance–increased ventilatory rate relationship
- Stimulation of J receptors
- Anxiety

Increased Heart Rate (Pulse) and Blood Pressure

Substernal or Intercostal Retractions

Cyanosis

Chest Assessment Findings

- Dull percussion note
- Bronchial breath sounds
- Crackles

CLINICAL DATA OBTAINED FROM LABORATORY TESTS AND SPECIAL PROCEDURES

Pulmonary Function Test Findings (Restrictive Lung Pathophysiology)

FORCED EXPIRATORY FLOW RATE FINDINGS

FVC	FEV_T	FEV_1/FVC ratio	$FEF_{25\%-75\%}$
↓	N or ↓	N or ↑	N or ↓

$FEF_{50\%}$	$FEF_{200-1200}$	PEFR	MVV
N or ↓	N or ↓	N or ↓	N or ↓

LUNG VOLUME AND CAPACITY FINDINGS

V_T	IRV	ERV	RV	
N or ↓	↓	↓	↓	
VC	IC	FRC	TLC	RV/TLC ratio
↓	↓	↓	↓	N

DECREASED DIFFUSION CAPACITY (Dlco)

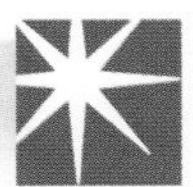

OVERVIEW of the Cardiopulmonary Clinical Manifestations Associated with Acute Respiratory Distress Syndrome—cont'd

Arterial Blood Gases

MILD TO MODERATE ACUTE RESPIRATORY DISTRESS SYNDROME
Acute Alveolar Hyperventilation with Hypoxemia
(Acute Respiratory Alkalosis)

pH	Pa_{CO_2}	HCO_3^-	Pa_{O_2}
↑	↓	↓ (slightly)	↓

SEVERE ACUTE RESPIRATORY DISTRESS SYNDROME
Acute Ventilatory Failure with Hypoxemia
(Acute Respiratory Acidosis)

pH*	Pa_{CO_2}	HCO_3^-*	Pa_{O_2}
↓	↑	↑ (slightly)	↓

*When tissue hypoxia is severe enough to produce lactic acid, the pH and HCO_3^- values will be lower than expected for a particular Pa_{CO_2} level.

Oxygenation Indices*

$\dot{Q}_S/\dot{Q}_T$	D_{O_2}†	$\dot{V}_{O_2}$	$C(a-\bar{v})_{O_2}$	O_2ER	$S\bar{v}_{O_2}$
↑	↓	N	N	↑	↓

†The D_{O_2} may be normal in patients who have compensated to the decreased oxygenation status with (1) an increased cardiac output, (2) an increased hemoglobin level, or (3) a combination of both. When the D_{O_2} is normal, the O_2ER is usually normal.

Hemodynamic Indices‡

Severe

CVP	RAP	$\overline{PA}$	PCWP	CO	SV
↑	↑	↑	N† or ↓	N or ↑‡	N or ↑‡

SVI‡	CI‡	RVSWI	LVSWI	PVR	SVR‡
N or ↑‡	N or ↑‡	↑	↓	↑	N or ↓‡

†A normal PCWP (<18 mm Hg) is the hallmark of ARDS, distinguishing it from cardiogenic pulmonary edema, in which the PCWP is elevated (see page 275).
‡If sepsis with systemic hypotension is present.

*$C(a-\bar{v})_{O_2}$, Arterial-venous oxygen difference; D_{O_2}, total oxygen delivery; O_2ER, oxygen extraction ratio; $\dot{Q}_S/\dot{Q}_T$, pulmonary shunt fraction; $S\bar{v}_{O_2}$, mixed venous oxygen saturation; $\dot{V}_{O_2}$, oxygen consumption.
‡*CO*, Cardiac output; *CVP*, central venous pressure; *LVSWI*, left ventricular stroke work index; *$\overline{PA}$*, mean pulmonary artery pressure; *PCWP*, pulmonary capillary wedge pressure; *PVR*, pulmonary vascular resistance; *RAP*, right atrial pressure; *RVSWI*, right ventricular stroke work index; *SV*, stroke volume; *SVI*, stroke volume index; *SVR*, systemic vascular resistance.

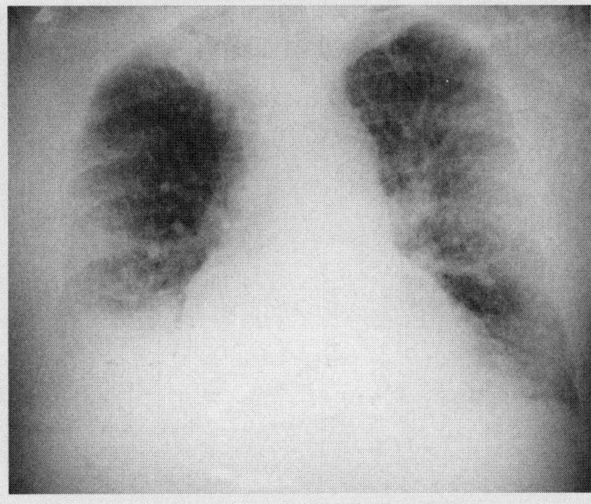

FIGURE 27-2 Chest x-ray film of a patient with moderately severe acute respiratory distress syndrome.

RADIOLOGIC FINDINGS

Chest Radiograph

- Increased opacity

The structural changes that develop in ARDS increase the radiodensity of the lungs. The increased lung density resists x-ray penetration and is revealed on the radiograph as increased opacity (i.e., whiter in appearance). Therefore the more severe the ARDS, the denser the lungs become and the "whiter" the radiograph (Figure 27-2). Ultimately, the lungs may have a **"ground-glass" appearance**.

General Management of Acute Respiratory Distress Syndrome

Respiratory Care Treatment Protocols

Oxygen Therapy Protocol

Oxygen therapy is used to treat hypoxemia, decrease the work of breathing, and decrease myocardial work. Because of the hypoxemia associated with ARDS, supplemental oxygen often is required. The hypoxemia that develops in ARDS most commonly is caused by widespread **alveolar consolidation, atelectasis, increased alveolar capillary thickening.** Hypoxemia caused by capillary shunting often is refractory to oxygen therapy (see Oxygen Therapy Protocol, Protocol 9-1).

Lung Expansion Therapy Protocol

Lung expansion measures (e.g., **positive end-expiratory pressure [PEEP]** or **continuous positive airway pressure [CPAP]**) may be administered to attempt to offset the alveolar consolidation and atelectasis associated with ARDS (see Lung Expansion Protocol, Protocol 9-3).

Mechanical Ventilation Protocol

Mechanical ventilation is often needed to provide and support alveolar gas exchange and eventually return the patient to spontaneous breathing. Continuous mechanical ventilation is justified when the acute ventilatory failure is thought to be reversible (see Protocols 9-5, 9-6, and 9-7).

Ventilation Strategy for Adult Respiratory Distress Syndrome*

Today, the ventilation strategy for most patients with ARDS entails **low tidal volumes and high respiratory rates.** The initial tidal volume is usually set at 5 to 7 mL/kg, and the rate is set at 20 to 25. Ventilatory rates as high as 35 breaths/min may be needed to maintain an adequate minute volume. The **plateau pressure** should be less than 30 cm H_2O. PEEP and CPAP are used with small tidal volumes to reduce atelectasis.

The patient's Pa_{CO_2} often is allowed to increase **(permissive hypercapnia)** as a tradeoff to protect the lungs from high airway pressures. In most cases, an increased ventilatory rate adequately offsets the decreased tidal volume used in the management of ARDS. The Pa_{CO_2}, however, should not be permitted to increase to the point of severe acidosis (e.g., a pH below 7.2).

The therapeutic goal of low tidal volume ventilation is to (1) decrease high **transpulmonary pressures,** (2) reduce overdistention of the lungs, and (3) decrease **barotrauma.** (See Mechanical Ventilation Protocols, Protocol 9-5, Protocol 9-6, and Protocol 9-7.)

*Over the past several decades, a number of ventilation strategies have been used, studied, and evaluated for the treatment of ARDS. Such ventilation strategies have included high-frequency ventilation (HFV), tracheal gas insufflation (TGI), inverse-ratio ventilation (IRV), airway pressure release ventilation (APRV), patient repositioning (including prone position), extracorporeal membrane oxygenation (ECMO), extracorporeal carbon dioxide removal ($ECCO_2R$), exogenous surfactant administration, liquid (perfluorocarbon) mechanical ventilation, inhaled nitric oxide (NO), and corticosteroid administration. Despite some encouraging results with some of these ventilation strategies, the safety, effectiveness, and survival benefits associated with these ventilation modes have not been established.

Medications and Procedures Commonly Prescribed by the Physician

Antibiotics

Antibiotics are commonly administered in an effort to treat secondary bacterial infections (see Appendix III).

Diuretic Agents

Diuretic agents frequently are ordered for patients with ARDS in an attempt to reduce interstitial edema. However, often their effects are poor (see Appendix VII).

CASE STUDY

Acute Respiratory Distress Syndrome (ARDS)

Admitting History and Physical Examination

This comatose 47-year-old woman was admitted to the emergency department of a small community hospital. Her husband found her lying in bed with an empty bottle of "sleeping pills" and a "goodbye note" on the bedside table. She had a long history of depression.

In the emergency department she was found to be in a moderately deep coma, responding to deep painful stimulation but otherwise nonresponsive. She was of average size and, according to the husband, had previously been in good physical health. She did not smoke or drink and was taking no other medication. Her blood pressure and pulse were within normal limits, but her respirations were shallow and noisy. The emergency department physician attempted to lavage her stomach. During the introduction of the nasogastric tube, the patient vomited and aspirated liquid gastric contents. At this time it was decided to transfer her by ambulance to a tertiary care medical center about 30 miles away. The pH of the gastric contents was not determined.

On arrival at the medical center, the patient was comatose but responsive to mild painful stimulation. Her weight was 50 kg and her rectal temperature was 101.5° F. Her blood pressure was 100/60, heart rate 114/min, and respirations 28/min. On auscultation, there were scattered crackles on the right side. A chest x-ray film showed bilateral moderate fluffy infiltrates, mostly on the right side. Blood gases on 5 L/min O_2 were pH 7.51, $Pa{CO_2}$ 29, HCO_3^- 23, and $Pa{O_2}$ 52. At the time the respiratory care practitioner recorded the following SOAP note.

Respiratory Assessment and Plan

S N/A

O Patient is comatose. BP 100/60; HR 114; RR 28; T 101.5° F; bilateral crackles; CXR: bilateral infiltrates, worse on right side; ABGs on 5 L/min O_2: pH 7.51, $Pa{CO_2}$ 29, HCO_3^- 23, and $Pa{O_2}$ 52.

A
- Sedative drug overdose with coma (history)
- Acute alveolar hyperventilation with moderate hypoxemia (ABGs)
  - Impending ventilatory failure
- Aspiration pneumonitis without previous history of pulmonary disease vs ARDS (history and x-ray film)

P **Oxygen Therapy Protocol:** (100% O_2 via nonrebreathing mask). Confer with physician regarding **Mechanical Ventilation Protocol**. Arterial line placement. Continuous oximetry. Repeat ABG 1 hour after intubation and prn.

The patient was admitted to the intensive care unit, intubated, and mechanically ventilated with these settings: V_T 500 mL, rate 12 breaths/min, $F{IO_2}$ 0.4, and 10 cm H_2O of PEEP. An arterial line was placed in her left radial artery, and an intravenous infusion was started with lactated Ringer's solution.

Over the next 72 hours, the patient's oxygenation status continued to deteriorate; in spite of a progressive increase in the delivered $F{IO_2}$, PEEP, and pressure-controlled mechanical ventilation. When the arterial oxygen tension did not improve appreciably on an $F{IO_2}$ of 1.0 and a PEEP of 20 cm H_2O, a Swan-Ganz catheter was placed in the pulmonary artery. In view of the PEEP, the pressure readings were difficult to interpret. A mean pulmonary artery pressure of 27 mm Hg, however, did suggest increased pulmonary vascular resistance.

A chest x-ray examination confirmed severe ARDS with extensive, diffuse infiltrates and atelectasis; worse on the right side. At this time, the respiratory practitioner immediately decreased the tidal volume on the ventilator to 350 mL (7 mL × 50 kg) and increased the rate to 20 breaths/min. The $F{IO_2}$ remained at 1.0, and the PEEP was still at 20 cm H_2O. The patient's arterial blood gas values 20 minutes later were pH 7.31, $Pa{CO_2}$ 49, HCO_3^- 25, and $Pa{O_2}$ 38. Her $Sp{O_2}$ was 70%. She had crackles, wheezes, and rhonchi in all lung fields. Moderate to large amounts of purulent sputum frequently were suctioned from the endotracheal tube. Her blood pressure was 90/60, and her heart rate was 130/min. Her temperature was 100.2° F. At this time, the respiratory care practitioner charted the following SOAP note:

Respiratory Assessment and Plan

S N/A (patient comatose)

O Patient remains comatose. BP 90/60, HR 130, T 100.2° F. Bilateral crackles, rhonchi, and wheezes. ABGs on decreased VT of 400 mL, rate 20, $F{IO_2}$ 1.0, and +20 PEEP: pH 7.31, $Pa{CO_2}$ 49, HCO_3^- 25, and $Pa{O_2}$ 38. $Sp{O_2}$: 70%. CXR: ARDS with bilateral infiltrates and atelectasis, worse on the right side. Purulent sputum. PA pressure (mean) 27 mm Hg.

A
- Persistent coma (physical exam)
- Aspiration pneumonitis progressing to ARDS with bilateral infiltrates and atelectasis (x-ray film)
- Increasing airway secretions with infection (fever, crackles, rhonchi, and purulent sputum)
- Acute ventilatory failure on present ventilator settings (acceptable hypercapnia)
  - Severe hypoxemia (ABGs)

P Call physician to discuss worsening $Pa{O_2}$ and to confirm an acceptable hypercapnia level and PEEP upper limit. **Bronchopulmonary Hygiene Therapy Protocol** and **Aerosolized Medication Protocol** (add 2 mL 10% acetylcysteine to 0.5 mL albuterol and aerosolize q2h; suction prn). Adjust **Mechanical Ventilation Protocol** (titrate tidal volume and rate to raise $Pa{CO_2}$ to permissive hypercapnia range). Gram stain and culture sputum. Closely monitor and reevaluate.

After 3 hours it was apparent that current management would not be successful; the physician decided to alert the extracorporeal membrane oxygenation (ECMO) team and place the patient on extracorporeal membrane oxygenation. This was done, and the patient was maintained on ECMO for 13 hours, when she developed ventricular tachycardia followed by ventricular fibrillation. Attempts to reestablish normal cardiac function were not successful, and the patient was pronounced dead 45 minutes later.

Discussion

This was possibly a preventable death. Gastric lavage *never* should be performed on an unconscious patient unless the airway is first protected with a cuffed endotracheal tube. This is one of the very few categoric imperatives in pulmonary medicine. The following three causative factors known to produce ARDS may have been operative in this patient: (1) drug overdose, (2) aspiration of gastric contents, and (3) breathing an excessive FIO_2 for a long period. As time progressed, the patient's lungs became stiffer and physiologically nonfunctional as a result of the anatomic alterations associated with ARDS. Careful measurement of the alveolar-arterial oxygen tension difference ($P[A-a]O_2$) would have detected this (see page 72).

As documented in the first assessment, her crackles, rhonchi, refractory hypoxemia, and x-ray findings all reflected the pathophysiologic changes seen in patients with **Atelectasis** (see Figure 9-8) and/or **Increased Alveolar-Capillary Membrane Thickening** (see Figure 9-10). Aggressive **Lung Expansion Therapy** (see Protocol 9-3), in the form of PEEP, was used with mechanical ventilation right from the start. When the chest radiograph confirmed severe ARDS after 72 hours of therapy, the immediate changes in the mechanical ventilator settings—the reduction in the patient's tidal volume to 350 mL, the increased respiratory rate of 20 breaths/min, and permissive hypercapnia—were all clearly indicated and appropriate. Unfortunately, these therapeutic techniques and use of ECMO to manage the condition were not enough in the final analysis.

SELF-ASSESSMENT QUESTIONS

evolve Answers to questions can be found on Evolve. To access additional student assessment questions and case studies for application of text material to real-life scenarios, visit **http://evolve.elsevier.com/DesJardins/respiratory.**

1. In response to injury, the lungs of an ARDS patient undergo which of the following changes?

1. Atelectasis
2. Decreased alveolar-capillary membrane permeability
3. Interstitial and intraalveolar edema
4. Hemorrhagic alveolar consolidation

   a. 1 and 3 only
   b. 2 and 4 only
   c. 1, 2, and 4 only
   d. 1, 3, and 4 only

2. Which of the following is or are recommended ventilation strategies for most patients with ARDS?

1. High tidal volumes
2. Low respiratory rates
3. High respirator rates
4. Low tidal volumes

   a. 1 only
   b. 3 only
   c. 2 and 4 only
   d. 1 and 3 only

3. Common chest assessment findings in ARDS include the following:

1. Diminished breath sounds
2. Dull percussion note
3. Bronchial breath sounds
4. Crackles

   a. 1 only
   b. 3 only
   c. 2 and 3 only
   d. 2, 3, and 4 only

4. During the early stages of ARDS, the patient commonly demonstrates which of the following arterial blood gas values?

1. Decreased pH
2. Increased HCO_3^-
3. Decreased $PaCO_2$
4. Normal PaO_2

   a. 2 only
   b. 3 only
   c. 2 and 3 only
   d. 3 and 4 only

5. Which of the following oxygenation indices is or are associated with ARDS?

1. Increased $\dot{V}O_2$
2. Decreased DO_2
3. Increased $S\bar{v}O_2$
4. Decreased $\dot{Q}_S/\dot{Q}_T$

   a. 1 only
   b. 2 only
   c. 3 only
   d. 2 and 3 only

PART X

Neurologic Disorders and Sleep Apnea

Guillain-Barré Syndrome 28

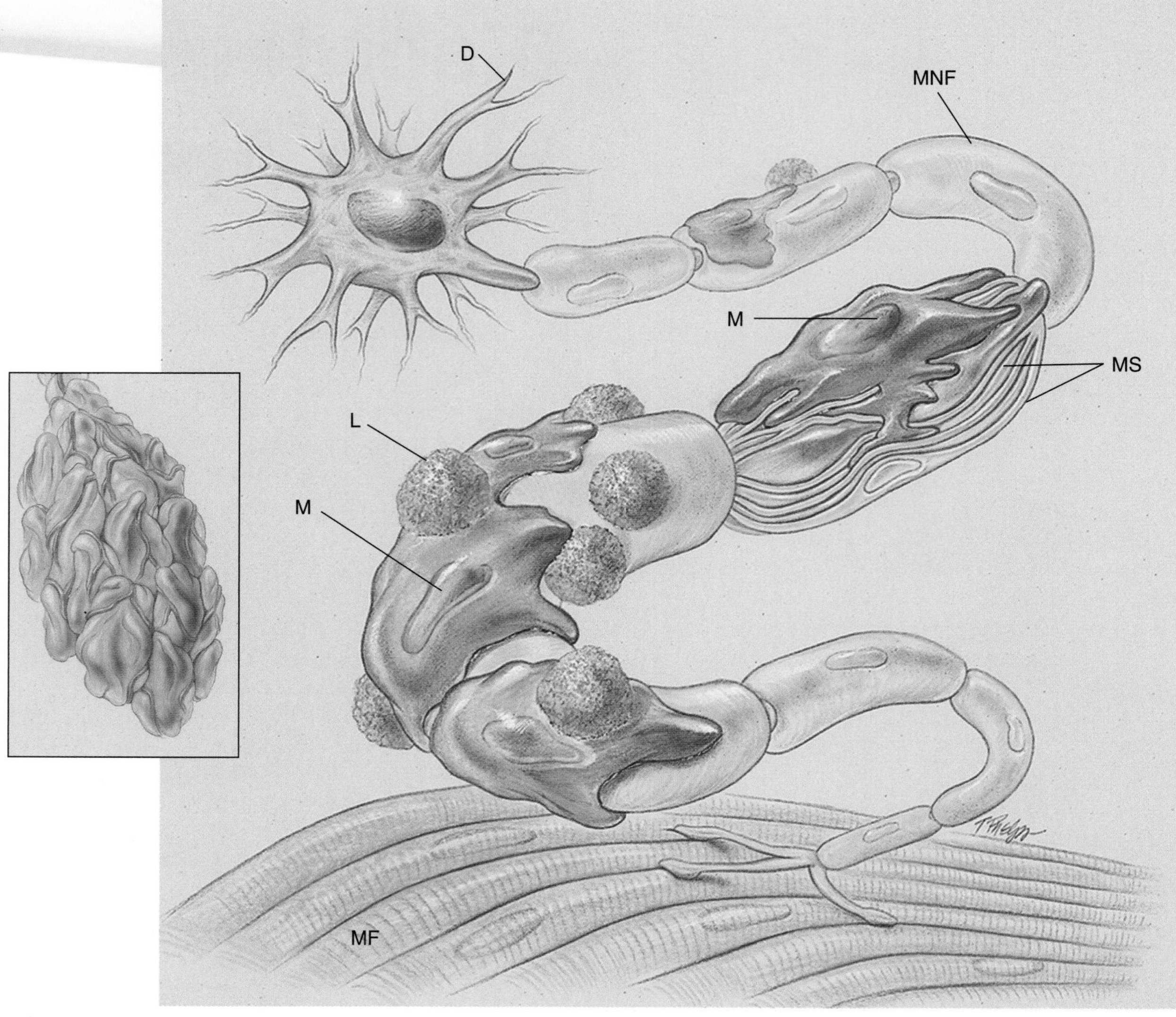

FIGURE 28-1 Guillain-Barré syndrome. Lymphocytes and macrophages attacking and stripping away the myelin sheath of a peripheral nerve. *D,* Dendrite; *L,* Lymphocyte; *M,* macrophage; *MF,* muscle fiber; *MNF,* myelinated nerve fiber; *MS,* myelin sheath (cross-sectional view; note the macrophage attacking the myelin sheath). *Inset,* Atelectasis, a common secondary anatomic alteration of the lungs.

Chapter Objectives

After reading this chapter, you will be able to:

- List the anatomic alterations of the lungs associated with Guillain-Barré syndrome.
- Describe the causes of Guillain-Barré syndrome.
- List the cardiopulmonary clinical manifestations associated with Guillain-Barré syndrome.
- Describe the general management of Guillain-Barré syndrome.
- Describe the clinical strategies and rationales of the SOAPs presented in the case study.
- Define key terms and complete self-assessment questions at the end of the chapter and on Evolve.

Key Terms

Albuminocytologic Dissociation
Ascending Paralysis
Autoimmune Disorder
Campylobacter jejuni
Demyelination
Electromyography (EMG)
High-Dose Immunoglobulin Therapy
Hydrotherapy (Whirlpool Therapy)
Immunoglobulin M (IgM)
Negative Inspiratory Force (NIF)
Paresthesia or Dysesthesias
Plasmapheresis

Chapter Outline

Anatomic Alterations of the Lungs Associated with Guillain-Barré Syndrome

Guillain-Barré syndrome is a relatively rare **autoimmune disorder** of the peripheral nervous system in which flaccid paralysis of the skeletal muscles and loss of reflexes develop in a previously healthy patient. In severe cases, paralysis of the diaphragm and ventilatory failure can develop. Clinically, this is a medical emergency. If the ventilatory failure is not properly managed, **mucous accumulation with airway obstruction, alveolar consolidation,** and **atelectasis** may develop.

Paralysis of the skeletal muscles develops in response to various pathologic changes in the peripheral nerves. Microscopically, the nerves show **demyelination,** inflammation, and edema. As the anatomic alterations of the peripheral nerves intensify, the ability of the neurons to transmit impulses to the muscles decreases, and eventually paralysis ensues (see Figure 28-1). Box 28-1 lists other names in the literature for Guillain-Barré syndrome.

The major pathologic or structural changes of the lungs associated with the ventilatory failure that may accompany Guillain-Barré syndrome are as follows:

- Mucous accumulation
- Airway obstruction
- Alveolar consolidation
- Atelectasis

Box 28-1 Other Names Found in the Literature for Guillain-Barré Syndrome

- Landry-Guillain-Barré-Strohl syndrome
- Acute idiopathic polyneuritis
- Postinfectious polyneuritis
- Landry's paralysis
- Acute postinfectious polyneuropathy
- Acute polyradiculitis
- Polyradiculoneuropathy

Etiology and Epidemiology

The annual incidence of Guillain-Barré syndrome is 1 to 2 per 100,000 people in the United States. The mortality rate is 4% to 6%, and the morbidity rate (permanent disabling weakness, imbalance, or sensory loss) is 5% to 10%. Although the condition is uncommon in early childhood, it may occur in all age groups and in either gender. A greater incidence has been noted among people 45 years of age and older, among male subjects, and among Caucasians (the condition is 50% to 60% more common in Caucasians). There is no obvious seasonal clustering of cases.

The precise cause of Guillain-Barré syndrome is not known. It is probably an immune disorder that causes inflammation and deterioration of the patient's peripheral nervous system. Elevated levels of **immunoglobulin M (IgM)** antibodies against myelin glycolipid have been found in the serum of patients with Guillain-Barré syndrome. Antibodies that are cell-mediated are thought to be responsible for peripheral nerve demyelination and inflammation. Lymphocytes and macrophages appear to attack and strip off the myelin sheath of the peripheral nerves and leave swelling and fragmentation of the neural axon (see Figure 28-1). It is believed that the myelin sheath covering the peripheral nerves (or the myelin-producing Schwann cell) is the actual target of the immune attack.

The onset of Guillain-Barré syndrome often occurs 1 to 4 weeks after a febrile episode caused by a mild respiratory or gastrointestinal viral or bacterial infection. In about 60% of the cases, ***Campylobacter jejuni*** is identified as the cause of the preceding infection. Other precipitating factors include infectious mononucleosis, parainfluenza 2, vaccinia, variola, measles, mumps, hepatitis A and B viruses, *Mycoplasma pneumoniae, Salmonella* Typhi, and *Chlamydia psittaci.* Although the significance of the association is controversial, during the nationwide immunization campaign in the United States in 1976, more than 40 million adults were vaccinated with swine influenza vaccine, and more than 500 cases of Guillain-Barré syndrome were reported among the vaccinated individuals, with 25 deaths.

Clinical Presentation

The general clinical history of patients with Guillain-Barré syndrome is (1) symmetric muscle weakness in the distal extremities accompanied by **paresthesia or dysesthesias** (tingling, burning, shocklike sensations), (2) pain (throbbing, aching, especially in the lower back, buttocks, and leg), and (3) numbness. The muscle paralysis then spreads upward **(ascending paralysis)** to the arms, trunk, and face. The muscle weakness and paralysis may develop within a single day or over several days. The muscle paralysis generally peaks in about 2 weeks. Deep tendon reflexes are commonly absent. The patient often drools and has difficulty chewing, swallowing, and speaking. The management of oral secretions may be a problem. Respiratory muscle paralysis, followed by acute ventilatory failure, occurs in 10% to 30% of cases.Although Guillain-Barré syndrome is typically an ascending paralysis—that is, moving from the lower portions of the legs and body upward—muscle paralysis may affect the facial and arm muscles first and then move downward. Although the weakness is commonly symmetric, a single arm or leg may be involved before paralysis spreads. The paralysis also may affect all four limbs simultaneously. Progression of the paralysis may stop at any point. After the paralysis reaches its maximum, it usually remains unchanged for a few days or weeks. Improvement generally begins spontaneously and continues for weeks or, in rare cases, months. About 10% of patients have permanent residual neurological deficits. About 90% of patients make a full recovery, but the recovery time may be as long as 3 years.If diagnosed early, patients with Guillain-Barré syndrome have an excellent prognosis. The diagnosis typically is based on the patient's clinical history (e.g., sudden ascending paralysis), cerebrospinal fluid (CSF) findings, and abnormal **electromyography (EMG)** results. The CSF in patients with Guillain-Barré syndrome shows an elevated protein level (500 mg/dL), without an increased lymphocyte count, called **albuminocytologic dissociation.** EMG helps to establish the diagnosis and the extent of neurologic involvement. The EMG measures the electrical activity of a muscle in response to nerve stimulation. It also measures the nature and speed of electrical conduction along a nerve.

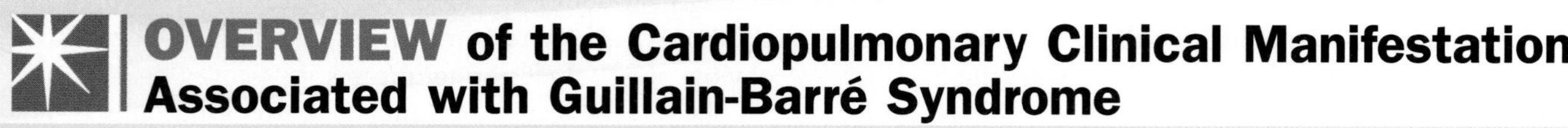

OVERVIEW of the Cardiopulmonary Clinical Manifestations Associated with Guillain-Barré Syndrome

The following clinical manifestations result from the pathologic mechanisms caused (or activated) by **Atelectasis** (see Figure 9-8), **Alveolar Consolidation** (see Figure 9-9), and **Excessive Bronchial Secretions** (see Figure 9-12)—the major anatomic alterations of the lungs associated with Guillain-Barré syndrome (when ventilatory failure is not properly managed) (see Figure 29-1).

CLINICAL DATA OBTAINED AT THE PATIENT'S BEDSIDE

The Physical Examination

Respiratory Rate

- Varies with the degree of respiratory muscle paralysis
- Apnea (in severe cases)

Cyanosis

Chest Assessment Findings

- Diminished breath sounds
- Crackles and rhonchi

Autonomic Nervous System Dysfunctions

- Heart rate and rhythm abnormalities
- Blood pressure abnormalities

Autonomic nervous system dysfunction develops in approximately 50% of all cases. The autonomic dysfunction involves the overreaction or underreaction of the sympathetic or parasympathetic nervous system. Clinically, the patient may manifest various cardiac arrhythmias, such as sinus tachycardia (the most common), bradycardia, ventricular tachycardia, atrial flutter, atrial fibrillation, and asystole.

Hypertension and hypotension also may be seen. Although the loss of bowel and bladder sphincter control is uncommon, transient sphincter paralysis may occur during the evolution of symptoms. The autonomic nervous system involvement may be transient or may persist throughout the duration of the disorder.

CLINICAL DATA OBTAINED FROM LABORATORY TESTS AND SPECIAL PROCEDURES

Pulmonary Function Test Findings*
(Restrictive Lung Pathology)

FORCED EXPIRATORY FLOW RATE FINDINGS

FVC	FEV_T	FEV_1/FVC ratio	$FEF_{25\%-75\%}$
↓	N or ↓	N or ↑	N or ↓
$FEF_{50\%}$	$FEF_{200-1200}$	PEFR	MVV
N or ↓	N or ↓	N or ↓	N or ↓

*Progressive worsening of these values is key to anticipating the onset of ventilatory failure.

OVERVIEW of the Cardiopulmonary Clinical Manifestations Associated with Guillain-Barré Syndrome—cont'd

LUNG VOLUME AND CAPACITY FINDINGS

V_T	IRV	ERV	RV	
↓	↓	↓	↓	
VC	IC	FRC	TLC	RV/TLC ratio
↓	↓	↓	↓	N

NEGATIVE INSPIRATORY FORCE (NIF) ↓

Arterial Blood Gases

MODERATE TO SEVERE GUILLAIN-BARRÉ SYNDROME

Acute Ventilatory Failure with Hypoxemia

(Acute Respiratory Acidosis)

pH*	Pa_{CO_2}	HCO_3^- *	Pa_{O_2}
↓	↑	↑ (slightly)	↓

*When tissue hypoxia is severe enough to produce lactic acid, the pH and HCO_3^- values will be lower than expected for a particular Pa_{CO_2} level.

Oxygenation Indices*

$\dot{Q}_S/\dot{Q}_T$	D_{O_2}†	$\dot{V}_{O_2}$	$C(a-\bar{v})_{O_2}$	O_2ER	$S\bar{v}_{O_2}$
↑	↓	N	N	↑	↓

†The D_{O_2} may be normal in patients who have compensated to the decreased oxygenation status with (1) an increased cardiac output, (2) an increased hemoglobin level, or (3) a combination of both. When the D_{O_2} is normal, the O_2ER is usually normal.

RADIOLOGIC FINDINGS

Chest Radiograph

- Normal, or
- Increased opacity (when atelectasis is present)

If the ventilatory failure associated with Guillain-Barré syndrome is properly managed, the chest x-ray film should be normal. However, if the bronchopulmonary hygiene and ventilatory failure are improperly managed, alveolar consolidation from secondary pneumonia and atelectasis may occur from excess secretion accumulation in the tracheobronchial tree. This increases the density of the lung segments affected.

*$C(a-\bar{v})_{O_2}$, Arterial-venous oxygen difference; D_{O_2}, total oxygen delivery; O_2ER, oxygen extraction ratio; $\dot{Q}_S/\dot{Q}_T$, pulmonary shunt fraction; $S\bar{v}_{O_2}$, mixed venous oxygen saturation; $\dot{V}_{O_2}$, oxygen consumption.

General Management of Guillain-Barré Syndrome

Guillain-Barré syndrome is a potential medical emergency, and patients must be monitored closely after the diagnosis has been made. The primary treatment should be directed at stabilization of vital signs and supportive care for the patient. Initially, such patients should be managed in an intensive care unit. Frequent measurements of the patient's vital capacity (VC), negative inspiratory force (NIF), blood pressure, oxygenation saturation, and arterial blood gases should be performed. Mechanical ventilation should be initiated when the clinical data demonstrate impending or acute ventilatory failure.

Good clinical indicators of acute ventilatory failure include the following:

- VC <20 mL/kg
- NIF <–25 cm H_2O—In other words, the patient is unable to generate a negative inspiratory pressure of 25 cm H_2O or more. For example, an NIF of only –15 would confirm severe muscle weakness and, important, that acute ventilatory failure was likely.
- pH <7.35 or Pa_{CO_2} >45 mm Hg

The **Bronchopulmonary Hygiene Protocol** and **Lung Expansion Therapy Protocol** should be instituted to prevent or treat mucous accumulation, airway obstruction, alveolar consolidation, and atelectasis.

As in any patient who is paralyzed, the risk of thromboembolism increases. Because of this danger, the patient commonly receives subcutaneously administered heparin, elastic stockings, and passive range-of-motion exercises (every 3 to 4 hours) for all extremities. To prevent skin breakdown, the patient should be turned frequently. A rotary bed or Stryker frame may be required. Blood pressure disturbances and cardiac arrhythmias require immediate attention. For example, nitroprusside (Nipride) or phentolamine (Regitine) are commonly administered during severe hypertensive episodes. Episodes of bradycardia are commonly treated with atropine.

Plasmapheresis

In severe cases, **plasmapheresis** (also known as *plasma exchange*) has been shown effective in decreasing the morbidity and shortening the clinical course of Guillain-Barré syndrome. Plasmapheresis entails the removal of damaged antibodies from the patient's blood plasma, followed by the retransfusion of the blood cells. It is believed that plasmapheresis removes the antibodies from the plasma that contribute to the immune system attack on the peripheral nerves. This procedure has been shown to reduce circulating antibody titers during the early stages of the disorder.

High-Dose Immunoglobulin Therapy

High-dose immunoglobulin therapy is another procedure used to reduce the severity and length of Guillain-Barré symptoms.

Corticosteroids

Corticosteroids have not been found to be effective in the treatment of Guillain-Barré syndrome. In fact, the administration of oral or intravenous corticosteroids may actually prolong the patient's recovery time.

Respiratory Care Treatment Protocols

Oxygen Therapy Protocol

Oxygen therapy is used to treat hypoxemia, decrease the work of breathing, and decrease myocardial work. Because of the hypoxemia that may develop in Guillain-Barré syndrome, supplemental oxygen may be required. However, because of the alveolar consolidation and atelectasis associated with Guillain-Barré syndrome, capillary shunting may be present. Hypoxemia caused by capillary shunting or alveolar hypoventilation is refractory to oxygen therapy (see Oxygen Therapy Protocol, Protocol 9-1).

Bronchopulmonary Hygiene Therapy Protocol

Because of the excessive mucous production and accumulation associated with Guillain-Barré syndrome, a number of bronchopulmonary hygiene modalities may be used to enhance the mobilization of bronchial secretions (see Bronchopulmonary Hygiene Therapy Protocol, Protocol 9-2).

Lung Expansion Therapy Protocol

Lung expansion measures are commonly administered to offset the alveolar consolidation and atelectasis associated with Guillain-Barré syndrome (see Lung Expansion Therapy Protocol, Protocol 9-3).

Mechanical Ventilation Protocol

Mechanical ventilation may be necessary to provide and support alveolar gas exchange and eventually return the patient to spontaneous breathing. Because acute ventilatory failure is seen in patients with severe Guillain-Barré syndrome, continuous mechanical ventilation is often required. Continuous mechanical ventilation is justified because the acute ventilatory failure is thought to be reversible (see Mechanical Ventilation Protocols, Protocol 9-5, Protocol 9-6, and Protocol 9-7).

Physical Therapy and Rehabilitation

Physical therapy usually begins long before the patient recovers from the effects of Guillain-Barré syndrome—often while the patient is still being mechanically ventilated. In long-term cases, for example, the patient's arms and legs will be manually moved on a regular basis to keep the muscles flexible and strong. After recovery, the patient frequently requires physical therapy to regain full strength and normal mobility. **Hydrotherapy (whirlpool therapy)** is commonly used to relieve pain and facilitate limb movement. Full recovery may require as little as a few weeks or as long as 3 years.

CASE STUDY

Guillain-Barré Syndrome

Admitting History and Physical Examination

A 48-year-old career U.S. Navy physician visited the hospital base clinic because of the acute onset of severe muscle weakness. He had joined the Navy immediately after medical school. Throughout his time in the service, he had the opportunity to pursue his passion—competitive water-ski jumping. For many years he was the first-place winner at most tournaments, including the nationals held yearly. For almost 25 years, he progressed through the age divisions, always remaining the top seed, always capturing the highest title.

The man was in outstanding physical condition. He was an avid runner and weightlifter, and during the off-season he often traveled to a warm climate to practice his water-ski jumping. He had never smoked and had never been hospitalized. He had an occasional "cold." About 2 years previously, he had begun to focus all his attention on his 19-year-old son, who was quickly following in his father's footsteps, having just captured the Men's Division I championship in collegiate ice hockey.

The man stated that he had felt good until 3 weeks before his admission, at which time he experienced a flulike syndrome for 3 days. About 10 days after returning to work, he noticed a tingling and burning sensation in his feet during his morning patient rounds. By dinner time that same day, the tingling and burning had radiated from his feet to about the level of his knees. Thinking that he was just tired from being on his feet all day, he went to bed early that evening. The next morning, however, his legs were completely numb, although he could still move them. Alarmed, he asked his son to drive him to the clinic. After examining him, his doctor (a personal friend) admitted him for a diagnostic workup and observation.

Over the next 3 days, the laboratory results showed that the patient's cerebrospinal fluid had an elevated protein concentration with a normal cell count. The electrodiagnostic studies showed a progressive ascending paralysis of the man's legs and arms. He began to have difficulty eating and swallowing his food. The respiratory care practitioners, who were monitoring his vital capacity, negative inspiratory pressure, pulse oximetry, and arterial blood gas values (ABGs), reported a progressive deterioration in all the values. A diagnosis of Guillain-Barré syndrome was recorded in the patient's chart.

When the man's ABGs showed pH 7.29, $Pa\text{CO}_2$ 53, HCO_3^- 23, and $Pa\text{O}_2$ 86 mm Hg (on a 2 L/min oxygen nasal cannula), the respiratory therapist called the attending physician and reported his assessment of acute ventilatory failure. The doctor transferred the patient to the intensive care unit (ICU), intubated him, and placed him on a mechanical ventilator. The initial ventilator settings were as follows: intermittent mechanical ventilation (IMV) mode, 12 breaths/min, tidal volume 0.75 L, and $F\text{IO}_2$ 0.40.

Approximately 15 minutes after the patient was committed to the ventilator, he appeared comfortable. No spontaneous breaths were noted between the 12 intermittent mandatory ventilations per minute. His vital signs were as follows: blood pressure 126/82 and heart rate 68 bpm. He was afebrile. A portable chest x-ray examination revealed that the endotracheal (ET) tube was in a good position and the lungs were adequately aerated. Normal vesicular breath sounds were auscultated over both lung fields. His ABGs were as follows: pH 7.51, $Pa\text{CO}_2$ 29, HCO_3^- 22, and $Pa\text{O}_2$ 204. His oxygen saturation measured by pulse oximetry ($Sp\text{O}_2$) was 98%. On the basis of these clinical data, the following SOAP was documented.

Respiratory Assessment and Plan

S N/A (intubated on ventilator)

O Vital signs: BP 126/82, HR 68, RR 12 (IMV); afebrile; no spontaneous breaths; CXR: normal; normal breath sounds; ABGs (on $F\text{IO}_2$ = 0.40): pH 7.51, $Pa\text{CO}_2$ 29, HCO_3^- 22, $Pa\text{O}_2$ 204; $Sp\text{O}_2$ 98%

A
- Acute alveolar hyperventilation with excessive oxygenation (ABGs)
- Excessive alveolar ventilation (increased pH and decreased $Pa\text{CO}_2$)
- $F\text{IO}_2$ too high (ABGs)

P Adjust mechanical ventilator settings (decrease tidal volume and $F\text{IO}_2$) according to **Mechanical Ventilation Protocol** and **Oxygen Therapy Protocol**. Monitor closely and reevaluate.

3 Days after Admission

The patient's cardiopulmonary status had been unremarkable. No improvement was seen in his muscular paralysis. No changes had been made in his ventilator settings over the previous 48 hours. His skin color appeared good. Palpation and percussion of the chest were unremarkable. On auscultation, however, crackles and rhonchi could be heard over both lung fields.

Moderate amounts of thick, whitish, clear secretions were being suctioned from the patient's endotracheal tube regularly. His vital signs were as follows: blood pressure 124/83, heart rate 74 bpm, and rectal temperature 37.7° C (99.8° F). A recent portable chest x-ray examination revealed no significant pathologic process. His ABGs on an $F\text{IO}_2$ of 0.40 were as follows: pH 7.44, $Pa\text{CO}_2$ 35, HCO_3^- 24, and $Pa\text{O}_2$ 98. His $Sp\text{O}_2$ was 97%. On the basis of these clinical data, the following SOAP was documented.

Respiratory Assessment and Plan

S N/A

O Skin color good; crackles and rhonchi over both lung fields; moderate amount of whitish, clear secretions being suctioned regularly; vital signs: BP 124/83, HR 74, T 37.7° C (99.8° F); CXR: unremarkable; ABGs (FIO_2 = 0.4): pH 7.44, $PaCO_2$ 35, HCO_3^- 24, and PaO_2 98; SpO_2 97%

A • Normal acid-base and oxygenation status on present ventilator settings (ABGs)
• Excessive sputum accumulation; possible progression to mucous plugging and atelectasis (crackles, rhonchi, whitish and clear secretions)

P Begin **Bronchopulmonary Hygiene Therapy Protocol** (vigorous tracheal suctioning and obtain sputum stain and culture). Begin **Lung Expansion Therapy Protocol** (10 cm H_2O positive end-expiratory pressure [PEEP] to offset any early development of atelectasis). Monitor and reevaluate (4 × per shift).

5 Days after Admission

The patient remained alert and comfortable, except for the ET tube. His muscular paralysis remained unchanged. His skin color appeared good, and no remarkable information was noted during palpation and percussion. Although crackles and rhonchi could still be heard over both lung fields, they were not as intense as they had been 48 hours earlier. A small amount of clear secretions was suctioned from the patient's ET tube. His vital signs were as follows: blood pressure 118/79, heart rate 68 bpm, and temperature normal. Results of a recent portable chest x-ray examination appeared normal. His ABGs on an FIO_2 of 0.40 were as follows: pH 7.42, $PaCO_2$ 37, HCO_3^- 24, and PaO_2 97 mm Hg. His SpO_2 was 97%. The sputum culture was unremarkable. On the basis of these clinical data, the following SOAP note was recorded.

Respiratory Assessment and Plan

S N/A

O Skin color good; crackles and rhonchi over both lung fields improving; small amount of clear secretions suctioned; vital signs: BP 118/79, HR 68, T normal; no spontaneous respirations; CXR: normal; ABGs (FIO_2 = 0.4): pH 7.42, $PaCO_2$ 37, HCO_3^- 24, PaO_2 97; SpO_2 97%

A • Normal acid-base and oxygenation status on present ventilator settings (ABGs)
• Respiratory insufficiency (no spontaneous respirations)
• Secretion control improving (crackles, rhonchi, clear secretions)

P Continue **Ventilator Management Protocol.** Continue **Bronchopulmonary Hygiene Therapy Protocol.** Continue **Lung Expansion Therapy Protocol.** Monitor and reevaluate (forced expiratory volume in 1 second [FEV_1], negative inspiratory force [NIF] 2 × per shift).

Discussion

Guillain-Barré syndrome is a neuromuscular paralysis that ensues after infection with a neurotropic virus. This patient had a classic history of ascending paralysis and paresthesias and the diagnostic finding of elevated protein concentration in the spinal fluid. In this setting, serial measurements of the patient's vital capacity (VC), negative inspiratory force (NIF), blood pressure, oxygen saturation, and arterial blood gases must be measured and charted. Once respiratory failure supervenes, intubation and respiratory support on a ventilator become necessary. As discussed in this chapter, good clinical indicators of acute ventilatory failure include the following: VC <20 mL/kg, NIF <–25 cm H_2O, pH <7.35, and $PaCO_2$ >45 mm Hg. As noted by the respiratory practitioner, a progressive deterioration was observed in all of these clinical indicators over a 3-day period.

As shown during the first assessment, when acute ventilatory failure developed, the patient was transferred to the ICU, intubated, and placed on a mechanical ventilator. Shortly after the patient was placed on the ventilator, his arterial blood gas values showed hyperoxia and acute alveolar hyperventilation—both of which were caused by the ventilator settings. The appropriate response was to immediately adjust the ventilator settings by reducing the tidal volume or frequency (or both) and the FIO_2. At the time of the assessment, the patient exhibited no evidence of airway obstruction or secretions. Therefore the **Bronchial Hygiene Therapy Protocol** (Protocol 9-2), was not indicated. Indeed, all that needed to be done at that time was to ensure adequate ventilation and oxygenation on the ventilator.

However, 3 days later, at the time of the second assessment, crackles and rhonchi were heard over all lung fields. Clearly the time had come to initiate the **Bronchial Hygiene Therapy Protocol** with suctioning and possibly even therapy with mucolytic agents. Because of the risk of atelectasis, the **Lung Expansion Therapy Protocol** (Protocol 9-3), in the form of PEEP on the ventilator, was indicated. In such a case the sputum should be cultured to see whether any infectious organisms are present.

At the time of the final assessment (2 days later), the clinical indicators for airway secretions had decreased—the rhonchi could no longer be heard over the lung fields, and the small amount of sputum suctioned appeared clear. At that point the down-regulation of the **Bronchial Hygiene Therapy Protocol** was indicated.

Serial VC or NIF measurements would continue to be made until the patient was ready to be extubated and thereafter for at least several days. Indeed, extubation occurred about 3 weeks after the initiation of mechanical ventilation. The patient recovered without incident and returned to his active lifestyle within a year.

SELF-ASSESSMENT QUESTIONS

evolve Answers to questions can be found on Evolve. To access additional student assessment questions and case studies for application of text material to real-life scenarios, visit **http://evolve.elsevier.com/DesJardins/respiratory.**

1. In Guillain-Barré syndrome, which of the following pathologic changes develop in the peripheral nerves?
1. Inflammation
2. Increased ability to transmit nerve impulses
3. Demyelination
4. Edema
   a. 2 and 3 only
   b. 3 and 4 only
   c. 2, 3, and 4 only
   d. 1, 3, and 4 only

2. Which of the following is associated with Guillain-Barré syndrome?
1. Alveolar consolidation
2. Mucous accumulation
3. Alveolar hyperinflation
4. Atelectasis
   a. 1 and 2 only
   b. 3 and 4 only
   c. 1, 2, and 4 only
   d. 2, 3, and 4 only

3. Guillain-Barré syndrome is more common in:
1. People older than 45 years of age
2. Blacks than in whites
3. Males than in females
4. Early childhood
   a. 1 only
   b. 4 only
   c. 1 and 3 only
   d. 3 and 4 only

4. Which of the following are possible precursors to Guillain-Barré syndrome?
1. Mumps
2. Swine influenza vaccine
3. Infectious mononucleosis
4. Measles
   a. 2 and 4 only
   b. 3 and 4 only
   c. 2, 3, and 4 only
   d. 1, 2, 3, and 4

5. Full recovery from Guillain-Barré syndrome is expected in approximately what percentage of cases?
   a. 30%
   b. 40%
   c. 50%
   d. 90%

6. Which of the following are indicators for intubation and mechanical ventilation in patients with Guillain-Barré syndrome?
1. pH < 7.40
2. $Paco_2 > 45$
3. FVC < 20 ml/kg
4. NIF < -25 cm H_2O
   a. 1 and 2 only
   b. 3 and 4 only
   c. 2, 3, and 4 only
   d. 1, 2, and 3 only

Myasthenia Gravis

29

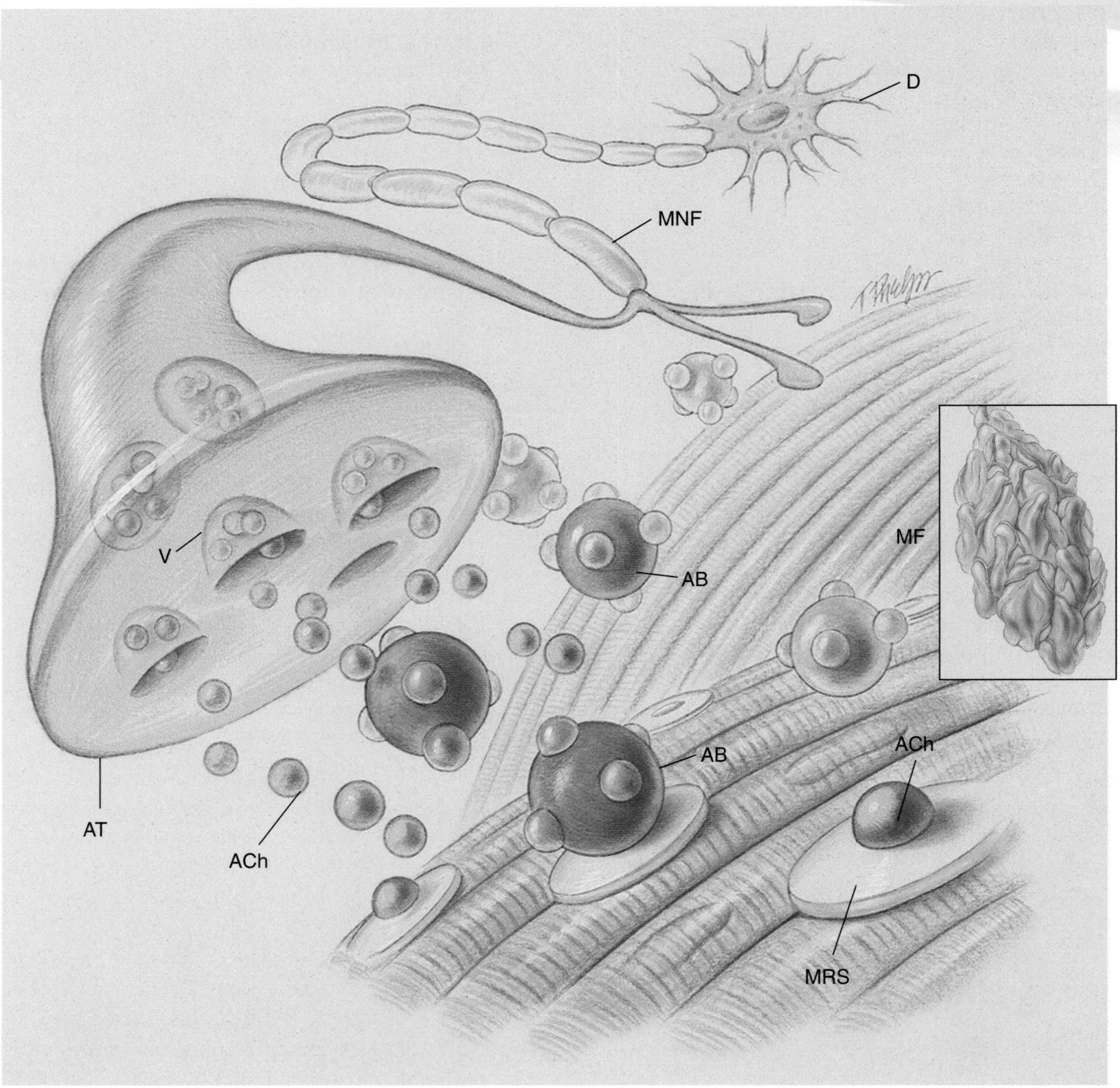

FIGURE 29-1 Myasthenia gravis, a disorder of the neuromuscular junction that interferes with the chemical transmission of acetylcholine. *AB,* Antibody; *ACh,* acetylcholine; *AT,* axonal terminal; *D,* dendrite; *MF,* muscle fiber; *MNF,* myelinated nerve fiber; *MRS,* muscle receptor site; *V,* vesicle. Note that the antibodies have a physical structure similar to that of ACh, which permits them to connect to (and block ACh from) the muscle receptor sites. *Inset,* Atelectasis, a common secondary anatomic alteration of the lungs.

Chapter Objectives

After reading this chapter, will be able to:

- List the anatomic alterations of the lungs associated with myasthenia gravis.
- Describe the causes of myasthenia gravis.
- List the cardiopulmonary clinical manifestations associated with myasthenia gravis.
- Describe the general management of myasthenia gravis.
- Describe the clinical strategies and rationales of the SOAPs presented in the case study.

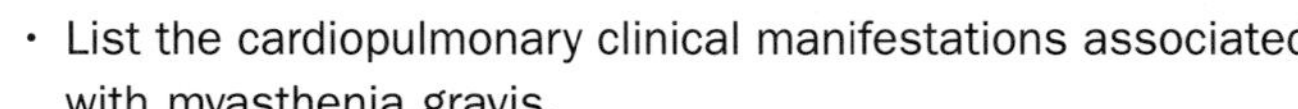

• Define key terms and complete self-assesment questions at the end of the chapter and on Evolve.

Key Terms

Acetylcholine (ACh)
Anticholinesterase Drugs
Aspiration of Gastric Contents
Azathioprine
Cyclosporine
Diplopia
Dynamometer
Edrophonium Test
Electromyography
Ice Pack Test
IgG Antibodies
Immunosuppressants
Mycophenolate Mofetil
Neostigmine (Prostigmin)
Neuromuscular Junction
Plasmapheresis
Prednisone
Ptosis
Pyridostigmine (Mestinon)
Sleep Test
Thymectomy
Thymoma

Chapter Outline

Anatomic Alterations of the Lungs Associated with Myasthenia Gravis

Myasthenia gravis is a chronic disorder of the **neuromuscular junction** that interferes with the chemical transmission of **acetylcholine (ACh)** between the axonal terminal and the receptor sites of voluntary muscles (see Figure 29-1). It is characterized by fatigue and weakness, with improvement following rest. Because the disorder affects only the myoneural (motor) junction, sensory function is not lost.

The abnormal weakness may be confined to an isolated group of muscles (e.g., the drooping of one or both eyelids), or it may manifest as a generalized weakness that in severe cases includes the diaphragm. When the diaphragm is involved, ventilatory failure can develop. If the ventilatory failure is not properly managed, mucous accumulation with airway obstruction, alveolar consolidation, and atelectasis may develop.

The major pathologic or structural changes of the lungs associated with the ventilatory failure that may accompany myasthenia gravis are as follows:

- Mucous accumulation
- Airway obstruction
- Alveolar consolidation
- Atelectasis

Etiology and Epidemiology

The cause of myasthenia gravis appears to be related to ACh receptor antibodies (the **IgG antibodies**) that block the nerve impulse transmissions at the neuromuscular junction. It is believed that the IgG antibodies disrupt the chemical transmission of ACh at the neuromuscular junction by (1) blocking the ACh from the receptor sites of the muscular cell, (2) accelerating the breakdown of ACh, and (3) destroying the receptor sites (see Figure 29-1). Receptor-binding antibodies are present in 85% to 90% of persons with myasthenia gravis. Although the specific events that activate the formation of the antibodies remain unclear, the thymus gland is almost always abnormal; it is generally presumed that the antibodies arise within the thymus or in related tissue.

About 30,000 people in the United States are affected by myasthenia gravis. It is most common in young women and older men. The disease usually has a peak age of onset in females of 15 to 35 years, compared with 40 to 70 years in males. The clinical manifestations associated with myasthenia gravis are often provoked by emotional upset, physical stress, exposure to extreme temperature changes, febrile illness, and pregnancy. Death caused by myasthenia gravis is possible, especially during the first few years after onset. After the disease has been in progress for 10 years, however, death from myasthenia gravis is rare.

Screening and Diagnosis

Screening methods and tests used to diagnosis myasthenia gravis include (1) the clinical history, (2) neurologic examination, (3) **electromyography,** (4) blood analysis, (5) **edrophonium** (Enlon) test, (6) **ice pack test,** (7) **sleep test,** and (8) computed tomography (CT) or magnetic resonance imaging (MRI) of the thymus.

Clinical Presentation

The hallmark of myasthenia gravis is chronic muscle fatigue. The muscles become progressively weaker during periods of activity and improve after periods of rest. Signs and symptoms include facial muscle weakness; **ptosis** (drooping of one or both eyelids); **diplopia** (double vision); difficulty in breathing, speaking, chewing, and swallowing; unstable gait; and weakness in arms, hands, fingers, legs, and neck brought on by repetitive motions. The muscles that control the eyes, eyelids, face, and throat are especially susceptible and are usually affected first. The respiratory muscles of the diaphragm and chest wall can become weak and impair the patient's ventilation. Impairment in deep breathing and coughing predispose the patient to excessive bronchial secretions, atelectasis, and pneumonia.

The signs and symptoms of myasthenia gravis during the early stages are often elusive. The onset can be subtle, intermittent, or sudden and rapid. The patient may (1) demonstrate normal health for weeks or months at a time, (2) show signs of weakness only late in the day or evening, or (3) develop a sudden and transient generalized weakness that includes the diaphragm. Because of this last characteristic, ventilatory failure is always a sinister possibility. In most cases, the first noticeable symptom is weakness of the eye muscles (droopy eyelids) and a change in the patient's facial expressions. As the disorder becomes more generalized, weakness develops in the arms and legs. The muscle weakness is usually more pronounced in the proximal parts of the extremities. The patient has difficulty in climbing stairs, lifting objects, maintaining balance, and walking. In severe cases the weakness of the upper limbs may be such that the hand cannot be lifted to the mouth. Muscle atrophy or pain is rare. Tendon reflexes almost always remain intact.

Neurologic Examination

Neurologic tests may include the evaluation of reflexes, muscle strength, muscle tone, senses of touch and sight, gait, posture, coordination, balance, and mental abilities.

Electromyography

Electromyography usually is performed to confirm the diagnosis of myasthenia gravis, identify the specific muscles involved, and determine the degree of fatigability. Electromyography entails the repetitive stimulation of a nerve, such as the ulnar nerve, with the simultaneous recording of the muscle response. Clinically, the degree of fatigability often is evaluated by having the patient use certain muscles for a sustained period. For example, the patient may be instructed to gaze upward for an extended period, blink continuously, hold both arms outstretched as long as possible, or count aloud as long as possible in one breath (normal is about 50). A **dynamometer** sometimes is used to measure the force of repetitive muscle contractions.

Blood Analysis

A blood test may reveal the presence of ACh receptor antibodies. About 85% to 90% of patients with myasthenia gravis have an elevated level of these antibodies.

Edrophonium Test

The diagnosis of myasthenia gravis is usually is confirmed with the injection of edrophonium (Enlon). Edrophonium, a short-acting drug, blocks cholinesterase from breaking down ACh after it has been released from the terminal axon. This action increases the myoneural concentration of ACh, which in turn offsets the influx of antibodies at the neuromuscular junction. When muscular weakness is caused by myasthenia gravis, a dramatic transitory improvement in muscle function (lasting about 10 minutes) is seen after the administration of edrophonium. A disadvantage of the edrophonium test is that it can be complicated by cholinergic side effects that include cardiopulmonary arrest.

Ice Pack Test

The ice pack test (Figure 29-2) is a very simple, safe, and reliable procedure for diagnosing myasthenia gravis in patients who have ptosis (droopy eye). In addition, the ice pack test does not require special medications or expensive equipment and is free of adverse effects. The test consists of the application of an ice pack to the patient's symptomatic eye for 3 to 5 minutes. The test is considered positive for myasthenia gravis when there is improvement of the ptosis (an increase of at least 2 mm in the palpebral fissure from before to after the test).

A major disadvantage of the ice pack test is that it is useful only when ptosis is present. Even though the symptoms associated with diplopia (double vision) may also improve with the ice pack test, the reliability of the ice pack test in patients with diplopia without ptosis is usually questionable because the patient's personal impression of the diplopia is subjective. Therefore caution should be exercised in patients with isolated diplopia without ptosis. The ice pack test may be especially useful in patients in whom the edrophonium test is contraindicated by either cardiac status or age.

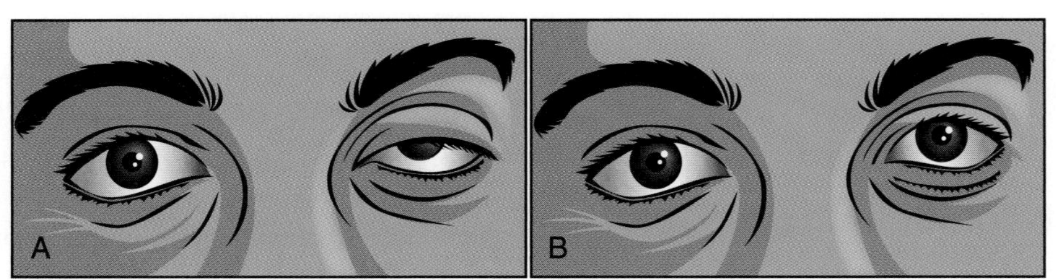

FIGURE 29-2 Ice pack test. **A**, Myasthenia gravis in patient who has ptosis (droopy left eye). **B**, Same patient after 5-minute application of an ice pack. Note the patient's left eye lid is no longer droopy.

Sleep Test

Because the signs and symptoms associated with myasthenia gravis increase with fatigue and improve after a period of rest, the **sleep test** is safe, moderately sensitive, and specific. Myasthenia gravis is indicated when ptosis improves after a 20- to 30-minute period of sleep. The reappearance of ptosis over the next 5 minutes further supports the diagnosis of myasthenia gravis. The sleep test is often not practical for the busy physician because it entails a dark room and quiet area to enhance sleep and is time-consuming.

Computed Tomography or Magnetic Resonance Imaging

A CT or MRI scan may be used to identify an abnormal thymus gland or the presence of a **thymoma** (a usually benign tumor of the thymus gland that may be associated with myasthenia gravis). A **thymectomy** has been shown to reduce symptoms in more than 70% of patients with myasthenia gravis. In fact, a thymectomy may be recommended even when there is no tumor. The removal of the thymus seems to improve the condition in many patients.

OVERVIEW of the Cardiopulmonary Clinical Manifestations Associated with Myasthenia Gravis

The following clinical manifestations result from the pathologic mechanisms caused (or activated) by **Atelectasis** (see Figure 9-8), **Alveolar Consolidation** (see Figure 9-9), and **Excessive Bronchial Secretions** (see Figure 9-12)—the major anatomic alterations of the lungs associated with myasthenia gravis (when ventilatory failure is not properly managed) (see Figure 29-1).

CLINICAL DATA OBTAINED AT THE PATIENT'S BEDSIDE

The Physical Examination

Respiratory Rate

- Varies with the degree of respiratory muscle paralysis
- Apnea (in severe cases)

Cyanosis (in Severe Cases)

Chest Assessment Findings

- Diminished breath sounds
- Crackles and rhonchi

CLINICAL DATA OBTAINED FROM LABORATORY TESTS AND SPECIAL

Pulmonary Function Test Findings*
(Restrictive Lung Pathology)

FORCED EXPIRATORY FLOW RATE FINDINGS

FVC	FEV_T	FEV_1/FVC ratio	$FEF_{25\%-75\%}$
↓	N or ↓	N or ↑	N or ↓

$FEF_{50\%}$	$FEF_{200-1200}$	PEFR	MVV
N or ↓	N or ↓	N or ↓	N or ↓

*Progressive worsening of these values is key to anticipating the onset of ventilatory failure.

LUNG VOLUME AND CAPACITY FINDINGS

V_T	IRV	ERV	RV	
↓	↓	↓	↓	
VC	IC	FRC	TLC	RV/TLC ratio
↓	↓	↓	↓	N

NEGATIVE INSPIRATORY FORCE (NIF) ↓

Arterial Blood Gases

MODERATE TO SEVERE MYASTHENIA GRAVIS
Acute Ventilatory Failure with Hypoxemia
(Acute Respiratory Acidosis)

pH*	Pa_{CO_2}	HCO_3^-*	Pa_{O_2}
↓	↑	↑ (slightly)	↓

*When tissue hypoxia is severe enough to produce lactic acid, the pH and HCO_3^- values will be lower than expected for a particular Pa_{CO_2} level.

Oxygenation Indices*

$\dot{Q}_S/\dot{Q}_T$	D_{O_2}†	$\dot{V}_{O_2}$	$C(a-\bar{v})_{O_2}$	O_2ER	$S\bar{v}_{O_2}$
↑	↓	N	N	↑	↓

†The D_{O_2} may be normal in patients who have compensated to the decreased oxygenation status with (1) an increased cardiac output, (2) an increased hemoglobin level, or (3) a combination of both. When the D_{O_2} is normal, the O_2ER is usually normal.

RADIOLOGIC FINDINGS

Chest Radiograph

- Normal in early stages
- Increased opacity (when atelectasis or consolidation is present)

**$C(a-\bar{v})_{O_2}$*, Arterial-venous oxygen difference; *D_{O_2}*, total oxygen delivery; *O_2ER*, oxygen extraction ratio; *$\dot{Q}_S/\dot{Q}_T$*, pulmonary shunt fraction; *$S\bar{v}_{O_2}$*, mixed venous oxygen saturation; *$\dot{V}_{O_2}$*, oxygen consumption.

General Management of Myasthenia Gravis

In the past, many patients with myasthenia gravis died within the first few years of diagnosis of the disease. Today, a number of therapeutic measures provide most patients with marked relief of symptoms and allow them to live a normal life. Frequent measurements of the patient's vital capacity (VC), negative inspiratory force (NIF), blood pressure, oxygen saturation, and arterial blood gases should be performed. Mechanical ventilation should be initiated when the clinical data demonstrate impending or acute ventilatory failure.

Good clinical indicators of acute ventilatory failure include the following:

- VC <20 mL/kg
- NIF <–25 cm H_2O—In other words, the patient is unable to generate a negative inspiratory pressure of 25 cm H_2O or more. For example, an NIF of only –15 would confirm severe muscle weakness and, important, that acute ventilatory failure was likely.
- pH <7.35 or Pa_{CO_2} >45 mm Hg

The **Bronchopulmonary Hygiene Protocol** and **Lung Expansion Therapy Protocol** should be instituted to prevent mucous accumulation, airway obstruction, alveolar consolidation, and atelectasis. During a myasthenic crisis, the treatment modalities described in the following paragraphs also may be used.

Cholinesterase Inhibitors

Cholinesterase inhibitors that enhance the action of ACh are used to treat myasthenia gravis. **Pyridostigmine** (Mestinon) is usually the first-line treatment for myasthenia gravis. **Neostigmine** (Prostigmin) is also available but not commonly used. These agents inhibit the function of cholinesterase. This action increases the concentration of ACh to compete with the circulating anti-ACh antibodies, which interfere with the ability of ACh to stimulate the muscle receptors. Although the **anticholinesterase drugs** are effective in mild cases of myasthenia gravis, they are not completely effective in severe cases.

Immunosuppressants

Corticosteroids and similar agents, such as **prednisone** (Deltasone), **cyclosporine** (Neoral), **mycophenolate mofetil** (CellCept), and **azathioprine** (Azathine) are used to suppress the immune system. These agents **(immunosuppressants)** usually are used for more severe cases. The patient's strength often improves strikingly with steroids. Patients receiving long-term steroid therapy, however, may develop serious complications such as diabetes, cataracts, steroid myopathy, gastrointestinal bleeding, infections, aseptic necrosis of the bone, osteoporosis, and psychoses.

Thymectomy

Although controversial, thymectomy has been helpful in many patients with myasthenia gravis, especially young adult females. The thymus gland in the myasthenic patient frequently appears to be the source of anti-ACh receptor antibodies. In some patients, muscle strength improves soon after surgery, whereas in others improvement takes months or years.

Plasmapheresis

Plasmapheresis is a blood plasma exchange procedure that is used to "filter" the blood of ACh receptor antibodies by replacing the patient's plasma with a donor's plasma. Plasmapheresis can be a life-saving intervention in the treatment of myasthenia gravis. However, it is time-consuming and associated with many side effects, such as low blood pressure, infection, and blood clots.

Respiratory Care Treatment Protocols

Oxygen Therapy Protocol

Oxygen therapy is used to treat hypoxemia, decrease the work of breathing, and decrease myocardial work. Because of the hypoxemia that may develop in myasthenia gravis, supplemental oxygen may be required. However, because of the alveolar consolidation and atelectasis associated with myasthenia gravis, capillary shunting may be present. Hypoxemia caused by capillary shunting is refractory to oxygen therapy (see Oxygen Therapy Protocol, Protocol 9-1).

Bronchopulmonary Hygiene Therapy Protocol

Because of the excessive mucous production and accumulation associated with myasthenia gravis, a number of bronchial hygiene treatment modalities may be used to enhance the mobilization of bronchial secretions (see Bronchopulmonary Hygiene Therapy Protocol, Protocol 9-2).

Lung Expansion Therapy Protocol

Lung expansion measures are commonly administered to prevent or offset the alveolar consolidation and atelectasis associated with myasthenia gravis (see Lung Expansion Therapy Protocol, Protocol 9-3).

Mechanical Ventilation Protocol

Mechanical ventilation may be needed to provide and support alveolar gas exchange and eventually return the patient to spontaneous breathing. Because acute ventilatory failure is often seen in patients with severe myasthenia gravis, continuous mechanical ventilation may be required. Continuous mechanical ventilation is justified when the acute ventilatory failure is thought to be reversible (see Mechanical Ventilation Protocols, Protocol 9-5, Protocol 9-6, and Protocol 9-7).

CASE STUDY

Myasthenia Gravis

Admitting History

A 35-year-old Spanish-American woman was a schoolteacher with a 3-year-old son and an unemployed husband who was still "finding his real place in life." The woman was a high achiever. She had recently received her doctoral degree in education, but she continued to work in the classroom with the grade-school children she loved so much. She was named Teacher of the Year in the large city where she lived. Her colleagues at school considered her a nonstop worker. She had never smoked.

At home, she was always on the move. She had just finished remodeling her kitchen and two bathrooms. She also did her own backyard landscaping on the weekends, a job she particularly enjoyed. She read and played with her son whenever they had time together. Although she enjoyed cooking (a skill she learned from her mother), she did not like to shop for groceries. Fortunately, this was a chore that her husband enjoyed.

Three weeks before the current admission, the woman noticed that her eyes "felt tired." She began to experience slight double vision. Thinking that she was working too hard, she slowed down a bit and went to bed earlier for about a week. However, she progressively felt weaker. Her legs quickly became tired, and she began having trouble chewing her food. Concerned, the woman finally went to see her doctor. After reviewing the woman's recent history and performing a careful physical examination, the physician admitted her to the hospital for further evaluation and treatment.

Over the next 48 hours, the woman's physical status declined progressively. At the patient's bedside, an ice pack test was positive for myasthenia gravis when her ptosis improved by 5 mm. She also indicated that her diplopia was better for about 10 minutes after the test. After the administration of edrophonium, her muscle strength increased significantly for about 10 minutes. Electromyography disclosed extensive muscle involvement and a high degree of fatigability in all the affected muscles. A diagnosis of myasthenia gravis was recorded in the patient's chart.

The woman began to choke and aspirate food during meals, and a nasogastric feeding tube was inserted. Her speech became more and more slurred. Both her upper eyelids drooped, and she was unable to hold her head off her pillow on request. The respiratory therapists who monitored her vital capacity, negative inspiratory pressure, pulse oximetry, and arterial blood gas values (ABGs) reported a progressive worsening in all parameters.

When the woman's ABGs were pH 7.32, Pa_{CO_2} 51, HCO_3^- 23, and Pa_{O_2} 59 (on room air), the respiratory therapist called the physician and reported an assessment of acute ventilatory failure. The doctor had the patient transferred to the intensive care unit, intubated (No. 7 endotracheal tube with a tube length charted at 23 cm at the lip), and placed on a mechanical ventilator. The initial ventilator settings were as follows: intermittent mechanical ventilation (IMV) mode, 10 breaths/min, tidal volume 0.6 L, F_{IO_2} 0.5, and positive end-expiratory pressure (PEEP) of 7 cm H_2O.

Approximately 25 minutes after the patient was placed on the ventilator, she appeared agitated. No spontaneous ventilations were seen. Her vital signs were as follows: blood pressure 132/86, heart rate 90 bpm, and rectal temperature 38° C (100.5° F). A portable chest x-ray film had been taken, but the image was still being processed. Normal vesicular breath sounds were auscultated over the right lung, and diminished-to-absent breath sounds were auscultated over the left lung. On an F_{IO_2} of 0.5, her ABG values were as follows: pH 7.28, Pa_{CO_2} 64, HCO_3^- 26, and Pa_{O_2} 52. Her oxygen saturation measured by pulse oximetry (Sp_{O_2}) was 80%. On the basis of these clinical data, the following SOAP was recorded.

Respiratory Assessment and Plan

S N/A (patient intubated)

O No spontaneous ventilations; vital signs: BP 132/86, HR 90, RR 10 (controlled), T 38° C (100.5° F); normal breath sounds over right lung; diminished-to-absent breath sounds over left lung; ABGs (on F_{IO_2} = 0.50): pH 7.28, Pa_{CO_2} 64, HCO_3^- 26, Pa_{O_2} 52; Sp_{O_2} 80%

A
- Endotracheal tube possibly placed in right main stem bronchi (diminished-to-absent breath sounds over left lung, ABGs)
- Acute ventilatory failure with moderate hypoxemia (ABGs)
- Condition likely caused by misplacement of endotracheal tube

P Notify physician stat. Check CXR. Pull endotracheal tube back until breath sounds can be auscultated over both lungs. Confirm initial placement of the endotracheal tube when x-ray image is available. **Mechanical Ventilation Protocol** (increase tidal volume and increase F_{IO_2}). Monitor and reevaluate immediately.

45 Minutes Later

After the patient's endotracheal tube was pulled back 3 cm to 20 cm at the lip, normal vesicular breath sounds could be auscultated over both lungs. The first chest x-ray examination confirmed that the endotracheal tube had been inserted too far into the patient's right main stem bronchus. A follow-up chest x-ray examination confirmed that the endotracheal tube was now appropriately positioned about 2 cm above the carina. Her vital signs were as follows: blood pressure 123/75, heart rate 74 bpm, and temperature normal. The ventilator settings were readjusted, and repeat ABGs were as follows: pH 7.53, Pa_{CO_2} 27, HCO_3^- 22, and Pa_{O_2} 176. Her Sp_{O_2} was 98%. On the basis of these clinical data, the following SOAP was written.

Respiratory Assessment and Plan

S N/A (patient intubated on ventilator)

O Vital signs: BP 123/75, HR 74, T normal; normal bronchovesicular breath sounds over both lung fields; CXR: #7 endotracheal tube in good position (20 cm @ lip); lungs adequately ventilated; ABGs: pH 7.53, Pa_{CO_2} 27, HCO_3^- 22, Pa_{O_2} 176; Sp_{O_2} 98%

A • Acute ventilator-induced alveolar hyperventilation (respiratory alkalosis) with overly corrected hypoxemia (ABGs)

P Adjust present settings per **Mechanical Ventilation Protocol** (decreasing tidal volume). Down-regulate **Oxygen Therapy Per Protocol** (decrease F_{IO_2} to 0.21). Monitor and reevaluate.

3 Days after Admission

No changes in the patient's ventilator settings were necessary over the previous 48 hours. No improvement was seen in her muscular paralysis. The woman appeared pale, and her vital signs were as follows: blood pressure 146/88, heart rate 92 bpm, and temperature 37.9° C (100.2° F). Large amounts of thick, yellowish sputum were being suctioned from her endotracheal tube approximately every 30 minutes.

Rhonchi were auscultated over both lung fields. A sputum sample was obtained and sent to the laboratory to be cultured. A portable chest x-ray examination revealed a new infiltrate in the right lower lobe consistent with pneumonia or atelectasis. The ABGs were as follows: pH 7.28, Pa_{CO_2} 36, HCO_3^- 17, and Pa_{O_2} 41. Her Sp_{O_2} was 69%. On the basis of these clinical data, the following SOAP was recorded.

Respiratory Assessment and Plan

S N/A

O No improvement seen in muscular paralysis; skin: pale; vital signs: BP 146/88, HR 92, T 37.9° C (100.2° F); large amounts of thick, yellowish sputum; rhonchi over both lung fields; CXR: pneumonia and atelectasis in right lower lobe; ABGs: pH 7.28, Pa_{CO_2} 36, HCO_3^- 17, Pa_{O_2} 41; Sp_{O_2} 69%

A
- Excessive bronchial secretions (rhonchi, sputum)
- Infection likely (yellow sputum, fever, CXR: pneumonia)
- Metabolic acidosis with moderate-to-severe hypoxemia (ABGs)
- Acidosis likely caused by lactic acid (ABGs)

P Up-regulate **Bronchopulmonary Hygiene Therapy Protocol** (med. neb. with 0.5 mL albuterol in 2 mL 10% acetylcysteine q4h; therapist to suction patient frequently; sputum culture check in 24 and 48 hours). Initiate **Lung Expansion Therapy Protocol** (add 10 cm H_2O PEEP to ventilator settings). Up-regulate **Oxygen Therapy Protocol** (increase F_{IO_2} to 0.6). Monitor closely and reevaluate (check ABGs in 30 minutes).

Discussion

As with the patient with Guillain-Barré syndrome, this case of myasthenia gravis provides another chance to discuss ventilatory failure secondary to neuromuscular disease. The presentation of this patient with double vision (diplopia), difficulty in swallowing (dysphagia), and progressive muscle weakness is classic for this condition. The positive endrophronium test noted in the history was necessary for a final diagnosis. Also important to note is that **aspiration of gastric contents** is not uncommon in such cases.

In the first assessment the therapist should have recognized that this case was more than simple respiratory failure. The reader sees that the patient was intubated and that breath sounds no longer were present in the entire left lung (inadvertent right main stem bronchus intubation). The therapist appropriately responded quickly and pulled the endotracheal tube back until breath sounds could be auscultated over both lung fields. The inappropriate positioning of the tube was confirmed 45 minutes later in the patient's chest x-ray film. The patient's respiratory status could have been seriously compromised if the therapist had waited a full 45 minutes before pulling the tube above the carina. This event further demonstrates the importance of good bedside assessment skills. In addition, because lactic acidosis was likely present at this time, oxygenating the patient was of primary importance. Increasing the F_{IO_2} to 0.80 to 1.0 would be appropriate in such a case. Any attempt to wean the patient at this early junction should not have proceeded.

The second assessment reflected that the patient was improving and was now hyperventilated and hyperoxygenated on the current ventilator settings. The therapist adjusted the ventilator therapy accordingly and began the process of longitudinal evaluation of forced vital capacity, forced expiratory volume in 1 second, and negative inspiratory force that is appropriate for this condition if weaning is to be accomplished successfully.

The final assessment suggested that the patient had taken another turn for the worse. The sputum was now purulent, rhonchi were heard over both lung fields, and a right lower lobe pneumonia or atelectasis had developed. The patient had an uncompensated metabolic acidemia that required evaluation. The fact that the patient's Pa_{O_2} was only 41 provided a significant clinical indicator that the cause of the metabolic acidosis was "lactic acid" generated from a low tissue oxygen level. It was clearly appropriate for the respiratory care practitioner to focus on the patient's oxygenation status. This was done by up-regulating the **Oxygen Therapy Protocol** (Protocol 9-1) (increasing the F_{IO_2} to 0.6) and starting the **Lung Expansion Therapy Protocol** (Protocol 9-3) (the addition of 10 cm H_2O PEEP to ventilator settings).

The therapist should have anticipated this development, obtained appropriate cultures, and, if not done before, prophylactically started the **Bronchopulmonary Hygiene Therapy Protocol** (Protocol 9-2) and **Aerosolized Medication Therapy Protocol** (Protocol 9-4)—with frequent suctioning, percussion, postural drainage, and possibly mucolytics. In addition to understanding lactic acidosis, the reader may wish to review other possible causes of metabolic acidemia at this time (e.g., diabetic ketoacidosis, renal failure).

Unfortunately the patient's pulmonary condition progressively deteriorated, and she died 3 weeks later.

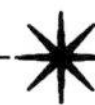

SELF-ASSESSMENT QUESTIONS

evolve Answers to questions can be found on Evolve. To access additional student assessment questions and case studies for application of text material to real-life scenarios, visit **http://evolve.elsevier.com/DesJardins/respiratory.**

1. The onset of the signs and symptoms myasthenia gravis is or are:
1. Slow and insidious
2. Sudden and rapid
3. Intermittent
4. Often elusive
   a. 1 only
   b. 2 only
   c. 2 and 4 only
   d. 1, 2, 3, and 4

2. Myasthenia gravis
1. Is more common in young men
2. Has a peak age of onset in females of 15 to 35 years
3. Is often provoked by emotional upset and physical stress
4. Is associated with receptor-binding antibodies
   a. 1 only
   b. 2 and 4 only
   c. 2, 3, and 4 only
   d. 1, 2, 3, and 4

3. Which of the following is associated with myasthenia gravis?
1. Bronchospasm
2. Mucous accumulation
3. Alveolar hyperinflation
4. Atelectasis
   a. 1 and 2 only
   b. 2 and 4 only
   c. 1, 2, and 4 only
   d. 2, 3, and 4 only

4. When monitoring the patient with myasthenia gravis, which of the following would indicators of acute ventilatory failure?
1. VC: 22 mL/kg
2. pH: 7.31
3. Pa_{CO_2}: 55 mm Hg
4. NIF: –15 cm H_2O
   a. 1 and 3 only
   b. 2 and 4 only
   c. 2, 3, and 4 only
   d. 1, 2, 3, and 4

5. Which of the following antibodies is believed to block the nerve impulse transmissions at the neuromuscular junction in myasthenia gravis?
   a. IgG
   b. IgE
   c. IgA
   d. IgM

Sleep Apnea

30

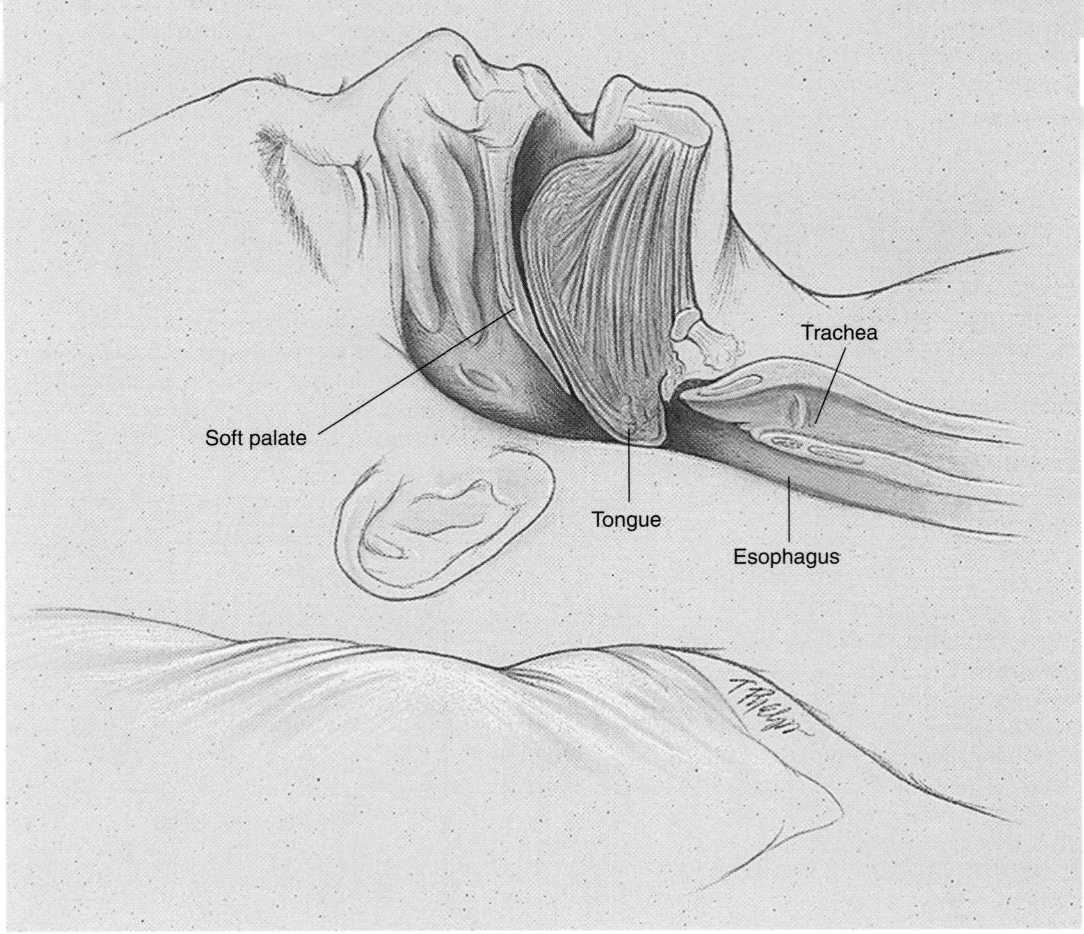

FIGURE 30-1 Obstructive sleep apnea. When the genioglossus muscle fails to oppose the force that tends to collapse the airway passage during inspiration, the tongue moves into the oropharyngeal area and obstructs the airway.

Chapter Objectives

After reading this chapter, you will be able to:

- List the anatomic alterations of the lungs associated with sleep apnea.
- Describe the causes of sleep apnea.
- Describe how a sleep study is performed.
- List the cardiopulmonary clinical manifestations associated with sleep apnea.
- Describe the meaning of the apnea-hypopnea index and oxygen desaturation index.
- Describe the general management of sleep apnea.
- Describe the clinical strategies and rationales of the SOAPs presented in the case study.
- Define key terms and complete self-assessment questions at the end of the chapter and on Evolve.

Key Terms

Active or Dreaming Sleep
Alpha Rhythm
Apnea-Hypopnea Index (AHI)
Autotitrating CPAP Device (AutoPap)
Basal Metabolic Index (BMI)
Bilevel Positive Airway Pressure (BiPAP)
Brady-Tachy Syndrome
Cardiopulmonary Complication of Sleep Apnea
Central Sleep Apnea (CSA)
Confusional Arousals
Continuous Positive Airway Pressure (CPAP)
CPAP Compliance
CPAP Titration Polysomnogram
Delta Waves

Electroencephalogram (EEG)
Electromyogram (EMG)
Electrooculogram (EOG)
Epoch
K Complexes
Laser-Assisted Uvulopalatoplasty (LAUP)
Metabolic Syndrome
Mixed Sleep Apnea
Neuropsychiatric Complications of Sleep Apnea
Nocturnal Low-Flow Oxygen Therapy
Non–Rapid Eye Movement (Non-REM) Sleep
Obstructive Sleep Apnea (OSA)
Oxygen Desaturation Index (ODI)
Pickwickian Syndrome
Polysomnogram (PSG)
Slow Wave Sleep
Rapid Eye Movement (REM) Sleep
Recording Oximetry
Saw-Toothed Waves
Sleep Density
Sleep Spindles
Sleep Stages
Slow Wave Sleep (SWS)
Split-Night Polysomogram
Theta Waves
Uvulopalatopharyngoplasty (UPPP)
Variable Positive Airway Pressure (VPAP)
Vertex Waves
Wake after Sleep Onset (WASO) Index

Chapter Outline

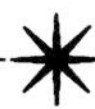

Despite the fact that the clinical characteristics of sleep apnea have been described in the literature for centuries, it was not until 1965 that this disorder became generally acknowledged by the medical community. Before this time, it was assumed that individuals who breathed normally while awake also did so during sleep. It also was assumed that patients with lung disorders were not likely to develop more severe respiratory problems when asleep than when awake. Indeed, the "rest cure" was an accepted treatment of tuberculosis for decades. Both of these assumptions are now recognized as incorrect. Nowadays, respiratory care practitioners (with additional training) are frequently employed in sleep disorder centers. Sleep apnea is a common condition that affects more than 12 million Americans.

Normal Sleep Stages

During normal sleep, the individual slips in and out of two major sleep stages: **non–rapid eye movement (non-REM) sleep** (also called *quiet* or *slow-wave sleep*) and **rapid eye movement (REM) sleep** (also called **active or dreaming sleep**). Each stage is associated with characteristic electroencephalographic, behavioral, and breathing patterns.

The following terminology (nosology) is now recommended to define the stages of sleep:

- stage W (wakefulness)
- stage N1 (non-REM 1)
- stage N2 (non-REM 2)
- stage N3 (non-REM 3)—represents **slow wave sleep**; replaces old stage 3 and stage 4 sleep.
- stage R (REM)

Non-REM Sleep

Non-REM sleep usually begins immediately after an individual dozes off. This phase consists of four separate stages, each progressing into a deeper sleep. During stages N1 and N2 the ventilatory rate and tidal volume continually increase and decrease, and brief periods of apnea may be seen. The **electroencephalogram (EEG)** shows increased slow-wave activity (**slow-wave sleep**) and loss of **alpha rhythm**. Alpha rhythm is defined as containing EEG signals at 8 to 13 Hz. Cheyne-Stokes respiration also is commonly seen in older male adults during non-REM sleep, especially at high altitudes.

During stage N3, ventilation becomes slow and regular. Minute ventilation is commonly 1 to 2 L/min less than during the quiet wakeful state. Typically, the Pa_{CO_2} levels are higher (4 to 8 mm Hg), the Pa_{O_2} levels are lower (3 to 10 mm Hg), and the pH is lower (0.03 to 0.05 units) during stage N3. Normally, non-REM sleep lasts for 60 to 90 minutes. Although an individual typically moves into and out of all four stages during non-REM sleep, most of the time is spent in stage N2. An individual may move into REM sleep at any time directly from any of the three non-REM sleep stages, although the lighter stages (N1 and N2) are commonly the levels of sleep just before REM sleep.

REM Sleep

During REM sleep a burst of fast alpha rhythms occurs in the electroencephalographic tracing. During this period the ventilatory rate becomes rapid and shallow. Sleep-related hypoventilation and apnea frequently are demonstrated during this period. Apneic periods occur in normal adults as often as five times per hour. These apneas may last 15 to 20 seconds without producing any discernible effects. In the normal infant, apneas are shorter (approximately 10 seconds in length), although even these may be cause for concern. A marked reduction in both the hypoxic ventilatory response and the hypercapnic ventilatory response occurs during REM sleep. The heart rate also becomes irregular, and the eyes move rapidly. Dreaming occurs mainly during REM sleep, and profound atonia (paralysis) of movement occurs. The skeletal muscle paralysis primarily affects the arms, legs, and intercostal and upper airway muscles. The activity of the diaphragm is maintained during REM sleep.

The muscle paralysis that occurs during REM sleep can affect an individual's ventilation in two major ways. First, because the muscle tone of the intercostal muscles is low during this period, the negative intrapleural pressure generated by the diaphragm often causes a paradoxic motion of the rib cage. In other words, during inspiration the tissues between the ribs move inward, and during expiration the tissues bulge outward. This paradoxic motion of the rib cage causes the functional residual capacity to decrease. During the wakeful state the intercostal muscle tone tends to stiffen the tissue between the ribs.

Second, the loss of muscle tone in the upper airway involves muscles that normally contract during each inspiration and hold the upper airway open. These muscles include the posterior muscles of the pharynx, the genioglossus (which normally causes the tongue to protrude), and the posterior cricoarytenoid (the major abductor of the vocal cords). The loss of muscle tone in the upper airway may result in airway obstruction. The negative pharyngeal pressure produced when the diaphragm contracts during inspiration tends to bring the vocal cords together, collapse the pharyngeal wall, and suck the tongue back into the oropharyngeal cavity.

REM sleep periods last 5 to 40 minutes and recur approximately every 60 to 90 minutes. The REM sleep periods lengthen and become more frequent toward the end of a night's sleep. REM sleep constitutes about 20% to 25% of the total sleep time. Most studies show that it is more difficult to awaken a subject during REM sleep. Table 30-1 provides an overview of the electroencephalographic findings in the various stages of sleep.

Types of Sleep Apnea

Apnea is defined as the cessation of breathing for a period of 10 seconds or longer. Sleep apnea is diagnosed in patients who have more than five episodes of apnea per hour that may occur in either or both non-REM and REM sleep, over a 6-hour period. Generally, the episodes of apnea per hour are more frequent and severe during REM sleep and in the supine body position. They last more than 10 seconds and occasionally may exceed 100 seconds in length. Often, patients with severe sleep apnea have more than 500 periods of apnea per night. Sleep apnea may occur in all age groups; in infants, it may play an important role in sudden infant death syndrome (SIDS). There are three primary types of sleep apnea: **obstructive sleep apnea (OSA), central sleep apnea (CSA),** and **mixed sleep apnea.** The most common type of apnea is OSA.

Obstructive Sleep Apnea

It is estimated that more than 12 million people in the United States have OSA.

OSA is caused by an anatomic obstruction of the upper airway in the presence of continued ventilatory effort (see Figure 30-1). During periods of obstruction, patients commonly appear quiet and still, as though they are holding their breath, followed by increasingly desperate efforts to inhale. Often the apneic episode ends only after an intense struggle. A snorting sound called "fricative breathing" may be heard at the end of the apneic periods. In severe cases, the patient may suddenly awaken, sit upright in bed, and gasp for air. These events are called **confusional arousals.** Patients with OSA usually demonstrate perfectly normal and regular breathing patterns during the wakeful period.

In fact, a large number of patients with OSA demonstrate what is commonly called the **Pickwickian syndrome** (named after a character in Charles Dickens's *The Posthumous Papers of the Pickwick Club,* published in 1837). Dickens's description of Joe, "the fat boy" who snored and had excessive daytime sleepiness, included many of the classic features of what is now recognized as the sleep apnea syndrome. Box 30-1 provides common signs and symptoms associated with OSA. However, many patients with sleep apnea are not obese, and therefore clinical suspicion should not be limited to this group. Table 30-2 provides the more common risk factors associated with OSA.

Cardiopulmonary and Other Conditions Associated with Obstructive Sleep Apnea

The morbidity associated with OSA is increased by an increased incidence of the following cardiovascular conditions: nocturnal angina and heart attacks, atrial fibrillation and other cardiac arrhythmias, hypertension, and congestive heart failure. The **metabolic syndrome** associated with OSA is composed of hypertension, hyperlipidemia, and centripetal (truncal) obesity. The **neuropsychiatric complications of sleep apnea** include morning headaches, cerebrovascular accidents, nocturnal seizures, depression, and short-term memory loss.

Central Sleep Apnea

CSA occurs when the respiratory centers of the medulla fail to send signals to the respiratory muscles. It is characterized by cessation of airflow at the nose and mouth along with cessation of inspiratory efforts (absence of diaphragmatic excursions), as opposed to OSA, which is characterized by the presence of heightened inspiratory efforts during apneic periods.

CSA is associated with cardiovascular, metabolic, and central nervous system disorders. A few brief central apneas normally occur with the onset of sleep or the onset of REM sleep. CSA, however, is diagnosed when the frequency of the apnea or hypopnea episodes is excessive (more than 30 in a 6-hour period). Box 30-2 provides a listing of clinical disorders associated with CSA.

TABLE 30-1 Stages of Sleep

Stage	Electroencephalogram (EEG)	Characteristics
Eyes open-wake (Stage W)		The EEG shows beta waves, and high-frequency, low-amplitude activity. The electrooculogram (EOG) looks very similar to REM sleep waves—low-amplitude, mixed-frequency, and saw-toothed waves. Electromyogram (EMG) activity is relatively high.
Eyes closed-wake (drowsy)		The EEG is characterized by prominent alpha waves (>50%). The EOG shows slow, rolling eye movements, and the EMG activity is relatively high.
Non-REM Sleep		
Stage N1 (light sleep)	Vertex Waves	The EEG shows low amplitude **alpha waves** (8-13 Hz) that may be replaced by mixed frequency activity and **theta waves** (4-7 Hz). **Vertex waves** commonly appear. Vertex wave are sharp upward deflection EEG waves. The amplitude of many of the vertex sharp waves is greater than 20 μv. Vertex waves are usually seen at the end of stage N1. The EOG shows slow, rolling eye movements. The EMG reveals decreased activity and muscle relaxation. Respirations become regular, and the heart rate and blood pressure decrease slightly. Snoring may occur. If awakened, the person may state that he or she was not asleep.
Stage N2 (light sleep)	K Complex	The EEG becomes more irregular and is composed predominantly of theta waves (4-7 Hz), intermixed with sudden bursts of sleep spindles (12-18 Hz), and one or more **K complexes. Sleep spindles** are a sudden burst of EEG activity in the 12-14 Hz frequency (6 or more distinct waves) with a duration of ≥ 0.5 to 1.5 seconds (not illustrated here). Vertex waves may also be seen during this stage. The EOG shows either slow eye movements or absence of slow eye movements. The EMG has low electrical activity. The heart rate, blood pressure, respiratory rate, and temperature decrease slightly. Snoring may occur. If awakened, the person may say he or she was thinking or daydreaming.
Stage N3 (slow wave sleep)	Medium Sleep	Slow wave activity 0.5 Hz-2.0 Hz and peak to peak amplitude > 75 μv. EOG shows little or no eye movement, and the EMG activity is low. Heart rate, blood pressure, respiratory rate, body temperature, and oxygen consumption continue to decrease. Snoring may occur, and there is no eye movement. Dreaming may occur, and the sleeper becomes more difficult to arouse.
(Deep sleep)		The EOG shows no eye movements, and the EMG has little or no electrical activity. The sleeper is very relaxed and seldom moves. The vital signs reach their lowest, normal level. Oxygen consumption is low. The patient is very difficult to awaken. Bed-wetting, night terrors, and sleepwalking may occur.
REM Sleep	Saw-Tooth Waves	About 90 minutes into the sleep cycle, there is an abrupt EEG pattern change. The EEG pattern resembles the wakeful state with low-amplitude, mixed frequency EEG activity. **Saw-toothed waves** are frequently seen. Alpha waves may be seen. The respiratory rate increases, and respiration is irregular and shallow. The heart rate and blood pressure increase. Rapid eye movement occurs, and there is paralysis of most skeletal muscles. Most dreams occur during REM sleep.

Mixed Sleep Apnea

Mixed sleep apnea is a combination of obstructive and CSAs. It usually begins as central apnea followed by the onset of ventilatory effort without airflow (obstructive apnea). Clinically, patients with predominantly mixed apnea are classified (and treated) as having OSA.

Figure 30-2 illustrates the patterns of airflow, respiratory effort (reflected through the esophageal pressure), and arterial oxygen saturation in central, obstructive, and mixed apneas.

Box 30-1 Signs and Symptoms Associated with Obstructive Sleep Apnea

- Loud snoring
- Observed episodes of breathing cessation during sleep
- Abrupt awakenings accompanied by shortness of breath
- Difficulty staying asleep (insomnia)
- Awakening with a dry mouth or sore throat
- Morning headache
- Nausea
- Excessive daytime sleepiness (hypersomnia)
- Intellectual and personality changes
- Depression
- Nocturnal enuresis
- Sexual impotence

Box 30-2 Clinical Disorders Associated with Central Sleep Apnea

- Congestive heart failure (Cheyne-Stokes respiration)
- Metabolic alkalosis
- Idiopathic hypoventilation syndrome
- Encephalitis
- Brain stem neoplasm
- Brain stem infarction
- Bulbar poliomyelitis
- Cervical cordotomy
- Spinal surgery
- Hypothyroidism

TABLE 30-2 Risk Factors Associated with Obstructive Sleep Apnea

Excess weight	More than 50% of the patients diagnosed with obstructive sleep apnea are overweight. It is suggested that fat deposits around the upper airway may obstruct breathing.
Neck size	Obstructive sleep apnea is often seen in the patients with large neck size. A neck circumference greater than 17 inches increases the risk for obstructive sleep apnea.
Hypertension	Obstructive sleep apnea is commonly seen in patients with high blood pressure.
Anatomic narrowing of upper airway	Common causes of anatomic narrowing of the upper airway include excessive pharyngeal tissue, enlarged tonsils or adenoids, deviated nasal septum, laryngeal stenosis, and vocal cord dysfunction.
Chronic nasal congestion	Obstructive sleep apnea occurs twice as often in patients with chronic nasal congestion from any cause.
Diabetes	Patients with diabetes are three times more likely to have obstructive sleep apnea than healthy individuals.
Male sex	Men are twice as likely to have obstructive sleep apnea as women.
Age older than 65 years	Obstructive sleep apnea is two to three times greater in people older than 65 years.
Age under 35 years, and black, Hispanic, or Pacific Islander heritage	Among individuals under the age of 35, the incidence of obstructive sleep apnea is greater in blacks, Hispanics, and Pacific Islanders.
Menopause	The risk of obstructive sleep apnea is greater after menopause.
Family history of sleep apnea	Individuals who have one or more family members who have obstructive sleep apnea are also at greater risk for developing obstructive sleep apnea.
Alcohol, sedatives, or tranquilizers	Depressive agents relax the muscles of the upper airway.
Smoking	Smokers are almost three times more likely to develop obstructive sleep apnea.

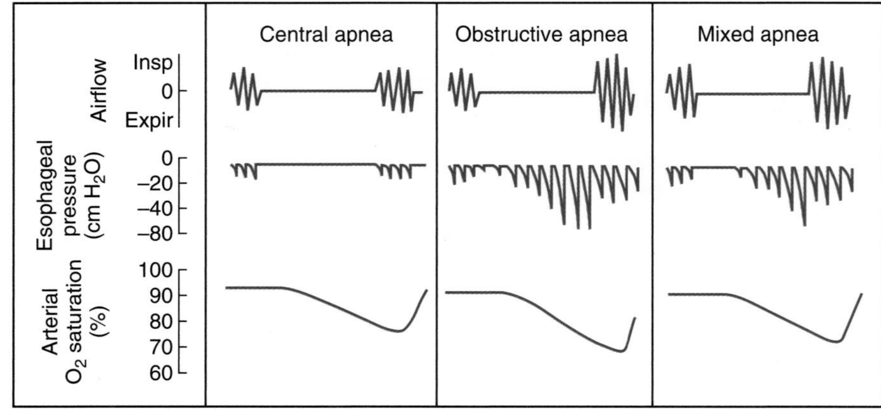

FIGURE 30-2 Patterns of airflow, respiratory efforts (reflected through the esophageal pressure), and arterial oxygen saturation produced by central, obstructive, and mixed apneas.

Diagnosis

The diagnosis of sleep apnea begins with a careful history from the patient and/or the patient's bed partner, especially noting the presence of snoring, sleep disturbance, and persistent daytime sleepiness. This is followed by a careful examination of the upper airway and perhaps by pulmonary function studies to determine whether upper airway obstruction is present.

The patient's blood is evaluated for the presence of polycythemia, reduced thyroid function, and bicarbonate retention. Arterial blood gas values are obtained to determine resting, wakeful oxygenation and acid-base status. When possible, a carboxyhemoglobin level should be obtained.

It should be noted that the pulse oximeter assumes that the patient has normal hemoglobin, Pa_{O_2}, and Sp_{O_2} relationships. If carboxyhemoglobin is present, it should be subtracted from the pulse oximeter reading. For example, if the pulse oximeter reads an Sp_{O_2} of 90% and the patient has 7% carboxyhemoglobin, the true O_2 saturation would be 83% (90% – 7% = 83%).

A chest x-ray examination, electrocardiogram (ECG), and echocardiogram are helpful in evaluating the presence of pulmonary hypertension, the state of right and left ventricular compensation, and the presence of any other cardiopulmonary disease.

The diagnosis and type of sleep apnea are confirmed with multichannel polysomnographic sleep studies, which include (1) an EEG, which measures the electrophysiologic changes in the brain; (2) an **electrooculogram (EOG),** which monitors the movement of the eyes and identifies the sleep stages; (3) an **electromyogram (EMG),** which monitors muscle activity; (4) the absence or presence of snoring; (5) nasal and oral air flow; (6) chest and/or abdominal movement; (7) oxygen saturation; and (8) an ECG. Figure 30-3 provides a representative period of a sleep study **polysomnogram (PSG)** (called an **epoch**) of REM sleep.

At many sleep lab centers, the diagnosis of OSA is commonly based on the **apnea-hypopnea index (AHI).** *Apnea* is defined as the cessation of airflow—a complete obstruction for at least 10 seconds—with a simultaneous 2% to 4% decrease in the patient's Sa_{O_2}. *Hypopnea* is defined as a reduction of airflow of 30% to 50%, with a concomitant drop in the patient's Sa_{O_2}. The AHI is defined as the average number of apneas and hypopneas the patient has per hour of sleep. The normal AHI is <5 episodes per hour. The AHI score provides the following three severity categories of sleep apnea:

- Mild—5 to 15 apnea-hypopnea episodes per hour
- Moderate—15 to 30 apnea-hypopnea episodes per hour
- Severe—more than 30 apnea-hypopnea episodes per hour*

*It is not uncommon for patients to have 100 to 150 episodes of apnea and hypopnea per hour of sleep during a polysomnographic sleep study. Transient nocturnal Sp_{O_2} desaturations to levels <30% are occasionally seen in the polysomnograms of individuals with severe sleep apnea. Fortunately, these episodes are self-limited when the patient wakens at the end of the apnea.

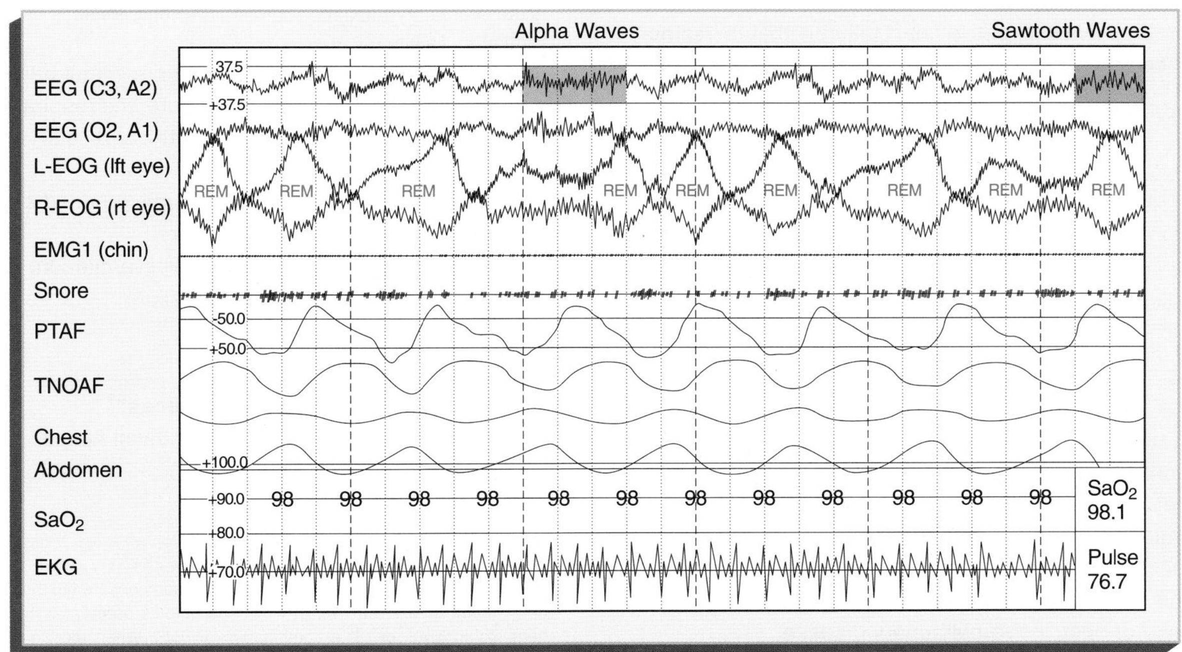

FIGURE 30-3 A 30-second epoch of REM sleep (each vertical line equals 1 second), resembling the eyes open-wake epoch. The electroencephalogram records low-voltage, mixed electroencephalographic activity, and frequent saw-toothed waves *(brown bar).* Alpha waves may be present *(purple bar).* The electrooculogram (EOG) records rapid eye movements (REM). The electromyogram (EMG) records low electrical activity and documents a temporary paralysis of most of the skeletal muscles (e.g., arms, legs). The breathing rate increases and decreases irregularly. During REM sleep, the heart rate becomes inconsistent, with episodes of increased and decreased rates. Snoring may or may not be present. REM is not as restful as non-REM sleep. REM is also known as *paradoxic sleep.* Most dreams occur during REM sleep. *PTAF,* Pneumotachograph air flow; *TNOAF,* thermistor nasal/oral air flow.

Other factors that also influence the severity of sleep apnea include the degree of oxygen desaturation; the presence of cardiac arrhythmias, tachycardia, and bradycardia; quality of life; and the severity of daytime sleepiness. The **oxygen desaturation index (ODI)** is a measure of the percentage of sleep time spent with an Sp_{O_2} <90%. Patients diagnosed as having OSA may also undergo a computed tomographic (CT) scan or a cephalometric head x-ray examination of the upper airway to determine the site (or sites) and severity of the pharyngeal narrowing. Patients diagnosed as having predominantly CSA are evaluated carefully for the presence of cardiac disease and lesions involving the cerebral cortex and the brain stem. **Sleep density** is derived from the arousals associated with sleep apnea. The **wake after sleep onset (WASO) index** is a measure of this. Sleep fragmentation results in nonrefreshing sleep and daytime sleepiness.

OVERVIEW of the Cardiopulmonary Clinical Manifestations Associated with Sleep Apnea

CLINICAL DATA OBTAINED AT THE PATIENT'S BEDSIDE

The Physical Examination (Also See Box 30-1 and Table 30-1)

Apnea or Hypopnea

Cyanosis

CLINICAL DATA OBTAINED FROM LABORATORY TESTS AND SPECIAL PROCEDURES

Pulmonary Function Test Findings

The following findings are expected in patients who are obese or who have congestive heart failure—that is, **restrictive pathophysiology**.

LUNG VOLUME AND CAPACITY FINDINGS

V_T	IRV	ERV*	RV
N or ↓	↓	↓	↓

VC	IC	FRC	TLC	RV/TLC ratio
↓	↓	↓	↓	N

*A decreased ERV is the hallmark of centripetal obesity.

Obviously, pulmonary function cannot easily be studied during sleep. However, patients with obstructive sleep apnea may demonstrate a sawtooth pattern on maximal inspiratory and expiratory flow-volume loops. Also characteristic of obstructive sleep apnea is a ratio of expiratory-to-inspiratory flow rates at 50% of the vital capacity ($FEF_{50\%}/FIF_{50\%}$) that exceeds 1.0 in the absence of obstructive pulmonary disease.

In addition, because the muscle tone of the intercostals muscles is low during periods of rapid eye movement (REM)–related apneas, the large swings in intrapleural pressure generated by the diaphragm often cause a magnified paradoxic motion of the rib cage—that is, during inspiration the tissue between the ribs moves inward, and during expiration the tissue bulges outward. This paradoxic motion of the rib cage may cause the vital capacity (VC), reserve volume (RV), functional residual capacity (FRC), and total lung capacity (TLC) to decrease further. This further contributes to the nocturnal hypoxemia seen in patients with sleep apnea syndrome.

Arterial Blood Gases

SEVERE OBSTRUCTIVE SLEEP APNEA

Chronic Ventilatory Failure with Hypoxemia (Compensated Respiratory Acidosis)

pH	Pa_{CO_2}	HCO_3^-	Pa_{O_2}
N	↑	↑ (significantly)	↓

Acute Ventilatory Changes Superimposed on Chronic Ventilatory Failure

Because acute ventilatory changes are frequently seen in patients with chronic ventilatory failure, the respiratory care practitioner must be familiar with and alert for the following:

- Acute alveolar hyperventilation superimposed on chronic ventilatory failure, and/or
- Acute ventilatory failure (acute hypoventilation) superimposed on chronic ventilatory failure

Oxygenation Indices*†

Severe Stage Obstructive Sleep Apnea

$\dot{Q}_S/\dot{Q}_T$	D_{O_2}‡	$\dot{V}_{O_2}$	$C(a-\bar{v})_{O_2}$	O_2ER	$S\bar{v}_{O_2}$
↑	↓	N	N	↑	↓

†The abnormal oxygenation indices may develop as a result of hypoventilation and/or atelectasis.

‡The D_{O_2} may be normal in patients who have compensated to the decreased oxygenation status with (1) an increased cardiac output, (2) an increased hemoglobin level, or (3) a combination of both. When the D_{O_2} is normal, the O_2ER is usually normal.

*$C(a-\bar{v})_{O_2}$, Arterial-venous oxygen difference; D_{O_2}, total oxygen delivery; O_2ER, oxygen extraction ratio; $\dot{Q}_S/\dot{Q}_T$, pulmonary shunt fraction; $S\bar{v}_{O_2}$, mixed venous oxygen saturation; $\dot{V}_{O_2}$, oxygen consumption.

OVERVIEW of the Cardiopulmonary Clinical Manifestations Associated with Sleep Apnea—cont'd

Hemodynamic Indices*†
Severe Obstructive Sleep Apnea

CVP	RAP	$\overline{PA}$	CO	PCWP	SV
↑	↑	↑	N or ↑	N or ↓	N or ↓

SVI	CI	RVSWI	LVSWI	PVR	SVR
↓	↓	↑	↑	↑	↑

†The presence of upper airway obstruction during apneic episodes often is accompanied by bradycardia and temporary reduction in CO. This is paradoxic, as hypoxemia usually causes tachycardia. In sleep apnea, oxygen transport ($\dot{Q}_T \times CaO_2 \times 10$) falls, and results in electrocardiographic "brady-tachy syndrome" episodes and swings in blood pressure secondary to surges of adrenalin in an attempt to compensate for tissue hypoxia.

During periods of apnea the heart rate decreases, then it increases after the termination of apnea. This phenomenon is known as the **brady-tachy syndrome**. It is believed that the carotid body peripheral chemoreceptors are responsible for this response—that is, when ventilation is kept constant or is absent (e.g., during an apneic episode), hypoxic stimulation of the carotid body peripheral chemoreceptors slows the cardiac rate. Therefore it follows that when the lungs are unable to expand (e.g., during periods of obstructive apnea), the depressive effect of the carotid bodies on the heart rate predominates. The increased heart rate noted when ventilation resumes is activated by the excitation of the pulmonary stretch receptors.

Although changes in cardiac output during periods of apnea have been difficult to study, several studies have reported a reduction in cardiac output (about 30%) during periods of apnea, followed by an increase (10% to 15% above controls) after the termination of apnea. Both pulmonary and systemic arterial blood pressures increase in response to the nocturnal oxygen desaturation that develops during periods of sleep apnea. The magnitude of the pulmonary hypertension is related to the severity of the alveolar hypoxia and hypercapnic acidosis. Repetition of these transient episodes of pulmonary hypertension many times a night every night for years may contribute to the development of the right ventricular hypertrophy, cor pulmonale, and eventual cardiac decompensation seen in such patients.

Episodic systemic vasoconstriction secondary to sympathetic adrenergic neural activity is believed to be responsible for the elevation in systemic blood pressure that is commonly seen during apneas. Sleep apnea is now recognized as one of the most frequent and correctable causes of systemic hypertension.

*CO, Cardiac output; CVP, central venous pressure; LVSWI, left ventricular stroke work index; PA, mean pulmonary artery pressure; PCWP, pulmonary capillary wedge pressure; PVR, pulmonary vascular resistance; RAP, right atrial pressure; RVSWI, right ventricular stroke work index; SV, stroke volume; SVI, stroke volume index; SVR, systemic vascular resistance.

RADIOLOGIC FINDINGS

Chest Radiograph

- Often normal
- Right- or left-sided heart failure

Because of the pulmonary hypertension and polycythemia associated with persistent periods of apnea, right- and/or left-sided heart failure may develop. This condition may be identified on a chest x-ray film and may help in diagnosis.

CARDIAC ARRHYTHMIAS

- Sinus arrhythmia
- Sinus bradycardia
- Sinus pauses
- Atrioventricular block (second degree)
- Premature ventricular contractions
- Ventricular tachycardia
- Atrial fibrillation

In severe cases of sleep apnea, sudden arrhythmia-related death is always possible. Periods of apnea commonly are associated with sinus arrhythmia, sinus bradycardia, and sinus pauses (greater than 2 seconds). The extent of sinus bradycardia is directly related to the severity of the oxygen desaturation. Obstructive apneas usually are associated with the greatest degrees of cardiac slowing. To a lesser extent, atrioventricular heart block (second degree), premature ventricular contractions, and ventricular tachycardia are seen. Apnea-related ventricular tachycardia is viewed as a life-threatening event.

Management of Sleep Apnea

Management of Obstructive Sleep Apnea

Continuous Positive Airway Pressure

The most common—and arguably the most effective—treatment for OSA is the use of a **continuous positive airway pressure (CPAP)** device. As discussed earlier, the cause of many OSAs is related to (1) an anatomic configuration of the pharynx and (2) the decreased muscle tone that normally develops in the pharynx during REM sleep. When the patient with OSA inhales, the pharyngeal muscles (and surrounding tissues) are sucked inward as a result of the negative airway pressure generated by the contracting diaphragm. Nocturnal CPAP therapy is useful in preventing the collapse of the hypotonic and obstructed airway and is the standard treatment for most cases of OSA (Figure 30-4). CPAP is not indicated in pure CSA.

A **CPAP titration polysomnogram** is usually obtained in the sleep disorder laboratory to determine the precise CPAP pressure that is needed to open and maintain the patient's airway. If the patient has lost or gained a significant amount of weight since the titration study, the critical CPAP pressure may not be correct. In hospitalized patients, another alternative is to use an **autotitrating CPAP device (AutoPap)** until the patient's condition is stable and the patient can be studied again.

Continuous Positive Airway Pressure Compliance. Despite the fact that CPAP efficiency is determined in the CPAP titration polysomnogram, its effectiveness over the long term (i.e., in the patient's home) is not without problems. The American Association of Sleep Medicine's suggestion for optimal **CPAP compliance** is only 5 hours per night. The patient's use of the device is both critical and problematic. There certainly is a "learning" curve for the patient to get used to the CPAP device, but once this critical acclimatization phase is over, the respiratory care practitioner must verify that the device is, indeed, being used as prescribed. Today, many CPAP devices have downloadable compliance features that provide periodic updates of patient compliance. Objective documentation of the patient's CPAP compliance is increasingly being required by third-party insurance agencies if payment for the CPAP device is to be made.

Management of Central Sleep Apnea

VPAP Adapt SV and Adaptive Servo-Ventilation*

With the recent development of the adaptive servo-ventilation algorithm and **variable positive airway pressure (VPAP),** the ResMed VPAP Adapt SV provides ventilatory support to treat all forms of CSA, mixed apnea, and periodic breathing (Cheyne-Stokes respirations). The VPAP Adapt SV responds to apnea by increasing pressure support. To determine the degree of pressure support needed to hold the patient's upper airway open, the VPAP Adapt SV algorithm continuously calculates a target ventilation. The algorithm uses the following three factors to achieve synchronization between the needed pressure support and the patient's breathing pattern:

1. The patient's recent average respiratory rate, including the inspiratory-expiratory ratio (I:E) and the time of any expiratory pause
2. The instantaneous direction of airflow, magnitude, and rate of change of airflow that are measured at specific points during each breath
3. A backup respiratory rate of 15 breaths per minute

The VPAP Adapt SV ensures that ventilatory support is synchronized with the patient's ventilatory efforts by means of numbers 1 and 2 in this list. When the patient experiences an episode of central apnea or hypopnea, the pressure support initially works to reflect the patient's recent ventilatory pattern. However, if the apnea or hypopnea persists, the VPAP Adapt SV increasingly uses the backup respiratory rate (number 3 in the list). Figure 30-5 illustrates this.

The VPAP Adapt SV has been widely accepted as a first-line treatment modality for CSA patients. Most patients with CSA do not tolerate conventional **bilevel positive airway pressure (BiPAP)** ventilatory support. This is because the pressure must be adjusted to a constant high pressure to adequately support the patient during periods of apnea and hypopnea. As a result, the patient is overventilated during periods of normal breathing or hyperpnea. This causes arousals and discomfort. It can even cause more CSA events. The VPAP Adapt SV (1) ventilates the patient appropriately during apnea and hypopnea periods, and (2) decreases ventilatory support during periods of hyperventilation or normal

*From ResMed Corporation; www.resmed.com.

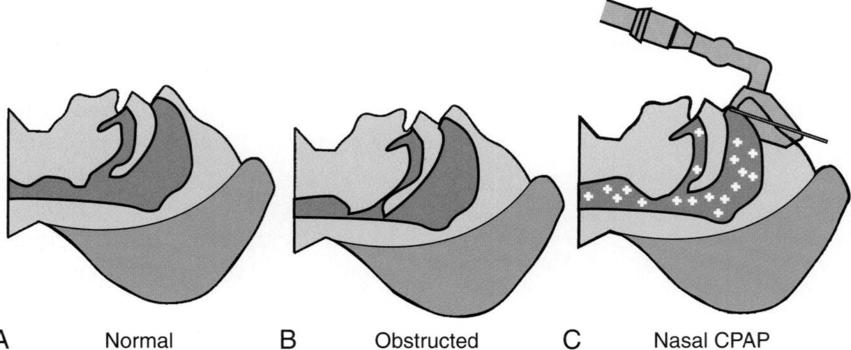

FIGURE 30-4 **A,** Normal airway. **B,** Obstructed airway during sleep. **C,** Nasal continuous positive airway pressure (CPAP) generates a positive pressure and holds the airway open during sleep.

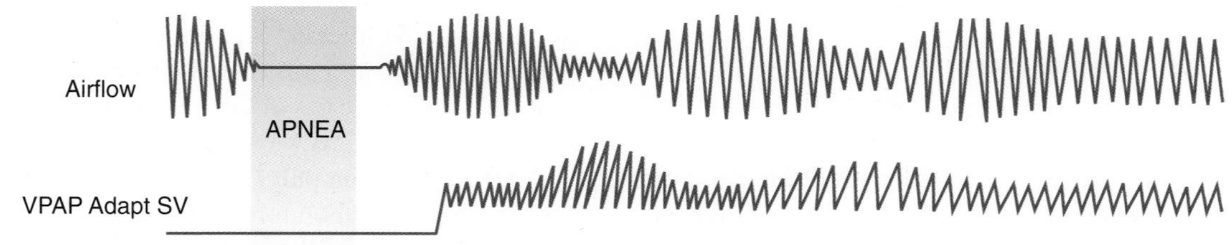

FIGURE 30-5 The VPAP Adapt SV responds to apnea by increasing pressure support. Note the progressive dampening of the Cheyne-Stokes cycles with the continued administration of VPAP.

breathing. These features minimize the discomfort and arousals commonly associated with BiPAP ventilatory support.

Therapeutic Strategies Used to Treat Sleep Apnea

Over the past few decades, it has become apparent that many pathologic conditions are associated with sleep apnea, including hypoxemia, fragmented sleep, cardiac arrhythmias, and neurologic and psychiatric disorders. In general, the prognosis is more favorable for obstructive and mixed apneas than for CSA. Table 30-3 provides an overview of the various therapeutic strategies used for sleep apnea. Table 30-4 summarizes the major therapeutic modalities described in this chapter for obstructive and central apnea and their effectiveness.

TABLE 30-3 Therapeutic Strategies Used to Treat Sleep Apnea

Weight reduction	Many patients with obstructive sleep apnea are overweight, and although the excess weight alone is not the cause of the apnea, weight reduction clearly leads to a reduction in apnea severity. The precise reason is not known. Weight reduction as a single form of therapy often fails.
Sleep posture	It is generally believed that most obstructive apnea is more severe in the supine position and, in fact, may be present only in this position (positional sleep apnea). Apnea and daytime hypersomnolence have significantly improved in some patients who have been instructed to sleep on their sides and avoid the supine posture. Others may benefit from sleeping in a head-up position (e.g., in a lounge chair). The effect of this change in sleeping habits can be documented by **recording oximetry** with the patient in the supine and lateral decubitus positions.
Oxygen therapy	Because of the hypoxemia-related cardiopulmonary complications of apnea (arrhythmias and pulmonary hypertension), **nocturnal low-flow oxygen therapy** is sometimes used to offset or minimize the oxygen desaturation, particularly in central sleep apnea (see Oxygen Therapy Protocol, Protocol 9-1). The reasoning behind the use of nasal oxygen therapy's effectiveness is that the airway is continually "flooded" with oxygen, which will be inspired during the nonapneic episodes—in effect, "preoxygenating" the patient in anticipation of the apnea events. Usually, no improvement in sleep fragmentation or hypersomnolence occurs with the use of supplemental oxygen.
Drug therapy	Drugs occasionally used to treat central sleep apnea include rapid eye movement (REM) inhibitors such as protriptyline (Vivactil). Acetazolamide (Diamox) is a carbonic anhydrase inhibitor that causes a bicarbonate diuresis and mild metabolic acidosis, which in turn stimulate respiration. It occasionally is also helpful in cases of central sleep apnea. Now that variable positive airway pressure (VPAP) therapy has become so successful in central sleep apnea, these drugs are rarely used.
Surgery	Some nonobese patients with obstructive sleep apnea benefit from surgical correction or bypass of the anatomic defect or obstruction that is responsible for the apneic episodes.
Uvulopalatopharyngoplasty	**Uvulopalatopharyngoplasty** (UPPP) is the surgical procedure most commonly used to treat snoring and sleep apnea. During this surgery, the soft palate tissue is shortened by removing the posterior third, including the uvula. The pillars of the palatoglossal arch and the palatopharyngeal arch are tied together, and the tonsils are removed if they are still present. As much excess lateral posterior wall tissue is removed as possible. The success rate of this type of surgery is 30% to 50%.
Laser-assisted uvulopalatoplasty	**Laser-assisted uvulopalatoplasty** (LAUP) is performed to eliminate snoring. This surgical procedure entails using a laser to remove tissue from the back of the throat.
Nasal surgery	Nasal surgery may be performed to remove nasal polyps or straighten a deviated nasal septum.
Tracheostomy	Tracheal intubation with or without tracheostomy is often the treatment of choice in emergency situations and in patients who do not respond satisfactorily to drug therapy or other treatment interventions.
Mandibular advancement surgery	Approximately 6% of patients with obstructive sleep apnea have a mandibular malformation. For example, patients who have obstructive sleep apnea because of retrognathia or mandibular micrognathia may benefit from surgical mandibular advancement. The surgery is not often performed and carries considerable risks.

Continued

TABLE 30-3 Therapeutic Strategies Used to Treat Sleep Apnea—cont'd

Mechanical ventilation	
Continuous mechanical ventilation	Intubation and continuous mechanical ventilation may be used for short-term therapy when acute ventilatory failure develops in central or obstructive sleep apnea.
Negative-pressure ventilation	In patients with central sleep apnea, negative-pressure ventilation without an endotracheal tube may be useful. For example, a negative-pressure cuirass, which is applied to the patient's chest and upper portion of the abdomen, may effectively control ventilation throughout the night. A negative-pressure cuirass is convenient for home use. It is contraindicated in obstructive sleep apnea.
Phrenic nerve pacemaker	An external phrenic nerve pacemaker may be useful in patients with central sleep apnea resulting from the absence of a signal from the central nervous system to the diaphragm by way of the phrenic nerve. This procedure has not received wide application.
Medical devices	Oral appliances that optimally position the tongue and jaw are the most successful alternatives to surgery and continuous positive airway pressure (CPAP) by mask or "nasal pillows." The devices are best used in patients with mild- to-moderate obstructive sleep apnea. Patients who have mandibular overbites, who clench or grind their teeth (bruxism), and who have temporomandibular joint (TMJ) dysfunction may benefit from these devices as well.
Neck collar	A small number of patients have used a collar (similar to those used to stabilize cervical fractures) to increase the diameter of the airway and reduce the apnea. The therapeutic success of this procedure is questionable.
Other therapeutic approaches	Patients should be advised to avoid alcohol and drugs that depress the central nervous system. Alcohol and sedatives have been shown to increase the severity and frequency of sleep apnea. All obese patients with sleep apnea should be encouraged to lose weight.

TABLE 30-4 Therapeutic Modalities for Obstructive Sleep Apnea and Central Sleep Apnea and their Effectiveness

	Type of Apnea	
Therapy	**Obstructive Sleep Apnea (OSA)**	**Central Sleep Apnea (CSA)**
Oxygen therapy	Rarely therapeutic, but is used in addition to CPAP in severe cases	Sometimes therapeutic
Carbonic anhydrase inhibitor drugs—acetazolamide	Contraindicated	Possibly indicated
Surgical		
Tracheostomy	Therapeutic (100%)	Not indicated by itself
Palatopharyngoplasty	Occasionally therapeutic	Not indicated
Mandibular advancement	Occasionally therapeutic	Not indicated
Mechanical ventilation		
Continuous positive airway pressure (CPAP)	Therapeutic	Not indicated
Mechanical ventilation	Short-term	Short-term
Negative-pressure ventilation	Contraindicated	Therapeutic
Adaptive servo-ventilation (variable positive airway pressure [VPAP])	Not indicated	Therapeutic
Phrenic nerve pacemaker	Not indicated	Experimental
Medical devices (e.g., mandibular advancement devices)	Possibly indicated	Not indicated

CASE STUDY

Obstructive Sleep Apnea

Admitting History

A 55-year-old Caucasian man had been in the U.S. Marine Corps for more than 25 years when he retired with honors at 46 years of age with the rank of sergeant. He had completed tours in Vietnam, Grenada, and Beirut. His last assignment had been in Iraq and Kuwait during Operation Desert Storm. During his military career he had received several medals, including a Purple Heart for a leg wound that he incurred in Vietnam when he pulled a fellow marine to safety. During his last 3 years in the service, he had been assigned to a desk job, working with new recruits as they progressed through various stages of boot camp.

Although it had not been mandatory that he retire, he had felt that "it was time". He had gained a great deal of weight over the years, and his ability to meet the physical challenge of being a Marine had become progressively more difficult. In addition, when he was doing paperwork at his office, he had become aware that he was "catnapping" while on the job. He knew that if he had observed a fellow Marine doing the same, he would have been quick to issue a severe reprimand. In view of these developments, the man had regretfully retired from the service.

For a few years after he retired, he had continued to work for the Marines as a volunteer at a local recruitment office. At first he had enjoyed this job a great deal. He had often found that his military experiences enhanced his ability to talk in a meaningful way to new recruits. Over the past few years, however, working had become progressively more difficult for him, and his attendance had become increasingly sporadic. He was often tardy for work. He told the other recruitment volunteers that he was always tired and was experiencing severe morning headaches. His co-workers frequently found him irritable and quick to anger.

The man was having trouble at home, too. Several months before the admission under discussion, his wife had begun sleeping in a room vacated by their daughter. His wife said that she no longer could sleep with her husband because of his loud snoring and constant thrashing in bed. At about this time, the man became clinically depressed and sexually impotent. Despite much discussion with and encouragement from his wife, he did not seek medical advice until a few hours before the admission under discussion, when he became extremely short of breath.

Physical Examination

On observation in the Emergency Room, the man appeared to be in severe respiratory distress. He was 5 feet 11 inches tall. He was obese, weighing more than 160 kg (355 lb) and was perspiring profusely. His **Basal Metabolic Index** (BMI) (BMI = weight [kg]/height [m^2]) was 50. His skin appeared cyanotic, and his neck veins were distended. He had +4 edema of his feet and legs, extending to midcalf. His blood pressure was 164/100, heart rate was 78 bpm, respiratory rate was 22/min, and temperature was normal. Although the man was in obvious discomfort, he stated that he was breathing "OK." His wife quickly piped up, "There's that damn Marine coming out again!"

The man's breath sounds were normal but diminished. The diminished breath sounds were believed to result primarily from the patient's obesity. Palpation of the chest was unremarkable, and percussion was unreliable because of the obesity. A chest x-ray film showed cardiomegaly; the lungs appeared unremarkable. To treat the presumed cor pulmonale, the treating physician immediately started the patient on diuretics. His awake arterial blood gas values (ABGs) on room air were as follows: pH 7.54, $Pa{CO_2}$ 58, HCO_3^- 48, and $Pa{O_2}$ 52. His oxygen saturation measured by pulse oximetry ($Sp{O_2}$) was 86%.

Because of the patient's history and present clinical manifestations, the respiratory therapist on duty suspected that the man had obstructive sleep apnea. The therapist suggested this possibility to the emergency room physician, who requested a polysomnographic study. The physician asked the respiratory therapist to document her assessment. The following SOAP was charted.

Respiratory Assessment and Plan

S "I'm breathing OK."

O Weight: 160 kg (355 lb); skin: flushed and cyanotic; distended neck veins and edema of feet and legs (4+) to midcalf; vital signs: BP 164/100, HR 78, RR 22, T normal; oropharyngeal exam typical for obstructive sleep apnea; diminished breath sounds, likely because of obesity; CXR: cor pulmonale; lungs appear normal; ABGs (on room air): pH 7.54, $Pa{CO_2}$ 58, HCO_3^- 48, $Pa{O_2}$ 52; $Sp{O_2}$ 86%

A
- Obstructive sleep apnea likely (history, cor pulmonale, ABGs, physical appearance)
- Acute alveolar hyperventilation superimposed on chronic ventilatory failure with moderate hypoxemia (ABGs and history)
- Impending ventilatory failure

P Place patient on alarming oximeter, set to alarm at 85%. Initiate **Oxygen Therapy Protocol** (venturi oxygen mask at $F{IO_2}$ = 0.28). If obstructive sleep apnea is confirmed, start **Continuous Positive Airway Pressure** (via CPAP mask). Monitor and reevaluate (vital signs, ECG, ABGs and $Sp{O_2}$ q4h).

Over the Next 72 Hours

A clinical diagnosis of severe obstructive sleep apnea was quickly established. Along with the patient's classic history of obstructive sleep apnea, the polysomnogram documented more than 325 periods of obstructive apnea or hypopnea in the study night. The continuous positive airway pressure (CPAP) titration study indicated that 12 cm H_2O CPAP was required to effectively treat the apneic syndrome. In addition to the patient's short, muscular neck and extreme obesity, an oropharyngeal examination revealed a small mouth and large tongue for his body size. The free margin of the soft palate hung low in the oropharynx, nearly obliterating the view behind it. The uvula was widened (4+) and elongated; the tonsillar pillars were widened (3+). Air entry through the nares was reduced bilaterally. The patient's hematocrit was 51%, and hemoglobin level was 17 g/dL.

A complete pulmonary function test (PFT) showed that the man had a severe restrictive disorder. In addition, a saw-toothed pattern was seen in the maximal inspiratory and expiratory flow-volume loops. A chest x-ray film obtained on the patient's second day of hospitalization showed reduction in heart size, and the lungs were clear. A brisk diuresis was in process. The patient stated that he was breathing much better.

On inspection the patient no longer appeared short of breath. Although he still appeared flushed, he did not look as cyanotic as he had on admission. His neck veins were no longer distended, and the peripheral edema of his legs and feet had improved. His breath sounds were clear but diminished. His room air ABGs were as follows: pH 7.38, Pa_{CO_2} 82, HCO_3^- 48, and Pa_{O_2} 66. His Sp_{O_2} was 91%. The physician again called for a respiratory care evaluation. On the basis of these clinical data, the following SOAP was recorded.

Respiratory Assessment and Plan

S "I'm breathing much better."

O Recent diagnosis: obstructive sleep apnea—more than 325 periods of obstructive apnea or hypopnea documented during sleep study; short muscular neck; narrow upper airway; obesity; Hct 51%; Hb 17 g/dL; PFTs: severe restrictive disorder; saw-tooth pattern seen on maximal inspiratory and expiratory flow-volume loops; no longer appearing short of breath; cyanotic appearance improved; clear but diminished breath sounds; ABGs (on room air): pH 7.38, Pa_{CO_2} 82, HCO_3^- 48, Pa_{O_2} 66; Sp_{O_2} 91%

A
- Severe obstructive sleep apnea confirmed (history, polysomnographic study, ABGs)
- Chronic ventilatory failure with mild hypoxemia

P Continue **Oxygen Therapy Protocol.** Start **Continuous Positive Airway Pressure** (12 cm H_2O via mask). Ensure that patient sleeps in the head-up position and refrains from sleeping on his back. Monitor and reevaluate.

Discussion

Although the diagnosis of obstructive sleep apnea is made most frequently in the outpatient setting, experience has shown that it often may be diagnosed in the course of an acute hospitalization. In the case under discussion, although the patient was first seen in the emergency room, it soon became clear that he was ill enough to be admitted, and his workup proceeded from there.

In the first assessment the therapist needed to perform a careful examination of the patient's nasopharynx and oropharynx, as well as his chest. The typical upper airway anatomy of obstructive sleep apnea was visible. While the patient's polysomnogram and CPAP titration study were in progress, the therapist appropriately ensured the patient's oxygenation (F_{IO_2} = 0.28 venturi oxygen mask) while attempting to prevent alveolar hypoventilation. In as classic a case as this, a **split night study** (half standard polysomnography, half CPAP titration) may be in order. Use of an autotitrating CPAP may be helpful in this setting. The autotitrating CPAP device senses the patient's airway resistance and up-regulates or down-regulates the CPAP pressure to optimize airflow during the apneic episode.

The patient's neck vein distention, polycythemia, cardiomegaly, and peripheral edema all suggested cor pulmonale. This condition would improve once the patient's overall hypoventilation and oxygenation were treated. Many physicians would go ahead and give the patient a bicarbonate-losing diuretic, watching for metabolic acidosis while this step were being done. The therapist (in the first assessment) correctly analyzed the situation as being potentially hazardous, and this assessment included impending ventilatory failure, which was a real possibility.

After the second assessment the diagnosis was made. Pulmonary function tests showed upper airway obstruction and a restrictive disorder. Based on the pH value of 7.38, the patient's Pa_{CO_2} appeared to be at its normal baseline level. It is not uncommon for patients with severe obstructive sleep apnea to have chronic ventilatory failure (compensated respiratory acidosis). The therapist elected to have the patient refrain from sleeping on his back and to sleep in the head-up position instead. In addition, the physician would likely ask for a nutrition consultation at that time because the patient needed to begin a drastic weight-loss program.

At the end of the case the patient's condition still was not markedly improved, and he awaited the benefits of CPAP therapy. Indeed, the CPAP therapy was eventually helpful. The patient had a 9-kg (20-lb) diuresis during the first week of its use, and good oxygenation was achieved with 10 cm H_2O CPAP pressure.

A diagnosis of obstructive sleep apnea often can complicate other primary respiratory disorders, such as chronic obstructive pulmonary disease (COPD), pneumonia, atelectasis, or chest wall deformity. In these settings, the care is more complicated and, if anything, should be even more data-driven, with careful examination of all subjective and objective data.

Patients with obstructive sleep apnea have a significant risk of cardiovascular and central nervous system morbidity and mortality (myocardial infarctions, arrhythmias, hypertension, and cerebrovascular accidents). Psychiatric effects such as depression, sleep-related job malperformance, and daytime motor vehicle accidents also are seen. Current evidence suggests that such patients need not experience these effects if the sleep disorder–related breathing problem is treated effectively. Compliance with CPAP therapy is important but difficult to achieve. Close clinical monitoring is important if good therapeutic outcomes are to be achieved consistently.

SELF-ASSESSMENT QUESTIONS

evolve Answers to questions can be found on Evolve. To access additional student assessment questions and case studies for application of text material to real-life scenarios, visit **http://evolve.elsevier.com/DesJardins/respiratory.**

1. What is or are another name(s) for non–rapid eye movement (non-REM) sleep?
1. Slow-wave sleep
2. Active sleep
3. Dreaming sleep
4. Quiet sleep
   a. 1 only
   b. 3 only
   c. 4 only
   d. 1 and 4 only

2. During non-REM sleep, ventilation becomes slow and regular during which stage(s)?
1. Stage 1
2. Stage 2
3. Stage 3
4. Stage 4
   a. 3 only
   b. 1 and 2 only
   c. 2 and 3 only
   d. 3 and 4 only

3. Moderate sleep apnea is said to be present when the apnea-hypopnea index (AHI) is:
   a. 3-5 episodes per hour
   b. 3-10 episodes per hour
   c. 15-30 episodes per hour
   d. 30-60 episodes per hour

4. During periods of apnea, the patient commonly demonstrates which of the following?
1. Systemic hypotension
2. Decreased cardiac output
3. Increased heart rate
4. Pulmonary hypertension
   a. 1 and 3 only
   b. 2 and 4 only
   c. 3 and 4 only
   d. 1, 2, and 3 only

5. Periods of severe sleep apnea are commonly associated with which of the following?
1. Ventricular tachycardia
2. Sinus bradycardia
3. Premature ventricular contraction
4. Sinus arrhythmia
   a. 2 and 3 only
   b. 3 and 4 only
   c. 2, 3, and 4 only
   d. 1, 2, 3, and 4

6. During REM sleep, there is paralysis of the:
1. Arm muscles
2. Upper airway muscles
3. Leg muscles
4. Intercostal muscles
5. Diaphragm
   a. 4 only
   b. 5 only
   c. 4 and 5 only
   d. 1, 2, 3, and 4 only

7. Normally, REM sleep constitutes about what percentage of the total sleep time?
   a. 5 to 10
   b. 10 to 20
   c. 20 to 25
   d. 25 to 30

8. Which of the following therapy modalities is or are therapeutic for obstructive apnea?
1. Phrenic pacemaker
2. CPAP
3. Theophylline
4. Negative-pressure ventilation
   a. 1 only
   b. 2 only
   c. 3 and 4 only
   d. 1 and 4 only

9. Which of the following therapy modalities is or are therapeutic for central sleep apnea?
1. Negative-pressure ventilation
2. CPAP
3. Tracheostomy
4. VPAP
   a. 1 only
   b. 3 only
   c. 1 and 4 only
   d. 2 and 3 only

10. How long do normal periods of apnea during REM sleep last?
   a. 0 to 5 seconds
   b. 5 to 10 seconds
   c. 10 to 15 seconds
   d. 15 to 20 seconds

11. While a formal polysomnographic diagnosis of the precise type of sleep apnea is being made (i.e., obstructive, central, or mixed sleep apnea), which of the following respiratory care modalities would be safely used?
   a. VPAP
   b. Low-flow nasal oxygen therapy
   c. CPAP
   d. AutoPap

PART XI

Newborn and Early Childhood Respiratory Disorders

Newborn and Early Childhood Respiratory Disorders

31

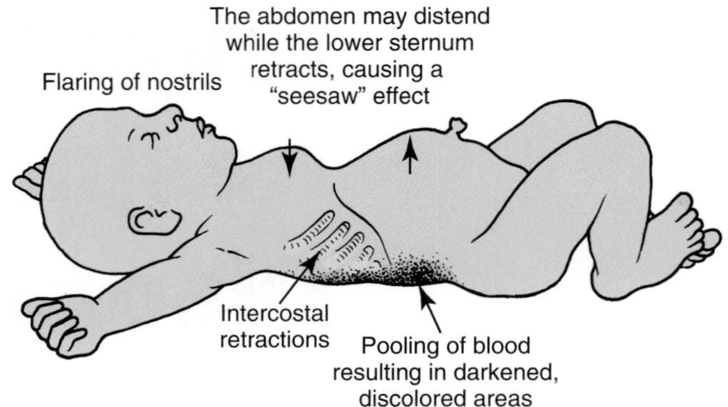

FIGURE 31-1 Clinical manifestations associated with increased negative intrapleural pressure during inspiration in infants. Common features include **flaring of the nostrils, cyanosis of the dependent portions of the thoracic and abdominal areas, susternal** and **intercostal retractions, abdominal distention**, and **seesaw movement.**

Chapter Objectives

After reading this chapter, you will be able to:

- List the clinical manifestations common with newborn and early childhood respiratory disorders, including the following:
  - Clinical manifestations associated with increased negative intrapleural pressures during inspiration
  - Flaring nostrils (or nasal flaring)
  - Expiratory grunting
- Describe the meaning of apnea of prematurity.
- List factors that trigger apnea in the premature infant.
- Describe persistent pulmonary hypertension of the newborn (PPHN).
- Describe the arterial blood gas values commonly associated with newborn respiratory disorders, and include the three major mechanisms responsible for the decreased Pa_{O_2} associated with newborn pulmonary disorders.
- Discuss the objective data, assessments, and treatment plans commonly associated with newborn respiratory disorders.
- Describe the major components of the Apgar score.
- Define key terms and complete self-assessment questions at the end of the chapter and on Evolve.

Key Terms

Apgar Score
Apnea of Prematurity
Bradykinin
Cyanosis of the Dependent Portions of the Thoracic and Abdominal Areas
Ductus Arteriosus
Endothelium-Derived Relaxing Factor (ERF)
Expiratory Grunting
Flaring Nostrils (or Nasal Flaring)
Foramen Ovale
Intercostal Retractions
Persistent Pulmonary Hypertension of the Newborn (PPHN)
Prostaglandins
Substernal and Intercostal Retraction and Abdominal Distention (Seesaw) Movement

Chapter Outline

Clinical Manifestations Common with Newborn and Early Childhood Respiratory Disorders

Respiratory disorders are the leading causes of admission to the neonatal intensive care unit (NICU). Essential to the understanding of respiratory distress of the neonate is the axiom "Oxygen is the primary nutrient of the human body." The clinical manifestations presented by a baby in *early* respiratory distress include lethargy, cyanosis, increased respiratory rate, nasal flaring, **expiratory grunting, intercostal retractions,** substernal retraction, tachycardia, increased blood pressure, and acute alveolar hyperventilation with hypoxemia. The *late*, ominous manifestations include a decreased respiratory rate, gasping respirations, apnea, bradycardia, decreased blood pressure, and acute ventilatory failure with both CO_2 retention and hypoxemia.

Although many of the pathophysiologic mechanisms and clinical manifestations presented by the newborn with a respiratory disorder are identical to those seen in the older child or adult, some of the pathophysiologic mechanisms and clinical manifestations are unique to the newborn. The more important clinical manifestations associated with neonatal respiratory disorders and the primary pathophysiologic mechanisms responsible for these clinical manifestations are outlined in this chapter.

Clinical Manifestations Associated with More Negative Intrapleural Pressures during Inspiration

The thorax of the newborn infant is quite flexible—that is, the compliance of the infant's thorax is high. This flexibility is a result of the large amount of cartilage found in the skeletal structure of newborns. Because of the structural alterations associated with many newborn respiratory disorders, however, the compliance of the infant's lungs is low. In an effort to offset the decreased lung compliance, the infant must generate more negative intrapleural pressures during inspiration. This condition causes the following (see Figure 31-1):

- The soft tissues between the ribs retract during inspiration.
- The substernal area retracts and the abdominal area protrudes in a seesaw fashion during inspiration. The substernal retraction is caused by high negative intrapleural pressure, and the abdominal distention is caused by the contraction (depression) of the diaphragm during inspiration.
- The blood vessels in the more dependent portions of the thoracic and abdominal areas dilate and pool blood, causing these areas to appear cyanotic.

Flaring Nostrils (or Nasal Flaring)

Flaring nostrils (or nasal flaring) frequently are observed in infants in respiratory distress. This clinical manifestation probably is a facial reflex to facilitate the movement of gas into the tracheobronchial tree. The dilator naris, which originates from the maxilla and inserts into the ala of the nose, is the muscle responsible for this movement. When activated, the dilator naris pulls the alae laterally and widens the nasal aperture, providing a larger orifice for gas to enter during inspiration (Figure 31-2).

Expiratory Grunting

An audible expiratory grunt frequently is heard in infants with respiratory problems. Depending on the listener's auditory perception, the expiratory grunt may sound like an expiratory cry. It often is first detected on auscultation. The expiratory grunt is a natural physiologic mechanism that generates high positive pressures in the alveoli, which, at least in part, counteracts the hypoventilation associated with the disorder (e.g., infant respiratory distress syndrome [RDS]). In short, as the gas pressure in the alveoli increases, the infant's P_{AO_2} increases. During exhalation the infant's epiglottis covers the glottis, which causes the intrapulmonary air pressure to increase. When the epiglottis abruptly opens, gas rushes past the infant's vocal cords and produces an expiratory grunt or cry.

Apnea of Prematurity

Periodic breathing frequently is seen in the newborn and is described as cycles of short pauses in respiration followed by

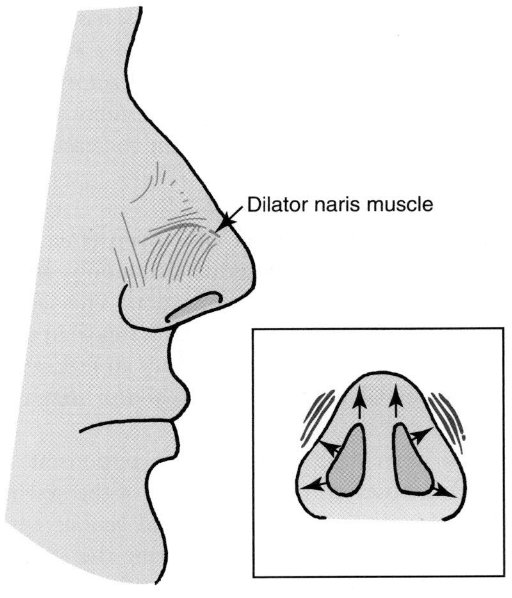

FIGURE 31-2 The dilator naris muscles cause the nostrils to dilate during a stressful inspiration.

an increased breathing rate. What is called **apnea of prematurity** also is a common form of apnea in the newborn. It is defined as a cessation of breathing effort that is longer than 20 seconds, or any respiratory pause that is long enough to cause bradycardia, cyanosis, or both to appear in a baby of less than 37 weeks' gestation. About 75% of premature babies weighing less than 1250 g experience severe apnea. More than 25% of infants weighing more than 1500 g manifest severe apnea. In general, the younger the infant, the greater the number of apneic episodes that may occur.

Premature infants are believed to be susceptible to apneic episodes because of immature functioning of the chemoreceptors, receptors in the airways, and central nervous system. Rapid eye movement (REM) sleep also is thought to play an important role in causing sleep apnea. Box 31-1 lists factors that trigger apneic episodes.

Box 31-1 Factors That Trigger Apnea in the Premature Infant

Control of Ventilation
- REM sleep
- Decreased hypoxic and hypercapnic response
- Ondine's curse (idiopathic alveolar hypoventilation)

Reflex Stimulation
- Suctioning of the nasopharynx and trachea
- Laryngeal stimulation
- Bowel movements (vagal response)
- Hiccups

Environmental Conditions
- Ambient temperature changes

Neurologic Disorders
- Seizures
- Intracranial hemorrhage
- Meningitis

Drug Depression
- Sedatives
- Analgesics
- Prostaglandins

Respiratory Diseases
- Respiratory distress syndrome (RDS)
- Pneumonia
- Transient tachypnea of the newborn (TTN)
- Meconium aspiration syndrome (MAS)
- Bronchopulmonary dysplasia (BPD)
- Diaphragmatic hernia

Cardiac Disorders
- Patent ductus arteriosus
- Congestive heart failure
- Right-to-left intracardiac shunting

Systemic Processes
- Hypothermia
- Hypoglycemia
- Hyponatremia
- Hypocalcemia
- Sepsis (group B *Streptococcus*)

Body Position
- Head flexion

Anatomic Abnormalities
- Micrognathia
- Choanal atresia
- Macroglossia

Persistent Pulmonary Hypertension of the Newborn

Persistent pulmonary hypertension of the newborn (PPHN) is commonly seen in infants with an underlying respiratory disorder such as pneumonia, meconium aspiration syndrome (MAS), or RDS. Box 31-2 lists disorders commonly associated with PPHN.

PPHN is caused in part by reflex pulmonary vasoconstriction, which can be activated by myriad stimuli, including alveolar hypoxia, hypercapnia, and decreased pH. As a result of the high pulmonary vascular resistance (PVR), right-to-left shunting develops—that is, mixed venous blood bypasses the infant's lungs via the **ductus arteriosus** and **foramen ovale** (see fetal circulation pathways, Figure 31-3).

After birth, approximately 80% of the PVR normally decreases within the first 24 hours in response to (1) increased Pa_{O_2} and pH; (2) lung expansion; and (3) release of vasoactive substances, including **prostaglandins, bradykinin,** and **endothelium-derived relaxing factor (ERF).** In infants with PPHN, however, the PVR stays high because of pulmonary vascular hyperreactivity to irritating stimuli. Clinically, PPHN usually appears within the first 12 hours of life with cyanosis, tachypnea, intercostal retractions, nasal flaring, and grunting. Arterial blood gases typically show what is termed *shunt physiology:* a low Pa_{O_2} that is refractory to oxygen therapy. Cardiomegaly may develop as a result of the increased right ventricular afterload caused by the increased PVR.

Arterial Blood Gases

Acute alveolar hyperventilation with hypoxemia and acute ventilatory failure with hypoxemia commonly are seen in newborn babies with pulmonary disorders. This is especially true for newborn infants who have MAS, transient tachypnea of the newborn (TTN), RDS, pulmonary air leak syndromes, respiratory syncytial virus infections, and/or diaphragmatic hernia.

There are three major mechanisms responsible for the decreased Pa_{O_2} observed in the disorders of the newborn just mentioned: (1) pulmonary shunting and venous admixture, (2) PPHN, and (3) infant fatigue. During the early or mild stages of the disorder, the infant commonly hyperventilates, causing the Pa_{CO_2} to decrease and the pH to increase. During the advanced or late stages of the disorder, the infant often goes into acute ventilatory failure. When this occurs, there is a progressive increase in the Pa_{CO_2}, a secondary increase in the HCO_3^-, and a decrease in the pH. The decreased pH also may result from the decreased Pa_{O_2} and the metabolic acidosis that results from anaerobic metabolism and lactic acid accumula-

Box 31-2 Factors Associated with Persistent Pulmonary Hypertension of the Newborn (PPHN)

Maternal Factors
- Diabetes
- Cesarean section
- Hypoxia

Cardiovascular Factors
- Systemic hypotension
- Congenital heart disease
- Shock

Hematologic Factors
- Increased hematocrit
- Septicemia
- Maternal-fetal blood loss
  - Abruptio placentae
  - Placenta previa
- Acute blood loss

Respiratory Diseases
- Meconium aspiration syndrome (MAS)
- Respiratory distress syndrome (RDS)
- Pneumonia

Fetal Factors
- Intrauterine stress
- Hypoxia
- Decreased pH
- Placental vascular abnormalities

Other Factors
- Central nervous system disorders
- Hypoglycemia
- Hypocalcemia
- Neuromuscular disorders

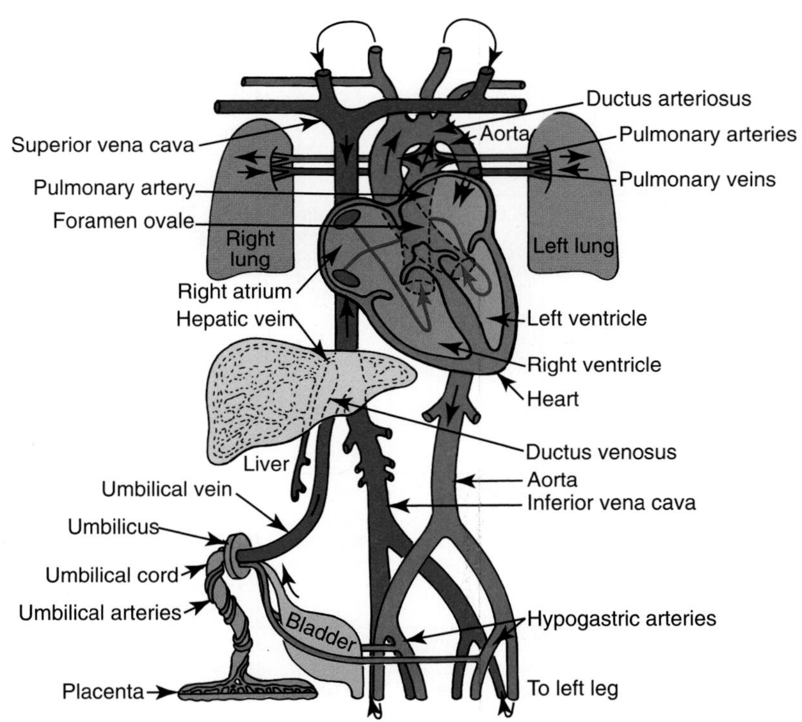

FIGURE 31-3 Fetal circulation. Red = oxygenated blood; blue = deoxygenated blood.

tion. If this is the case, the calculated HCO_3^- reading and pH will be lower than expected for a particular $PaCO_2$ level.

Assessment of the Newborn

As already discussed in Chapter 10, good assessment skills include (1) the systematic collection of clinical data, (2) the evaluation of the data, and (3) the formulation of an appropriate treatment plan. As with the older child or adult, the newborn with respiratory disease must be evaluated frequently. To enhance this process, Figure 31-4 illustrates objective data, assessments, and treatment plans commonly associated with newborn respiratory disorders. Another common assessment tool for the newborn is the **Apgar score.**

Apgar Score

The Apgar score is a rating system for the rapid identification of infants requiring immediate intervention or transfer to an NICU. The Apgar evaluation is performed 1 minute after birth and again 5 minutes later. It is based on a rating of five factors that reflect the infant's ability to adjust to extrauterine life. As shown in Figure 31-5, the infant's heart rate, respiratory effort, muscle tone, reflex irritability, and color are scored from a low value of 0 to a normal value of 2. The five scores are combined and the totals at 1 minute and 5 minutes are recorded. For example, Apgar 8/10 is a score of 8 at 1 minute and 10 at 5 minutes.

A score of 0 to 3 represents severe distress, a score of 4 to 6 indicates moderate distress, and a score of 7 to 10

A HISTORY	OBJECTIVE DATA Clinical manifestations that commonly develop in response to respiratory disease				ASSESSMENT	PLAN
	Inspection	Auscultation	ABGs/ Pulse Oximetry	Chest Radiograph	COMMON CAUSES OF CLINICAL INDICATORS	
Prematurity, maternal diabetes,C-section, multiple births, sibling with RDS	• Retractions • Nasal flaring • Paradoxical (see-saw) respirations • Cyanosis or pallor	• Expiratory grunting • Poor air entry • May have crackles	↓PO_2/SpO_2 while on ↑FIO_2 (Note: premature infants need PO_2 in 60-80 range) Avoid SpO_2 >95%	Reticulogranular, ground glass appearance with air bronchograms	RESPIRATORY DISTRESS SYNDROME (RDS) • Surfactant deficiency • Atelectasis	• Oxygen therapy • Hyperinflation therapy (CPAP/PEEP) • Mechanical ventilation • Surfactant administration
Prematurity, history of RDS, mechanical ventilation	• Decreased chest movement	• Diminished or distant breath sounds	Further ↓PO_2/SpO_2 while on ↑FIO_2	Small cystic areas with possibly flattened diaphragms	PULMONARY INTERSTITIAL EMPHYSEMA (PIE) • Air trapping	• Oxygen therapy • Decrease ventilator pressures • Permissive hypercapnia • Possibly high frequency ventilation and/or selective mainstem intubation • Monitor for barotrauma
Low birth weight, RDS, prolonged mechanical oxygen, slow growth	• Cyanosis if off O_2 • Barrel chest	• Wheezes • Crackles • Rhonchi	↑PCO_2 with normal pH, ↓PO_2/SpO_2	Cystic pattern	BRONCHOPULMONARY DYSPLASIA (BPD) • Airtrapping • Bronchospasm	• Oxygen therapy • Bronchodilator therapy • Bronchial hygiene therapy • Permissive hypercapnia • Fluid management • Increased calorie intake
Usually full term, possibly C-section, perinatal complications	• Tachypnea • Retractions	• Crackles	↓PCO_2, ↓PO_2/SpO_2	Perihilar streaking with enlarged cardiac silhouette	TRANSIENT TACHYPNEA OF THE NEWBORN • Airway fluid	• Oxygen therapy
Stress and/or asphyxia in utero, meconium noted in amniotic fluid, usually full term to post term	• Dyspnea • Meconium-stained umbilical cord or fingernails	• Crackles • Rhonchi	↓PCO_2 (May increase as patient fatigues), ↓PO_2/SpO_2	Hyperaeration	MECONIUM ASPIRATION SYNDROME (MAS) • Airway secretions • Air trapping	• Suction oropharynx and trachea before delivery • Oxygen therapy • Bronchial hygiene therapy • Possible hyperventilation (to further ↓PCO_2 and ↑pH) if hypertension likely • May need to consider ECMO, HFV, etc. • Monitor for barotrauma
Possible underlying problem with meconium aspiration, congenital heart disease, or perinatal asphyxia. Minimal ↑PO_2 with 100% O_2 challenge	• Persistent cyanosis disproportionate to degree of pulmonary disease on CXR • Tachypnea	• Corresponds to underlying cardiopulmonary disorder	Fluctuations in PO_2 /SpO_2	Normal to mild pulmonary parenchymal disease	PERSISTENT PULMONARY HYPERTENSION OF THE NEWBORN (PPHN) • Pulmonary vasoconstriction • Reopening of fetal circulation pathways	• Oxygen therapy • Mechanical ventilation • Treat underlying cause • May need to consider ECMO, HFV, nitric oxide, etc.
May have normal pregnancy and delivery (full term), may have dusky, cyanotic episodes. Minimal ↑PO_2 with 100% O_2 challenge.	• May be normal in appearance if Left→Right shunt present • Cyanotic if Right→Left shunt present	• Heart murmur may be present	PO_2 may vary widely depending on heart lesion: low with Right→Left shunt; more normal with Left→Right	May have irregular heart shape (e.g., boot or egg) depending on lesion	CONGENITAL HEART DISEASE • Pulmonary shunting	• Evaluation to identify problem • Cardiac catheterization • Surgery; pre and post-op supportive care
Problems with breathing; difficulty with eating and breathing (e.g., dusky with feeding), noisy breathing	• Varies with lesion • Respiratory distress, drooling, gastric distension	• Varies with lesion	Usually ↓PCO_2 and ↓PO_2, extent of which varies with lesion	Normal to highly irregular, depending on lesion	CONGENITAL ANOMALIES of the respiratory system • Airway obstruction	• Evaluation to identify problem • Radiographic procedures/operative procedures to diagnose and treat • Pre and post-op supportive care

NEONATAL RESPIRATORY CARE POCKET CARD

Used with permission of author, Terry Des Jardins, WindMist LLC.

FIGURE 31-4 Common neonatal clinical manifestations (objective data), assessments, and treatment plans.

B

PEDIATRIC RESPIRATORY CARE POCKET CARD

HISTORY	OBJECTIVE DATA Clinical manifestations that commonly develop in response to respiratory disease				ASSESSMENT	PLAN
	Inspection	Auscultation	ABGs/ Pulse Oximetry	Chest Radiograph	COMMON CAUSES OF CLINICAL INDICATORS	
Infant or young child (usually newborn–3y.o.), upper respiratory infection, barking cough	• Tachypnea • Retractions • Nasal flaring • May have cyanosis	• Barking cough • Stridor	$\downarrow PCO_2$ and $\downarrow PO_2/SpO_2$	Subglottic edema on neck radiograph–*steeple* sign	LARYNGOTRACHEO-BRONCHITIS (CROUP) (*typically parainfluenza viruses, occasionally bacterial in origin*) • Laryngeal edema	• Oxygen therapy • Cool mist • Racemic epinephrine • Steroids
Toddler or school age child (usually 2y.o. or >), acute onset of fever and respiratory distress	• Stridor • Dyspnea • Drooling • May have cyanosis	• Stridor	$\downarrow PCO_2$ and $\downarrow PO_2/SpO_2$	Epiglottis appears as large, round, soft tissue density on neck radiograph–*thumb* sign	EPIGLOTTITIS (*H. influenzae Type B; vaccine available*) • Edema	• Emergency attention • Oxygen therapy • Intubation in OR or tracheostomy in OR • Antibiotics
Upper respiratory infection, apnea (newborn–2y.o. or older child with chronic cardiopulmonary condition)	• Tachypnea, retractions, nasal flaring, nasal secretions • Cyanosis if severe	• Wheezes • Rhonchi	$\downarrow PO_2/SpO_2$	May vary from normal to streaky infiltrates or hyperaeration	BRONCHIOLITIS (*typically RSV organism*) • Airway secretions • Bronchospasm	• Supportive • Oxygen therapy • Mist hood/tent • Bronchial hygiene therapy • Trial of bronchodilator therapy • Mechanical ventilation rare • Possible ribavirin via SPAG if critically ill)
Upper respiratory infection, late onset of fever, may c/o earache	• Tachypnea, retractions, nasal flaring, nasal secretions • Cyanosis if severe	• Crackles • Wheezes • Bronchial sounds	$\downarrow PO_2/SpO_2$	Infiltrates and/or consolidation	PNEUMONIA • Consolidation • Airway secretions	• Supportive as above if viral • Antibiotics if bacterial with supportive care also provided
Wheezing, family history of asthma/allergies, frequent respiratory infections, or chronic unexplained cough	• Accessory muscle use • Decreased chest excursion • Pursed-lip breathing	• Wheezes, • Prolonged expiration • Crackles	$\downarrow PCO_2$ (increasing PCO_2 is an ominous sign), $\downarrow PO_2/SpO_2$	May be normal or show hyperaeration	ASTHMA (*most common chronic disease in childhood; see Expert Guidelines ref. below*) • Inflammation • Reversible airway obstruction/bronchospasm	(*See Expert Guidelines ref. below*) • Plan varies with severity • Inhaled β_2 agonists, steroids, anticholinergics, mast cell stabilizers, leukotriene modifiers, PEF or FEV_1 assessments, oxygen therapy, possible mechanical ventilation • Discharge teaching of med use, peakflow self-monitoring, and school management plan
Meconium ileus at birth, excessive thick respiratory secretions, frequent respiratory infections, failure to thrive	• Accessory muscle use • Barrel chest • Clubbed fingertips	• Rhonchi • Wheezes • Crackles	May have $\downarrow PO_2/SpO_2$	Hyperaeration, peribronchial thickening, bronchiectasis, increased AP diameter	CYSTIC FIBROSIS (*one of the most common hereditary disorders*) • Excessive secretions • Air trapping	• Bronchial hygiene therapy (postural drainage and percussion, PEP mask therapy, mucoloytics) • Bronchodilators • Antibiotics if indicated • Oxygen therapy • Nutritional support • May need to consider lung transplant
Previously healthy, acute onset of choking, coughing. Occasionally chronic unexplained cough	• Drooling • Stridor • May have cyanosis	• Asymmetrical breath sounds • Wheezes	May be normal, May have $\downarrow PO_2/SpO_2$	Asymmetrical expansion of chest with forced expiratory film	FOREIGN BODY OBSTRUCTION • Airway obstruction	Rigid bronchoscopy with anesthesia, followed by bronchial hygiene therapy and bronchodilator therapy
Presence of underlying disorder such as shock, sepsis, near drowning, aspiration	• Dyspnea • Tachypnea progressing to cyanosis • Irritability	• Crackles • Rhonchi • Bronchial sounds	$\downarrow PCO_2$ (PCO_2 increases as disease progresses), $\downarrow PO_2/SpO_2$, which continues to worsen despite treatment	Normal early in course, progressively shows fluffy infiltrates and patchy, nodular densities	ADULT RESPIRATORY DISTRESS SYNDROME (ARDS) • Increased alveolar-capillary membrane • Atelectasis • Consolidation	• Oxygen therapy • Hyperinflation therapy (CPAP) • Mechanical ventilation • May need to consider HFV, ECMO • Monitor for barotrauma

Used with permission of author, Terry Des Jardins, WindMist LLC.

FIGURE 31-4, cont'd

	0	1	2	1 Minute	5 Minute
Heart rate	Absent	Slow, irregular	More than 100 beats per minute		
Respiratory effort	Apnea	Irregular, slow, shallow, gasping	Strong cry		
Muscle tone	Flaccid/limp	Some flexion of extremities	Well flexed		
Reflex irritability	None-no response to stimulus	Grimace (withdraws)	Crying		
Skin color	Pale blue (shock)	Blue hands and feet, body pink	Pink all over		

FIGURE 31-5 Apgar score interpretation (add the points in the 1-minute and 5-minute columns): 0 to 3 = severe distress; 4 to 6 = moderate distress; 7 to 10 = mild to no distress.

represents an absence of difficulty in adjusting to extrauterine life. The 5-minute score is normally higher than the 1-minute score. A low 1-minute score requires immediate intervention, including the administration of oxygen and oral and nasal suctioning. A baby with a low score that remains low after 5 minutes requires expert care, which may include transfer to the NICU, continuous positive airway pressure (CPAP), umbilical catheterization, and mechanical ventilation.

In the newborn who is lethargic, apneic, pale, blue, and bradycardic at birth, assessments to verify that resuscitation efforts are being done correctly and effectively typically follow this order: First, the heart rate returns to normal. This is followed by spontaneous respiratory movements and improved color. The last assessment to be made is that of the baby's tone and reflex irritability.

SELF-ASSESSMENT QUESTIONS

evolve Answers to questions can be found on Evolve. To access additional student assessment questions and case studies for application of text material to real-life scenarios, visit **http://evolve.elsevier.com/DesJardins/respiratory.**

1. Which of the following trigger(s) apneic episodes?
1. Hypoglycemia
2. Nasotracheal suctioning
3. Head flexion
4. MAS
   a. 4 only
   b. 2 and 3 only
   c. 2, 3, and 4 only
   d. 1, 2, 3, and 4

2. Clinically, PPHN usually manifests within the first:
   a. 3 hours of life
   b. 6 hours of life
   c. 12 hours of life
   d. 24 hours of life

3. When resuscitation of the newborn is being done correctly, which of the following begins to improve first?
   a. Tone
   b. Heart rate
   c. Reflex irritability
   d. Respiratory movements

4. Which of the following is associated with PPHN?
1. Hypoglycemia
2. Decreased pH
3. Hypercalcemia
4. Systemic hypotension
   a. 1 only
   b. 3 only
   c. 2 and 4 only
   d. 1, 2, and 4 only

5. The Apgar evaluation is performed 1 minute after birth, and again:
   a. 3 minutes after birth
   b. 5 minutes after birth
   c. 10 minutes after birth
   d. 15 minutes after birth

Meconium Aspiration Syndrome

32

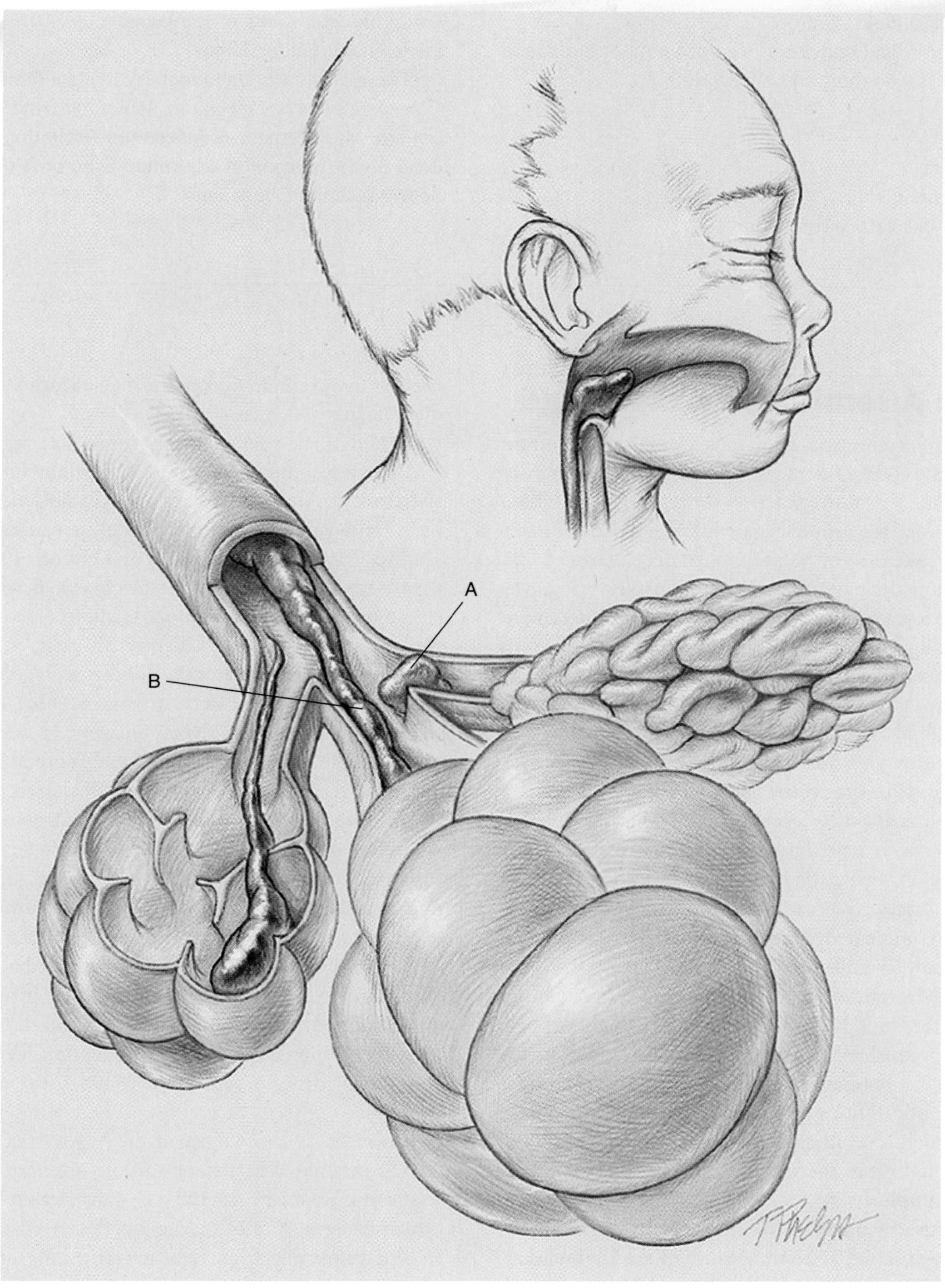

FIGURE 32-1 Meconium aspiration syndrome. **A,** Total obstruction with meconium causing alveolar atelectasis. **B,** Partial obstruction causing air trapping and alveolar hyperinflation.

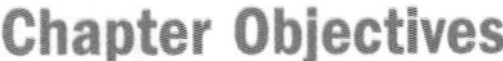

Chapter Objectives

After reading this chapter, you will be able to:

- List the anatomic alterations of the lungs associated with meconium aspiration.
- Describe the causes of meconium aspiration.
- List the cardiopulmonary clinical manifestations associated with meconium aspiration syndrome (MAS).
- Describe the general management of meconium aspiration.
- Describe the clinical strategies and rationales of the SOAPs presented in the case study.
- Define key terms and complete self-assessment questions at the end of the chapter and on Evolve.

Key Terms

"Ball-Valve" Effect
Chemical Pneumonitis
High Frequency Oscillatory Ventilation
Jet Ventilation
Meconium
Meconium Aspiration Syndrome (MAS)
Meconium Staining
Persistent Pulmonary Hypertension of the Neonate (PPHN)
Pneumomediastinum
Pneumothorax

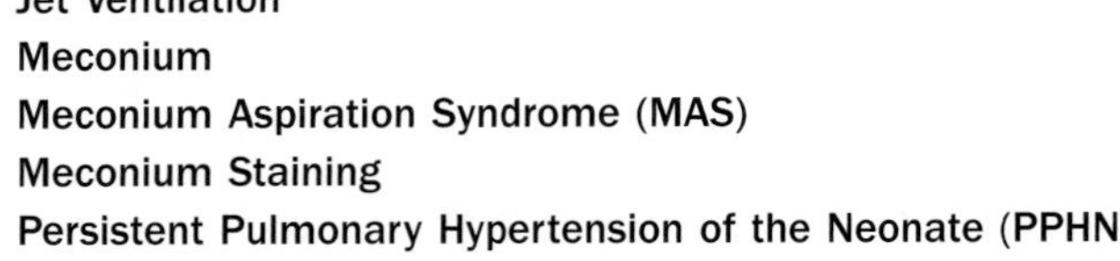

Chapter Outline

Anatomic Alterations of the Lungs

During normal intrauterine fetal development, the infant periodically demonstrates normal rapid, shallow respiratory chest movements. This normal action moves pulmonary fetal fluid into and out of the oropharynx while the glottis remains closed. During periods of fetal hypoxemia, however, the infant may demonstrate very deep, gasping inspiratory movements that may force the contents of the naso-oropharynx to pass through the glottis into the airways. The aspiration of minimal amounts of clear amniotic fluid usually is not associated with serious anatomic or functional problems of the lungs. During fetal hypoxemia, however, the aspirate may contain **meconium** and amniotic fluid—hence the phrase **meconium aspiration syndrome (MAS).**

MAS is a clinical entity seen primarily in full-term or postterm infants who have had some degree of hypoxemia either prenatally or during the birth process. When the fetus experiences in utero hypoxia, the intestinal response is vasoconstriction, increased gastrointestinal peristalsis, anal sphincter relaxation, and passage of meconium into the amniotic fluid. Meconium is the material that collects in the intestine of the fetus and forms the first stools of the newborn. Meconium is an odorless, thick, sticky, blackish green material. Meconium is a heterogeneous mixture of intestinal tract secretions, amniotic fluid, pulmonary fetal fluid, and intrauterine debris such as epithelial cells, mucus, lanugo, blood, and vernix. Aspiration of meconium leads to one or more of the following complications.

First, the physical presence of the meconium results in upper airway obstruction at birth because of the high viscosity of the meconium. Shortly after birth (within 1 hour), and especially if gasping inspirations are present, clumps of meconium rapidly migrate past the glottis and penetrate the smaller airways (see Figure 32-1). In cases of severe intrauterine hypoxemia, meconium may already be present in the distal airways at birth.

When thick particulate meconium is aspirated into the small airways, the meconium can partially or totally obstruct the airways. Airways that are partially obstructed are affected by a **"ball-valve" effect,** in which air can enter but cannot readily leave the distal airways and alveoli. This condition in turn leads to air trapping and alveolar hyperinflation. Excessive hyperinflation commonly leads to alveolar rupture and air leak syndromes (see Chapter 35) such as **pneumomediastinum** or **pneumothorax.** Totally obstructed airways lead to alveolar shrinkage and atelectasis. This combination of areas of overexpanded alveoli adjacent to areas of atelectasis creates both an increased functional residual capacity (FRC) and a decrease in air flow during exhalation.

The second chain of events that can develop from MAS is **chemical pneumonitis,** which is characterized by an acute inflammatory reaction and edema of the bronchial mucosa and alveolar epithelium. This reaction commonly leads to excessive bronchial secretions and alveolar consolidation. Meconium also promotes the growth of bacteria, which in turn augments the development of alveolar pneumonitis and consolidation. Meconium aspiration can also interfere with alveolar pulmonary surfactant production. When this occurs, respiratory distress syndrome (RDS) also may complicate MAS.

Third, as a consequence of the hypoxemia associated with MAS, infants with the condition often develop hypoxia-induced pulmonary arterial vasoconstriction and vasospasm, which cause a state of pulmonary hypertension. This results in blood shunting from right to left through the ductus arteriosus and the foramen ovale; intrapulmonary shunts occasionally are seen also. As a consequence, the blood flow is diverted away from the lungs (pulmonary hypoperfusion), which worsens the hypoxemia. Clinically, this condition is referred to as **persistent pulmonary hypertension of the neonate (PPHN),** previously called *persistent fetal circulation* (PFC).

The major pathologic or structural changes associated with MAS are as follows:

- Physical presence of the meconium leading to:
  - Partially obstructed airways, air trapping, and alveolar hyperinflation
  - Pulmonary air leak syndromes (pneumomediastinum or pneumothorax)
  - Totally obstructed airways and absorption atelectasis
- Edema of the bronchial mucosa and alveolar epithelium
- Excessive bronchial secretions
- Alveolar consolidation
- Decreased pulmonary surfactant production
- Hypoxia-induced pulmonary vasospasm and vasoconstriction:
  - Pulmonary hypertension
  - Right-to-left shunting
  - Worsening hypoxia
  - Pulmonary hypoperfusion

Etiology and Epidemiology

About 10,000 to 15,000 infants are diagnosed with MAS annually. From this group, about 30% of the infants with MAS require mechanical ventilation, and 10% and 15% of the infants with MAS will develop a pneumothorax. The overall mortality rate is about 4%. As discussed earlier, the fetal passage of meconium is caused by fetal hypoxemia and stress. Fetal hypoxemia causes a vagal response that relaxes anal sphincter tone and allows meconium to move into the amniotic fluid.

MAS rarely is seen in infants younger than 36 weeks' gestation because the release of meconium requires strong peristalsis and sphincter tone, which usually are not present among preterm infants. Thus, postterm infants (infants older than 42 weeks' gestation) are especially at risk for MAS, because both strong peristalsis and sphincter tone are present in babies of this age. Other infants who are at high risk for MAS are those who are small for gestational age, those who are delivered in the breech position, and those whose mothers are toxemic, hypertensive, or obese.

OVERVIEW of the Cardiopulmonary Clinical Manifestations Associated with Meconium Aspiration Syndrome

The following clinical manifestations result from the pathologic mechanisms caused (or activated) by **Atelectasis** (see Figure 9-8), **Alveolar Consolidation** (see Figure 9-9), **Excessive Bronchial Secretions** (see Figure 9-12), and **Airway Obstruction**—the major anatomic alterations of the lungs associated with meconium aspiration syndrome (MAS) (see Figure 32-1).

CLINICAL DATA OBTAINED AT THE PATIENT'S BEDSIDE

The Physical Examination

Vital Signs

Increased Respiratory Rate (Tachypnea)

Normally, a newborn infant's respiratory rate is about 40 to 60 breaths per minute. In MAS the respiratory rate generally is well over 60 breaths per minute. Several pathophysiologic mechanisms operating simultaneously may lead to an increased ventilatory rate:

- Stimulation of the peripheral chemoreceptors (hypoxemia)
- Decreased lung compliance–increased ventilatory rate relationship
- Stimulation of the central chemoreceptors

Increased Heart Rate (Pulse) and Blood Pressure

Apnea

Clinical Manifestations Associated with More Negative Intrapleural Pressure during Inspiration

- Intercostal retractions
- Substernal retraction and abdominal distention (seesaw movement)
- Cyanosis of the dependent portion of the thoracic and abdominal areas
- Flaring nostrils

Chest Assessment Findings

- Wheezes
- Rhonchi
- Crackles

Expiratory Grunting

Cyanosis

Common General Appearance Clinical Manifestations

- Meconium staining (brownish-yellow color) on:
  - Skin
  - Nails
  - Umbilical cord
  - Wrinkles and creases in the skin
- Barrel chest (when airways are partially obstructed)

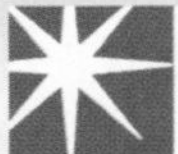

OVERVIEW of the Cardiopulmonary Clinical Manifestations Associated with Meconium Aspiration Syndrome—cont'd

CLINICAL DATA OBTAINED FROM LABORATORY TESTS AND SPECIAL PROCEDURES

Pulmonary Function Test Findings (Extrapolated Data for Instructional Purposes) (Primarily Restrictive Lung Pathophysiology)

FORCED EXPIRATORY FLOW RATE FINDINGS

FVC	FEV_T	FEV_1/FVC ratio	$FEF_{25\%-75\%}$
↓	N or ↓	N or ↑	N or ↓

$FEF_{50\%}$	$FEF_{200-1200}$	PEFR	MVV
N or ↓	N or ↓	N or ↓	N or ↓

LUNG VOLUME AND CAPACITY FINDINGS

V_T	IRV	ERV	RV*
N or ↓	↓	↓	↓

VC	IC	FRC*	TLC	RV/TLC ratio
↓	↓	↓	↓	N

*↑ When airways are partially obstructed.

Arterial Blood Gases

MILD TO MODERATE MECONIUM ASPIRATION SYNDROME
Acute Alveolar Hyperventilation with Hypoxemia
(Acute Respiratory Alkalosis)

pH	Pa_{CO_2}	HCO_3^-	Pa_{O_2}
↑	↓	↓ (slightly)	↓

SEVERE MECONIUM ASPIRATION SYNDROME
Acute Ventilatory Failure with Hypoxemia
(Acute Respiratory Acidosis)

pH*	Pa_{CO_2}	HCO_3^- *	Pa_{O_2}
↓	↑	↑ (slightly)	↓

*When tissue hypoxia is severe enough to produce lactic acid, the pH and HCO_3^- values will be lower than expected for a particular Pa_{CO_2} level.

Oxygenation Indices*

$\dot{Q}_S/\dot{Q}_T$	D_{O_2}[†]	$\dot{V}_{O_2}$	$C(a-\bar{v})_{O_2}$	O_2ER	$S\bar{v}_{O_2}$
↑	↓	N	N	↑	↓

[†]The D_{O_2} may be normal in patients who have compensated to the decreased oxygenation status with (1) an increased cardiac output, (2) an increased hemoglobin level, or (3) a combination of both. When the D_{O_2} is normal, the O_2ER is usually normal.

RADIOLOGIC FINDINGS

Chest Radiograph

When alveolar atelectasis and consolidation are present, the chest x-ray film shows irregular densities throughout the lungs. Although the chest x-ray picture clearly is different from that seen in respiratory distress syndrome, it is difficult to differentiate the x-ray appearance of MAS from that of pneumonia (Figure 32-2).

The chest x-ray film may show local or generalized problem areas. When significant partial airway obstruction, air trapping, and alveolar hyperinflation are present, the chest x-ray film appears hyperlucent and the diaphragms may be depressed. The practitioner should be alert for the sudden development of a pneumothorax or pneumomediastinum in infants with MAS (Figure 32-3).

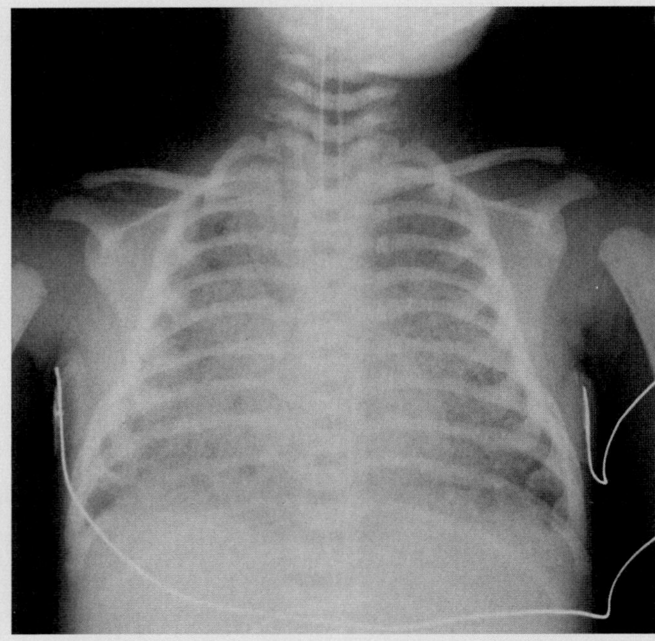

FIGURE 32-2 Chest radiograph of an infant with meconium aspiration syndrome (MAS). Patchy areas of increased density are observed in both lungs. (From Taussig LM, Landau LI: *Pediatric respiratory medicine,* ed 2, St Louis, 2008, Elsevier.)

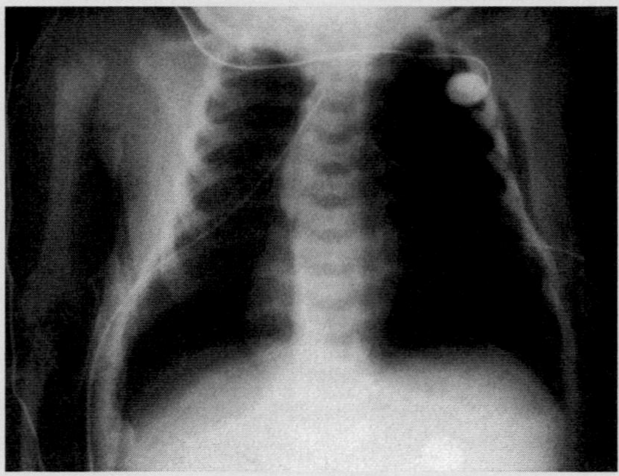

FIGURE 32-3 Meconium aspiration with bilateral pneumothorax.

*$C(a-\bar{v})_{O_2}$, Arterial-venous oxygen difference; D_{O_2}, total oxygen delivery; O_2ER, oxygen extraction ratio; $\dot{Q}_S/\dot{Q}_T$, pulmonary shunt fraction; $S\bar{v}_{O_2}$, mixed venous oxygen saturation; $\dot{V}_{O_2}$, oxygen consumption.

General Management of Meconium Aspiration Syndrome

The respiratory care practitioner should be proactive whenever an infant is at risk for meconium aspiration. In other words, when the amniotic fluid is found to be stained with meconium—and when the infant is not actively breathing or crying immediately after delivery—the infant should be intubated and the upper airways should be suctioned until all the meconium has been cleared. This measure should be routine for all infants born through particulate meconium, even if meconium is not visualized in the oropharynx. *Positive-pressure ventilation should not be administered until a thorough suctioning of the upper airways has been completed,* because any particulate meconium remaining in the upper airways likely will be forced into the lower airways in response to positive-pressure ventilation.

After the infant is stabilized and has been transported to the neonatal intensive care unit, vigorous **bronchial hygiene** (e.g., postural drainage, percussion, suctioning) of the airways should be performed per protocol. Appropriate **oxygen therapy** should be administered per protocol; in severe cases, **mechanical ventilation** may be necessary. As already mentioned, however, mechanical ventilation should be avoided or applied cautiously to prevent the possibility of dislodging unseen particulate meconium and pushing it further down the infant's airways. In addition, a high incidence of pneumothorax is associated with MAS. If some mechanical ventilation is necessary, an inspiration/expiration ratio that permits a long exhalation time (to allow expired gas enough time to flow past partially obstructed airways) should be used. Finally, the infant should be monitored closely for possible superimposed infection. Antibiotics may be indicated and steroids may be required to offset the inflammatory response in chemical pneumonitis. Because a decreased production of pulmonary surfactant is associated with MAS, exogenous pulmonary surfactant may be administered to infants with MAS.

CASE STUDY

Meconium Aspiration Syndrome (MAS)

Admitting History and Physical Examination

A 38-week-gestation newborn male infant was delivered by emergency cesarean section because of sudden maternal vaginal hemorrhage. The mother was a primigravida Caucasian 19-year-old with a history of no prenatal care. She was a heavy smoker and had an uncertain history of recreational psychopharmaceutical drug use during pregnancy. Rupture of membranes was believed to have occurred about 18 hours before delivery.

At delivery, the infant's umbilical cord was wrapped once around his neck. He was covered with meconium. He was limp and blue and did not show any spontaneous movement or respiratory effort when he was handed to the neonatologist, who was heading the resuscitation team of one registered nurse and a registered respiratory therapist. While receiving 100% free-flow oxygen to the oral and nasal area, the infant was dried and warmed. With the aid of a laryngoscope, several clumps of meconium were suctioned from the infant's oral and pharyngeal areas. On two separate passes below the vocal cords, no meconium was visualized or suctioned.

In spite of these efforts, the infant demonstrated no spontaneous respirations, and his heart rate was less than 60 bpm. Because of this, manual ventilation could no longer be avoided. At this time, the respiratory therapist started to ventilate the infant with a bag-valve-mask resuscitation bag, at an F_{IO_2} of 1.0 and a respiratory rate of 30/min. The nurse started chest compressions at about 90 per minute, with a rhythm of three compressions to one breath. Bilateral crackles and rhonchi were auscultated.

At 1 minute, the Apgar score was 1 for the heart rate. By the third minute, the baby's heart rate was 80/min. The infant was gasping occasionally and demonstrated some central pinkness. Although compressions were stopped, bagging continued at 40 breaths per minute. At the fifth minute, the Apgar score was 6 (heart rate 2, respirations 1, tone 1, reflex irritability 0, and color 2). The neonatologist decided at this time to intubate the baby with a 3.5-mm endotracheal tube. The respiratory therapist confirmed the correct position of the endotracheal tube by means of (1) careful auscultation, and (2) the appearance of a "yellow" color on the CO_2 detector (i.e., a yellow color confirms CO_2 and a purple color indicates no CO_2). The respiratory therapist then taped the tube at the 8.5-cm mark at the infant's lips. The baby was transferred to the neonatal intensive care unit (NICU) and placed on a ventilator. Initial ventilator settings were respiratory rate (RR) 40, inspiratory time (TI) 0.35 sec, F_{IO_2} 100%, positive inspiratory pressure (PIP) +25, positive end-expiratory pressure (PEEP) +5, and flow 8 L/min. A chest x-ray examination was ordered. At that time the respiratory therapist documented the following in the infant's chart.

Respiratory Assessment and Plan

S N/A

O Apneic at birth, hypoactive, cyanotic, covered with meconium. 1 minute Apgar 1, 5 minute Apgar 6. Bilateral crackles and rhonchi. Meconium suctioned from oral and pharyngeal areas.

A
- Possible MAS (meconium in airway)
- Airway secretions (meconium?) (crackles and rhonchi)
- Probable asphyxic episode; likely combined respiratory and metabolic acidosis (history, cyanosis)

P **Mechanical Ventilation Protocol** in combination with **Oxygen Therapy** and **Hyperinflation Therapy Protocol** (RR 40, F_{IO_2} 100%, PIP +25, flow 8 L/min, and PEEP 5). **Bronchopulmonary Hygiene Protocol** (suction prn and CPT qid). Assist physician with surfactant administration. Monitor closely (oximetry, vital signs, watch for signs of acute air leak, pulmonary hemorrhage).

Over the next hour, an umbilical artery catheter (UAC) was inserted; it showed a pH of 7.19, Pa_{CO_2} 37, HCO_3^- 14, Pa_{O_2} 87, and Sp_{O_2} 94%. Although the infant's skin was now completely pink, bilateral crackles and rhonchi were still present. The chest x-ray film revealed hyperinflation in both the right and left lungs. There was whiteout of the right upper and middle lobes, most likely caused by atelectasis. Clumps of white patches of atelectasis (resembling small popcorn balls) were seen throughout the remainder of the lungs. The endotracheal tube tip was at the clavicle level, and the UAC tip was appropriately positioned at T-8. The following SOAP note was recorded at this time:

Respiratory Assessment and Plan

S N/A

O Pink skin. Bilateral crackles and rhonchi. Atelectasis in the right upper and middle lobes. Air trapping right and left lower lobes. ABGs: pH 7.19, Pa_{CO_2} 37, HCO_3^- 14, Pa_{O_2} 87, and Sp_{O_2} 94% (on F_{IO_2} 1.0).

A
- Airway secretions (crackles and rhonchi)
- Atelectasis (CXR)
- Uncompensated metabolic acidosis (ABG)

P Continue **Mechanical Ventilation Protocol** in combination with **Oxygen Therapy** and **Hyperinflation Therapy Protocols** (RR 40, F_{IO_2} 100%, PIP +30 cm H_2O, and PEEP +5 cm H_2O). Continue **Bronchopulmonary Hygiene Protocol** (suction prn and CPT qid). Monitor closely (vital signs, watch for signs of acute air leak, pulmonary hemorrhage).

Because the infant's mechanical ventilation was adequate (confirmed by a normal Pa_{CO_2} of 37), the neonatologist administered sodium bicarbonate to correct the baby's metabolic acidosis. The baby progressively improved over the next 4 days. On the fifth day, the baby was off the ventilator; on the seventh, he was discharged from the hospital. The mother was scheduled to see Social Services on a weekly basis.

Discussion

Inspection—the first step in the assessment process—was of the utmost importance in this case. The umbilical cord wrapped around the infant's neck, the presence of meconium, the blue skin, and the absence of spontaneous respirations all were important clinical indicators demonstrating the severity of the baby's condition. Paramount in this case is the fact that the baby was not manually ventilated—in spite of the fact that the baby had no spontaneous respirations—until after several clumps of meconium were suctioned from the infant's oral and laryngeal areas. Great care must be taken not to blow any meconium, blood, or amniotic fluid deeper down the tracheobronchial tree. The neonatal team must always be alert for the presence of a ball-valve meconium obstruction and the possibility of a pneumothorax. A ball-valve obstruction was verified in this case by the identification of alveolar hyperinflation on the chest x-ray film. Fortunately, a pneumothorax did not develop.

As with adult subjects, several of the clinical manifestations in this case can be traced back through the "clinical scenarios" associated with **Atelectasis** (see Figure 9-8) and **Excessive Bronchial Secretions** (see Figure 9-12). For example, the increased lung density caused by the atelectasis was revealed on the chest x-ray film, and the crackles and rhonchi were produced by the excessive airway secretions recorded in the second SOAP.

Although it was not used in this case, high-frequency oscillatory ventilation or jet ventilation is often used with these babies. Either ventilator management approach appears to benefit the patient equally. The therapeutic effect of these ventilator techniques is that they ventilate by air streams that flow down the center of the airways while gas leaving the lungs moves along the peripheral walls of the airways, thus moving meconium and secretions out of the lungs.

These babies are very sensitive to external stimuli. Great caution should be taken not to overstimulate them. They should be suctioned only as needed. When suctioning is necessary, the respiratory therapist should not prolong the suctioning process but should get in and out of the infant's trachea as fast as possible. Often, these babies are given eye patches and earplugs to decrease external sensory stimulation. Occasionally, they will be paralyzed to minimize their reactions to stimuli and resistance to ventilation.

SELF-ASSESSMENT QUESTIONS

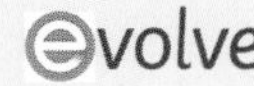

Answers to questions can be found on Evolve. To access additional student assessment questions and case studies for application of text material to real-life scenarios, visit **http://evolve.elsevier.com/DesJardins/respiratory.**

1. When the fetus experiences in utero hypoxia, which of the following occur(s)?
1. Vasoconstriction
2. Inspiratory gasping
3. Sphincter constriction
4. Increased intestinal peristalsis
   a. 1 only
   b. 2 only
   c. 1, 2, and 4 only
   d. 2, 3, and 4 only
   e. 1, 2, 3, and 4

2. Aspiration of meconium may lead to which of the following?
1. Ball-valve effect
2. Atelectasis
3. Total airway obstruction
4. Alveolar hyperinflation
5. Chemical pneumonitis
   a. 2 only
   b. 1, 2, and 4 only
   c. 2, 3, and 4 only
   d. 1, 2, 3, 4, and 5

3. Meconium-stained amniotic fluid is seen in approximately what percentage of all births?
   a. 1
   b. 3
   c. 10
   d. 15

4. Which of the following clinical manifestations are associated with meconium aspiration syndrome?
1. Apnea
2. Intercostal retractions
3. Barrel chest
4. Expiratory grunting
   a. 2 only
   b. 1, 2, and 4 only
   c. 2, 3, and 4 only
   d. 1, 2, 3, and 4

5. What percentage of the infants with MAS who require mechanical ventilation will likely develop a pneumothorax?
   a. 1% to 5%
   b. 5% to 10%
   c. 10% to 15%
   d. 15% to 20%

Transient Tachypnea of the Newborn

33

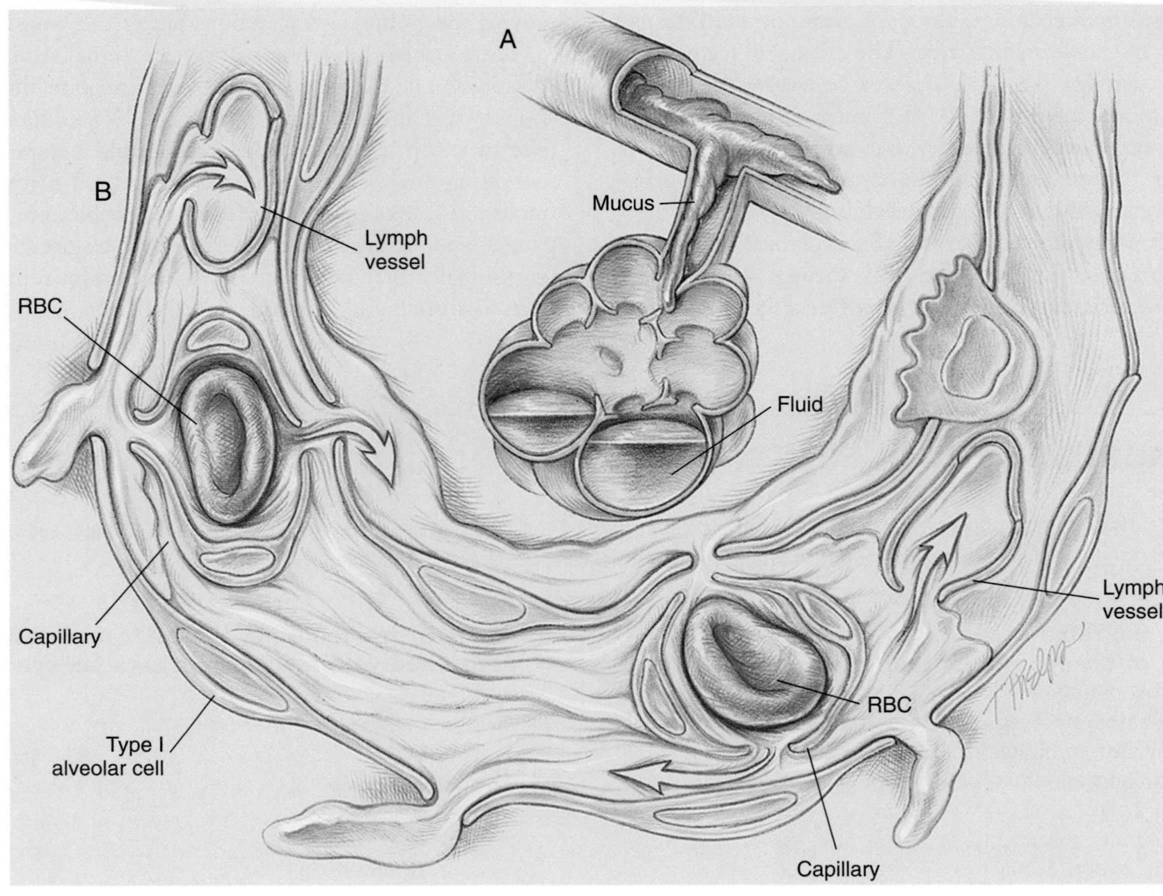

FIGURE 33-1 Transient tachypnea of the newborn. **A**, Excessive bronchial secretions and pulmonary capillary congestion. **B**, Cross-section of alveolus with interstitial edema.

Chapter Objectives

After reading this chapter, you will be able to:

- List the anatomic alterations of the lungs associated with transient tachypnea of the newborn.
- Describe the causes of transient tachypnea of the newborn.
- List the cardiopulmonary clinical manifestations associated with transient tachypnea of the newborn.
- Describe the general management of transient tachypnea of the newborn.
- Describe the clinical strategies and rationales of the SOAP presented in the case study.
- Define key terms and complete self-assessment questions at the end of the chapter and on Evolve.

Key Terms

Interstitial Edema
Macrosomia
Perihilar Streaking (Starbursts or Sunbursts)
Pulmonary Capillary Congestion
Rapid and Shallow Breathing Pattern (Hallmark Clinical Manifestation)
Type II Respiratory Distress Syndrome
Wet Lung Syndrome

Chapter Outline

Overview of the Cardiopulmonary Clinical Manifestations Associated with Transient Tachypnea of the Newborn
General Management of Transient Tachypnea of the Newborn
Respiratory Care Treatment Protocols
Case Study: Transient Tachypnea of the Newborn
Self Assessment Questions

Anatomic Alterations of the Lungs

Transient tachypnea of the newborn (TTN) (also called *type II respiratory distress syndrome* and *"wet lung" syndrome*) was first described in the literature in 1965. Within the first 4 to 6 hours after birth, TTN produces clinical signs very similar to those associated with the early stages of respiratory distress syndrome (see Chapter 34). However, the anatomic alterations of the lungs associated with TTN are much different from the pulmonary pathology seen in respiratory distress syndrome.

As shown in Figure 33-1, the infant with TTN has a delay in the pulmonary fluid absorption by the lymphatic system and pulmonary capillaries. It is thought that this condition results, in part, from the infant's hypoxemia and inadequate inspiratory effort, producing a delay in clearance of pulmonary fluid. As this condition worsens, the infant develops pulmonary capillary congestion, interstitial edema, decreased lung compliance, decreased tidal volume, and increased dead space. Because the swallowing and cough efforts of infants with TTN are commonly depressed, the clearance of bronchial secretions is compromised. This condition often leads to air trapping and alveolar hyperinflation.

In severe cases, the excessive fluid accumulation throughout the alveolar-capillary interstitial tissue may also compress the bronchial airways. As a general rule, however, the abnormal anatomic alterations of the lungs associated with TTN usually begin to resolve about 48 to 72 hours after birth.

The major pathologic or structural changes associated with TTN are as follows:

- Excessive bronchial secretions and incomplete absorption of pulmonary fetal fluid
- Air trapping and alveolar hyperinflation
- Decreased removal of fluid by pulmonary lymphatics
- Pulmonary capillary congestion
- Interstitial edema
- Compressed bronchial airways (from excessive alveolar-capillary interstitial fluid)

Etiology and Epidemiology

TTN affects 1% to 2% of all newborns. Classically, TNN is most often seen in full-term infants. Risk factors include elective cesarean section, excessive administration of fluids to the mother during labor, male gender, and macrosomia (a newborn with excessive birth weight). The infant's history often includes maternal analgesia or anesthesia during labor and delivery or episodes of intrauterine hypoxia. TTN is also commonly associated with maternal bleeding, maternal diabetes, and prolapsed cord. TTN is occasionally seen in very small infants.

Although the precise mechanism is not known, it is believed that TTN results from a delayed absorption of fetal lung fluid. The delayed absorption of lung fluid is thought to be caused by any condition that increases the central venous pressure, which in turn slows the clearance of lung fluid by the lymphatic system. Infants with TTN are often lethargic at birth, resulting in a depressed cough effort and accumulation of airway secretions and mucus. The typical baby with TTN usually has good Apgar scores at birth. During the next few hours, however, signs of respiratory distress develop. Early clinical manifestations include tachypnea, retractions nasal flaring, grunting, and cyanosis. It is common to see respiratory rates of 80 to 120 breaths/minute. In fact, the rapid and shallow breathing pattern often is considered a hallmark clinical manifestation of TTN. In addition, the infant may demonstrate a barrel chest and coarse breath sounds. Within 24 to 48 hours, the clinical manifestations of respiratory distress usually disappear.

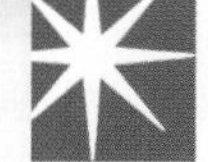

OVERVIEW of the Cardiopulmonary Clinical Manifestations Associated with Transient Tachypnea of the Newborn

The following clinical manifestations result from the pathologic mechanisms caused (or activated) by **Increased Alveolar-Capillary Membrane Thickness** (see Figure 9-10), **Excessive Bronchial Secretions** (see Figure 9-12), and **Airway Obstruction**—the major anatomic alterations of the lungs associated with transient tachypnea of the newborn (TTN) (see Figure 33-1).

CLINICAL DATA OBTAINED AT THE PATIENT'S BEDSIDE

The Physical Examination

Vital Signs

Increased Respiratory Rate (Tachypnea)

Infants with TTN frequently breathe rapidly and shallowly. In fact, this rapid and shallow breathing pattern often is consid-

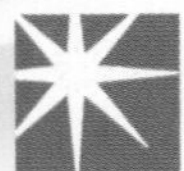

OVERVIEW of the Cardiopulmonary Clinical Manifestations Associated with Transient Tachypnea of the Newborn—cont'd

ered a hallmark clinical manifestation of TTN. Normally, a newborn infant's respiratory rate is about 40 to 60 breaths per minute. During the early stages of TTN, the respiratory rate is often 60 to 100 breaths per minute. Several pathophysiologic mechanisms operating simultaneously may lead to an increased ventilatory rate:

- Stimulation of the peripheral chemoreceptors (hypoxemia)
- Decreased lung compliance–increased ventilatory rate relationship
- Stimulation of the central chemoreceptors

Increased Heart Rate (Pulse) and Blood Pressure

Clinical Manifestations Associated with More Negative Intrapleural Pressure during Inspiration

Intercostal Retractions

- Substernal retraction and abdominal distention (seesaw movement)
- Cyanosis of the dependent portions of the thoracic and abdominal areas
- Flaring nostrils

Chest Assessment Findings

- Wheezes
- Rhonchi
- Crackles

Expiratory Grunting

Cyanosis

CLINICAL DATA OBTAINED FROM LABORATORY TESTS AND SPECIAL PROCEDURES

Pulmonary Function Test Findings (Extrapolated Data for Instructional Purposes) (Restrictive Lung Pathophysiology)

FORCED EXPIRATORY FLOW RATE FINDINGS

FVC	FEV_T	FEV_1/FVC ratio	$FEF_{25\%-75\%}$
↓	N or ↓	N or ↑	N or ↓
$FEF_{50\%}$	$FEF_{200-1200}$	PEFR	MVV
N or ↓	N or ↓	N or ↓	N or ↓

LUNG VOLUME AND CAPACITY FINDINGS

V_T	IRV	ERV	RV*	
N or ↓	↓	↓	↓	
VC	IC	FRC*	TLC*	RV/TLC ratio*
↓	↓	↓	↓	N

*↑ When airways are partially obstructed.

Arterial Blood Gases

MILD TO MODERATE TRANSIENT TACHYPNEA OF THE NEWBORN

Acute Alveolar Hyperventilation with Hypoxemia

(Acute Respiratory Alkalosis)

pH	Pa_{CO_2}	HCO_3^-	Pa_{O_2}
↑	↓	↓ (slightly)	↓

SEVERE TRANSIENT TACHYPNEA OF THE NEWBORN*

Acute Ventilatory Failure with Hypoxemia

(Acute Respiratory Acidosis)

pH*	Pa_{CO_2}	HCO_3^- †	Pa_{O_2}
↓	↑	↑ (slightly)	↓

*The clinical manifestations of TTN usually disappear in the first 24 to 48 hours. Severe TTN is rare.

†When tissue hypoxia is severe enough to produce lactic acid, the pH and HCO_3^- values will be lower than expected for a particular Pa_{CO_2} level.

Oxygenation Indices*

$\dot{Q}_S/\dot{Q}_T$	D_{O_2}†	$\dot{V}_{O_2}$	$C(a-\bar{v})_{O_2}$	O_2ER	$S\bar{v}_{O_2}$
↑	↓	N	N	↑	↓

†The D_{O_2} may be normal in patients who have compensated to the decreased oxygenation status with (1) an increased cardiac output, (2) an increased hemoglobin level, or (3) a combination of both. When the D_{O_2} is normal, the O_2ER is usually normal.

RADIOLOGIC FINDINGS

Chest Radiograph

Initially, the chest radiograph appears normal. Over the next 4 to 6 hours, however, signs of pulmonary vascular congestion develop. These are revealed on the chest radiograph as prominent perihilar streaking (commonly called *starbursts* or *sunbursts*), air bronchograms, and fluid in the interlobular fissures. Air trapping and hyperinflation may occur and are manifested by peripheral hyperlucency, flattened diaphragms, and bulging intercostal spaces. Patches of infiltrates may be seen in some infants. Mild cardiomegaly and pleural effusions also may be seen (Figure 33-2).

*$C(a-\bar{v})_{O_2}$, Arterial-venous oxygen difference; D_{O_2}, total oxygen delivery; O_2ER, oxygen extraction ratio; $\dot{Q}_S/\dot{Q}_T$, pulmonary shunt fraction; $S\bar{v}_{O_2}$, mixed venous oxygen saturation; $\dot{V}_{O_2}$, oxygen consumption.

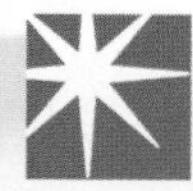

OVERVIEW of the Cardiopulmonary Clinical Manifestations Associated with Transient Tachypnea of the Newborn—cont'd

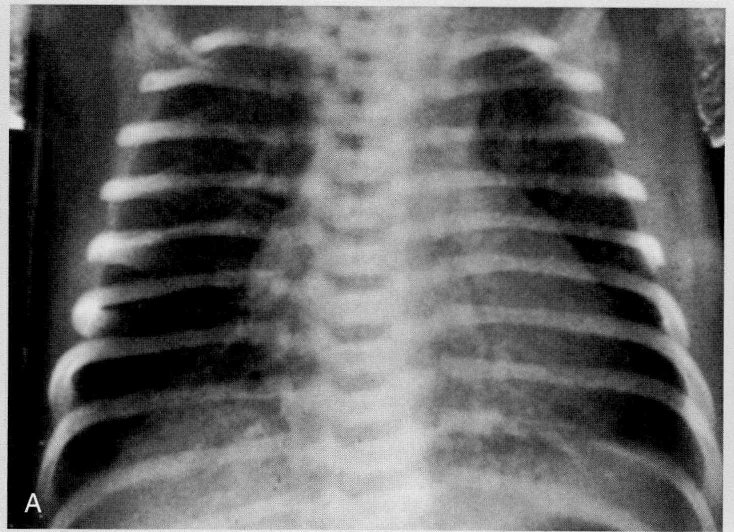

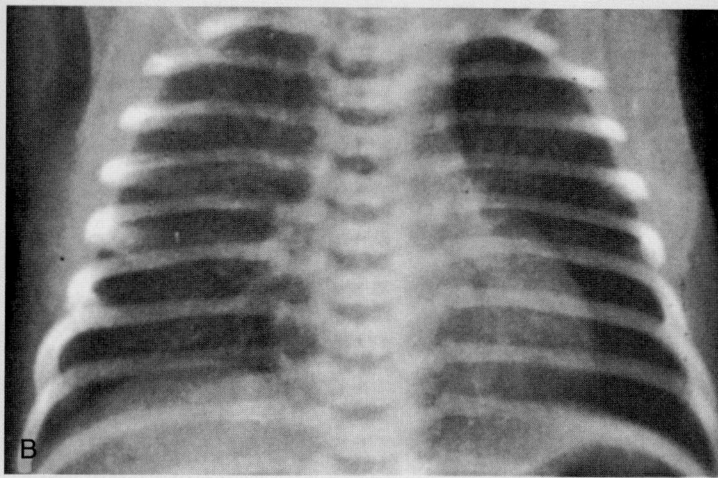

FIGURE 33-2 The large cardiovascular silhouette, air bronchogram, and streaky lung fields were seen at 2 hours of age (**A**) but had cleared by 24 hours of age (**B**), typical of transient tachypnea of the newborn or delayed clearance of lung liquid. (From Taeusch WH, Ballard RA, Gleason CA: *Avery's diseases of the newborn,* ed 8, Philadelphia, 2005, Saunders.)

General Management of Transient Tachypnea of the Newborn

Because of the relatively short course of TTN, the treatment consists mostly of proper stabilization, close monitoring, and frequent and thorough evaluations to rule out other, more serious conditions that may develop. Oxygen therapy is provided to maintain adequate oxygenation, and bronchopulmonary hygiene therapy may be administered to keep the airways clear of bronchial secretions. Lung expansion therapy is often used as a preventative measure, but mechanical ventilation is usually not required. Fluid restriction is usually ordered until the signs associated with TTN resolve. Oral feedings are usually started as soon as the infant is able tolerate them. Diuretics do not affect the clinical course of the TTN. In cases in which pneumonia is suspected, the use of antibiotics is indicated.

Respiratory Care Treatment Protocols

Oxygen Therapy Protocol

Oxygen therapy is used to treat hypoxemia, decrease the work of breathing, and decrease myocardial work. Because of the hypoxemia that often develops in TTN, supplemental oxygen may be required (see Oxygen Therapy Protocol, Protocol 9-1).

Bronchopulmonary Hygiene Therapy Protocol

Because of the excessive airway secretions and accumulation associated with TTN, a number of bronchial hygiene treatment modalities may be used to enhance the mobilization of bronchial secretions (see Bronchopulmonary Hygiene Therapy Protocol, Protocol 9-2).

Lung Expansion Therapy Protocol

Lung expansion measures commonly are performed to offset the pulmonary capillary congestion and interstitial edema associated with TTN (see Lung Expansion Therapy Protocol, Protocol 9-3).

Mechanical Ventilation Protocol

Mechanical ventilation may occasionally be necessary to provide and support alveolar gas exchange and eventually return the patient to spontaneous breathing. Patients with TTN rarely require mechanical ventilation (see Mechanical Ventilation Protocols, Protocol 9-5, Protocol 9-6, and Protocol 9-7).

CASE STUDY

Transient Tachypnea of the Newborn

Admitting History and Physical Examination

A 27-year-old woman in the thirty-fifth week of her second pregnancy awakened at 2 AM with sudden lower abdominal pain and some bleeding. She had no contractions at the time. She woke her husband, who in turn called the obstetrician. The doctor instructed him to bring his wife to the hospital. On arrival at the hospital, she was immediately taken to the labor and delivery room. The nurse on duty placed an oxygen mask on the patient's face and started an intravenous (IV) line. The patient's vital signs were monitored closely. An ultrasound Doppler belt also was placed around the mother's lower abdominal area to monitor the baby's heart rate. Over the next 20 minutes, the mother continued to bleed (saturating two pads with numerous blood clots), her blood pressure fell, and her heart rate increased. The baby's heart rate had increased from 155/min to 170/min.

The obstetrician called the operating room and asked the staff to prepare for an emergency cesarean section. The doctor also called for the neonatal resuscitation team (which consisted of a neonatologist, nurse, and respiratory therapist) and asked that they be on standby. The cesarean section was uneventful. The baby was a 7-pound girl. The neonatologist assessed the baby and gave a 1-minute Apgar score of 8 (2 heart rate, 2 respiratory rate, 1 tone, 1 reflex irritability, and 2 skin color). The baby, however, was clearly having difficulty breathing. Auscultation revealed mild bilateral rhonchi and crackles. The baby was transferred to the neonatal intensive care unit (NICU).

In the NICU, the baby was placed in a warmed isolette, and an umbilical artery catheter was inserted. An IV line and nasogastric tube also were inserted. Warm, humidified oxygen was started via a high-flow nasal cannula (HFNC)* at 4 L/min and an F_{IO_2} of 0.5. Ten minutes later the infant's vital signs were as follows: heart rate 155 bpm, blood pressure 75/40, and respiratory rate 75/min. The infant's ventilatory pattern was described by the neonatologist as fast and shallow. In other words, even though the infant was breathing fast and not very deeply, she did not appear to be working hard to breathe. She had no intercostal retractions or nasal flaring at this time. Arterial blood gas values were as follows: pH 7.33, Pa_{CO_2} 31, HCO_3^- 21, and Pa_{O_2} 42. The baby's Sp_{O_2} was 75%.

About 2 hours later, however, the baby started to show signs of distress. Her vital signs were as follows: heart rate 170 bpm, blood pressure 75/45, and respiratory rate 110/min. She demonstrated abdominal movements and nasal flaring. Her skin appeared pale and blue. Auscultation revealed moderate to severe bilateral rhonchi and crackles. On the same HFNC settings (4 L/min and an F_{IO_2} of 0.5), her Sp_{O_2} was 58%. Arterial blood gas values were as follows: pH 7.52, Pa_{CO_2} 28, HCO_3^- 22, and Pa_{O_2} 35.

*Also called high-humidity nasal cannula (HHNC).

A chest x-ray film showed areas of infiltrates and microatelectasis throughout both lung fields, as well as prominent white-lined lung fissures (indicating fluid in the fissures). A starburst pattern was seen at the hilum of the lungs (indicating increased lymphatic fluid). The chest x-ray film also showed air trapping and hyperinflation in the lower lobes (indicating fluid in the airways). The infant's diaphragms were flattened. The neonatologist charted a diagnosis of TTN in the baby's progress notes. The doctor also stated that he did not want to mechanically ventilate the baby at this time. The respiratory therapist entered the following assessment in the baby's chart.

Respiratory Assessment and Treatment Plan

S N/A

O Vital signs: HR 170/min, BP 75/45, and RR 110/min. Chest retractions, nasal flaring. Skin pale and blue. Moderate to severe bilateral rhonchi and crackles. CXR: Infiltrates and microatelectasis over both lungs, generalized hyperinflation. ABGs on HFNC at 4 L/min and F_{IO_2} 0.50: pH 7.52, Pa_{CO_2} 28, HCO_3^- 22, Pa_{O_2} 35, Sp_{O_2} 58%.

A
- TTN (neonatologist, CXR, history)
- Infiltrates and atelectasis (CXR film)
- Air trapping (CXR film)
- Excessive bronchial secretions (rhonchi and crackles)
- Acute alveolar hyperventilation with severe hypoxemia (ABGs)

P **Lung Expansion Therapy Protocol** (nasal CPAP at +2 cm H_2O). Increase **Oxygen Therapy Protocol** (F_{IO_2} 0.60 via CPAP at +2 cm H_2O setup). **Bronchopulmonary Hygiene Therapy Protocol** (CPT q2h). Continue to monitor closely.

Over the next 48 hours, the baby's condition progressively improved. She no longer required oxygen therapy, and her breath sounds were normal. Her last room air arterial blood gas values showed a pH of 7.38, Pa_{CO_2} 39, HCO_3^- 24, Pa_{O_2} 73, and Sa_{O_2} 94%. Her chest x-ray film was normal. The baby was discharged the next day.

Discussion

This case reinforces the importance of observation and inspection in the assessment process. The respiratory care practitioner must continuously inspect and analyze infants with TTN. This baby, for example, born at 35 weeks, may have had respiratory distress syndrome (RDS; see Chapter 34), but the clinical symptoms ruled out the diagnosis. For example, babies with RDS have alveolar collapse and consolidation, whereas babies with TTN have airway trapping and alveolar hyperinflation. In addition, babies with RDS generally breathe hard, quickly, and deeply, whereas infants with TTN usually breathe rapidly and shallowly. In fact, this rapid and shallow breathing pattern often is considered a hallmark of TTN. Certainly, the rapid shallow breathing seen in this baby was caused, in part, by the **Increased Alveolar-Capillary Membrane Thickness** (Figure 9-10)—and decreased lung compliance—associated with TTN.

Although apnea may occur in these babies, it is not common. Therapeutically, most do quite well with just oxygen via an HFNC. Occasionally, nasal continuous positive airway pressure (CPAP) may be used. Caution, however, must be taken not to give the baby too much CPAP. The lungs of these babies are usually already hyperinflated. Too much CPAP expands the baby's lungs even more and may cause a tension pneumothorax. CPAP at +3 to +4 cm H_2O is usually safe. Mechanical ventilation rarely is needed for babies with TTN.

SELF-ASSESSMENT QUESTIONS

evolve Answers to questions can be found on Evolve. To access additional student assessment questions and case studies for application of text material to real-life scenarios, visit **http://evolve.elsevier.com/DesJardins/respiratory.**

1. Which of the following is or are associated with TTN?

1. Rapid and shallow breathing pattern
2. PPHN
3. Clinical signs similar to those of infant respiratory distress syndrome
4. Reduced Do_2
   a. 1 and 3 only
   b. 2 and 4 only
   c. 2, 3, and 4 only
   d. 1, 2, 3, and 4

2. The clinical manifestations associated with TTN usually disappear within:

a. 10 to 24 hours after birth
b. 24 to 48 hours after birth
c. 48 to 72 hours after birth
d. 2 weeks after birth

3. Which of the following is the hallmark clinical manifestation of TTN?

a. PPHN
b. Rapid and shallow breathing pattern
c. Substernal retraction and abdominal distention (seesaw movement)
d. Expiratory grunting

4. Which of the following pulmonary function testing findings is or are associated with TTN?

1. Normal or decreased FEV_T
2. Normal or increased FEV_1/FVC ratio
3. Normal or decreased $FEF_{25\%-75\%}$
4. Normal or increased PEFR
   a. 1 and 3 only
   b. 2 and 4 only
   c. 1, 2, and 3 only
   d. 1, 2, 3, and 4

5. Which of the following is or are the major anatomic alterations of the lungs associated with TTN?

1. Consolidation
2. Bronchospasm
3. Increased alveolar-capillary membrane thickness
4. Atelectasis
5. Excessive bronchial secretions
   a. 3 and 5 only
   b. 2 and 4 only
   c. 3, 4, and 5 only
   d. 1, 3, 4, and 5 only

Respiratory Distress Syndrome

34

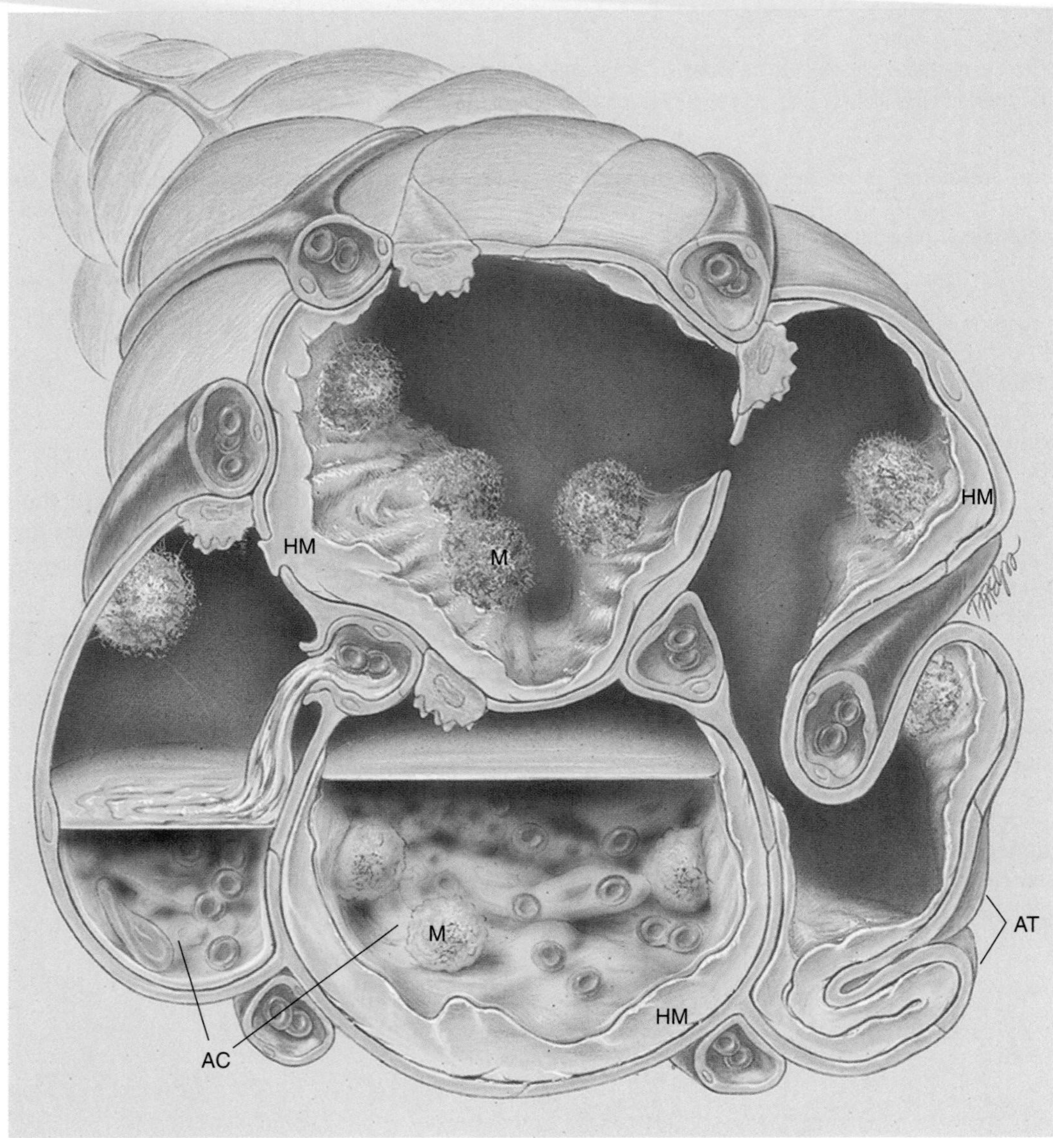

FIGURE 34-1 Respiratory distress syndrome. Cross-sectional view of alveoli in infant respiratory distress syndrome. *AC,* Alveolar consolidation; *AT,* atelectasis; *HM,* hyaline membrane; *M,* macrophage.

Chapter Objectives

After reading this chapter, you will be able to:

- List the anatomic alterations of the lungs associated with respiratory distress syndrome.
- Describe the causes of respiratory distress syndrome.
- List the cardiopulmonary clinical manifestations associated with respiratory distress syndrome.
- Describe the general management of respiratory distress syndrome.
- Describe the clinical strategies and rationales of the SOAP presented in the case study.
- Define key terms and complete self-assessment questions at the end of the chapter and on Evolve.

Key Terms

Alveolar Type II Cells (Granular Pneumocytes)
Beractant (Survanta)
Calfactant (Infasurf)
Continuous Positive Airway Pressure (CPAP)
Ground-Glass Appearance (Chest Radiograph)
Hard, Fast, and Deep Breathing Pattern
Hyaline Membrane Disease
Idiopathic Respiratory Distress Syndrome
Infant Respiratory Distress Syndrome
Lecithin/Sphingomyelin Ratio (L : S Ratio)
Neonatal Respiratory Distress Syndrome
Phosphatidylglycerol (PG)
Poractant Alfa (Curosurf)
Pulmonary Hyperperfusion
Pulmonary Hypoperfusion
Respiratory Distress Syndrome of the Newborn
Surfactant/Albumin Ratio (S : A Ratio)
Transient Pulmonary Hypertension
Volutrauma

Chapter Outline

Respiratory distress syndrome (RDS) is the most common cause of respiratory failure in the preterm infant. Over the past several decades, a number of names have been used to identify infants with RDS (Box 34-1). A common thread running through most of the names is the term "respiratory distress," which characterizes an immature lung disorder in a preterm infant caused by inadequate pulmonary surfactant. RDS is a major cause of morbidity and mortality in the premature infant born after less than 37 weeks' gestation. The introduction of exogenous surfactant therapy has greatly improved the clinical course of this disorder and reduced the morbidity and mortality rates.

Anatomic Alterations of the Lungs

On gross examination, the lungs of an infant with RDS are dark red and liver-like. Under the microscope the lungs appear solid because of countless areas of alveolar collapse. The pulmonary capillaries are congested, and the lymphatic vessels are distended. Extensive interstitial and intraalveolar edema and hemorrhage are evident.

In what appears to be an effort to offset alveolar collapse, the respiratory bronchioles, alveolar ducts, and some alveoli dilate. As the disease intensifies, the alveolar walls become lined with a dense, rippled **hyaline membrane** identical to the hyaline membrane that develops in acute respiratory distress syndrome (ARDS) of the adult patient (see Chapter 27). The membrane contains fibrin and cellular debris.

During the later stages of the disease, leukocytes are present, and the hyaline membrane is often fragmented and partially ingested by macrophages. Type II cells begin to proliferate, and secretions begin to accumulate in the tracheobronchial tree. The anatomic alterations in RDS produce a restrictive type of lung disorder (see Figure 34-1).

As a consequence of the anatomic alterations associated with RDS, babies with this disorder often develop hypoxia-induced pulmonary arterial vasoconstriction and vasospasm, causing a state of **transient pulmonary hypertension.** This results in blood shunting from right to left through the ductus arteriosus and foramen ovale. Occasionally, intrapulmonary shunting may also occur. As a consequence, the blood flow is diverted away from the lungs **(pulmonary hypoperfusion),** which worsens the hypoxemia. It should be noted that if this condition does not resolve within 24 hours or so, shunting will begin to flow from left to right through the patent ductus arteriosus. This condition can lead to excessive lung fluid, **pulmonary hyperperfusion,** and pulmonary edema.

The major pathologic or structural changes associated with RDS are as follows:

- Interstitial and alveolar edema and hemorrhage
- Alveolar consolidation
- Intraalveolar hyaline membrane
- Pulmonary surfactant deficiency or qualitative abnormality
- Atelectasis
- Hypoxia-induced vasospasm and vasoconstriction:
    - Transient pulmonary hypertension
    - Right-to-left shunting
    - Left-to-right shunting in cases lasting longer than 24 hours
    - Worsening hypoxia
- Hyperperfusion (in cases lasting longer than 24 hours; leads to excessive lung fluid and pulmonary edema)

Box 34-1 Names Used to Identify Respiratory Distress Syndrome

- Infant respiratory distress syndrome
- Idiopathic respiratory distress syndrome
- Neonatal respiratory distress syndrome
- Respiratory distress syndrome of the newborn
- Hyaline membrane disease

Etiology and Epidemiology

Although the exact cause of RDS is controversial, the most popular theory suggests that the early stages of RDS develop as a result of (1) a pulmonary surfactant abnormality or defi-

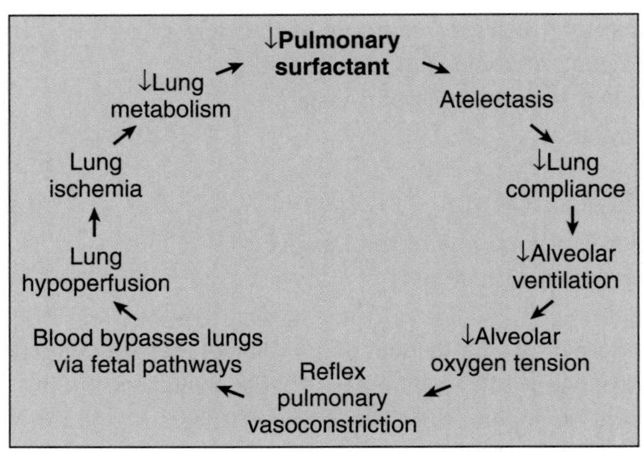

FIGURE 34-2 Early stages of respiratory distress syndrome.

ciency, and (2) pulmonary hypoperfusion evoked by hypoxia. The pulmonary hypoperfusion evoked by hypoxia is probably a secondary response to the surfactant abnormality. The probable sequence of steps in the development of RDS is as follows:

1. Because of the pulmonary surfactant abnormality, alveolar compliance decreases, resulting in alveolar collapse.
2. The pulmonary atelectasis causes the infant's work of breathing to increase.
3. Alveolar ventilation decreases in response to the decreased lung compliance and infant fatigue, causing the alveolar oxygen tension (P_{AO_2}) to decrease.
4. The decreased P_{AO_2} (alveolar hypoxia) stimulates a reflex pulmonary vasoconstriction.
5. Because of the pulmonary vasoconstriction, blood bypasses the infant's lungs through fetal pathways—the patent ductus and the foramen ovale.
6. The lung hypoperfusion in turn causes lung ischemia and decreased lung metabolism.
7. Because of the decreased lung metabolism, the production of pulmonary surfactant is reduced even further, and a vicious cycle develops (Figure 34-2).

It is estimated that approximately 30,000 cases of RDS occur annually in the United States. RDS is the leading cause of death in preterm infants. About 50% of the neonates born at 26 to 28 weeks' gestation develop RDS. About 25% of the babies born at 30 to 31 weeks' gestation develop RDS. RDS occurs more often in male babies and is usually more severe than in female babies. The higher incidence and severity of RDS in male infants is explained by the increased circulating androgens in males—which, in turn, slows the maturation of the infant's lung. The delayed lung maturation results in immature **alveolar type II cells (granular pneumocytes)** and a decreased pulmonary surfactant production.

RDS is also more commonly seen in infants of diabetic mothers (the high fetal insulin levels decrease lung surfactant and structural maturation), white preterm babies compared with black preterm infants, and infants delivered by cesarean. RDS is also associated with low birth weight (1000 to 1500 g), multiple births, prenatal asphyxia, prolonged labor, maternal bleeding, and second-born twins.

Diagnosis

There are three primary tests that can be performed to determine the lung maturity of the fetus: the **lecithin/sphingomyelin ratio,** the presence of **phosphatidylglycerol (PG),** and, more recently, the **surfactant/albumin ratio.**

The lecithin/sphingomyelin ratio (L : S ratio) is commonly used to test lung maturity. Lecithin, also called *dipalmitoyl phosphatidylcholine,* is the most abundant phospholipid found in surfactant. When the concentration of lecithin is two times greater than that of sphingomyelin—an L : S ratio of 2 : 1—the infant's lung maturity is likely great enough that the lungs will produce adequate pulmonary surfactant at birth. Most infants with an L : S ratio less than 1 : 1 develop RDS. The L : S ratio is not reliable in pregnancies associated with diabetes and Rh isoimmunization.

PG is the second most abundant phospholipid found in surfactant. Because the PG level normally increases toward term, the presence of PG in the amniotic fluid indicates a low risk for RDS. When the amniotic fluid reveals an L : S ratio less than 2 : 1 and a lack of PG, the infant has more than an 80% risk for the development of RDS. However, when the amniotic fluid shows an L : S greater than 2 : 1 and when PG is present, the risk drops to almost zero.

The surfactant/albumin ratio (S : A ratio) is reported as milligrams of surfactant per gram of protein. An S : A ratio <35 indicates immature lungs. An S : A ratio of 35 to 55 indicates uncertain lung maturity. When the S : A ratio is >55, adequate lung maturity is present.

OVERVIEW of the Cardiopulmonary Clinical Manifestations Associated with Respiratory Distress Syndrome

The following clinical manifestations result from the pathologic mechanisms caused (or activated) by **Atelectasis** (see Figure 9-8), **Alveolar Consolidation** (see Figure 9-9), and **Increased Alveolar-Capillary Membrane Thickness** (see Figure 9-10)—the major anatomic alterations of the lungs associated with respiratory distress syndrome (RDS) (see Figure 34-1).

CLINICAL DATA OBTAINED AT THE PATIENT'S BEDSIDE

The Physical Examination

Vital Signs

Increased Respiratory Rate (Tachypnea)

Normally, a newborn infant's respiratory rate is about 40 to 60 breaths per minute. During the early stages of RDS, the respiratory rate is generally well over 60 breaths per minute. The respiratory pattern of the baby with RDS commonly is described as **"hard, fast, and deep breathing."** Several pathophysiologic mechanisms operating simultaneously may lead to an increased ventilatory rate:

- Stimulation of peripheral chemoreceptors (hypoxemia)
- Decreased lung compliance–increased ventilatory rate relationship
- Stimulation of central chemoreceptors

Increased Heart Rate (Pulse) and Blood Pressure

Apnea (See Table 31-1)

Clinical Manifestations Associated with More Negative Intrapleural Pressures during Inspiration

- Intercostal retractions
- Substernal retraction and abdominal distention (seesaw movement)
- Cyanosis of the dependent portions of the thoracic and abdominal areas
- Flaring nostrils

Chest Assessment Findings

- Bronchial (or harsh) breath sounds
- Fine crackles

Expiratory grunting

Cyanosis

CLINICAL DATA OBTAINED FROM LABORATORY TESTS AND SPECIAL PROCEDURES

Pulmonary Function Test Findings (Extrapolated Data for Instructional Purposes) (Restrictive Lung Pathophysiology)

FORCED EXPIRATORY FLOW RATE FINDINGS

FVC	FEV_T	FEV_1/FVC ratio	$FEF_{25\%-75\%}$
↓	N or ↓	N or ↑	N or ↓

$FEF_{50\%}$	$FEF_{200-1200}$	PEFR	MVV
N or ↓	N or ↓	N or ↓	N or ↓

LUNG VOLUME AND CAPACITY FINDINGS

V_T	IRV	ERV	RV
N or ↓	↓	↓	↓

VC	IC	FRC	TLC	RV/TLC ratio
↓	↓	↓	↓	N

Arterial Blood Gases

MILD TO MODERATE RESPIRATORY DISTRESS SYNDROME

Acute Alveolar Hyperventilation with Hypoxemia

(Acute Respiratory Alkalosis)

pH	$Paco_2$	HCO_3^-	Pao_2
↑	↓	↓ (slightly)	↓

SEVERE RESPIRATORY DISTRESS SYNDROME

Acute Ventilatory Failure with Hypoxemia

(Acute Respiratory Acidosis)

pH*	$Paco_2$	HCO_3^- *	Pao_2
↓	↑	↑ (slightly)	↓

*When tissue hypoxia is severe enough to produce lactic acid, the pH and HCO_3^- values will be lower than expected for a particular $Paco_2$ level.

Oxygenation Indices*

$\dot{Q}_S/\dot{Q}_T$	Do_2†	$\dot{V}o_2$	$C(a-\bar{v})o_2$	O_2ER	$S\bar{v}o_2$
↑	↓	N	N	↑	↓

†The Do_2 may be normal in patients who have compensated to the decreased oxygenation status with (1) an increased cardiac output, (2) an increased hemoglobin level, or (3) a combination of both. When the Do_2 is normal, the O_2ER is usually normal.

RADIOLOGIC FINDINGS

Chest Radiograph

- Increased opacity (ground-glass appearance)

On chest x-ray film of infants with RDS, the air-filled tracheobronchial tree typically stands out against a dense

*$C(a-\bar{v})o_2$, Arterial-venous oxygen difference; Do_2, total oxygen delivery; O_2ER, oxygen extraction ratio; $\dot{Q}_S/\dot{Q}_T$, pulmonary shunt fraction; $S\bar{v}o_2$, mixed venous oxygen saturation; $\dot{V}o_2$, oxygen consumption.

OVERVIEW of the Cardiopulmonary Clinical Manifestations Associated with Respiratory Distress Syndrome—cont'd

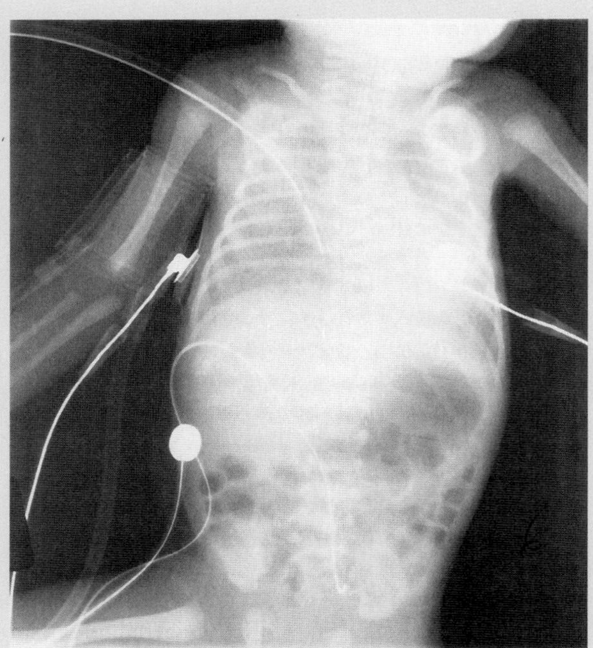

FIGURE 34-3 Whole body x-ray film of an infant with respiratory distress syndrome. Note the "whiteout," particularly of the left lower and right upper lobes.

opaque (or white) lung. This white density is often described as having a fine **ground-glass appearance** throughout the lung fields. Because of the pathologic processes, the density of the lungs is increased. Increased lung density resists x-ray penetration and is revealed on the x-ray film as increased opacity. Therefore the more severe the RDS, the whiter the x-ray image (Figure 34-3).

General Management of Respiratory Distress Syndrome

During the early stages of RDS, **continuous positive airway pressure (CPAP)** is the treatment of choice. Mechanical ventilation usually is avoided as long as possible. CPAP generally works well with these patients because it (1) increases the functional residual capacity, (2) decreases the work of breathing, and (3) works to increase the Pa_{O_2} through alveolar recruitment while the infant is receiving a lower inspired concentration of oxygen. **A Pa_{O_2} of 40 to 70 mm Hg is normal for newborn infants.** No effort should be made to get an infant's Pa_{O_2} within the normal adult range (80 to 100 mm Hg). Special attention should be given to the thermal environment of the infant with RDS because the infant's oxygenation can be further compromised if the body temperature is above or below normal.

Finally, because of the decreased pulmonary surfactant associated with RDS, the administration of exogenous surfactant preparations such as **beractant (Survanta), calfactant (Infasurf),** and **poractant alfa (Curosurf)** is helpful. The term *exogenous,* used to describe these artificial surfactant agents, indicates that these preparations are from outside the patient's body. Exogenous surfactant preparations originate from other humans, from animals, or from laboratory synthesis. These agents replace the missing pulmonary surfactant of the premature or immature lungs of the baby with

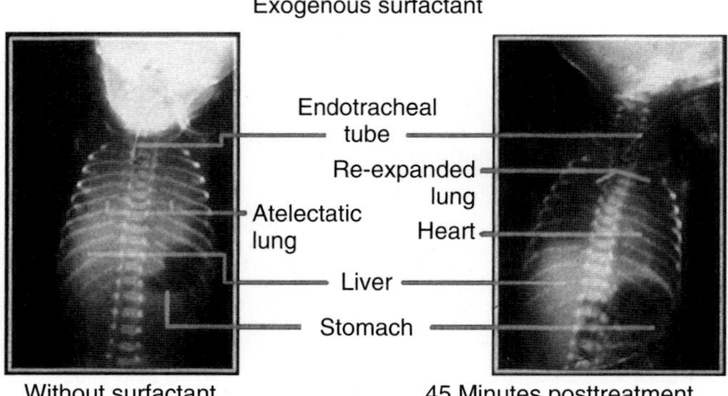

FIGURE 34-4 Chest x-ray films of an infant with respiratory distress syndrome before and after exogenous surfactant treatments.

RDS until the lungs are mature enough to provide adequate pulmonary surfactant. Figure 34-4 provides comparison chest radiographs of an infant without exogenous surfactant and the same infant 45 minutes after treatment.

Respiratory Care Treatment Protocols

Oxygen Therapy Protocol

Oxygen therapy is used to treat hypoxemia, decrease the work of breathing, and decrease myocardial work. Because of the hypoxemia that often develops in RDS, supplemental oxygen is usually required (see Oxygen Therapy Protocol, Protocol 9-1).

Lung Expansion Therapy Protocol

Lung expansion measures commonly are performed to offset the pulmonary capillary congestion and interstitial edema and atelectasis associated with RDS (see Lung Expansion Therapy Protocol, Protocol 9-3).

Mechanical Ventilation Protocol

Mechanical ventilation may be necessary to provide and support alveolar gas exchange and eventually return the patient to spontaneous breathing. (See Mechanical Ventilation Protocols, Protocol 9-5, Protocol 9-6, and Protocol 9-7).

CASE STUDY

Respiratory Distress Syndrome

Admitting History and Physical Examination

A premature male infant was delivered after 30 weeks' gestation. The mother was a 19-year-old, unmarried primigravida patient who claimed to be in good health during the entire pregnancy until 6 hours before admission. At that time, she noticed the onset of painless vaginal bleeding. She called her obstetrician, who told her he would meet her in the emergency department of the medical center.

On examination she was found to be a healthy young woman, approximately 30 weeks pregnant, in early labor, and bleeding slightly from the vagina. Her vital signs were stable and within normal limits. A diagnosis of premature separation of the placenta was made. Because bleeding was minimal and both mother and fetus seemed to be doing well, it was decided to deliver the baby vaginally. She was monitored very closely, and labor progressed satisfactorily for about 8 hours, at which time she delivered the infant under epidural anesthesia without any obstetric complications. The baby weighed 2100 g. The Apgar scores were 7 after 1 minute and 9 after 5 minutes. Physical examination findings were entirely normal for an infant of this size.

On admission to the newborn nursery 30 minutes after delivery, the infant was noted to have some moderate respiratory distress. His respiratory rate was 40/min. There was flaring of the nostrils. A chest x-ray film obtained at this time suggested the presence of left upper lobe atelectasis, but no other pulmonary abnormality was noted.

During the next 5 hours, the infant deteriorated rapidly and the respiratory distress became markedly accentuated. The baby was cyanotic, retracting, and using the accessory muscles of respiration. The respiratory rate was 64/min, and respirations were described as "grunting." His heart rate was 165 bpm. Crackles were heard bilaterally. A chest x-ray film taken at this time revealed generalized haziness that one radiologist described as "ground glass." Arterial blood gases on an F_{IO_2} of 0.30 via an oxygen hood were pH 7.25, Pa_{CO_2} 52, HCO_3^- 21, and Pa_{O_2} 35. The Sa_{O_2} was 60%. At this time, the respiratory therapist working with the baby recorded the following assessment and plan.

Respiratory Assessment and Plan

S N/A (newborn)

O Dyspneic and cyanotic. Retracting and using accessory muscles. Flaring of nostrils. RR 64 with "grunting." HR 165. Bilateral crackles. CXR: Bilateral "ground-glass" haziness. ABGs on 30% O_2: pH 7.25, Pa_{CO_2} 52, HCO_3^- 21, Pa_{O_2} 35, and Sa_{O_2} 60%.

A
- **Infant respiratory distress syndrome** (history)
- Alveolar hyaline membrane, atelectasis (CXR)
- Acute ventilatory failure with severe hypoxemia (ABGs)
  - Lactic acidosis likely (pH and HCO_3^- lower than expected)

P **Mechanical Ventilation Protocol:** Intubate, ventilate, positive end-expiratory pressure (PEEP) per neonatal intensive care unit (NICU) protocol. **Oxygen Therapy Protocol:** Continuous transcutaneous oximetry. Exogenous surfactant per protocol.

The baby was intubated by the therapist and put on a ventilator. The initial ventilator settings were respiratory rate (RR) of 40, inspiratory time (TI) 0.35, F_{IO_2} 0.40, positive inspiratory pressure (PIP) +25 cm H_2O, positive end-expiratory pressure (PEEP) +5 cm H_2O, and flow 8 L/min. Artificial surfactant (Exosurf) therapy was begun. Fluid and electrolyte balance was maintained within normal levels. On this management the baby was weaned from PEEP in 72 hours, and from artificial ventilation in 96 hours. Chest x-ray examination on the seventh day was unremarkable. The baby was discharged on the fifteenth day and has been healthy ever since.

Discussion

RDS is a fascinating disorder in which meticulous respiratory care of the infant is crucial. Most respiratory therapy students greatly look forward to and enjoy their NICU rotation. In these units the expertise of the respiratory care practitioner is crucial to the functioning of the unit because the majority of patients there have respiratory disorders. Indeed, many of the first reports of therapist-driven protocols came from this setting.

Many of the clinical manifestations seen in this case are associated with **Atelectasis** (see Figure 9-8) and **Increased Alveolar-Capillary Membrane Thickness** (see Figure 9-10). For example, the use of accessory muscles of inspiration was likely a compensatory mechanism activated to offset the increased stiffness of the lungs (decreased lung compliance) caused by the atelectasis and alveolar hyaline membrane. The atelectasis and alveolar hyaline membrane were objectively verified by the chest x-ray film. In addition, the severity level of the anatomic alterations and clinical manifestations seen in this case was very high. This was objectively confirmed by the arterial blood gas analysis that identified the acute ventilatory failure with severe hypoxemia.

Thus the aggressive implementation of mechanical ventilation and use of artificial surfactant were certainly justified. Neonatal intensive care units usually are staffed by an in-house neonatologist, who can guide the respiratory therapist through the intricacies of therapy. Artificial surfactant has markedly improved the outlook for these infants. However, the respiratory care practitioner should be on the alert for sudden changes in lung compliance that often occurs shortly after the administration of artificial surfactant. If the infant is on a pressure-cycled ventilator, this is especially important to avoid **volutrauma.*** As in adults with ARDS, in which the pathology is very similar, constant attention must be given to the possibility of nosocomial infection, fluid overload, and cardiovascular instability. In addition, lung protection strategies such as PEEP, permissive hypercapnia, and use of small ventilator tidal volumes are commonly used in RDS cases.

*Volutrauma is defined as damage to the lung caused by overdistention by a mechanical ventilator set for an excessively high tidal volume.

SELF-ASSESSMENT QUESTIONS

evolve Answers to questions can be found on Evolve. To access additional student assessment questions and case studies for application of text material to real-life scenarios, visit **http://evolve.elsevier.com/DesJardins/respiratory.**

1. When transient pulmonary hypertension exists in RDS, blood bypasses the infant's lungs through which of the following structures?

1. Ductus venosus
2. Umbilical vein
3. Ductus arteriosus
4. Foramen ovale
   a. 1 and 2 only
   b. 1 and 3 only
   c. 2 and 3 only
   d. 3 and 4 only

2. It is suggested that RDS is a result of which of the following?

1. Vernix membrane
2. Decreased perfusion of the lungs
3. Pulmonary surfactant abnormality
4. Congenital alveolar dysplasia
   a. 1 and 3 only
   b. 2 and 3 only
   c. 1 and 4 only
   d. 2, 3, and 4 only

3. When an infant with RDS creates more negative intrapleural pressure during inspiration, which of the following occur(s)?

1. The soft tissue between the ribs bulges outward.
2. The substernal area protrudes.
3. The abdominal area retracts.
4. The dependent blood vessels dilate and pool blood.
   a. 2 only
   b. 4 only
   c. 2 and 3 only
   d. 1, 3, and 4 only

4. Infants with severe RDS often have which of the following?

1. Diminished breath sounds
2. Bronchial breath sounds
3. Hyperresonant percussion notes
4. Fine crackles
   a. 1 and 4 only
   b. 3 and 4 only
   c. 2 and 3 only
   d. 2 and 4 only

5. Continuous positive airway pressure (CPAP) often is administered to infants with RDS in an effort to do which of the following?

1. Increase the infant's FRC
2. Decrease the infant's work of breathing
3. Increase the infant's Pa_{O_2}
4. Decrease the F_{IO_2} necessary to oxygenate the infant
   a. 1 and 3 only
   b. 2 and 4 only
   c. 2, 3, and 4 only
   d. 1, 2, 3, and 4

Pulmonary Air Leak Syndromes

35

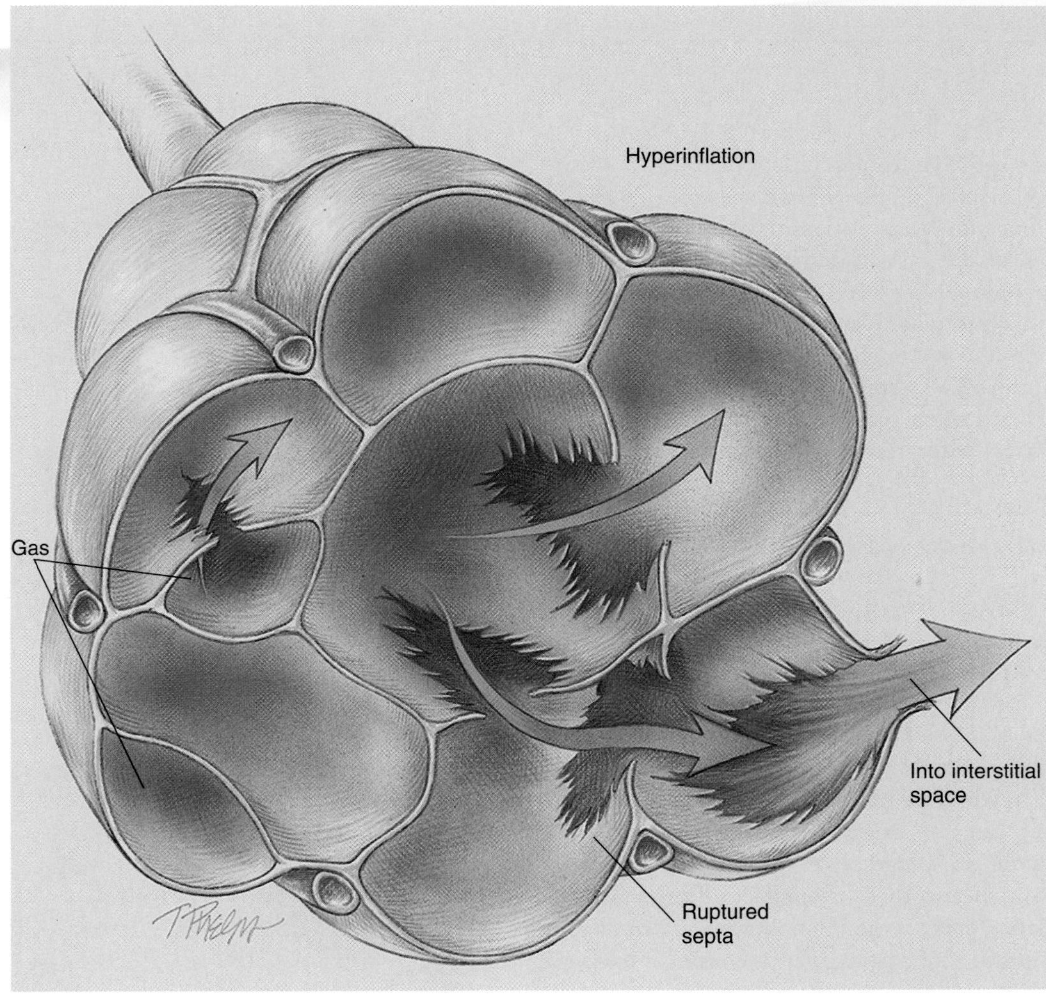

FIGURE 35-1 Pulmonary air leak syndromes.

Chapter Objectives

By the end of this chapter, the reader will be able to:

- List the anatomic alterations of the lungs associated with pulmonary air leak syndrome.
- Describe the causes of pulmonary air leak syndrome.
- List the cardiopulmonary clinical manifestations associated with pulmonary air leak syndrome.
- Describe the general management of pulmonary air leak syndrome.
- Describe the clinical strategies and rationales of the SOAP presented in the case study.
- Define key terms and complete self-assessment questions at the end of the chapter and on Evolve.

Key Terms

Air Embolism
Blebs (Emphysema-Like)
Bronchopulmonary Dysplasia
High-Frequency Ventilation
High Levels of Positive End-Expiratory Pressure (PEEP)
Iatrogenic Pneumathorax
Peak Inspiratory Pressures (PIPs)
Pneumomediastinum
Pneumopericardium
Pneumoperitoneum
Pneumothorax
Point of Maximum Impulse (PMI)

Prolonged Inspiratory Times (ITs)
Pulmonary Air Leak Syndromes
Pulmonary Interstitial Emphysema (PIE)
Subcutaneous Emphysema
Syndrome of Inappropriate Antidiuretic Hormone (SIADH)
Transillumination of the Chest

Chapter Outline

Pulmonary air leak syndromes (also called *air block syndromes*) in the infant comprise a large spectrum of clinical entities, including **pulmonary interstitial emphysema (PIE),** followed by, in severe cases, **pneumomediastinum, pneumothorax, pneumopericardium, pneumoperitoneum,** and, in rare cases, **intravascular air embolism.** Pulmonary air leak syndromes are common complications of mechanical ventilation in premature infants, especially when very high pressures are used. They are often seen in infants being treated for respiratory distress syndrome (see Chapter 34).

Anatomic Alterations of the Lungs

Pulmonary Interstitial Emphysema

Virtually all pulmonary air leak syndromes begin with some degree of PIE. When high airway pressures are applied to an infant's lungs (e.g., during mechanical ventilation), the distal airways and alveoli often become overdistended—that is, they develop bleb or emphysema-like areas—and rupture (see Figure 35-1). In addition, gas trapping from an insufficient expiratory time can also cause alveolar overdistention and rupture. Once the gas escapes, it is forced into (1) the loose connective tissue sheaths that surround the airways and pulmonary capillaries, and (2) the interlobular septa containing pulmonary veins. In severe cases, the gas continues to spread peripherally by dissecting along the peribronchial and perivascular spaces to the hilum of the lung, producing the classic radiographic appearance of PIE that shows bubbles of air in the interstitial cuffs (Figure 35-2 and Figure 35-3).

The overdistention associated with PIE forces the lungs into a full inflation position and thereby decreases lung compliance (remember that static lung compliance is reduced at *both* very low and very high lung volumes). Moreover, air trapped within the interstitial cuffs compresses the airways and increases airway resistance. In addition, the trapped air in the interstitial spaces impairs lymphatic function, resulting in fluid accumulation in the interstitial cuffs and alveoli. Once the interstitial gas reaches the hilum of the lung, it either (1) coalesces to form large hilar blebs, or (2) tracks beneath the visceral pleura to form large subpleural pockets of air. In either case, the accumulation of gas can be large enough to significantly compress the lung or mediastinal structures.

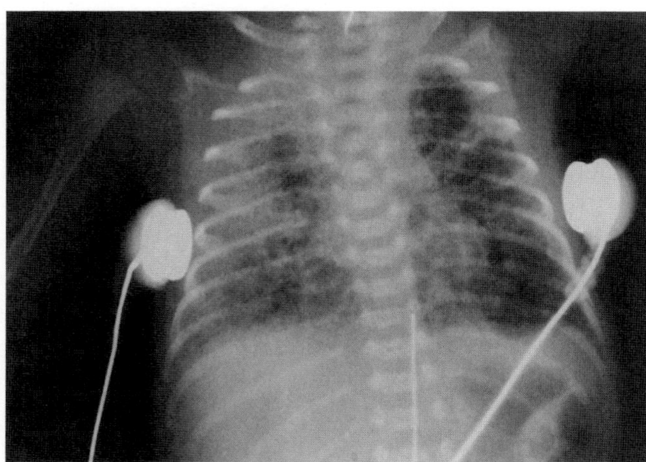

FIGURE 35-2 Pulmonary interstitial emphysema (PIE). Fine, bubbly appearance of the lungs in an infant with severe respiratory distress syndrome (RDS). (From Taussig LM, Landau LI: *Pediatric respiratory medicine,* ed 2, St Louis, 2008, Elsevier.)

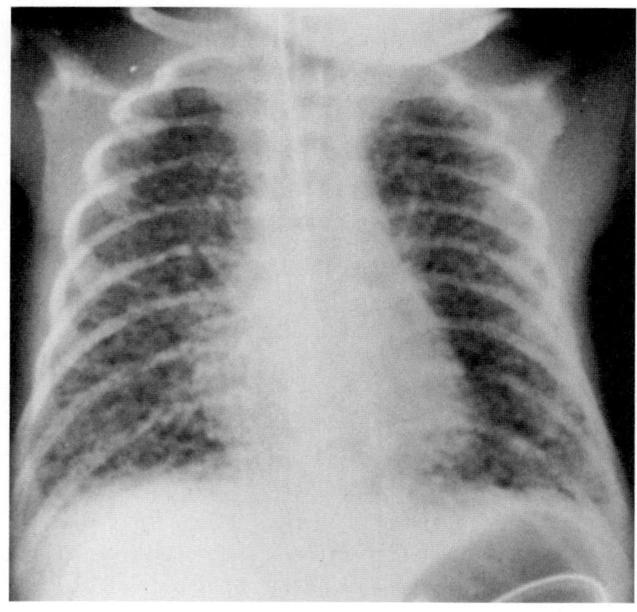

FIGURE 35-3 Pulmonary interstitial emphysema. The lung is grossly hyperinflated, with coarse radiolucencies extending from the pleura to the hilum. These radiolucencies represent bubbles of air in the perivascular and peribronchial interstitial cuffs. (From Taeusch WH, Ballard RA, Gleason CA: *Avery's diseases of the newborn,* ed 8, Philadelphia, 2005, Saunders.)

A pneumomediastinum may occur when the excessive air associated with a PIE continues to track—and accumulate—through the perivascular and peribronchial cuffs and causes the gas in the hilum area to rupture into the mediastinum. In addition, the high gas pressures associated with a pneumomediastinum may also dissect into the pleural space and the fascial planes of the neck and skin, resulting in the condition known as **subcutaneous emphysema.**

A pneumothorax may occur because of the alveolar overdistention and subsequent rupture commonly associated with a PIE (Figure 35-4). A pneumopericardium can develop from direct tracking of interstitial air along the great vessels into the pericardial sac (Figure 35-5). Gas pressure in the pericardium restricts atrial and ventricular filling, resulting in a decreased stroke volume and, ultimately, a reduced cardiac output and systemic hypotension. During the late stages, inflammatory changes of the airways lead to increased capillary leakage and excessive bronchial secretions.

A pneumoperitoneum may develop from the tracking of gas along the sheaths of the aorta and vena cava and eventually may burst into the peritoneal cavity. Clinically, the infant with a pneumoperitoneum manifests a sudden onset of abdominal distention. The pneumoperitoneum may be large enough to block the descent of the diaphragm and may require drainage. Finally, the excessive gas accumulation associated with a pneumoperitoneum may end up in the scrotum in male babies or the labia in females.

In very rare cases, an intravascular air embolism may be seen. It is hypothesized that the air is actually pumped under high pressure through the pulmonary lymphatics into the systemic venous circulation. Intravascular air causes an abrupt cardiovascular collapse and is frequently diagnosed when air is observed in vessels on chest radiographs taken to establish the cause of cardiovascular collapse.

The major pathologic changes associated with pulmonary air leak syndromes are as follows:

- Atelectasis, caused by the following:
    - Alveoli adjacent to overdistended alveoli (e.g., blebs or emphysema-like area)
    - Pneumothorax
    - Pneumomediastinum
    - Pneumoperitoneum
- Airway compression (caused by interstitial air accumulation)
- Excessive bronchial secretions (late stages)

Etiology and Epidemiology

Preterm infants who weigh less than 1000 g at birth have an increased risk for the early occurrence of pulmonary air leak syndromes (often within the first 24 to 48 hours of life), especially because of the weak noncartilaginous structures of their distal airways. The most frequent causative factor resulting in pulmonary air leak syndromes in preterm infants is the use of mechanical ventilation. Pulmonary air leak syndromes commonly result from the use of **high levels of positive end-expiratory pressure (PEEP)**, high peak inspiratory pressures (PIPs), and **prolonged inspiratory times (ITs).** Occasionally, full-term babies will develop a spontaneous tension pneumothorax.

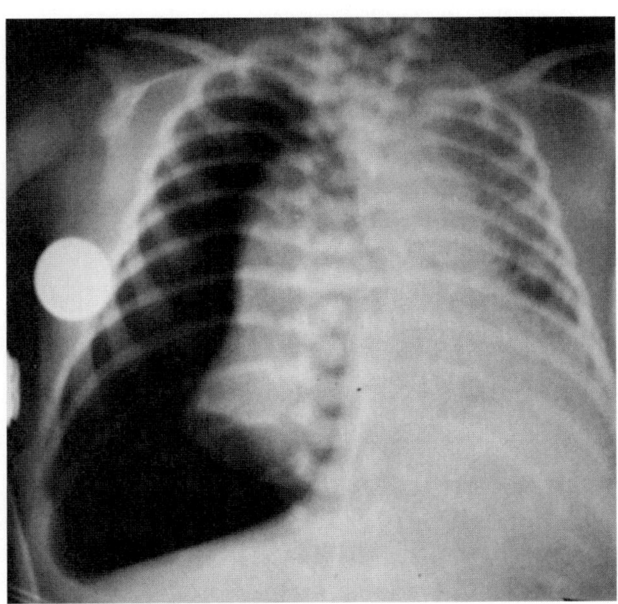

FIGURE 35-4 Tension pneumothorax. The lung on the involved (right) side is collapsed, and the mediastinum is shifted to the opposite side. Pleura can be seen bulging into the intercostal spaces. (From Taeusch WH, Ballard RA, Gleason CA: *Avery's diseases of the newborn,* ed 8, Philadelphia, 2005, Saunders.)

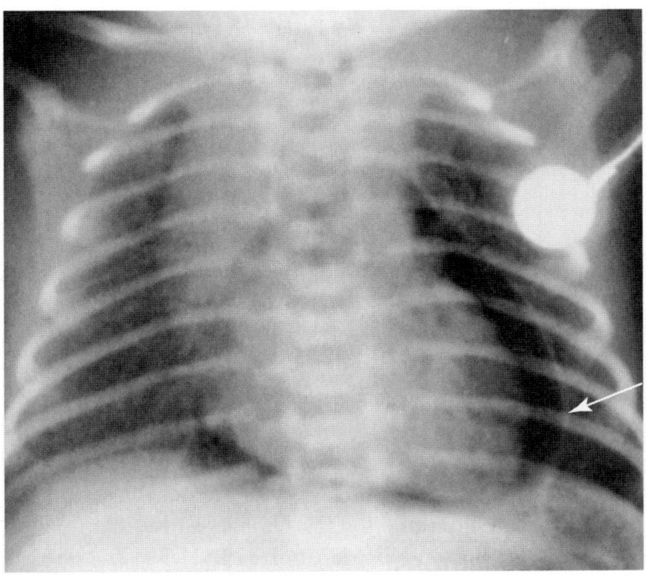

FIGURE 35-5 Pneumopericardium. A thin rim of pericardium (arrow) is visible and clearly separated from the heart by air within the pericardial sac. (From Taeusch WH, Ballard RA, Gleason CA: *Avery's diseases of the newborn,* ed 8, Philadelphia, 2005, Saunders.)

OVERVIEW of the Cardiopulmonary Clinical Manifestations Associated with Pulmonary Air Leak Syndromes

The following clinical manifestations result from the pathologic mechanisms caused (or activated) by **Atelectasis** (see Figure 9-8)—the major anatomic alteration of the lungs associated with pulmonary air leak syndromes (see Figure 35-1).

CLINICAL DATA OBTAINED AT THE PATIENT'S BEDSIDE

The Physical Examination

Vital Signs

Increased Respiratory Rate (Tachypnea)

Normally, a newborn's respiratory rate is about 40 to 60 breaths/min. During the early stages of pulmonary air leak syndromes, the respiratory rate generally is well over 60 breaths/min. Several pathophysiologic mechanisms operating simultaneously may lead to an increased ventilatory rate:

- Stimulation of peripheral chemoreceptors (hypoxemia)
- Decreased lung compliance–increased ventilatory rate relationship
- Stimulation of central chemoreceptors

Increased Heart Rate (Pulse) and Blood Pressure

Apnea (See Table 31-1)

Clinical Manifestations Associated with More Negative Intrapleural Pressures during Inspiration

- Intercostal retractions
- Substernal retraction and abdominal distention (seesaw movement)
- Cyanosis of the dependent portions of the thoracic and abdominal areas
- Flaring nostrils

Chest Assessment Findings

- Wheezes
- Rhonchi
- Crackles
- Change in **point of maximum impulse (PMI)**

The PMI is defined as the point at which the impulse of the left ventricle can be felt most strongly (normally over the fifth intercostal space).* When gas accumulates in the chest, the heart is pushed to the unaffected side, and the position of the PMI changes. Often the presence of a pneumothorax can be identified by PMI changes long before a chest x-ray can be obtained.

Expiratory Grunting

Cyanosis

*Some practitioners use the stethoscope to determine the point at which the heart sounds are most audible.

CLINICAL DATA OBTAINED FROM LABORATORY TESTS AND SPECIAL PROCEDURES

Pulmonary Function Test Findings
(Extrapolated Data for Instructional Purposes)
(Primarily Restrictive Lung Pathophysiology)

FORCED EXPIRATORY FLOW RATE FINDINGS

FVC	FEV_T	FEV_1/FVC ratio	$FEF_{25\%-75\%}$
↓	N or ↓	N or ↑	N or ↓

$FEF_{50\%}$	$FEF_{200-1200}$	PEFR	MVV
N or ↓	N or ↓	N or ↓	N or ↓

LUNG VOLUME AND CAPACITY FINDINGS

V_T	IRV	ERV	RV*
N or ↓	↓	↓	↓

VC	IC	FRC*	TLC	RV/TLC ratio
↓	↓	↓	↓	N

*↑ When airways are partially obstructed.

Arterial Blood Gases

MILD TO MODERATE PULMONARY AIR LEAK SYNDROMES
Acute Alveolar Hyperventilation with Hypoxemia
(Acute Respiratory Alkalosis)

pH	Pa_{CO_2}	HCO_3^-	Pa_{O_2}
↑	↓	↓ (slightly)	↓

SEVERE PULMONARY AIR LEAK SYNDROMES
Acute Ventilatory Failure with Hypoxemia
(Acute Respiratory Acidosis)

pH*	Pa_{CO_2}	HCO_3^- *	Pa_{O_2}
↓	↑	↑ (slightly)	↓

*When tissue hypoxia is severe enough to produce lactic acid, the pH and HCO_3^- values will be lower than expected for a particular Pa_{CO_2} level.

Oxygenation Indices*

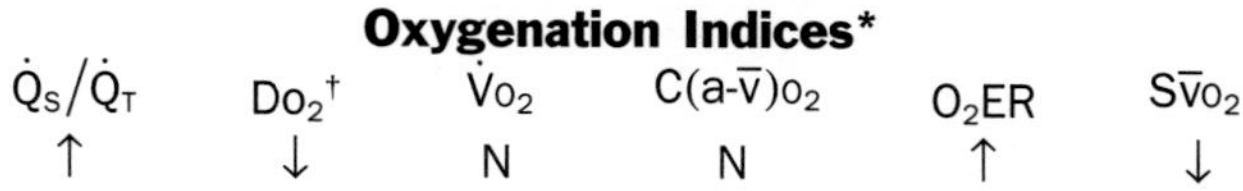

$\dot{Q}_S/\dot{Q}_T$	D_{O_2}†	$\dot{V}_{O_2}$	$C(a-\bar{v})_{O_2}$	O_2ER	$S\bar{v}_{O_2}$
↑	↓	N	N	↑	↓

†The D_{O_2} may be normal in patients who have compensated to the decreased oxygenation status with (1) an increased cardiac output, (2) an increased hemoglobin level, or (3) a combination of both. When the D_{O_2} is normal, the O_2ER is usually normal.

Increased Transillumination

Transillumination of the chest is performed by placing a high-intensity fiberoptic light source against the infant's chest in a dark room. When air is present in the chest cavity, an increased illumination is seen on the affected side.

**$C(a-\bar{v})_{O_2}$*, Arterial-venous oxygen difference; *D_{O_2}*, total oxygen delivery; *O_2ER*, oxygen extraction ratio; *$\dot{Q}_S/\dot{Q}_T$*, pulmonary shunt fraction; *$S\bar{v}_{O_2}$*, mixed venous oxygen saturation; *$\dot{V}_{O_2}$*, oxygen consumption.

OVERVIEW of the Cardiopulmonary Clinical Manifestations Associated with Pulmonary Air Leak Syndromes—cont'd

RADIOLOGIC FINDINGS

Chest Radiograph

The chest x-ray film may show focal or generalized problem areas. When significant partial airway obstruction, air trapping, and alveolar hyperinflation are present, the chest x-ray film appears hyperlucent and the diaphragms may be depressed. The diagnosis of pulmonary interstitial emphysema (PIE) is commonly confirmed when the x-ray film reveals lung hyperinflation and a fine, bubbly appearance (emphysema-like blebs) extending from the hilum to the pleura (Figures 35-2 and 35-3).

The respiratory care practitioner should always be alert for the sudden development of a pneumomediastinum or pneumothorax in infants with pulmonary air leak syndromes. When the excessive air associated with a PIE continues to track—and accumulate—through the perivascular and peribronchial cuffs, it may cause the gas in the hilum area to rupture into the mediastinum, resulting in a pneumomediastinum. A pneumothorax may occur because of the alveolar overdistention and subsequent rupture commonly associated with PIE (Figure 35-4). Figure 35-5 shows an infant with a pneumopericardium, which develops from the direct tracking of interstitial gas along the great vessels of the pericardial sac.

General Management of Pulmonary Air Leak Syndromes

Prevention is the best treatment for pulmonary air leak syndromes. These syndromes may be prevented by the use of low mechanical ventilator pressures and the maintenance of good ventilation and oxygenation. Selective intubation of the unaffected or less affected lung may allow the injured lung time to heal. **High-frequency ventilation** has been successful in treating infants with pulmonary air leak syndromes. Survivors of pulmonary air leak syndromes often develop **bronchopulmonary dysplasia** (see Chapter 37) as a result of overly vigorous mechanical ventilation. Finally, the respiratory care practitioner must always be on alert for signs and symptoms of subcutaneous emphysema, pneumothorax, pneumopericardium, pneumoperitoneum, and intravascular air embolism. Mechanical removal of free air from the intrathoracic cavity, pericardium, or mediastinum may sometime be necessary, especially if vascular collapse is present.

Respiratory Care Treatment Protocols

Oxygen Therapy Protocol

Oxygen therapy is used to treat hypoxemia, decrease the work of breathing, and decrease myocardial work. Because of the hypoxemia that often develops in pulmonary air leak syndromes, supplemental oxygen may be required (see Oxygen Therapy Protocol, Protocol 9-1).

Bronchopulmonary Hygiene Therapy Protocol

Because of the excessive airway secretions and mucous accumulation associated with pulmonary air leak syndromes, a number of bronchial hygiene treatment modalities may be used to enhance the mobilization of bronchial secretions (see Bronchopulmonary Hygiene Therapy Protocol, Protocol 9-2).

Lung Expansion Therapy Protocol

Cautious use of lung expansion measures commonly are administered to offset the pulmonary capillary congestion and interstitial edema and atelectasis associated with pulmonary air leak syndromes (see Lung Expansion Therapy Protocol, Protocol 9-3).

Mechanical Ventilation Protocol

Mechanical ventilation may be necessary to provide and support alveolar gas exchange and eventually return the patient to spontaneous breathing. As previously mentioned, prevention is the best treatment for pulmonary air leak syndromes. Selective intubation of the unaffected or less affected lung may allow the injured lung time to heal. High-frequency ventilation has been successful in treating infants with pulmonary air leak syndromes (see Mechanical Ventilation Protocols, Protocol 9-5, Protocol 9-6, and Protocol 9-7).

CASE STUDY

Pulmonary Air Leak Syndromes

Admitting History and Physical Examination

A 32-week-gestation, preterm female infant was delivered by emergency cesarean section to a healthy 25-year-old mother. The infant weighed 2750 g. The mother's admitting history showed her to be a primigravida with normal prenatal care and no history of illness during her pregnancy. The cesarean section was performed because of repeated and prolonged fetal heart rate decelerations that did not improve with maternal positioning or oxygen administration. At delivery, the infant was found to have the umbilical cord twice wrapped tightly around her neck. She was limp, appeared pale and cyanotic, and was apneic. She showed no response to tactile stimuli, and her heart rate was 65 bpm. Her 1-minute Apgar score was 1 (color 0, pulse 1, grimace 0, reflex irritability 0, muscle tone 0, respiratory 0).

Immediately the neonatologist, nurse, and respiratory therapist started cardiopulmonary resuscitation (CPR) procedures, including ventilation with a bag-valve-mask at an F_{IO_2} of 1.0 and vigorous chest compressions. The 5-minute Apgar was 5 (color 1, pulse 2, grimace 0, reflex irritability 0, muscle tone 1, respiratory 1). Despite the fact that the baby's condition had started to improve, she suddenly took a turn for the worse. Her heart rate started to drop; she again appeared cyanotic, and her muscle tone decreased.

At this time, the respiratory therapist noted that the baby's breath sounds were absent over the right lung and severely decreased over the left upper and middle lobes. Her heart sounds were muffled and faint, and the **point of maximum impulse (PMI)** was displaced to the left. Transillumination showed a large right pneumothorax. This was later confirmed by chest x-ray examination as a right tension pneumothorax. The neonatologist inserted a chest tube, and the baby was placed on a mechanical ventilator with the following settings: intermittent mandatory ventilation (IMV) 30, F_{IO_2} 1.0, positive inspiratory pressure (PIP) +25 cm H_2O, positive end-expiratory pressure (PEEP) +5 cm H_2O, inspiratory time (TI) 0.35, and flow 6 L/min.

Moments later, an umbilical artery catheter (UAC) was inserted; it showed the following values: pH 7.19, Pa_{CO_2} 77, HCO_3^- 19, Pa_{O_2} 31, and Sa_{O_2} 47%. The ventilator rate was increased immediately to 40 breaths/min. ABG values 20 minutes later were as follows: pH 7.33, Pa_{CO_2} 43, HCO_3^- 21, Pa_{O_2} 47, and Sa_{O_2} 83%.

A second chest x-ray examination an hour later showed that the right lung had reexpanded, with segmental atelectasis throughout. At this time, the infant appeared pink and her vital signs were stable, with a heart rate of 155 bpm and blood pressure of 68/35. Breath sounds revealed bilateral crackles and rhonchi. ABG values were as follows: pH 7.34, Pa_{CO_2} 42, HCO_3^- 22, and Pa_{O_2} 53. The Sa_{O_2} was 89%. The respiratory therapist recorded the following in the baby's chart:

Respiratory Assessment and Plan

S N/A

O Skin: Pink. HR 155 bpm, BP 68/35. Crackles and rhonchi throughout. ABGs: pH 7.34, Pa_{CO_2} 42, HCO_3^- 22, Pa_{O_2} 53, and Sa_{O_2} 89%. CXR: Reexpanded right lung with segmental atelectasis.

A
- Preterm infant in severe respiratory distress
- Right tension pneumothorax, treated
- Atelectasis—right lung (CXR)
- Adequate ventilation and oxygenation on present ventilator settings (ABGs)
- Excessive airway secretions (crackles and rhonchi)

P Continue **Mechanical Ventilation Protocol.** Attempt to reduce F_{IO_2} per **Oxygen Therapy Protocol.** Continue **Lung Expansion Therapy Protocol** (PEEP +5 cm H_2O). Start **Bronchopulmonary Hygiene Therapy Protocol** (chest physical therapy [CPT] qid). Monitor closely (vital signs, color, ABGs, transillumination).

Discussion

An **iatrogenic tension pneumothorax** caused by a resuscitation effort is not uncommon during resuscitation of the newborn. This is especially true when the staff is inexperienced or performs resuscitation too aggressively because of the anxiety and urgency of the situation. Respiratory care practitioners must be prepared to attend deliveries, manage the airways, and provide ventilatory support as requested by the other members of the health-care team. Such members of the respiratory care department are often called *designated neonatal resuscitators.*

Because of the risk of cerebral interventricular hemorrhage (IVH), many centers would not perform CPT on the infant. Proper positioning of the infant for CPT (head down) would increase the risk for IVH. Since the advent of surfactant therapy, pneumothoraces in mechanically ventilated infants in neonatal intensive care units (NICUs) have decreased. Tension pneumothorax is a potentially life-threatening emergency, and the respiratory therapist should always be alert for any signs or symptoms associated with this condition.

In this case the clinical manifestations associated with **Atelectasis** (see Figure 9-8) were quickly identified when the respiratory therapist noted the possibility of a pneumothorax by pointing out that the baby's breath sounds were absent over the right lung and severely decreased over the left upper and middle lobes. Transillumination further supported the presence of a pneumothorax. The chest radiograph confirmed a right lung pneumothorax. To help in the monitoring and the identification of a possible pneumothorax, the respiratory care practitioners often make a simple ballpoint pen mark at the PMI on the chests of infants at risk for pneumothorax. The PMI is the point at which the impulse of the left ventricle is felt most strongly. If the PMI moves away from the mark, the practitioner has a good and timely clinical indication that the baby has developed a pneumothorax—even before a chest x-ray examination can be performed.

Finally, it is not uncommon for infants with pulmonary air leak syndromes to develop fluid in their lungs shortly after a pneumothorax has resolved (i.e., the chest tube is no longer sucking any air out of the baby's chest). When this occurs, these infants gain weight, demonstrate rhonchi and crackles, and require a higher FIO_2 to maintain their desired PaO_2 levels. The reason for this is that babies who have iatrogenic tension pneumothoraces often develop what is called a transient **syndrome of inappropriate antidiuretic hormone (SIADH).** In other words, the pneumothorax causes the release of antidiuretic hormone, which inhibits urination. Some of the retained fluid accumulates in the baby's lungs. Often, a diuretic (such as furosemide), a little more airway pressure, an increased FIO_2, or an increased ventilator rate may be administered to offset this transient problem. The condition usually lasts only about 24 hours. The respiratory practitioner should expect this condition and should not be overly concerned.

SELF-ASSESSMENT QUESTIONS

evolve Answers to questions can be found on Evolve. To access additional student assessment questions and case studies for application of text material to real-life scenarios, visit **http://evolve.elsevier.com/DesJardins/respiratory.**

1. The most frequent etiologic factor causing air leak syndromes in preterm infants is:

a. Infants who weigh less than 1000 g
b. Mechanical ventilation
c. Excessive bronchial secretions
d. Increased expiratory grunting

2. During the advanced stages of pulmonary air leak syndromes, the infant demonstrates a(n):

1. Increased $PaCO_2$
2. Decreased HCO_3^-
3. Increased pH
4. Decreased PaO_2

a. 1 and 4 only
b. 2 and 3 only
c. 1, 3, and 4 only
d. 1, 2, 3, and 4

3. Infants with pulmonary air leak syndromes often have:

1. Reduced urine output
2. Increased transillumination
3. Hypoxia-induced pulmonary arterial vasoconstriction
4. A change in the PMI

a. 1 and 3 only
b. 2 and 4 only
c. 2, 3, and 4 only
d. 1, 2, 3, and 4

4. Which of the following are the major pathologic changes associated with pulmonary air leak syndromes?

1. Airway obstruction
2. Consolidation
3. Increased alveolar-capillary membrane thickness
4. Atelectasis
5. Excessive bronchial secretions

a. 3 and 5 only
b. 1, 4, and 5 only
c. 3, 4, and 5 only
d. 1, 3, 4, and 5 only

5. In pulmonary air leak syndromes, if the high interstitial lung pressure persists, the gas may:

1. Continue to spread peripherally
2. Remain localized and restrict the airway lumen
3. Cause a pneumomediastinum or pneumopericardium
4. Rupture the visceral pleura

a. 1 and 3 only
b. 2 and 4 only
c. 2, 3, and 4 only
d. 1, 2, 3, and 4

Respiratory Syncytial Virus Infection (Bronchiolitis or Pneumonitis)

36

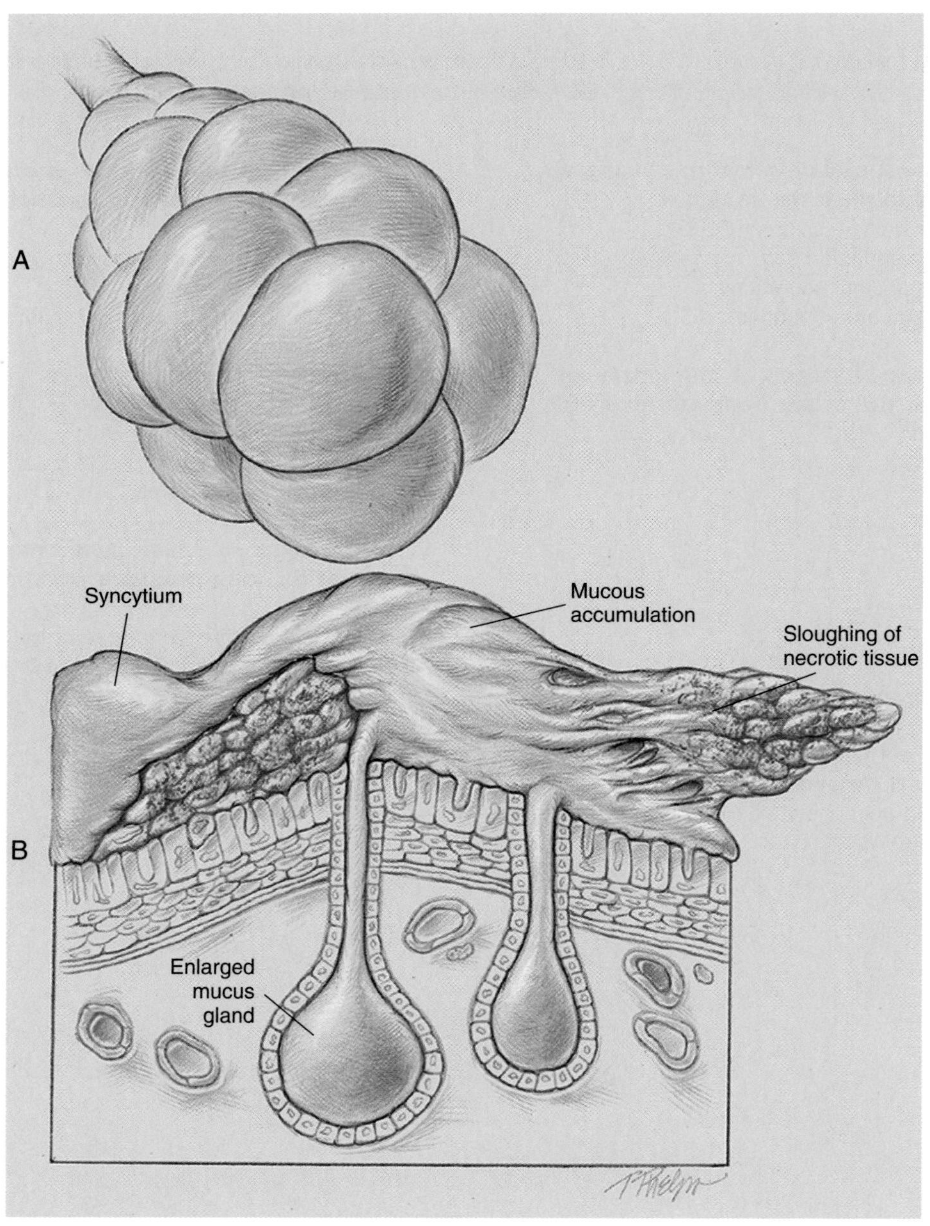

FIGURE 36-1 Bronchiolitis caused by respiratory syncytial virus. **A,** Partial airway obstruction and alveolar hyperinflation. **B,** Cross-section of inflamed airway.

Chapter Objectives

After reading this chapter, you will be able to:

- List the anatomic alterations of the lungs associated with respiratory syncytial virus (RSV) infection.
- Describe the causes of respiratory syncytial virus infection.
- List the cardiopulmonary clinical manifestations associated with respiratory syncytial virus infection.
- Describe the general management of respiratory syncytial virus infection.
- Describe the clinical strategies and rationales of the SOAP presented in the case study.
- Define key terms and complete self-assessment questions at the end of the chapter and on Evolve.

Key Terms

Antigen Assay Tests
Ball-Valve Mechanism
Bronchiolitis
Nasopharygeal Culture
Palivizumab (Synagis)
Pneumonitis
Reverse Transcriptase–Polymerase Chain Reaction (RT-PCR) Assays
Ribavirin (Virazole)
Small Particle Aerosol Generator (SPAG)
Sputum culture
Syncytium

Chapter Outline

Anatomic Alterations of the Lungs

The respiratory syncytial virus (RSV) moves down the respiratory tract by means of cell-to-cell transfer, causing **bronchiolitis** and, later, atelectasis and pneumonia in the child. The **syncytium** is defined as a "multinucleate mass of protoplasm produced by the merging of cells." At the level of the bronchioles the virus causes neighboring cells to fuse to form a syncytium, hence the name *respiratory syncytial virus.* The lower airways may also become infected when secretions from RSV-infected upper airways are aspirated.

RSV infection causes peribronchiolar mononuclear infiltration and necrosis of the epithelium of the small airways. This condition leads to edema of the small airways and increased production of mucus. As the condition worsens, the epithelium of the small airways becomes necrotic and proliferates into the airway lumen. The combination of sloughing necrotic tissue, airway edema, and accumulation of mucus leads to (1) a decreased airway lumen, (2) a partially obstructed airway, or (3) a completely obstructed airway. Partial airway obstruction leads to alveolar hyperinflation as a result of a **"ball-valve" mechanism** (see Figure 36-1). Complete airway obstruction leads to alveolar collapse or atelectasis. Pneumonic consolidation is common. RSV is also referred to as *bronchiolitis* or **pneumonitis.**

The following major pathologic or structural changes are associated with RSV infection:

- Inflammation and swelling of the peripheral airways
- Excessive airway secretions
- Sloughing of necrotic airway epithelium
- Partial airway obstruction and alveolar hyperinflation
- Complete airway obstruction and atelectasis
- Consolidation

Etiology and Epidemiology

RSV is the most common viral respiratory pathogen seen in infancy and early childhood. Although RSV infection can occur at any age, it is most commonly seen in young children. Almost all children will be infected with RSV by their second birthday. At highest risk for severe respiratory distress syndrome (RDS) are premature infants, children less than 1 year of age, and children with weakened immune systems as a result of a medical condition or medical treatment. Adults with compromised immune systems and those 65 years of age and older are also at increased risk of severe RDS.

RSV is commonly transmitted by young children who are infected with RSV and demonstrate the signs and symptoms of a mild upper respiratory tract infection or a cold—for example, coughing, sneezing, runny nose, decreased appetite, irritability, decreased activity, and respiratory distress. RSV is easily transmitted when droplets containing the virus are coughed or sneezed into the air. Infection occurs when the particles touch the nose, mouth, or eyes of uninfected individuals in the immediate area. RSV can also spread from direct or indirect contact with nasal or oral secretions from an infected person. For example, RSV can be contracted by kissing the face or hands of a child infected with RSV who has a runny nose. Indirect contact may occur when touching the hard surface of a table, crib rail, or doorknob that has been touched by a person infected with RSV. RSV can survive several hours on a hard surface. Common areas of RSV transmission include elementary schools and day care centers. Frequent hand washing and wiping the hard surfaces with a disinfectant may help stop the spread of RSV.

Infants and children infected with RSV usually develop symptoms within 4 to 6 days of infection (range: 2 to 8 days). Most will recover in 1 to 2 weeks. Infected individuals are

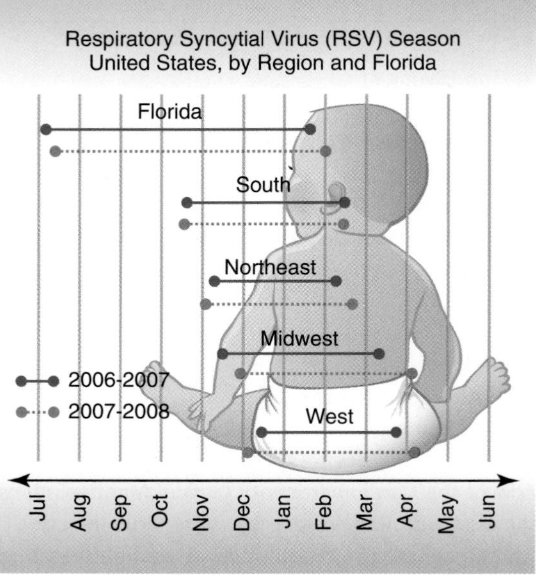

FIGURE 36-2 Respiratory syncytial virus (RSV) season in the United States by region and in Florida. (Image and data from Centers for Disease Control and Prevention: www.cdc.gov/Features/dsRSV/.)

usually contagious for 3 to 8 days. However, even after recovery an infected person can spread the virus for 1 to 3 weeks. Some patients with a weakened immune system may be contagious for as long as 4 weeks.

Most otherwise healthy children with RSV do not require hospitalization. However, according to the Centers for Disease Control and Prevention, 75,000 to 125,000 children under the age of 1 year are hospitalized each year in the United States because of RSV infection. Of this group, most of the children hospitalized because of RSV are under 6 months old.

Although the outbreak of RSV cases varies by location each year, the number of RSV cases typically increases during the fall, winter, and early spring months. It is not fully known why RSV outbreaks occur in certain regions more than in others, but temperature, climate, and humidity appear to play a role. Figure 36-2 shows the typical RSV season in the United States by region and in Florida according to the Centers for Disease Control and Prevention.

Laboratory Testing for Respiratory Syncytial Virus

RSV infection should be suspected when the clinical manifestations correlate to the time of year, the presence of a local outbreak, the age of the patient, and the history of the illness. Through use of an oropharyngeal or nasopharyngeal secretion sample, RSV is most commonly diagnosed with commercially available **antigen assay tests.** RSV can also be confirmed with a **nasopharyngeal culture.** Both the antigen assay test and the nasopharyngeal culture are usually reliable in young children but are less sensitive in older children and adults. Highly sensitive **reverse transcriptase–polymerase chain reaction (RT-PCR) assays** are also available. The RT-PCR assay may be used to test adults.

OVERVIEW of the Cardiopulmonary Clinical Manifestations Associated with Respiratory Syncytial Virus Infection

The following clinical manifestations result from the pathologic mechanisms caused (or activated) by **Atelectasis** (see Figure 9-8), **Alveolar Consolidation** (see Figure 9-9), and **Excessive Bronchial Secretions** (see Figure 9-12)—the major anatomic alterations of the lungs associated with respiratory syncytial virus (RSV) infection (see Figure 36-1).

CLINICAL DATA OBTAINED AT THE PATIENT'S BEDSIDE

The Physical Examination

Vital Signs

Increased Respiratory Rate (Tachypnea)

Normally a newborn's respiratory rate is about 40 to 60 breaths/min. During the early stages of RSV infection the respiratory rate generally is well over 60 breaths/min. Several pathophysiologic mechanisms operating simultaneously may lead to an increased ventilatory rate:

- Stimulation of peripheral chemoreceptors (hypoxemia)
- Decreased lung compliance–increased ventilatory rate relationship
- Stimulation of central chemoreceptors

Increased Heart Rate (Pulse) and Blood Pressure

Apnea

Clinical Manifestations Associated with More Negative Intrapleural Pressures during Inspiration

- Intercostal retractions
- Substernal retraction and abdominal distention (seesaw movement or paradoxic chest motion)
- Cyanosis of the dependent portions of the thoracic and abdominal areas
- Flaring nostrils

Chest Assessment Findings

- Wheezes
- Rhonchi
- Crackles

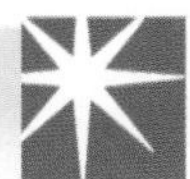

OVERVIEW of the Cardiopulmonary Clinical Manifestations Associated with Respiratory Syncytial Virus Infection—cont'd

Respiratory Secretions (Copious)
Expiratory Grunting
Cyanosis

CLINICAL DATA OBTAINED FROM LABORATORY TESTS AND SPECIAL PROCEDURES

Pulmonary Function Test Findings (Extrapolated Data for Instructional Purposes) (Restrictive Lung Pathophysiology)

FORCED EXPIRATORY FLOW RATE FINDINGS

FVC	FEV_T	FEV_1/FVC ratio	$FEF_{25\%-75\%}$
↓	N or ↓	N or ↑	N or ↓

$FEF_{50\%}$	$FEF_{200-1200}$	PEFR	MVV
N or ↓	N or ↓	N or ↓	N or ↓

LUNG VOLUME AND CAPACITY FINDINGS

V_T	IRV	ERV	RV*
N or ↓	↓	↓	↓

VC	IC	FRC*	TLC*	RV/TLC ratio*
↓	↓	↓	↓	N

*↑ When airways are partially obstructed.

Arterial Blood Gases

MILD TO MODERATE RESPIRATORY SYNCYTIAL VIRUS INFECTION
Acute Alveolar Hyperventilation with Hypoxemia
(Acute Respiratory Alkalosis)

pH	$Paco_2$	HCO_3^-	Pao_2
↑	↓	↓ (slightly)	↓

SEVERE RESPIRATORY SYNCYTIAL VIRUS INFECTION
Acute Ventilatory Failure with Hypoxemia
(Acute Respiratory Acidosis)

pH*	$Paco_2$	HCO_3^- *	Pao_2
↓	↑	↑ (slightly)	↓

*When tissue hypoxia is severe enough to produce lactic acid, the pH and HCO_3^- values will be lower than expected for a particular $Paco_2$ level.

Oxygenation Indices*

$\dot{Q}_S/\dot{Q}_T$	Do_2†	$\dot{V}o_2$	$C(a-\bar{v})o_2$	O_2ER	$S\bar{v}o_2$
↑	↓	N	N	↑	↓

†The Do_2 may be normal in patients who have compensated to the decreased oxygenation status with (1) an increased cardiac output, (2) an increased hemoglobin level, or (3) a combination of both. When the Do_2 is normal, the O_2ER is usually normal.

RADIOLOGIC FINDINGS

Chest Radiograph

RSV infection appears as both bronchiolitis and bronchopneumonia in infants and young children. The chest radiograph commonly shows streaky peribronchial opacities associated with air trapping and hyperinflation. Lobar atelectasis frequently is seen, and alveolar and lobar pneumonic consolidation occasionally may be seen also (Figure 36-3).

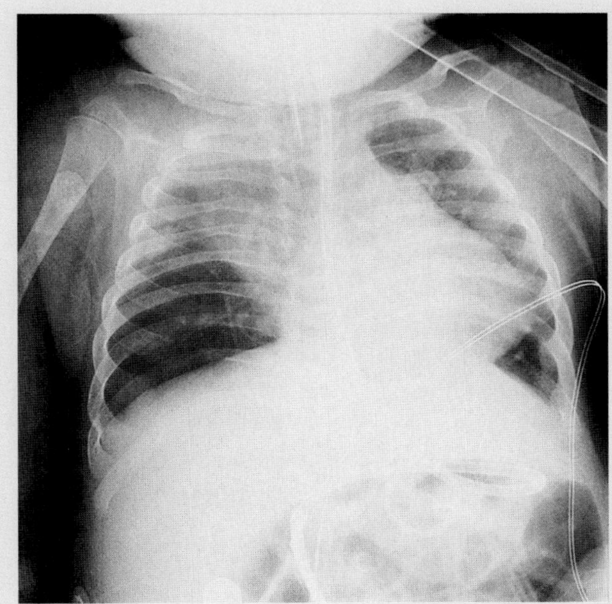

FIGURE 36-3 Chest x-ray film of a 6-month-old child with respiratory syncytial virus infection.

*$C(a-\bar{v})o_2$, Arterial-venous oxygen difference; Do_2, total oxygen delivery; O_2ER, oxygen extraction ratio; $\dot{Q}_S/\dot{Q}_T$, pulmonary shunt fraction; $S\bar{v}o_2$, mixed venous oxygen saturation; $\dot{V}o_2$, oxygen consumption.

General Management of Respiratory Syncytial Virus Infection (Bronchiolitis, Pneumonitis)

Respiratory Care Treatment Protocols

Oxygen Therapy Protocol

Oxygen therapy is used to treat hypoxemia, decrease the work of breathing, and decrease myocardial work. The hypoxemia that develops in RSV most commonly is caused by the excessive airway fluid, atelectasis, and consolidation associated with the disorder. Hypoxemia caused by capillary shunting is often partially refractory to oxygen therapy (see Oxygen Therapy Protocol, Protocol 9-1).

Bronchopulmonary Hygiene Therapy Protocol

Because of the excessive airway secretions associated with RSV infection, bronchial hygiene treatment modalities often are used to enhance the mobilization of bronchial secretions (see Bronchopulmonary Hygiene Therapy Protocol, Protocol 9-2).

Aerosolized Medication Protocol

Both sympathomimetic and parasympatholytic agents may be used to induce bronchial smooth muscle relaxation (see Aerosolized Medication Protocol, Protocol 9-4).

Antiviral Aerosols

Ribavirin. Although ribavirin was widely used when it was first introduced, the routine use of nebulized **ribavirin (Virazole)** in infants and children with RSV is no longer recommended. This is because the efficacy of ribavirin in this population has not been clearly confirmed. Major drawbacks of ribavirin are that the decision to use the drug must be made early and importantly, must be based on other clinical data, such as underlying congenital heart disease, lung disease, immunosuppression, or the need for mechanical ventilation. In addition, ribavirin is expensive, requires special equipment, and is associated with concerns regarding occupational exposure. A continuous medication nebulizer for administration of ribavirin is known as a **small particle aerosol generator (SPAG).**

Palivizumab. As a preventive measure against RSV infection, health-care guidelines recommend that some high-risk babies (e.g., premature babies, infants on long-term ventilator care) be injected with an agent called **palivizumab (Synagis)**—an immune globulin prophylaxis—once a month for 5 months.*

Corticosteroids

Some practitioners routinely administer steroids to patients with severe RSV infection. However, steroids are not recommended as standard treatment for RSV infection.

---

*Over the last several years, research has shown that the use of palivizumab has significantly reduced the number of hospitalizations and the duration of hospitalization in high-risk babies.

CASE STUDY

Respiratory Syncytial Virus (RSV) Infection

Admitting History and Physical Examination

A premature baby boy was born in mid-November at 31 weeks' gestation. He weighed 1300 g at birth and immediately demonstrated respiratory distress that rapidly progressed into respiratory distress syndrome (RDS; see Chapter 34). During the first hour after delivery, the baby was intubated, placed on a mechanical ventilator, and given a dose of pulmonary surfactant. An umbilical artery line was inserted, and antibiotics were given for several days. Over the next 10 days, the baby was slowly weaned off the ventilator and started on oral feedings. Both the umbilical artery and intravenous (IV) lines were discontinued. Over the next week, the baby gained weight and appeared to be doing well.

Two days later, however, the baby started to demonstrate more periods of apnea and signs of respiratory distress. His vital signs were as follows: heart rate 165 bpm, blood pressure 85/55, respiratory rate 65, and temperature 37° C. He demonstrated nasal flaring and intercostal retractions. Wheezing and rhonchi could be auscultated over both lung fields. His skin appeared cyanotic, and his oxygen saturation by pulse oximetry decreased from 90% to 83%. A chest x-ray examination revealed bilateral streaky infiltrates and scattered areas of atelectasis.

Because of the baby's history, the time of year, and the increased number of colds and flu reported throughout the medical community, the neonatologist suspected RSV infection. The baby was placed in an oxygen hood at an FIO_2 of 0.50, and a nasopharyngeal swab was obtained and sent to the laboratory. The smear was positive for RSV. Because apnea is sometimes associated with RSV infection, the baby was reintubated and placed back on the ventilator for support. The ventilator settings were as follows: intermittent mandatory ventilation (IMV) mode 15, positive inspiratory pressure (PIP) +20 cm H_2O, positive end-expiratory pressure (PEEP) +4 cm H_2O, flow 6 L/min, and FIO_2 0.4. His saturation increased to 88%. At this time, the respiratory therapist charted the following SOAP note.

Respiratory Assessment and Plan

S N/A

O Apnea. Positive RSV smear. Vital signs: HR 165 bpm, BP 85/55, RR 65, T 37° C. Nasal flaring, intercostal retractions, and cyanosis. Wheezing and rhonchi. CXR: Atelectasis. SpO_2 on FIO_2 0.40: 88%. Ventilator settings: IMV rate 15, PIP +20, PEEP +4, flow 6 L/min.

A
- Atelectasis (CXR)
- Bronchospasm (wheezing)
- Excessive airway secretions (rhonchi)
- Hypoxemia (SpO_2 and cyanosis)

P Continue **Mechanical Ventilation Protocol.** Begin **Bronchopulmonary Hygiene Therapy Protocol** (CPT and suction prn). Begin **Aerosolized Medication Therapy** Protocol (0.25 mg albuterol per kg with 2 mL normal saline q3h, in-line with the ventilator). Oxygen therapy per **Mechanical Ventilation Protocol.** Continue to monitor closely. Obtain ABGs via capillary heel stick and reevaluate.

Because the neonatologist preferred to use ribavirin only as a last resort (because of the potential environmental pollutant hazards associated with the agent), he fully agreed with the respiratory therapist's assessment. Over the next 7 days, the baby was slowly weaned off the bronchopulmonary hygiene therapy, bronchodilator therapy, oxygen therapy, and mechanical ventilator. The baby was monitored closely over the next week and discharged in good health.

Discussion

The value of routine bronchodilator therapy has been questioned in the treatment of RSV. Many centers implement a short trial period of bronchodilator therapy and then reassess. Respiratory care practitioners must recognize their potential role in transmitting RSV. Any infected health-care practitioners or family members can easily transmit the virus through aerosolized sprays generated by a cough or a sneeze or even through the secretions from the mucous membranes of the eyes (when the eyes have been rubbed, the virus can be transmitted by hand to the infant). Therefore the mainstay of treatment for RSV infection clearly is *prevention.*

Medical personnel who can recognize infants at risk for RSV (e.g., premature babies, babies on ventilators for long periods, babies on oxygen, babies who have bronchopulmonary dysplasia) also can easily take extra preventive measures, including the use of hand washing, gloves, gowns, and masks. As previously mentioned in the treatment section, babies at high risk for RSV are injected with a dose of palivizumab—an immune globulin prophylaxis—once a month.

In most cases, however, the anatomic alterations of the lung and the clinical manifestations that ensue can be effectively treated by good respiratory therapy (i.e., appropriate oxygen therapy, bronchopulmonary hygiene therapy, and bronchodilator therapy). For example, the implementation of the **Bronchopulmonary Hygiene Therapy Protocol** to offset the **Excessive Bronchial Secretions** (see Figure 9-12) and the administration of the **Aerosolized Medication Therapy Protocol** (albuterol) to offset the **Bronchospasm** (see Figure 9-11) demonstrated in this case were clearly justified.

SELF-ASSESSMENT QUESTIONS

evolve Answers to questions can be found on Evolve. To access additional student assessment questions and case studies for application of text material to real-life scenarios, visit **http://evolve.elsevier.com/DesJardins/respiratory.**

1. Which of the following are associated with RSV infection?
   1. Alveolar hyperinflation
   2. Atelectasis
   3. Excessive bronchial secretions
   4. Pneumonic consolidation
      a. 2 and 4 only
      b. 3 and 4 only
      c. 2, 3, and 4 only
      d. 1, 2, 3, and 4

2. Although the outbreak of RSV cases varies, the number of patients with RSV typically increase during:
   1. Summer
   2. Fall
   3. Winter
   4. Early spring
      a. 1 only
      b. 3 only
      c. 2, 3, and 4 only
      d. 1, 2, 3, and 4

3. How long may RSV typically remain contagious?
   a. 1 to 2 days
   b. 3 to 8 days
   c. 2 weeks
   d. 1 month

4. Although RSV infection can occur at any age, children younger than what age tend to be more severely affected?
   a. Less than 1 year old
   b. Less than 2 years old
   c. Less than 3 years old
   d. Less than 4 years old

5. Which of the following agents is or are used to prevent RSV infection in high-risk babies?
   1. Virazole
   2. Synagis
   3. Streptomycin
   4. Ribavirin
      a. 1 only
      b. 2 only
      c. 3 only
      d. 1 and 4 only

Bronchopulmonary Dysplasia

37

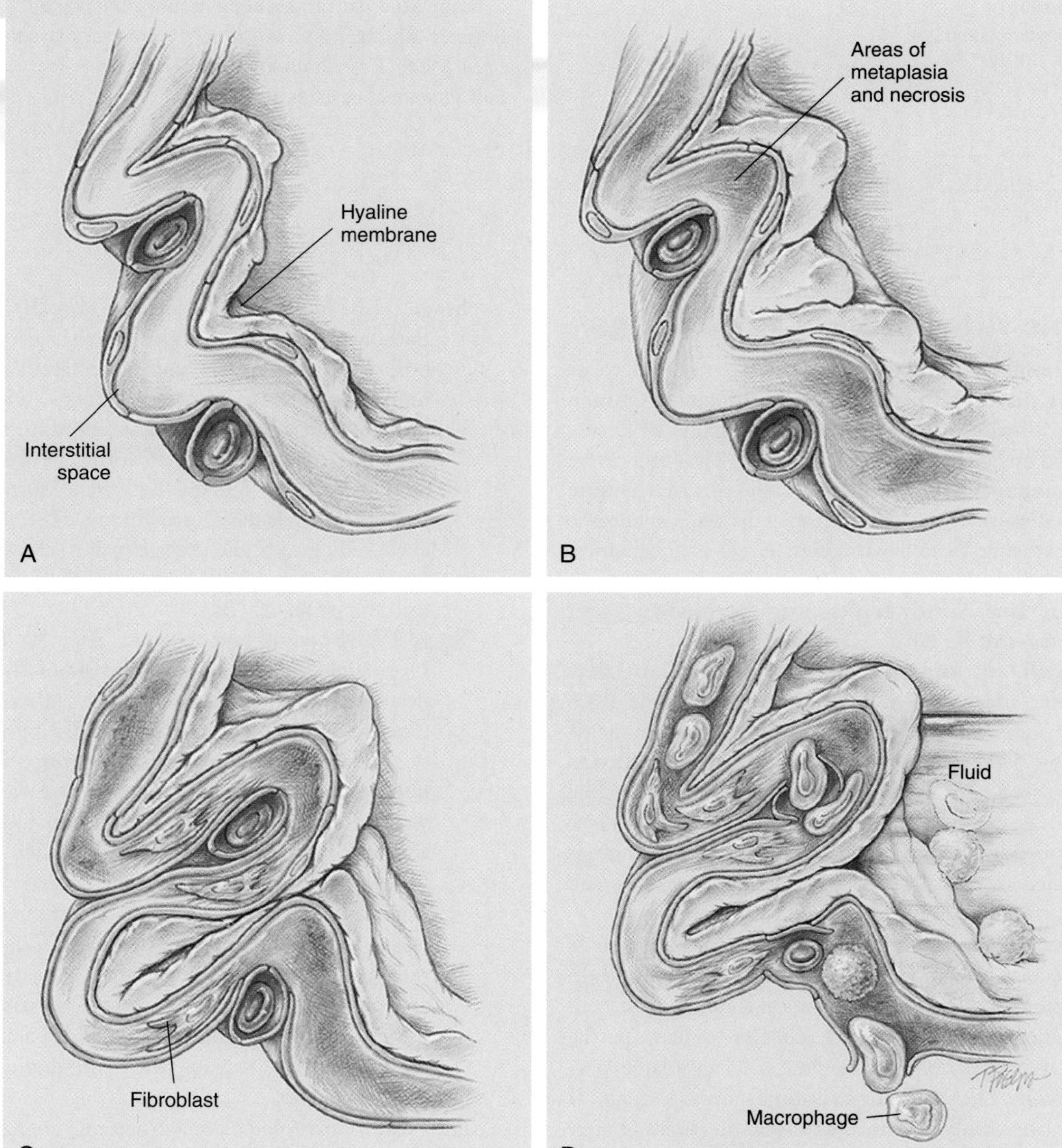

FIGURE 37-1 Alveolar changes during the four stages of bronchopulmonary dysplasia. **A,** Stage I, the formation of hyaline membrane. **B,** Stage II, the development areas of metaplasia and necrosis. **C,** Stage III, extensive metaplasia, hyperplasia, and interstitial fibrosis. **D,** Stage IV, progressive destruction of alveoli and airways.

Chapter Objectives

After reading this chapter, you will be able to:

- List the anatomic alterations of the lungs associated with bronchopulmonary dysplasia.
- Describe the causes of bronchopulmonary dysplasia.
- List the cardiopulmonary clinical manifestations associated with bronchopulmonary dysplasia.
- Describe the general management of bronchopulmonary dysplasia.

- Describe the clinical strategies and rationales of the SOAP presented in the case study.
- Define key terms and complete self-assessment questions at the end of the chapter and on Evolve.

Key Terms

Alveolar Hypoplasia
Bronchopulmonary Dysplasia (BPD)
Chronic Lung Disease of Prematurity
Gentle Ventilation
Hyaline Membrane Disease
"New" BPD
Stage I BPD
Stage II BPD
Stage III BPD
Stage IV BPD

Chapter Outline

Anatomic Alterations of the Lungs

Bronchopulmonary dysplasia (BPD), also referred to as **chronic lung disease of prematurity,** is the most common chronic lung disease of prematurity. Historically, BPD was first described by Northway and colleagues in 1967 as a severe chronic lung injury in premature infants who survived **hyaline membrane disease** (i.e., respiratory distress syndrome [RDS]) after being treated with high levels of mechanical ventilation and oxygen exposure for prolonged periods of time. At that time Northway described the following four pathologic stages of BPD:

Stage I BPD was said to occur during the first 2 to 3 days of life. This stage is often indistinguishable from RDS. During this period, alveolar hyaline membranes, patches of atelectasis, and lymphatic dilation were seen. In addition, early signs of bronchial mucosal necrosis appeared during this time (see Figure 37-1, *A*). The chest radiographic findings revealed ground glass-like granular patterns and small lung volumes (Figure 37-2, *A*).

Stage II BPD was said to occur 4 to 10 days after birth. Atelectasis was more extensive during this period. In addition, metaplasia of the normal lung tissue cells caused bronchial necrosis, cellular debris, partial airway obstruction, air trapping, and alveolar hyperinflation. The pathologic findings during Stage II were commonly described as alternating areas of atelectasis and of emphysema (see Figure 37-1, *B*). These changes appeared on chest x-ray films as patchy opaque areas with bronchograms (areas of atelectasis) next to areas of dark translucency (areas of hyperinflation) (see Figure 37-2, *B*).

It is interesting to note that at the time of this description in 1967, the therapeutic usefulness of continuous positive airway pressure (CPAP) or positive end-expiratory pressure (PEEP), as we know it today, had not yet been described. During this time period, the ventilation of these infants was with zero CPAP or PEEP—factors that contributed to severe atelectasis.

Stage III BPD was said to occur at 11 to 30 days of age. Pathologic findings included extensive bronchial and bronchiolar metaplasia and hyperplasia (an increased number of cells), interstitial fibrosis, and excessive bronchial airway secretions. In addition, the alveolar hyperinflation continued to form circular groups of emphysematous bullae that were surrounded by patches of atelectasis (see Figure 37-1, *C*). On the chest radiograph, the lungs began to show circular or cystic areas surrounded by patches of irregular density (see Figure 37-2, *C*).

Stage IV BPD was said to occur after 30 days of life. During this stage, massive fibrosis of the lung and destruction of the bronchial airways, alveoli, and pulmonary capillaries occured. Areas of emphysematous, or cystlike, areas continued to increase in size and number. Thin strands of atelectasis and normal alveoli were interspersed around emphysematous areas. In addition, pulmonary hypertension often developed, lymphatic and bronchial mucous gland deformation occurred, and excessive bronchial secretions continued to be a problem (see Figure 37-1, *D*). The chest radiographs revealed fibrosis and edema with areas of consolidation adjacent to areas of overinflation (see Figure 37-2, *D*). Table 37-1 provides a summary of the original BPD stages, with pathologic and radiologic correlates.

The major pathologic or structural changes of the lungs associated with earlier descriptions of BPD are as follows:

- Hyaline membrane formation
- Atelectasis
- Bronchial mucosal necrosis
- Excessive bronchial secretions
- Chronic alveolar fibrosis and bronchial smooth muscle hypertrophy
- Bronchial mucosal metaplasia and hyperplasia
- Alveolar hyperinflation
- Emphysematous areas surrounded by areas of atelectasis and normal alveoli

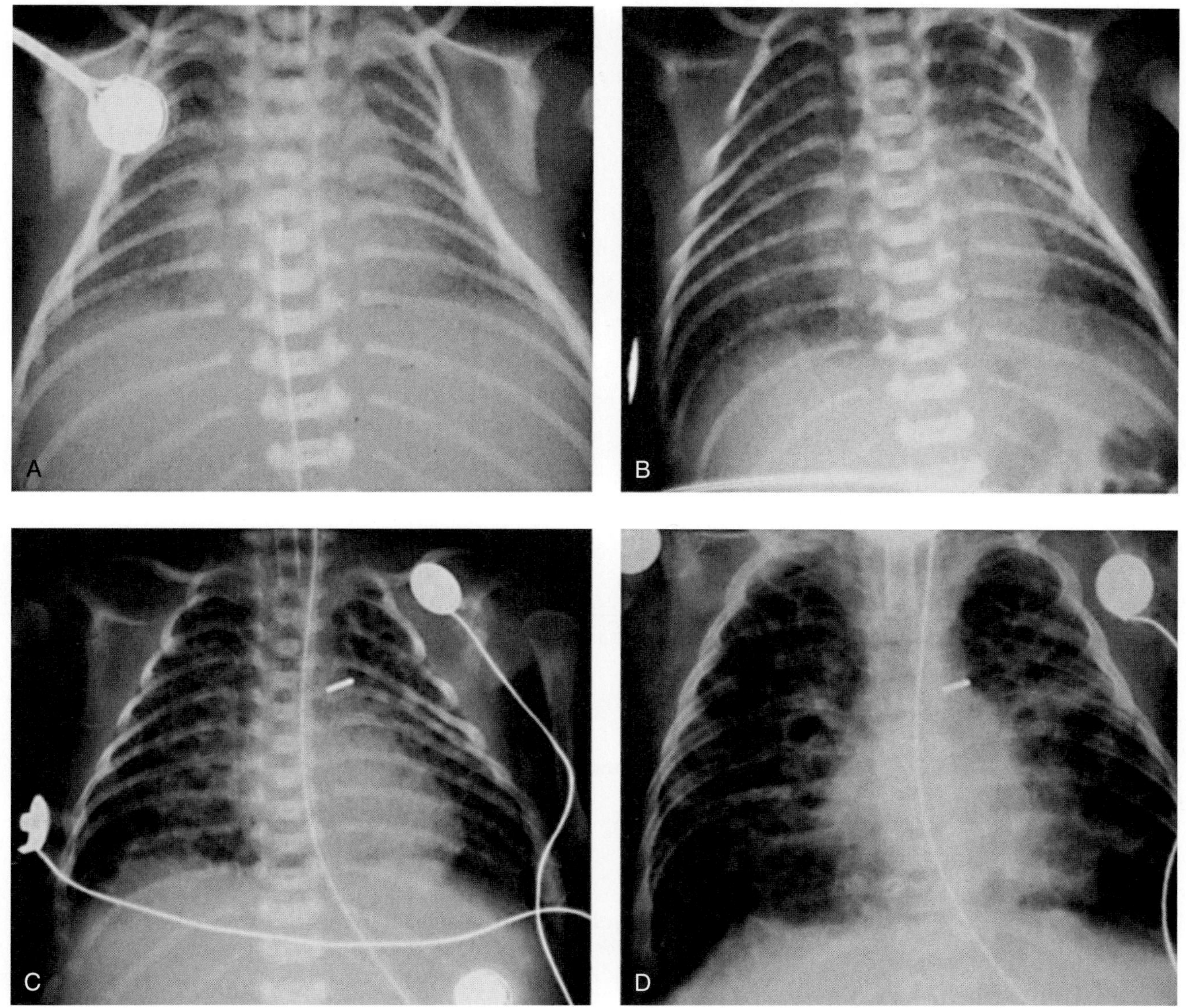

FIGURE 37-2 **A**, Stage I; occurs during the first 2 to 3 days of life. The chest radiographic findings show ground glass–like granular patterns and small lung volumes. **B**, Stage II; occurs 4 to 10 days after birth. The chest x-ray film shows patchy opaque areas with bronchograms (areas of atelectasis) next to areas of dark translucency (areas of hyperinflation). **C**, Stage III; occurs at 11 to 30 days of age. The chest radiograph shows circular or cystic areas surrounded by patches of irregular density. **D**, Stage IV; occurs after 30 days of life. The chest radiographs shows fibrosis and edema with areas of consolidation adjacent to areas of overinflation. (From Taeusch WH, Ballard RA, Gleason CA: *Avery's diseases of the newborn,* ed 8, Philadelphia, 2005, Saunders.)

The "New" Bronchopulmonary Dysplasia—Anatomic Alterations of the Lungs

Much has been learned about BPD since it was first described in 1967. During the late 1960s, BPD occurred predominantly in larger preterm infants born at 30 to 34 weeks' gestation, with a history of severe respiratory distress necessitating aggressive ventilatory support and high oxygen concentrations for prolonged periods of time. Today, BPD as it was originally described has virtually disappeared. The infants who more commonly develop BPD today are those of very low birth weights and born at less than 26 weeks' gestation. These infants are now usually managed with several new and improved therapeutic techniques—including prenatal maternal steroids, the use of postnatal exogenous surfactant, gentle ventilation techniques, low oxygen concentrations, nasal CPAP, fluid restriction, vitamin A, diuretics, bronchodilator therapy, bronchial hygiene therapy, postnatal corticosteroids, and inhaled nitric oxide.

In the **"new" BPD,** the pathologic findings of the lungs are described as "more uniformly inflated with minimal airway injury or fibrosis." The major anatomic pathology is a decrease in alveolar number, called **alveolar hypoplasia.** In the very preterm infant with the "new" BPD, the lung is just completing the canalicular stage of development at the time of birth. It is believed that the interruption of the canalicular stage significantly disrupts the progress of alveolar growth and likely contributes to the development of the "new" BPD.

TABLE 37-1 Bronchopulmonary Dysplasia Staging (Northway)

Stage	Days after Birth	Radiologic Findings	Pathologic Findings
I	2-3	Ground-glass granular pattern; small lung volume	Atelectasis Hyaline membranes Lymphatic dilation
II	4-10	Patchy opaque areas with bronchograms (areas of atelectasis) adjacent to areas of dark translucency (areas of hyperinflation)	Widespread necrosis of alveolar epithelium Persistent alveolar hyaline membranes and atelectasis Metaplasia of bronchiolar smooth muscles Bronchial necrosis Emphysematous coalescence of alveoli
III	11-20	Circular or cystlike areas of hyperlucency, surrounded by patches of irregular density caused by atelectasis	Persisting injury to alveoli Interstitial edema and septal thickening Bronchial mucosal metaplasia and hyperplasia Emphysematous areas surrounded by atelectasis Excessive airway secretions
IV	>30	Increased size and numbers of cystlike areas of hyperlucency, surrounded by thinner stands of radiodensity	Increased size and numbers of emphysematous areas, next to collapsed alveoli and normal alveoli Septal fibrosis Pulmonary hypertension, lymphatic and bronchial mucous gland deformation Excessive airway secretions

Northway WH Jr, Rosan RC, Porter DY: Pulmonary disease following respiratory therapy of hyaline-membrane disease: bronchopulmonary dysplasia, *N Engl J Med* 276:357-368, 1967.

TABLE 37-2 Diagnostic Criteria for the "New" Bronchopulmonary Dysplasia (BPD)

Gestational Age	<32 Weeks	≥32 weeks
Time point of assessment	36 weeks PMA or discharge to home, whichever comes first	>28 days but <56 days postnatal age or discharge to home, whichever comes first
	Treatment with Oxygen >21% for at Least 28 Days, PLUS	
Mild BPD	Breathing room air at 36 weeks PMA or discharge, whichever comes first	Breathing room air by 56 days postnatal age or discharge, whichever comes first
Moderate BPD	Need* for <30% oxygen at 36 weeks PMA or discharge, whichever comes first	Need* for <30% oxygen at 56 days postnatal age or discharge, whichever comes first
Severe BPD	Need* for ≥30% oxygen and/or PPV or NCPAP at 36 weeks PMA or discharge, whichever comes first	Need* for ≥30% oxygen and/or PPV or NCPAP at 56 postnatal age or discharge, whichever comes first

Modified from Jobe AH, Bancalari E: Bronchopulmonary dysplasia, *Am J Respir Crit Care Med* 163:1723-1729, 2001.

BPD, Bronchopulmonary dysplasia; *NCPAP,* nasal continuous positive airway pressure; *PMA,* postmenstrual age; *PPV,* positive-pressure ventilation.

*A physiologic test confirming that the oxygen requirement at the time point of assessment has not yet been defined. This assessment may include a pulse oximetry saturation range.

OVERVIEW of the Cardiopulmonary Clinical Manifestations Associated with Bronchopulmonary Dysplasia

The following clinical manifestations result from the pathologic mechanisms caused (or activated) by **Atelectasis** (see Figure 9-8), **Increased Alveolar-Capillary Membrane Thickness** (see Figure 9-10), and **Excessive Bronchial Secretions** (see Figure 9-12)—the major anatomic alterations of the lungs associated with bronchopulmonary dysplasia (BPD) (see Figure 37-1).

CLINICAL DATA OBTAINED AT THE PATIENT'S BEDSIDE

The Physical Examination

Vital Signs

Increased Respiratory Rate (Tachypnea)

Normally, a newborn's respiratory rate is about 40 to 60 breaths/min. During the early stages of BPD, the respiratory rate is generally well over 60 breaths/min. Several pathophysiologic mechanisms operating simultaneously may lead to an increased ventilatory rate:

- Increased stimulation of peripheral chemoreceptors (hypoxemia)
- Decreased lung compliance–increased ventilatory rate relationship
- Stimulation of central chemoreceptors

Increased Heart Rate (Pulse) and Blood Pressure

Clinical Manifestations Associated with More Negative Intrapleural Pressures during Inspiration

- Intercostal retractions
- Substernal retraction and abdominal distention (seesaw movement)
- Cyanosis of the dependent portions of the thoracic and abdominal areas
- Flaring nostrils

Chest Assessment Findings

- Wheezes
- Rhonchi
- Crackles

Expiratory Grunting

Cyanosis

CLINICAL DATA OBTAINED FROM LABORATORY TESTS AND SPECIAL PROCEDURES

Pulmonary Function Test Findings (Extrapolated Data for Instructional Purposes) (Primarily Restrictive Physiology)

FORCED EXPIRATORY FLOW RATE FINDINGS

FVC	FEV_T	FEV_1/FVC ratio	$FEF_{25\%-75\%}$
↓	N or ↓	N or ↑	N or ↓

$FEF_{50\%}$	$FEF_{200-1200}$	PEFR	MVV
N or ↓	N or ↓	N or ↓	N or ↓

Pulmonary Function Test Findings (Extrapolated Data for Instructional Purposes) (Primarily Restrictive Physiology)—cont'd

LUNG VOLUME AND CAPACITY FINDINGS

V_T	IRV	ERV	RV*
N or ↓	↓	↓	↓

VC	IC	FRC*	TLC*	RV/TLC ratio*
↓	↓	↓	↓	N

*↑ When airways are partially obstructed and/or bullae and/or emphysematous changes are present (e.g., in stage IV BPD).

Arterial Blood Gases

MILD TO MODERATE BRONCHOPULMONARY DYSPLASIA

Acute Alveolar Hyperventilation with Hypoxemia (Acute Respiratory Alkalosis)

pH	$Paco_2$	HCO_3^-	Pao_2
↑	↓	↓ (slightly)	↓

SEVERE BRONCHOPULMONARY DYSPLASIA

Chronic Ventilatory Failure with Hypoxemia (Compensated Respiratory Acidosis)

pH	$Paco_2$	HCO_3^-	Pao_2
N	↑	↑ (significantly)	↓

Acute Ventilatory Changes Superimposed on Chronic Ventilatory Failure

Because acute ventilatory changes are frequently seen in patients with chronic ventilatory failure, the respiratory care practitioner must be familiar with and alert for the following:

- Acute alveolar hyperventilation superimposed on chronic ventilatory failure, and/or
- Acute ventilatory failure (acute hypoventilation) superimposed on chronic ventilatory failure

Oxygenation Indices*

$\dot{Q}_S/\dot{Q}_T$	Do_2†	$\dot{V}o_2$	$C(a-\bar{v})o_2$	O_2ER	$S\bar{v}o_2$
↑	↓	N	N	↑	↓

†The Do_2 may be normal in patients who have compensated to the decreased oxygenation status with (1) an increased cardiac output, (2) an increased hemoglobin level, or (3) a combination of both. When the Do_2 is normal, the O_2ER is usually normal.

*$C(a-\bar{v})o_2$, Arterial-venous oxygen difference; Do_2, total oxygen delivery; O_2ER, oxygen extraction ratio; $\dot{Q}_S/\dot{Q}_T$, pulmonary shunt fraction; $S\bar{v}o_2$, mixed venous oxygen saturation; $\dot{V}o_2$, oxygen consumption.

OVERVIEW of the Cardiopulmonary Clinical Manifestations Associated with Bronchopulmonary Dysplasia—cont'd

RADIOLOGIC FINDINGS

Chest Radiograph

During Stage I, the radiologic findings are analogous to those of severe respiratory distress syndrome (RDS), showing a ground-glass granular pattern and small lung volume (Figure 37-2, *A*). During Stage II, patchy opaque areas with bronchograms (atelectasis) adjacent to areas of dark translucency (hyperinflation) appear. Identifying the precise cause of the haziness, whether pulmonary edema, alveolar consolidation, or atelectasis, is usually difficult (Figure 37-2, *B*).

The radiologic findings during Stage III are more specific to BPD. Circular or cystlike areas of hyperlucency begin to appear that are surrounded by patches of irregular density areas caused by atelectasis. This condition generates a spongelike appearance of the lungs on the chest x-ray film (Figure 37-2, *C*). Stage IV shows an increase in the size and number of cystlike areas of hyperlucency (emphysematous bullae), surrounded by thin strands of radiodensity (atelectasis and interstitial fibrosis). The emphysematous bullae and interstitial fibrosis around the bullae create a honeycomb appearance on the chest x-ray. Cor pulmonale may be seen during the advanced stages of BPD (Figure 37-2, *D*).

TABLE 37-3 Causative Factors of Bronchopulmonary Dysplasia (BPD)

Host susceptibility and genetic predisposition	The single most important causative factor associated with the development of BPD is prematurity. In addition, the retardation or restriction of intrauterine growth and a family history of RDS and asthma also put the infant at a higher risk for BPD.
Oxygen toxicity	Even in the first cases of BPD reported by Northway and colleagues in 1967, it was clear that exposure to high concentrations of oxygen was a factor in causing BPD. Subsequent reports continue to show that prolonged exposure to high levels of supplemental oxygen puts infants at risk for BPD.
Inflammation	A severe inflammatory response also plays a major role in the development of BPD.
Neonatal infection	The development of postnatal bacterial sepsis puts the infant at risk for BPD. Even airway microbial colonization without frank sepsis may increase the risk of BPD.
Mechanical ventilation	The development of BPD is strongly associated with mechanical ventilation. The major causative factors linked to mechanical ventilation are (1) high peak inspiratory pressures, (2) high mean airway pressures, and (3) overdistention of the lungs. Overinflation of the lungs causes stress fractures of the capillary endothelium, epithelium, and basement membranes. This mechanical injury in turn causes leakage of fluid into the alveolar spaces, with additional inflammation.
Pulmonary edema and patent ductus arteriosus	Abnormalities of lung fluid volume are associated with BPD. Several reports have shown that patency of the ductus arteriosus has a high correlation with the incidence of BPD.
Poor nutrition	All of the above causative factors are intensified by a poor nutritional status.

In response to the awareness of the "new" BPD, the National Institutes of Health sponsored a workshop on BPD, providing a new definition of BPD.* The new definition outlines specific diagnostic criteria, including the need for oxygen, positive pressure ventilation, and/or CPAP. The definition also includes the postnatal age to better assess the severity of BPD. Table 37-2 provides an overview of the new diagnostic criteria for the "new" BPD.

Etiology and Epidemiology

BPD is the most common form of chronic lung disease in children. It is estimated that 10,000 to 12,000 infants are diagnosed with BPD in the United States annually. The current understanding of BPD indicates that there are multiple causative factors associated with BPD. Table 37-3 provides an overview of the primary causes of BPD.

General Management of Bronchopulmonary Dysplasia

Today a number of preventive methods are used to avert or treat BPD. Such measures include prenatal maternal steroid administration, the use of postnatal exogenous surfactant, gentle ventilation techniques, low oxygen concentrations, nasal CPAP, fluid restriction, vitamin A, diuretics, bronchodilator therapy, bronchial hygiene therapy, postnatal corticosteroids, and

*Jobe AH, Bancalari E: Bronchopulmonary dysplasia, *Am J Respir Crit Care Med* 163:1723-1729, 2001.

TABLE 37-4 Therapeutic Measures Used to Prevent or Manage Infants with Bronchopulmonary Dysplasia (BPD)

Prenatal steroids	A single course of prenatal glucocorticoids administered to women who are at high risk for premature delivery results in a significant decrease in the mortality rate and in the morbidity associated with prematurity.
Gentle ventilation	In spite of the development of numerous sophisticated ventilators for the newborn, there is still no clear advantage to any one approach. The general approach is a ventilatory mode that prevents atelectasis, sustains or maintains FRC, uses a minimal tidal volume, and permits the infant to trigger his or her own ventilation as much as possible. Every effort should be made to minimize high peak inspiratory pressures, high mean airway pressures (MAPs), and overdistention of the lungs. For example, high-frequency ventilation and low tidal volumes (with the goal of maintaining the $Paco_2$ above 55 mm Hg) are commonly used.
Low inspired oxygen concentrations	Every effort should be made to administer only the lowest concentration of oxygen that is necessary.
Nasal continuous positive airway pressure (CPAP)	The early application of nasal CPAP in high-risk respiratory distress syndrome (RDS) and BPD infants is highly recommended during postnatal care.
Fluid restriction	Because fluid overload is a causative factor associated with BPD, the limitation of fluids may be helpful. However, care should be taken to not be too aggressive in the limitation of fluid administration, because undernutrition is also associated with the development of BPD.
Vitamin A	Vitamin A is an essential nutrient for maintaining the epithelial cells of the tracheobronchial tree.
Diuretics	In infants with severe BPD, pulmonary edema is a major component of the disorder. There is clear evidence that either daily or alternate-day therapy with furosemide improves lung mechanics and gas exchange in infants with established BPD.
Bronchodilator therapy	Increased airway resistance is highly associated with BPD. Short-term therapy with inhaled or parenteral $beta_2$-adrenergic agonists is frequently administered to infants with BPD. Inhaled albuterol has been the most widely used agent.
Bronchial hygiene therapy	Because of the high incidence of mucous plugging of the airways and endotracheal tubes, adequate humidification of the inspired gas is important. Postural drainage, percussion, and vigorous suctioning also are extremely beneficial.
Postnatal corticosteroids	The administration of postnatal corticosteroids to preterm infants has been shown to reduce lung inflammation and the incidence of BPD. Postnatal corticosteroids are also believed to increase surfactant synthesis, enhance beta-adrenergic activity, increase antioxidant production, stabilize cell and lysosomal membranes, and inhibit prostaglandin and leukotriene synthesis.
Inhaled nitric oxide	The administration of inhaled nitric oxide (iNO) may prevent BPD or benefit infants with evolving BPD. It is suggested that preterm infants with early BPD may have a deficiency of endogenous NO. It is hypothesized that the administration of iNO causes both pulmonary vasodilation and bronchial dilation and therefore reduces the need for oxygen and ventilatory support.

inhaled nitric oxide. In general, the management of infants who are at high risk for development of BPD or who have evolving BPD is directed at (1) minimizing the need for ventilatory support, (2) using low inspiratory pressures, (3) avoiding high mean airway pressures (MAPs), (4) minimizing the administration of high concentrations of oxygen, and (5) supporting and maintaining an adequate functional residual capacity (FRC) with PEEP or CPAP. Table 37-4 provides an overview of the therapeutic measures used to prevent or manage infants with BPD.

CASE STUDY

Bronchopulmonary Dysplasia

Admitting History and Physical Examination

An 1100-g baby boy was born at 28 weeks' gestation to a mother who received no prenatal care. The mother had used cocaine and marijuana and may have had a vaginal infection during her pregnancy. Because of the baby's history and condition, mechanical ventilation was started moments after birth. Pulmonary surfactant was given. Within 24 hours the baby developed respiratory distress syndrome (RDS); needed numerous lines for vascular access (i.e., feeding tube, intravenous [IV] line, and umbilical artery catheter); and required high concentrations of oxygen, positive end-expiratory pressure (PEEP), and continuous positive airway pressure (CPAP). Over the next 4½ weeks, he developed pneumonia and was aggressively treated for atelectasis and excessive bronchial secretions. At that time the baby was considered to have a chronic case of bronchopulmonary dysplasia (BPD).

At 5 weeks the baby was still on a pressure-cycled mechanical ventilator with the following settings: peak inspiratory pressure (PIP) +25 cm H_2O, respiratory rate (RR) 35/min, inspiratory time (Ti) 0.5 sec, F_{IO_2} 0.60, and PEEP +7 cm H_2O. His pulmonary mechanics showed increased airway resistance and decreased lung compliance. He demonstrated coarse bilateral rhonchi and some wheezes. His chest radiograph had the classic Stage III BPD appearance, with bilateral patches of bullae and areas of atelectasis. The chest x-ray film also showed interstitial emphysema and areas of pulmonary fibrosis. His arterial blood gases on an F_{IO_2} of 0.4 were pH 7.36, Pa_{CO_2} 55, HCO_3^- 30, Pa_{O_2} 50, and Sa_{O_2} of 84%. The doctor wrote the following order in the baby's chart: "Respiratory therapy to assess patient and begin to wean from ventilator." The respiratory care practitioner charted the following assessment at this time.

Respiratory Assessment and Plan

S N/A

O Marginal pulmonary mechanics—decreased compliance and increased airway resistance. Coarse rhonchi and wheezes. CXR: BPD—interstitial emphysema and fibrosis. ABGs on ventilator and 40% oxygen: pH 7.36, Pa_{CO_2} 55, HCO_3^- 30, Pa_{O_2} 50, Sa_{O_2} 84%.

A
- Stiff lung with airway obstruction (pulmonary mechanics)
- Chronic ventilatory failure with moderate hypoxemia (ABGs)
- Excessive bronchial secretions (rhonchi and suctioning results)
- Possible bronchospasm (wheezes—maybe caused by bronchial secretions)
- Appears ready for slow weaning trial

P Wean slowly per **Mechanical Ventilation Protocol** (decrease mandated respiratory rate slowly—decrease need for pressure and rate). Continue **Oxygen Therapy Protocol** (do not attempt to wean from oxygen therapy until ventilator mandated rate is down to about 5 breaths/min). Continue aggressive bronchopulmonary hygiene therapy per **Bronchopulmonary Hygiene Therapy Protocol** (CPT q2h and suction prn). Continue **Bronchodilator Therapy Protocol** (in-line neb with 0.15 mL albuterol in 2 mL normal saline q4h). Continue to monitor closely and assess frequently.

Over the next 10 weeks, the baby slowly improved. Five days before discharge, the mother was trained on several respiratory and nursing procedures for home care. Over the following 4 years, the child's lungs continued to improve even though he often had pneumonia and was unstable during the first 6 months. On one occasion, he was readmitted to the hospital for a week. However, he recovered and currently is doing well. He now is of normal weight and height for his age, runs and plays well with other children, and is about to enter preschool.

Discussion

Several comments should be made regarding this challenging pulmonary disorder of the newborn. First, infants with BPD have limited pulmonary reserves. Their lungs are seriously damaged, scarred, and fibrotic. They have increased airway resistance and decreased lung compliance. Because their lung tissues are constantly being bombarded by inflammatory stimuli, their hearts and lungs have a limited ability to recover from stress. These infants may require hours to recover from such procedures as tracheal or nasal suctioning, chest physical therapy, or pulmonary surfactant administration. Therefore health-care personnel should perform all therapeutic procedures as quickly and efficiently as possible.

Second, every attempt should be made to wean the baby off the ventilator because the ventilator pressures, rates, and high oxygen concentrations are the main factors causing the pulmonary damage. The longer the baby is on the ventilator, the more the lungs are being damaged. Also, because chronic ventilatory failure with hypoxemia commonly occurs in infants with chronic BPD, the respiratory therapist should not hurry to decrease the infant's Pa_{CO_2} to the "normal" 35 to 45 mm Hg range. Infants in the acute and chronic stages of BPD often have a high Pa_{CO_2} and normal pH (compensated). A Pa_{CO_2} of 60 or 70 mm Hg is often tolerated well. Therefore the therapist must be prepared to accept chronically high Pa_{CO_2} levels. As the baby's lungs deteriorate, moreover, the ability of blood to flow easily through the lungs progressively declines. As the condition worsens, the work of the right side of the heart increases. If the BPD does not resolve, cor pulmonale may develop.

BPD is a disorder that requires a great deal of parental education and support at the time of the baby's discharge from the hospital. The respiratory therapist can be instrumental in working with the family both in the hospital and in the home to ensure that the parents are prepared to support the child's respiratory care needs. For example, the parents must understand the procedures of tracheal and nasal suctioning, chest physical therapy, and aerosolized medication administration at home. Infants with BPD who have been discharged from the hospital commonly return to the hospital once or twice a year in acute respiratory distress. Therefore the importance of aggressive, long-term respiratory care in the home must be stressed to the family. For example, the value of good bronchopulmonary hygiene therapy at home to offset the clinical manifestations associated with the accumulation of **Excessive Bronchial Secretions** (see Figure 9-12) cannot be over emphasized.

SELF-ASSESSMENT QUESTIONS

evolve Answers to questions can be found on Evolve. To access additional student assessment questions and case studies for application of text material to real-life scenarios, visit **http://evolve.elsevier.com/DesJardins/respiratory.**

1. Which of the following is or are associated with the cause of bronchopulmonary dysplasia?

1. History of RDS
2. Low positive pressure mechanical ventilation
3. High concentrations of oxygen
4. Infant's weight greater than 2000 g

a. 2 and 4 only
b. 1 and 3 only
c. 2, 3, and 4 only
d. 1, 3, and 4 only

2. The anatomic alterations of the lungs associated with bronchopulmonary dysplasia are:

1. Increased alveolar-capillary membrane thickness
2. Atelectasis
3. Excessive bronchial secretions
4. Consolidation

a. 2 and 4 only
b. 3 and 4 only
c. 1, 2, and 3 only
d. 1, 2, 3, and 4

3. Stage IV bronchopulmonary dysplasia usually occurs after:

a. 10 days
b. 20 days
c. 30 days
d. 40 days

4. Which of the following arterial blood gas values are associated with severe bronchopulmonary dysplasia?

1. Decreased pH
2. Increased $Paco_2$
3. Normal pH
4. Decreased HCO_3^-

a. 2 and 3 only
b. 1 and 4 only
c. 2, 3, and 4 only
d. 1, 2, and 4 only

5. Which of the following clinical manifestations are associated with bronchopulmonary dysplasia?

1. Rhonchi
2. Intercostal retractions
3. Normal or decreased FEV_T
4. Increased $C(a-\bar{v})o_2$

a. 1 and 4 only
b. 2 and 3 only
c. 1, 2, and 3 only
d. 1, 2, 3, and 4

Congenital Diaphragmatic Hernia

38

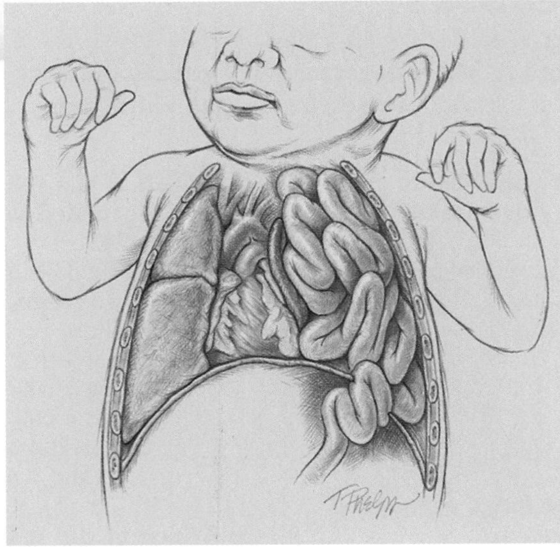

FIGURE 38-1 Diaphragmatic hernia.

Chapter Objectives

After reading this chapter, you will be able to:

- List the anatomic alterations of the lungs associated with congenital diaphragmatic hernia.
- Describe the causes of congenital diaphragmatic hernia.
- List the cardiopulmonary clinical manifestations associated with congenital diaphragmatic hernia.
- Describe the general management of congenital diaphragmatic hernia.
- Describe the clinical strategies and rationales of the SOAP presented in the case study.
- Define key terms and complete self-assessment questions at the end of the chapter and on Evolve.

Key Terms

Atelectasis
Bochdalek Foramen
Bochdalek Hernia
Congenital Diaphragmatic Eventration
Congenital Diaphragmatic Hernia (CDH)
Dextrocardia
Extracorporeal Membrane Oxygenation (ECMO)
Hemothorax
Inhaled Nitric Oxide (iNO)
Morgagni's Hernia
Pneumothorax
Posterior-Lateral Diaphragmatic Hernia
Pulmonary Hypertension
Pulmonary Hypoplasia
Scaphoid Abdomen

Chapter Outline

Anatomic Alterations of the Lungs

During normal fetal development, the diaphragm first appears anteriorly between the heart and liver and then progressively grows posteriorly. Between the eighth and tenth week of gestation, the diaphragm normally completely closes at the left **Bochdalek foramen,** which is located posteriorly and laterally on the left diaphragm. At about the tenth week of gestation (close to the same time the Bochdalek foramen is closing), the intestines and stomach normally migrate from the yolk sac. If, however, the bowels reach this area before the Bochdalek foramen closes, a hernia results—a **congenital diaphragmatic hernia (CDH)** (also called a **Bochdalek hernia** or **posterior-lateral diaphragmatic hernia**). In other words, a Bochdalek hernia is an abnormal hole in the posterolateral corner of the left diaphragm that allows the intestines—and in some cases the stomach—to move directly into the chest cavity and compress the developing lungs.*

As shown in Figure 38-1, the effects of a diaphragmatic hernia are similar to the effects of a **pneumothorax** or **hemothorax**—the lungs are compressed. As the condition becomes more severe, **atelectasis** and complete lung collapse may occur. When this happens, the heart and mediastinum are pushed to the right side of the chest—called **dextrocardia.** In addition, long-term lung compression in utero causes **pulmonary hypoplasia**, which is most severe on the affected (ipsilateral) side but also occurs on the unaffected (contralateral) side.

This pathologic process causes a marked reduction in the number of bronchial generations and alveoli per acinus. The concomitant increased muscularity of the small pulmonary arteries may contribute to the increased pulmonary vascular resistance and **pulmonary hypertension** commonly seen in these patients. Respiratory distress usually develops soon after birth. As the infant struggles to inhale, the increased negative intrathoracic pressure generated during each inspiration causes more bowel to be sucked into the thorax. Further compression of the heart occurs as the infant cries and swallows air, causing the intestine and stomach to distend further.

Finally, as a consequence of the hypoxemia associated with a diaphragmatic hernia, these babies often develop hypoxia-induced pulmonary arterial vasoconstriction and vasospasm, which produces a state of pulmonary hypertension. As a general rule, however, these babies only have a transient state of pulmonary hypertension until the diaphragmatic hernia is repaired. This is different from persistent pulmonary hypertension of the newborn (PPHN) (see Chapter 31).

The major pathologic or structural changes associated with diaphragmatic hernia may include the following:

- Failure of the Bochdalek foramen of the diaphragm to close
- Migration of intestines and stomach into the thorax
    - Atelectasis
    - Complete lung collapse
    - Mediastinum shift to the unaffected side of the thorax
    - Reduction in the number of bronchial generations and alveoli per acinus
    - Pulmonary hypoplasia
    - Transient pulmonary hypertension

*Most CDHs are Bochdalek hernias (about 95%). Rare CDHs include **Morgagni's hernia** and **congenital diaphragmatic eventration** of the diaphragm. A **Morgagni's hernia** is characterized by herniation through the foramina of Morgagni, which are located immediately adjacent to the xyphoid process of the sternum. The majority of Morgagni's hernias occur on the right side of the body and are asymptomatic. A congenital diaphragmatic eventration is when there is abnormal elevation of part or all of an otherwise intact diaphragm into the chest cavity. This rare form of CDH occurs when a region of the diaphragm is thinner (commonly caused by an incomplete muscularization of the diaphragm), which in turn allows the abdominal viscera to protrude upward.

Etiology and Epidemiology

A CDH occurs in an overall incidence ranging from 1 in 2000 to 4000 live births. The baby is usually mature, and two thirds of affected infants are male. About 95% of CDHs occur on the left side through the Bochdalek foramen. The mortality rate is about 40%. The prognosis depends on (1) the size of the defect, (2) the degree of hypoplasia, (3) the condition of the lung on the unaffected side, and (4) the success of the surgical diaphragmatic closure.

OVERVIEW of the Cardiopulmonary Clinical Manifestations Associated with Congenital Diaphragmatic Hernia

The following clinical manifestations result from the pathologic mechanisms caused (or activated) by **Atelectasis** (see Figure 9-8)—the major anatomic alteration of the lungs associated with diaphragmatic hernia (see Figure 38-1).

CLINICAL DATA OBTAINED AT THE PATIENT'S BEDSIDE

The Physical Examination

Vital Signs

Increased Respiratory Rate (Tachypnea)

Normally, a newborn's respiratory rate is about 40 to 60 breaths/min. When a diaphragmatic hernia is present, the respiratory rate is generally well over 60 breaths/min. Several pathophysiologic mechanisms operating simultaneously may lead to an increased ventilatory rate:

- Stimulation of peripheral chemoreceptors (hypoxemia)
- Decreased lung compliance–increased ventilatory rate relationship
- Stimulation of central chemoreceptors

OVERVIEW of the Cardiopulmonary Clinical Manifestations Associated with Congenital Diaphragmatic Hernia—cont'd

Increased Heart Rate (Pulse) and Blood Pressure

Clinical Manifestations Associated with More Negative Intrapleural Pressures during Inspiration

- Intercostal retraction
- Substernal retraction
- Cyanosis of the dependent portions of the thoracic and abdominal areas
- Flaring nostrils

Chest Assessment Findings

- Diminished or absent breath sounds over the affected side
- Bowel sounds over the affected side
- Apical heartbeat heard over the unaffected side (usually right)

Expiratory Grunting

Cyanosis

Barrel Chest

When the intestines are in the chest and distended with gas, the baby often demonstrates a barrel chest.

Scaphoid Abdomen

Depending on the degree of intestinal displacement into the thorax, the infant's abdomen often appears flat or concave.

CLINICAL DATA OBTAINED FROM LABORATORY TESTS AND SPECIAL PROCEDURES

Pulmonary Function Test Findings (Extrapolated Data for Instructional Purposes) (Restrictive Lung Pathophysiology)

FORCED EXPIRATORY FLOW RATE FINDINGS

FVC	FEV_T	FEV_1/FVC ratio	$FEF_{25\%-75\%}$
↓	N or ↓	N or ↑	N or ↓

$FEF_{50\%}$	$FEF_{200-1200}$	PEFR	MVV
N or ↓	N or ↓	N or ↓	N or ↓

LUNG VOLUME AND CAPACITY FINDINGS

V_T	IRV	ERV	RV
N or ↓	↓	↓	↓

VC	IC	FRC	TLC	RV/TLC ratio
↓	↓	↓	↓	N

Arterial Blood Gases

MILD TO MODERATE DIAPHRAGMATIC HERNIA

Acute Alveolar Hyperventilation with Hypoxemia (Acute Respiratory Alkalosis)

pH	$Paco_2$	HCO_3^-	Pao_2
↑	↓	↓ (slightly)	↓

SEVERE DIAPHRAGMATIC HERNIA

Acute Ventilatory Failure with Hypoxemia (Acute Respiratory Acidosis)

pH*	$Paco_2$	HCO_3^- *	Pao_2
↓	↑	↑ (slightly)	↓

*When tissue hypoxia is severe enough to produce lactic acid, the pH and HCO_3^- values will be lower than expected for a particular $Paco_2$ level.

Oxygenation Indices*

$\dot{Q}_S/\dot{Q}_T$	Do_2†	$\dot{V}o_2$	$C(a-\bar{v})o_2$	O_2ER	$S\bar{v}o_2$
↑	↓	N	N	↑	↓

†The Do_2 may be normal in patients who have compensated to the decreased oxygenation status with (1) an increased cardiac output, (2) an increased hemoglobin level, or (3) a combination of both. When the Do_2 is normal, the O_2ER is usually normal.

*$C(a-\bar{v})o_2$, Arterial-venous oxygen difference; Do_2, total oxygen delivery; O_2ER, oxygen extraction ratio; $\dot{Q}_S/\dot{Q}_T$, pulmonary shunt fraction; $S\bar{v}o_2$, mixed venous oxygen saturation; $\dot{V}o_2$, oxygen consumption.

RADIOLOGIC FINDINGS

Chest Radiograph

- Increased opacity (ground-glass appearance of compressed lung)

A typical radiograph shows fluid- and air-filled loops of intestine in the chest and a shift of the heart and mediastinum to the unaffected side. Atelectasis and complete lung collapse may be present. The lungs may appear hyoplastic and may not expand to meet the chest wall. A nasogastric tube (in the patient's stomach, it is hoped) may be seen on the chest radiograph. It is used to decompress the abdominal viscera. The presence of a diaphragmatic hernia on a chest x-ray film usually confirms the need for surgery (Figure 38-2).

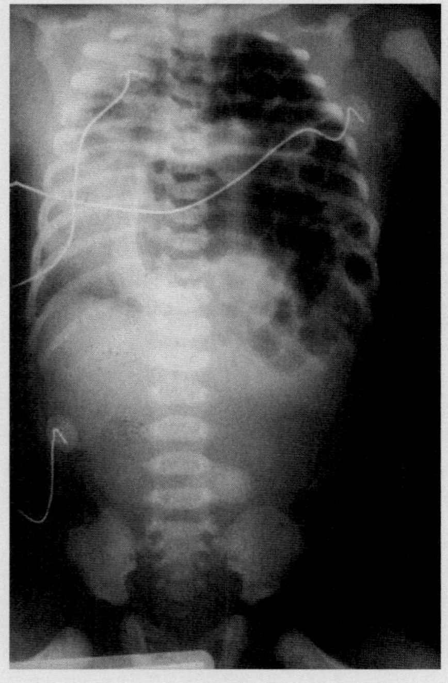

FIGURE 38-2 Chest x-ray film of left diaphragmatic hernia.

General Management of a Congenital Diaphragmatic Hernia

Severe diaphragmatic hernia is one of the most urgent neonatal surgical emergencies. Although prompt surgical repair is imperative, a number of therapeutic measures may be instituted until the baby is stabilized for surgery. The baby may not be stable enough for surgery for several days.

As soon as the diagnosis of a diaphragmatic hernia is made, a double-lumen oral gastric tube should be inserted with intermittent or low continuous suction. This reduces the amount of gas in the stomach and bowels and thereby reduces lung compression. Oxygen therapy should be started immediately. The infant also may be placed in the semi-Fowler's position, which reduces the intrathoracic pressure and facilitates the downward positioning of the abdominal viscera. Placing the infant on the affected side aids expansion of the good lung. *The infant must not be manually ventilated with a bag and mask, because of the danger of air swallowing.*

The infant must, however, be intubated and ventilated. Mechanical ventilation should be applied with low peak airway pressures (<30 cm H_2O) and rapid respiratory rates. A typical set of ventilator parameters would be as follows: peak inspiratory pressure (PIP) +18 to +20 cm H_2O, respiratory rate (RR) 40, F_{IO_2} 100%, positive end-expiratory pressure (PEEP) +2 to +3 cm H_2O, and inspiratory time (TI) 0.4. High-frequency oscillatory ventilation and jet ventilation are sometimes successful. Because the infant's lungs are fragile and rupture easily, the incidence of pneumothorax is high. Therefore the physician may need to insert one or more chest tubes during mechanical ventilation. Paralysis with pancuronium and sedation with morphine are helpful at times. Paralysis eliminates the swallowing of air, which helps to keep the bowels compressed. These infants are usually treated with **extracorporeal membrane oxygenation (ECMO)** as long as the diaphragmatic hernia is present. While on ECMO, the infant is usually ventilated only three or four times per minute to keep the lung inflated.

The surgical procedure entails repositioning the abdominal contents into the abdomen and closing the diaphragmatic defect. In some infants the peritoneal cavity may be too small to contain the abdominal contents. In these cases the surgeon leaves the fascia open and closes only the skin. This results in a ventral hernia that is repaired several months after the initial surgery. After surgery the baby is placed back on the ventilator and weaned per ventilator protocol. Mechanical ventilation with PEEP and continuous positive airway pressure (CPAP) commonly are required to offset the atelectasis and hypoplasia associated with the disorder. Often, the lung on the affected side is hypoplastic, and days or weeks of therapy may be required for full expansion to occur.

Occasionally, certain pharmacologic agents may be administered to offset the infant's pulmonary hypertension. Such drugs include tolazoline, digitalis agents, diuretics, nitroglycerin, and **inhaled nitric oxide (iNO).** The physiologic action of iNO is believed to be similar to that of the vasoactive substance endothelium-derived relaxing factor (ERF). The use of iNO has significantly reduced the need for ECMO therapy.

ECMO may be indicated to treat circulatory and respiratory complications after surgery for infants who do not respond favorably to conventional medical therapy. Pulmonary surfactant usually is administered because the lungs are immature and hypoplastic. The administration of pulmonary surfactant may not only offset the infant's surfactant deficiency and improve compliance but may also lower pulmonary vascular resistance and improve pulmonary blood flow.

CASE STUDY

Diaphragmatic Hernia

Admitting History and Physical Examination

A full-term baby boy was delivered at 2:25 AM with no remarkable problems to a mother who had received no prenatal care. After delivery, however, the baby made one cry and quickly became blue and limp, started to have bradycardia, and became apneic. The baby's 1-minute Apgar score was 3 (heart rate 1, respiration 0, tone 1, reflex irritability 1, color 0). The nurse handed the baby to a student intern, who immediately began to ventilate the baby manually. Both the respiratory therapist and the nurse noted that the baby's abdomen was scaphoid; the therapist stated that the baby might have a diaphragmatic hernia and that bagging should be stopped immediately. Moments later, the neonatologist entered the room, confirmed the **scaphoid abdomen,** noted that the lungs were very stiff in response to the bagging, and ordered a stat intubation with a 3.5-mm tube and a chest x-ray examination.

The infant was then transferred to the neonatal intensive care unit (NICU). The chest x-ray film confirmed a left diaphragmatic hernia and hypoplastic left lung. At this time, a nasogastric tube was inserted, and suction was begun. The baby was sedated and placed on a pressured cycled mechanical ventilator. An intravenous (IV) line and umbilical artery catheter were then secured. The initial ventilatory settings were respiratory rate (RR) 30/min, inspiratory time (TI) 0.6, positive end-expiratory pressure (PEEP) +4, positive inspiratory pressure (PIP) + 25, and FIO_2 1.0. Initial arterial blood gases were pH 7.19, $PaCO_2$ 63, HCO_3^- 21, PaO_2 24, and SaO_2 38%. No breath sounds could be heard over the infant's left lung. The neonatologist diagnosed pulmonary hypertension of the neonate. The respiratory therapist then adjusted the ventilatory settings as follows: RR 35/min, TI 0.6 second, PEEP +5, PIP +28 cm H_2O, and FIO_2 1.0. A second set of arterial blood gases taken 15 minutes later showed pH 7.29, $PaCO_2$ 49, HCO_3^- 23, PaO_2 44, and SaO_2 74%.

The baby was placed on extracorporeal membrane oxygenation (ECMO), with the ventilator set to minimal settings. Even though the ECMO was doing all the oxygenation, the baby's lungs were expanded by the ventilator about four times a minute. Four days later, the baby's pulmonary artery pressure was determined to be low enough for surgery. The diaphragmatic hernia was repaired, and the baby was returned to the NICU with a chest tube in the left side of the chest. The baby was again placed on a ventilator.

The ventilator settings 3 days later were RR 8/min, TI 0.6, PIP +20, PEEP and CPAP +4, and FIO_2 0.45. His vital signs were heart rate 145 bpm, blood pressure 70/45, RR 65 (between ventilator breaths), and temperature 37° C (96.8° F). His skin was pink and normal. Good breath sounds were auscultated over the right lung, and rhonchi and crackles could be heard over the left lung.

Arterial blood gas values at this time were as follows: pH 7.36, $PaCO_2$ 44, HCO_3^- 23, PaO_2 73, and SaO_2 94%. The baby's chest x-ray film showed good lung expansion on the right side. Although the upper half of the left lung was well expanded, atelectasis and hypoplasia were still seen over the lower half of the left lung. Bubbles were no longer coming from the left-sided chest tube. A small amount of thin, clear secretions was suctioned from the baby's endotracheal tube three or four times an hour. At that time the respiratory therapist wrote the following assessment in the infant's chart.

Respiratory Assessment and Plan

S N/A

O Vital signs: On ECMO HR 145, BP 70/45, RR 65 (8 mechanical breaths), T 37° C (96.8° F). Skin: Pink and normal. Breath sounds: Right lung—normal; left lung—rhonchi and crackles. No chest tube bubbles. ABGs: pH 7.36, $PaCO_2$ 44, HCO_3^- 23, PaO_2 73, SaO_2 94%. CXR: Right lung normal; atelectasis and hypoplasia in left lower lung.

A
- On ECMO, ventilator-dependent, but improving (vital signs, skin color, ABGs)
- Mild amount of large and small airway secretions (crackles, rhonchi)
- Atelectasis and hypoplasia of the left lower lobe (CXR)
- May be ready to wean from ECMO—check with physician

P Mechanical Ventilation Protocol (continue to wean per protocol—wean pressures first, then FIO_2). **Lung Expansion Therapy Protocol** (continue PEEP or CPAP per **Mechanical Ventilator Protocol**). **Bronchopulmonary Hygiene Therapy Protocol** (continue suction and CPT prn). **Oxygen Therapy Protocol** (keep SpO_2 at 97% or more as the FIO_2 is decreased. Do not decrease FIO_2 more than 10% per hour).

ECMO was discontinued. The baby continued to improve over the next 5 days. On day 6, the baby was off the ventilator. The baby was discharged from the hospital 1 week later. The baby continued to develop normally over the next 4 years; at the time of this writing, he was about to enter kindergarten.

Discussion

This case nicely illustrates the importance of good assessment skills. Most diaphragmatic hernias are identified before the baby is born by abdominal ultrasound of the abdomen during routine prenatal care. Unfortunately, this mother had no prenatal care, and as a result, the baby's diaphragmatic hernia was a surprise. Fortunately, the respiratory care practitioner and nurse in this case quickly and correctly identified the possibility of the diaphragmatic hernia by noting the scaphoid abdomen. Had the student intern continued to bag the baby manually, more gas would have entered the stomach and intestines, compressing and compromising the infant's lungs even more. The **Atelectasis** (see Figure 9-8) caused by the enlarged intestines was objectively confirmed on the chest radiograph. The **Lung Expansion Therapy Protocol** was clearly justified to offset the atelectasis after the diaphragmatic hernia was repaired.

This case further illustrates that the first objective in the management of the infant born with a diaphragmatic hernia is the correction of the transient pulmonary hypertension. Often, as in this case, treatment requires that the infant be treated with ECMO for 3 or 4 days before surgery. After the pulmonary hypertension is controlled, the second objective is surgical repair of the hernia. Mechanical ventilation with PEEP and CPAP are usually required after surgery to correct the atelectasis and hypoplasia associated with the disorder. Typically, weaning involves decreasing the F_{IO_2} while monitoring the baby's pulse oximetry. Ideally, the ventilator pressures are decreased first, and then the ventilatory rates are decreased. A target Pa_{CO_2} of 40 mm Hg or less is commonly used. An infant on a ventilatory rate of 12/min, a peak inspiratory pressure of +15 cm H_2O or less, and a PEEP of +3 cm H_2O or less is usually ready for a weaning trial.

SELF-ASSESSMENT QUESTIONS

evolve Answers to questions can be found on Evolve. To access additional student assessment questions and case studies for application of text material to real-life scenarios, visit **http://evolve.elsevier.com/DesJardins/respiratory.**

1. The Bochdalek foramen closes at the:
- a. Fourth to sixth week of gestation
- b. Sixth to eighth week of gestation
- c. Eighth to tenth week of gestation
- d. Tenth to twelfth week of gestation

2. Which of the following are associated with a congenital diaphragmatic hernia?
1. Females are affected more than males
2. Left side (90%)
3. A scaphoid abdomen at birth
4. Bowel sounds on the affected side of chest
- a. 1 and 3 only
- b. 2 and 4 only
- c. 2, 3, and 4 only
- d. 1, 2, 3, and 4

3. Which of the following arterial blood gas values is or are associated with mild to moderate congenital diaphragmatic hernia?
1. Increased pH
2. Increased Pa_{CO_2}
3. Increased Pa_{O_2}
4. Increased HCO_3^-
- a. 1 only
- b. 1 and 4 only
- c. 2, 3, and 4 only
- d. 1, 2, and 4 only

4. Which of the following clinical manifestations is or are associated with a congenital diaphragmatic hernia?
1. Diminished or absent breath sounds
2. Intercostal retractions
3. Normal or decreased FEV_T
4. Increased $C(a-\bar{v})_{O_2}$
- a. 3 and 4 only
- b. 1 and 2 only
- c. 1, 2, and 3 only
- d. 1, 2, 3, and 4

5. Which of the following is or are associated with a congenital diaphragmatic hernia?
1. Increased alveolar-capillary membrane thickness
2. Atelectasis
3. Excessive bronchial secretions
4. Pulmonary consolidation
- a. 2 only
- b. 3 only
- c. 1, 2, and 3 only
- d. 1, 2, 3, and 4

Croup Syndrome: Laryngotracheobronchitis and Acute Epiglottitis

39

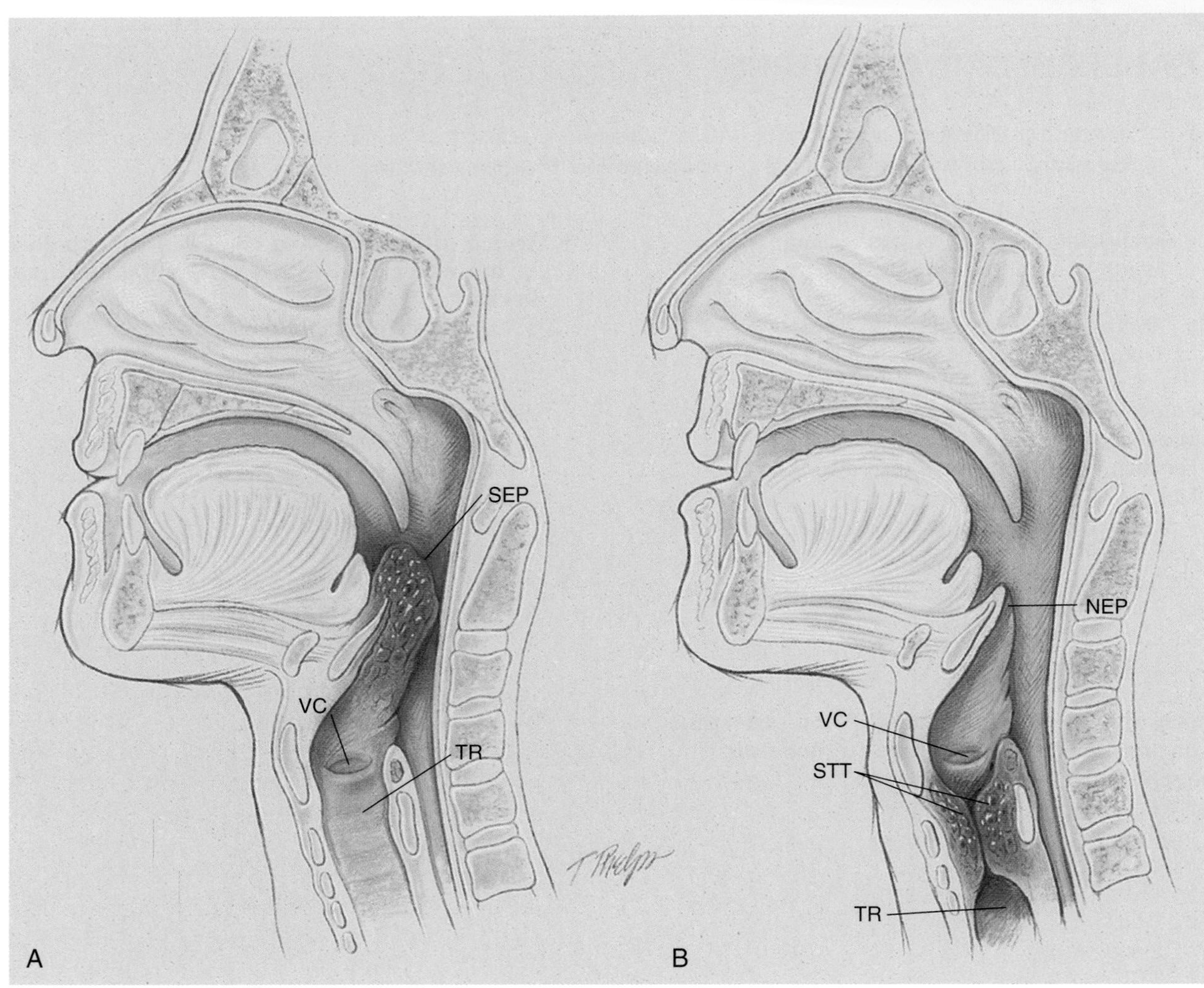

FIGURE 39-1 Laryngotracheobronchitis and acute epiglottitis. **A**, Acute epiglottitis. **B**, Laryngotracheobronchitis. *NEP,* Normal epiglottis; *SEP,* swollen epiglottis; *STT,* swollen tracheal tissue; *TR,* trachea. *VC,* vocal cords.

Chapter Objectives

After reading this chapter, you will be able to:

- List the anatomic alterations of the lungs associated with croup syndrome.
- Describe the causes of croup syndrome.
- List the cardiopulmonary clinical manifestations associated with croup syndrome.
- Describe the general management of croup syndrome.
- Describe the clinical strategies and rationales of the SOAPs presented in the case studies.
- Define key terms and complete self-assessment questions at the end of the chapter and on Evolve.

Key Terms

Acute Epiglottitis
Cool Aerosol Mist

Croup
Haemophilus influenzae type B
Inspiratory Stridor
Laryngotracheobronchitis (LTB)
Parainfluenza Viruses
Racemic Epinephrine (MicroNefrin, Vaponefrin)
Steeple Point or Pencil Point (Lateral Neck X-Ray Film—LTB)
Subglottic Airway Obstruction
Subglottic Croup
Supraglottic Airway Obstruction
Supraglottic Croup
"Thumb Sign" (Lateral Neck X-Ray Film—Epiglottis)

Chapter Outline

The word **croup** is a general term used to describe the inspiratory, barking or brassy sound associated with a partial upper airway obstruction. In other words, croup is actually a clinical sign (objective data) or a clinical manifestation—that is, the "barking or brassy sound" associated with a partial upper airway obstruction. Clinically, the inspiratory barking sound heard in a patient with a partial upper airway obstruction is called **inspiratory stridor**.

Most experts treat **laryngotracheobronchitis (LTB)**—which is a **subglottic airway obstruction**—and the term *croup* interchangeably, and **acute epiglottitis**—which is a **supraglottic airway obstruction**—as two entirely separate disease entities (see Figure 39-1). Historically, this is likely a result, in part, of the fact that the inspiratory stridor (i.e., the croup sound) associated with a patient with LTB is usually a loud and high-pitched brassy sound, whereas the inspiratory stridor associated with a patient with acute epiglottis is often lower in pitch or muffled, or even absent.

In addition, some sources refer to LTB as a **subglottic croup** and to acute epiglottis as a **supraglottic croup.** In essence, these phrases (*subglottic croup* versus *supraglottic croup*) simply mean that the inspiratory stridor sound originates from either the subglottic area (i.e., in LTB) or the supraglottic area (i.e., in acute epiglottis).

Thus, in view of the confusing nature of the term *croup* and the two types of partial upper airway disorders—LTB and acute epiglottis—the phrase *inspiratory stridor* will always be used in place of the term *croup* throughout this chapter to enhance the clarity of the subject matter.

Anatomic Alterations of the Upper Airway

Laryngotracheobronchitis

Because laryngotracheobronchitis can affect the lower laryngeal area, trachea, and occasionally the bronchi, the term *laryngotracheobronchitis* is used as a synonym for "classic" subglottic croup. Pathologically, LTB is an inflammatory process that causes edema and swelling of the mucous membranes. Although the laryngeal mucosa and submucosa are vascular, the distribution of the lymphatic capillaries is uneven or absent in this region. Consequently, when edema develops in the upper airway, fluid spreads and accumulates quickly throughout the connective tissues, which causes the mucosa to swell and the airway lumen to narrow. The inflammation also causes the mucous glands to increase their production of mucus and the cilia to lose their effectiveness as a mucociliary transport mechanism.

Because the subglottic area is the narrowest region of the larynx in an infant or small child, even a slight degree of edema can cause a significant reduction in cross-sectional area of the airway. The edema in this area is further aggravated by the rigid cricoid cartilage, which surrounds the mucous membrane and prevents external swelling as fluid engorges the laryngeal tissues. The edema and swelling in the subglottic region decrease the ability of the vocal cords to abduct (move apart) during inspiration. This further reduces the cross-sectional area of airway in this region.

Acute Epiglottitis

Acute epiglottitis is a life-threatening emergency. In contrast to LTB, epiglottitis is an inflammation of the supraglottic region, which includes the epiglottis, aryepiglottic folds, and false vocal cords (see Figure 39-1). Epiglottitis does not involve the pharynx, trachea, or other subglottic structures. As the edema in the epiglottis increases, the lateral borders curl and the tip of the epiglottis protrudes posteriorly and inferiorly. During inspiration the swollen epiglottis is pulled (or sucked) over the laryngeal inlet. In severe cases, this may completely block the laryngeal opening. Clinically, the classic finding is a swollen, cherry-red epiglottis.

The major pathologic or structural changes associated with croup are as follows:

- LTB—Airway obstruction caused by tissue swelling just *below* the vocal cords
- Epiglottitis—Airway obstruction caused by tissue swelling just *above* the vocal cords

TABLE 39-1 General History and Physical Findings of Laryngotracheobronchitis (LTB) and Epiglottitis

	LTB	Epiglottitis
Age	6 months-5 years (with the peak prevalence in the second year)	2-6 years
Onset	Usually slow or gradual (24-48 hours)	Abrupt (2-4 hours)
Fever	Absent	Present
Drooling	Absent	Present
Lateral neck x-ray findings	Haziness in subglottic area	Haziness in supraglottic area
Inspiratory stridor	High-pitched, brassy, loud sound	Low-pitched and muffled, or absent
Cough	Present (barking or brassy cough)	Absent
Hoarseness	Present	Absent
Swallowing difficulty	Absent	Present
White blood count	Normal (viral—parainfluenza viruses 1, 2, and 3; influenza A and B; respiratory syncytial virus)	Elevated (bacterial—*Haemophilus influenza* type B)

Etiology and Epidemiology

Laryngotracheobronchitis

The **parainfluenza viruses** cause most cases of LTB, with type 1 being the most common type, type 3 less common, and type 2 infrequent. LTB also may be caused by influenza A and B, respiratory syncytial virus (RSV), herpes simplex virus, *Mycoplasma pneumoniae,* rhinovirus, and adenoviruses. LTB is primarily seen in children 6 months to 5 years of age, with peak prevalence in the second year of life. Boys are affected slightly more often than girls. The onset of LTB is slow (i.e., symptoms progressively increase over 24 to 48 hours), and it is most common during the fall and winter. A brassy or barking cough is commonly present. The child's voice is hoarse, and the inspiratory stridor is typically loud and high in pitch. The patient usually does not have a fever, drooling, swallowing difficulties, or a toxic appearance.

*It is of interest to note that George Washington, the first president of the United States, died in the winter of 1799 from acute epiglottitis during an epidemic of influenza. The details of the illness were fully recorded by his secretary, Tobias Lear, and this is the first published description in English of this condition. An account is given of the medical treatment and controversies that arose in criticism of the attendant doctors. (From Cohen B: The death of George Washington 1732-99: the history of "cynanchum," *J Med Biogrid* Nov;13(4):225-31, 2005.)

Acute Epiglottitis*

Acute epiglottitis is a bacterial infection that is almost always caused by ***Haemophilus influenzae* type B.** It is transmitted via aerosol droplets. Since 1985, when vaccinations with *H. influenzae* type B vaccine became widespread, the number of reported cases of epiglottitis has decreased by over 95%. *H. influenzae* type B, however, is still responsible for 75% of the epiglottitis cases. Other causes of epiglottitis include aspiration of hot liquid and trauma from repeated intubation attempts.

Epiglottitis has no clear-cut geographic or seasonal incidence. Although acute epiglottitis may develop in all age groups (neonatal to adulthood), it most often occurs in children 2 to 6 years of age. Boys are affected more often than girls. The onset of epiglottitis is usually abrupt. Although the initial clinical manifestations are usually mild, they progress rapidly over a 2- to 4-hour period. A common scenario includes a sore throat or mild upper respiratory problem that quickly progresses to a high fever, lethargy, and difficulty in swallowing and handling secretions. The child usually appears pale. As the supraglottic area becomes swollen, breathing becomes noisy, the tongue is often thrust forward during inspiration, and the child may drool. Compared with LTB, the inspiratory stridor is usually softer and lower in pitch. A cough is usually not associated with acute epiglottis. The voice and cry are usually muffled rather than hoarse. Older children commonly complain of a sore throat during swallowing. A cough is usually absent in patients with epiglottitis. Acute epiglottitis in adults is typically seen in patients with neck trauma (e.g., blunt force neck injury or aspiration of hot liquid), in those who have been intubated repeatedly, and in drug abuse (crack cocaine) cases.

The general history and physical findings of LTB and epiglottitis are compared and contrasted in Table 39-1.

OVERVIEW of the Cardiopulmonary Clinical Manifestations Associated with Laryngotracheobronchitis and Epiglottitis

The following clinical manifestations result from the pathologic mechanisms caused (or activated) by an **Upper Airway Obstruction**—the major anatomic alteration of the lungs associated with laryngotracheobronchitis (LTB) and epiglottitis (see Figure 39-1).

(Upper airway obstruction is not one of the major clinical scenarios discussed in Chapter 9.)

CLINICAL DATA OBTAINED AT THE PATIENT'S BEDSIDE

The Physical Examination

Vital Signs

Increased Respiratory Rate (Tachypnea)

Several pathophysiologic mechanisms operating simultaneously may lead to an increased ventilatory rate:

- Increased stimulation of peripheral chemoreceptors
- Anxiety

Increased Heart Rate (Pulse) and Blood Pressure

Chest Assessment Findings

- Diminished breath sounds

Inspiratory Stridor

Under normal circumstances the slight narrowing of the upper (extrathoracic) airway that naturally occurs during inspiration is insignificant. Because the upper airway is relatively small in infants and children, however, even a slight degree of edema may become significant. Thus when the cross-section of the upper airway is reduced because of the edema, the child will generate stridor during inspiration, when the upper airway naturally becomes smaller. It also should be noted that if the edema becomes severe, the patient may generate both inspiratory and expiratory stridor.

Cyanosis

Use of Accessory Muscles During Inspiration

Substernal and Intercostal Retraction

CLINICAL DATA OBTAINED FROM LABORATORY TESTS AND SPECIAL PROCEDURES

Arterial Blood Gases

MILD TO MODERATE LARYNGOTRACHEOBRONCHITIS OR EPIGLOTTITIS

Acute Alveolar Hyperventilation with Hypoxemia

(Acute Respiratory Alkalosis)

pH	Pa_{CO_2}	HCO_3^-	Pa_{O_2}
↑	↓	↓ (slightly)	↓

SEVERE LARYNGOTRACHEOBRONCHITIS OR EPIGLOTTITIS

Acute Ventilatory Failure with Hypoxemia

(Acute Respiratory Acidosis)

pH*	Pa_{CO_2}	HCO_3^- *	Pa_{O_2}
↓	↑	↑ (slightly)	↓

*When tissue hypoxia is severe enough to produce lactic acid, the pH and HCO_3^- values will be lower than expected for a particular Pa_{CO_2} level.

Oxygenation Indices*

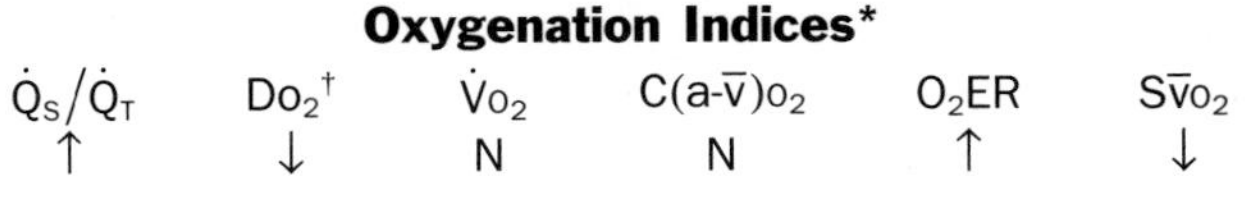

$\dot{Q}_S/\dot{Q}_T$	D_{O_2}†	$\dot{V}_{O_2}$	$C(a-\bar{v})_{O_2}$	O_2ER	$S\bar{v}_{O_2}$
↑	↓	N	N	↑	↓

†The D_{O_2} may be normal in patients who have compensated to the decreased oxygenation status with (1) an increased cardiac output, (2) an increased hemoglobin level, or (3) a combination of both. When the D_{O_2} is normal, the O_2ER is usually normal.

* *$C(a-\bar{v})_{O_2}$*, Arterial-venous oxygen difference; *D_{O_2}*, total oxygen delivery; *O_2ER*, oxygen extraction ratio; *$\dot{Q}_S/\dot{Q}_T$*, pulmonary shunt fraction; *$S\bar{v}_{O_2}$*, mixed venous oxygen saturation; *$\dot{V}_{O_2}$*, oxygen consumption.

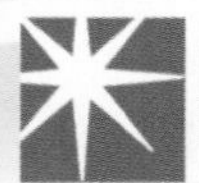

OVERVIEW of the Cardiopulmonary Clinical Manifestations Associated with Laryngotracheobronchitis and Epiglottitis—cont'd

LATERAL NECK RADIOGRAPH

- Haziness in the subglottic area (LTB)
- **"Steeple point"** or **"pencil point"** narrowing of the upper airway (LTB)
- Haziness in the supraglottic area (epiglottitis)
- Classic **"thumb sign"** (epiglottitis)

Although the diagnosis of epiglottitis or LTB can generally be made on the basis of the patient's clinical history, a lateral neck x-ray examination sometimes is used to confirm the diagnosis. When the patient has LTB, a white haziness is demonstrated in the subglottic area. When the patient has acute epiglottitis, a white haziness is evident in the supraglottic area. In addition, epiglottitis often appears on a lateral neck x-ray film as the classic "thumb sign." The epiglottis is swollen and rounded, giving it an appearance of the distal portion of a thumb (Figure 39-2). Figure 39-3 shows a lateral neck radiograph of a 27-year-old man with severe epiglottitis caused by crack cocaine abuse and neck and head trauma from a motorcycle accident.

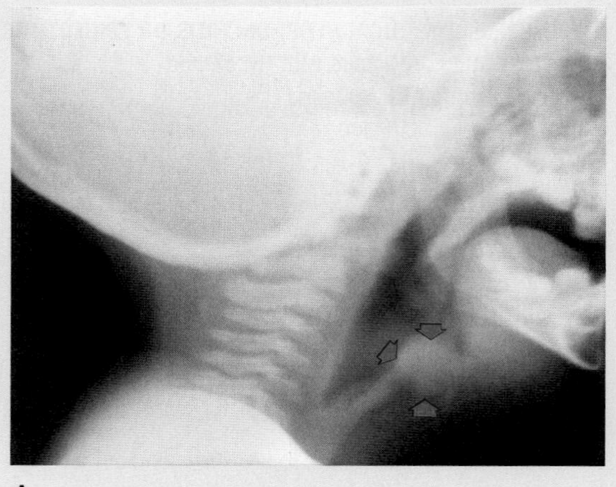

A

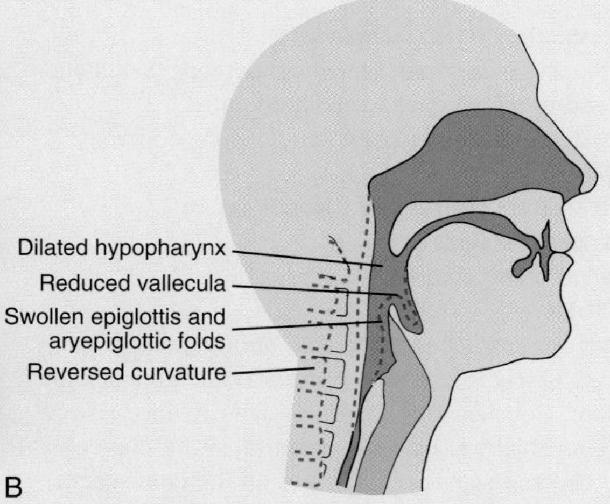

B

FIGURE 39-2 The classic **"thumb sign"** of an edematous epiglottis is evident in this lateral neck film (see arrows in **A**). The schematic illustrates the findings to look for in a lateral film of a patient with suspected epiglottitis (**B**). Such films are unnecessary in a child with the classic history, signs, and symptoms of epiglottitis; they can be of tremendous help, however, in diagnosing mild or questionable cases and explaining to parents the need for aggressive treatment. (From Ashcraft CK, Steele RW: Epiglottitis—a pediatric emergency, *J Respir Dis* 9:48, 1988.)

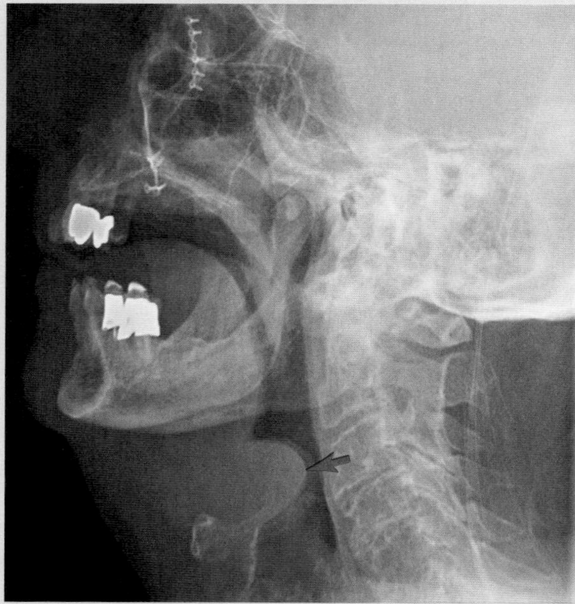

FIGURE 39-3 A 27-year-old man with severe epiglottitis *(red arrow)* caused by crack cocaine abuse and upper neck and head trauma from a motorcycle accident. (Used with permission from the author: T. Des Jardins, Wind-Mist LLC.)

General Management of Laryngotracheobronchitis and Epiglottitis

The treatment of mild cases of LTB primarily is supportive. Care includes temperature control, adequate hydration, and humidification of inspired air. The patient's vital signs, degree of intercostal retractions, mental status, and ventilatory and oxygenation status are closely monitored. Early recognition of epiglottitis may save a patient's life. A history of upper airway obstruction requires a general examination as soon as possible. *Under no circumstances should the mouth or throat be examined unless personnel and equipment are available to rapidly intubate or tracheostomize the patient.*

In cases of suspected epiglottitis, examination or inspection of the pharynx and larynx is absolutely contraindicated, except in the operating room with a fully trained team. This is because direct examination of the throat (even though depression of the tongue may reveal a bright red epiglottis and confirm the diagnosis) often results in a sudden and complete closure of the upper airway. A lateral neck radiograph may be necessary to differentiate LTB from epiglottitis or some other upper airway obstruction. The patient with a confirmed diagnosis of acute epiglottis is intubated immediately! After the diagnosis is established, the general management of LTB and acute epiglottitis is as follows:

Supplemental Oxygen

Because hypoxemia is associated with both LTB and epiglottitis, supplemental oxygen is required (see Oxygen Therapy Protocol, Protocol 9-1).

Cool Aerosol Mist

Cool aerosol mist therapy (with oxygen) either by face mask or tent is the primary mode of treatment for LTB. It liquefies thick secretions and cools and reduces subglottic edema. Generations of mothers have learned this homespun therapy, and it usually (although not always) works. Warm aerosols also are often effective.

Racemic Epinephrine (MicroNefrin, Vaponefrin)

Aerosolized **racemic epinephrine (MicroNefrin, Vaponefrin)** usually is administered to children with LTB. This adrenergic agent is used for its mucosal vasoconstriction and is recognized as an effective and safe aerosol decongestant (see Aerosolized Medication Protocol, Protocol 9-4).

Corticosteroids

Corticosteroids have been shown to reduce the severity and duration of LTB. They generally are prescribed when the patient does not respond to cool mist and racemic epinephrine therapy (see Appendix II).

Antibiotic Therapy

Because acute epiglottitis almost always is caused by *H. influenzae* type B, appropriate antibiotic therapy should be part of the treatment plan. Ampicillin and chloramphenicol often are prescribed to cover the most common organisms that cause acute epiglottitis.

Endotracheal Intubation or Tracheostomy

In the patient with a suspected acute epiglottis, the examination or inspection of the pharyngeal and laryngeal areas is only to be performed in the operating room with a trained surgical team in attendance. This is because the epiglottis may obstruct completely in response to even the slightest touch during inspection. The physician, nurse, and respiratory care practitioner should not leave the patient's bedside until the endotracheal tube is secured. If the patient is anxious, restless, or uncooperative, restraints and sedation may be needed to prevent accidental extubation. After intubation, the patient should be transferred to the intensive care unit (ICU) and placed on continuous positive airway pressure (CPAP).

CASE STUDY 1

Laryngotracheobronchitis

Admitting History and Physical Examination

A 3-year-old boy had a mild viral upper respiratory infection and some hoarseness; at 10 PM on the third day of his illness, he rapidly developed a brassy cough and high-pitched inspiratory stridor. He became moderately dyspneic. The child was restless and appeared frightened. Rectal temperature was 37° C. The mother claimed that the child was "blue" on two occasions during this episode. She was going to take the child to the emergency room, but the grandmother suggested that she try steam inhalation first. Accordingly, the child was taken to the bathroom, where the hot shower was turned on full force. The child was comforted by the grandmother and urged to breathe slowly and deeply. As the bathroom became filled with steam, the respiratory distress abated and within a few minutes the child was free of stridor, breathing essentially normally. The next day the same symptoms recurred, and the patient was taken to the emergency department.

Cough and inspiratory stridor were noted. Vital signs were: blood pressure 90/60, pulse 160 bpm, respiratory rate 50/minute. The room air Sp_{O_2} was 92%. A chest x-ray film and cross-table soft tissue x-ray examination of the neck suggested laryngotracheobronchitis (LTB). The chest x-ray findings were otherwise normal. The respiratory therapist documented the following assessment and plan.

Respiratory Assessment and Plan

S Mother reports patient had cough and inspiratory stridor.

O Confirms above. Lungs clear except for stridor and tracheal breath sounds throughout. Vital signs: BP: 90/60, P: 160/minute, RR 50/min. Pallor noted. O_2 sat. 92% on room air. CXR and soft tissue x-ray film of neck suggest laryngotracheobronchitis.

A LTB, moderate (history and inspiratory stridor)

P Notify the physician. Start cool mist aerosol treatment and **Aerosolized Medication Protocol** (med. neb. treatment with racemic epinephrine per protocol). Will obtain throat culture when physician is present.

Over the next 8 hours, the patient progressively improved. At his discharge the next morning, the patient's mother was instructed in home treatment of LTB, using aerosolized racemic epinephrine prn.

Discussion

Home remedies sometimes do work. Any parent who has had a child with LTB will find this scenario familiar. What may not be as widely recognized is that sometimes warm and sometimes cool aerosols improve this syndrome. When this approach failed, the parents were wise to bring their son to the emergency department for prompt vasoconstrictive therapy accompanied by a cool mist aerosol. This resulted in prompt improvement. In most pediatric units, decongestant aerosol therapy and mist inhalation are part of the **Aerosolized Medication Protocol** (see Protocol 9-4). Note the emphasis on family education, including the prn use of racemic epinephrine aerosolization for outpatients. These instructions may have kept the patient from ever returning again to the emergency department to be treated for such an episode.

CASE STUDY 2

Acute Epiglottitis

Admitting History and Physical Examination

A 2-year-old girl appeared quite well in the evening and was put to bed at the usual time. She woke up 2 hours later, and her parents were immediately aware that she was in serious respiratory distress. She was sitting up in bed, drooling, unable to speak or cry, and breathing noisily. The parents wrapped the child in warm blankets and drove her to the emergency department of the nearest hospital.

On inspection, the child demonstrated a puffy face, drooling, inspiratory stridor, and cyanotic nail beds. At this time, she was placed on a 4 L/min nasal cannula. The emergency physician looked at the girl and listened to her chest but did not examine her mouth. Respiratory rate was 42/min, blood pressure was 80/50, and pulse was 140 bpm. The rectal temperature was 100.6° F. The physician ordered a lateral soft tissue x-ray examination of the neck, but while waiting for the x-ray examination, the child became increasingly dyspneic and more cyanotic. Her Spo_2 on room air was 70%. At this time, the following respiratory SOAP note was charted.

Respiratory Assessment and Plan

S Mother states that patient is in severe respiratory distress.

O RR 42/min, BP 80/50, P 140 regular. T 100.6° F. Child's face puffy, drooling. Inspiratory stridor (worsening). Nail beds cyanotic. On a 4 L/min nasal cannula: Spo_2 70%. Soft tissue x-ray exam of neck pending.

A
- Probable acute epiglottitis. No history of foreign body aspiration (general history).
- Impending acute ventilatory failure (history, drooling, inspiratory stridor, and cyanosis)

P STAT page for anesthesiologist and ENT surgeon. Up-regulate the **Oxygen Therapy Protocol** and add **Aerosolized Medication Protocol** pending their arrival (cool mist aerosol with 100% oxygen, with an in-line med-treatment with racemic epinephrine).

While the emergency page for the anesthesiologist and the ENT surgeon went out, a nonrebreathing oxygen mask was immediately "lightly" held to the child's face by the respiratory therapist. As soon as the physicians arrived (after about 10 minutes), the child was taken to the operating room. The surgeon stood by to perform an emergency cricothyrotomy while the anesthesiologist attempted to intubate the child.

Fortunately, the anesthesiologist was successful in spite of an enlarged, cherry-red epiglottis partially obstructing the larynx. As soon as the endotracheal tube was in place, the child relaxed and soon went to sleep. She was admitted to the intensive care unit (ICU), sedated, and placed on +5 cm H_2O continuous positive airway pressure (CPAP). She was extubated the next day and discharged on the third hospital day. A throat culture taken in the ICU was positive for *H. influenzae* type B. She was treated orally with amoxicillin.

Discussion

Acute epiglottitis is a life-threatening condition. The key point to remember is to refrain from examining the throat until a staff member qualified in pediatric intubation is nearby. Such manipulation often is unsuccessful, and unless qualified assistance is at hand, the child may asphyxiate. The treatment suitably selected here was placement of a nonrebreathing oxygen mask while the appropriate team was assembled. Typical of this disease is its abrupt onset and, under appropriate therapy, the rapid manner in which it subsides.

SELF-ASSESSMENT QUESTIONS

evolve Answers to questions can be found on Evolve. To access additional student assessment questions and case studies for application of text material to real-life scenarios, visit **http://evolve.elsevier.com/DesJardins/respiratory.**

1. The onset of LTB is usually:

a. 2 to 4 hours
b. 5 to 10 hours
c. 12 to 24 hours
d. 24 to 48 hours

2. Which of the following is or are associated with epiglottitis?

1. Parainfluenza viruses
2. *Haemophilus influenza* type B
3. RSV
4. Influenza A and B

a. 1 only
b. 2 only
c. 3 and 4 only
d. 1, 3, and 4 only

3. Which of the following is or are clinical manifestations associated with LTB?

1. Haziness in supraglottic area on x-ray film
2. High-pitched and loud inspiratory stridor
3. Swallowing difficulty
4. Drooling

a. 2 only
b. 3 only
c. 1 and 3 only
d. 1, 3, and 4 only

4. The signs and symptoms associated with acute epiglottitis usually develop within:

a. 1 to 2 hours
b. 2 to 4 hours
c. 8 to 10 hours
d. 12 to 24 hours

5. Which of the following arterial blood gas values is or are associated with mild to moderate LTB or epiglottitis?

1. Decreased pH
2. Decreased Pa_{CO_2}
3. Increased HCO_3^-
4. Increased pH

a. 1 only
b. 4 only
c. 2 and 4 only
d. 1 and 3 only

PART XII

Other Important Topics

Near Drowning

40

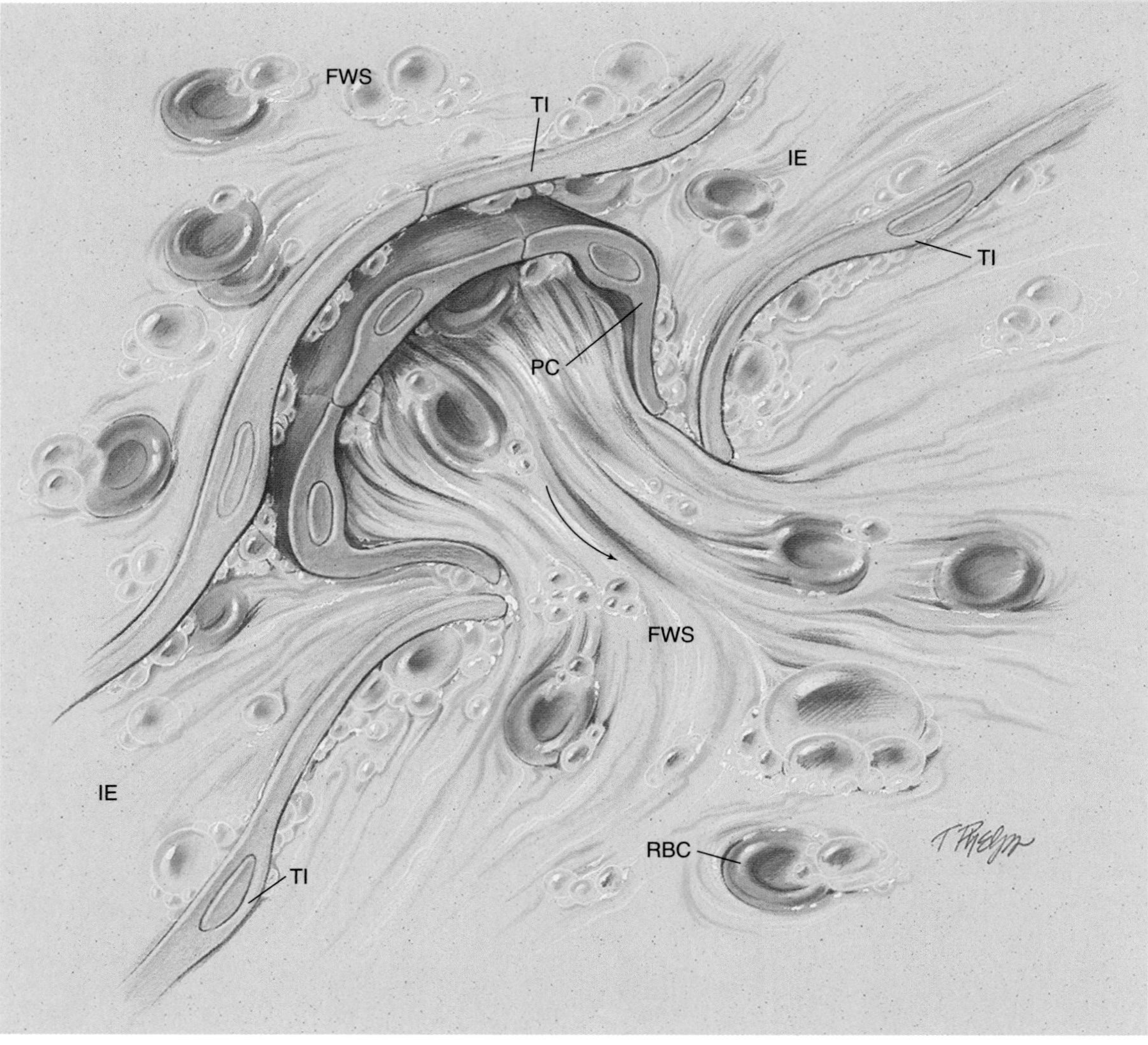

FIGURE 40-1 Near wet drowning. Cross-sectional, microscopic view of the alveolar-capillary unit. Illustration shows fluid moving from a pulmonary capillary to an alveolus. *FWS*, Frothy white secretions; *IE*, interstitial edema; *PC*, pulmonary capillary; *RBC*, red blood cell; *TI*, type I alveolar cell.

Chapter Objectives

After reading this chapter, you will be able to:

- List the anatomic alterations of the lungs associated with near drowning.
- Describe the causes of near drowning.
- List the cardiopulmonary clinical manifestations associated with near drowning.
- Describe the general management of near drowning.
- Describe the clinical strategies and rationales of the SOAPs presented in the case study.
- Define key terms and complete self-assessment questions at the end of the chapter and on Evolve.

Key Terms

Dry Drowning
First Responder
Laryngospasm
Near Drowning
Noncardiogenic Pulmonary Edema
Wet Drowning

Chapter Outline

Anatomic Alterations of the Lungs

Drowning is defined as suffocation and death as a result of submersion in liquid. Drowning may be classified further as **near drowning, dry drowning,** and **wet drowning.** *Near drowning* refers to the situation in which a victim survives a liquid submersion, at least temporarily. In dry drowning the glottis spasms and prevents water from passing into the lungs. The lungs of dry drowning victims are usually normal.

In wet drowning the glottis relaxes and allows water to flood the tracheobronchial tree and alveoli. When fluid initially is inhaled, the bronchi constrict in response to a parasympathetic-mediated reflex. As fluid enters the alveoli, the pathophysiologic processes responsible for **noncardiogenic pulmonary edema** begin—that is, fluid from the pulmonary capillaries moves into the perivascular spaces, peribronchial spaces, alveoli, bronchioles, and bronchi. As a consequence of this fluid movement, the alveolar walls and interstitial spaces swell, pulmonary surfactant concentration decreases, and the alveolar surface tension increases.

As this condition intensifies, the alveoli shrink and **atelectasis** develops. Excess fluid in the interstitial spaces causes the lymphatic vessels to dilate and the lymph flow to increase. In severe cases the fluid that accumulates in the tracheobronchial tree is churned into a frothy, white (sometimes blood-tinged) sputum as a result of air moving into and out of the lungs (generally by means of mechanical ventilation).

Finally, if the victim was submerged in unclean water (e.g., swamp, pond, sewage, or mud), a number of pathogens (e.g., *Pseudomonas*) and solid material may be aspirated. When this happens, pneumonia may occur, and in severe cases, acute respiratory distress syndrome (ARDS) may develop. Although the theory has been controversial in the past, it is now believed that the major pathologic changes of the lungs are essentially the same in fresh water and sea water wet drownings; both result in a reduction in pulmonary surfactant, alveolar injury, atelectasis, and pulmonary edema (see Figure 40-1).

The major pulmonary pathologic and structural changes associated with wet drowning are as follows:

- **Laryngospasm**
- Interstitial edema, including engorgement of the perivascular and peribronchial spaces, alveolar walls, and interstitial spaces
- Decreased pulmonary surfactant with increased surface tension of alveolar fluid
- Frothy, white and pink secretions throughout the tracheobronchial tree
- Alveolar shrinkage and atelectasis
- Alveolar consolidation
- Bronchospasm

Etiology and Epidemiology

Each year 6000 to 8000 people drown in the United States. Drowning is the third leading cause of accidental death in the United States. Drowning is the second leading cause of accidental death in people 5 to 44 years of age. About 15% of children experience near drowning by middle-school age. Drowning is most common in teenagers and in children younger than 4 years of age. More than 40% of drownings are in the under-4 age group. Swimming pools with poor adult supervision are the most common sites of drownings. Up to 33% of adults have experienced near drowning at some time. Alcohol use is present in about 50% of adult drownings. African-American children drown at a rate of 4.5 per 100,000 annually, usually in freshwater lakes and ponds. Caucasian children drown at a rate of 2.5 per 100,000 annually, usually in home pools.

Box 40-1 summarizes the general sequence of events that occurs in drowning or near drowning. Victims submerged in cold water generally demonstrate a much higher survival rate than victims submerged in warm water. Table 40-1 lists favorable prognostic factors in cold-water near drowning.

Box 40-1 Drowning or Near Drowning Sequence

1. Panic and violent struggle to return to the surface
2. Period of calmness and apnea
3. Swallowing of large amounts of fluid, followed by vomiting
4. Gasping inspirations and aspiration
5. Convulsions
6. Coma
7. Death

OVERVIEW of the Cardiopulmonary Clinical Manifestations Associated with Near Wet Drowning

The following clinical manifestations result from the pathologic mechanisms caused (or activated) by **Atelectasis** (see Figure 9-8), **Alveolar Consolidation** (see Figure 9-9), **Increased Alveolar-Capillary Membrane Thickness** (see Figure 9-10), **Bronchospasm** (see Figure 9-11), and **Excessive Bronchial Secretions** (see Figure 9-12)—the major anatomic alterations of the lungs associated with near wet drowning (see Figure 40-1).

CLINICAL DATA OBTAINED AT THE PATIENT'S BEDSIDE

The Physical Examination

Apnea

Apnea is directly related to the length of time the victim is submerged. The longer the submersion, the more likely it is that the victim will not have spontaneous respiration. When spontaneous breathing is present, the respiratory rate is usually increased.

Vital Signs

Increased Respiratory Rate (Tachypnea)

Several pathophysiologic mechanisms operating simultaneously may lead to an increased ventilatory rate:

- Stimulation of peripheral chemoreceptors (hypoxemia)
- Decreased lung compliance–increased ventilatory rate relationship
- Stimulation of J receptors
- Anxiety (conscious patient)

Increased Heart Rate (Pulse) and Blood Pressure

Cyanosis

Cough and Sputum Production (Frothy, White or Pink, Stable Bubbles)

Chest Assessment Findings

- Crackles and rhonchi

CLINICAL DATA OBTAINED FROM LABORATORY TESTS AND SPECIAL PROCEDURES

Pulmonary Function Test Findings
(Extrapolated Data for Instructional Purposes)
(Primary Restrictive Lung Pathophysiology)

FORCED EXPIRATORY FLOW RATE FINDINGS

FVC	FEV_T	FEV_1/FVC ratio	$FEF_{25\%-75\%}$
↓	N or ↓	N or ↑	N or ↓

$FEF_{50\%}$	$FEF_{200-1200}$	PEFR	MVV
N or ↓	N or ↓	N or ↓	N or ↓

LUNG VOLUME AND CAPACITY FINDINGS

V_T	IRV	ERV	RV
N or ↓	↓	↓	↓

VC	IC	FRC	TLC	RV/TLC ratio
↓	↓	↓	↓	N

DECREASED DIFFUSION CAPACITY (DLCO)

Arterial Blood Gases

EARLY AND ADVANCED STAGES OF NEAR DROWNING
Acute Ventilatory Failure with Hypoxemia
(Acute Respiratory Acidosis)

pH*	Pa_{CO_2}	HCO_3^- *	Pa_{O_2}
↓	↑	↑ (slightly)	↓

*When tissue hypoxia is severe enough to produce lactic acid, the pH and HCO_3^- values will be lower than expected for a particular Pa_{CO_2} level.

Oxygenation Indices*

$\dot{Q}_S/\dot{Q}_T$	D_{O_2}†	$\dot{V}_{O_2}$	$C(a-\bar{v})_{O_2}$	O_2ER	$S\bar{v}_{O_2}$
↑	↓	N	N	↑	↓

†The D_{O_2} may be normal in patients who have compensated to the decreased oxygenation status with (1) an increased cardiac output, (2) an increased hemoglobin level, or (3) a combination of both. When the D_{O_2} is normal, the O_2ER is usually normal.

*$C(a-\bar{v})_{O_2}$, Arterial-venous oxygen difference; D_{O_2}, total oxygen delivery; O_2ER, oxygen extraction ratio; $\dot{Q}_S/\dot{Q}_T$, pulmonary shunt fraction; $S\bar{v}_{O_2}$, mixed venous oxygen saturation; $\dot{V}_{O_2}$, oxygen consumption.

RADIOLOGIC FINDINGS

Chest Radiograph

- Fluffy infiltrates

The initial appearance of the radiograph may vary from being completely normal to showing varying degrees of pulmonary edema and atelectasis (Figure 40-2). It should be emphasized, however, that an initially normal chest radiograph still may be associated with significant hypoxemia, hypercapnia, and acidosis. In any case, radiographic deterioration may occur in the first 48 to 72 hours.

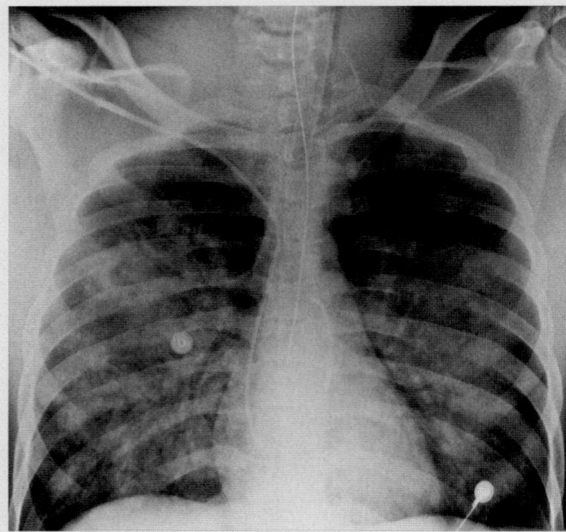

FIGURE 40-2 This radiograph of a young man, taken just after an episode of near drowning, shows a pulmonary edema pattern. Note the air bronchograms in both lungs reflecting atelectasis. (From Hansell DM, Armstrong P, Lynch DA, McAdams HP, eds: *Imaging of diseases of the chest,* ed 4, Philadelphia, 2005, Elsevier.)

TABLE 40-1 Favorable Prognostic Factors in Cold-Water Near Drowning

Age	The younger, the better
Submersion time	The shorter, the better (60 minutes appears to be the upper limit in cold-water submersions)
Water temperature	The colder, the better (range, 27° F to 70° F)
Water quality	The cleaner, the better
Other injuries	None serious
Amount of struggle	The less struggle, the better
Cardiopulmonary resuscitation (CPR) quality	Good CPR technique increases the survival rate
Suicidal intent	Lower survival rate among victims who attempted suicide than among victims of accidental submersion

General Management

The First Responder

For the **first responder,** the first objectives in treating a drowning victim are to remove the person from the water and, if the patient has no spontaneous ventilation and pulse, to call for help and immediately initiate cardiopulmonary resuscitation (CPR). When the patient has been submerged for less than 60 minutes in cold water, fixed and dilated pupils do not necessarily indicate a poor prognosis. Because water is an excellent conductor of body heat (cold water can cool the body 25 times faster than air at the same temperature) and because evaporation further reduces an individual's body heat, the victim's wet clothing should immediately be removed and replaced with warm, dry coverings.

Management during Transport

The primary goal in treating near drowning victims during transport is high-quality CPR with 100% oxygen. The victim's body heat should be conserved by removing any wet garments and covering high heat-loss areas with warm, dry coverings. High heat-loss areas of the body include the head and neck, axillae, and inguinal areas. The victim's vital signs, including rectal temperature, should be monitored closely during travel to the hospital. The victim's body temperature frequently falls during transport, and measures to conserve the patient's body heat are extremely important. Victims with spontaneous ventilation should be monitored with pulse oximetry during transport, if at all possible.

Management at the Hospital

Treatment at the hospital is an extension of prehospital management. Virtually every near drowning victim suffers from hypoxemia, hypercapnia, and acidosis (acute ventilatory failure). Hypoxemia generally persists after aspiration of fluids in the airway (wet drowning) because of alveolar capillary damage and continued intrapulmonary shunting. The degree of hypoxemia is directly related to the amount of alveolar-capillary damage. A chest radiograph should be obtained to help evaluate the magnitude of the alveolar-capillary injury. However, a normal chest radiograph does not rule out the possibility of alveolar-capillary deterioration during the first 24 hours.

Intubation and mechanical ventilation should be performed immediately for any victim with no spontaneous ventilations and for victims who are breathing spontaneously but are unable to maintain a Pa_{O_2} of 60 mm Hg with an F_{IO_2} of 0.5 or lower. Because of the nature of the alveolar-capillary injury seen in most wet drowning victims, mechanical ventilation with positive end-expiratory pressure (PEEP) or continuous positive airway pressure (CPAP) should be administered. It should be noted, however, that barotrauma is a common complication of ventilator therapy in these patients. Low tidal volume ventilation and permissive hypercapnia are ventilator management techniques to consider when appropriate. The patient also may benefit from inotropic agents and diuretics.

Finally, warming the victim should progress concomitantly with all the other treatment modalities. Nearly all near drowning victims are hypothermic to some degree. Depending on the severity of the hypothermia and on the available resources, a number of warming techniques may be employed. For example, the body temperature can be increased by the intravenous administration of heated solutions; by heated lavage of the gastric, intrathoracic, pericardial, and peritoneal spaces; or by the administration of heated lavage to the bladder and rectum. Additional external heating techniques include warming of the patient's inspired air or gas mixtures, heating blankets, warm baths, and immersion in a heated Hubbard tank. In rare cases, extracorporeal circulation, with complete cardiopulmonary bypass and blood warming, has been successful.

CASE STUDY

Near Drowning

Admitting History and Physical Examination

A 12-year-old boy had a history of a seizure disorder but had not taken his medication for almost a year. On the morning of admission, he participated in a regular swimming class in the junior high school pool. According to the coach on duty, there had been a "pool check" 30 seconds before the patient's partner reported that the patient seemed to stay under water "too long."

When taken from the water, he was unconscious and "blue." He was given mouth-to-mouth resuscitation, and by the time the emergency medical technician (EMT) squad arrived about 20 minutes later, he was breathing at a rate of 10 breaths/min, although his lips and fingers were still cyanotic. He remained comatose and was taken to the nearest hospital.

On admission the patient's blood pressure was 100/60 and his pulse was 140 bpm. Auscultation of his chest revealed fine crackles bilaterally. Clear secretions were suctioned from his oral airway. An x-ray showed bilateral, diffuse increase in density, which suggested pulmonary edema or possible hemorrhage. His oxygen saturation on 5 L/min O_2 was 72%. Plans were made to transfer him to a nearby tertiary care medical center. The respiratory therapist in the emergency department entered the following assessment moments before the patient transfer.

Respiratory Assessment and Plan

S N/A (patient comatose). History of near drowning.

O Comatose. Spontaneous breathing at 10/min, BP 100/60, P 140. Crackles bilaterally. Nasotracheal suctioning yields clear fluid. Cyanotic. Sp_{O_2} on 5 L/min O_2 per nasal cannula: 72%.

A
- Near drowning. R/O seizure disorder (history)
- Increased airway secretions (suctioning of clear fluid)
- Poor oxygenation (cyanosis, Sp_{O_2})
- Pulmonary edema (CXR)

P Stat ABG on 100% oxygen, then titrate per **Oxygen Therapy Protocol.** Have equipment to intubate on standby. Bag-mask ventilate, and suction. Provide continuous pulse oximetry. Continue nasotracheal suctioning. Take seizure precautions. Will accompany on transfer.

After transfer to the tertiary care medical center, the patient was described as a well-developed, slightly obese adolescent in obvious respiratory distress. He was now alert, oriented, but extremely apprehensive. His vital signs were: temperature (rectal) 100.8° F, blood pressure 112/70, pulse 140 bpm, and respirations 60/min. The lips and fingertips were cyanotic. The respirations were paradoxic. There was marked substernal retraction. Breath sounds were diminished bilaterally, and loud crackles were heard over both lungs anteriorly.

Laboratory examination revealed a leukocytosis of 21,000/mm^3 and 2+ albumin in the urine, but findings were otherwise within normal limits. There was no evidence of hemolysis. On bag-mask ventilation with an F_{IO_2} of 0.8, the arterial blood gas (ABG) values were pH 7.29, Pa_{CO_2} 52, HCO_3^- 25, and Pa_{O_2} 38. The patient's condition was rapidly deteriorating, and he developed even more severe crackles. He now had a spontaneous cough with frothy sputum production. The chest x-ray revealed pulmonary edema and nearly complete opacification of both lungs. The following was entered in the patient's chart.

Respiratory Assessment and Plan

S Anxious, dyspneic, crying. "I can't get my breath. Where am I? Am I going to die?"

O Afebrile. BP 112/70, P 140/min, RR 60/min. Cyanotic. Paradoxic chest/abdomen movements, sternal retraction. Crackles in both lungs anteriorly. Spontaneous cough with frothy sputum production, WBC 21,000/mm^3. On 80% oxygen: pH 7.29, Pa_{CO_2} 52, HCO_3^- 25, Pa_{O_2} 38. CXR: "White-out."

A
- Pulmonary edema secondary to near drowning (frothy sputum)
- Acute ventilatory failure with metabolic acidosis (likely lactic acid) with severe hypoxemia (ABGs)

P Place on 100% O_2 and bag-mask ventilate. Page physician stat. Obtain intubation equipment and prepare to place patient on ventilator. Follow oximetry. Prepare to assist in placement of Swan-Ganz catheter.

The patient was intubated and paralyzed with succinylcholine. As soon as he was intubated, copious pink foam was aspirated from the endotracheal tube. He was alternately suctioned and ventilated with an Ambu bag. He was given 7 mg of morphine for sedation and was mechanically ventilated in continuous mechanical ventilation (CMV) mode at a rate of 10 breaths/min. On an F_{IO_2} of 0.6 and PEEP of 10 cm H_2O, his blood gases were pH 7.44, Pa_{CO_2} 43, HCO_3^- 24, and Pa_{O_2} 109. Because he was still fighting the respirator, he was paralyzed with pancuronium.

After several hours, the lungs were clear, the secretions were no longer present, and his blood gas values returned to normal on an F_{IO_2} of 0.5 and PEEP of 10 cm H_2O (pH 7.42, Pa_{CO_2} 42, HCO_3^- 24, and Pa_{O_2} 98). His hemodynamic status was normal. The chest x-ray revealed considerable clearing of the earlier noted bilateral pulmonary infiltrates.

Respiratory Assessment and Plan

S N/A (patient sedated, paralyzed)

O Lungs clear. No secretions. On 50% O_2 and +10 PEEP: pH 7.42, Pa_{CO_2} 42, HCO_3^- 24, and Pa_{O_2} 98. CXR: Considerable improvement in bilateral infiltrates.

A • Considerable improvement on CMV and PEEP (general improvement of clinical indicators)
• Acceptable ventilation and oxygenation status on present ventilatory settings (ABG)
• Frothy airway secretions no longer present (clear lungs and no secretions)

P Contact physician to wean from muscle relaxant. Wean from mechanically ventilated breaths, F_{IO_2}, and PEEP per **Mechanical Ventilation Protocol.** Change ventilator mode to synchronized intermittent mandatory ventilation (SIMV).

The patient was weaned from the ventilator over a period of 6 hours, after which he was extubated. The following morning, arterial blood gases on a 28% HAFOE oxygen mask were as follows: pH 7.37, Pa_{CO_2} 35, HCO_3^- 23, and Pa_{O_2} 158. X-ray examination of the lungs was normal. An oxygen titration protocol was performed. He was discharged 2 days later.

Discussion

This case demonstrates initial worsening of the near drowning victim despite intensive respiratory care. The initial ABG values showed severe hypoxemia as a result of **Increased Alveolar-Capillary Membrane Thickness** and alveolar flooding (see Figures 9-10 and 40-1), as well as acute ventilatory failure and metabolic (probably lactic) acidosis. Bronchospasm never developed, and aggressive respiratory care prohibited the development of atelectasis and aspiration pneumonia.

When suctioning, supplemental oxygen, and bag ventilation were no longer successful, the patient was intubated and mechanical ventilation with PEEP was begun. Even on these modalities, the patient remained anxious and was ultimately paralyzed to allow better respiratory synchrony and diminish the chance for barotrauma. Morphine was used for its sedative qualities and as a vascular afterload reducer. The fact that the patient was fighting the ventilator some time after succinylcholine had been administered reflects the fact that it is a very short-acting paralyzing agent. Pancuronium has a much longer half-life, and its use is standard in settings where longer effectiveness is required. Once the abnormal pathology of the lungs associated with this case improved, the patient's cardiopulmonary status quickly returned to normal and the respiratory practitioner was able wean the patient from the ventilation in a relatively short period of time.

This case demonstrates again the necessity for frequent reassessment of the patient and therapeutic adjustments to follow the findings so observed.

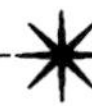

SELF-ASSESSMENT QUESTIONS

evolve Answers to questions can be found on Evolve. To access additional student assessment questions and case studies for application of text material to real-life scenarios, visit **http://evolve.elsevier.com/DesJardins/respiratory.**

1. In the United States, drowning is the:
a. Leading cause of accidental death
b. Second leading cause of accidental death
c. Third leading cause of accidental death
d. Fourth leading cause of accidental death

2. Drowning is most common in teenagers and in children younger than:
a. 18 years of age
b. 12 years of age
c. 8 years of age
d. 4 years of age

3. Which of the following are the major anatomic alterations of the lungs associated with near drowning victims?
1. Consolidation
2. Bronchospasm
3. Increased alveolar-capillary membrane thickness
4. Atelectasis
5. Excessive bronchial secretions
a. 3 and 5 only
b. 2 and 4 only
c. 3, 4, and 5 only
d. 1, 2, 3, 4, and 5

4. Which of the following clinical manifestations are associated with near drowning victims?
1. Frothy, pink sputum
2. Crackles
3. Increased pH
4. Increased $S\bar{v}_{O_2}$
a. 1 and 2 only
b. 3 and 4 only
c. 2, 3, and 4 only
d. 1, 2, 3, and 4 only

5. Which of the following pulmonary function testing values are associated with near drowning victims?
1. N or ↓ FEV_T
2. ↓ FVC
3. ↓ RV
4. N or ↑ FEV_1/FVC ratio
a. 1 and 2 only
b. 3 and 4 only
c. 2, 3, and 4 only
d. 1, 2, 3, and 4

Smoke Inhalation and Thermal Injuries

41

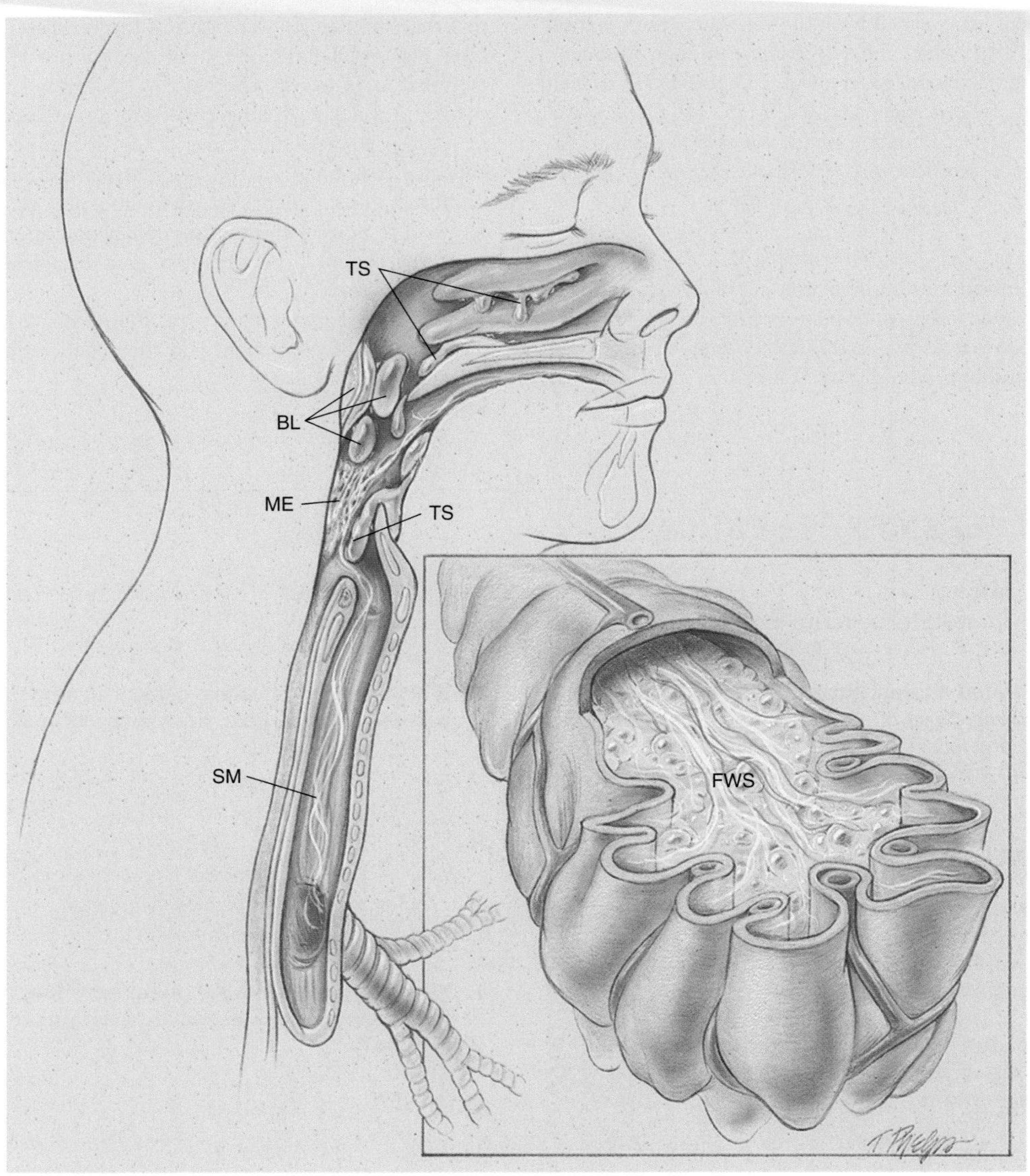

FIGURE 41-1 Smoke inhalation and thermal injuries. *BL,* Airway blister; *FWS,* frothy white secretions (pulmonary edema); *ME,* mucosal edema; *SM,* smoke (toxic gas); *TS,* thick secretions.

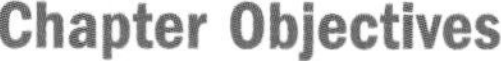

Chapter Objectives

After reading this chapter, you will be able to:

- List the anatomic alterations of the lungs associated with smoke inhalation and thermal injuries.
- Describe the causes of smoke inhalation and thermal injuries.
- List the cardiopulmonary clinical manifestations associated with smoke inhalation and thermal injuries.
- Describe the general management of smoke inhalation and thermal injuries.
- Describe the clinical strategies and rationales of the SOAPs presented in the case study.
- Define key terms and complete self-assessment questions at the end of the chapter and on Evolve.

Key Terms

Acute Respiratory Distress Syndrome
Body Surface Burns
Bronchospasm
Burn Stages
Carbon Monoxide Poisoning
Carbonaceous Sputum
Carboxyhemoglobin
Cyanide Poisoning
Cryptogenic Organizing Pneumonia (COP)
First Degree Burn
Hyperbaric Oxygenation (HBO) Therapy
Noncardiogenic Pulmonary Edema
Parkland Formula (Fluid Resuscitation)
Second Degree Burn
Smoke Inhalation Injury
Steam Inhalation
Thermal Injury
Third Degree Burn

Chapter Outline

Anatomic Alterations of the Lungs

The inhalation of smoke and hot gases and **body surface burns**—in any combination—continue to be a major cause of morbidity and mortality among fire victims and firefighters. In general, fire-related pulmonary injuries can be divided into thermal and smoke (toxic gases) injuries.

Thermal Injury

Thermal injury refers to injury caused by the inhalation of hot gases. Thermal injuries are usually confined to the upper airway—the nasal cavity, oral cavity, nasopharynx, oropharynx, and larynx. The distal airways and the alveoli are usually spared serious injury because of (1) the remarkable ability of the upper airways to cool hot gases, (2) reflex laryngospasm, and (3) glottic closure. The upper airway is an extremely efficient "heat sink." In fact, in 1945, Moritz and associates demonstrated that the inhalation of hot gases alone did not produce significant damage to the lung. Anesthetized dogs were forced to breathe air heated to 500° C through an insulated endotracheal tube. The researchers' results showed that the air temperature dropped to 50° C by the time it reached the level of the carina. No histologic damage was noticed in the lower trachea or lungs.

Even though thermal injury may occur with or without surface burns, the presence of facial burns is a classic predictor of thermal injury. Thermal injury to the upper airway results in blistering, mucosal edema, vascular congestion, epithelial sloughing, and accumulation of thick secretions. An acute upper airway obstruction (UAO) occurs in about 20% to 30% of hospitalized patients with thermal injury and is usually most marked in the supraglottic structures. When body surface burns require the rapid administration of resuscitative fluids, a UAO may develop rapidly (see Figure 41-1).

It should be noted that the inhalation of steam at 100° C or greater usually results in severe damage at all levels of the respiratory tract. This damage occurs because steam has about 500 times the heat energy content of dry gas at the same temperature. Thermal injury to the distal airways results in mucosal edema, vascular congestion, epithelial sloughing, **cryptogenic organizing pneumonia (COP)**—also known as *bronchiolitis obliterans organizing pneumonia* (BOOP)—atelectasis, and pulmonary edema.

Therefore, direct thermal injuries usually do not occur below the level of the larynx, except in the rare instance of **steam inhalation**. Damage to the distal airways is mostly caused by a variety of harmful products found in smoke.

Smoke Inhalation Injury

The pathologic changes in the distal airways and alveoli are mainly caused by the irritating and toxic gases, suspended soot particles, and vapors associated with incomplete combustion and smoke. Many of the substances found in smoke are extremely caustic to the tracheobronchial tree and poisonous to the body. The progression of injuries that develop from smoke inhalation and burns is described as the early stage, intermediate stage, and late stage.

Early Stage (0 to 24 Hours after Inhalation)

The injuries associated with smoke inhalation do not always appear right away, even when extensive body surface burns are evident. During the first 24 hours—the early stage (0 to 24 hours after smoke inhalation)—however, the patient's pulmonary status often changes markedly. Initially, the tracheobronchial tree becomes more inflamed, resulting in **bronchospasm**. This process causes an overabundance of bronchial secretions to move into the airways, resulting in further airway obstruction. In addition, the toxic effects of smoke often slow the activity of the mucosal ciliary transport mechanism, causing further retention of mucus.

Smoke inhalation also may cause **acute respiratory distress syndrome (ARDS)**, noncardiogenic high-permeability pulmonary edema—commonly referred to in smoke inhalation cases as "leaky alveoli." **Noncardiogenic pulmonary edema** also may be caused by overhydration resulting from overzealous fluid resuscitation (see insert panel in Figure 41-1). In severe cases, ARDS also may occur early in the course of the pathology.

Intermediate Stage (2 to 5 Days after Inhalation)

Whereas upper airway thermal injuries usually begin to improve during the intermediate stage (2 to 5 days after smoke inhalation), the pathologic changes deep in the lungs associated with smoke inhalation usually peak. Production of mucus continues to increase, whereas mucosal ciliary transport activity continues to decrease. The mucosa of the tracheobronchial tree frequently becomes necrotic and sloughs (usually at 3 to 4 days). The necrotic debris, excessive production of mucus, and retention of mucus lead to mucous plugging and atelectasis. In addition, the mucous accumulation often leads to bacterial colonization, bronchitis, and pneumonia. Organisms commonly cultured include gram-positive *Staphylococcus aureus* and gram-negative *Klebsiella, Enterobacter, Escherichia coli,* and *Pseudomonas.* If not already present, ARDS may develop at any time during this period.

When chest wall (thorax) burns are present, the situation may be further aggravated by the patient's inability to breathe deeply and cough as a result of (1) pain, (2) the use of narcotics, (3) immobility, (4) increased airway resistance, and (5) decreased lung and chest compliance.

Late Stage (5 or More Days after Inhalation)

Infections resulting from burn wounds on the body surface are the major concern during the late stage (5 or more days after smoke inhalation). These infections often lead to sepsis and multiorgan failure. Sepsis-induced multiorgan failure is the primary cause of death in seriously burned patients during this stage.

Pneumonia continues to be a major problem during this period. Pulmonary embolism also may develop within 2 weeks after serious body surface burns. Pulmonary embolism may develop from deep venous thrombosis secondary to a hypercoagulable state and prolonged immobility.

Finally, the long-term effects of smoke inhalation can result in restrictive and obstructive lung disorders. In general, a restrictive lung disorder develops from alveolar fibrosis and chronic atelectasis. An obstructive lung disorder generally is caused by increased and chronic bronchial secretions, bronchial stenosis, bronchial polyps, bronchiectasis, and bronchiolitis.

The major pathologic and structural changes of the respiratory system caused by thermal or smoke inhalation injuries are as follows:

Thermal injury (upper airway—nasal cavity, oral cavity, and pharynx):

- Blistering
- Mucosal edema
- Vascular congestion
- Epithelial sloughing
- Thick secretions
- Acute UAO

Smoke inhalation injury (tracheobronchial tree and alveoli):

- Inflammation of the tracheobronchial tree
- Bronchospasm
- Excessive bronchial secretions and mucous plugging
- Decreased mucosal ciliary transport
- Atelectasis
- Alveolar edema and frothy secretions (pulmonary edema)
- ARDS (severe cases)
- COP (also called *bronchiolitis obliterans organizing pneumonia* [BOOP])
- Alveolar fibrosis, bronchial stenosis, bronchial polyps, bronchiolitis, and bronchiectasis (severe cases)

Pneumonia (Chapter 15) and pulmonary embolism (Chapter 20) often complicate smoke inhalation injury.

Etiology and Epidemiology

According to the National Fire Protection Association (NFPA), public fire departments responded to an estimated 1,557,500 fires in the United States in 2007. There were about 530,500 structure fires (85% were residential fires), 258,000 vehicle fires, and 769,000 outside and other fires. This means that every 20 seconds a fire department responded to a fire somewhere in the nation. A fire occurs in a structure at the rate of once every 59 seconds, and in particular, a residential fire occurs every 76 seconds. Fires occur in vehicles at the rate of 1 every 122 seconds, and there is a fire in an outside property every 41 seconds. In addition, there were 3430 civilian fire deaths (1 every 153 minutes) and 17,675 civilian injuries (1 every 30 minutes) according to the NFPA in 2007. The NFPA estimated that more than 14 billion dollars in property damage occurred as a result of fires in 2007.

The prognosis of fire victims usually is determined by the (1) extent and duration of smoke exposure, (2) chemical composition of the smoke, (3) size and depth of body surface burns, (4) temperature of gases inhaled, (5) age (the prognosis worsens in the very young or old), and (6) preexisting health status. When smoke inhalation injury is accompanied by a full-thickness or third-degree skin burn, the mortality rate almost doubles.

Smoke can result from either pyrolysis (smoldering in a low-oxygen environment) or combustion (burning, with visible flame, in an adequate-oxygen environment). Smoke is composed of a complex mixture of particulates, toxic gases, and vapors. The composition of smoke varies according to the chemical makeup of the material that is burning and the amount of oxygen being consumed by the fire. Table 41-1 lists some of the more common toxic substances produced by burning products that frequently are found in office, industrial, and residential buildings.

Although in some instances the toxic components of the smoke may be obvious, in most cases the precise identification of the inhaled toxins is not feasible. In general, the inhalation of smoke with toxic agents that have high water solubility (e.g., ammonia, sulfur dioxide, and hydrogen fluoride) affects the structures of the upper airway. In contrast, the inhalation of toxic agents that have a low water solubility (e.g., hydrogen chloride, chlorine, phosgene, and oxides of nitrogen) affects the distal airways and alveoli. Many of the substances in smoke are caustic and can cause significant injury to the tracheobronchial tree (e.g., aldehydes [especially acrolein], hydrochloride, and oxides of sulfur).

TABLE 41-1 Toxic Substances and Sources Commonly Associated with Fire and Smoke

Substance	Source
Aldehydes (acrolein, acetaldehyde, formaldehyde)	Wood, cotton, paper
Organic acids (acetic and formic acids)	
Carbon monoxide, hydrogen chloride, phosgene	Polyvinylchloride (PVC)
Hydrogen cyanide, isocyanate	Polyurethanes
Hydrogen fluoride, hydrogen bromide	Fluorinated resins
Ammonia	Melamine resins
Oxides of nitrogen	Nitrocellulose film, fabrics
Benzene	Petroleum products
Carbon monoxide, carbon dioxide	Organic material
Sulfur dioxide	Sulfur-containing compounds
Hydrogen chloride	Fertilizer, textiles, rubber manufacturing
Chlorine	Swimming pool water
Ozone	Welding fumes
Hydrogen sulfide	Metal works, chemical manufacturing

Body Surface Burns

Because the amount and severity of body surface burns play a major role in the patient's risk of mortality and morbidity, an approximate estimate of the percentage of the body surface area burned is important. Table 41-2 lists the approximate percentage of surface area for various body regions of adults and infants. The severity and depth of burns usually are defined as follows:

First degree (minimal depth in skin): Superficial burn, damage limited to the outer layer of epidermis. This burn is characterized by reddened skin, tenderness, and pain. Blisters are not present. Healing time is about 6 to 10 days. The result of healing is normal skin.

Second degree (superficial to deep thickness of skin): Burns in which damage extends through the epidermis and into the dermis but is not of sufficient extent to interfere with regeneration of epidermis. If secondary infection results, the damage from a second-degree burn may be equivalent to that of a third-degree burn. Blisters usually are present. Healing time is 7 to 21 days. The result of healing ranges from normal to a hairless and depigmented skin with a texture that is normal, pitted, flat, or shiny.

Third degree (full thickness of skin including tissue beneath skin): Burns in which both epidermis and dermis are destroyed, with damage extending into underlying tissues. Tissue may be charred or coagulated. Healing may occur after 21 days or may never occur without skin grafting if the burned area is large. The resultant damage heals with hypertrophic scars (keloids) and chronic granulation.

TABLE 41-2 The Approximate Percentage of Body Surface Area (BSA) for Various Body Regions of Adults and Infants

Anatomic Region	Percent of BSA in Adults	Percent of BSA in Infants
Entire head and neck	9	18
Each arm	9	9
Anterior trunk	18	18
Posterior trunk	18	18
Genitalia	1	1
Each leg	18	13.5

Note: The "rule of nines" is used to estimate percentage of injury; each of the areas listed here represents about 9% or 18% of the body surface area. This rule does not apply to the legs of infants.

OVERVIEW of the Cardiopulmonary Clinical Manifestations Associated with Smoke Inhalation and Thermal Injuries

The following clinical manifestations result from the pathologic mechanisms caused (or activated) by **Atelectasis** (see Figure 9-8), **Alveolar Consolidation** (see Figure 9-9), **Increased Alveolar-Capillary Membrane Thickness** (see Figure 9-10), **Bronchospasm** (see Figure 9-11), and **Excessive Bronchial Secretions** (see Figure 9-12)—the major anatomic alterations of the lungs associated with smoke inhalation and thermal injuries (see Figure 41-1).

CLINICAL DATA OBTAINED AT THE PATIENT'S BEDSIDE

The Physical Examination

Vital Signs

Increased Respiratory Rate (Tachypnea)

Several pathophysiologic mechanisms operating simultaneously may lead to an increased ventilatory rate:

- Stimulation of peripheral chemoreceptors (hypoxemia)
- Decreased lung compliance–increased ventilatory rate relationship
- Stimulation of J receptors
- Pain, anxiety

Increased Heart Rate (Pulse) and Blood Pressure

Assessment of Acute Upper Airway Obstruction (Thermal Injury)

- Obvious pharyngeal edema and swelling
- Inspiratory stridor
- Hoarseness
- Altered voice
- Painful swallowing

Because the inhalation of hot gases often results in severe upper airway edema, the respiratory care practitioner always should be alert for any clinical manifestations of acute upper airway obstruction, even when the patient shows no remarkable upper airway problems or upper body burns at admission.

Cyanosis

Cough and Sputum Production

When the patient experiences upper airway thermal injuries, an excessive amount of thick secretions usually is present. During the early stage of recovery from smoke inhalation, the patient generally expectorates a small amount of black, sooty sputum (**carbonaceous sputum**). During the intermediate stage the patient may produce moderate to large amounts of frothy secretions. During the late stage, purulent mucus is common.

Chest Assessment Findings

- Usually normal breath sounds (early stage)
- Wheezing
- Crackles
- Rhonchi

CLINICAL DATA OBTAINED FROM LABORATORY TESTS AND SPECIAL PROCEDURES

Pulmonary Function Test Findings (Extrapolated Data for Instructional Purposes) (Primarily Restrictive Lung Pathophysiology)

FORCED EXPIRATORY FLOW RATE FINDINGS

FVC	FEV_T	FEV_1/FVC ratio	$FEF_{25\%-75\%}$
↓	N or ↓	N or ↑	N or ↓

$FEF_{50\%}$	$FEF_{200-1200}$	PEFR	MVV
N or ↓	N or ↓	N or ↓	N or ↓

LUNG VOLUME AND CAPACITY FINDINGS

V_T	IRV	ERV	RV*
N or ↓	↓	↓	↓

VC	IC	FRC*	TLC	RV/TLC ratio
↓	↓	↓	↓	N

DECREASED DIFFUSION CAPACITY (Dlco)

*↑ when airways are partially obstructed.

Arterial Blood Gases

EARLY STAGES OF SMOKE INHALATION

Acute Alveolar Hyperventilation with Hypoxemia (Acute Respiratory Alkalosis)

pH	$Paco_2$	HCO_3^-	Pao_2
↑	↓	↓ (slightly)	↓ or Normal

SEVERE SMOKE INHALATION AND BURNS WITH METABOLIC ACIDOSIS

COHb[†]	pH*	$Paco_2$	HCO_3^- *	Pao_2
↑	↓ (lactic acidemia)	↓	↓	↓ or N (but tissue hypoxemia)

*When tissue hypoxia is severe enough to produce lactic acid, the pH and HCO_3^- values will be lower than expected for a particular $Paco_2$ level.
[†]Carboxyhemoglobin.

When carbon monoxide or cyanide poisoning is present, the pH may be decreased during the early stages of smoke inhalation. This decrease in pH occurs because patients with severe carbon monoxide or cyanide poisoning commonly have lactic acidemia as a result of tissue hypoxia—even in the presence of a normal Pao_2. Therefore when carbon monoxide or cyanide poisoning is present, the patient may demonstrate the following arterial blood gas values.

SEVERE SMOKE INHALATION AND BURNS WITH METABOLIC ACIDOSIS

Acute Ventilatory Failure with Hypoxemia (Acute Respiratory Acidosis)

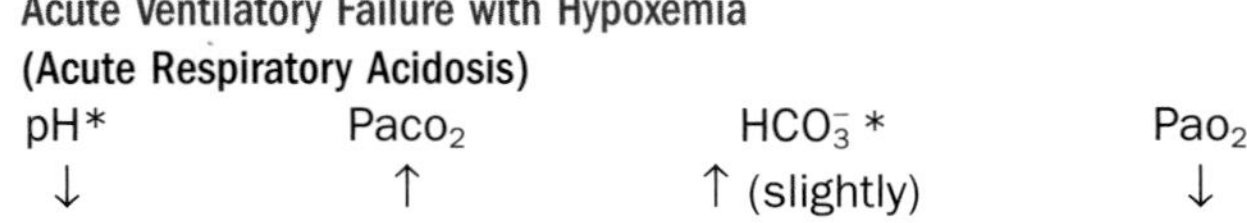

pH*	$Paco_2$	HCO_3^- *	Pao_2
↓	↑	↑ (slightly)	↓

*When tissue hypoxia is severe enough to produce lactic acid, the pH and HCO_3^- values will be lower than expected for a particular $Paco_2$ level.

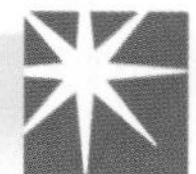

OVERVIEW of the Cardiopulmonary Clinical Manifestations Associated with Smoke Inhalation and Thermal Injuries—cont'd

Oxygenation Indices
Smoke Inhalation and Burns

	Early and Intermediate Stages	Late Stage
Do_2	↓	↓
$\dot{V}o_2$	↑	↓
$C(a-\bar{v})o_2$	↑	↓
O_2ER	↑	↓
$S\bar{v}o_2$	↓	↓

When carbon monoxide or cyanide poisoning is present, the oxygenation indices are unreliable because the Pao_2 often is normal in the presence of carbon monoxide poisoning, and when cyanide poisoning is present, the tissue cells are prevented from consuming oxygen. Both of these conditions cause false oximeter readings. For example, when carbon monoxide is present, a normal Do_2 value may be calculated when, in reality, the patient's oxygen transport status is extremely low. When cyanide poisoning is present, the patient's $\dot{V}o_2$ may appear normal or increased when in actuality the tissue cells are extremely hypoxic. Typically these problems are not present during the intermediate and late stages in the presence of appropriate treatment.

Hemodynamic Indices*
Cardiogenic Pulmonary Edema

	Early Stage	Intermediate Stage	Late Stage
CVP	↓	Normal	↓
RAP	↓	Normal	↓
$\overline{PA}$	↓	Normal	↓
PCWP	↓	Normal	↓
CO	↓	Normal	↓
SV	↓	Normal	↓
SVI	↓	Normal	↓
CL	↓	Normal	↓
RVSWI	↓	Normal	↓
LVSWI	↓	Normal	↓
PVR	Normal	Normal	↑
SVR	↑	Normal	↑

**CO*, Cardiac output; *CVP,* central venous pressure; *LVSWI,* left ventricular stroke work index; *$\overline{PA}$,* mean pulmonary artery pressure; *PCWP,* pulmonary capillary wedge pressure; *PVR,* pulmonary vascular resistance; *RAP,* right atrial pressure; *RVSWI,* right ventricular stroke work index; *SV,* stroke volume; *SVI,* stroke volume index; *SVR,* systemic vascular resistance.

In general, the hemodynamic profile seen in patients with body surface burns relates to the amount of intravascular volume loss (hypovolemia) that occurs as a result of third-space fluid shifts. For example, during the early stage, the decreased values shown for the CVP, RAP, $\overline{PA}$, CWP, CO, SV, SVI, CI, RVSWI, and LVSWI reflect the reduction in pulmonary intravascular and cardiac filling volumes. Hypovolemia causes a generalized peripheral vasoconstriction, which is reflected in an elevated SVR. When appropriate fluid resuscitation is administered, the patient's hemodynamic indices usually are normal during the intermediate stage.

CARBON MONOXIDE POISONING

When a patient has been exposed to smoke, *carbon monoxide (CO) poisoning must be assumed.* Although CO has no direct injurious effect on the lungs, it can greatly reduce the patient's oxygen transport because CO has an affinity for hemoglobin that is about 210 times greater than that of oxygen. CO attached to hemoglobin is called **carboxyhemoglobin (COHb).** Breathing CO at a partial pressure of less than 2 mm Hg can result in a COHb of 40% or more. In other words, 40% or more of the oxygen transport system is inactivated.

In addition, high concentrations of COHb cause the oxyhemoglobin dissociation curve to move markedly to the left, which makes it more difficult for oxygen to leave the hemoglobin at the tissue sites. In essence, the tissue cells are better oxygenated when 40% of the hemoglobin is absent (anemia) than when a COHb of 40% is present. Thus, it should be stressed that Pao_2 and SpO_2 measurements are misleading and unreliable in the presence of COHb. Arterial blood gas measurements, however, do provide important information regarding the presence of hypoxemia, widened alveolar-arterial oxygen gradient, and acid-base status.

A COHb level in excess of 20% is usually considered CO poisoning, and a COHb level of 40% or greater is considered severe. A COHb level in excess of 50% may cause irreversible damage to the central nervous system (CNS). If available, hyperbaric oxygen (HBO) therapy is usually used at a COHb >10%.

Table 41-3 lists the clinical manifestations associated with carbon monoxide poisoning.

CYANIDE POISONING

When smoke contains cyanide, oxygen transport may be further impaired. Cyanide poisoning should be suspected in comatose patients who have inhaled fumes from burning plastic (polyurethane) or other synthetic materials. Inhaled cyanide is easily

TABLE 41-3 Blood Carboxyhemoglobin (COHb) Levels and Clinical Manifestations

COHb (%)	Clinical Manifestations
0-10	Usually no symptoms
10-20	Mild headache, dilation of cutaneous blood vessels Cherry red skin—but not always
20-30	Throbbing headache, nausea, vomiting, impaired judgment
30-50	Throbbing headache, possible syncope, increased respiratory and pulse rates
50-60	Syncope, increased respiratory and pulse rates, coma, convulsions, Cheyne-Stokes respiration
60-70	Coma, convulsions, cardiovascular and respiratory depression, and possible death
70-80	Cardiopulmonary failure and death

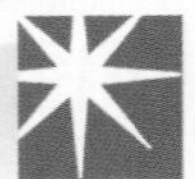

OVERVIEW of the Cardiopulmonary Clinical Manifestations Associated with Smoke Inhalation and Thermal Injuries—cont'd

transported in the blood to the tissue cells, where it bonds to the cytochrome oxidase enzymes of the mitochondria. This inhibits the metabolism of oxygen and causes the tissue cells to shift to an inefficient anaerobic form of metabolism. The end product of anaerobic metabolism is lactic acid. Cyanide poisoning may result in lactic acidemia, which is caused by an inadequate *tissue* oxygen level, even though the Pa_{O_2} is normal or above normal. Clinically, cyanide concentrations are easily measured with commercially available kits. A cyanide blood level in excess of 1 mg/L usually is fatal.

RADIOLOGIC FINDINGS

Chest Radiograph

- Usually normal (early stage)
- Pulmonary edema, acute respiratory distress syndrome (ARDS) (intermediate stage)
- Patchy or segmental infiltrates (late stage)

During the early stage, the radiograph is generally normal. Signs of pulmonary edema and ARDS may be seen during the intermediate and late stages. The chest x-ray film reveals dense, fluffy opacities and patchy or segmental infiltrates (Figure 41-2).

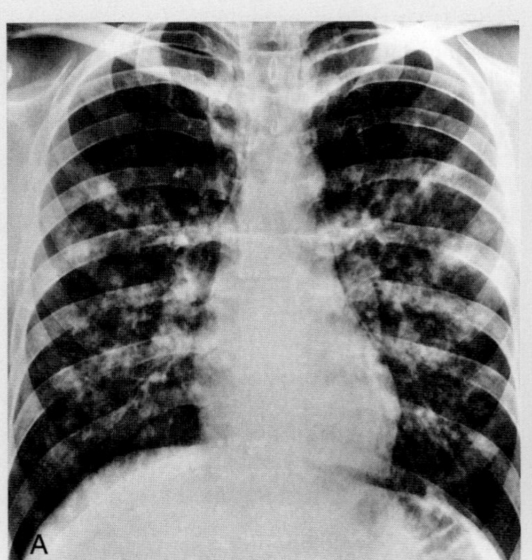

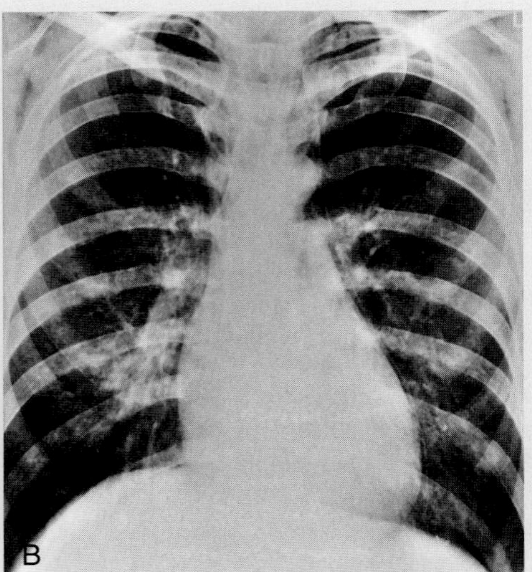

FIGURE 41-2 **A**, Radiograph of a young man admitted after accidentally setting his kitchen on fire while intoxicated. **B**, Prompt recovery after 72 hours. (From Hansell DM, Armstrong P, Lynch DA, McAdams HP, eds: *Imaging of diseases of the chest,* ed 4, Philadelphia, 2005, Elsevier.)

General Management Smoke Inhalation and Thermal Injuries

General Emergency Care

The principal goals in the initial care of patients with smoke inhalation injury and burns include the immediate assessment of the patient's airway, respiratory status, and cardiovascular status, the percentage of body burned, and the depth of burns. An intravenous line should be started immediately to administer medications and fluids. Easily separated clothing should be removed. Any remaining clothing should be soaked thoroughly before removing. When present, burn wounds should be covered to prevent shock, fluid loss, heat loss, and pain. Infection control includes isolation, room pressurization, air filtration, and wound coverings.

Fluid resuscitation with Ringer's lactate solution is usually initiated according to the **Parkland Formula**—4 mL/kg of body weight for each percent of body surface area burned (see Table 41-2) over a 24-hour period. The patient's hemodynamic status will usually remain stable at this fluid replacement rate, with an average urine output target of 30 to 50 mL/hr and a central venous pressure (CVP) target of 2 to 6 mm Hg. Because this process often leads to overhydration and acute UAO and pulmonary edema, the patient's fluid and electrolyte status (weight, input and output, and laboratory values) must be monitored carefully.

Finally, knowledge of the exposure characteristics of the fire-related accident may be helpful in assessing the potential clinical complications. For example, did the accident involve a closed-space setting or entrapment? The amount and concentration of smoke usually are much greater under these conditions. What type of material was burning in the fire? Are the inhaled toxins known? Was carbon monoxide (CO) or cyanide produced by the burning substances? Was the patient unconscious before entering the hospital?

Airway Management

Early elective endotracheal intubation should be performed on the patient who has inhaled hot gases and demonstrates any signs of impending UAO (e.g., upper airway edema, blisters, inspiratory stridor, thick secretions). *This is a medical emergency.* Even though acute UAO is considered one of the most treatable complications of smoke inhalation, death still occurs from UAO (hence the well-supported clinical guideline that states "When in doubt, intubate").

Securing an endotracheal tube often is difficult in the presence of facial burns (typically wet wounds). Adhesive tape may cause further trauma to the burn wounds. The ingenuity and creativity of the respiratory care practitioner may be required. Securing the endotracheal tube without traumatizing the patient has been successful with the use of umbilical tape and a variety of helmets, halo traction devices, and Velcro straps.

Because of the infections associated with body surface burns and smoke inhalation, a tracheostomy should be reserved for conditions in which an airway cannot be established otherwise, or for the patient who will require prolonged mechanical ventilation.

Bronchoscopy

Therapeutic bronchoscopy often is used to clear the airways of mucous plugs and eschar. In addition, early bronchoscopy often is performed for inspection and evaluation of the upper airways. Mucosal changes distal to the larynx serve as good predictors of subsequent respiratory problems.

Hyperbaric Oxygen Therapy

Hyperbaric oxygenation (HBO) therapy is useful in the rapid elimination of CO and the enhancement of skin graft viability. Although a Pa_{O_2} greater than 1500 mm Hg can be achieved with a hyperbaric chamber, it often is not possible or practical to institute this therapy. The chamber may not be immediately available. Can the patient be transported safely? Will the interruption of immediate therapy be detrimental?

Treatment for Cyanide Poisoning

The treatment for **cyanide poisoning** includes amyl nitrite inhalation and intravenous sodium thiosulfate.

Antibiotic Agents

Antibiotics may be used to treat burn wounds and pulmonary infections (see Appendix III).

Expectorants

Expectorants may be administered to facilitate expectoration (see Appendix V).

Analgesic Agents

Analgesics generally are ordered when surface burns are present.

Prophylactic Anticoagulants

Heparin and other anticoagulants often are administered to patients with severe, long-term fire-related injuries to reduce the risk of pulmonary embolism. Immobile patients also are treated with this therapy.

Respiratory Care Treatment Protocols

Oxygen Therapy Protocol

Oxygen therapy is used to treat hypoxemia, decrease the work of breathing, and decrease myocardial work. Because of the hypoxemia and **carbon monoxide (CO) poisoning** associated with smoke inhalation, a high concentration of oxygen always should be administered immediately. The carboxyhemoglobin (COHb) half-life when a patient is breathing room air at 1 atmosphere is approximately 5 hours. In other words, a 40% COHb decreases to about 20% in 5 hours and about 10% in another 5 hours. Breathing 100% oxygen at 1 atmosphere reduces the COHb half-life to less than 1 hour. If available, HBO therapy is in order, especially in comatose smoke inhalation victims with COHb levels >10%.

See Oxygen Therapy Protocol, Protocol 9-1.

Bronchopulmonary Hygiene Therapy Protocol

Because of the excessive mucous production and accumulation in the intermediate and late stages of smoke inhalation injuries, a number of respiratory therapy modalities may be used to enhance the mobilization of bronchial secretions. However, even though chest physical therapy is an excellent treatment modality to mobilize secretions, patients with severe chest burns or recent skin grafts do not tolerate chest percussion and vibration (see Bronchopulmonary Hygiene Therapy Protocol, Protocol 9-2).

Lung Expansion Therapy Protocol

Lung expansion techniques commonly are used to offset the alveolar atelectasis and consolidation associated with smoke inhalation injuries. The administration of continuous positive airway pressure (CPAP) via an endotracheal tube or mask (when the patient has no facial or neck burns) may help minimize the development of pulmonary edema. CPAP also supports the edematous airway and maintains or increases the patient's functional residual capacity (see Lung Expansion Therapy Protocol, Protocol 9-3).

Aerosolized Medication Protocol

Both sympathomimetic and parasympatholytic agents commonly are used to produce vasoconstriction of the mucosa and to offset bronchial smooth muscle constriction. Bland (saline) aerosols may be helpful. Mucolytics and antiinflammatory agents also may be administered as part of the Aerosolized Medication Protocol (see Protocol 9-4).

Mechanical Ventilation Protocol

Mechanical ventilation with positive end-expiratory pressure (PEEP) usually is required for patients who develop pulmonary edema, ARDS, and pneumonia. Mechanical ventilation should be implemented in the presence of acute or impending ventilatory failure (see Mechanical Ventilation Protocols, Protocol 9-5, Protocol 9-6, and Protocol 9-7).

CASE STUDY

Smoke Inhalation and Thermal Injury

Admitting History and Physical Examination

A 21-year-old man, after smoking marijuana and falling asleep, suffered second- and third-degree burns on his face, chest, and abdomen as a result of his bed catching fire. The extent of second- and third-degree burns was only 6% to 8% of his total body surface area. He had previously been in excellent health.

Shortly after admission, he developed respiratory distress and pulmonary edema. His blood pressure was 110/60, pulse 100 bpm, and respiratory rate 30/min. His oral temperature was 98.8° F. Bilateral crackles, rhonchi, and occasional wheezing were present. Spontaneous cough produced large amounts of thick, whitish-grey sputum. The chest radiograph revealed bilateral patchy infiltrates and consolidation. On 4 L/min oxygen, his arterial blood gas values were pH 7.51, Pa_{CO_2} 28, HCO_3^- 21, and Pa_{O_2} 45. A COHb level was not obtained.

The patient was treated conservatively. He was placed on a oxygen mask, and the pulmonary edema progressively cleared over the next 48 hours. However, the respiratory distress and hypoxemia persisted, even on 60% oxygen by high-flow oxygen enrichment (HAFOE) mask. Three days after his admission, the patient's condition was worsening. The patient was agitated and he complained of a productive cough, worsening shortness of breath, and substernal chest pain with deep breathing and coughing. Thick whitish-grey secretions were noted. Auscultation revealed bilateral crackles, rhonchi, and expiratory wheezing. His vital signs were as follows: temperature 98.6° F (rectal), blood pressure 120/65, pulse 119 (regular sinus rhythm), respiratory rate 35/min. On an F_{IO_2} of 0.60 his ABG values were as follows: pH 7.54, Pa_{CO_2} 25, HCO_3^- 20, and Pa_{O_2} 38. His chest x-ray showed patchy infiltrates and some segmental consolidation. Fiberoptic bronchoscopy revealed extensive thermal damage and eschar in the trachea and large bronchi. At that time, the following respiratory assessment was documented.

Respiratory Assessment and Plan

S Complains of productive cough, substernal chest pain when coughing, and dyspnea.

O Afebrile. BP 120/65, P 119 and regular, RR 35. Bilateral crackles, rhonchi, and expiratory wheezing. On 60% O_2 by HAFOE mask: pH 7.54, Pa_{CO_2} 25, HCO_3^- 20, and Pa_{O_2} 38. CXR: Bilateral patchy infiltrates and consolidation. No cardiomegaly. Bronchoscopy—blackish eschar in oropharynx; reddened and inflamed larynx, trachea, and large airways. Thick, whitish-grey secretions noted.

A
- Smoke inhalation with thermal burns of the oropharynx, larynx, and large airways (history and bronchoscopy)
- Alveolar infiltrates and consolidation (CXR)
- Acute alveolar hyperventilation with severe hypoxemia (ABGs)
- Impending ventilatory failure (general history and clinical trend)
- Excessive and thick airway secretions (sputum)

P Confer with attending physician to intubate and initiate mechanical ventilation care per **Mechanical Ventilation Protocol. Oxygen Therapy Protocol:** F_{IO_2} at 1.0 via nonrebreather mask. **Aerosolized Medication Protocol** and **Bronchopulmonary Hygiene Protocol:** albuterol premix 2.0 mL via med. neb. q2h (alternate with epinephrine 6 drops in 2.0 mL normal saline). Gentle nasotracheal and oral suctioning after med. neb. treatments and prn. Check I&O status and daily weights. If physician commits patient to ventilator, consider in-line ultrasonic nebulizer treatments, for 30 min q4h.

The patient was intubated and started on intravenously administered steroids. He was ventilated with an F_{IO_2} of 0.60, rate of 12, and PEEP of +10 cm H_2O. Because of the upper body burns, chest physical therapy and postural drainage were prohibited. The bronchial secretions, however, were loosened and mobilized adequately with an in-line ultrasonic nebulizer and frequent endotracheal suctioning. In-line aerosolized steroids also were administered at this time.

The patient's vital signs and blood gas values improved on this regimen. After 12 days of respiratory care, he was weaned to room air and extubated. He continued to complain of exertional dyspnea with transfer activities but denied dyspnea at rest. Crackles were improved but still easily auscultated throughout all lung fields when the patient took deep breaths. Occasional expiratory wheezes also were heard.

Three days after extubation, on an F_{IO_2} of 0.35 via a HAFOE mask, his pH was 7.46, Pa_{CO_2} 38, HCO_3^- 24, and Pa_{O_2} 63. On exercise, the Sp_{O_2} fell to 85%. His peak expiratory flow rate (PEFR) was 40% of predicted. The infiltrates previously noted on chest x-ray were much improved. At that time, the respiratory therapist recorded the following assessment in the patient's chart.

Respiratory Assessment and Plan

S Complains of shortness of breath with any activity.

O Vital signs stable. Crackles heard over both lung bases. Some expiratory prolongation. ABGs (spontaneous breathing) (F_{IO_2} = 0.35 by HAFOE): pH 7.46, Pa_{CO_2} 38, HCO_3^- 24, and Pa_{O_2} 63. Sp_{O_2} falls to 85% with exercise. PEFR 40% of predicted. CXR: Improvement in patchy lung infiltrates.

A
- Mild to moderate hypoxemia secondary to thermal injury to lung (ABGs and history)
- Moderate obstructive pulmonary disease (PEFR)

P Complete pulmonary function tests ordered. Up-regulate **Oxygen Therapy Protocol** (increase F_{IO_2} to 0.40 via a HAFOE). If obstructive pulmonary disease is confirmed, restart **Bronchial Hygiene Protocol** and **Aerosolized Medication Protocol.**

Pulmonary function studies showed severely reduced expiratory flows and a sharply decreased diffusion capacity. Chest x-rays taken at regular intervals thereafter began to show emphysematous changes. The diaphragms were flattened, and bilateral coarse reticular infiltrates were evident. In spite of vigorous therapy over the next 6 weeks, the patient's cardiopulmonary status continued to worsen. The patient died on day 59, 2 months after his original thermal and inhalational injury. The postmortem diagnosis at autopsy was cryptogenic organizing pneumonia (COP)—also known as *bronchiolitis obliterans organizing pneumonia* (BOOP).

Discussion

At the time of the first assessment, the patient demonstrated most of the pathophysiologic correlates of smoke inhalation and thermal injuries to the lung. His dyspnea reflected the increased work of breathing associated with **Bronchospasm** (see Figure 9-11), **Increased Alveolar-Capillary Membrane Thickness** (see Figure 9-10), and **Excessive Bronchial Secretions** (see Figure 9-12). The bronchospasm was treated with the vigorous use of both bronchodilator (albuterol) and decongestant (epinephrine) aerosols. The excessive bronchial secretions were treated with ultrasonic bland aerosols and airway suctioning. No specific treatment was available for the changes that occurred in the alveolar-capillary membrane

This interesting case is instructive for these reasons. The first is that all patients with burns of the upper chest, neck, or face should have a careful oropharyngeal examination to determine whether burns have indeed occurred in the upper airway. The presence of soot or eschar in the oropharynx is diagnostic of this problem; respiratory distress almost certainly will ensue if such findings are present, although this does not happen immediately. A 24- to 72-hour lag may occur between the burn and clinical obstruction of the airway. Second, a dreaded complication of smoke and heat inhalation is COP, which developed in this patient and ultimately was responsible for his demise.

Today, this patient might be considered a candidate for lung transplantation. This case study should remind the respiratory care practitioner that immediate intubation over the diagnostic bronchoscope may be necessary and that he or she should prepare accordingly.

SELF-ASSESSMENT QUESTIONS

evolve Answers to questions can be found on Evolve. To access additional student assessment questions and case studies for application of text material to real-life scenarios, visit **http://evolve.elsevier.com/DesJardins/respiratory.**

1. About what percentage of hospitalized patients with thermal injury have an acute upper airway obstruction (UAO)?

a. 0% to 10%
b. 10% to 20%
c. 20% to 30%
d. 30% to 40%

2. Except for the rare instance of steam inhalation, direct thermal injuries usually do not occur below the level of which of the following structures?

a. Oral pharynx
b. Larynx
c. Carina
d. Bronchi

3. When chest wall burns are present, the patient's pulmonary condition may be further aggravated by which of the following?

1. Decreased lung and chest compliance
2. Increased airway resistance
3. The use of narcotics
4. Immobility

a. 2 and 3 only
b. 1 and 3 only
c. 2 and 4 only
d. 1, 2, 3, and 4

4. Which of the following is or are the pulmonary-related pathologic change(s) associated with smoke inhalation?

1. Alveolar hyperinflation
2. Bronchospasm
3. Pulmonary edema
4. Pulmonary embolism

a. 1 only
b. 2 only
c. 3 and 4 only
d. 2, 3, and 4 only

5. Which of the following produce carbon monoxide when burned?

1. Polyurethanes
2. Wood, cotton, paper
3. Organic material
4. Polyvinylchloride (PVC)

a. 1 only
b. 2 only
c. 3 and 4 only
d. 1, 2, and 3 only

6. Which of the following oxygenation indices is or are associated with smoke inhalation and burns during the early and intermediate stages?

1. Increased $\dot{V}O_2$
2. Decreased $C(a-\bar{v})O_2$
3. Increased DO_2
4. Decreased $S\bar{v}O_2$
   a. 2 only
   b. 4 only
   c. 2 and 3 only
   d. 1 and 4 only

7. Which of the following hemodynamic indices is or are associated with body surface burns during the early stage?

1. Decreased CO
2. Increased SVR
3. Decreased $\overline{PA}$
4. Increased PCWP
   a. 1 only
   b. 3 only
   c. 2 and 4 only
   d. 1, 2, and 3 only

8. If an adult's entire right arm, right leg, and anterior trunk have been burned, approximately what percentage of the patient's body surface area is burned?

a. 15%
b. 25%
c. 35%
d. 45%

9. Healing time for a second-degree burn is:

a. 1 to 7 days
b. 7 to 21 days
c. 21 to 31 days
d. 1 to 2 months

10. Breathing 100% oxygen at 1 atmosphere reduces the carboxyhemoglobin (COHb) half-life to less than:

a. 1 hour
b. 2 hours
c. 3 hours
d. 4 hours

Postoperative Atelectasis

42

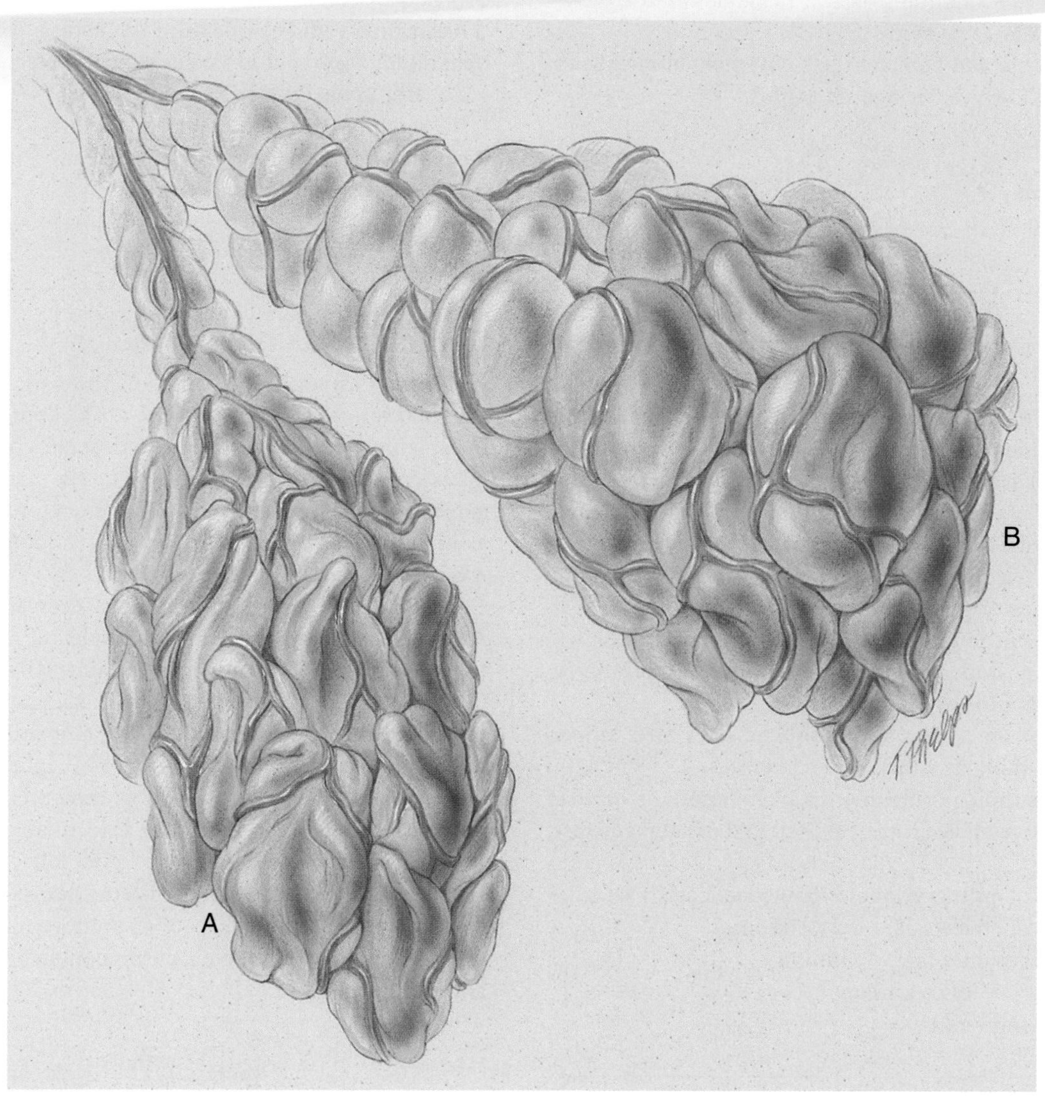

FIGURE 42-1 Alveoli in postoperative atelectasis. **A**, Total alveolar collapse. **B**, Partial alveolar collapse.

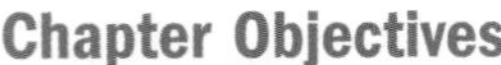

Chapter Objectives

After reading this chapter, you will be able to:

- List the anatomic alterations of the lungs associated with postoperative atelectasis.
- Describe the causes of postoperative atelectasis.
- List the cardiopulmonary clinical manifestations associated with postoperative atelectasis.
- Describe the general management of postoperative atelectasis.
- Describe the clinical strategies and rationales of the SOAP presented in the case study.
- Define key terms and complete self-assessment questions at the end of the chapter and on Evolve.

Key Terms

Air Bronchograms
Alveolar Degassing

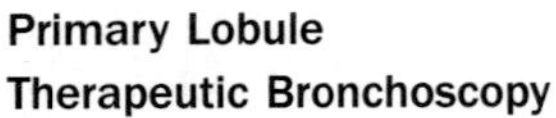

Primary Lobule
Therapeutic Bronchoscopy

Chapter Outline

Anatomic Alterations of the Lungs

Atelectasis, in the strict sense of the term, is defined as the condition in which the lungs of the newborn remain unexpanded (airless) at birth. In the clinical setting, however, the meaning of *atelectasis* in all age groups generally is broadened to include partial or total collapse of previously expanded lung regions. Atelectasis may be limited to the smallest lung unit (i.e., alveolus or **primary lobule***; see Figure 42-1), or it may involve an entire lung or a segment or lobe of the lung. In this chapter, postoperative atelectasis is used as a prototype of the atelectasis process.

Postoperative atelectasis commonly is seen after upper abdominal and thoracic surgical procedures.

The major pathologic and anatomic alterations associated with postoperative atelectasis include partial or total collapse of the following:

- Alveoli of primary lobules (microatelectasis or subsegmental atelectasis)—very common
- Lung segment—fairly common
- Lung lobe—less common
- Entire lung—rare

Etiology and Epidemiology

Postoperative atelectasis develops when lung expansion is decreased or when excess airway secretions cause mucous plugs, which in turn produce distal "degassing" of lung units.

*A primary lobule is a cluster of alveoli that originates from a single terminal bronchiole. Each primary lobule is about 3.5 mm in diameter and contains about 2000 alveoli. Each lung contains about 150,000 primary lobules. A primary lobule also is called an *acinus, terminal respiratory unit,* or *functional lung unit.* The lung parenchyma consists of the terminal respiratory units.

Decreased Lung Expansion

Good lung expansion depends on the patient's intact chest cage and his or her ability to generate an appropriate negative intrapleural pressure. Thoracic and upper abdominal procedures often result in a reduction in the patient's ability to generate good lung expansion and therefore are considered as high-risk factors for subsequent development of postoperative atelectasis.

Other precipitating factors that decrease the patient's ability to generate a negative intrapleural pressure include (1) anesthesia, (2) postoperative pain, (3) supine position, (4) obesity, (5) advanced age, (6) inadequate tidal volumes during mechanical ventilation, (7) malnutrition, (8) free fluid in the abdominal cavity (ascites), (9) diaphragmatic apraxia (e.g., topical cooling of the left phrenic nerve often occurs during cardiac surgery and may lead to an inadequate diaphragmatic movement and left lower lobe atelectasis), and (10) the presence of restrictive lung disorders (e.g., pleural effusion, pneumothorax, acute respiratory distress syndrome [ARDS], pulmonary edema, chronic interstitial lung disease, and pleural masses).

Alveolar Degassing Distal to Airway Secretions and Mucous Plugs (Airway Obstruction)

Postoperative atelectasis often is associated with retained airway secretions and mucous plugs. Precipitating factors for retained secretions include (1) decreased mucociliary transport, (2) excessive secretions, (3) inadequate hydration, (4) weak or absent cough, (5) general anesthesia, (6) smoking history, (7) gastric aspiration, and (8) certain preexisting conditions (e.g., bronchiectasis, chronic bronchitis, cystic fibrosis, asthma). When total airway obstruction develops, alveolar oxygen is absorbed into the pulmonary circulation and **alveolar degassing** ensues. The breathing of high oxygen concentrations favors this pathologic process.

OVERVIEW of the Cardiopulmonary Clinical Manifestations Associated with Postoperative Atelectasis

The following clinical manifestations result from the pathologic mechanisms caused (or activated) by **Atelectasis** (see Figure 9-8)—the major anatomic alterations of the lungs associated with postoperative atelectasis (see Figure 42-1).

CLINICAL DATA OBTAINED AT THE PATIENT'S BEDSIDE

The Physical Examination

Vital Signs

Increased Respiratory Rate (Tachypnea)

Several pathophysiologic mechanisms operating simultaneously may lead to an increased ventilatory rate:

- Stimulation of peripheral chemoreceptors (hypoxemia)
- Decreased lung compliance–increased ventilatory rate relationship
- Stimulation of J receptors
- Pain, anxiety, fever

Increased Heart Rate (Pulse) and Blood Pressure

Cyanosis

Chest Assessment Findings

- Increased tactile and vocal fremitus
- Dull percussion note
- Bronchial breath sounds
- Diminished breath sounds (common when atelectasis in caused by mucous plugs)
- Crackles (usually heard initially in the dependent lung regions and during late inspiration)
- Whispered pectoriloquy

CLINICAL DATA OBTAINED FROM LABORATORY TESTS AND SPECIAL PROCEDURES

Pulmonary Function Test Findings
(Extrapolated Data for Instructional Purposes)
(Primarily Restrictive Lung Pathophysiology)

FORCED EXPIRATORY FLOW RATE FINDINGS

FVC	FEV_T	FEV_1/FVC ratio	$FEF_{25\%-75\%}$
↓	N or ↓	N or ↑	N or ↓

$FEF_{50\%}$	$FEF_{200-1200}$	PEFR	MVV
N or ↓	N or ↓	N or ↓	N or ↓

LUNG VOLUME AND CAPACITY FINDINGS

V_T	IRV	ERV	RV	
N or ↓	↓	↓	↓	
VC	**IC**	**FRC**	**TLC**	**RV/TLC ratio**
↓	↓	↓	↓	N

DECREASED DIFFUSION CAPACITY (DLCO)

Arterial Blood Gases

SMALL OR LOCALIZED POSTOPERATIVE ATELECTASIS
Acute Alveolar Hyperventilation with Hypoxemia
(Acute Respiratory Alkalosis)

pH	$Paco_2$	HCO_3^-	Pao_2
↑	↓	↓ (slightly)	↓

WIDESPREAD POSTOPERATIVE ATELECTASIS
Acute Ventilatory Failure with Hypoxemia
(Acute Respiratory Acidosis)

pH*	$Paco_2$	HCO_3^- *	Pao_2
↓	↑	↑ (slightly)	↓

*When tissue hypoxia is severe enough to produce lactic acid, the pH and HCO_3^- values will be lower than expected for a particular $Paco_2$ level.

Oxygenation Indices*

$\dot{Q}_S/\dot{Q}_T$	Do_2†	$\dot{V}o_2$	$C(a-\bar{v})o_2$	O_2ER	$S\bar{v}o_2$
↑	↓	N	N	↑	↓

†The Do_2 may be normal in patients who have compensated to the decreased oxygenation status with (1) an increased cardiac output, (2) an increased hemoglobin level, or (3) a combination of both. When the Do_2 is normal, the O_2ER is usually normal.

*$C(a-\bar{v})o_2$, Arterial-venous oxygen difference; Do_2, total oxygen delivery; O_2ER, oxygen extraction ratio; $\dot{Q}_S/\dot{Q}_T$, pulmonary shunt fraction; $S\bar{v}o_2$, mixed venous oxygen saturation; $\dot{V}o_2$, oxygen consumption.

RADIOLOGIC FINDINGS

Chest Radiograph

- Increased density in areas of atelectasis
- Air bronchograms
- Elevation of the hemidiaphragm on the affected side
- Mediastinal shift toward the affected side

Areas of increased density generally appear initially in dependent lung regions, such as the lower lobes, or posteriorly in patients who must recline in the supine position. **Air bronchograms** can be seen when large areas of atelectasis are present. An elevation of the hemidiaphragm or mediastinal shift toward the affected side often is seen when large areas of atelectasis exist. Figure 42-2, *A* shows left lung atelectasis caused by a misplaced endotracheal tube in the right main stem bronchus. Figure 42-2, *B* shows the same patient 20 minutes after the endotracheal tube was pulled back above the carina.

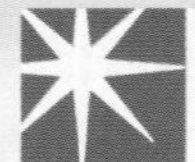

OVERVIEW of the Cardiopulmonary Clinical Manifestations Associated with Postoperative Atelectasis—cont'd

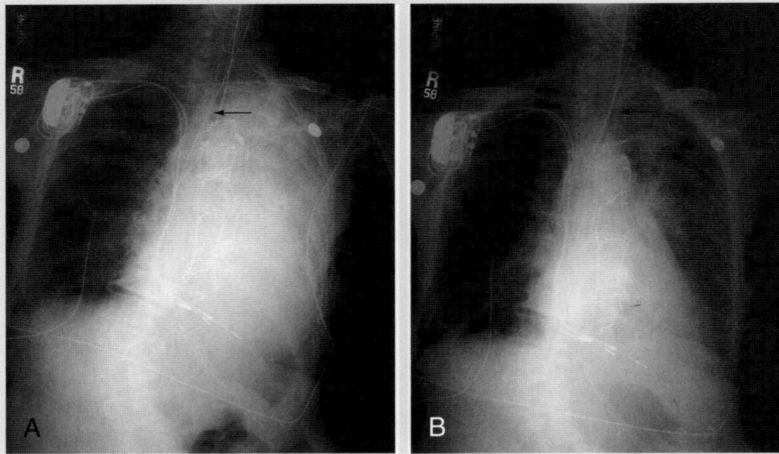

FIGURE 42-2 **A**, Endotracheal tube tip misplaced in the right main stem bronchus *(arrow)*. Note that the left lung has collapsed completely (i.e., white fluffy appearance in the left lung). **B**, The same patient 20 minutes after the endotracheal tube was pulled back above the carina *(arrow)*. Note that the left lung is better ventilated (i.e., appears darker). Used with permission from the author: WindMist LLC.)

General Management of Postoperative Atelectasis

Precipitating factors for postoperative atelectasis should be identified during the preoperative and postoperative assessments (see the previous section on etiology). High-risk patients should be monitored closely. For example, bedside spirometry (vital capacity and inspiratory capacity) is useful in the early detection of atelectasis. Preventive measures often are prescribed for high-risk patients. For example, incentive spirometry frequently is prescribed to encourage good lung expansion. Chest physical therapy also may be given to the patient with mild to moderate preoperative or postoperative bronchial secretions to offset the development of mucous plugs and atelectasis. Patients who demonstrate combined obstructive and restrictive pulmonary disease preoperatively generally are thought to be at extremely high risk for atelectasis. When the diagnosis of postoperative atelectasis has been made, the following respiratory care procedures may be prescribed.

General Considerations

Whenever possible, treatment of the underlying cause of the postoperative atelectasis should be prescribed immediately (e.g., medication for pain, correction of inadequate tidal volumes during mechanical ventilation, repositioning of an endotracheal tube in the right main stem bronchus, or withdrawal of air or fluid from the pleural cavity).

Respiratory Care Treatment Protocols

Oxygen Therapy Protocol

Oxygen therapy is used to treat hypoxemia, decrease the work of breathing, and decrease myocardial work. Because of the hypoxemia that may develop in atelectasis, supplemental oxygen may be required. However, the hypoxemia that develops in postoperative atelectasis is caused by capillary shunting and therefore is often refractory to oxygen therapy (see Oxygen Therapy Protocol, Protocol 9-1).

Bronchopulmonary Hygiene Therapy Protocol

When atelectasis is caused by mucous accumulation and mucous plugs, a number of bronchial hygiene treatment modalities may be used to enhance the mobilization of airway secretions (see Bronchopulmonary Hygiene Therapy Protocol, Protocol 9-2).

Lung Expansion Therapy Protocol

Lung expansion therapy measures commonly are administered to offset atelectasis and reinflate collapsed lung areas (see Lung Expansion Therapy Protocol, Protocol 9-3).

Mechanical Ventilation Protocol

Short-term mechanical ventilation often is prescribed after major surgery, especially if the patient demonstrates one or more high-risk factors for postoperative atelectasis. For example, in patients undergoing cardiac surgery, mechanical ventilation generally is maintained until the cardiopulmonary parameters are stable (see Mechanical Ventilation Protocols, Protocol 9-5, Protocol 9-6, and Protocol 9-7).

CASE STUDY

Postoperative Atelectasis

Admitting History and Physical Examination

A 62-year-old man with a 35-pack/year smoking history had his left lower lobe resected because of small-cell carcinoma. Anesthesia had been performed using a right-sided double-lumen endotracheal tube. At the end of the procedure, the patient was breathing well and the tube was removed.

In the recovery room 30 minutes after arrival, his respiratory rate increased from 22/min to 34/min. His pulse increased from 70 to 130 bpm with regular rhythm, and his blood pressure decreased from 115/85 to 100/60 mm Hg. His peripheral oxygen saturation dropped from 97% to 85% while he was on 2 L/min O_2 per cannula. Breath sounds were decreased in the left lower anterior chest. A chest x-ray film showed atelectasis of the left lower lobe. Arterial blood gas values (on 2 L/min O_2 per cannula) were pH 7.29, $Pa\text{CO}_2$ 63, HCO_3^- 25, and $Pa\text{O}_2$ 55. At that time the respiratory therapist recorded the following SOAP note.

Respiratory Assessment and Plan

S N/A. Patient still sedated from anesthesia.

O RR 34/min, P 130 and regular, BP 100/60. Breath sounds decreased in left lower chest anteriorly. CXR: Left lower lobe atelectasis. On 2 L/min O_2 per cannula: pH 7.29, $Pa\text{CO}_2$ 63, HCO_3^- 25, and $Pa\text{O}_2$ 55.

A
- Left lower lobe atelectasis; rule out mucous plugs (CXR and decreased breath sounds)
- Acute ventilatory failure with moderate hypoxemia (ABGs)

P Contact physician regarding intubation and **Mechanical Ventilation Protocol** (SIMV mode). **Oxygen Therapy Protocol** ($F\text{IO}_2$ 0.5). **Bronchopulmonary Hygiene Therapy Protocol** (encourage cough and deep breathing, suction frequently, discuss with physician the possibility of respiratory therapist assistance with therapeutic bronchoscopy). **Lung Expansion Therapy Protocol** after intubation (PEEP based on titration study). **Aerosolized Medication Therapy Protocol** (in-line albuterol 0.5 mL in 2.0 mL 20% acetylcysteine q2h, then decrease or increase according to reassessment). Repeat ABGs in 30 minutes, and reevaluate. Monitor $Sp\text{O}_2$ for next 72 hours.

The patient was reintubated, ventilated, and oxygenated according to protocol. A mucolytic (acetylcysteine) was aerosolized and also directly instilled into the patient's endotracheal tube. Aggressive tracheobronchial suctioning was performed. This produced small amounts of secretions with little or no benefit to the patient.

In view of this, a fiberoptic bronchoscope was inserted through the endotracheal tube, and a large mucous plug was identified in the orifice of the left lower lobe bronchus. The plug was removed under direct vision. After the bronchoscopy, the patient improved rapidly and could be extubated after about 60 minutes. A chest x-ray film taken before that time showed full expansion of the left lower lobe. The patient was discharged on the sixth postoperative day.

Discussion

Care of a patient with postoperative **Atelectasis** (see Figure 9-8) is one of the day-to-day responsibilities of the respiratory care practitioner. Accordingly, the respiratory care practitioner must be extremely adept in the assessment and management of such patients. The development of immediate postoperative atelectasis almost always is related to **Excessive Bronchial Secretions** (see Figure 9-12)—in this case caused by a large mucous plug obstructing the left lower lobe. Because such patients (in the immediate postoperative period) often cannot cough vigorously, particularly after thoracotomy, the decision to initiate **therapeutic bronchoscopy** immediately rather than to rely on physical therapy and mucolytics was certainly in order.

In patients who have undergone abdominal surgery or those who develop atelectasis later, the simpler approaches should certainly be tried first. Atelectasis has a tendency to recur, and these patients need to be followed at least 72 hours postoperatively to ensure that this has not happened. Therefore the therapist's suggestion to follow pulse oximetry is entirely appropriate.

As important as treatment is, prevention is better. In this regard, the **Bronchopulmonary Hygiene Protocol** and the **Lung Expansion Protocol** were very important. Indeed, the application of these simple protocols often prevents the late development of atelectasis in postoperative patients.

SELF-ASSESSMENT QUESTIONS

evolve Answers to questions can be found on Evolve. To access additional student assessment questions and case studies for application of text material to real-life scenarios, visit **http://evolve.elsevier.com/DesJardins/respiratory.**

1. Which of the following clinical manifestations are associated with postoperative atelectasis?

1. Frothy, pink sputum
2. Crackles
3. Air bronchograms
4. Increased $S\bar{v}O_2$
    a. 1 and 2 only
    b. 2 and 3 only
    c. 3, and 4 only
    d. 2, 3, and 4 only

2. Which of the following pulmonary function testing values are associated with postoperative atelectasis?

1. N or ↑ FEV_T
2. ↑ FVC
3. ↓ RV
4. N or ↑ FEV_1/FVC ratio
    a. 1 and 2 only
    b. 3 and 4 only
    c. 2, 3, and 4 only
    d. 1, 2, 3, and 4 only

3. A primary lobule is a cluster of alveoli. About how many alveoli does a primary lobule contain?

a. 500 alveoli
b. 1000 alveoli
c. 1500 alveoli
d. 2000 alveoli

4. Which of the following are precipitating factors of postoperative atelectasis?

1. Obesity
2. Anesthesia
3. Postoperative pain
4. Ascites
    a. 1 and 3 only
    b. 2 and 4 only
    c. 2, 3, and 4 only
    d. 1, 2, 3, and 4

5. Which of the following arterial blood gas values are associated with small or localized postoperative atelectasis?

1. Increased Pa_{O_2}
2. Decreased Pa_{CO_2}
3. Increased pH
4. Decreased HCO_3^- (slightly)
    a. 1 and 3 only
    b. 2 and 4 only
    c. 2, 3, and 4 only
    d. 1, 2, 3, and 4

Symbols and Abbreviations Commonly Used in Respiratory Physiology

I

Primary Symbols	
Gas Symbols	**Blood Symbols**
P Pressure	Q Blood volume
V Gas volume	$\dot{Q}$ Blood flow
$\dot{V}$ Gas volume per unit of time, or flow	C Content in blood
F Fractional concentration of gas	S Saturation
Secondary Symbols	
Gas Symbols	**Blood Symbols**
I Inspired	a Arterial
E Expired	c Capillary
A Alveolar	v Venous
T Tidal	$\bar{v}$ Mixed venous
D Deadspace	

Abbreviations

Lung Volumes	
VC	Vital capacity
IC	Inspiratory capacity
IRV	Inspiratory reserve volume
ERV	Expiratory reserve volume
FRC	Functional residual capacity
RV	Residual volume
TLC	Total lung capacity
RV/TLC (%)	Residual volume–to–total lung capacity ratio, expressed as a percentage
V_T	Tidal volume
V_A	Alveolar volume
V_D	Dead-space volume
V_L	Actual lung volume
Respiratory Gas Flows and Rates	
$\dot{V}_A$	Alveolar ventilation
$\dot{V}_D$	Dead-space ventilation
f	Frequency (i.e., respiratory rate)

Continued

Abbreviations—cont'd

Spirometry	
FVC	Forced vital capacity with maximally forced expiratory effort
FEV_T	Forced expiratory volume, timed
$FEF_{50\%}$	Forced expiratory flow at 50%
FEV_1	Forced expiratory volume in 1 second
FEV_2	Forced expiratory volume in 2 second
FEV_3	Forced expiratory volume in 3 second
FEV_1/FVC	Forced expiratory volume in 1 second/forced vital capacity ratio
$FEV_{1\%}$	Forced expiratory volume in 1 second (percentage)
$FEF_{200\text{-}1200}$	Average rate of airflow between 200 and 1200 ml of the FVC
$FEF_{25\%\text{-}75\%}$	Forced expiratory flow during the middle half of the FVC (*formerly called the maximal midexpiratory flow [MMF]*)
PEFR	Peak expiratory flow rate
$\dot{V}_{max}$	Forced expiratory flow related to the actual volume of the lungs as denoted by the subscript *x*, which refers to the amount of lung volume remaining when measurement is made (e.g., $\dot{V}_{50}$ = flow at 50% of FVC)
MVV	Maximal voluntary ventilation as the volume of air expired in a specified interval
Mechanics	
C_L	Lung compliance, volume change per unit of pressure change
CL_{dyn}	Dynamic lung compliance (lung compliance with flow)
CL_{stat}	Static lung compliance (lung compliance without flow)
R_{aw}	Airway resistance, pressure per unit of flow
Diffusion	
D_{LCO}	Diffusing capacity of carbon monoxide
Blood Gases	
P_{AO_2}	Alveolar oxygen tension
P_{CO_2}	Pulmonary capillary oxygen tension
P_{aO_2}	Arterial oxygen tension
$P_{\bar{v}O_2}$	Mixed venous oxygen tension
P_{ACO_2}	Alveolar carbon dioxide tension
P_{cCO_2}	Pulmonary capillary carbon dioxide tension
P_{aCO_2}	Arterial carbon dioxide tension
S_{aO_2}	Arterial oxygen saturation
$S_{\bar{v}O_2}$	Mixed venous oxygen saturation
pH	Negative logarithm of the H^1 concentration, expressed as a positive number
HCO_3^-	Plasma bicarbonate concentration
mEq/L	The number of grams of solute contained in 1 ml of a normal solution
C_{aO_2}	Oxygen content of arterial blood
C_{cO_2}	Oxygen content of capillary blood
$C_{\bar{v}O_2}$	Oxygen content of mixed venous blood
$\dot{V}/\dot{Q}$	Ventilation-perfusion ratio
$\dot{Q}_S/\dot{Q}_T$	Shunt fraction
$\dot{Q}_T$ or CO	Total cardiac output

Agents Used to Treat Bronchospasm and Airway Inflammation

Agents Used to Treat Bronchospasm and Airway Inflammation—Controller Medications

Generic Name	Brand Name	Dose and Administration
Inhaled Corticosteroids (ICSs)		
Beclomethasone dipropionate	QVAR	MDI: 2 puffs, 40 μg/puff or 80 μg/puff, bid
Triamcinolone acetonide	Azmacort	MDI: 2 puffs, 100 μg/puff, tid, qid
Flunisolide	Aerobid, Aerobid-M	MDI: 2 puffs, 250 μg/puff, bid
Flunisolide hemihydrate	Aerospan	MDI: 2 puffs, 80 μg/puff, bid
Fluticasone propionate	Flovent HFA	MDI: 2 puffs, 44 μg/puff, 110 μg/puff, 220 μg/puff, bid
	Flovent Diskus	DPI: 50 μg, 100 μg, 250 μg, 100-1000 μg, bid
Ciclesonide	Alvesco	MDI: 1-2 puffs, 80 μg/puff abd 160 μg/puff, daily
Budesonide	Pulmicort Turbuhaler	DPI: 200 μg/actuation, 200-800 μg, bid
	Pulmicort Respules	SVN: 0.25 mg/2 mL, 0.5 mg/2 mL, once daily or bid
Mometasone furoate	Asmanex Twisthaler	DPI: 220 μg/actuation, 220-880 μg, q day
Systemic Corticosteroids		
Prednisone	Deltasone	Tablets and syrups: For acute attacks 40-60 mg daily in 1 or 2 divided doses for adults or 1-2 mg/kg daily in children
Methylprednisolone	Medrol	
	Solu-Medrol	
Hydrocortisone	Solu-Cortef	
Prednisolone	Orapred	
Long-Acting Beta$_2$ Agents (LABAs)		
Salmeterol	Serevent	DPI: 50 μg/inhalation, bid
Formoterol	Foradil	DPI: 12 μg/inhalation, bid
Arformoterol	Brovana	SVN: 15 μg/2 mL unite dose, bid
Inhaled Corticosteroids and Long-Acting Beta$_2$ Agents		
Fluticasone propionate and salmeterol	Advair Diskus	DPI: 100 μg, 250 μg, or 500 μg fluticasone with 50 μg salmeterol, 1 inhalation bid
	Advair HFA	MDI: 45 μg, 115 μg, or 230 μg, 1-2 inhalations bid
Budesonide and formoterol fumarate	Symbicort	MDI: 80 μg and 160 μg budesonide with 4.5 μg formoterol, 1-2 inhalations bid
Mast Cell–Stabilizing Agents		
Cromolyn sodium	Intal	SVN: 1 ampule, 20 mg/2 mL qid
		MDI: 2 puffs, 800 μg/puff, qid
Nedocromil sodium	Tilade	MDI: 2 puffs, 1.75 mg/puff, qid

Continued

Agents Used to Treat Bronchospasm and Airway Inflammation—Controller Medications—cont'd

Generic Name	Brand Name	Dose and Administration
Leukotriene Inhibitors (Antileukotrienes)		
Zafirlukast	Accolate	Tablet: 10 and 20 mg Adults and children ≥12 yr: 20 mg twice daily, without food Children 5-11 yr: 10 mg twice daily
Montelukast	Singulair	Tablets: 10 mg and 4- and 5-mg cherry-flavored chewable; 4-mg packet of granules Adults and children ≥15 yr: one 10 mg tablet daily Children 6-14 yr: one 5-mg chewable tablet daily Children 2-5 yr: one 4-mg chewable tablet or one 4-mg packet of granules daily 6-24 months: one 4-mg packet of granules daily
Zileuton	Zyflo	Tablets: 600 mg Adults and children ≥12 yr: one 600-mg tablet 4 times per day
Monoclonal Anti–Immunoglobulin E (IgE) Antibody		
Omalizumab	Xolair	Adults and children ≥12 yr: Subcutaneous injection every 4 weeks; dose dependent on weight and serum immunoglobulin E (IgE) level
Xanthine Derivatives		
Theophylline	Slo-phyllin, Theolair, Quibron-T/SR Dividose, Bronkodyl, Elixophyllin, Theo-Dur, Uniphyl	Dose formulations are based on individual metabolism Tablets, capsules, syrup, elixir, extended-release tablets, capsules, injection
Oxtriphylline	Choledyl SA	Dose formulations are based on individual metabolism Tablets, syrup, elixir, sustained-release tablets
Aminophylline	Aminophylline	Dose formulations are based on individual metabolism Tablets, oral liquid, injection, suppositories
Dyphylline	Dylix, Lufyllin	Dose formulations are based on individual metabolism Tablets, elixir

Data from Global Initiative for Asthma (GINA): *Global strategy for asthma management and prevention*, updated 2008. The GINA reports are available at www.ginasthma.org; and Gardenshire DS: *Rau's repiratory care pharmacology*, ed 7, St. Louis, 2008, Elsevier.
DPI, Dry powder inhaler; *MDI,* metered dose inhaler; *SVN,* small-volume nebulizer.

Reliever Medications (Rescue Medications) Commonly Used to Treat Bronchospasm

Medication	Trade Name	Adult Dosage
Ultra-Short–Acting Bronchodilator Agents		
Epinephrine	Adrenaline CL, Epinephrine Mist, Primatene Mist	SVN: 1% solution (1:100), 0.25-0.5 mL (2.5-5.0 mg) qid MDI: 0.22 mg/puff, puffs as ordered or needed
Racemic epinephrine	MicroNefrin, Nephron, S2	SVN: 2.25% solution, 0.25-0.5 mL (5.63-11.25 mg) qid
Isoetharine	Isoetharine (HCL)	SVN: 1% solution, 0.5 mL (5.0 mg) q4h
Short-Acting Adrenergic Bronchodilator Agents (SABAs) (Beta$_2$ Agents)		
Metaproterenol	Alupent	SVN: 0.4%, 0.6%, 5% solution, 0.3 mL (15 mg) tid, qid MDI: 650 µg/puff, 2 or 3 puffs tid, qid Tab: 10 mg and 20 mg, tid, qid Syrup: 10 mg/5 mL
Albuterol	Proventil	SVN: 0.5% solution, 0.5 mL (2.5 mg), 0.63 mg, 1.25 mg, and 2.5 mg unit dose, tid, qid
	Ventolin	MDI: 90 µg/puff, 2 puffs tid, qid
	AccuNeb	Tab: 2 mg, 4 mg, and 8 g, bid, tid, qid
	ProAir	Syrup: 2 mg/5 mL, 1-2 tsp tid, qid
Pirbuterol	Maxair Autohaler	MDI: 200 µg/puff, 2 puffs q4-6h
Levalbuterol	Xopenex, Xopenex HFA	SVN: 0.31 mg/3 mL tid, 0.63 mg/3 mL tid, or 1.25 mg/3 mL tid; concentrate 1.25 mg/0.5 mL, tid MDI: 45 µg/puff, 2 puffs q4-6h

Reliever Medications (Rescue Medications) Commonly Used to Treat Bronchospasm—cont'd

Medication	Trade Name	Adult Dosage
Anticholinergics (Chronic Obstructive Pulmonary Disease [COPD])		
Ipratropium bromide	Atrovent	MDI: 18 μg/puff, 2 puffs qid
	Atrovent HFA	HFA MDI: 17 μg/puff, 2 puffs qid
		SVN: 0.02% solution (0.2 mg/mL) 500 μg tid, qid
Tiotropium	Spiriva	DPI: 18 μg/inhalation, 1 inhalation daily (one capsule)
$Beta_2$ Agents and Anticholinergic Agents		
Ipratropium and albuterol	Combivent	MDI: ipratropium 18 μg/puff and albuterol 90 μg/puff, 2 puffs qid
	DuoNeb	SVN: ipratropium 0.5 mg and albuterol 2.5 mg

Data from Global Initiative for Asthma (GINA): *Global strategy for asthma management and prevention*, updated 2008. The GINA reports are available at www.ginasthma.org; and Gardenshire DS: Rau's *repiratory care pharmacology*, ed 7, St. Louis, 2008, Elsevier.

Antibiotics

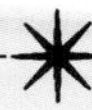

Antibiotics are used to treat the infective agents that cause bacterial pneumonia. The following table provides an overview of the commonly encountered organisms responsible for pneumonia and the therapeutic agents currently used to treat them.

Commonly Encountered Organisms Responsible for Pneumonia and the Therapeutic Agents Used to Treat Them

Organism Responsible for Pneumonia	Common Treatment Choices
Gram-Positive Organisms	
Staphylococcus aureus	Methicillin-susceptible strains: nafcillin or oxacillin with or without rifampin Methicillin-resistant strains: vancomycin with or without rifampin Alternative choices: cephalosporins, clindamycin
Streptococcus	Penicillins: procaine penicillin G or aqueous penicillin G, amoxicillin Alternative choices: macrolides, cephalosporins, doxycycline, quinolones cefotaxime or ceftriaxone; antipseudomonal fluoroquinolones (levofloxacin, gatifloxacin, moxifloxacin)
Gram-Negative Organisms	
Haemophilus influenzae	Ampicillin, third- or fourth-generation cephalosporins, macrolides (azithromycin, clarithromycin), fluoroquinolones
Klebsiella pneumoniae	Third- and/or fourth-generation cephalosporins (cefotaxime, ceftriaxone) plus aminoglycoside, antipseudomonal penicillin, monobactam (aztreonam), or quinolones
Pseudomonas aeruginosa	Tobramycin (TOBI), aminoglycoside and antipseudomonal agents (ticarcillin, piperacillin, mezlocillin, ceftazidime)
Atypical Organisms	
Mycoplasma pneumoniae	Doxycycline, macrolides or fluoroquinolones
Legionella pneumophila	Erythromycin ± rifampin (in severely compromised patient) or clarithromycin, or a macrolide (azithromycin), or a fluoroquinolone (ofloxacin, levofloxacin, sparfloxacin)
Chlamydia pneumoniae	Tetracycline, erythromycin, macrolide, quinolone
Anaerobic Bacterial Infections	
Peptostreptococcus species *Bacteroides melaninogenica* *Fusobacterium necrophorum* *Bacteroides asaccharolyticus* *Porphyromonas endodontalis* *Porphyromonas gingivalis*	Most of these organisms are oral contaminants. For anaerobic coverage use metronidazole (Flagyl) or clindamycin; or metronidazole + ceftriaxone; or penicillin + amoxicillin. Infections respond slowly; 4-6 weeks of therapy is generally recommended. Most of the problem with aspiration pneumonia is secondary to the acid present in stomach contents, causing a chemical pneumonia. Quinolones, penicillins are also useful. Aspiration fluid should be cultured immediately (even with bronchoscopy and special culture), with the patient started on coverage medication while culture results are awaited. If the culture is negative, stop the antibiotics. Then reculture if chest x-ray findings or patient's condition worsens. Monitor closely for superinfections such as with *Candida,* other yeasts. May add vancomycin and diflucan to cover nosocomial superinfections.
Viral Causes	
Influenza virus	Type A: Amantadine and rimantadine Type A/B: Zanamivir, oseltamivir phosphate
Respiratory syncytial virus	Ribavirin (Virazole), palivizumab (Synagis)

Commonly Encountered Organisms Responsible for Pneumonia and the Therapeutic Agents Used to Treat Them—cont'd

Organism Responsible for Pneumonia	Common Treatment Choices
Other Common Causes	
Pneumocystis carinii	Pentamidine
	Trimethoprim-sulfamethoxazole (TMP-SMZ), dapsone-trimethoprim, primaquine plus clindamycin
Fungal infections	Amphotericin B, itraconazole, fluconazole, ketoconazole
Tuberculosis *(Mycobacterium tuberculosis)*	Isoniazid (INH), rifampin, pyrazinamide, ethambutol, streptomycin, ethionamide

Antifungal Agents

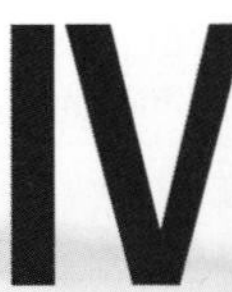

The antifungal agents are the first line of defense in treating fungal lung infections. In general, the drug of choice for most fungal infections is the intravenous administration of the polyene amphotericin B. Although ketoconazole was used as a first line agent against common fungal organisms, it has largely been replaced by the triazoles fluconazole and itraconazole. The echinocandins, a relatively new class of antifungal agents, are now available.

Agents	Common Uses (Microorganisms)
Polyenes	
Amphotericin B (Fungizone)	*Cryptococcus neoformans, Histoplasma capsulatum, Blastomyces dermatitidis, Coccidioides immitis, Candida* species, *Aspergillus* species
Amphotericin B colloidal dispersion (Amphotec)	*Candida* species, *Aspergillus* species, mucormycosis, *C. neoformans*
Azoles	
Ketoconazole (Nizoral)	*Candida* species, *C. neoformans, H. capsulatum, B. dermatitidis*
Fluconazole (Diflucan)	*Candida* species, *C. neoformans*
Itraconazole (Sporanox)	*Candida* species, *Aspergillus* species, *C. neoformans, H. capsulatum, B. dermatitidis, C. immitis, Sporothrix schenckii*
Echinocandins	
Caspofungin (Cancidas)	*Aspergillus* species, *Candida* species
Micafungin (Mycamine)	
Anidulafungin (Eraxis)	
Other Antifungals	
Flucytosine (Ancobon)	*Aspergillus* species, *Candida* species, *C. neoformans*
Griseofulvin (Fulvicin)	Tinea corporis, tinea cruris, tinea barbae
Terbinafine (Lamisil)	Tinea corporis, tinea pedis, tinea manuum

Modified from Gardenhire DS: *Rau's respiratory care pharmacology,* ed 7, St Louis, 2008, Elsevier.

Mucolytic and Expectorant Agents

V

Mucolytics

Mucolytic agents are used to enhance the mobilization and thinning of thick bronchial secretions

Agent	Trade Name	Adult Dosage
N-acetylcysteine	10% Mucomyst 20% Mucomyst	Small-volume nebulizer: 3-5 mL
Dornase alfa	Pulmozyme	Small-volume nebulizer: 2.5 mg/ampule, one ampule daily
Aqueous aerosols: water, saline	N/A	Small-volume nebulizer: 3-5 mL, as ordered Ultrasonic nebulizer: 3-5 mL, as ordered

Expectorants

Expectorants are agents used to increase bronchial submucous gland secretion, which in turn decreases viscosity of mucus. This facilitates the mobilization and expectoration of bronchial secretions.

Agents

Iodide-containing agents
Sodium bicarbonate (2%)
Guaifenesin (Robitussin, Naldecon Senior EX, Humibid LA)
Dissociating solvents (urea)
Oligosaccharides (dextran, mannitol, lactose)

Positive Inotropes and Vasopressors

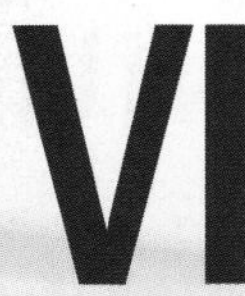

Positive inotropes are drugs that increase the strength of the cardiac muscular contraction. Vasopressors are agents that cause contraction of the capillaries and arteries.

Agent	Alpha Stimulation (Capillary Constriction)	Beta-1 Stimulation (Heart Contractility)
Dopamine (Inotropin)	+ to +++*	+++*
Dobutamine (Dobutrex)	0 to +*	0 to +*
Epinephrine (Adrenalin)	+++*	+++
Isoproterenol (Isuprel)	0	+++
Norepinephrine (Levophed)	+++	++
Phenylephrine (Neo-Synephrine)	+++	0

Modified from Gardenhire DS: *Rau's respiratory care pharmacology,* ed 7, St Louis, 2008, Elsevier.
*At higher doses: 0 effect; + slight effect; ++ moderate effect; +++ pronounced effect.

Diuretic Agents

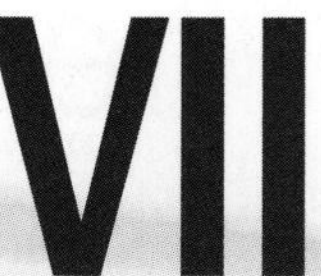

The primary purpose of diuretics is to lower the extracellular fluid volume in order to decrease blood pressure and/or clear the body of excess interstitial fluid.

Agents

Osmotic Diuretics

- Glycerin
- Isosorbide
- Mannitol
- Urea

Thiazide Diuretics

- Bendroflumethiazide
- Benzthiazide
- Chlorothiazide
- Chlorthalidone
- Hydrochlorothiazide
- Hydroflumethiazide
- Indapamide
- Methylclothiazide
- Metolazone
- Polythiazide
- Quinethazone
- Trichlormethiazide

Loop Diuretics

- Bumetanide
- Ethacrynic acid
- Furosemide
- Torsemide

Potassium-Sparing Diuretics

- Amiloride
- Spironolactone
- Triamterene

The Ideal Alveolar Gas Equation

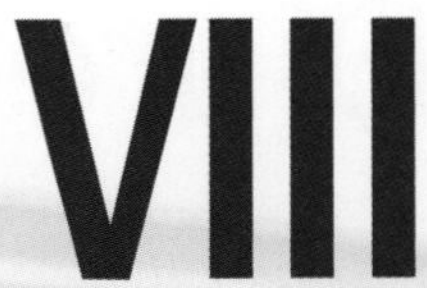

Clinically, the alveolar oxygen tension can be computed from the ideal alveolar gas equation. A useful clinical approximation of the ideal alveolar gas equation is as follows:

$$P_{AO_2} = [P_B - P_{H_2O}]\, F_{IO_2} - P_{aCO_2}\,(1.25)$$

where PB is barometric pressure, P_{AO_2} is the partial pressure of oxygen within the alveoli, P_{H_2O} is the partial pressure of water vapor in the alveoli (at body temperature and at sea level P_{H_2O} in the alveoli is 47 mm Hg), F_{IO_2} is the fractional concentration of inspired oxygen, and P_{aCO_2} is the partial pressure of arterial carbon dioxide. The number 1.25 is a factor that adjusts for alterations in oxygen tension resulting from variations in the respiratory exchange ratio. The respiratory exchange ratio indicates that less carbon dioxide is transferred into the alveoli (about 200 cc/min) than the amount of oxygen that moves into the pulmonary capillary blood (about 250 ml/min). This ratio is normally about 0.8.

Therefore if a patient is receiving an F_{IO_2} of 40% on a day when the barometric pressure is 755 mm Hg and the P_{aCO_2} is 55 mm Hg, the patient's alveolar oxygen tension (P_{aO_2}) can be calculated as follows:

$$\begin{aligned} P_{AO_2} &= [P_B - P_{H_2O}]\, F_{IO_2} - P_{aCO_2}\,(1.25) \\ &= (755 - 47)\, 0.40 - 55\,(1.25) \\ &= (708)\, 0.40 - 68.75 \\ &= (283.2) - 68.75 \\ &= 214.45 \end{aligned}$$

The ideal alveolar gas equation is part of the clinical information needed to calculate the degree of pulmonary shunting (see Chapter 4).

Physiologic Dead Space Calculation

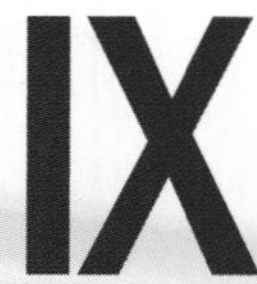

The amount of physiologic dead space (V_D) in the tidal volume (V_T) can be estimated by using the dead space–to–tidal volume ratio (V_D/V_T) equation. The equation is arranged as follows:

$$V_D/V_T = \frac{PaCO_2 - P\bar{E}CO_2}{PaCO_2}$$

For example, in a patient whose $PaCO_2$ is 40 mm Hg and whose $P\bar{E}CO_2$ is 28 mm Hg:

$$\begin{aligned} V_D/V_T &= \frac{40-28}{40} \\ &= \frac{12}{40} \\ &= 0.3 \end{aligned}$$

In this case, approximately 30% of the patient's ventilation is dead–space ventilation. This is within the normal range.

Units of Measure

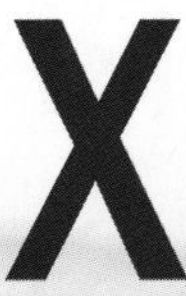

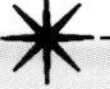

Metric Weight

Grams	Centigrams	Milligrams	Micrograms	Nanograms
1	100	1000	1,000,000	1,000,000,000
0.01	1	10	10,000	10,000,000
0.001	0.1	1	1000	1,000,000
0.000001	0.0001	0.001	1	1000
0.000000001	0.0000001	0.000001	0.001	1

Weight

Metric	Approximate Apothecary Equivalents
Grams	*Grains*
0.0002	1/300
0.0003	1/200
0.0004	1/150
0.0005	1/120
0.0006	1/100
0.001	1/60
0.002	1/30
0.005	1/12
0.010	1/6
0.015	1/4
0.025	3/8
0.030	1/2
0.050	3/4
0.060	1
0.100	1 1/2
0.120	2
0.200	3
0.300	5
0.500	7 1/2
0.600	10
1	15
2	30
4	60

Liquid Measure

Metric	Approximate Apothecary Equivalents
Milliliters	
1000	1quart
750	1½ pints
500	1 pint
250	8 fluid ounces
200	7 fluid ounces
100	3½ fluid ounces
50	1¾ fluid ounces
30	1 fluid ounce
15	4 fluid drams
10	2½ fluid drams
8	2 fluid drams
5	1¼ fluid drams
4	1 fluid dram
3	45 minims
2	30 minims
1	15 minims
0.75	12 minims
0.6	10 minims
0.5	8 minims
0.3	5 minims
0.25	4 minims
0.2	3 minims
0.1	1½ minims
0.06	1 minim
0.05	¾ minim
0.03	½ minim

Metric Liquid

Liter	Centiliter	Milliliter	Microliter	Nanoliter
1	100	1000	1,000,000	1,000,000,000
0.01	1	10	10,000	10,000,000
0.001	0.1	1	1000	1,000,000
0.000001	0.0001	0.001	1	1000
0.000000001	0.0000001	0.000001	0.001	1

Metric Length

Meter	Centimeter	Millimeter	Micrometer	Nanometer
1	100	1000	1,000,000	1,000,000,000
0.01	1	10	10,000	10,000,000
0.001	0.1	1	1000	1,000,000
0.000001	0.0001	0.001	1	1000
0.000000001	0.0000001	0.000001	0.001	1

Weight Conversions (Metric and Avoirdupois)

Grams	Kilograms	Ounces	Pounds
1	0.001	0.0353	0.0022
1000	1	35.3	2.2
28.35	0.02835	1	1⁄16
454.5	0.4545	16	1

Weight Conversions (Metric and Apothecary)

Grams	Milligrams	Grains	Drams	Ounces	Pounds
1	1000	15.4	0.2577	0.0322	0.00268
0.001	1	0.0154	0.00026	0.0000322	0.00000268
0.0648	64.8	1	1/60	1/480	1/5760
3.888	3888	60	1	1/8	1/96
31.1	31104	480	8	1	1/12
363.25	373248	5760	96	12	1

Approximate Household Measurement Equivalents (volume)

						1 tsp =	5 ml
					1 tbsp =	3 tsp =	15 ml
				1 fl oz =	2 tbsp =	6 tsp =	30 ml
			1 cup =	8 fl oz =			240 ml
		1 pt =	2 cups =	16 fl oz =			480 ml
	1 qt =	2 pt =	4 cups =	32 fl oz =			960 ml
1 gal =	4 qt =	8 pt =	16 cups =	128 fl oz =			3840 ml

Volume Conversions (Metric and Apothecary)

Milliliters	Minims	Fluid Drams	Fluid Ounces	Pints	Liters	Gallons	Fluid Quarts	Ounces	Pints
1	16.2	0.27	0.0333	0.0021	1	0.2642	1.057	33.824	2.114
0.0616	1	1/60	1/480	1/7680	3.785	1	4	128	8
3.697	60	1	1/8	1/128	0.946	1/4	1	32	2
29.58	480	8	1	1/16	0.473	1/8	1/2	16	1
473.2	7680	128	16	1	0.0296	1/128	1/32	1	1/16

Length Conversions (Metric and English System)

	Millimeters	Centimeters	Inches	Feet	Yards	Meters
1 Å =	$\frac{1}{10{,}000{,}000}$	$\frac{1}{100{,}000{,}000}$	$\frac{1}{254{,}000{,}000}$	$\frac{1}{3{,}050{,}000{,}000}$	$\frac{1}{9{,}140{,}000{,}000}$	$\frac{1}{10{,}000{,}000{,}000}$
1 nm =	$\frac{1}{1{,}000{,}000}$	$\frac{1}{10{,}000{,}000}$	$\frac{1}{25{,}400{,}000}$	$\frac{1}{305{,}000{,}000}$	$\frac{1}{914{,}000{,}000}$	$\frac{1}{1{,}000{,}000{,}000}$
1 µm =	$\frac{1}{1000}$	$\frac{1}{10{,}000}$	$\frac{1}{25{,}400}$	$\frac{1}{305{,}000}$	$\frac{1}{914{,}000}$	$\frac{1}{1{,}000{,}000}$
1 mm =	1	0.1	0.03937	0.00328	0.0011	0.001
1 cm =	10	1	0.3937	0.03281	0.0109	0.01
1 in =	25.4	2.54	1	0.0833	0.0278	0.0254
1 ft =	304.8	30.48	12	1	0.333	0.3048
1 yd =	914.40	91.44	36	3	1	0.9144
1 m =	1000	100	39.37	3.2808	1.0936	1

Poiseuille's Law

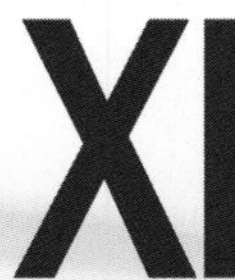

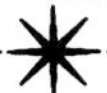

Poiseuille's Law for Flow Rearranged to a Simple Proportionality

$\dot{V} \simeq \Delta P r^4$, or rewritten as $\frac{\dot{V}}{r^4} \simeq \Delta P$

When ΔP remains constant, then

$$\frac{\dot{V}}{r_1^4} \simeq \frac{\dot{V}}{r_2^4}$$

Example 1—If the radius (r_1) is decreased to half its previous radius ($r_2 = \frac{1}{2}r_1$), then

$$\frac{\dot{V}}{r_1^4} \simeq \frac{\dot{V}}{(\frac{1}{2}r_1)^4}$$

$$\frac{\dot{V}_1}{r_1^4} \simeq \frac{\dot{V}_2}{(\frac{1}{16})r_1^4}$$

$$(\cancel{r_1^4})\frac{\dot{V}_1}{\cancel{r_1^4}} \simeq (\cancel{r_1^4})\frac{\dot{V}_2}{(\frac{1}{16})\cancel{r_1^4}}$$

$$\dot{V}_1 \simeq \frac{\dot{V}_2}{\frac{1}{16}}$$

$$(\tfrac{1}{16})\dot{V}_1 \simeq (\tfrac{1}{16})\frac{\dot{V}_2}{\frac{1}{16}}$$

$$(\tfrac{1}{16})\dot{V}_1 \simeq \dot{V}_2$$

The gas flow ($\dot{V}_1$) is reduces to $\frac{1}{16}$ its original flow rate [$\dot{V}_2 \simeq (\frac{1}{16})\dot{V}_1$].

Example 2—If the radius (r_1) is decreased by 16% ($r_2 = r_1 - 0.16r_1 = 0.84r_1$), then

$$\frac{\dot{V}_1}{r_1^4} \simeq \frac{\dot{V}_2}{r_2^4}$$

$$\frac{\dot{V}_1}{r_1^4} \simeq \frac{\dot{V}_2}{(0.84r_1)^4}$$

$$\dot{V}_2 \simeq \frac{(0.84r_1)^4\,\dot{V}_1}{r_1^4}$$

$$\dot{V}_2 \simeq \frac{0.4979\,\cancel{r_1^4}\,\dot{V}_1}{\cancel{r_1^4}}$$

$$\dot{V}_2 \simeq \tfrac{1}{2}\dot{V}_1$$

The flow rate ($\dot{V}_1$) decreases to half the original flow rate ($\dot{V}_2 \simeq \frac{1}{2}\dot{V}_1$).

Poiseuille's Law for Pressure Rearranged to a Simple Proportionality

$P \simeq \frac{\dot{V}}{r^4}$ or rewritten as $P \cdot r^4 \simeq \dot{V}$

When $\dot{V}$ remains constant, then

$$P_1 \cdot r_1^4 \simeq P_2 \cdot r_2^4$$

Example 1—If the radius (r_1) is decreased to half its original radius [$r_2 = (1/2)r_1$], then

$$P_1 \cdot r_1^4 \simeq P_2 \cdot r_2^4$$

$$P_1 \cdot r_1^4 \simeq P_2[(1/2)r_1]^4$$

$$P_1 \cdot r_1^4 \simeq P_2 \cdot (1/16)r_1^4$$

$$\frac{P_1 \cdot \cancel{r_1^4}}{\cancel{r_1^4}} \simeq \frac{P_2 \cdot (1/16)\,\cancel{r_1^4}}{\cancel{r_1^4}}$$

$$P_1 \simeq P_2 \cdot (1/16)$$

$$16 P_1 \simeq 16 \cdot P_2 \cdot (1/16)$$

$$16 P_1 \simeq P_2$$

The pressure (P_1) increases to 16 times its original level ($P_2 \simeq 16 \cdot P_1$).

Example 2—If the radius (r_1) is decreased by 16% ($r_2 = r_1 - 0.16r_1 = 0.84r_1$), then

$$P_1 \cdot r_1^4 \simeq P_2 \cdot r_2^4$$

$$P_1 \cdot r_1^4 \simeq P_2(0.4979) \cdot r_1^4$$

$$\frac{P_1\,\cancel{r_1^4}}{(0.4979\,\cancel{r_1})^4} = P_2$$

$$2 \cdot P_1 = P_2$$

The pressure (P_1) increases to twice its original level ($P_2 \simeq 2 \cdot P_1$).

$Pco_2/HCO_3^-/pH$ Nomogram

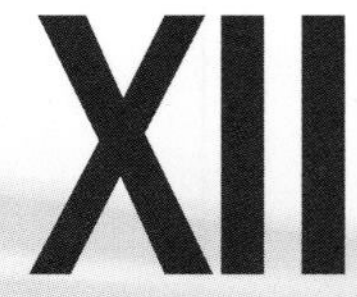

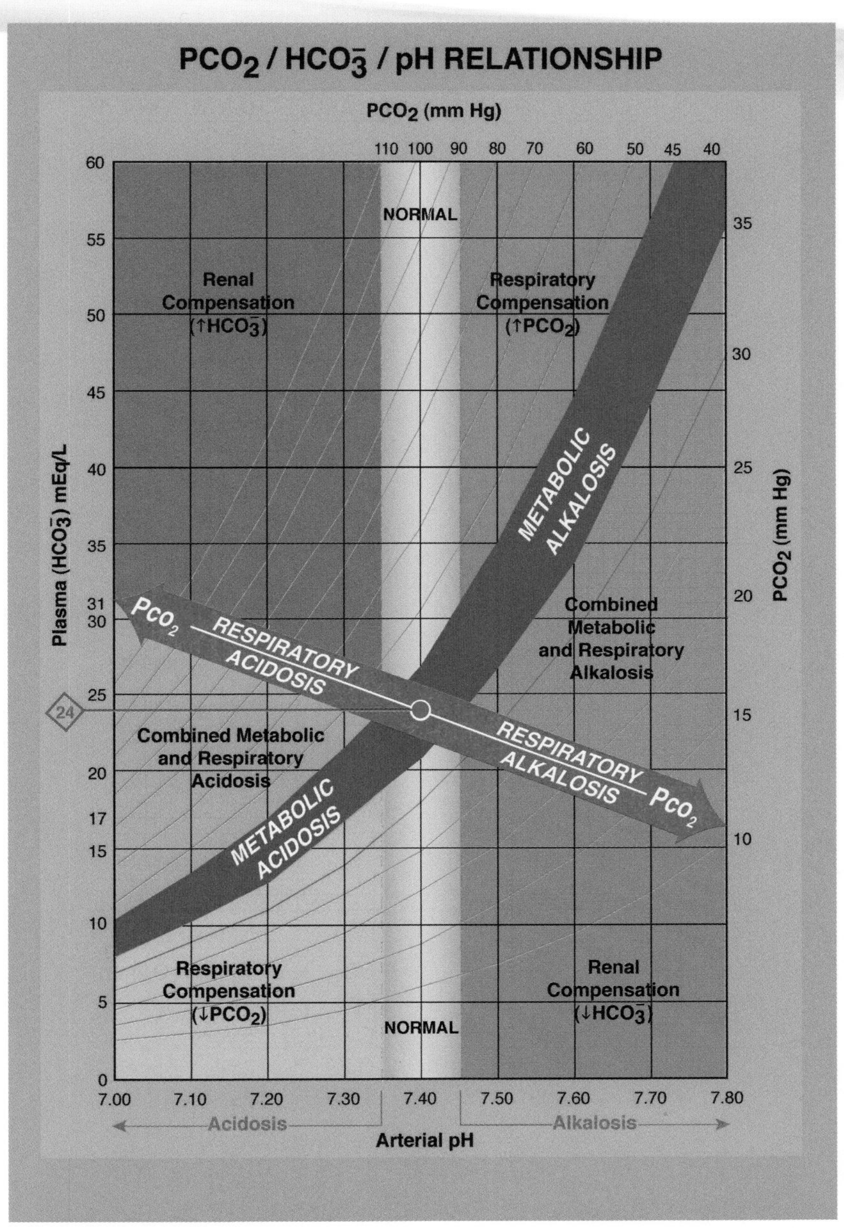

Used with permission from author, Terry DesJardins, WindMist LLC.

pH, PCO_2, HCO_3 RELATIONSHIP

$PaCO_2$		pH	HCO_3
100	≈	7.10	30
80	≈	7.20	28
60	≈	7.30	26
40	≈	7.40	24
30	≈	7.50	22
20	≈	7.60	20
10	≈	7.70	18

EX: ACUTE CHANGES ON CVF

	AVF on CVF		CVF Baseline		AAH on CVF
pH	7.21	⟵	7.39	⟶	7.53
$PaCO_2$	110	⟵	76	⟶	51
HCO_3	43	⟵	41	⟶	37
PaO_2	34	⟵	61	⟶	46

CVF: Chronic ventilatory failure
AVF: Acute ventilatory failure
AAH: Acute alveolar hyperventilation

PaO_2 & SaO_2 RELATIONSHIP

	PaO_2	SaO_2
Normal	97	97
Range	> 80–100	> 95
Hypoxemia	< 80	< 95
Mild	60–80	90–95
Moderate	40–60	75–90
Severe	< 40	< 75

PaO_2 & SaO_2 RELATIONSHIP

PO_2 30 ≈ 60% saturated

PO_2 40 ≈ 75% saturated

PO_2 50 ≈ 85% saturated

PO_2 60 ≈ 90% saturated

FIO_2 & PaO_2 RELATIONSHIP

FIO_2		PaO_2
0.30	≈	150
0.40	≈	200
0.50	≈	250
0.80	≈	400
1.00	≈	500

O_2 TRANSPORT

	Normal Values
DO_2	1000 ml O_2/min
$\dot{V}O_2$	250 ml O_2/min
$C(a-\bar{v})O_2$	5 vol%
O_2ER	25%
$S\bar{v}O_2$	75%

Used with permission from author, Terry DesJardins, WindMist LLC.

Cut out the above two-sided $PCO_2/HCO_3^-/pH$ nomogram and have it laminated for use as a handy, pocket-sized reference tool. See Chapter 4 for information about how to use the nomogram in the clinical setting.

Calculated Hemodynamic Measurements

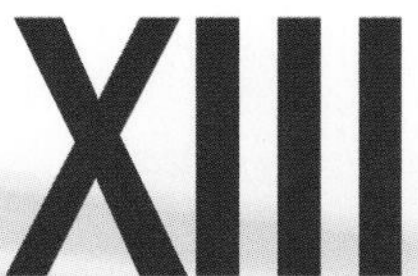

The following are the major hemodynamic values that can be calculated from the direct hemodynamic measurements listed in Table 6-1. The calculated hemodynamic values are easily obtained from a programmed calculator or by using the specific hemodynamic formula and a calculator. Because the calculated hemodynamic measurements vary with the size of an individual, some hemodynamic values are "indexed" by body surface area (BSA). Clinically, the BSA is obtained from a height-weight nomogram (see Appendix XIV). In the normal adult, the BSA is 1.5 to 2 m^2.

Stroke Volume

The stroke volume (SV) is the volume of blood ejected by the ventricles with each contraction. The preload, afterload, and myocardial contractility are the major determinants of SV. SV is derived by dividing the cardiac output (CO) by the heart rate (HR):

$$SV = \frac{CO}{HR}$$

For example, if an individual has a cardiac output of 4 L/min (4000 ml/min) and a heart rate of 80 beats/min, the SV is calculated as follows:

$$\begin{aligned} SV &= \frac{CO}{HR} \\ &= \frac{4000 \text{ ml/min}}{80 \text{ beats/min}} \\ &= 50 \text{ ml/beat} \end{aligned}$$

Stroke Volume Index

The stroke volume index (SVI), also known as stroke index, is calculated by dividing the SV by the BSA:

$$SVI = \frac{SV}{BSA}$$

For example, if a patient has an SV of 50 ml and a BSA of 2 m^2, the SVI is determined as follows:

$$\begin{aligned} SVI &= \frac{SV}{BSA} \\ &= \frac{50 \text{ ml/beat}}{2 \text{ m}} \\ &= 25 \text{ ml/beat/m}^2 \end{aligned}$$

Assuming that the HR remains the same, as the SVI increases or decreases, the cardiac index also increases or decreases. The SVI reflects the (1) contractility of the heart, (2) overall blood volume status, and (3) amount of venous return.

Cardiac Index

The cardiac index (CI) is calculated by dividing the cardiac output (CO) by the BSA:

$$CI = \frac{CO}{BSA}$$

For example, if a patient has a CO of 6 L/min and a BSA of 2 m^2, the CI is computed as follows:

$$\begin{aligned} CI &= \frac{CO}{BSA} \\ &= \frac{6 \text{ L/min}}{2 \text{ m}^2} \\ &= 3 \text{ L/min/m}^2 \end{aligned}$$

Right Ventricular Stroke Work Index

The right ventricular stroke work index (RVSWI) measures the amount of work done by the right ventricle to pump blood. The RVSWI is a reflection of the contractility of the right ventricle. In the presence of normal right ventricular contractility, increases in afterload (such as those caused by pulmonary vascular constriction) cause the RVSWI to increase until a plateau is reached. When the contractility of the right ventricle is diminished by disease states, however, the RVSWI does not appropriately increase. The RVSWI is derived from the following formula:

$$RVSWI = SVI \times (\overline{PA} - CVP) \times 0.0136 \text{ g/ml}$$

where SVI is stroke volume index, $\overline{PA}$ is mean pulmonary artery pressure, and CVP is central venous pressure. The density of mercury factor 0.0136 g/ml is needed to convert the equation to the proper units of measurement—i.e., gram meters/m^2 (g m/m^2).

For example, if a patient has an SVI of 40 ml, a $\overline{PA}$ of 20 mm Hg, and a CVP of 5 mm Hg, the RVSWI is calculated as follows:

$$\begin{aligned} RVSWI &= SVI\,(\overline{PA} - CVP) \times 0.0136 \text{ g/mL} \\ &= 40 \text{ ml/beat/m}^2 = (15 \text{ mm Hg} - 5 \text{ mm Hg}) \times 0.0136 \text{ g/ml} \\ &= 40 \text{ ml/beat/m}^2 \times 10 \text{ mm Hg} \times 0.0136 \text{ g/ml} \\ &= 5.44 \text{ g m/m}^2 \end{aligned}$$

Left Ventricular Stroke Work Index

The left ventricular stroke work index (LVSWI) measures the amount of work done by the left ventricle to pump blood. The LVSWI is a reflection of the contractility of the left ventricle. In the presence of normal left ventricular contractility, increases in afterload (such as those caused by systemic vascular constriction) cause the LVSWI to increase until a plateau is reached. When the contractility of the left ventricle is diminished by disease states, however, the LVSWI does not increase appropriately. The following formula is used for determining this hemodynamic variable:

$$LVSWI = SVI \times (MAP - PCWP) \times 0.0136 \text{ g/ml}$$

where SVI is stroke volume index, MAP is mean arterial pressure, and PCWP is pulmonary capillary wedge pressure. The density of mercury factor 0.0136 g/ml is needed to convert the equation to the proper units of measurement—i.e., gram meters/m^2 (g m/m^2).

For example, if a patient has an SVI of 40 ml, an MAP of 110 mm Hg, and a PCWP of 5 mm Hg, the patient's LVSWI is calculated as follows:

$$\begin{aligned} LVSWI &= SVI \times (MAP - PCWP) \times 0.0136 \text{ g/ml} \\ &= 40 \text{ ml/beat/m}^2 \times (110 \text{ mm Hg} - 5 \text{ mm Hg}) \times 0.0136 \text{ g/ml} \\ &= 40 \text{ ml/beat/m}^2 \times (105 \text{ mm Hg}) \times 0.0136 \text{ g/ml} \\ &= 59.84 \text{ g m/m}^2 \end{aligned}$$

Vascular Resistance

As blood flows through the pulmonary and systemic vascular systems, resistance to flow occurs. The pulmonary vascular system is a low-resistance system. The systemic vascular system is a high-resistance system.

Pulmonary Vascular Resistance (PVR)

The PVR measurement reflects the afterload of the right ventricle. It is calculated by the following formula:

$$PVR = \overline{PA} - \frac{PCWP}{CO} \times 80$$

where $\overline{PA}$ is the mean pulmonary artery pressure, PCWP is the capillary wedge pressure, CO is the cardiac output, and 80 is a conversion factor for adjusting to the correct units of measurement (dyne × sec × cm^{-5}).

For example, if a patient has a $\overline{PA}$ of 20 mm Hg, a PCWP of 5 mm Hg, and a CO of 6 L/min, the patient's PVR is calculated as follows:

$$\begin{aligned} PVR &= \overline{PA} - \frac{PCWP}{CO} \times 80 \\ &= \frac{20 \text{ mm Hg} - 5 \text{ mm Hg}}{6 \text{ L/min}} \times 80 \\ &= \frac{15 \text{ mm Hg}}{6 \text{ L/min}} \times 80 \\ &= 200 \text{ dynes} \times \text{sec} \times \text{cm}^{-5} \end{aligned}$$

Systemic or Peripheral Vascular Resistance (SVR)

The SVR measurement reflects the afterload of the left ventricle. It is calculated by the following formula:

$$SVR = \frac{MAP - CVP}{CO} \times 80$$

where MAP is the mean arterial pressure, CVP is the central venous pressure, CO is the cardiac output, and 80 is a conversion factor for adjusting to the correct units of measurement (dyne × sec × cm^{-5}). (NOTE: The right atrial pressure [RAP] can be used in place of the CVP value.)

For example, if a patient has an MAP of 90 mm Hg, a CVP of 5 mm Hg, and a CO of 4 L/min, the patient's SVR is calculated as follows:

$$\begin{aligned} SVR &= \frac{MAP - CVP}{CO} \times 80 \\ &= \frac{90 \text{ mm Hg} - 5 \text{ mm Hg}}{4 \text{ L/min}} \times 80 \\ &= \frac{85 \text{ mm Hg}}{4 \text{ L/min}} \times 80 \\ &= 1700 \text{ dynes} \times \text{sec} \times \text{cm}^{-5} \end{aligned}$$

Note: For normal values of all these hemodynamic measurements, see Chapter 6 and Appendix XV.

DuBois Body Surface Area Chart

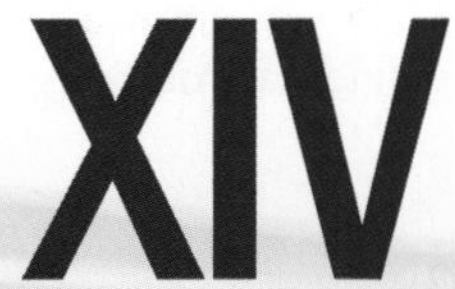

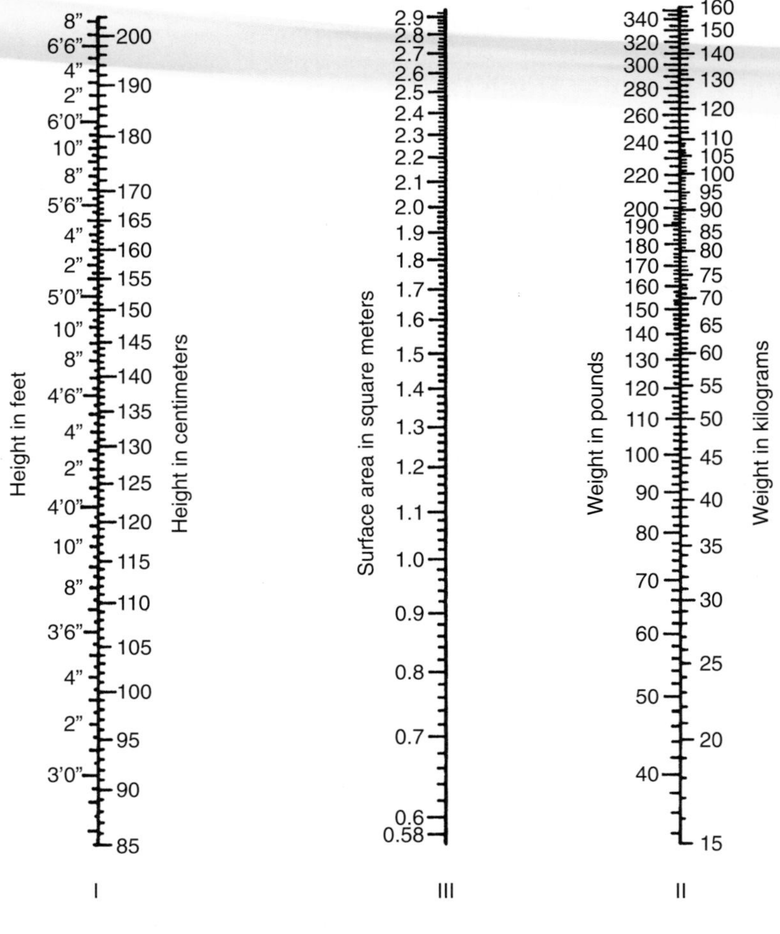

To find the body surface area of a patient, locate the height in inches (or centimeters) on Scale I and the weight in pounds (or kilograms) on Scale II, and place a straightedge (ruler) between these two points, which will intersect Scale III at the patient's surface area.

Cardiopulmonary Profile

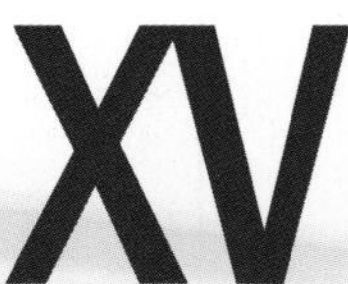

A representative example of cardiopulmonary profile sheets used to monitor a critically ill patient.

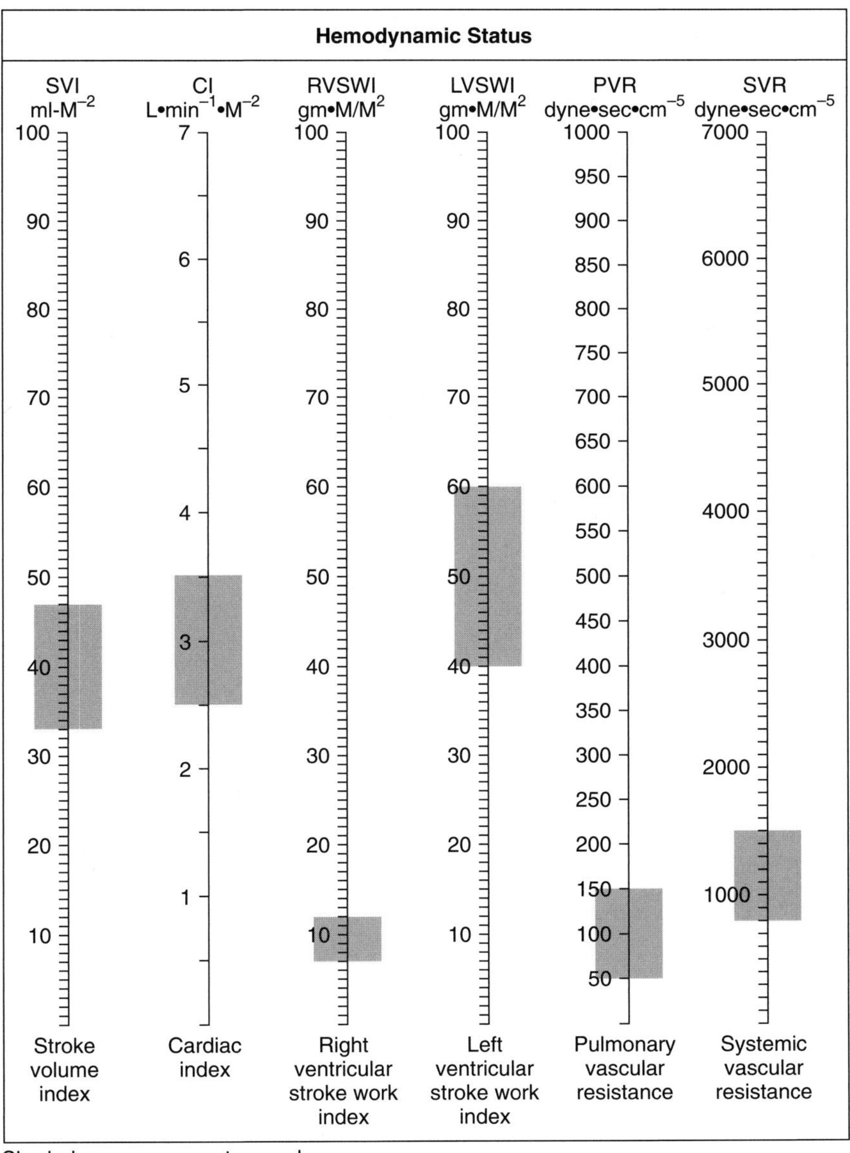

Shaded areas represent normal range.

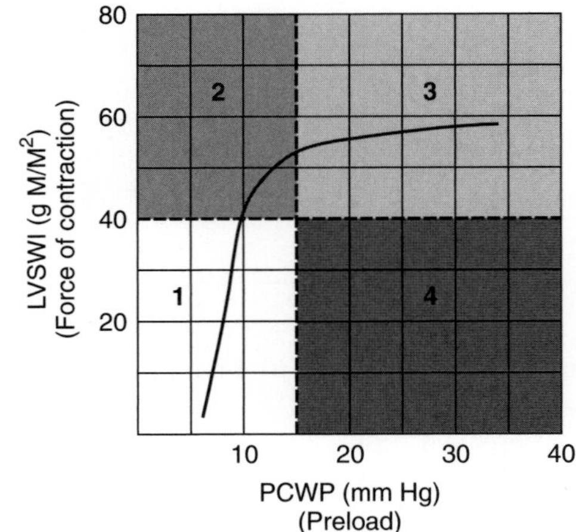

Quadrant 1: Hypovolemia
Quadrant 2: Optimal function
Quadrant 3: Hypervolemia
Quadrant 4: Cardiac failure

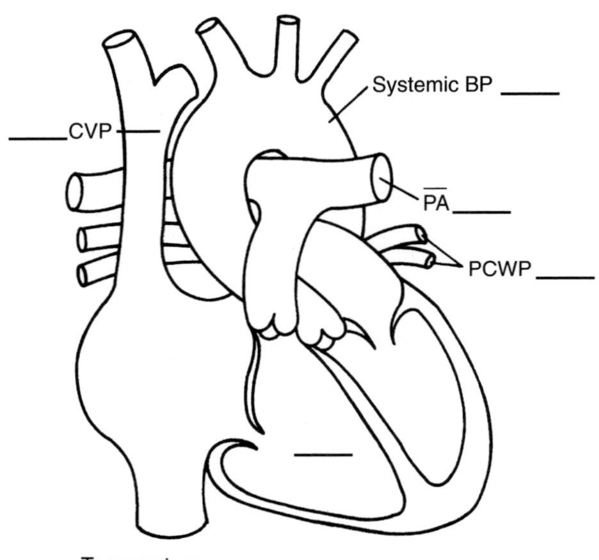

Temperature: ______________________________

Heart rate: ________________________________

Cardiac output: ____________________________

Medications: ______________________________

____

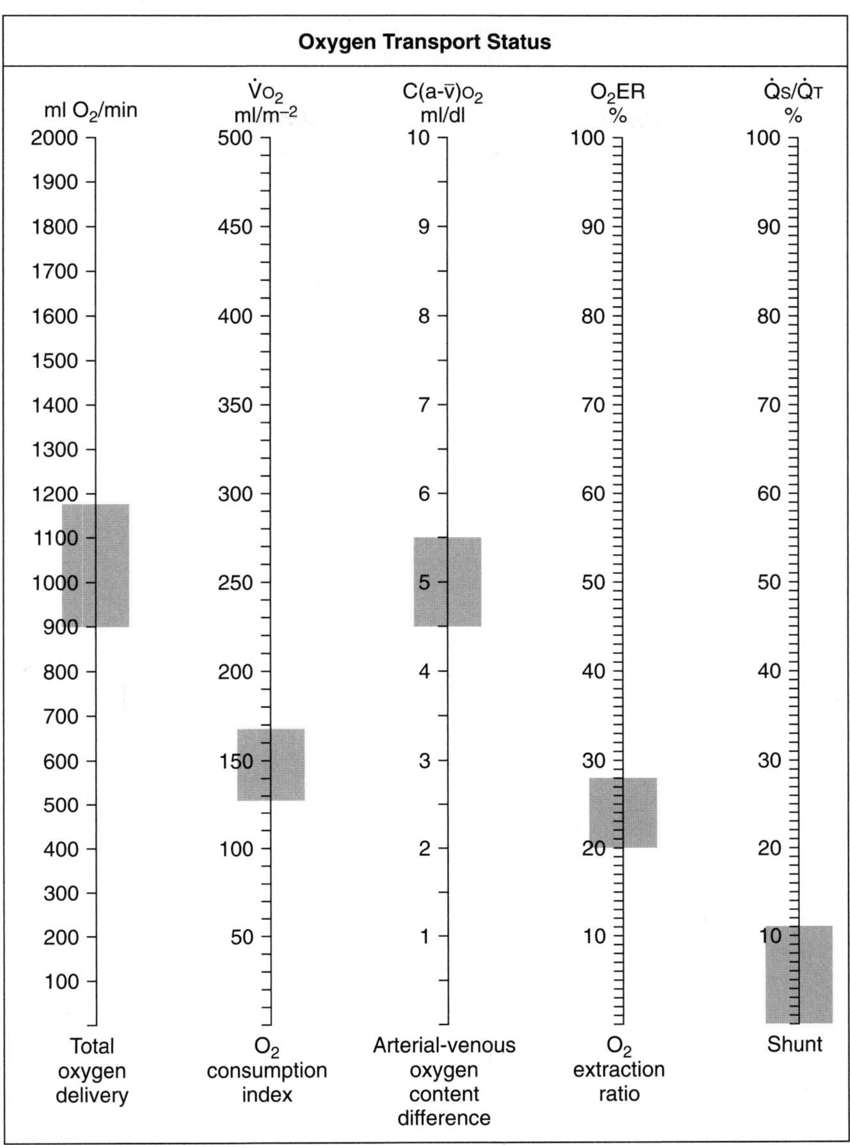

Shaded area represents normal range.

Blood Gas Values

pH ______________

Paco$_2$ ______________

HCO$_3^-$ ______________

Pao$_2$ ______________ **P$\bar{v}$o$_2$** __________

Sao$_2$ ______________% **S$\bar{v}$o$_2$** __________%

Fio$_2$ ______________ **Hb** __________

Mode(s) of Ventilatory Support: ______________________________

____

____

____

____

Patient's Name ______________________________

Date ______________________________

Time ______________________________

GLOSSARY

abscess Localized collection of pus that results from disintegration or displacement of tissue in any part of the body.

accessory muscles of expiration The accessory muscles of exhalation are often recruited when airway resistance becomes significantly elevated. When these muscles actively contract, intrapleural pressure increases and offsets the increased airway resistance. The major accessory muscles of exhalation are as follows: rectus abdominis, external oblique, internal oblique, transversus abdominis.

accessory muscles of inspiration During the advanced stages of chronic obstructive pulmonary disease, the accessory muscles of inspiration are activated when the diaphragm becomes significantly depressed by the increased residual volume and functional residual capacity. The accessory muscles assist or largely replace the diaphragm in creating subatmospheric pressure in the pleural space during inspiration. The major accessory muscles of inspiration are as follows: scalene, sternocleidomastoid, pectoralis major, trapezius.

acetylcholine (ACh) A direct-acting cholinergic neurotransmitter agent widely distributed in body tissues, with a primary function of mediating synaptic activity of the nervous system and skeletal muscles. Its half-life and duration of activity are short because it is rapidly destroyed by acetylcholinesterase. Its activity also can be blocked by atropine at junctions of nerve fibers with glands and smooth muscle tissue. It is a stimulant of the vagus and parasympathetic nervous system and functions as a vasodilator and cardiac depressant.

acidemia Decreased pH or an increased hydrogen ion concentration of the blood.

acidosis Pathologic condition resulting from accumulation of acid or loss of base from the body.

acinus Smallest division of a gland, a group of secretory cells surrounding a cavity; the functional part of an organ. (The respiratory acinus includes terminal [respiratory] bronchioles, alveolar ducts, alveoli, and all other structures therein.)

acquired bronchiectasis Destruction and widening of the large airways. If the condition is present at birth, it is called congenital bronchiectasis. If it develops later in life, it is called acquired bronchiectasis.

acute alveolar hyperventilation A condition marked by low levels of carbon dioxide, and a high pH in the blood, due to breathing excessively. Also called acute respiratory alkalosis.

acute alveolar hyperventilation with partial renal compensation A condition marked by low levels of carbon dioxide and a high pH in the blood due to hyperventilation, which is partly corrected by the excretion of HCO_3^- via the renal system.

acute epiglottitis A very rapidly progressive infection causing inflammation of the epiglottis (the flap that covers the trachea) and tissues around the epiglottis that may lead to abrupt blockage of the upper airway and death.

acute respiratory acidosis A condition marked by high levels of carbon dioxide, and a low pH in the blood, due to hypoventilation. Also called acute ventilatory failure.

acute respiratory alkalosis A condition marked by low levels of carbon dioxide, and a high pH in the blood, due to hyperventilation. Also called acute alveolar hyperventilation.

acute ventilatory failure A condition marked by high levels of carbon dioxide, and a low pH in the blood, due to hypoventilation. Also called acute ventilatory failure.

acute ventilatory failure with partial renal compensation A condition marked by high levels of carbon dioxide and a low pH in the blood resulting from hypoventilation, which is partly corrected by the retention of HCO_3^- via the renal system and/or the administration of HCO_3^-.

acute Sharp, severe; of rapid onset and characterized by severe symptoms and a short course; not chronic.

adenocarcinoma Any one of a large group of malignant epithelial cell tumors of the glandular tissue. Specific tumors are diagnosed and named by cytologic identification of the tissue affected; for example, an adenocarcinoma of the uterine cervix is characterized by tumor cells resembling the glandular epithelium of the cervix. **—adenocarcinomatous,** *adj.*

adenovirus Any one of the 49 medium-sized viruses of the Adenoviridae family, pathogenic to humans, that cause conjunctivitis, upper respiratory tract infection, cystitis, or GI infection. After the acute and symptomatic period of illness, the virus may persist in a latent stage in the tonsils, adenoids, and other lymphoid tissue.

adhesion Fibrous band that holds together parts that are normally separated.

adolescent One in the state or process of adolescence; a teenager.

adrenergic Term applied to nerve fibers that, when stimulated, release epinephrine at their endings. Includes nearly all sympathetic postganglionic fibers except those innervating sweat glands.

adrenocorticotropic hormone (ACTH) A hormone secreted by the anterior pituitary. It is regulated by the corticotropin-releasing factor (CRF) from the hypothalamus and is essential to growth, development, and continued function of the adrenal cortex.

adventitious (abnormal) breath sounds Additional or different sounds that are not *normally* heard over a particular area of the thorax.

aerosol Gaseous suspension of fine solid or liquid particles.

afebrile Without fever.

afferent Carrying impulses toward a center.

afferent nerves Nerves that transmit impulses from the peripheral to the central nervous system.

afterload reduction The load, or resistance, against which the left ventricle must eject its volume of blood during contraction. The resistance is produced by the volume of blood already in the vascular system and by the constriction of the vessel walls.

air bronchogram When air can be visualized in the more peripheral intrapulmonary bronchi, this is known as the "air-bronchogram sign." This abnormality is usually caused by an infiltrate/consolidation that surrounds the bronchi.

air cyst Nonspecific term usually used to describe the presence in the lung of a thin-walled, well-defined and well-circumscribed lesion, greater than 1 cm in diameter. Cysts may contain either air or fluid, but this term is usually used to refer to an air-containing lesion, or air-filled cyst.

air trapping Trapping of alveolar gas during exhalation.

airway resistance A measure of the impedance to airflow through the bronchopulmonary system. It is the reciprocal of airway conductance.

alkalemia Increased pH or decreased hydrogen ion concentration of the blood.

allergen Any substance that causes manifestations of allergy. It may or may not be a protein.

allergy Acquired hypersensitivity to a substance (allergen) that normally does not cause a reaction. An allergic reaction is essentially an antibody-antigen reaction, but in some cases the antibody cannot be demonstrated. The reaction is caused by the release of histamine or histamine-like substances from injured cells.

α_1-antitrypsin Inhibitor of trypsin that may be deficient in persons with emphysema.

α-receptor Site in the autonomic nerve pathways where excitatory responses occur when adrenergic agents such as norepinephrine and epinephrine are released.

alpha waves One of the four brain waves, characterized by a relatively high voltage or amplitude and a frequency of 8-13 Hz. Alpha waves are known as the "relaxed waves" of the brain. They are commonly recorded when the individual is awake, but in a drowsy state and when the eyes are closed. Alpha waves are commonly seen during Stage N1 sleep. Bursts of Alpha waves are also seen during brief awakenings from sleep-called arousals. Alpha waves may also be seen during REM sleep.

alpha$_1$-antitrypsin deficiency Blood test useful for individuals with a family history of emphysema, since a familial tendency to have a deficiency of alpha$_1$-antitrypsin antienzyme exists. A similar deficiency also exists in children with liver disease.

alteplase A tissue plasminogen activator.

alveolar hypoplasia Underdevelopment of the alveolar tissue.

anaerobic organisms Pertaining to the absence of air or oxygen.

anaerobic Metabolic pathway that does not require oxygen; such processes usually produce lactic acid.

anaphylaxis Allergic hypersensitivity reaction of the body to a foreign protein or drug.

anemia Condition in which there is a reduction in the number of circulating red blood cells per cubic millimeter, the amount of hemoglobin per 100 ml, or the volume of packed red cells per 100 ml of blood.

anemic hypoxia The $Pa{O_2}$ is normal, but the oxygen-carrying capacity of the hemoglobin is inadequate.

aneurysm Localized dilation of a blood vessel, usually an artery.

angiogram Serial roentgenograms of a blood vessel taken in rapid sequence after injection of a radiopaque substance into the vessel.

angiography Roentgenography of blood vessels after injection of a radiopaque substance.

anion gap The balance between acids and bases in the blood plasma. Normally it results in a slightly alkaline state with an excess of hydroxyl ions in comparison to hydrogen. The balance is achieved by the offset of the ingestion and production of acidic and basic material by the amount of acidic and basic material metabolized and excreted by the body.

anoxia Absence of oxygen.

anterior axillary line An imaginary vertical line on the body wall continuing the line of the anterior axillary fold with the upper arm.

anterolateral In front and to one side.

anteroposterior radiograph Chest x-ray from the front to the back of the body.

antibody Protein substance that develops in response to and interacts with an antigen. The antigen-antibody reaction forms the basis of immunity. Antibodies are produced by plasma cells in lymphoid tissue. Antibodies may be present because of previous infection, vaccination, or transfer from the mother to the fetus in utero or may occur without known antigenic stimulus, usually as a result of unknown, accidental exposure.

antidysrhythmic agents Drugs used to treat irregularity or loss of heart rhythm.

antigen assay tests A laboratory assessment of the amounts of components in multimolecular antigen-antibody complexes. The assay is used in various diagnostic tests for collagen-vascular disorders, glomerulonephritis, vasculitis, hepatitis, and neoplastic diseases.

antigen Substance that induces the formation of antibodies that interact specifically with it. An antigen may be introduced into the body or may be formed within the body.

aortic valve Valve between the left ventricle and the ascending aorta that prevents regurgitation of blood into the left ventricle.

aperture Opening or orifice.

apex Top, end, or tip of a structure.

apical pulse The heartbeat as heard with a stethoscope placed on the chest wall adjacent to the apex cordi.

apnea Complete absence of spontaneous ventilation.

apnea-hypopnea index (AHI) At many sleep lab centers, the diagnosis of OSA is commonly based on the apnea-hypopnea index (AHI). *Apnea* is defined as the cessation of airflow—a complete obstruction for at least 10 seconds—with a simultaneous 2% to 4% decrease in the patient's Sa_{O_2}. *Hypopnea* is defined as a reduction of airflow of 30% to 50%, with a concomitant drop in the patient's Sa_{O_2}. The AHI is defined as the average number of apneas and hypopneas the patient has per hour of sleep.

aponeurosis Flat, fibrous sheet of connective tissue that attaches muscle to bone or other tissues. May sometimes serve as a fascia.

arrhythmia Irregularity or loss of heart rhythm.

arterial catheter A tubular instrument that can be inserted into an artery either to draw blood or to measure blood pressure directly.

arteriole Minute artery that, at its distal end, leads into a capillary.

arthralgia Any pain that affects a joint.

ascending paralysis A condition in which there is successive flaccid paralysis of the legs, then the trunk and arms, and finally the muscles of respiration. Causes include poliomyelitis, Guillain-Barré syndrome, and exposure to toxic chemicals, for example, botulinum toxin.

asepsis The absence of germs; sterile.

asphyxia Condition caused by an insufficient uptake of oxygen.

aspiration Inhalation of pharyngeal contents into the pulmonary tree.

asymmetric Unequal correspondence in shape, size, and relative position of parts on opposite sides of the midline.

asystole (cardiac standstill) Absence of contractions of the heart.

atelectasis Collapsed or airless lung. May be caused by obstruction of the airways by foreign bodies, mucous plugs, or excessive secretions or by compression from without, as by tumors, aneurysms, or enlarged lymph nodes.

atmospheric pressure Pressure of air on the earth at mean sea level—approximately 14.7 pounds to the square inch (760 mm Hg).

atopic Of or pertaining to a hereditary tendency to develop immediate allergic reactions because of the presence of an antibody in the skin and sometimes the bloodstream.

atrial fibrillation Irregular and rapid randomized contractions of the atria working independently of the ventricles.

atrial flutter Extremely rapid (200 to 400/min) contractions of the atrium. In pure flutter a regular rhythm is maintained; in impure flutter the rhythm is irregular.

atrophy A wasting or decrease in size of an organ or a tissue.

atropine An alkaloid obtained from belladonna. It is a parasympatholytic agent.

auscultation The act of listening for sounds within the body to evaluate the condition of the heart, blood vessels, lungs, pleura, intestines, or other organs or to detect the fetal heart sound. Auscultation may be performed directly with the unaided ear, but most commonly a stethoscope is used to determine the frequency, intensity, duration, and quality of the sounds.

autoimmune disorder A condition in which a patient exhibits symptoms of at least two of a group of diseases, including Addison's disease, autoimmune thyroid disease, mucocutaneous candidiasis, hypoparathyroiditis, and insulin-dependent diabetes.

autosomal recessive trait Pattern of inheritance in which the transmission of a recessive gene results in a carrier state if the person is heterozygous for the trait and in an affected state if the person is homozygous for the trait. Males and females are affected with equal frequency.

bacillus Any rod-shaped bacterium.

bacteria Unicellular ovoid or rod-shaped organisms existing in free-living or parasitic forms. They display a wide range of biochemical and pathogenic properties.

Bacteroides fragilis A pleomorphic gram-negative bacillus and an obligate anaerobe of the gut.

Bacteroides melaninogenicus a normal flora found in the upper respiratory tract.

Ball-valve effect (and/or mechanism) The intermittent opening and closing of an orifice by a buoyant, ball-shaped mass, which acts as a valve. Some kinds of objects that may act in this manner are kidney stones, gallstones, and blood clots.

barotrauma Physical damage to body tissues caused by a difference in pressure between an air space inside or beside the body and the surrounding fluid.

basophils The least common of the granulocytes, representing about 0.01% to 0.3% of circulating white blood cells.

benign tumors Noncancerous and therefore not an immediate threat, even though treatment eventually may be required for health or cosmetic reasons.

beta waves Waves are known as the "busy waves" of the brain. They are recorded when the patient is awake and alert with eyes open. They are also seen during stage N1 sleep.

β-receptor Site in autonomic nerve pathways wherein inhibitory responses occur when adrenergic agents such as norepinephrine and epinephrine are released.

bicarbonate Any salt containing the HCO_3^- anion.

bifurcation A separation into two branches; the point of forking.

Bilevel positive airway pressure (BiPAP) BiPAP is the brand name of a machine manufactured by Respironics (Pittsburgh, Pa.), which became popular in the 1980s as a home care device for treating sleep apnea. When BiPAP is administered, the patient receives both an inspiratory positive airway pressure (IPAP) and an expiratory positive airway pressure (EPAP). The IPAP is higher than EPAP when applied to patients. The term *BiPAP* has become so commonly used, it often is applied to any device that provides bilevel pressure control. Other names for BiPAP include the following: bilevel airway pressure, bilevel positive pressure, bilevel positive airway pressure, bilevel CPAP (continuous positive airway pressure), bilevel PEEP (positive end-expiratory pressure), bilevel pressure assist, and bilevel pressure support.

bi-lobectomy Removal of two lung lobes.

biopsy Excision of a small piece of living tissue for microscopic examination; usually performed to establish a diagnosis.

Biot's An abnormal respiratory pattern characterized by short episodes of rapid, uniformly deep inspirations followed by 10 to 30 seconds of apnea. Biot's respiration is symptomatic of meningitis or increased intracranial pressure.

bleb Blister or bulla. Blebs may vary in size from that of a bean to that of a goose egg and may contain serous, seropurulent, or bloody fluid.

blood pressure The pressure exerted by circulating blood on the walls of blood vessels, and is one of the principal vital signs. During each heartbeat, BP varies between a maximum (systolic) and a minimum (diastolic) pressure. The mean BP decreases as the circulating blood moves away from the heart through arteries, has its greatest decrease in the small arteries and arterioles, and continues to decrease as the blood moves through the capillaries and back to the heart through veins.

blood urea nitrogen (BUN) A measure of the amount of nitrogen in the blood in the form of urea, and a measurement of renal function. *Urea* is a substance secreted by the liver, and removed from the blood by the kidneys.

Bochdalek foramen A posterolateral opening in the fetal diaphragm. Its failure to close leaves a congenital posterolateral defect that may become a site for a congenital diaphragmatic hernia. Also called pleuroperitoneal hiatus.

body plethysmography A very sensitive lung measurement used to detect lung pathology that might be missed with conventional pulmonary function tests. This method of obtaining the absolute volume of air within one's lungs may also be used in situations where several repeated trials are required or where the patient is unable to perform the multibreath tests. The technique requires moderately complex coaching and instruction for the subject. In the United States, such tests are usually performed by Certified or Registered Pulmonary Function Technologists (CPFT or RPFT) who are credentialed by the National Board for Respiratory Care (NBRC).

body surface burns An assessment measure of burns of the skin. In adults, the "rule of nines" is used to determine the total percentage of area burned for each major section of the body. In some cases, the burns may cover more than one body part, or may not fully cover such a part—in these cases, burns are measured by using the casualty's palm as a reference point for 1% of the body.

body temperature Also known as normothermia or euthermia, is a concept that depends upon the place in the body at which the measurement is made, and the time of day and level of activity of the body. Although the value 37.0° C (98.6° F) is the commonly accepted average core body temperature, the value of 36.8 ± 0.7° C, or 98.2 ± 1.3° F is an average oral (under the tongue) measurement. Rectal measurements, or measurements taken directly inside the body cavity, are typically slightly higher.

brachial pulse The pulse of the brachial artery is palpable on the anterior aspect of the elbow, medial to the tendon of the biceps, and, with the use of a stethoscope and sphygmomanometer (blood pressure cuff) often used to measure the blood pressure.

brachytherapy Radiation treatment given by placing radioactive material directly in or near the target, which is often a tumor.

bradycardia A slow heart rate, usually defined as less than 60 beats/min. The word bradycardia is logically derived from two Greek roots: *bradys*, slow + *cardia*, heart = slow heart.

bradypnea Abnormally slow breathing. A respiratory rate that is too slow. The normal rate of respirations (breaths per minute) depends on a number of factors, including the age of the individual and the degree of exertion.

brady-tachy syndrome During periods of apnea the heart rate decreases, then it increases after the termination of apnea.

bronchial Pertaining to the bronchi or bronchioles.

bronchial breath sounds A normal sound heard with a stethoscope over the main airways of the lungs, especially the trachea. An abnormal breath sound transmitted through consolidated lungs in pneumonia; they are similar to the sounds heard normally over the larger bronchi and are louder and harsher than vesicular breath sounds.

bronchiolitis Inflammation of the bronchioles, the airways that extend beyond the bronchi and terminate in the alveoli. Bronchiolitis is due to viral infections such as parainfluenza, influenza, adenovirus, and, especially, respiratory syncytial virus (RSV).

bronchoconstriction Constriction of the bronchial tubes.

bronchodilation Dilation of a bronchus.

bronchogenic carcinoma One of the more than 90% of malignant lung tumors that originate in bronchi.

bronchogram Film of the airways after a radiopaque substance has been injected into them.

bronchography An x-ray examination of the bronchi after they have been coated with a radiopaque substance.

bronchopulmonary dysplasia (formerly *chronic lung disease of infancy*) A chronic lung disorder that is most common among children who were born prematurely, with low birth weights and who received prolonged mechanical ventilation to treat respiratory distress syndrome.

bronchoscopy A visual examination of the tracheobronchial tree with the bronchoscope.

bronchospasm Involuntary sudden movement or convulsive contraction of the muscular layer of the bronchus.

bronchovesicular Pertaining to the bronchi, bronchioles, and alveoli.

bulla Blister, cavity, or vesicle filled with air or fluid; a bleb.

calcification Process in which organic tissue becomes hardened by the deposition of calcium salts in tissue.

cannulation Placement of a tube or sheath enclosing a trocar to allow the escape of fluid after the trocar is withdrawn from the body.

capillary stasis Stagnation of the normal flow of fluids or blood in capillaries.

carbon dioxide (CO_2) Colorless, odorless, incombustible gas formed during respiration and combustion; normally constitutes only 0.03% of the atmosphere. Concentrations above 5% in inspired air stimulate respiration. CO_2 retention occurs in end-stage pulmonary disease.

carbon monoxide (CO) A product of incomplete combustion of fossil fuels. Also found in tobacco smoke, and highly toxic at high levels. Also used in pulmonary function testing to detect diffusion abnormalities.

carbon monoxide poisoning A toxic condition in which carbon monoxide gas has been inhaled and binds to hemoglobin molecules, thus displacing oxygen from the red blood cells and decreasing the capacity of the blood to carry oxygen to the cells of the body.

carcinoma Malignant tumor that occurs in epithelial tissue. These neoplasms tend to infiltrate and give rise to metastases.

cardiac diastole The period between contractions of the atria or the ventricles during which blood enters the relaxed chambers from the systemic circulation and the lungs. Ventricular diastole begins with the onset of the second heart sound and ends with the first heart sound.

cardiac output (CO) The volume of blood expelled by the ventricles of the heart with each beat (the stroke volume) multiplied by the heart rate. Cardiac output is commonly measured by the thermodilution technique. A normal, resting adult has a cardiac output of 4 to 8 L/min.

cardiac systole The contraction of the heart, driving blood into the aorta and pulmonary arteries. The occurrence of systole is indicated by the first heart sound heard on auscultation, by the palpable apex beat, and by the peripheral pulse.

cardiogenic Originating in the heart.

cardiotonic drugs Drugs that increase the tonicity (contraction strength) of the heart.

carotid pulse The pulse of the carotid artery, palpated by gently pressing a finger in the area between the larynx and the sternocleidomastoid muscle in the neck.

carotid sinus baroreceptors Sensory nerve endings located in the carotid sinus. Changes in pressure stimulate the nerve endings.

cartilage Dense, firm, compact connective tissue capable of withstanding considerable pressure and tension; located in all true joints, the outer ear, bronchi, and movable sections of the ribs.

caseous tubercles Cottage cheeselike mixture of fat and protein that appears in some body tissues undergoing necrosis. Also described as a nodule or a small eminence. For example, a small rounded nodule produced by infection with *Mycobacterium tuberculosis* is commonly described as a gray translucent mass of small spheric cells surrounded by connective cells.

catecholamines Biologically active amines that behave as epinephrine and norepinephrine. Catecholamines have marked effects on the nervous and cardiovascular systems, metabolic rate, temperature, and smooth muscle.

cavitation The formation of cavities or hollow spaces within the body such as those formed in the lung by tuberculosis.

cavity A hollow space within a larger structure, such as the peritoneal cavity or the oral cavity.

central sleep apnea (CSA) A form of sleep apnea resulting from decreased respiratory center output. It may involve primary brainstem medullary depression resulting from a tumor of the posterior fossa, poliomyelitis, or idiopathic central hypoventilation.

central venous pressure (CVP) Pressure within the superior vena cava. The pressure under which the blood is returned to the right atrium.

centriacinar emphysema One of the types of emphysema, characterized by enlargement of air spaces in the proximal part of the acinus, primarily at the level of the respiratory bronchioles. Also called *centrilobular emphysema, focal emphysema.*

centrilobular emphysema One of the types of emphysema, characterized by enlargement of air spaces in the proximal part of the acinus, primarily at the level of the respiratory bronchioles. Also called *centriacinar emphysema, focal emphysema.*

cerebrospinal fluid (CSF) Liquid cushion protecting the brain and spinal cord from shock.

chemoreceptor Sense organ or sensory nerve ending that is stimulated by and reacts to chemical stimuli and that is located outside the central nervous system. Chemoreceptors are found in the large arteries of the thorax and neck (carotid and aortic bodies), the taste buds, and the olfactory cells of the nose.

chemotherapy The treatment of cancer, infections, and other diseases such as cancer with chemical agents. The term has been applied over the centuries to a variety of therapies, including malaria therapy with herbs and use of mercury for syphilis. In modern usage, chemotherapy usually entails the use of chemicals to destroy cancer cells on a selective basis.

Cheyne-Stokes An abnormal pattern of respiration, characterized by alternating periods of apnea and deep, rapid breathing. The respiratory cycle begins with slow, shallow breaths that gradually become abnormally rapid and deep. Breathing gradually becomes slower and shallower and is followed by 10 to 20 seconds of apnea before the cycle is repeated. Each episode may last from 45 seconds to 3 minutes.

Chlamydia Genus of viruslike microorganisms that causes disease in humans and birds. Some *Chlamydia* infections of birds can be transmitted to humans (e.g., ornithosis, parrot disease). The organisms resemble bacteria but are of similar size to viruses and are obligate parasites.

chronic Denoting a process that shows little change and slow progression and is of long duration.

chronotropic Agent that increases heart rate.

chylothorax A condition marked by the effusion of chyle from the thoracic duct into the pleural space. The cause is usually a traumatic injury to the neck or a tumor that invades the thoracic duct. Treatment is directed at repairing damage to the duct.

cilia Small, hairlike projections on the surface of epithelial cells. In the bronchi, they propel mucus and foreign particles in a whiplike movement toward the throat.

clinical manifestations Symptoms or signs demonstrated by a patient; may be subjective or objective.

coagulation Process of clotting. Coagulation requires the presence of several substances, the most important of which are prothrombin, thrombin, thromboplastin, calcium in ionic form, and fibrinogen.

coalesce To fuse, run, or grow together.

coccobacillus Short, thick bacterial rod in the shape of an oval or slightly elongated coccus.

coccus Bacterium with a spherical shape.

collagen Fibrous insoluble protein found in connective tissue, including skin, bone, ligaments, and cartilage. Collagen represents about 30% of the total body protein.

colloid Type of solution; a gluelike substance such as protein or starch whose particles (molecules or aggregates of molecules), when dispersed in a solvent to the greatest degree, remain uniformly distributed and fail to form a true solution.

compromise A blending of the qualities of two different things; an unfavorable change.

congenital Existing at and usually before birth; referring to conditions that are present at birth, regardless of their cause.

congestion Excessive amount of blood, tissue, or fluid in an organ or in tissue.

consolidation The process of becoming solid; a mass that has solidified.

continuous positive airway pressure (CPAP) The application of pressures above ambient to improve oxygenation in a spontaneously breathing patient.

contusion Injury in which the skin is not broken; a bruise. Symptoms are pain, swelling, and discoloration.

convex Having a rounded, somewhat elevated surface resembling a segment of the external surface of a sphere.

cor pulmonale Hypertrophy or failure of the right ventricle resulting from disorders of the lungs, pulmonary vessels, or chest wall.

core temperature The temperature of deep structures of the body, such as the liver, as compared to that of peripheral tissues.

corticosteroids Any of a number of hormonal steroid substances obtained from the cortex of the adrenal gland.

costophrenic angle The junction of the rib cage and the diaphragm.

cuirass A chest covering; breastplate, as in cuirass ventilator.

cyanide poisoning Poisoning resulting from the ingestion or inhalation of cyanide from such substances as bitter almond oil, wild cherry syrup, prussic acid, hydrocyanic acid, or potassium or sodium cyanide. Characterized by tachycardia, drowsiness, seizures, headache, apnea, and cardiac arrest, it may cause death within 1 to 15 minutes.

cyclic adenosine monophosphate (cAMP) Cyclic nucleotide participating in the activities of many hormones, including catecholamines, adrenocorticotropin, and vasopressin. It is synthesized from adenosine triphosphate and is stimulated by the enzyme adenylate cyclase.

cyst Closed pouch or sac with a definite wall that contains fluid, semifluid, or solid material.

cytoplasm Protoplasm of a cell exclusive of the nucleus.

D-dimer blood test A simple and confirmatory test for disseminated intravascular coagulation that can also indicate when a clot is lysed by thrombolytic therapy. The fragment D-dimer assesses both thrombin and plasmin activity.

deep venous thrombi (DVT) A disorder involving a thrombus in one of the deep veins of the body, most commonly the iliac or femoral vein. Symptoms include tenderness, pain, swelling, warmth, and discoloration of the skin. A deep vein thrombus is potentially life threatening. Treatment—including bed rest and use of thrombolytic and anticoagulant drugs—is directed to preventing movement of the thrombus toward the lungs.

delta waves Amplitude (>75 μV) broad waves. Although delta EEG activity is usually defined as <4 Hz, in human sleep scoring, the slow-wave activity used for staging is defined as EEG activity <2 Hz (>0.5 second duration) and a peak-to-peak amplitude of >75 μV. Delta waves are called the "deep-sleep waves." They are associated with a dreamless state from which an individual is not easily aroused. Delta waves are seen primarily during Stage N3.

demarcate To set or mark boundaries or limits.

demyelination The destruction or removal of the myelin sheath from a nerve or nerve fiber.

density Mass of a substance per unit of volume, the relative weight of a substance compared with a reference standard.

deoxyribonucleic acid (DNA) Type of nucleic acid containing deoxyribose as the sugar component and found principally in the nuclei of animal and vegetable cells, usually loosely bound to protein (hence termed *deoxyribonucleoprotein*).

depolarize To reduce to a nonpolarized condition. To reduce the amount of electrical charge between oppositely charged particles.

desensitization Prevention of anaphylaxis.

dextrocardia The location of the heart in the right hemithorax, either as a result of displacement by disease or as a congenital defect.

diabetes mellitus Chronic disease of pancreatic origin that is characterized by insulin deficiency or functional abnormality and a subsequent inability to process carbohydrates. This condition results in excess sugar in the blood and urine; excessive thirst, hunger, urination, weakness, and emaciation; and imperfect combustion of fats. If untreated, diabetes mellitus leads to acidosis, coma, and death.

diagnostic Pertaining to the use of scientific methods to establish the cause and nature of disease.

diastole Period in the heart cycle during which the muscle fibers lengthen, the heart dilates, and the cavities fill with blood.

diastolic blood Pressure The minimum level of blood pressure measured between contractions of the heart. It may vary with age, gender, body weight, emotional state, and other factors.

digitalis A general term for cardiac glycoside.

dilation Expansion of an organ, orifice, or vessel.

dimorphism The quality of existing in two distinct forms.

diplopia Double vision caused by defective function of the extraocular muscles or a disorder of the nerves that innervate the muscles. It occurs when the object of fixation falls on the fovea in one eye and a nonfoveal point in the other eye or when the object of fixation falls on two noncorresponding points.

disseminate Scatter or distribute over a considerable area; when applied to disease organisms, scattered throughout an organ or the body.

distal Farthest from the center, from a medial line, or from the trunk.

double pneumonia Acute lobar pneumonia affecting both lungs.

driving pressure Pressure difference between two areas.

ductus arteriosus Vessel between the pulmonary artery and the aorta. It bypasses the lungs in the fetus.

duplex ultrasonography A combination of real-time and Doppler ultrasonography.

dynamometer An instrument for measuring the force of muscular contractions. For example, a squeeze dynamometer is one by which the grip of the hand is measured.

dysphagia Difficulty in swallowing, commonly associated with obstructive or motor disorders of the esophagus. Patients with obstructive disorders such as esophageal tumor or lower esophageal ring are unable to swallow solids but can tolerate liquids. Persons with motor disorders, such as achalasia, are unable to swallow solids or liquids. Diagnosis of the underlying condition is made through barium studies, the observed clinical signs, and evaluation of the patient's symptoms.

dysplasia Abnormal development of tissues or cells.

dyspnea Air hunger resulting in labored or difficult breathing, sometimes accompanied by pain. Symptoms include audible labored breathing, distressed anxious expression, dilated nostrils, protrusion of the abdomen with an expanded chest, and gasping.

edema A local or generalized condition in which the body tissues contain an excessive amount of fluid.

edrophonium chloride A cholinesterase inhibitor that acts as an antidote to curare and other nondepolarizing neuromuscular blockers and is an aid in the diagnosis of **myasthenia gravis**.

efferent nerves Nerves that carry impulses having the following effects: motor, causing contraction of the muscles; secretory, causing glands to secrete; and inhibitory, causing some organs to become quiescent.

efferent Away from a central organ or section. Efferent nerves conduct impulses from the brain or spinal cord to the periphery.

effusion Seeping or serous, purulent, or bloody fluid into a cavity, the result of such a seeping.

elastase Enzyme that dissolves elastin.

electrocardiogram (ECG) Record of the electrical activity of the heart.

electrodiagnostic Use of electric and electronic devices for diagnostic purposes.

electroencephalogram (EEG) Record of the electrical activity of the brain.

electrolyte Substance that, in solution, conducts an electrical current and is decomposed by the passage of an electrical current. Acids, bases, and salts are electrolytes.

electromyogram (EMG) A graphic record of the contraction of a muscle as a result of electrical stimulation.

Electromyography (EMG) The electrical recording of muscle action potentials.

electrophoresis Movement of charged colloidal particles through the medium in which they are dispersed as a result of changes in electrical potential.

embolus Mass of undissolved matter present in blood or lymphatic vessels to which it has been brought by the blood or lymph current. Emboli may be solid, liquid, or gaseous.

empathy The ability to recognize and to some extent share the emotions and states of mind of another and to understand the meaning and significance of that person's behavior. It is an essential quality for effective psychotherapy.

empyema Pus in a body cavity, especially in the pleural cavity; usually the result of a primary infection in the lungs.

encapsulated Enclosed in a fibrous or membranous sheath.

encephalitis Inflammation of the brain.

endemic A disease that occurs continuously in a particular population but has low mortality, such as measles.

endocarditis Inflammation of the endocardium. It may involve only the membrane covering the valves, or it may involve the general lining of the chambers of the heart.

endothelium The layer of epithelial cells that lines the cavities of the heart, blood and lymph vessels, and the serous cavities of the body; it originates from the mesoderm.

enuresis Involuntary discharge of urine, usually referring to involuntary discharge of urine during sleep at night or bed-wetting beyond the age when bladder control should have been achieved.

enzyme Complex protein capable of inducing chemical changes in other substances without being changed itself. Enzymes speed chemical reactions.

eosinophil Cell or cellular structure that stains readily with the acid stain eosin. Specifically refers to a granular leukocyte.

epidemiology Scientific discipline concerned with defining and explaining the interrelationships of factors that determine disease frequency and distribution.

epinephrine Hormone secreted by the adrenal medulla in response to splanchnic stimulation.

epithelium Covering of the internal and external organs of the body, including the lining of vessels. It consists of cells bound together by connective material and varies in the number of layers and the kinds of cells.

epoch A period marked by distinctive character or reckoned from a fixed point or event

erythema multiforme A hypersensitivity syndrome characterized by polymorphous eruptions of the skin and mucous membranes.

erythropoiesis Formation of red blood cells.

etiology Cause of disease.

exocrine gland Gland whose secretion reaches an epithelial surface either directly or through a duct.

expectoration To clear out the chest and lungs by coughing up and spitting out matter.

expiratory reserve volume (ERV) The maximum volume of gas that can be exhaled after a resting volume exhalation.

extracorporeal membrane oxygenator (ECMO) A device that oxygenates a patient's blood outside the body and returns the blood to the patient's circulatory system. The technique may be used to support an impaired respiratory system.

extravascular Outside a vessel.

exudate Accumulation of a fluid in a cavity; matter that penetrates through vessel walls into adjoining tissue.

facilitation The enhancement or reinforcement of any action or function so that it can be performed more easily.

fascia Fibrous membrane covering, supporting, and separating muscles.

febrile Pertaining to a fever.

femoral pulse The pulse of the femoral artery, palpated in the groin.

fibrin Whitish, filamentous protein formed by the action of prothrombin on fibrinogen. The conversion of fibrinogen into fibrin is the basis for blood clotting. Fibrin is deposited as fine interlacing filaments in which are entangled red and white blood cells and platelets, the whole forming a coagulum or clot.

fibrinolytic Pertaining to the splitting of fibrin.

fibroelastic Composed of fibrous and elastic tissue.

fibrosis Formation of scar tissue in the connective tissue framework of the lungs.

first responder The first emergency person to arrive at the scene of a traumatic or medical situation. This person is trained according to a national standard curriculum set up by the U.S. Department of Transportation.

fissure Cleft or groove on the surface of an organ, often marking the division of the organ into parts, as the lobes of the lung.

fistula Abnormal passage or communication, usually between two internal organs or leading from an internal organ to the surface of the body; designated according to the organs or parts with which it communicates.

flaccid paralysis Paralysis in which there is loss of muscle tone, loss or reduction of tendon reflexes, and atrophy and degeneration of muscles.

flare Flush or spreading area of redness that surrounds a line made by drawing a pointed instrument across the skin. It is the second reaction in the triple response of skin to injury and is caused by dilation of the arterioles.

flash burn A lesion caused by exposure to an extremely intense source of radiant energy or heat. Flash burn commonly occurs on the corneas of arc welders.

flow-volume loop A graph of the rate of airflow as a function of lung volume during a complete respiratory cycle consisting of a forced inspiration followed by a forced expiration. The plotted curve appears as a loop and is used in assessing pulmonary function.

fluorescent antibody microscopy Microscopic examination of antibodies tagged with fluorescent material for the diagnosis of infections.

fluoroscopy The visual examination of a part of the body or the function of an organ with a fluoroscope. The technique offers continuous imaging of the motion of internal structures and immediate serial images. It is invaluable in many clinical procedures, such as intrauterine fetal transfusion and cardiac catheterization.

focal emphysema Centriacinar emphysema associated with inhalation of environmental dusts, producing dilation of the terminal and respiratory bronchioles.

foramen ovale Opening between the atria of the heart in the fetus. This opening normally closes shortly after birth.

forced expiratory flow (FEF) The average volumetric flow rate during any stated volume interval while a forced expired vital capacity test is performed. It is usually expressed as a percentage of vital capacity.

forced expiratory flow$_{200\text{-}1200}$ (FEF$_{200\text{-}1200}$) The average flow rate between 200 and 1200 mL of a forced vital capacity measurement.

forced expiratory flow$_{25\%\text{-}75\%}$ (FEF$_{25\%\text{-}75\%}$) The average flow rate generated by the patient during the middle 50% of a forced vital capacity measurement.

forced expiratory flow$_{50\%}$ (FEF$_{50\%}$) The flow rate generated by the patient at the point in which 50% of a forced vital capacity has been exhaled.

forced expiratory volume in 1 second (FEV$_1$) The maximum volume of gas that can be exhaled in 1 second.

forced expiratory volume 1 second percentage (FEV$_{1\%}$) Compares the amount of air exhaled in 1 second with the total amount exhaled during a forced vital capacity maneuver. Also called *forced expiratory volume time (FEV$_T$).*

forced expiratory volume time (FEV$_T$) The maximum volume of gas that can be exhaled over a specific period is the forced expiratory volume timed.

forced expiratory volume in 1 second/forced vital capacity ratio (FEV$_1$/FVC ratio) Compares the amount of air exhaled in 1 second with the total amount exhaled during an forced vital capacity maneuver. Also called *forced expiratory volume 1 second percentage (FEV$_{1\%}$).*

forced vital capacity (FVC) The maximum volume of gas that can be forcibly and rapidly exhaled after a full inspiration.

fossa Hollow or depression, especially on the surface of the end of a bone.

functional residual capacity (FRC) The volume of gas in the lungs at the end of a normal tidal volume exhalation. The functional residual capacity is equal to the residual volume plus the expiratory reserve volume.

fungal infection Any inflammatory condition caused by a fungus. Most fungal infections are superficial and mild, though persistent and difficult to eradicate. Some, particularly in older, debilitated, or immunosuppressed or immunodeficient people, may become systemic and life threatening.

gastric juice (or gastric secretions) Fluid produced by the gastric glands of the stomach. It contains pepsin, hydrochloric acid, mucin, small quantities of inorganic salts, and the intrinsic antianemic principle. Gastric juice is strongly acid, having a pH of 0.9 to 1.5.

gastroesophageal reflux disease (GERD) A backflow of contents of the stomach into the esophagus that is often the result of incompetence of the lower esophageal sphincter. Gastric juices are acidic and therefore produce burning pain in the esophagus. Repeated episodes of reflux may cause esophagitis, peptic esophageal stricture, or esophageal ulcer. In uncomplicated cases, treatment consists of elevation of the head of the bed, avoidance of acid-stimulating foods, and regular administration of antacids. In complicated cases, surgical repair may provide relief.

genus In natural history classification, the division between the family or tribe and the species; a group of species alike in the broad features of their organization but different in detail.

globulin One of a group of simple proteins insoluble in pure water but soluble in neutral solutions of salts of strong acids; the fraction of the blood serum with which antibodies are associated.

glossopharyngeal nerve Ninth cranial nerve. Function: special sensory (taste), visceral sensory, and motor. Distribution: pharynx, ear, meninges, posterior third of the tongue, and parotid gland.

glycolysis Breakdown of sugar by enzymes in the body. This occurs without oxygen.

glycoprotein Any of a class of conjugated proteins consisting of a compound of protein with a carbohydrate group.

gram-negative organisms Having the pink color of the counterstain used in Gram's method of staining microorganisms. This property is a primary method of characterizing organisms in microbiology. Some of the most common gram-negative pathogenic bacteria are *Bacteroides fragilis, Brucella abortus, Escherichia coli, Haemophilus influenzae, Klebsiella pneumoniae, Neisseria gonorrhoeae, Proteus vulgaris, Pseudomonas aeruginosa, Salmonella typhi, Shigella dysenteriae, and Yersinia pestis.*

gram-positive organisms Retaining the violet color of the stain used in Gram's method of staining microorganisms. This property is a primary method of characterizing organisms in microbiology. Some of the most common kinds of gram-positive pathogenic bacteria are *Bacillus anthracis, Clostridium sp., Mycobacterium leprae, Mycobacterium tuberculosis, Staphylococcus aureus, Streptococcus pneumoniae, and Streptococcus pyogenes.*

granuloma A chronic inflammatory lesion most commonly caused by histoplasmosis, a fungal infection. It is characterized by an accumulation of macrophages; epithelioid macrophages, with or without lymphocytes; and giant cells into a discrete granule. Granulomas most often occur in the lungs. They may resolve spontaneously, remain static, become gangrenous, spread, or act as a focus of infection. Treatment depends on the cause and probable course of the particular granuloma.

Harrington rod One of the rigid, contoured metal rods inserted surgically, along with metal hooks, in the posterior elements of the spine to provide distraction and compression in treatment of scoliosis and other deformities.

hematocrit Volume of erythrocytes packed by centrifugation in a given volume of blood. Hematocrit is expressed as a percentage of the total blood volume that consists of erythrocytes or as the volume in cubic centimeters of erythrocytes packed by centrifugation of the blood.

hematocrit (Hct) A measure of the packed cell volume of red cells, expressed as a percentage of the total blood volume. The normal range is between 43% and 49% in men and between 37% and 43% in women.

hematology The scientific study of blood and blood-forming tissues.

hematopoietic Pertaining to the production and development of blood cells.

hemoglobin (Hb) A complex protein-iron compound in the blood that carries oxygen to the cells from the lungs and carbon dioxide away from the cells to the lungs. Each erythrocyte contains 200 to 300 molecules of hemoglobin, each molecule of hemoglobin contains four groups of heme, and each group of heme can carry one molecule of oxygen.

hemoptysis Expectoration of blood.

hemorrhage Abnormal internal or external discharge of blood; may be venous, arterial, or capillary.

hemothorax An accumulation of blood and fluid in the pleural cavity, between the parietal and visceral pleura, usually the result of trauma. Blood can also accumulate in the thorax cavity as a result of erosion of pulmonary vessels, the rupture of blebs, or granulomas. Hemothorax also may be caused by the rupture of small blood vessels resulting from inflammation caused by pneumonia, tuberculosis, or tumors. Shock from hemorrhage, pain, and respiratory failure follow if emergency care is not available. Also spelled *haemothorax.*

heparin Polysaccharide that has been isolated from the liver, lung, and other tissues. It is produced by the mast cells of the liver and by basophil leukocytes. It inhibits coagulation by preventing conversion of prothrombin to thrombin and blocking the liberation of thromboplastin from blood platelets.

hepatosplenomegaly Enlargement of both the liver and spleen.

Hering-Breuer reflex A neural mechanism that terminates inspiration and initiates expiration. The reflex is triggered by impulses that originate in stretch receptors of the bronchi and bronchioles in response to distension of the airway, increased intratracheal pressure, or pulmonary inflation. The impulses travel via afferent fibers of the vagus nerves to the medullary respiratory center. The Hering-Breuer reflex is well developed at birth and is hyperactive in conditions of restrictive ventilatory insufficiency.

heterozygote Individual with different alleles for a given characteristic.

high-frequency ventilation A technique for providing ventilatory support to patients at a rate of at least 60 breaths/min with small tidal volumes. Types of HFV include high-frequency jet ventilation (HFJV) and high-frequency oscillation (HFO). HFJV uses a high-pressure gas source that can produce short, rapid jets of gas through a small-bore cannula into the airway above the carina at a rate of 100 to 400/min. HFO forces small impulses of gas into and out of the airway at a rate of 400 to 4000/min.

hilus Root of the lungs at the level of the fourth and fifth dorsal vertebrae.

histamine Substance normally present in the body; it exerts a pharmacologic action when released from injured cells. The red flush of a burn is caused by the local production of histamine. It is produced from the amino acid histidine.

Homans' sign Pain in the calf with dorsiflexion of the foot, indicating thrombophlebitis or thrombosis.

homozygote Individual developing from gametes with similar alleles and thus possessing like pairs of genes for a given hereditary characteristic.

horizontal fissure of the right lung A cleft that marks the separation of the upper and middle lobes of the right lung.

hormone Substance originating in an organ or gland that is conveyed through the blood to another part of the body where, by chemical action, it stimulates increased functional activity and increased secretion.

humoral Pertaining to body fluids or substances contained in them.

hyaline membrane A fibrous covering of the alveolar membranes in infants, caused by a lack of pulmonary surfactant associated with prematurity and low-birth-weight delivery.

hydralazine A vasodilator used in hypertension.

hydrostatic Pertaining to the pressure of liquids in equilibrium and to the pressure exerted on liquids by other forces.

hydrotherapy The use of water in the treatment of various disorders. Hydrotherapy may include continuous tub baths, wet sheet packs, or shower sprays.

hydrous Containing water, usually chemically combined.

hyperbaric oxygenation (HBO) The administration of oxygen at greater than normal atmospheric pressure. Also called *hyperbaric oxygen therapy.*

hypercarbia, hypercapnea Excess carbon dioxide in the blood; indicated by an elevated $Pa{CO_2}$.

hypercoagulation Greater than normal clotting.

hyperinflation Distention of a part by air, gas, or liquid.

hyperplasia Excessive proliferation of normal cells in the normal tissue arrangement of an organ.

hyperpnea Increased depth (volume) of breathing with or without an increased frequency.

hyperpyrexia An extremely elevated temperature that sometimes occurs in acute infectious diseases, especially in young children.

hypersecretion Secretion from glands or cells.

hypersensitivity Abnormal sensitivity to a stimulus of any kind.

hypertension Higher than normal blood pressure; greater than normal tension or tonus.

hyperthermia A much higher than normal body temperature induced therapeutically or iatrogenically.

hypertrophy Increase in size of an organ or structure that does not involve tumor formation.

hyperventilation Increased rate and/or depth of breathing, which in turn causes an increased alveolar ventilation and a decreased $Pa{CO_2}$.

hypochromic microcytic anemia A group of anemias characterized by a decreased concentration of hemoglobin in the red blood cells; a form of anemia in which the hemoglobin is deficient in proportion to the size of erythrocytes or the individual erythrocyte has the capacity to contain more hemoglobin, as in iron deficiency anemia.

hypoperfusion Deficiency of blood coursing through the vessels of the circulatory system.

hypoproteinemia Decrease in the amount of protein in the blood.

hypotension An abnormal condition in which the blood pressure is not adequate for normal perfusion and oxygenation of the tissues. An expanded intravascular space, hypovolemia, or diminished cardiac output may be the cause.

hypoventilation Decreased rate and/or depth of breathing, which in turn causes a decreased alveolar ventilation and an increased $Pa{CO_2}$.

hypoxemia Refers to an abnormally low arterial oxygen tension ($Pa{CO_2}$) and is frequently associated with hypoxia, which is an inadequate level of tissue oxygenation .

hypoxia Refers to low or inadequate oxygen for aerobic cellular metabolism.

iatrogenic pneumothorax A condition in which air or gas is present in the pleural cavity as a result of mechanical ventilation, tracheostomy tube placement, or other therapeutic intervention.

iatrogenic Any adverse mental or physical condition induced in a patient by the effects of treatment by a physician or by the patient himself.

idiopathic pulmonary fibrosis A disorder of unknown cause characterized by fibrosis of the lungs. It may follow an earlier inflammation or disease, such as tuberculosis or pneumoconiosis.

idiopathic Disease or condition without a recognizable cause.

IgG antibodies An immunoglobulin produced by lymphocytes in response to bacteria, viruses, or other antigenic substances. An antibody is specific to an antigen. Each class of antibody is named for its action. Antibodies include **agglutinins, bacteriolysins, opsonins,** and **precipitin.**

immunoglobin E (IgE) An α-globulin produced by cells of the lining of the respiratory and intestinal tract. IgE is important in forming reagin antibodies.

immunoglobulin One of a family of closely related but not identical proteins that are capable of acting as antibodies. Five major types of immunoglobulins are normally present in the human adult: IgG, IgA, IgM, IgD, and IgE.

immunoglobulin M (IgM) One of the five classes of antibodies produced by the body and the largest in molecular structure. It is found in circulating fluids and is the first immunoglobulin produced when the body is challenged by antigens. IgM triggers the increased production of immunoglobulin G and the complement fixation required for effective immune response. It is the dominant antibody in ABO blood group incompatibilities. The normal concentration of IgM in serum is 40 to 120 mg/dL.

immunologic mechanism Reaction of the body to substances that are foreign or are interpreted as foreign.

immunotherapy Production or enhancement of immunity.

incubation period Development of an infection in a person from the time of entry into an organism up to the time of the first appearance of signs or symptoms.

infarction Necrosis of tissue after cessation of blood supply.

inferior vena cava (IVC) Venous trunk draining the lower extremities, the pelvis, and the abdominal viscera.

infiltrate v. To penetrate the interstices of a tissue or substance; *n*, the material or solution so deposited.

inflammation Localized heat, redness, swelling, and pain as a result of irritation, injury, or infection.

inotropic (positive) Increasing myocardial contractility.

insertion Manner or place of attachment of a muscle to the bone.

inspiratory capacity (IC) The maximum volume of gas that can be inhaled from the end of a resting exhalation. Equal to the sum of the tidal volume and the inspiratory reserve volume, it is measured with a spirometer.

inspiratory-to-expiratory ratio (I : E ratio) The ratio of the duration of inspiration to the duration of expiration. A range of 1 : 1.5 to 1 : 2 for an adult is considered acceptable for mechanical ventilation. Ratios of 1 : 1 or higher may cause hemodynamic complications, whereas ratios lower than 1 : 2 indicate lower mean airway pressure and fewer associated hazards.

inspiratory reserve volume (IRV) The maximum volume of gas that can be inhaled beyond a normal resting inspiration.

intercostal retraction Retraction of the chest. Sinking-in of the soft tissues of the chest is visible between and around the cartilaginous and bony ribs.

intermittent fever A fever that recurs in cycles of paroxysms and remissions, such as in malaria.

internal oblique One of a pair of anterolateral muscles of the abdomen, lying under the external oblique muscle in the lateral and ventral part of the abdominal wall. It is smaller and thinner than the external oblique muscle. It functions to compress the abdominal contents and assists in micturition, defecation, emesis, parturition, and forced expiration. Both muscles acting together serve to flex the vertebral column, drawing the costal cartilages toward the pubis. One side acting alone bends the vertebral column laterally and rotates it, drawing the shoulder of the opposite side downward.

interstitial edema The abnormal accumulation of fluid in interstitial spaces of tissues, such as in the pericardial sac, intrapleural space, peritoneal cavity, or joint capsules.

interstitial Placed or lying between; pertaining to interstices or spaces within an organ or tissue.

intrapleural pressure Pressure within the pleural cavity.

iodine Nonmetallic element belonging to the halogen group.

ion Atom, group of atoms, or molecule that has acquired a net electrical charge by gaining or losing electrons.

ischemia Deficiency of blood supply caused by obstruction of the circulation to a part.

isosorbide An antianginal agent. Its prototype is nitroglycerin.

isotope One of a series of chemical elements that have nearly identical chemical properties but differ in their atomic weights and electrical charges. Many isotopes are radioactive.

K complexes K complexes are intermittent high-amplitude, biphasic waves of at least 0.5 second duration that signal the start of stage N2 sleep. A K complex consists of a sharp negative wave (upward deflection), followed immediately by a slower positive wave (downward deflection), that is >0.5 second. K complexes are usually seen during stage N2 sleep. They are sometimes seen in stage N3. Sleep spindles are often superimposed on K complexes.

Kartagener's syndrome An inherited disorder characterized by bronchiectasis, chronic paranasal sinusitis, and transposed viscera, usually dextrocardia.

Kerley A and B lines Thickening of the interlobular septa as seen in chest roentgenography; may be caused by cellular infiltration or edema associated with pulmonary venous hypertension.

ketoconazole An antifungal agent.

kinetic Pertaining to or consisting of motion.

Klebsiella A genus of diplococcal bacteria that appear as small, plump rods with rounded ends. Several respiratory diseases, including bronchitis, sinusitis, and some forms of pneumonia, are caused by infection by species of *Klebsiella.*

Kulchitsky cell A cell containing serotonin-secreting granules that stain readily with silver and chromium; also known as an *argentaffin cell.*

Kussmaul breathing Abnormally deep, very rapid sighing respirations characteristic of diabetic ketoacidosis.

lactic acid Acid formed in muscles during activity by the breakdown of sugar without oxygen.

lactic acidosis A disorder characterized by an accumulation of lactic acid in the blood, resulting in a lowered pH in muscle and serum. The condition occurs most commonly in tissue hypoxia but may also result from liver impairment, respiratory failure, burn trauma, neoplasms, and cardiovascular disease.

laryngospasm A spasmodic closure of the larynx.

latency State of being concealed, hidden, inactive, or inapparent.

lecithin-to-sphingomyelin ratio (L : S ratio) The ratio of two components of amniotic fluid, used for predicting fetal lung maturity. The normal ratio in amniotic fluid is 2 : 1 or greater when fetal lungs are mature.

Legionella pneumophila A small gram-negative rod-shaped bacterium that is the causative agent in *Legionnaires' disease.*

lesion A wound, injury, or pathologic change in body tissue.

lethargy The state or quality of being indifferent, apathetic, or sluggish; stupor.

leukocytes White blood corpuscles, including cells both with and without granules within their cytoplasm.

leukopenia An abnormal decrease in the number of white blood cells to fewer than 5000 cells/mm^3.

linea alba White line of connective tissue in the middle of the abdomen from sternum to pubis.

lipid Any of numerous fats generally insoluble in water that constitute one of the principal structural materials of cells.

lobectomy The surgical excision of one or more lobes of a lung. It is performed to remove a malignant tumor or large benign tumor and to treat uncontrolled bronchiectasis, trauma with hemorrhage, congenital anomalies, or intractable tuberculosis.

longitudinal Parallel to the long axis of the body or part.

lubricant Agent, usually a liquid oil, that reduces friction between parts that brush against each other as they move. Joints are lubricated by synovial fluid.

lumen Inner open space of a tubular organ such as a blood vessel or intestine.

lung and chest topography The anatomic description of the lung and chest in terms of the region in which it is located.

lung biopsy A test to obtain a specimen of pulmonary tissue for histologic examination to diagnose pulmonary parenchymal disease, including carcinoma, granuloma, lung diseases caused by toxic exposure, sarcoidosis, and infection.

lung capacity A lung volume that is the sum of two or more of the four primary, nonoverlapping lung volumes. Lung capacities are **functional residual capacity, inspiratory capacity, total lung capacity,** and **vital capacity.**

lung compliance A measure of the ease of expansion of the lungs and thorax, determined by pulmonary volume and elasticity. A high degree of compliance indicates a loss of elastic recoil of the lungs, as in old age or emphysema. Decreased compliance means that a greater change in pressure is needed for a given change in volume, as in atelectasis, edema, fibrosis, pneumonia, or absence of surfactant. Dyspnea on exertion is the main symptom of diminished lung compliance.

lymph node Rounded body consisting of accumulations of lymphatic tissue. Found at intervals in the course of lymphatic vessels.

lymphangitis carcinomatosa The condition of having widespread dissemination of carcinoma in lymphatic channels or vessels.

lymphatic vessels Thin-walled vessels conveying lymph from the tissues. Similar to veins, they possess valves ensuring one-way flow and eventually empty into the venous system at the junction of the internal jugular and subclavian veins.

macrocytic anemia A disorder of the blood characterized by impaired erythropoiesis and the presence of large red blood cells in the circulation. Macrocytic anemia is most often the result of a deficiency of folic acid or vitamin B_{12}.

macrophage Cell whose major function is phagocytosis of foreign matter.

malaise A vague feeling of body weakness, fatigue, or discomfort that often marks the onset of disease.

malignant tumor A neoplasm that characteristically invades surrounding tissue, metastasizes to distant sites, and contains anaplastic cells. A malignant tumor may cause death if treatment does not intervene.

malleolus The protuberance on both sides of the ankle joint, the lower extremity of the fibula being known as the *lateral malleolus* and the lower end of the tibia as the *medial malleolus.*

mannitol A poorly metabolized sugar used as an osmotic diuretic and in kidney function tests.

mast cell Connective tissue cells that contain heparin and histamine in their granules; important in cellular defense mechanisms, including blood coagulation; needed during injury or infection.

maximum voluntary ventilation (MVV) The maximum volume of gas that a person can inhale and exhale by voluntary effort per minute by breathing as quickly and deeply as possible. It is measured in pulmonary function tests.

mechanoreceptor Receptor that receives mechanical stimuli, such as pressure from sound or touch.

meconium A material that collects in the intestines of a fetus and forms the first stools of a newborn. It is thick and sticky, usually greenish to black, and composed of secretions of the intestinal glands, some amniotic fluid, and intrauterine debris, such as bile pigments, fatty acids, epithelial cells, mucus, lanugo, and blood. With ingestion of breast milk or formula and proper functioning of the GI tract, the color, consistency, and frequency of the stools change by the third or fourth day after the initiation of feedings. The presence of meconium in the amniotic fluid during labor may indicate fetal distress and may lead to a lack of oxygen and developmental delays.

meconium aspiration syndrome (MAS) The inhalation of meconium by a fetus or newborn. It can block the air passages and cause failure of the lungs to expand or other pulmonary dysfunction, such as pneumonia or emphysema.

meconium ileus Obstruction of the small intestine in the newborn by impaction of thick, dry, tenacious meconium, usually at or near the ileocecal valve. The condition results from a deficiency in pancreatic enzymes and is the earliest manifestation of cystic fibrosis.

mediastinoscopy An examination of the mediastinum through an incision in the suprasternum, by using an endoscope with light and lenses.

Mendelson's syndrome A respiratory condition caused by the aspiration of acidic gastric contents into the lungs. It usually occurs when a person vomits while inebriated, stuporous from anesthesia, or unconscious, as during a seizure. It is marked by bronchoconstriction and destruction of the tracheal mucosa, progressing to a syndrome resembling acute respiratory distress syndrome.

meningitis Any infection or inflammation of the membrane covering the brain and spinal cord.

mesothelioma A rare, malignant tumor of the meso-thelium of the pleura or peritoneum; associated with early exposure to asbestos.

metabolic acidosis Acidosis in which excess acid is added to the body fluids or bicarbonate is lost from them. Acidosis is indicated by a pH of blood below 7.4. In starvation and in uncontrolled diabetes mellitus, glucose is not present or is not available for oxidation for cellular nutrition.

metabolic alkalosis An abnormal condition characterized by the significant loss of acid in the body or by increased levels of base bicarbonate. Loss of acid may be caused by excessive vomiting, insufficient replacement of electrolytes, hyperadrenocorticism, or Cushing's disease.

metabolism Sum of all physical and chemical changes that take place within an organism; all energy and material transformations that occur within living cells.

metaplasia Conversion of one kind of tissue into a form that is not normal for that tissue.

microvilli Minute cylindrical processes on the free surface of a cell, especially cells of the proximal convoluted renal tubule and the intestinal epithelium; they increase the surface area of the cell.

mitosis A type of cell division of somatic cells in which each daughter cell contains the same number of chromosomes as the parent cell.

mitral valve Bicuspid valve between the left atrium and the left ventricle.

mixed sleep apnea A condition marked by signs and symptoms of both central sleep apnea and obstructive sleep apnea. It often begins as central sleep apnea and develops into the obstructive form. Mixed sleep apnea may also result from obstructive sleep apnea as hypoxia and hypercapnia induce signs and symptoms of the central form.

mononucleosis Presence of an abnormally high number of mononuclear leukocytes in the blood.

motile Having the power to move spontaneously.

mucous Pertaining to or resembling mucus; also glands secreting mucus.

mucus The free slime of the mucous membranes. It is composed of secretions of the glands along with various inorganic salts, desquamated cells, and leukocytes.

myelin Insulating material covering the axons of many neurons; increases the velocity of the nerve impulse along the axon.

myeloma Tumor originating in cells of the hematopoietic portion of bone marrow.

myocardial infarction Development of an area(s) of cellular death in the myocardium, the result of myocardial ischemia following occlusion of a coronary artery.

myocarditis Inflammation of the myocardium.

myocardium Middle layer of the walls of the heart, composed of cardiac muscle.

myopathy An abnormal condition of skeletal muscle characterized by muscle weakness, wasting, and histologic changes within muscle tissue.

necrosis Death of areas of tissue.

neoplasm New and abnormal formation of tissue, such as a tumor or growth. It serves no useful function but grows at the expense of the healthy organism.

nephritis Inflammation of the kidney. The glomeruli, tubules, and interstitial tissue may be affected.

nephrotic syndrome An abnormal condition of the kidney characterized by marked proteinuria, hypoalbuminemia, and edema.

neuroendocrine Pertaining to the nervous and endocrine systems as an integrated functioning mechanism.

neuromuscular junction The area of contact between the ends of a large myelinated nerve fiber and a fiber of skeletal muscle.

nitrogen oxides Automotive air pollutant. Depending on concentration, these gases cause respiratory irritation, bronchitis, and pneumonitis. Concentrations greater than 100 ppm usually cause pulmonary edema and result in death.

nocturnal Pertaining to or occurring in the night.

nodule A small aggregation of cells; a small node.

nomogram Graph consisting of three lines or curves (usually parallel) graduated for different variables in such a way that a straight line cutting the three lines gives the related values of the three variables.

non–small cell lung carcinoma (NSCLC) A general term comprising all lung carcinomas except small cell carcinoma, including adenocarcinoma of the lung, large cell carcinoma, and squamous cell carcinoma.

norepinephrine Hormone produced by the adrenal medulla, similar in chemical and pharmacologic properties to epinephrine.

normal flora Naturally occurring bacteria found in specific bodily areas. Normal flora has no detrimental effect.

oblique fissure The groove marking the division of the lower and the middle lobes in the right lung; the groove marking the division of the upper and the lower lobes in the left lung.

occlude To close, obstruct, or join together.

olfactory Pertaining to the sense of smell.

oncotic pressure Osmotic pressure resulting from the presence of colloids in a solution.

opacity Opaque spot or area; the condition of being opaque.

opaque Impervious to light rays or, by extension, to roentgen rays or other electromagnetic vibrations; neither transparent nor translucent.

open pneumothorax The presence of air or gas in the chest as a result of an open wound in the chest wall.

orbicularis oculi The muscular body of the eyelid; it is composed of the palpebral, orbital, and lacrimal parts.

orifice Mouth, entrance, or outlet to any aperture.

origin The more fixed attachment (usually proximal or central) part of a muscle.

orthopnea Respiratory complaint of discomfort in any but an erect sitting or standing position.

osmotic pressure Pressure that develops when two unequally osmolar solutions are separated by a semipermeable membrane.

osteoporosis Increased brittleness of bone seen most often in elderly persons.

ozone Formed by the action of sunlight on oxygen in which three atoms form the molecule O_3. It is an irritant to the respiratory tract.

P wave The component of the cardiac cycle shown on an electrocardiogram as an inverted U-shaped curve that follows the T wave and precedes the QRS complex. It represents atrial depolarization.

palatine arches Vault-shaped muscular structures forming the soft palate between the mouth and the nasopharynx.

palpation A technique used in physical examination in which the examiner feels the texture, size, consistency, and location of certain body parts with the hands.

panacinar emphysema One of the principal types of emphysema, characterized by relatively uniform enlargement of air spaces throughout the terminal bronchioles and alveoli. It is an inherited condition. Also called *panlobular emphysema.*

pancreas Fish-shaped, grayish pink gland that stretches transversely across the posterior abdominal wall in the epigastric region of the body. It secretes various substances, such as digestive enzymes, insulin, and glucagon.

pancreatic juice Clear alkaline pancreatic secretion that contains at least three different enzymes (trypsin, amylopsin, and lipase). It is poured into the duodenum, where, mixed with bile and intestinal juices, it furthers the digestion of food.

panlobular emphysema One of the principal types of emphysema, characterized by relatively uniform enlargement of air spaces throughout the terminal bronchioles and alveoli. It is an inherited condition. Also called *panacinar emphysema.*

paracentesis A procedure in which fluid is withdrawn from the abdominal cavity.

paradoxical Occurring at variance with the normal rule.

paramyxovirus Subgroup of viruses including parainfluenza, measles, mumps, German measles, and respiratory syncytial viruses.

parasite Any organism that grows, feeds, and is sheltered on or in a different organism while contributing nothing to the survival of the host.

parenchyma Essential parts of an organ that are concerned with its function.

paroxysmal nocturnal dyspnea (PND) A disorder characterized by sudden attacks of respiratory distress that awaken the person, usually after several hours of sleep in a reclining position. This occurs because of increased fluid central circulation with reclining position. It is most commonly caused by pulmonary edema resulting from congestive heart failure. The attacks are often accompanied by coughing, a feeling of suffocation, cold sweat, and tachycardia with a gallop rhythm. Sleeping with the head propped up on pillows may prevent PND, but treatment of the underlying cause is required to prevent fluid from accumulating in the lungs.

paroxysmal Concerning the sudden, periodic attack or recurrence of symptoms of a disease.

particulate Made up of particles.

patent ductus Open, narrow, tubular channel.

pathogen Any agent causing disease, especially a microorganism.

peak expiratory flow rate (PEFR) The greatest rate of airflow that can be achieved during forced expiration, beginning with the lungs fully inflated. Also called *peak expiratory flow rate.*

pectoralis major A large muscle of the upper chest wall that acts on the joint of the shoulder. Thick and fan-shaped, it arises from the clavicle, the sternum, the cartilages of the second to the sixth ribs, and the aponeurosis of the obliquus externus abdominis. It serves to flex, adduct, and medially rotate the arm in the shoulder joint.

pendelluft Shunting of air from one lung to another.

percussion A technique in physical examination of tapping the body with the fingertips or fist to evaluate the size, borders, and consistency of some of the internal organs and to discover the presence of and evaluate the amount of fluid in a body cavity. **Immediate** or **direct percussion** is percussion performed by striking the fingers directly on the body surface. **Indirect, mediate,** or **finger percussion** involves striking a finger of one hand on a finger of the other hand (normally the second phalanx of the third digit) as it is placed over the organ.

perforation Hole made through a substance or part.

peribronchial Located around the bronchi.

peripheral airways Small bronchi on the outer portion of the lung where most gas transfer takes place.

peritoneal dialysis Removal of toxic substances from the body by perfusing specific warm sterile chemical solutions through the peritoneal cavity.

perivascular Located around a vessel, especially a blood vessel.

permeability The quality of being permeable.

permeable Capable of allowing the passage of fluids or substances in solution.

permissive hypercapnia Ventilation that allows Pa_{CO_2} to rise slowly over time as the pH becomes normalized. The goal is to reduce tidal volume and rate while preventing volutrauma during mechanical ventilation. Patients may need to be sedated during this.

pH Symbol for the logarithm of the reciprocal of the hydrogen ion concentration.

phagocytosis Envelopment and digestion of bacteria or other foreign bodies by cells.

phalanges Bones of the fingers or toes.

phenotype Physical makeup of an individual Some phenotypes, such as the blood groups, are completely determined by heredity, whereas others, such as stature, are readily altered by environmental agents.

phenylketonuria Abnormal presence of phenylketone in the urine.

phlegmasia alba dolens Acute edema, especially of the leg, from lymphatic or venous obstruction, usually a thrombosis.

phosgene Carbonyl chloride ($COCl_2$), a poisonous gas causing nausea and suffocation.

phosphodiesterase Enzyme that catalyzes the breakdown of the second messenger cyclic adenosine monophosphate to adenosine monophosphate.

Pickwickian syndrome An abnormal condition characterized by obesity, decreased pulmonary function, somnolence, and polycythemia.

plaque A flat, often raised patch on the skin mucous surface or any other organ of the body. A patch of atherosclerosis. Also called *dental plaque*, usually a thin film on the teeth.

plasmapheresis The removal of plasma from previously withdrawn blood by centrifugation, reconstitution of the cellular elements in an isotonic solution, and reinfusion of this solution into the donor or another client who needs red blood cells rather than whole blood.

platelets The smallest cells in the blood. They are formed in the red bone marrow, and some are stored in the spleen. Platelets are disk-shaped, contain no hemoglobin, and are essential for the coagulation of blood and in maintenance of hemostasis. Normally between 200,000 and 300,000 platelets are found in 1 mL^3 of blood.

pleomorphic Multiform; occurring in more than one form.

pleural Friction rub An abnormal coarse, grating sound heard on auscultation of the lungs during late inspiration and early expiration. It occurs when the visceral and parietal pleural surfaces rub against each other. The sound is not affected by coughing. A pleuropericardial rub indicates primary inflammatory, neoplastic, or traumatic pleural disease or inflammation secondary to infection or neoplasm.

pleurisy Inflammation of the pleura.

pleuritis Inflammation of the pleura.

pneumomediastinum The presence of air or gas in the mediastinal tissues. In infants it may lead to pneumothorax or pneumopericardium, especially in those with respiratory distress syndrome or aspiration pneumonitis. In older children the condition may result from bronchitis, acute asthma, pertussis, cystic fibrosis, or bronchial rupture from cough or trauma.

pneumonectomy The surgical removal of all or part of a lung.

pneumonitis Inflammation of the lung. Pneumonitis may be caused by a virus or may be a hypersensitivity reaction to chemicals or organic dusts, such as bacteria, bird droppings, or molds. It is usually an interstitial, granulomatous, fibrosing inflammation of the lung, especially of the bronchioles and alveoli. Dry cough is a common symptom. Treatment depends on the cause but includes removal of any offending agents and administration of corticosteroids to reduce inflammation.

pneumopericardium The presence of air or gas in the pericardial sac.

pneumoperitoneum The presence of air or gas within the peritoneal cavity of the abdomen. It may be spontaneous, such as from rupture of a hollow, gas-containing organ, or induced for diagnostic or therapeutic purposes.

pneumothorax The presence of air or gas in the pleural space, causing a lung to collapse. Pneumothorax may be the result of an open chest wound that permits the entrance of air, the rupture of an emphysematous vesicle on the surface of the lung, or a severe bout of coughing. It may also occur spontaneously without apparent cause.

point of maximum impulse (PMI) The place where the apical pulse is palpated as strongest, often in the fifth intercostal space of the thorax, just medial to the left midclavicular line.

polyarteritis nodosa Necrosis and inflammation of small and medium-sized arteries and subsequent involvement of tissue supplied by these arteries.

polycythemia Excess of red blood cells.

polymorphonuclear leukocyte Subclass of white blood cells, including neutrophils, eosinophils, and basophils.

polyneuritis Inflammation of two or more nerves at once.

polyneuropathy Term applied to any disorder of peripheral nerves, but particularly used to describe those of a noninflammatory nature.

polyradiculitis Inflammation of nerve roots, especially those of spinal nerves as found in Guillain-Barré syndrome.

polyradiculoneuropathy Guillain-Barré syndrome.

popliteal pulse The pulsation of the popliteal artery, behind the knee, best palpated with the patient lying prone with the knee flexed.

positive inotropic agent A substance that influences the force of muscular contractions. An agent that increases the force of muscular contractions of the heart.

positron emission tomography (PET) A computerized radiographic technique that uses radioactive substances to examine the metabolic activity of various body structures. The patient either inhales or is injected with a metabolically important substance such as glucose, carrying a radioactive element that emits positively charged particles, or positrons. When the positrons combine with electrons normally found in the cells of the body, gamma rays are emitted. The electronic circuitry and computers of the PET device detect the gamma rays and construct color-coded images that indicate the intensity of metabolic activity throughout the organ involved. The radioactive isotopes used in PET are very short-lived, so that patients undergoing a PET scan are exposed to very small amounts of radiation. Researchers use PET to examine blood flow and the metabolism of the heart and blood vessels, to study and diagnose cancer, and to investigate the biochemical activity of the brain.

postpartum Occurring after childbirth.

postural drainage Drainage of secretions from the bronchi or a cavity in the lung by positioning the patient so that gravity will allow drainage of the particular lobe or lobes of the lung involved.

primigravida A woman pregnant for the first time.

prognostic Related to prediction of the outcome of a disease.

proliferation Increasing or spreading at a rapid rate; the process or results of rapid reproduction.

prophylactic Any agent or regimen that contributes to the prevention of infection and disease.

prostration A condition of extreme exhaustion.

proteolytic An enzyme producing proteolysis.

protocol(s) A standard way of performing work. Usually consists of algorithms involving diagnostic and therapeutic components (e.g., Mechanical Ventilation Protocol).

proximal Nearest the point of attachment, center of the body, or point of reference.

Pseudomonas aeruginosa A species of gram-negative, non–spore-forming, motile bacteria that may cause various human diseases ranging from purulent meningitis to nosocomial infected wounds.

ptosis An abnormal condition of one or both upper eyelids in which the eyelid droops because of a congenital or acquired weakness of the levator muscle or paralysis of the third cranial nerve. The condition may be treated surgically by shortening the levator muscle.

pulmonary alveolar proteinosis A condition in which the air sacs of the lungs become filled with protein and lipids, progressing to respiratory failure. The cause is unknown.

pulmonary angiography The radiographic examination of the blood vessels of the lungs after the injection of radiopaque contrast medium into the pulmonary circulation. It is used to detect pulmonary emboli.

pulmonary artery catheter Any of various cardiac catheters for measuring pulmonary arterial pressures, introduced into the venous system through a large vein and guided by blood flow into the superior vena cava, the right atrium and ventricle, and the pulmonary artery.

pulmonary blood vessels Vessels that transport blood from the heart to the lungs and then back to the heart.

pulmonary circulation Passage of blood from the heart to the lungs and back again for gas exchange. The blood flows from the right ventricle to the lungs, where it is oxygenated and carbon dioxide is removed. The blood then flows back to the left atrium.

pulmonary embolectomy A surgical incision into a pulmonary artery for the removal of an embolus or clot, performed as emergency treatment for arterial embolism. The operation is done as soon as possible after a decrease in perfusion is detected. Before surgery, heparin may be administered, and an arteriogram may be used to identify the affected artery. A longitudinal incision is made in the artery, and the embolus is removed. After surgery the blood pressure is maintained close to the level of the preoperative baseline, as a decrease might predispose to new clot formation.

pulmonary Concerning or involving the lungs.

pulse The regular, recurrent expansion and contraction of an artery, produced by waves of pressure caused by the ejection of blood from the left ventricle of the heart as it contracts. The pulse is easily detected on superficial arteries, such as the radial and carotid arteries, and corresponds to each beat of the heart.

pulse oximetry (Spo_2) A device that measures the amount of saturated hemoglobin in the tissue capillaries by transmitting a beam of light through the tissue to a receiver. This noninvasive method of measuring the saturated hemoglobin is a useful screening tool for determining basic respiratory function. This cliplike device may be used on either the earlobe or the fingertip. As the amount of saturated hemoglobin alters the wavelengths of the transmitted light, analysis of the received light is translated into a percentage of oxygen saturation (SO_2) of the blood. Also called (informally) *pulse ox.*

pulsus alternans A pulse characterized by a regular alternation of weak and strong beats without changes in the pulse rate.

pulsus paradoxus An exaggeration of the normal variation in the pulse volume with respiration. The pulse becomes weaker with inspiration and stronger with expiration. Pulsus paradoxus is characteristic of constrictive pericarditis and pericardial effusion. The changes are independent of changes in pulse rate.

purulent Containing or forming pus.

pyrexia An elevation of body temperature above the normal circadian range as a result of an increase in the body's core temperature.

radial pulse The pulse of the radial artery palpated at the wrist over the radius. The radial pulse is the one most often taken because of the ease with which it is palpated.

radiation therapy The treatment of neoplastic disease by using x-rays or gamma rays to deter the proliferation of malignant cells by decreasing the rate of mitosis or impairing DNA synthesis.

radiodensity The ability to stop or reduce the passage of x-rays. Bones have relative radiopacity and therefore display as white areas on an exposed x-ray film. Lead has marked radiopacity and therefore is widely used to shield x-ray equipment and atomic power sources.

radiolucency The ability of materials of relatively low atomic number to allow most x-rays to pass through them, producing dark images on x-ray film.

radiopaque Impenetrable to x-radiation or other forms of radiation.

rapid eye movement (REM) sleep The stage of sleep that can be detected with electrodes placed on the skin around the eyes so that tiny electric discharges from contractions of the eye muscles are transmitted to recording equipment. The REM sleep periods, lasting from a few minutes to half an hour, alternate with the NREM periods. Dreaming occurs during REM time. Individual sleep patterns normally change throughout life because daily requirements for sleep gradually diminish from as much as 20 hours a day in infancy to as little as 6 hours a day in old age. Infants tend to begin a sleep period with REM sleep, whereas REM activity usually follows the four stages of NREM sleep in adults.

rectus abdominis One of a pair of anterolateral muscles of the abdomen, extending the whole length of the ventral aspect of the abdomen. The pair is separated by the linea alba. Each rectus arises in a lateral tendon from the crest of the pubis and is interlaced by a medial tendon with the muscle of the opposite side. The rectus abdominis inserts into the fifth, sixth, and seventh ribs. It functions to flex the vertebral column, tense the anterior abdominal wall, and assist in compressing the abdominal contents.

recumbent Lying down or leaning backward.

red blood cell (RBC) count A count of the erythrocytes in a specimen of whole blood, commonly made with an electronic counting device. The normal RBC concentrations in the whole blood of males are 4.6 to 6.2 million/mm^3. In females the concentrations are 4.2 to 5.4 million/mm^3.

red blood cell indices A test routinely performed as part of a complete blood count to obtain information about the size, weight, and hemoglobin concentration of red blood cells.

refractory Resistant to ordinary treatment; obstinate, stubborn.

remission Lessening of severity or abatement of symptoms; the period during which symptoms abate.

remittent fever Diurnal variations of an elevated temperature with exacerbations and remissions but never a return to normal.

residual volume (RV) The amount of air remaining in the lungs at the end of a maximum expiration.

residual volume/total lung capacity ratio The amount of air remaining in the lungs at the end of a maximum expiration/the volume of gas in the lungs at the end of a maximum inspiration. It equals the vital capacity plus the residual capacity.

respiration The molecular exchange of oxygen and carbon dioxide within the body's tissues.

reteplase A recombinant form of tissue plasminogen activator used intravenously as a thrombolytic agent in treatment of myocardial infarction.

reticular formation Located in the brain stem, it acts as a filter from sense organs to the conscious brain. It analyzes incoming information for importance and influences alertness, waking, sleeping, and some reflexes.

rheumatoid arthritis A chronic, inflammatory, destructive, and sometimes deforming collagen disease that has an autoimmune component. It is characterized by symmetric inflammation of synovial membranes and increased synovial exudate, leading to thickening of the membranes and swelling of the joints. Rheumatoid arthritis usually first appears when patients, most often women, are between 36 and 50 years of age. The course of the disease is variable but is most frequently marked by alternating periods of remission and exacerbation.

ribonucleic acid (RNA) Nucleic acid occurring in the nucleus and cytoplasm of cells that is involved in the synthesis of proteins. The RNA molecule is a single strand made up of nucleotides.

roentgenogram Film produced by roentgenography. Also referred to as an *x-ray*.

roentgenography Process of obtaining x-rays by the use of roentgen rays.

sawtooth waves Notched-jagged waves of frequency in the theta range (3 to 7 Hz). They are commonly seen during REM sleep. Although sawtooth waves are not part of the criteria for REM sleep, their presence is a clue that REM sleep is present.

scalene Pertaining to one of the scalenous muscles.

scaphoid abdomen An abdomen with a sunken anterior wall.

scintillation camera Camera used to photograph the emissions that come from radioactive substances injected into the body.

segmentectomy Removal of a lung segment or segments of the lung.

semilunar valves Valves separating the left ventricle and aorta and right ventricle and pulmonary artery. Also referred to as the *aortic and pulmonary valves*.

semipermeable Permitting diffusion or flow of some liquids or particles but preventing the transmission of others, usually used in reference to a membrane.

septicemia Systemic disease caused by pathogenic organisms or toxins in the blood; may be a late development of any purulent infection.

septum Wall dividing two cavities.

serotonin Chemical present in platelets, gastro-intestinal mucosa, mast cells, and carcinoid tumors; a potent vasoconstrictor.

serum (1) Clear, watery fluid, especially that moistening surfaces of serous membranes; (2) fluid exuded in inflammation of any of those membranes; (3) the fluid portion of the blood obtained after removal of the fibrin clot and blood cells; (4) sometimes used as a synonym for *antiserum*.

sibilant Hissing or whistling; applied to sounds heard in a certain crackle (or rhonchus).

sign Any objective evidence or manifestation of an illness or disordered function of the body. Signs are more or less definitive, obvious, and, apart from the patient's impressions, in contrast to symptoms, which are subjective.

silence Absence of noise or a state of producing no detectable signs or symptoms.

silica Silicon dioxide, an inorganic compound occurring in nature as agate, sand, amethyst, flint, quartz, and other stones. It is one of the major constituents of dental porcelain and a common filler in resin composites. In granular form it serves as a dental abrasive and polishing agent.

silicate Salt of silicic acid.

sinus arrhythmia An irregular cardiac rhythm in which the heart rate usually increases during inspiration and decreases during expiration. It is common in children and young adults and has no clinical significance except in elderly patients.

sinus bradycardia Beating of the sinus node at a rate below 60/min.

sinus tachycardia Uncomplicated tachycardia when sinus cardiac rhythm is faster than 100 beats/min.

sleep spindles Sleep spindles are sudden bursts of EEG activity in the 12 to 14 Hz frequency (6 or more distinct waves) and duration of 0.5 to 1.5 seconds. Sleep spindles mark the onset of stage N2. They may be seen in stage N3, but usually do not occur in REM sleep.

small cell (or oat-cell carcinoma) A malignant, usually bronchogenic epithelial neoplasm consisting of small, tightly packed round, oval, or spindle-shaped epithelial cells that stain darkly and contain neurosecretory granules and little or no cytoplasm. Tumors produced by these cells do not form bulky masses but usually spread along submucosal lymphatics. Many malignant tumors of the lung are of this type. Usually surgical resection is not possible and chemotherapy and radiation therapy are not effective in treatment; thus the long-term prognosis is poor.

small cell lung carcinoma (SCLC) A malignant, usually bronchogenic epithelial neoplasm consisting of small, tightly packed round, oval, or spindle-shaped epithelial cells that stain darkly and contain neurosecretory granules and little or no cytoplasm. Tumors produced by these cells do not form bulky masses but usually spread along submucosal lymphatics. Many malignant tumors of the lung are of this type. Usually surgical resection is not possible and chemotherapy and radiation therapy are not effective in treatment; thus the long-term prognosis is poor.

smooth muscle Muscle tissue that lacks cross-striations on its fibers; involuntary in action and found principally in visceral organs.

SOAP In a problem-oriented medical record, an abbreviation for *subjective, objective, assessment,* and *plan,* the four parts of a written account of the health problem. In taking and charting the patient history and physical examination, a SOAP statement is made for each syndrome, problem, symptom, or diagnosis. Charting by this method is said to be "soaped," and charts produced by using it are called "soap charts."

somatic nerve Nerve that innervates somatic structures (i.e., those constituting the body wall and extremities).

spasm Involuntary sudden movement or convulsive muscular contraction. Spasms may be clonic or tonic.

sphygmomanometer Instrument for determining arterial blood pressure indirectly.

spinal fusion The fixation of an unstable segment of the spine, accomplished sometimes by skeletal traction or immobilization of the patient in a body cast but most frequently by a surgical procedure. Operative ankylosis may be performed in the treatment of spinal fractures or after diskectomy or laminectomy for the correction of a herniated vertebral disk. Surgical fusion involves the stabilization of a spinal section with a bone graft or synthetic device introduced through a posterior incision in the lumbar region; in the less frequently fused cervical region the incision may be anterior or posterior.

spontaneous pneumothorax The presence of air or gas in the pleural space as a result of a rupture of the lung parenchyma and visceral pleura with no demonstrable cause.

sputum culture A test for pathogenic bacteria in the sputum of patients with respiratory infections.

sputum Substance expelled by coughing or clearing the throat. It may contain cellular debris, mucus, blood, pus, caseous material, and microorganisms.

squamous cell carcinoma A slow-growing malignant tumor of squamous epithelium, frequently found in the lungs and skin and occurring also in the anus, cervix, larynx, nose, and bladder. The neoplastic cells characteristically resemble prickle cells and form keratin pearls.

staging The classification of phases, quantity, or periods of a disease or other pathologic process, as in the TMN clinical method of assigning numerical values to various stages of tumor development.

stasis Stagnation of the normal flow of fluids, as of the blood, urine, or intestinal mechanism.

status asthmaticus Persistent and intractable asthma.

sternocleidomastoid A muscle of the neck that is attached to the mastoid process of the temporal bone and to the superior nuchal line and by separate heads to the sternum and clavicle. They function together to flex the head.

stridor An abnormal, high-pitched musical sound caused by an obstruction in the trachea or larynx. It is usually heard during inspiration. Stridor may indicate several neoplastic or inflammatory conditions, including glottic edema, asthma, diphtheria, laryngospasm, and papilloma.

stroke volume (SV) Amount of blood ejected by the ventricle at each beat.

subarachnoid space Space occupied by cerebrospinal fluid beneath the arachnoid membrane surrounding the brain and spinal cord.

subcutaneous emphysema The presence of air or gas in the subcutaneous tissues. The air or gas may originate in the rupture of an airway or alveolus and migrate through the subpleural spaces to the mediastinum and neck. The face, neck, and chest may appear swollen. Skin tissues can be painful and may produce a crackling or popping sound as air moves under them. The patient may experience dyspnea and appear cyanotic if the air leak is severe. Treatment may require an incision to release the trapped air.

subcutaneous Beneath the skin.

sulfur dioxide Common industrial air pollutant; causes bronchospasm and cell destruction.

superficial Confined to the surface.

superior vena cava syndrome A condition of edema and engorgement of the veins of the upper body caused by obstruction of the superior vena cava by thrombi or primary pulmonary tumors. Signs and symptoms include a nonproductive cough, breathing difficulty, cyanosis, central nervous system disorders, and edema of the conjunctiva, trachea, and esophagus.

superior vena cava Venous trunk draining blood from the head, neck, upper extremities, and chest. It begins by union of the two brachiocephalic veins, passes directly downward, and empties into the right atrium of the heart.

surface tension Condition at the surface of a liquid in contact with a gas or another liquid. It is the result of the mutual attraction of molecules to produce a cohesive state, which causes liquids to assume a shape presenting the smallest surface area to the surrounding medium. It accounts for the spherical shape assumed by fluids such as drops of oil or water.

surfactant Phospholipid substance important in controlling the surface tension of the air-liquid emulsion in the lungs; an agent that lowers the surface tension.

symmetric Equal correspondence in shape, size, and relative position of parts on opposite sides of the body.

sympathomimetic Producing effects resembling those resulting from stimulation of the sympathetic nervous system, such as the effects following the injection of epinephrine.

symptom Any perceptible change in the body or its functions that indicates disease or the phases of a disease. Symptoms may be classified as objective, subjective, cardinal, and sometimes constitutional. However, another classification considers all symptoms as being subjective, with objective indications being called *signs*.

syncope Transient loss of consciousness resulting from inadequate blood flow to the brain.

syncytial Group of cells in which the protoplasm of one cell is continuous with that of adjoining cells.

Syncytium a group of cells in which the cytoplasm of one cell is continuous with that of adjoining cells, resulting in a multinucleate unit.

systemic reaction Whole-body response to a stimulus.

systemic Pertaining to the whole body rather than to one of its parts.

systole Part of the heart cycle in which the heart is in contraction.

systolic blood pressure Maximum blood pressure; occurs during contraction of the ventricle.

T wave The component of the cardiac cycle shown on an electrocardiogram as a short, inverted, U-shaped curve after the S-T segment. It represents membrane repolarization phase 3 of the cardiac action potential.

tachycardia Abnormal rapidity of heart action, usually defined as a heart rate greater than 100 beats/min.

tachypnea A rapid breathing rate.

tactile fremitus A tremulous vibration of the chest wall during speaking that is palpable on physical examination. Tactile fremitus may be decreased or absent when vibrations from the larynx to the chest surface are impeded by chronic obstructive pulmonary disease, obstruction, pleural effusion, or pneumothorax. It is increased in pneumonia.

talc A native, hydrous magnesium silicate, sometimes containing a small proportion of aluminum silicate, used as a dusting powder and adsorbent in clarifying liquids.

temporal pulse The pulse points over the temporal artery in front of the ear.

tenacious Adhering to; adhesive; retentive.

tension of gas Gas pressure measured in millimeters of mercury (mm Hg).

tension pneumothorax Presence of air in the pleural space when pleural pressure exceeds alveolar pressure, caused by a rupture through the chest wall or lung parenchyma associated with the valvular opening. Air passes through the valve during coughing but cannot escape on exhalation. Unrelieved pneumothorax can lead to respiratory arrest.

theta waves Of the several types of brain waves, characterized by a relatively low frequency of 4 to 7 Hz and a low amplitude of 10 μV. Theta waves are the "drowsy waves" of the temporal lobes of the brain and appear in electroencephalograms when the individual is awake but relaxed and sleepy. Also called **theta rhythm.**

third degree In third-degree burns, the entire thickness of the epidermis and dermis is destroyed.

thoracentesis The surgical perforation of the chest wall and pleural space with a needle to aspirate fluid for diagnostic or therapeutic purposes or to remove a specimen for biopsy. The procedure is usually performed using local anesthesia, with the patient in an upright position. Thoracentesis may be used to aspirate fluid to treat pleural effusion or to collect fluid samples for culture or examination.

thoracentesis Puncture of the chest wall for removal of fluid.

thrombocytopenia Abnormal decrease in the number of blood platelets.

thromboembolism Blood clot caused by an embolus obstructing a vessel.

thrombophlebitis Inflammation of a vein in conjunction with the formation of a thrombus; usually occurs in an extremity, most frequently a leg.

thrombus Blood clot that obstructs a blood vessel or a cavity of the heart.

thymectomy Surgical removal of the thymus gland.

thymoma A usually benign tumor of the thymus gland that may be associated with myasthenia gravis or an immune deficiency disorder.

thymus Ductless gland situated in the anterior mediastinal cavity that reaches maximum development during early childhood and then undergoes involution. It usually has two longitudinal lobes. An endocrine gland, the thymus is now thought to be a lymphoid body. It is a site of lymphopoiesis and plays a role in immunologic competence.

tidal volume (V_T) The amount of air inhaled and exhaled during normal ventilation. Inspiratory reserve volume, expiratory reserve volume, and tidal volume make up vital capacity.

titer A measurement of the concentration of a substance in a solution.

tone The state of a body or any of its organs or parts in which the functions are healthy and normal. In a more restricted sense, the resistance of muscles to passive elongation or stretch; normal tension or responsiveness to stimuli.

total lung capacity (TLC) The volume of gas in the lungs at the end of a maximum inspiration. It equals the vital capacity plus the residual capacity.

toxemia The condition resulting from the spread of bacterial products via the bloodstream; toxemic condition resulting from metabolic disturbances.

toxin Poisonous substance of animal or plant origin.

trachea Largest airway; a fibroelastic tube found at the level of the sixth cervical vertebra to the fifth thoracic vertebra; carries air to and from the lungs. At the carina it divides into two bronchi, one leading to each lung. The trachea is lined with mucous membrane, and its inner surface is lined with ciliated epithelium.

tracheobronchial clearance Mechanisms by which the airways are cleared of foreign substances; the act of clearing the airways by mucociliary action, coughing, or macrophages.

tracheostomy Operation entailing cutting into the trachea through the neck, usually for insertion of a tube to overcome upper airway obstruction.

tracheotomy Incision of the skin, muscles, and trachea.

transfusion Injection of blood or a blood component into the bloodstream; transfer of the blood of one person into the blood vessels of another.

transillumination The passage of light through body tissues for the purpose of examining a structure interposed between the observer and the light source. A diaphanoscope is an instrument introduced into a body cavity to transilluminate tissues.

translucent Transmitting light, but diffusing it so that objects beyond are not clearly distinguishable.

transmission Transference of disease or infection.

transpulmonary pressure The pressure difference between the mouth and intrapleural pressure.

transudate A fluid passed through a membrane or squeezed through a tissue or into the space between the cells of a tissue. It is thin and watery and contains few blood cells or other large proteins.

transverse Describing the state of something that is lying across or at right angles to something else; lying at right angles to the long axis of the body.

trauma Physical injury or wound caused by external forces.

tricuspid valve Right atrioventricular valve separating the right atrium from the right ventricle.

trypsin Proteolytic enzyme of the pancreas.

tuberculosis Infectious disease caused by the tubercle bacillus *Mycobacterium tuberculosis* and characterized by inflammatory infiltrations, formation of tubercles, caseation, necrosis, abscesses, fibrosis, and calcification. It most commonly affects the respiratory system.

ulcerate To produce or become affected with an open sore or lesion of the skin.

underventilation Reduced rate and depth of breathing.

uremia Toxic condition associated with renal insufficiency that is produced by retention in the blood of nitrogenous substances normally excreted by the kidney.

vaccinia A contagious disease of cattle that is produced in humans by inoculation with cowpox virus to confer immunity against smallpox.

vagus Pneumogastric or tenth cranial nerve. It is a mixed nerve, having motor and sensory functions and a wider distribution than any of the other cranial nerves.

varicella Chickenpox.

Vasoactive substances tending to cause vasodilation or vasoconstriction.

vasoconstriction Constriction of the blood vessels.

Vasodilation An increase in the diameter of a blood vessel. It is caused by a relaxation of the smooth muscles in the vessel wall.

venous stasis Stagnation of the normal flow of blood caused by venous congestion.

ventilation Mechanical movement of air into and out of the lungs in a cyclic fashion. The activity is autonomic and voluntary and has two components—an inward flow of air, called *inhalation* or *inspiration*, and an outward flow, called *exhalation* or *expiration*.

ventilatory rate The volume of air passing into and out of the lungs per minute.

ventricle Either of the two lower chambers of the heart. The right ventricle forces blood into the pulmonary artery, the left into the aorta.

ventricular fibrillation A cardiac arrhythmia marked by rapid depolarizations of the ventricular myocardium. The condition is characterized by a complete lack of organized electric activity and of ventricular ejection. Blood pressure falls to zero, resulting in unconsciousness. Death may occur within 4 minutes. Cardiopulmonary resuscitation must be initiated immediately, with defibrillation and resuscitative medications given according to advanced cardiac life support protocol.

ventricular flutter A condition of very rapid contractions of the ventricles of the heart. Electrocardiograms show poorly defined QRS complexes occurring at a rate of 250 beats/min or higher. Cardiac output is severely compromised or absent. The condition is fatal if untreated.

ventricular tachycardia Tachycardia of at least three consecutive ventricular complexes with a rate greater than 100 beats/min. It usually originates in a focus distal to the branching of the atrioventricular bundle.

verapamil A calcium channel blocker.

vernix Protective fatty deposit covering the fetus.

vertex waves Sharp negative (upward deflection) EEG waves, often in conjunction with high amplitude and short (2 to 7 Hz) activity. The amplitude of many of the vertex sharp waves are greater than 20 μV and, occasionally, they may be as high as 200 μV. Vertex waves are usually seen at the end of stage N1.

vesicular breath sound A normal sound of rustling or swishing heard with a stethoscope over the lung periphery. It characteristically has a higher pitch during inspiration and fades rapidly during expiration.

visceral pleura Pleura that invests the lungs and enters into and lines the interlobar fissures.

viscosity Stickiness or gumminess; resistance offered by a fluid to change of form or relative position of its particles caused by the attraction of molecules to one another.

viscous Sticky; gummy; gelatinous.

viscus Any internal organ enclosed within a cavity such as the thorax or abdomen.

vital capacity (VC) The maximum volume of air that can be expelled at the normal rate of exhalation after a maximum inspiration, representing the greatest possible breathing capacity.

vocal fremitus The vibration of the chest wall as a person speaks or sings that allows the person's voice to be heard by auscultation of the chest with a stethoscope.

volume percent (vol%) The number of cubic centimeters (milliliters) of a substance contained in 100 cc (or mL) of another substance.

walking pneumonia The phrase "walking pneumonia" has no clinical significance; it is often used to describe a mild case of pneumonia. For example, patients infected with *Mycoplasma pneumoniae*, who generally have mild symptoms and remain ambulatory, are sometimes told that they have walking pneumonia.

wedge resection The surgical excision of part of an organ, such as part of an ovary containing a cyst. The segment excised may be wedge-shaped.

wheal More or less round and evanescent elevation of the skin, white in the center, with a red periphery. It is accompanied by itching and is seen in urticaria, insect bites, anaphylaxis, and angioneurotic edema.

wheeze A form of rhonchus, characterized by a high-pitched or low-pitched musical quality. It is caused by a high-velocity flow of air through a narrowed airway and is heard during both inspiration and expiration. It may be caused by bronchospasm, inflammation, or obstruction of the airway by a tumor or foreign body. Wheezes are associated with asthma and chronic bronchitis. Unilateral wheezes are characteristic of bronchogenic carcinoma, foreign bodies, and inflammatory lesions. In asthma, expiratory wheezing is more common, although inspiratory and expiratory wheezes are heard.

whispering pectoriloquy The term used to describe the unusually clear transmission of the whispered voice of a patient as heard through the stethoscope.

white blood cell count (WBC) An examination and enumeration of the distribution of leukocytes in a stained blood smear. The different kinds of white cells are counted and reported as percentages of the total examined. Differential white blood cell count provides more specific information related to infections and diseases. Also called **differential leukocyte count.**

xenon 133 Radioactive isotope of xenon used in photoscanning studies of the lung.

Index

Page numbers with "t" denote tables; those with "f " denote figures; and those with "b" denote boxes.

B

G

H

I

M

P

S

T

W

X

Y

Z